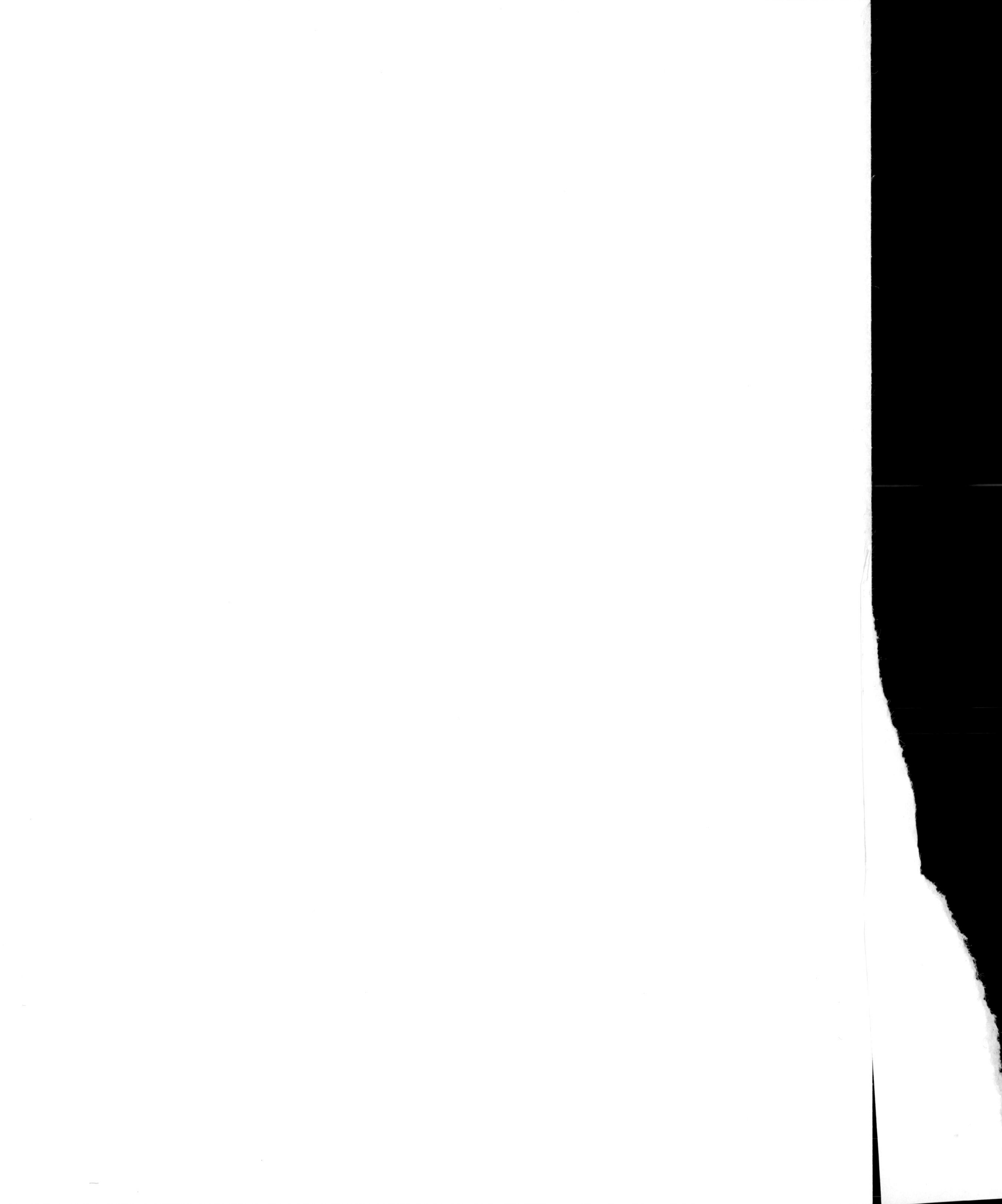

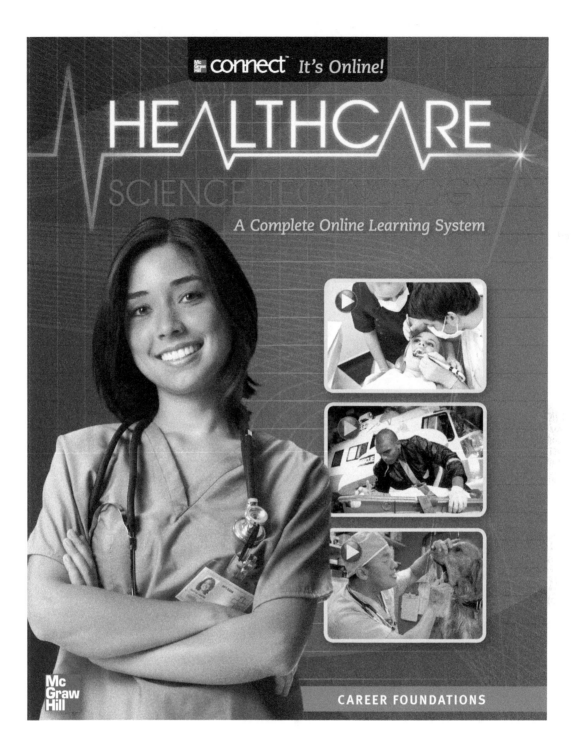

connect It's Online!

HEALTHCARE

SCIENCE TECHNOLOGY

A Complete Online Learning System

CAREER FOUNDATIONS

Kathryn A. Booth, R.N., M.S.

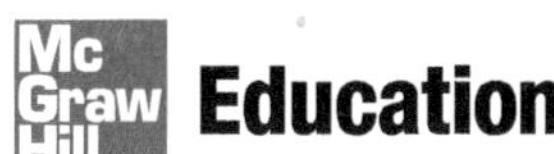

Bothell, WA • Chicago, IL • Columbus, OH • New York, NY

About the Author

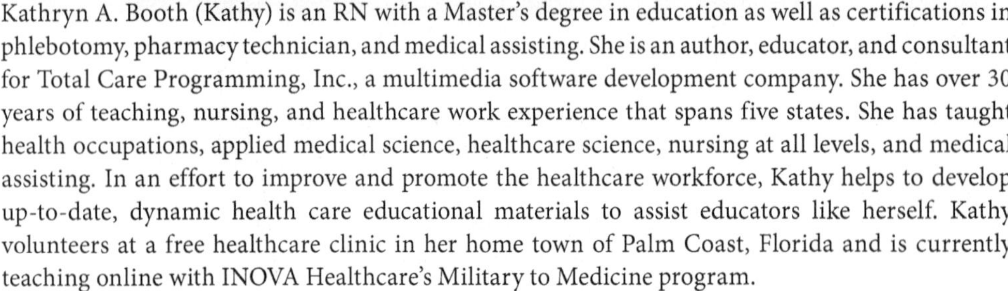

Kathryn A. Booth (Kathy) is an RN with a Master's degree in education as well as certifications in phlebotomy, pharmacy technician, and medical assisting. She is an author, educator, and consultant for Total Care Programming, Inc., a multimedia software development company. She has over 30 years of teaching, nursing, and healthcare work experience that spans five states. She has taught health occupations, applied medical science, healthcare science, nursing at all levels, and medical assisting. In an effort to improve and promote the healthcare workforce, Kathy helps to develop up-to-date, dynamic health care educational materials to assist educators like herself. Kathy volunteers at a free healthcare clinic in her home town of Palm Coast, Florida and is currently teaching online with INOVA Healthcare's Military to Medicine program.

Safety Notice: The reader is expressly advised to consider and use all safety precautions described in this book and online program, or that might also be indicated by undertaking the activities described herein. In addition, common sense should be exercised to help avoid all potential hazards, and, in particular, to take relevant safety precautions concerning any known or likely hazards involved in healthcare, or in use of the procedures described in Healthcare Science Technology: Career Foundations, such as the risk of infection.

Publisher and Authors assume no responsibility for the activities of the reader or for the subject matter experts who prepared this book. Publisher and Authors make no representation or warranties of any kind, including but not limited to, the warranties of fitness for particular purpose or merchantability, nor for any implied warranties related thereto, or otherwise. Publisher and Authors will not be liable for damages of any types, including any consequential, special or exemplary damages resulting, in whole or in part, from reader's use or reliance upon the information, instructions, warnings, or other matter contained in this book.

Internet Disclaimer: The Internet listings in this product are a source for extended information related to this title. We have made every effort to recommend sites that are informative and accurate. However, these sites are not under the control of McGraw-Hill Education, and, therefore, McGraw-Hill Education makes no representation concerning the content of these sites. We strongly encourage teachers to preview Internet sites before students use them. Many sites may eventually contain links to other sites that could lead to inappropriate material. Internet sites are sometimes "under construction" and may not always be available. Sites may also move or have been discontinued completely by the time you or your students attempt to access them.

Notice: Information on featured companies, organizations, and their products and services is included for educational purposes only and does not present or imply endorsement of the *Healthcare Science Technology* program.

Front Cover (l)Rubberball/Getty Images, (tr)gehringj/the Agency Collection/Getty Images, (cr)Corbis, (br)Stewart Cohen/Pam Ostrow/Blend Images/Getty Images; **Back Cover** Brand X/ Getty Images.

MHEonline.com

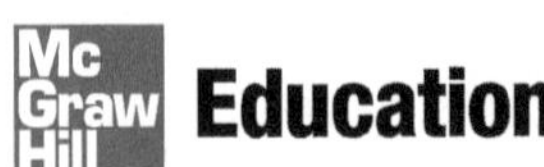

Printed in the United States of America.

Send all inquiries to:
McGraw-Hill Education
4400 Easton Commons, Suite 200
Columbus, OH 43219

ISBN: 978-0-07-878092-9 (Student Edition)
MHID: 0-07-878092-6 (Student Edition)

9 10 11 12 13 14 QVS 22 21 20 19 18

Contributors and Reviewers

Contributors

Emilee Anderson Shelton RD, LD
Mobile, AL

Meaghan Eckert, Spectacle/Contact Lens Licensed Optician
Westerville, OH

Pearce Eckert, Spectacle Licensed Optician
Westerville, OH

Wesley Hellums RT(R)AART
Dunedin, FL

Megan Hess
Galloway, OH

Amanda L. Jones MBA, NR-CMA, NCPT, CPC
Program Director- Medical Assisting
Central Florida Institute

Thomas E. O'Brien, AS, CST, CCT, CRAT
Cardiovascular Basic Studies
Central Florida Institute

Kathy Ozols, RT
Dunedin, FL

Amy L. Richards, RVT
Columbus, OH

Susan Dunn, Box 12 Communications
Cary, NC

Ellen Stadler
Westerville, OH

Acknowledgements

The following individuals and companies were instrumental in completion of this project. Many thanks to their extraordinary efforts and time spent.

Jody James

Lynn Egler

Buzz Machines Studios

Otterstream, Inc.

Scott McKenzie

Anastasia Nectar

Justin Parente

Reviewers

Sarah D. Andrews, BS, RN, MS
Ohio Hi-Point Career Center
Bellefontaine, OH

Robert Bundy
Clay High School
Oregon, OH

Carol (Cookie) Cealey, RN
Richwoods High School
Peoria, IL

Rachel Clothier
East High School
Salt Lake City, UT

Deborah Dubendorff, RN
George Jenkins High School
Lakeland, FL

Janet Hodge
Academy of Technology and Academics
Conway, CS

Karen Kropp
Grand Island Senior High
Grand Island, NE

Michelle Maskulinski, MA, BSN, RN
Fairfield Career Center
Carroll, OH

Keri Ray, RN, BS
Temple High School
Temple, TX

Judy Smith
Stadium High School
Tacoma, WA

Karen Ziemke
R.G. Drage Career Technical Center
Massilon, OH

Brief Contents

Contents

Photo: Dr. P. Marazzi/Science Photo Library/Photo Researchers

Contents

Photos: (t to b)Biophoto Associates/Science Source/Photo Researchers, Prof. P. Motta, Dept. of Anatomy, University "La Sapienza," Rome/Science Photo Library/Photo Researchers, Biophoto Associates/Photo Researchers, Michael Abbey/Photo Researchers, Doug Martin

Contents

Photos: (t)PhotoDisc/Getty Images, (b)CORBIS

Contents

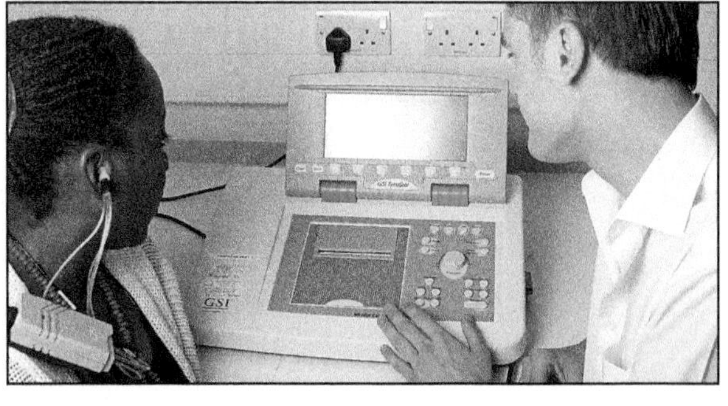

Photos: (t)Kenneth Murry/Photo Researchers, (b)adam james/Alamy

Contents

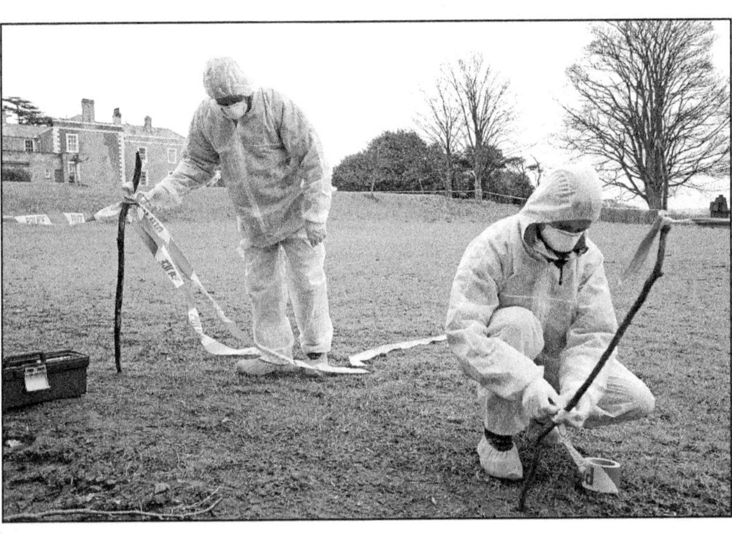

Contents

Photo: Laurent/Photo Researchers

Contents

Connect

ONLINE PROCEDURES

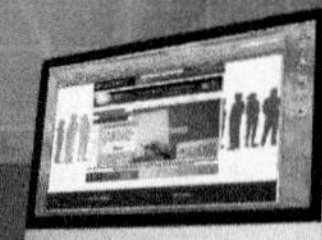

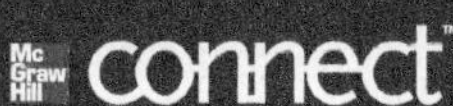

ONLINE PROCEDURES

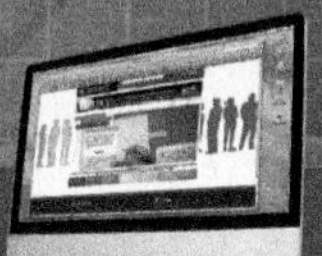

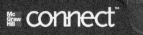

connect ONLINE PROCEDURES

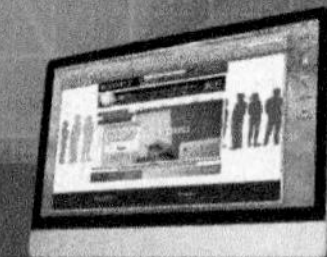

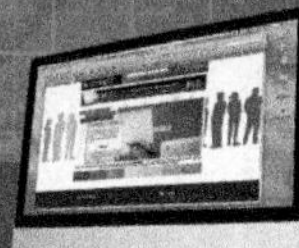

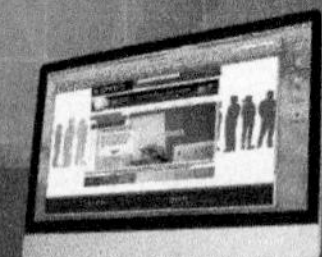

connect ONLINE PROCEDURES

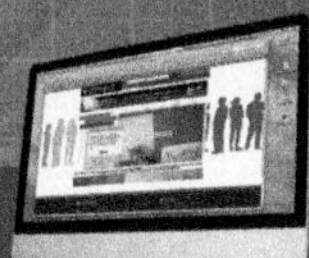

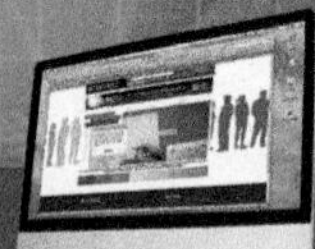

connect

ONLINE PROCEDURES

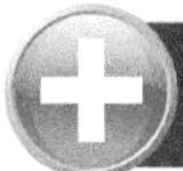

Safety

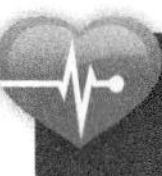

Preventive
Care & Wellness

Online Features Connect

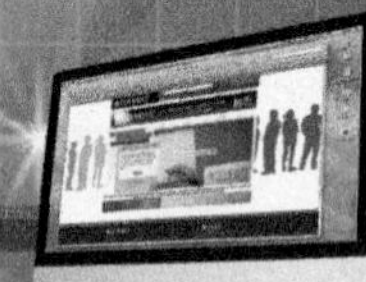

VIRTUAL LAB:

ANATOMY ACTIVITY

Ethics in Action

Medical Math

Medical Science

How to Use the *Healthcare Science Technology* Program

Healthcare Science Technology is a hybrid program in which the Student Edition and online content are fully integrated and designed to work together. The Student Edition introduces you to key healthcare science concepts. Connect allows you to extend and apply your healthcare skills with activities and projects.

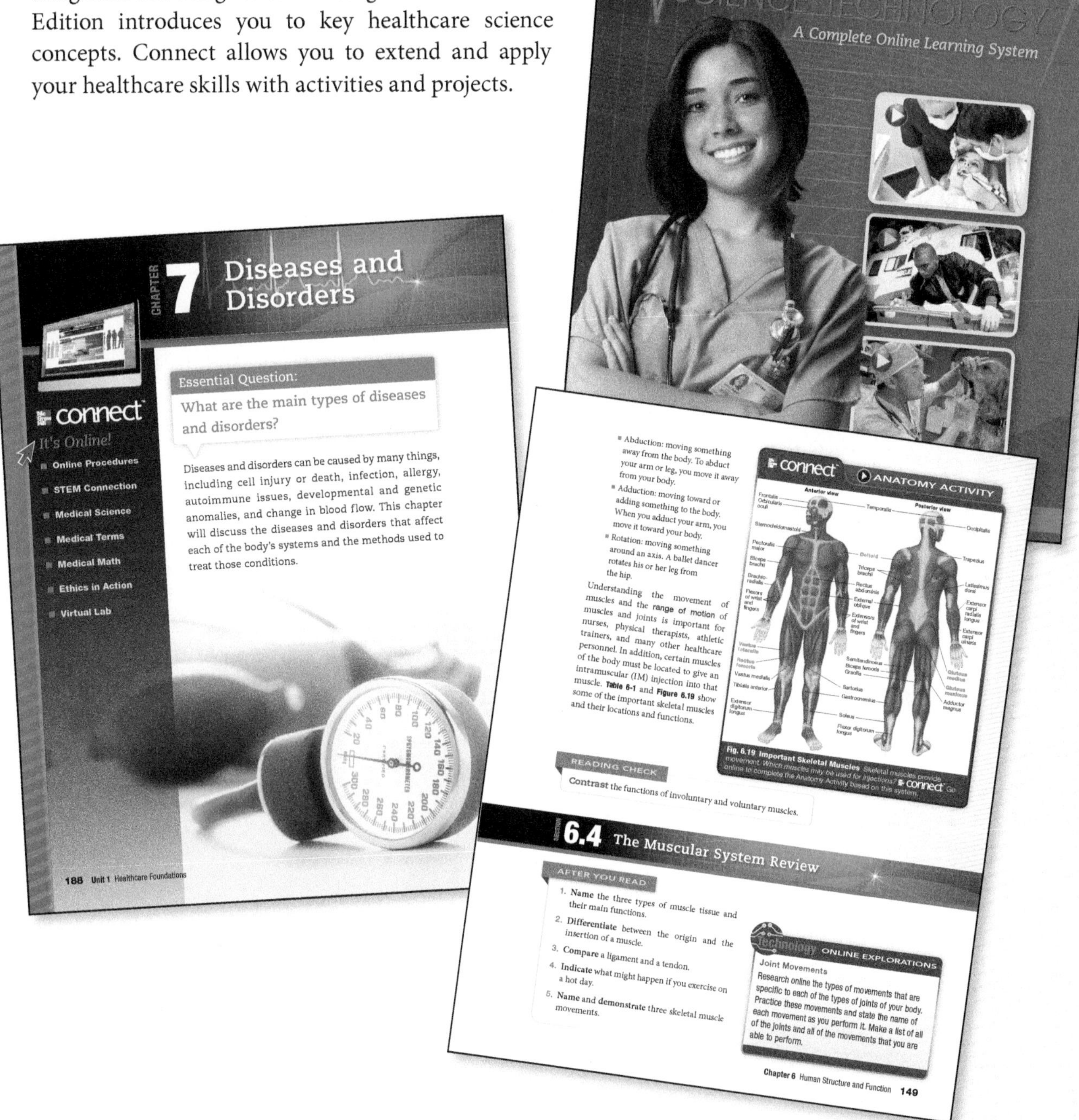

connect It's Online!

HEALTHCARE SCIENCE TECHNOLOGY

A Complete Online Learning System

CHAPTER 7 Diseases and Disorders

connect It's Online!

- Online Procedures
- STEM Connection
- Medical Science
- Medical Terms
- Medical Math
- Ethics in Action
- Virtual Lab

Essential Question:

What are the main types of diseases and disorders?

Diseases and disorders can be caused by many things, including cell injury or death, infection, allergy, autoimmune issues, developmental and genetic anomalies, and change in blood flow. This chapter will discuss the diseases and disorders that affect each of the body's systems and the methods used to treat those conditions.

188 Unit 1 Healthcare Foundations

- Abduction: moving something away from the body. To abduct your arm or leg, you move it away from your body.
- Adduction: moving toward or adding something to the body. When you adduct your arm, you move it toward your body.
- Rotation: moving something around an axis. A ballet dancer rotates his or her leg from the hip.

Understanding the movement of muscles and the **range of motion** of muscles and joints is important for nurses, physical therapists, athletic trainers, and many other healthcare personnel. In addition, certain muscles of the body must be located to give an intramuscular (IM) injection into that muscle. **Table 6-1** and **Figure 6.19** show some of the important skeletal muscles and their locations and functions.

connect ANATOMY ACTIVITY

Fig. 6.19 Important Skeletal Muscles Skeletal muscles provide movement. *Which muscles may be used for injections?* connect Go online to complete the Anatomy Activity based on this system.

READING CHECK

Contrast the functions of involuntary and voluntary muscles.

SECTION 6.4 The Muscular System Review

AFTER YOU READ

1. **Name** the three types of muscle tissue and their main functions.
2. **Differentiate** between the origin and the insertion of a muscle.
3. **Compare** a ligament and a tendon.
4. **Indicate** what might happen if you exercise on a hot day.
5. **Name** and **demonstrate** three skeletal muscle movements.

Technology ONLINE EXPLORATIONS

Joint Movements

Research online the types of movements that are specific to each of the types of joints of your body. Practice these movements and state the name of each movement as you perform it. Make a list of all of the joints and all of the movements that you are able to perform.

Chapter 6 Human Structure and Function 149

Learning for Everyone

What Are Standards?

Being prepared for college or a career includes developing a wide range of skills that you will need to meet future educational and employment needs and expectations. Standards are an established and agreed-upon set of measures or guidelines for the knowledge, processes, and practices that you as a student should know or be able to do to succeed in your academic and professional careers.

Healthcare Science Technology meets key academic and professional standards. The Reading Guide at the beginning of each chapter contains a list of the standards that are covered in that chapter. With these standards as your foundation, you will have a better understanding of healthcare science principles, and you will continue to develop your academic skills, too.

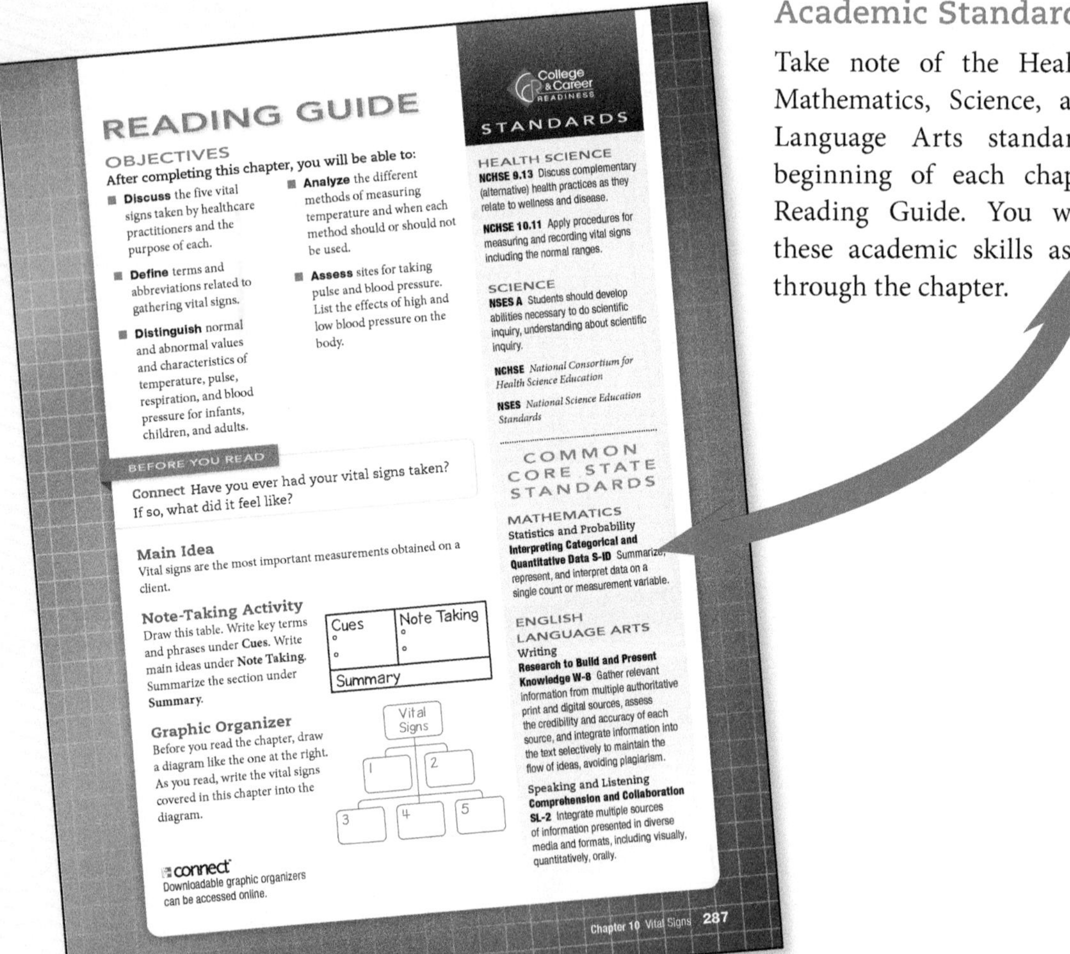

READING GUIDE

OBJECTIVES

After completing this chapter, you will be able to:

- **Discuss** the five vital signs taken by healthcare practitioners and the purpose of each.
- **Define** terms and abbreviations related to gathering vital signs.
- **Distinguish** normal and abnormal values and characteristics of temperature, pulse, respiration, and blood pressure for infants, children, and adults.
- **Analyze** the different methods of measuring temperature and when each method should or should not be used.
- **Assess** sites for taking pulse and blood pressure. List the effects of high and low blood pressure on the body.

BEFORE YOU READ

Connect Have you ever had your vital signs taken? If so, what did it feel like?

Main Idea
Vital signs are the most important measurements obtained on a client.

Note-Taking Activity
Draw this table. Write key terms and phrases under **Cues**. Write main ideas under **Note Taking**. Summarize the section under **Summary**.

Cues	Note Taking
∘ ∘	∘ ∘
Summary	

Graphic Organizer
Before you read the chapter, draw a diagram like the one at the right. As you read, write the vital signs covered in this chapter into the diagram.

connect
Downloadable graphic organizers can be accessed online.

College & Career READINESS

STANDARDS

HEALTH SCIENCE

NCHSE 9.13 Discuss complementary (alternative) health practices as they relate to wellness and disease.

NCHSE 10.11 Apply procedures for measuring and recording vital signs including the normal ranges.

SCIENCE

NSES A Students should develop abilities necessary to do scientific inquiry, understanding about scientific inquiry.

NCHSE *National Consortium for Health Science Education*

NSES *National Science Education Standards*

COMMON CORE STATE STANDARDS

MATHEMATICS
Statistics and Probability
Interpreting Categorical and Quantitative Data S-ID Summarize, represent, and interpret data on a single count or measurement variable.

ENGLISH LANGUAGE ARTS
Writing
Research to Build and Present Knowledge W-8 Gather relevant information from multiple authoritative print and digital sources, assess the credibility and accuracy of each source, and integrate information into the text selectively to maintain the flow of ideas, avoiding plagiarism.

Speaking and Listening
Comprehension and Collaboration SL-2 Integrate multiple sources of information presented in diverse media and formats, including visually, quantitatively, orally.

Chapter 10 Vital Signs 287

Academic Standards

Take note of the Health Science, Mathematics, Science, and English Language Arts standards at the beginning of each chapter in the Reading Guide. You will practice these academic skills as you move through the chapter.

Integrating the Student Edition and McGraw-Hill connect™

For *Healthcare Science Technology*, McGraw-Hill's Connect houses animated healthcare procedures and resources for students and instructors, as well as the eBook.

McGraw-Hill Connect is a Web-based assignment and assessment platform that links students with their coursework.

The eBook is the electronic version of the textbook. It is only available on Connect.

After students have been registered in a McGraw-Hill Connect course, they may sign in at the course's Web address or http://connect.mcgraw-hill.com/k12 to access the corresponding program materials.

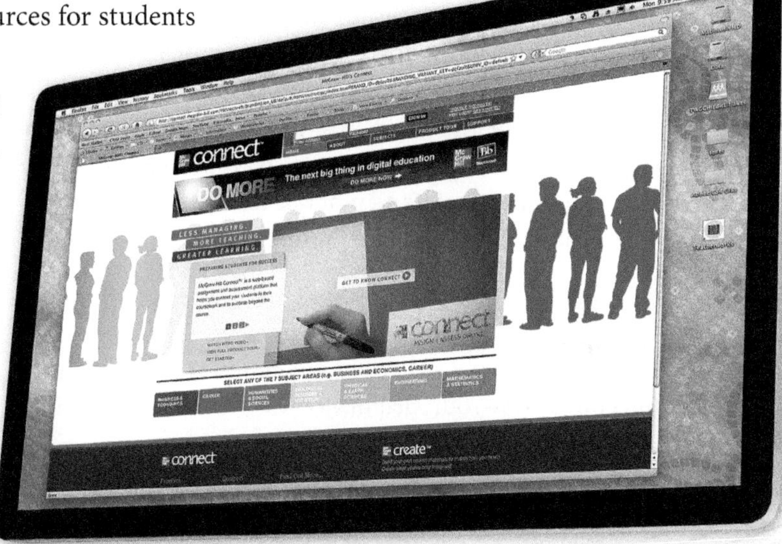

McGraw-Hill Connect

The course homepage provides links to these and other resources, as assigned by the teacher. This is where students will find course procedures, assignments, and activities.

Healthcare Science Technology features procedures that allow students to apply the concepts they have learned in the textbook. They can be completed using animations and the Lab Procedure Assessments within Connect. 150 lab procedures are animated online, allowing students to view them as often as necessary. Procedure recording sheets are available online for each lab procedure.

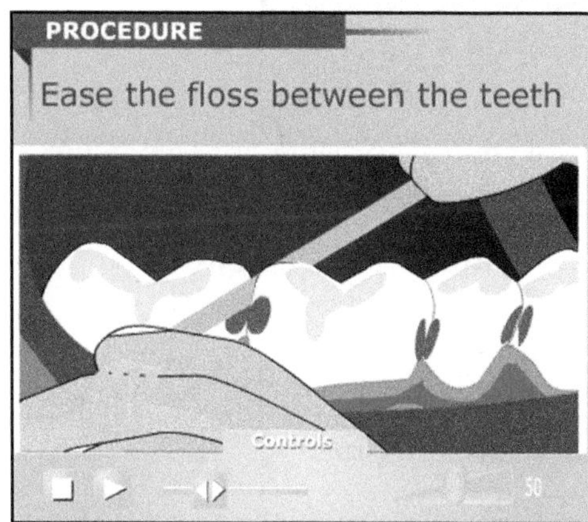

In Connect, students can move seamlessly between the eBook and other resources by following these steps:

1. Open the eBook in Connect.
2. When you encounter a feature with a blue launch button, click on it to launch the assignment. You can return to the eBook at any time.

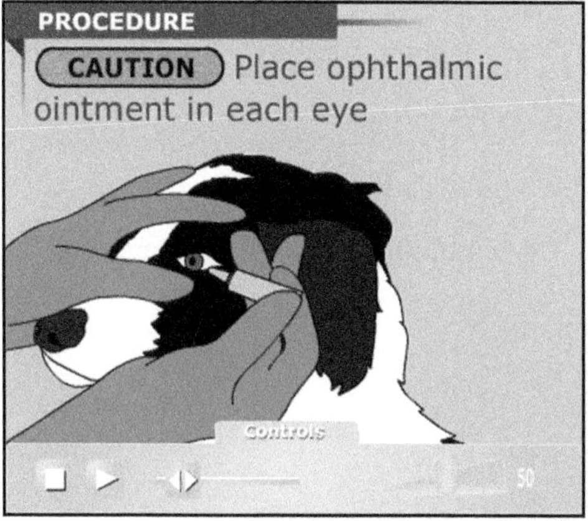

Hybrid Program Overview

Mc Graw Hill **connect**™

McGraw-Hill's *Healthcare Science Technology* is the first truly integrated text and online healthcare science program. Reading the textbook will introduce you to the core principles of healthcare science and will help you to understand the knowledge, skills, and vocabulary needed in this field. At various points throughout the text, you will be directed to apply what you have learned in online activities, hands-on projects, and practice tests. Become familiar with the key icons shown below to know when to complete an assignment online:

Connect

Use Connect to access your *Healthcare Science Technology* course.

Access Your Materials

- Watch videos and complete assignments.
- Complete hands-on Lab Procedures and interact with class members.

Learn

Access additional resources

- Online Procedures (pre-procedure, procedure, and post-procedure)
- Virtual Lab animations
- Medical Math
- Medical Science
- Medical Terms
- Anatomy Activities

Access Your eBook Anywhere

- Store class notes.
- Highlight and bookmark material online.

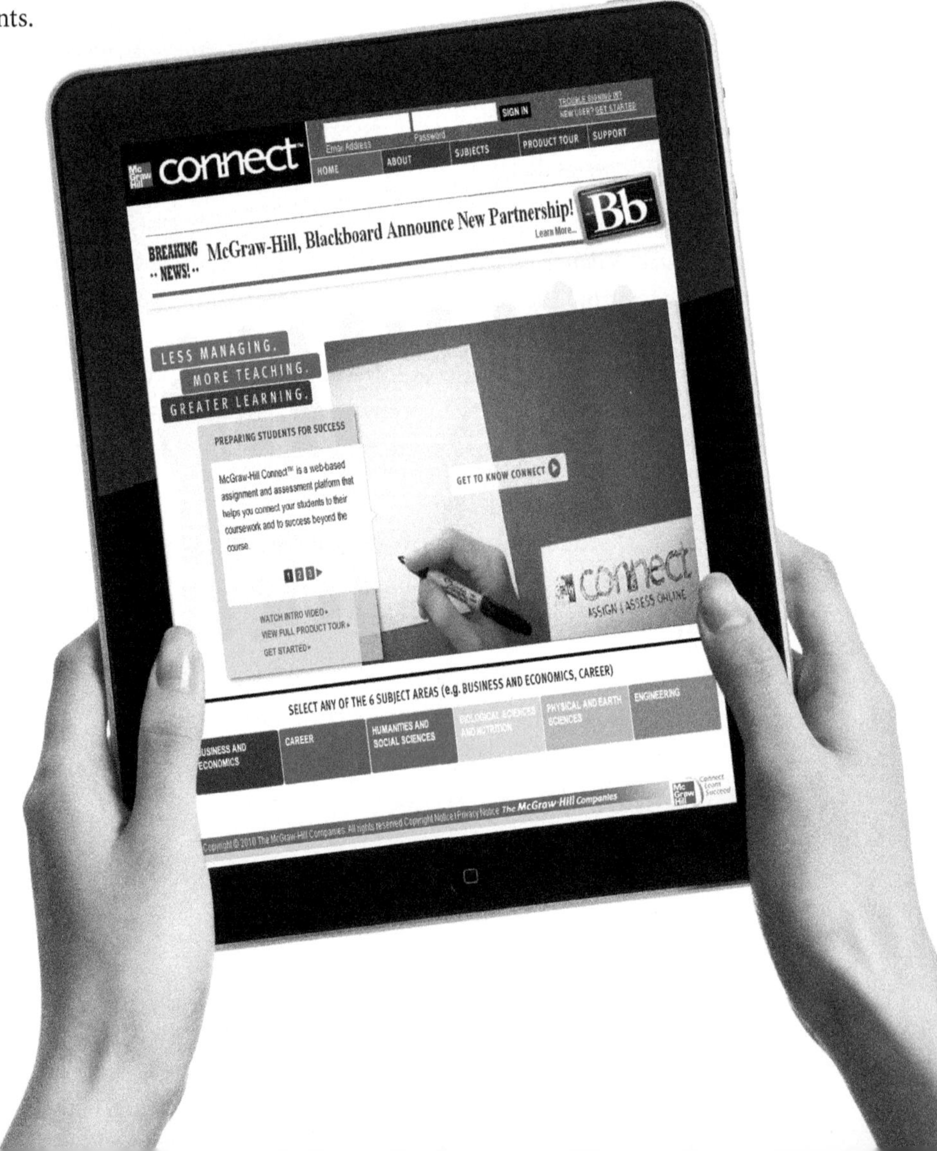

Hybrid Program Overview

Assess

- Complete Procedure Assessments online.
- Medical Terminology practice online.

Succeed

- Complete your homework online.
- Get immediate feedback on your work.
- Link back to sections of the book to review core healthcare concepts.
- Review online procedures.

Easy to access! Easy to use!

Connect to McGraw-Hill *Healthcare Science Technology* at connect.mcgraw-hill.com/k12

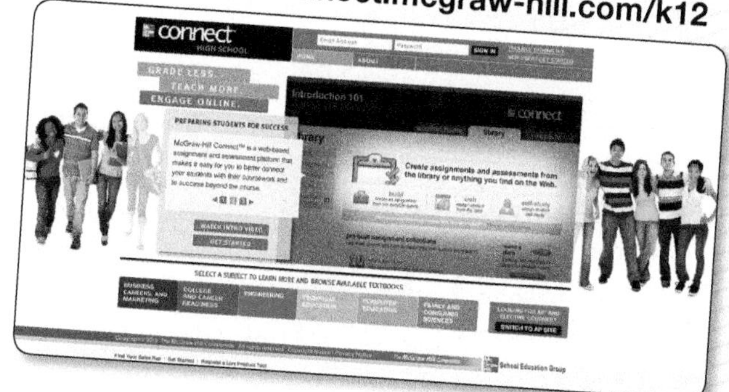

Icon Key

connect™

McGraw-Hill Connect™ is a web-based assignment and assessment platform that helps you connect to your course and success beyond the course. Every time you see the Connect logo, your assignment will involve watching a video or animation online, working in the lab manual, or completing another activity.

Procedures

The *Online Procedures* bring healthcare concepts to life through animation.

Medical Math

The *Medical Math* features help you learn about and practice important math concepts.

Medical Science

The *Medical Science* features will help you understand the different science concepts you'll need to know in the healthcare field.

Virtual Lab

The *Virtual Lab* features help you practice healthcare-related science concepts.

Online Activities

The *Online Activities* include review questions, medical terminology practice flash cards, and procedure assessment sheets.

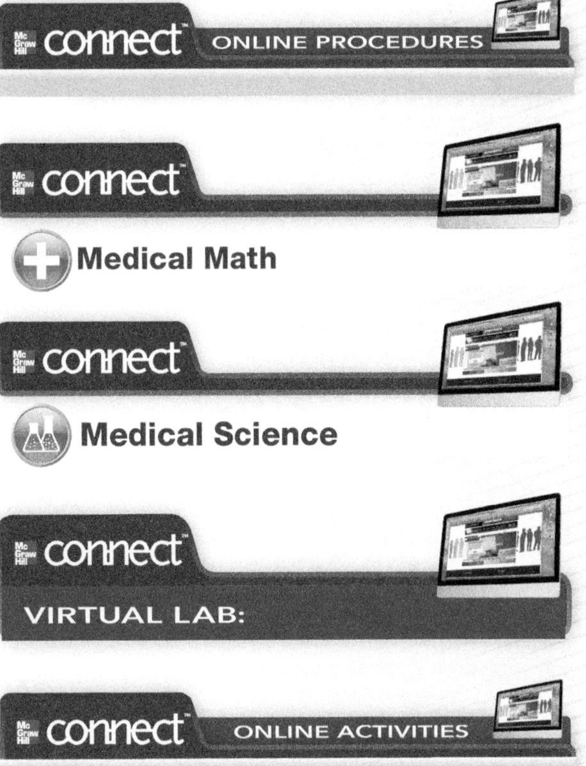

UNIT 1 Healthcare Foundations

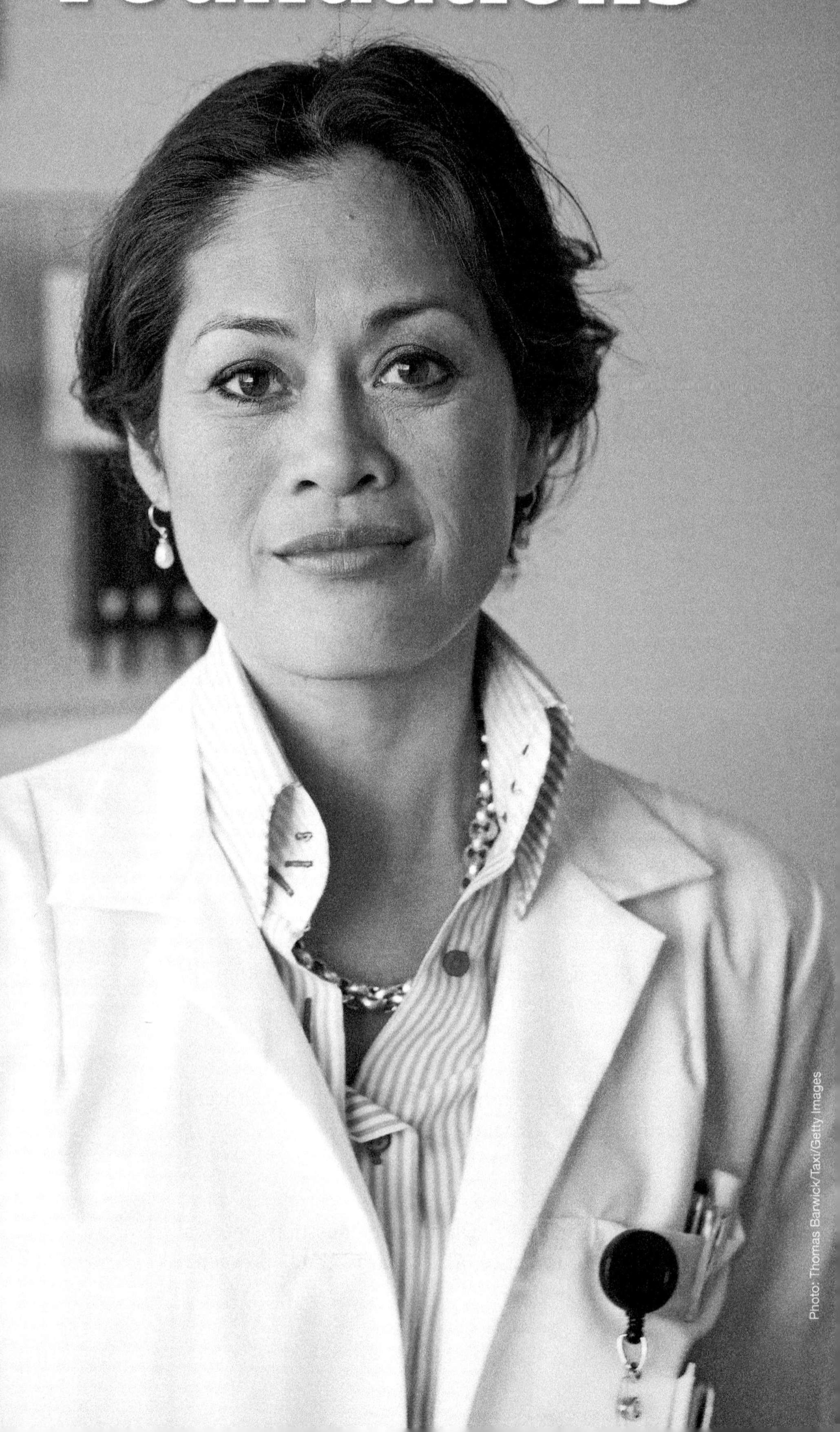

Photo: Thomas Barwick/Taxi/Getty Images

CHAPTER 1 Healthcare Career Clusters

Essential Question:

How will you determine which area of healthcare to pursue in your career?

Welcome! You are about to embark on an exciting adventure into the healthcare profession. The chapters of this book will introduce you to a variety of health careers. Some health careers are stepping stones to other careers in healthcare. Because the healthcare field is growing so rapidly, there may even be health careers in your future that do not currently exist! Health career opportunities are many. There are more than 300 career possibilities waiting for you!

This course can help you decide whether the healthcare field is right for you. It can also help you choose the right health career.

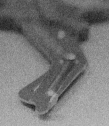

McGraw-Hill connect™

It's Online!

- Online Procedures
- STEM Connection
- Medical Science
- Medical Terms
- Medical Math
- Ethics in Action
- Virtual Lab

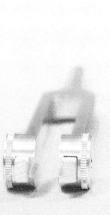

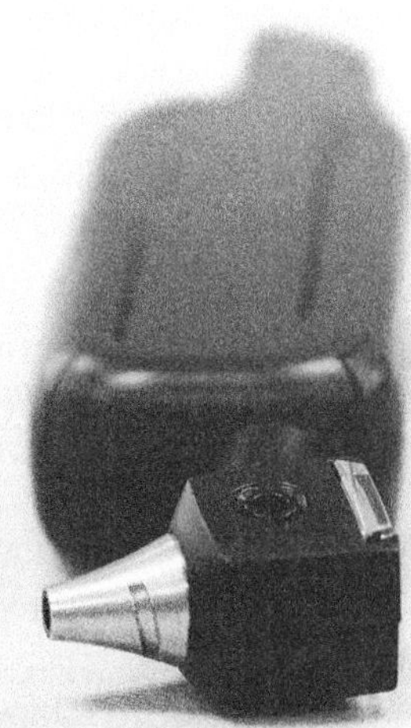

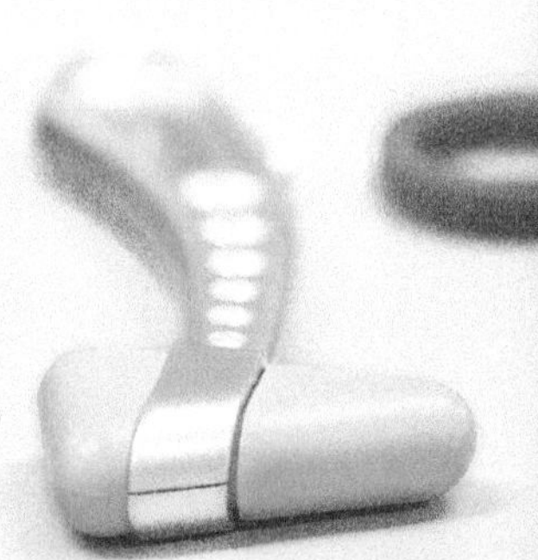

Photo: The McGraw-Hill Companies Inc.

READING GUIDE

OBJECTIVES

After completing this chapter, you will be able to:

- **Discuss** the importance of the National Healthcare Skill Standards.
- **Identify** two reasons for maintaining standards for the healthcare industry.
- **Explain** the five career pathways in healthcare employment.
- **Identify** opportunities for employment and entrepreneurship in the healthcare field.
- **Carry out** a career assessment.
- **Summarize** the importance of professional student organizations and outline how meetings should be conducted.

BEFORE YOU READ

Connect Do you know what career options you have in the healthcare industry?

Main Idea

The five career pathways in healthcare are therapeutic services, diagnostic services, health informatics, support services, and biotechnology research and development.

Note-Taking Activity

Draw this table. Write key terms and phrases under **Cues**. Write main ideas under **Note Taking**. Summarize the section under **Summary**.

Cues	Note Taking
o	o
o	o
Summary	

Graphic Organizer

Before you read the chapter, draw a diagram like the one below. As you read, write the main opportunities covered in the chapter into the diagram.

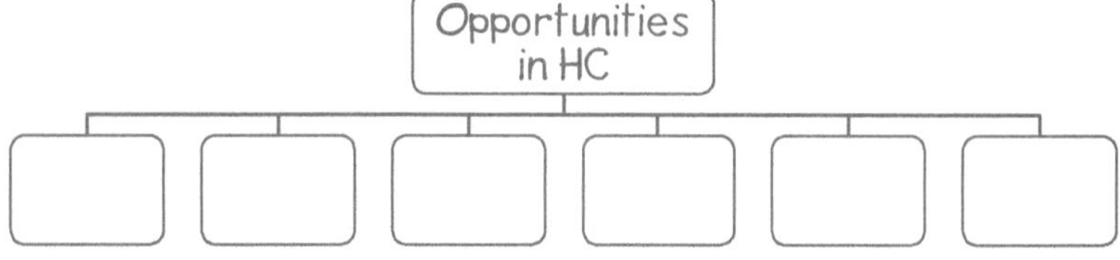

connect
Downloadable graphic organizers can be accessed online.

STANDARDS

HEALTH SCIENCE

NCHSE 4.31 Discuss levels of education, credentialing requirements, and employment trends in healthcare.

NCHSE 4.32 Compare careers within the health science career pathways (diagnostic services, therapeutic services, health informatics, support services, or biotechnology research and development).

SCIENCE

NSES F Develop understanding of personal and community health; population growth; natural resources; environmental quality; natural and human-induced hazards; science and technology in local, national, and global challenges.

NCHSE *National Consortium for Health Science Education*

NSES *National Science Education Standards*

COMMON CORE STATE STANDARDS

MATHEMATICS

Number and Quantity

Quantities N–Q Reason quantitatively and use units to solve problems.

ENGLISH LANGUAGE ARTS

Reading

Key Ideas and Details R-1 Cite specific textual evidence to support analysis of science and technical texts, attending to the precise details of explanations or descriptions.

Writing

Production and Distribution of Writing W-4 Produce clear and coherent writing in which the development, organization, and style are appropriate to task, purpose, and audience.

SECTION

1.1 Careers in Healthcare

National Healthcare Skill Standards

How do I enter the field of healthcare?

The **National Consortium for Health Science Education** has set forth National Standards that identify the knowledge and skills that a healthcare worker needs if he or she is to deliver quality healthcare. This framework of **standards** guides educators as they work to produce quality entry-level healthcare professionals. In **Table 1.1** on page 6, you will see a list of the healthcare skill foundation standards. This table shows the basic knowledge and skills you must attain in order to enter the field of healthcare. If you know the standards, you will be better prepared for the job, and your chances for advancement will increase. When you and your coworkers are familiar with the standards, you will have clear goals and will become more valuable as healthcare employees.

All members of a healthcare system need to be in agreement regarding the quality of patient care. When each member of the healthcare team follows a set of high standards, the care given to the patient is of the highest quality. We will look at each of the standards, their importance, and what they mean to your employment in the field of healthcare.

Academic Foundation

A strong academic foundation is vital to any type of career. A person cannot perform a task if he or she has not learned how to perform it. As a healthcare professional, you will need to know about human structure, body systems and functions, diseases and disorders, and medical mathematics.

Communication

Communication, whether it is reading, writing, speaking, or listening, is a part of life as well as a part of patient care. As a healthcare professional, you must be able to interact with, and relate to, the patient and other healthcare team members. For example, you may need to read a patient's chart, record information, educate a patient, or listen to your supervisor's instructions. Or you may need to spend time listening to your patients and determining their needs. Knowledge of medical terminology is a must. See Chapter 5, Medical Terminology.

Vocabulary

Content Vocabulary

You will learn these content vocabulary terms in this section

- **National Consortium for Health Science Education**
- **standards**
- **therapeutic services**
- **diagnostic services**
- **health informatics**
- **support services**
- **biotechnology**

Academic Vocabulary

You will see these words in your reading and on your tests. Find their meanings in the Glossary in the back of the book.

- **foundation**
- **communication**
- **ethics**
- **technology**

Table 1.1 Healthcare Skill Standards

NATIONAL HEALTHCARE SKILL STANDARD	INTERPRETATION
Academic foundation	Healthcare professionals will know the academic subject matter required for proficiency within their area. They will use this knowledge as needed in their role. These include: human structure and function, diseases and disorders, and medical mathematics.
Communication	Healthcare professionals will know the various methods of giving and obtaining information. They will communicate effectively, both orally and in writing, and have knowledge of medical terminology.
Systems	Healthcare professionals will understand how their roles fit into their departments, their organizations, and the overall health-care environment. They will be able to identify how healthcare delivery systems affect the services they perform and quality of care they provide.
Employability skills	Healthcare professionals will understand how employability skills enhance their employment opportunities and job satis-faction. They will demonstrate personal traits and behaviors, such as decision-making abilities and preparation, that enhance their employability.
Legal responsibilities	Healthcare professionals will understand the legal responsibilities, limitations, and implications of their actions within the healthcare delivery setting. They will perform their duties according to regulations, policies, laws, and the legislated rights of patients.
Ethics	Healthcare professionals will understand accepted ethical practices with respect to cultural, social, and ethnic differences within the healthcare environment. They will perform quality healthcare delivery.
Safety practices	Healthcare professionals will understand the existing and potential hazards to patients, coworkers, and themselves. They will prevent injury or illness through safe work practices and will follow health and safety policies and procedures.
Teamwork	Healthcare professionals will understand the roles and responsibilities of individual members as part of a healthcare team, including their ability to promote the delivery of quality healthcare. They will interact effectively and sensitively with all members of the healthcare team.
Health maintenance practices	Healthcare professionals will understand the fundamentals of wellness and the process of preventing disease. They will practice preventive health behaviors among the patients.
Technical skills	Healthcare professionals will apply technical skills required for all career specialties. They will demonstrate skills and knowledge as appropriate.
Information technology skills	Healthcare professionals will use information technology applications required within all career specialties. They will demonstrate the use of information technology as appropriate to healthcare applications.

ADMINISTRATION

Hospital Board
Physicians
Administrator

HOSPITAL DEPARTMENTS

Nursing
Pharmacy
Laboratory
Dietary
Biomedical
Radiology
Business Office
Rehabilitation
Central Supply
Physical Therapy
Occupational Therapy

NURSING DEPARTMENT OF HOSPITAL

Director of Nursing
Surgery
Emergency
Inpatient
Nursing Education
Clinic
Nursing Supervisor
Head or Charge Nurse
R.N.
L.P.N./L.V.N.
Assistants/Aides
Orderlies
Unit or Ward Clerk
Volunteers

CLINIC OR MEDICAL OFFICE ORGANIZATION

Physician
Office Manager
Laboratory
R.N.
Housekeeping/Maintenance
Business Office
L.P.N./L.V.N.
Clinical Medical Assistants
Clerical Reception
Billing Insurance

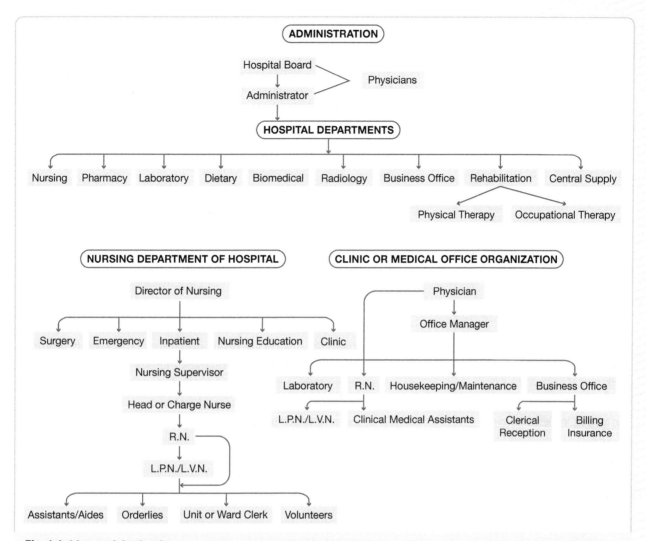

Fig. 1.1 Lines of Authority Organizational structures help define responsibilities. *Can you determine the lines of authority in these organizations?*

Systems

As a healthcare professional, you must learn how all the systems in a healthcare facility work together to provide patient care. You should also be aware of how your facility fits into the overall healthcare environment and relates to other facilities. In addition, you should know what services each department within the facility provides for patient care. For example, a physician sees a patient in his or her office or in a hospital, depending upon the patient's needs. A laboratory must draw blood, and an X-ray department may do an X-ray before surgery. A coordinated effort is required for ideal care.

Employability Skills

To be employable, which means to be able to get and keep a job, you must develop certain traits and behaviors. For example, you should arrive on time and complete each task with attention to detail. Otherwise, you may lose your job. Chapter 13, Communication and Employability Skills, gives more details about such skills.

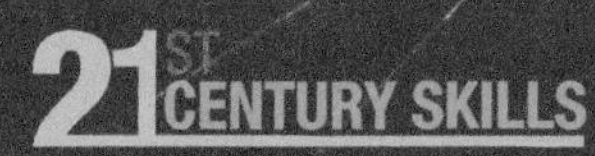

Teamwork and the Organizational Structure

All facilities have an organizational structure that contribute to the efficient operation of the facility. It identifies the relationships among departments or individuals and the line of authority. It also defines areas of responsibility. **Figure 1.1** shows sample structures. Healthcare professionals must know the organizational structure of their place of employment. You should know and follow the line of authority leading from you upward through the levels of supervision.

 connect 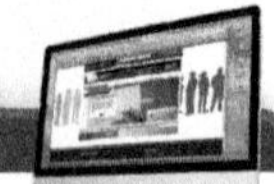

Ethics in Action

Cloning

A stem cell is a primitive type of cell that can be made to develop into most of the 220 types of cells found in the human body, such as blood cells, heart cells, and brain cells. Some researchers regard stem cells as offering the greatest potential for the lessening of human suffering since the development of antibiotics. More than 100 million Americans suffer from diseases that may eventually be treated more effectively, or may even be cured, with stem cells. Duplicating stem cells is called cloning. When this is done with the objective of finding cures for diseases, it is called therapeutic cloning.

Go to connect to learn more about the ethics of cloning and complete the related Group Workspace discussion activity.

Legal Responsibilities

Knowing what you are and are not allowed to do according to law is a requirement for healthcare employees. You must follow the rules and regulations of the career field you choose. For example, a nursing assistant may give a patient a bath but is not allowed to give an injection.

Ethics

Ethics is defined as a set of principles that determines what is morally right or wrong. Healthcare professional organizations define the ethics by which their field is governed. Professionals are expected to know these ethical standards, and they are expected to practice according to those principles. Ethical dilemmas often arise in the field of healthcare. Legal and ethical responsibilities are discussed in Chapter 12.

Safety Practices

The patient and the healthcare professional must stay safe throughout the patient care process. Safety practices include fire safety training, electrical safety training, infection control, prevention of injury, and emergency preparedness. You should know how to clean up spills, handle blood and other bodily fluids, and lift and move patients in a safe manner so as not to cause injury or spread disease. See Chapter 3, Safety and Infection Control Practices.

Teamwork

Teams are groups of people working together for a common goal. Teamwork is crucial to quality healthcare. As a healthcare professional, you must understand your role and know how to interact effectively with others. For example, as a nurse, you may need to call the laboratory to find out the results of a test, or you may work side by side with a physician who is sewing up a wound.

Health Maintenance Practices

Prevention of disease means engaging in behaviors that help you maintain an optimal state of health, which is known as wellness. Have you ever been told to "eat right, exercise, and get plenty of rest"? These are examples of health practices that you should engage in—and should encourage your patients to practice.

Technical Skills

Healthcare professionals should learn the skills related to their career field. For example, a laboratory technician needs the skills to draw blood safely and efficiently.

Information Technology Skills

Today you may learn how to use one machine to take blood pressure. Tomorrow you may need to learn how to use a more technical or advanced machine to take blood pressure. Systems of computers connect departments within one facility. Wireless connections provide high-speed communication. Technology change is constant in healthcare. The challenge for you is to stay informed.

READING CHECK

Identify three parts of the academic foundations for healthcare professionals.

Healthcare Career Pathways

Which career pathway do you think is the best fit for you?

The National Healthcare Skill Standards were created for the benefit of all students in the field of healthcare. No matter what healthcare career you choose, these standards apply.

Healthcare careers are divided into five career pathways. Learning about the pathways will help you make an educated decision about which healthcare career to enter. The five pathways are:

- Therapeutic Service Careers
- Diagnostic Service Careers
- Health Informatics Careers
- Support Services Careers
- Biotechnology Research and Development Careers

Table 1.2 on page 10, which was developed by the National Consortium for Health Science Education, lists sample career specialties and occupations in each of the five pathways. Note that each pathway includes a wide variety of careers. This book will focus on the most common careers. It will include more detailed information about the types of careers, the education needed, and the procedures employed.

Therapeutic Service Careers

Healthcare professionals in a career in **therapeutic services** provide a service to the patient over time. Some career options in this pathway are in the areas of clinical medical assisting, nursing, home healthcare, respiratory care, rehabilitation, and pharmacy. The amount of education required within this pathway depends on the level of achievement the student chooses within his or her career. Skills needed in this pathway include data collection, treatment planning, implementing procedures, and patient status evaluation. **Figure 1.2** shows a nursing assistant, one of the careers in therapeutic services.

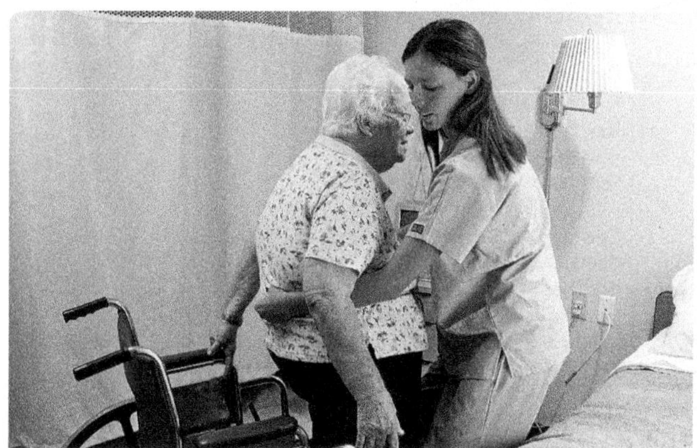

Fig. 1.2 Career Pathways A nursing assistant is one career in therapeutic services. *Why is the position of nursing assistant included in the therapeutic career pathway?*

Table 1.2 Healthcare Career Pathways

Pathways	THERAPEUTIC SERVICES	DIAGNOSTICS SERVICES	HEALTH INFORMATICS	SUPPORT SERVICES	BIOTECHNOLOGY RESEARCH AND DEVELOPMENT
Sample Career Specialties/Occupations	Acupuncturist Anesthesiologist/Assistant Anesthesia Technologist/Technician Art/Music/Dance Therapist(s) Athletic Trainer Audiologist Certified Nursing Assistant Chiropractor Chiropractic Assistant Dental Assistant/Hygienist Dental Lab Technician Dietitian/Nutritionist Dosimetrist EMT/Paramedic Endodontist Exercise Physiologist Home Health Aide Kinesiotherapist Licensed Practical Nurse Massage Therapist Medical Assistant Mental Health Counselor Naturopathic Doctor Nurse Anesthetist Nurse Midwife Nurse Practitioner Occupational Therapist/Assistant Oral Surgeon Orientation/Mobility Specialist Orthodontist Orthoptist Orthotist/Prosthetist/Technician Pedorthist Perfusionist Pharmacist Pharmacy Technician Physical Therapist/Assistant Physician (MD/DO) Physician Assistant Podiatrist Psychologist Psychiatrist Radiation Therapist Recreation Therapist Registered Nurse Rehabilitation Counselor Respiratory Therapist Speech-Language Therapist Surgical Technician Veterinarian Veterinarian Assistant/Technician Vision Rehabilitation Therapist Wellness Coach	Audiologist Blood Bank Technology Specialist Cardiovascular Technologist Clinical Lab Technician Clinical Laboratory/Technologist Computer Tomography (CT) Technologist Cytogenetic Technologist Cytotechnologist Dentist Diagnostic Medical Sonographer Electrocardiographic (ECG) Technician Electroneurodiagnostic Technologist Electronic Diagnostic (EEG) Technologist Exercise Physiologist Geneticist Geriatrician Histotechnician Histotechnologist Magnetic Resonance Technologist Mammographer Medical Technologist/Clinical Laboratory Scientist Nuclear Medicine Technologist Optician Ophthalmologist Ophthalmic Assistant/Technologist Optometrist Pathologist Pathologists' Assistant Phlebotomist Polysomnographic Technologist Positron Emission Tomography (PET) Technologist Radiologic Technologist Radiologist Speech-Language Pathologist	Admitting Clerk Applied Researcher Compliance Technician Clinical Account Manager Clinical Account Technician Clinical Data Specialist Community Services Specialists Data Quality Manager Epidemiologist Ethicist Health Educator Health Information Mgmt. Administrator Health Information Mgmt. Technician Healthcare Access Manager Healthcare Administrator Healthcare Finance Informatician Information Privacy Officer Managed Care Contract Analyst Medical Coder Medical Historian Medical Illustrator Medical Information Technologist Medical Librarian Medical Transcriptionist Patient Account Manager Patient Account Technician Patient Advocate Patient Information Coordinator Project Manager Public Health Educator Quality Management Specialist Quality Data Analyst Research and Decision Support Specialist Reimbursement Specialist Risk Manager Unit Coordinator Utilization Manager Utilization Review Manager	Animal Behaviorist Biomedical/Clinical Engineer Biomedical/Clinical Technician Clinical Simulator Technician Central Service Manager Central Service Technician Community Health Worker Dietary Manager Dietetic Technician Environmental Health Advocate Environmental Health Practitioner Environmental Services/Specialist Facilities Manager Food Safety Specialist Health Advocate Hospital Maintenance Engineer Industrial Hygienist Interpreter/Translator Marital, Couple, Family Counselor/Therapist Materials Manager Medical Health Counselor Mortician/ Funeral Director Nurse Educator Occupational Health Nurse Occupational Health & Safety Expert Social Worker Transport Technician	Biochemist Bioinformatics Scientist Biomedical Chemist Biomedical Manufacturing Technician Biostatistician Cancer Registrar Cell Biologist Clinical Data Management Specialist Clinical Pharmacologist Clinical Trials Monitor Clinical Trials Research Coordinator Crime Scene Investigator Diagnostic Molecular Scientist Forensic Biologist Forensic Chemist Forensic Odontologist Forensic Pathologist Genetic Counselor Geneticist-Lab Assistant Lab Technician Medical Editor/Writer Microbiologist Molecular Biologist Nurse Researcher Packaging Technician Patent Lawyer Pharmaceutical/Clinical Project Manager Pharmaceutical Sales Representative Pharmaceutical Scientist Pharmacokineticist Pharmacologist Product Safety Scientist Process Development Scientist Processing Technician Quality Assurance Technician Quality Control Technician Regulatory Affairs Specialist Research Assistant Research Scientist Toxicologist
Cluster K & S	**Cluster Knowledge and Skills** • Academic Foundation • Communications • Systems • Employability Skills • Legal Responsibilities• Ethics • Safety Practices • Teamwork• Health Maintenance Practices • Technical Skills• Information Technology Applications				

Diagnostic Service Careers

People in **diagnostic service** careers create a "picture" of the health status of a patient at one point in time. For example, if a patient has blood drawn, the results reported are only for the point in time at which the blood was drawn. If the patient were in an accident the next day, the results might be different. Skills needed within this pathway include planning, preparation, procedure, evaluation, and reporting. Some careers in this pathway are in the areas of cardiology, imaging, and radiology. The technician shown in **Figure 1.3** has a career in diagnostic services.

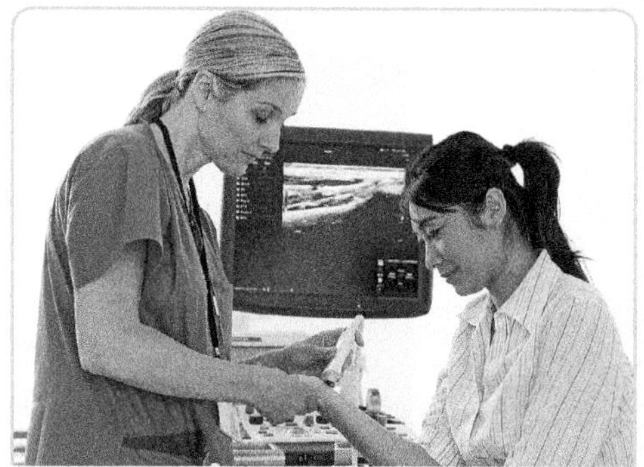

Fig. 1.3. Diagnostic Services Careers in this field create a "picture" of a client's health status. *What is the basic function of diagnostic services?*

Health Informatics Careers

People employed in **health informatics** careers record the patient's valuable healthcare information. Skills needed are analysis, abstracting and coding, informatics systems, documentation, and operations. Some career options in informatics services are in medical records and unit coordination. **Figure 1.4** shows a health informatics technician at work.

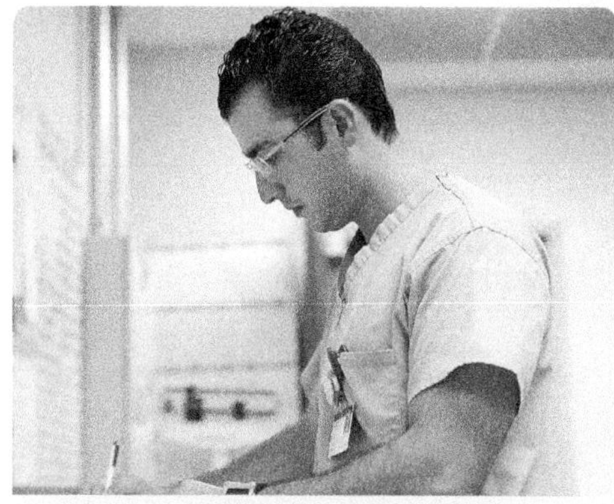

Fig. 1.4 Health Informatics Careers in this field record a client's healthcare information. *Why is a career in computerized medical records considered to be in the health informatics career category?*

Support Services Careers

People in careers in **support services** create a safe and healthful environment for the patient and other healthcare professionals. In support services, knowledge of aseptic procedures and an understanding of the importance of an esthetically appealing environment are important. Examples of careers in this field are biomedical engineer and central supply technician. The central supply technician shown in **Figure 1.5** has a career in support services.

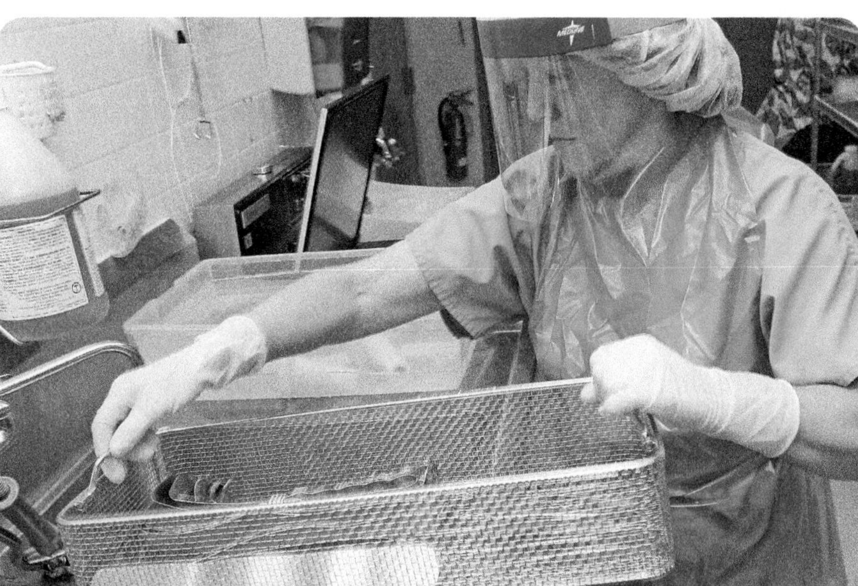

Fig. 1.5 Support Services Biomedical engineer and central supply technician are careers in support services. *Why is a central supply technician in the support services career category?*

Photos: (t)Echo/Cultura/Getty Images, (c)Helen King/CORBIS, (b)David Grossman/Alamy

Biotechnology Research and Development Careers

The fifth pathway for health careers is **biotechnology** research and development. These careers are highly scientific. Biotechnology is a field of applied biology that involves living organisms and bioprocesses such as engineering, technology, and medicine. In general, people in these careers work in laboratories. However, they may also travel to various locations to study and explore elements in the environment. They are biologists and chemists. A strong background in and enjoyment of science is necessary. Your high school course work for a career of this kind should include biology, chemistry, physics, computer science, and mathematics. Working in a summer research program at a local college also will be good experience if you have an interest in this field. You may also want to find a mentor or someone who is currently in the field to provide additional information.

It is exciting to choose a career in healthcare because you have so many careers from which to choose. Choosing a career means matching your needs and interests with a career. Your choice will depend on many things, such as the education necessary and the jobs available. Section 1.2 will discuss education, employment, and entrepreneurial opportunities, along with the value of a career assessment.

READING CHECK

List the five career pathways in healthcare.

SECTION 1.1 Careers in Healthcare Review

AFTER YOU READ

1. **Illustrate** why the National Healthcare Skill Standards are important in pursuing a career in the healthcare industry.
2. **Examine** one of the National Healthcare Skill Standards and explain why it is important. Give an example of how the standard is used in a healthcare profession.
3. **Identify** a job opportunity in each of the healthcare career pathways.
4. **Classify** each of the following professional careers by pathway: physician assistant, biomedical engineer, veterinary technician, electrocardiographic technician, geneticist, and unit coordinator.
5. **Select** five courses you should take in high school as a foundation for a career in biotechnology.

Technology ONLINE EXPLORATIONS

Career Information

Choose a health career that interests you and find out about it by accessing the Occupational Outlook Handbook at www.bls.gov. This is a U.S. Department of Labor website, and it will give you valuable information regarding all types of careers. Print out the information on your chosen career and share the information with your class.

SECTION

1.2 Opportunities in Healthcare

Education

How much time do you plan to spend on career education?

Opportunities in healthcare are increasing. According to the Bureau of Labor Statistics, about 26 percent of new jobs until 2018 will be in the healthcare and social assistance industry. This industry, which includes public and private hospitals, nursing and residential care facilities, and individual and family services, is expected to grow by 24 percent, adding 4 million new jobs. This growth is driven by an aging population and longer life expectancies.

Some high schools offer programs in the health sciences and certificates for completion of the programs. After high school, you might receive on-the-job training, or you might attend a career or technical school, a community college, or a university. The levels of education and the jobs for which they will prepare you are quite varied. These educational paths include:

- **High school health science or health occupations courses.** These programs can prepare you for entry-level employment.
- **On-the-job training.** During or after high school, you may receive training to advance your career while working. This training provides experience and education. However, advancement in most health career fields comes through formal education.
- **Technical or career schools.** These institutions provide training for specific health careers during and beyond high school.
- **Community college.** Community colleges and some technical and career schools offer two-year **associate's degrees.**
- **University or four-year college.** Students spend four or more years to earn a **bachelor's degree.** Afterwards, they may spend one or more years to earn a **master's degree.** Some high-level positions require a **doctorate,** which takes two to six more years.
- **Continuing education.** Once you have achieved a career goal, your education will continue in the workplace. This is called **continuing education.** In many health careers, continuing education is required to maintain professional status. The amount of education required varies by state and career. Continuing education can be obtained at your place of employment, at a school or college, online, or through reading professional publications. You are responsible for knowing the requirements regarding continuing education in your field.

Vocabulary

Content Vocabulary

You will learn these content vocabulary terms in this section.

- **associate's degree**
- **bachelor's degree**
- **master's degree**
- **doctorate**
- **continuing education**
- **entrepreneurs**
- **career**
- **career assessment**
- **parliamentary procedure**

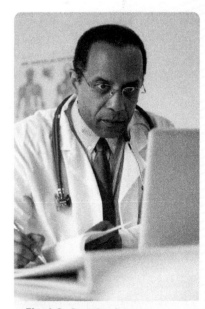

Fig. 1.6 Continuing Education Most healthcare careers require continuing education. *How might that study take place?*

Photo: Hero Images/Getty Images

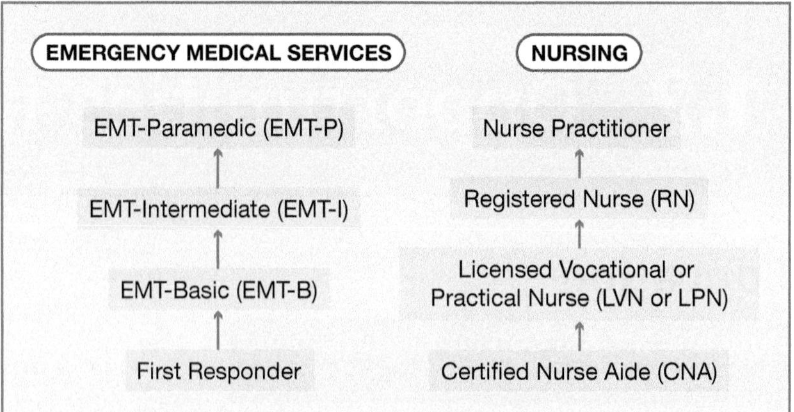

Fig. 1.7 Career Ladders These are career ladders for emergency medical services and nursing. *What is the highest level in the Nursing career ladder?*

READING CHECK

Explain when a healthcare professional is finished with his or her education.

Levels of Employment

Have you ever considered continuing education as a way to develop your career?

The learning process should never stop. Many students receive a two-year degree and return to school later for a four-year degree.

You can enter the healthcare field at various levels, depending upon your education, experience, and training. You might enter as an aide and move to assistant, technician, or technologist. The idea of climbing a career ladder applies to all these positions. See **Figure 1.7** for examples of career ladders for nursing and emergency medical services. **Table 1.3** shows healthcare career levels with an example at each level.

READING CHECK

Describe career ladder steps for emergency medical services.

Table 1.3 Levels of Employment

LEVEL	EDUCATIONAL REQUIREMENTS	CAREER EXAMPLE
Professional	Four-year degree, advanced degree, and clinical training	Pathologist
Technologist	Three to four years of college and work experience	Laboratory technologist
Technician	Usually two years of training	Laboratory technician
Assistant	Up to one year of classroom and clinical preparation	Laboratory assistant
Aide	High school diploma; on-the-job training	Laboratory aide

Entrepreneurs

Does an entrepreneurial career in healthcare appeal to you?

Entrepreneurs organize, manage, and take on the responsibilities and risks of a business or enterprise. They work independently. They may be associated with a facility, but they are usually their own bosses.

Many healthcare professionals become entrepreneurs. Some of these entrepreneurs can be massage therapists, veterinarians, physicians, dentists, and medical transcriptionists. A massage therapist may start a business traveling to clients' homes. Veterinarians, physicians, and dentists may open offices to practice their skills. A medical transcriptionist may prepare doctors' reports and patient records at home.

READING CHECK

List three careers in healthcare that are especially suitable for entrepreneurs.

Mc Graw Hill connect™ ONLINE PROCEDURES

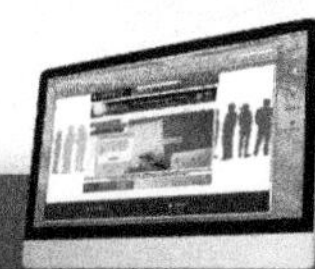

PROCEDURE 1-1

Recalling Healthcare Career Standards

All members of the healthcare team must adhere to high standards. These standards ensure that high quality care is provided to patients. Knowing these standards will prepare you for a career in healthcare.

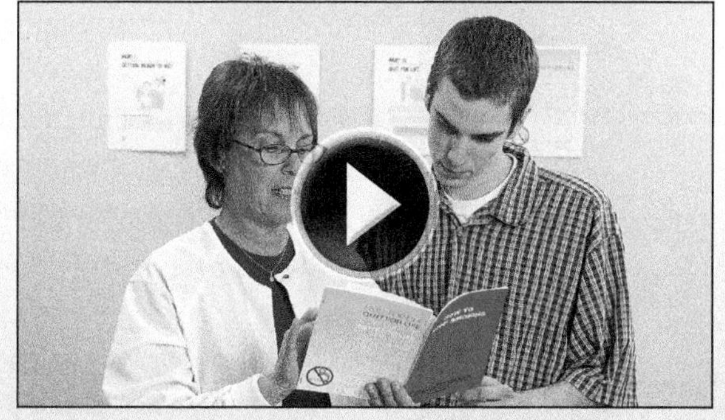

PROCEDURE 1-2

Identifying Healthcare Career Cluster Pathways

Healthcare careers are divided into five pathways. Learning about the pathways will help you make an educated decision about which healthcare career to enter.

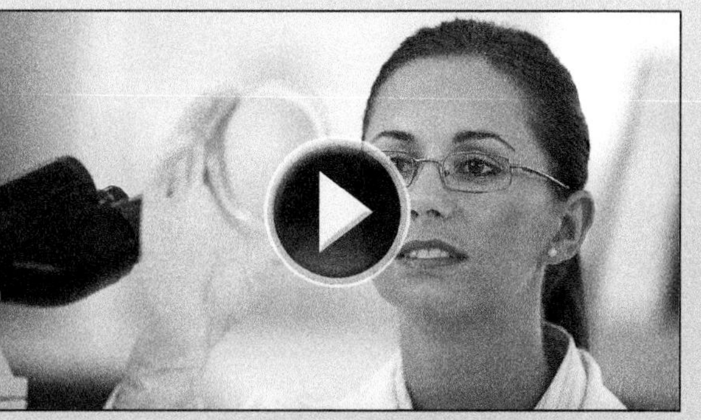

Photos: (t)Colin Young-Wolff/PhotoEdit, (b)Adam Gault/Getty Images

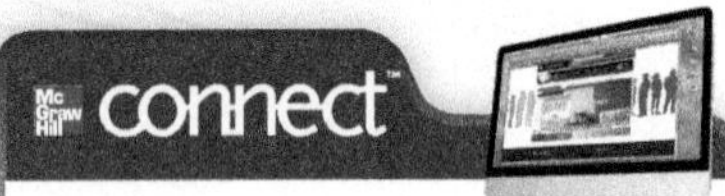

STEM CONNECTION

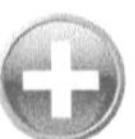

Medical Math

Managing Finances
Whether you are an entrepreneur or employee, you will need enough income to meet your expenses. Developing a budget can help. To stay on budget, you must determine what your monthly or weekly expenses will be and compare them to your income for that period. Use the steps in this activity to determine your monthly or weekly expenses and the amount of money you will make to meet the expenses.

Go to connect to complete the Managing Finances STEM Activity and worksheet.

Choosing a Career

Do you think the job that appeals most to you today will change in the future?

Before you choose a **career** path, think about what you might like to do in one, five, or ten years. Learn your needs and interests. Identify careers that best fit your personality and aptitudes.

In addition to a **career assessment,** get help from resources such as teachers, counselors, professionals, or websites. Talk with friends and family. Take it seriously, but remember that many people change professions several times in a lifetime. Your goal is to find a place to start.

READING CHECK

Describe how to make an informed career choice.

Professional Organizations

Does your school have a chapter of a healthcare student organization?

A professional student organization gives you a link to others who share your interests. As a member, you will gain knowledge of health careers. Student organizations will help you

- develop leadership abilities, citizenship skills, social competencies, and a wholesome attitude.
- strengthen creativity, thinking skills, decision-making abilities, and self-confidence.
- enhance the quality and relevance of your education by developing the knowledge, skills, and attitudes that lead to successful employment and encourage the pursuit of continuing education.
- promote quality of work and pride in occupational excellence through competitive activities.

READING CHECK

Describe the benefits of participation in professional student organizations.

Parliamentary Procedure

Have you ever been to a meeting that uses parliamentary procedure?

As part of your responsibility to a professional organization, you will attend or conduct meetings. **Parliamentary procedure** is a set of rules to follow in order to conduct a meeting in an efficient manner.

General Henry M. Robert wrote the book *Robert's Rules of Order* to help protect democratic procedures in organizations. Published in 1876, it aimed to ensure that everyone had the right to present business, discuss issues, and vote. The book's basic principles are:

1. Take up business one item at a time.
2. The majority rules.
3. Protect the rights of the minority to speak and to vote.

Robert's Rules of Order, Newly Revised, still serves as a guideline for conducting meetings. Organizations using these rules usually follow a fixed order of business. Here are examples:

1. Call to order
2. Roll call of members present
3. Reading and approval of minutes of last meeting
4. Officers' reports
5. Unfinished business
6. New business
7. Announcements
8. Adjournment

Procedures for Motions

Issues that membership is to discuss are presented as "motions." A motion is a proposal for action. The membership considers the motion and votes on it. See Appendix A for detailed procedures for motions.

1. Obtain the floor.
2. Make your motion.
3. Another member will second your motion, or the Chairman will call for a second.
4. If there is no second to your motion, it is lost.
5. If your motion is seconded, the Chairman states your motion.
6. Expand on your motion.
7. The question of whether or not to vote is put to the membership.

Voting on a motion will depend upon the organization or the motion requiring a vote. There are five methods most often used to vote:

1. By Voice—The Chairman asks those in favor to say "aye" and those opposed to say "no." Any member may move for an exact count.
2. By Roll Call—Each member answers "aye" or "no" as his or her name is called. This method is used when a record of each person's vote is required.
3. By General Consent—When a motion is not likely to be opposed, the Chairman says, "If there is no objection..." The membership shows agreement by silence. However, if one member says, "I object," the item must be put to a vote.
4. By Division—This is a slight variation of a voice vote. It does not require a count unless the Chairman so desires. Members raise their hands or stand.
5. By Ballot—Members write their vote on a slip of paper. This method is used when secrecy is desired.

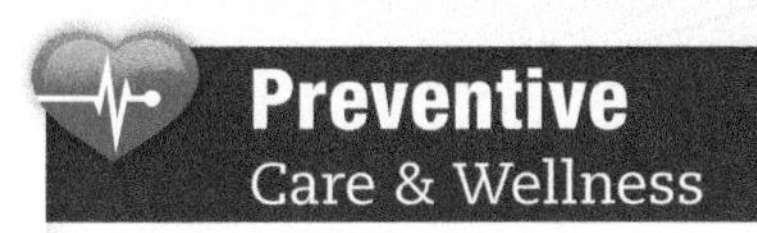

Reflect on Your Health

As you enter the field of healthcare, you should consider your own health. Healthcare professionals should be good role models. Do you eat well? Did you have breakfast this morning? How about exercise? How many times a week do you exercise? When did you go to bed last night? Are you getting enough sleep? Proper nutrition, enough sleep, and exercising most days of the week are part of a healthy lifestyle that will help prevent illness and improve your state of wellness.

Go to connect to complete the personal nutrition inventory.

Relating to Others in a Meeting

Have you ever been in a meeting in which someone constantly interrupts when things are not going their way? Do you know someone in charge who believes they have complete control over all things? These situations can occur even when parliamentary procedure is being used. Some suggestions for conducting a successful meeting include:

1. Always have a purpose for the meeting. Ask yourself: "What do we want to accomplish?" Write it down. If you have several things that you want to get done, list them in order of importance.
2. Put these items in the form of an agenda. Stick to the agenda and the topic under discussion. If someone wants to stray off the subject, remind the member to stick to the topic.
3. Do not allow everyone to speak at once. The person conducting the meeting should state who is to speak. For example, the presiding officer states, "It is Amber's turn to speak."
4. If members keep rehashing the same points, ask, "Is there anything new someone wants to add?" If not, restate the points, take a vote, and get on with the next subject on the agenda.

READING CHECK

Identify the three basic principles of Robert's Rules of Order.

SECTION 1.2 Opportunities in Healthcare Review

AFTER YOU READ

1. **Choose** what kind of school you would most likely attend to obtain an associate's degree. To obtain a bachelor's degree?
2. **Indicate** the level of education you would need to become a technician.
3. **Examine** the three factors that determine your entry point into a career.
4. **Explain** why it is important to do continuing education.
5. **Define** the word "entrepreneur" and give one example of an entrepreneur.
6. **Describe** a professional student organization.
7. **Identify** a professional student organization at your school.
8. **Explain** why parliamentary procedure was developed.

Technology ONLINE EXPLORATIONS

Career Inventory

Obtain a copy of a career assessment from your teacher or search the Internet using terms such as "career assessment" or "career inventory." Some websites charge a fee, but free assessments are also available at sites such as careeronestop.org. Follow the directions carefully and answer each question honestly. Once you have completed the assessment, evaluate your career match. Do you think that it is correct? Why or why not?

CHAPTER
1 Review

Chapter Summary

SECTION 1.1

- The entry-level healthcare professional should be proficient in each of the following eleven National Healthcare Skill Standards: academic foundation, communications, systems, employability skills, legal responsibilities, ethics, safety practices, teamwork, health maintenance practices, technical skills, and information technology skills. **(pg. 5)**
- National Healthcare Skill Standards were established to communicate the importance of the knowledge and skills needed by all healthcare professionals. **(pg. 5)**
- The five career pathways identified within the National Healthcare Skill Standards are therapeutic, diagnostic, health informatics, support, and biotechnology research and development. **(pg. 9)**

SECTION 1.2

- Entry into a healthcare profession requires varying amounts of education, experience, and clinical training. Continuing education is necessary for career advancement. **(pg. 13)**
- Entrepreneurship involves working independently when practicing healthcare skills such as massage therapy or medical transcription. **(pg. 15)**
- Choosing a career takes time and requires an understanding of your interests and aptitudes. A career assessment is a good starting point to help you determine your career. **(pg. 16)**
- Professional student organizations assist with career advancement and the development of character and leadership qualities. **(pg. 16)**
- The book *Robert's Rules of Order* explains parliamentary procedure, which provides for organized and efficient meetings. **(pg. 16)**

Mc Graw Hill connect™ ONLINE ACTIVITIES

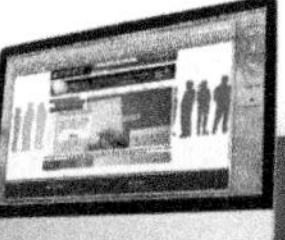

Complete our HST online activities for Chapter 1, which include Concept Check review questions, Reference Flash Cards, and Online Procedures assessment sheets.

- **Concept Check** review questions
- **Reference Flash Cards** medical terminology practice
- **Online Procedures** assessment sheets

CHAPTER 1 Assessment

Critical Thinking/Problem Solving

1. A nurse practitioner works daily with a plastic surgeon. He is expected to be at the hospital for scheduled surgeries at 7 A.M. After assisting the physician in the operating room, he performs follow-up visits to all of their clients who are still in the hospital. He is back at the office by 2 P.M. At the office, he sees clients until 5:30 P.M. Review the National Healthcare Skill Standards and explain in detail how this nurse practitioner uses each of these skills in his professional work.
2. During a meeting of your professional student organization, one student keeps interrupting and repeating information. If you were conducting the meeting, how would you handle this student?

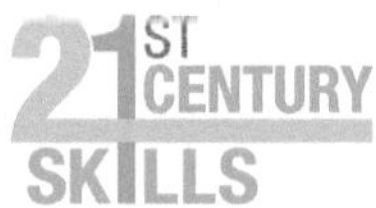

3. **Teamwork** Your teacher will divide the class into groups of five or more students, with each student in a group representing a different healthcare career. The groups should stand in a circle. Then each student reaches into the center of the circle and grasps one hand of two other students. Students should not grasp the hand of the person next to them or grasp both hands of the same person. Now, without letting go of hands, the group unwinds to form a full circle. Ask each student which health career he or she represents. Then each class member should find out how his or her career and the careers of the two other students might work together in real life.
4. **Problem Solving** In a small group, practice parliamentary procedures using this textbook, *Robert's Rules of Order, Newly Revised,* or another source. Choose a chairman and other officers and then role-play a meeting. During your meeting, practice obtaining the floor to make a motion, phrasing a motion correctly, and voting on a motion. Role-play different situations that may occur to disrupt a meeting, and then discuss how they can be corrected.
5. **Information Literacy** Search the Internet for professional healthcare organizations. Find an organization that matches your health career interest and review the information given on the website. Obtain the following information: name of the organization, web address, physical address, phone number, and title of current newsletter or other informational publication (if available).
6. **Information Literacy** Search the Internet for the website of a local healthcare facility of your choice. Visit the healthcare facility's careers or help wanted page to see the kinds of jobs that are currently available there. Write a paragraph explaining how those careers do or do not match up with what you expect to learn in this course.

CHAPTER

2 Healthcare Systems

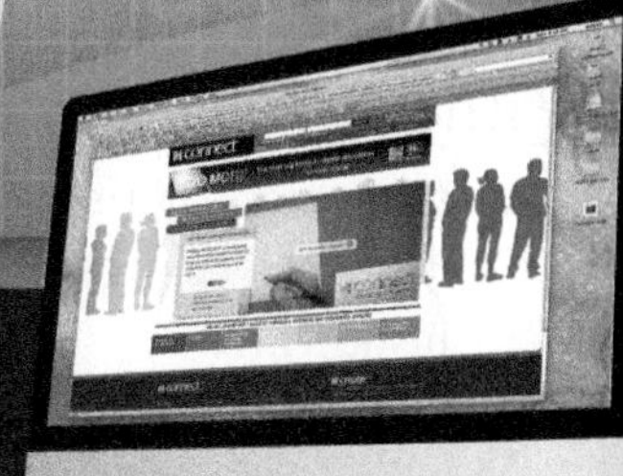

Essential Question:

How has healthcare changed from prehistoric times to today?

"Fresh air, exercise, and healthy food." We have all heard this "prescription" as a way to stay healthy. Is this a new idea? Not at all. During the fourth century BCE, **Hippocrates,** known as the father of Western medicine, advised these practices both to prevent and to cure illness. Native Americans used hundreds of different plants to treat illness. The value of these resources is beginning to be recognized today in Western medicine and is practiced in the form of herbal therapy.

Mc Graw Hill connect™

It's Online!

- Online Procedures
- STEM Connection
- Medical Science
- Medical Terms
- Medical Math
- Ethics in Action
- Virtual Lab

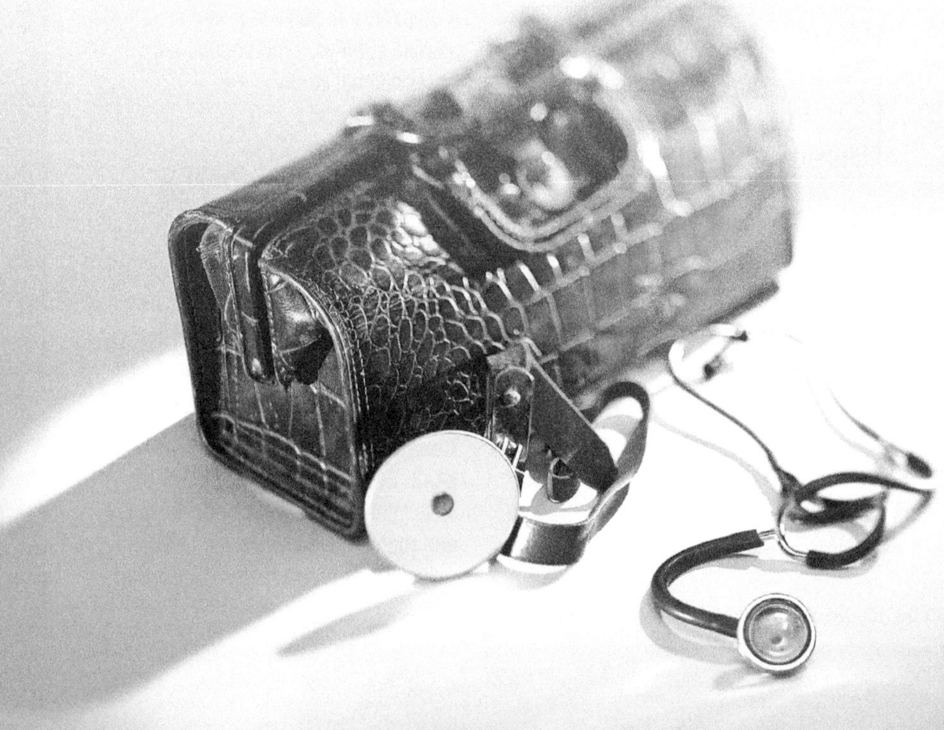

Photo: Comstock Images/Getty Images

READING GUIDE

OBJECTIVES

After completing this chapter, you will be able to:

- **Describe** significant historical changes in healthcare.
- **Illustrate** the reasons for the importance of the scientific method in healthcare.
- **Compare** ancient and current medical practices.
- **Examine** major trends in healthcare.
- **Classify** the types of healthcare facilities and the services provided in each.
- **Assess** how healthcare facilities, government agencies, and nonprofit volunteer agencies contribute to the health of a community and the world.
- **Identify** the clients served by Medicare and Medicaid.
- **Discuss** the impact of healthcare reform.
- **Compare** two types of managed care organizations.
- **Explain** the purpose of workers' compensation.

BEFORE YOU READ

Connect Can you think of some significant events and developments in the past that have formed the foundation for modern healthcare careers?

Main Idea

The healthcare industry has undergone dramatic changes through history, and continues to develop today.

Note-Taking Activity

Draw this table. Write key terms and phrases under **Cues**. Write main ideas under **Note Taking**. Summarize the section under **Summary**.

Cues	Note Taking
o	o
o	o
Summary	

Graphic Organizer

Before you read the chapter, draw a diagram like the one below. As you read, write the topics covered in the chapter into the diagram.

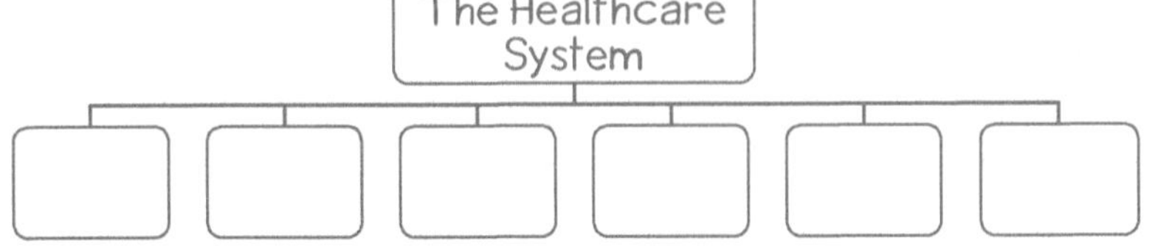

Downloadable graphic organizers can be accessed online.

STANDARDS

HEALTH SCIENCE

NCHSE 3.11 Understand the healthcare delivery system (public, private, government, and non-profit).

NCHSE 6.31 Understand religious and cultural values as they impact healthcare.

SCIENCE

NSES F Develop understanding of personal and community health; population growth; natural resources; environmental quality; natural and human-induced hazards; science and technology in local, national, and global challenges.

NCHSE *National Consortium for Health Science Education*

NSES *National Science Education Standards*

COMMON CORE STATE STANDARDS

MATHEMATICS

Statistics and Probability

Making Inferences and Justifying Conclusions S-IC Make inferences and justify conclusions from sample surveys, experiments, and observational studies.

ENGLISH LANGUAGE ARTS

Writing

Text Types and Purposes W-3 Write narratives to develop real or imagined experiences or events using effective technique, well-chosen details, and well-structured event sequences.

Speaking and Listening

Comprehension and Collaboration SL-3 Evaluate a speaker's point of view, reasoning, and use of evidence and rhetoric, identifying any fallacious reasoning or exaggerated or distorted evidence.

SECTION

2.1 History of Healthcare

Prehistory and the Ancient World

When did medical ethics as we know it begin?

Although ideas about the causes of health and illness, diagnostics, and treatments have changed since ancient times, some things remain the same.

For as long as human beings have lived on this planet, we have practiced medicine in some form. Some cultures credited health and illness to the moods of the gods. Others used reason to attempt to explain the causes of disease. Archaeological and anthropological findings tell us that many so-called primitive cultures practiced healing in a variety of ways. Healers in ancient times used natural remedies such as diet, rest, and medications made from herbs and other plants. They even performed surgery.

Religion played an important role in healthcare as well. Many cultures combined the use of medications or surgery with religious rites. **Figure 2.2** on pages 24 and 25 gives you an overview of the history of healthcare.

An important symbol still linked with medicine began in ancient times. Asclepius was the Greek god of healing, and people went to his temple to pray for cures. His symbol was the snake. In time, priest healers adopted the symbol of Asclepius. It is possible that this symbol evolved into an insignia called the caduceus, which, even today, is the symbol for the physician. **Figure 2.1** shows a **caduceus,** two snakes entwined around a pole.

The doctor's code of ethics is rooted in ancient Greek history. **Hippocrates** practiced and taught medicine around 400 BCE. He and his students left scores of manuscripts advising doctors on the examination and treatment of patients. His students followed a strict ethical code. Followers of Hippocrates swore that they would maintain their patients' privacy and never deliberately harm them. This code of ethics, the Hippocratic Oath, continues today.

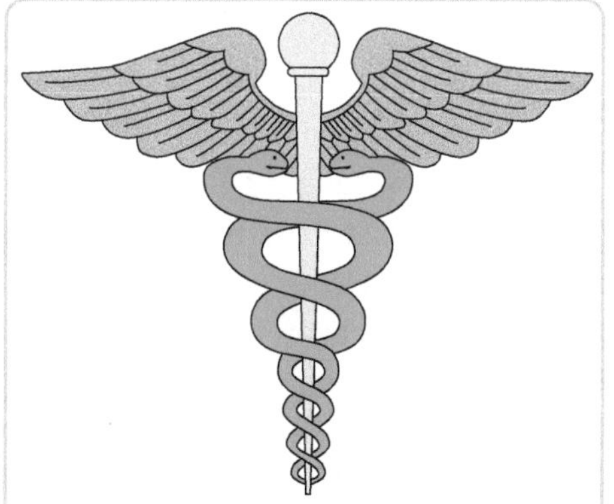

Fig. 2.1 Caduceus The caduceus is a symbol that originated in Ancient Greece. *What does this symbol represent?*

Vocabulary

Content Vocabulary

You will learn these content vocabulary terms in this section.

- caduceus
- Hippocrates
- Industrial Revolution
- medical asepsis
- pathogens
- electronic health records (EHR)

Academic Vocabulary

You will see these words in your reading and on your tests. Find their meanings in the Glossary in the back of the book.

- professionals
- adapting

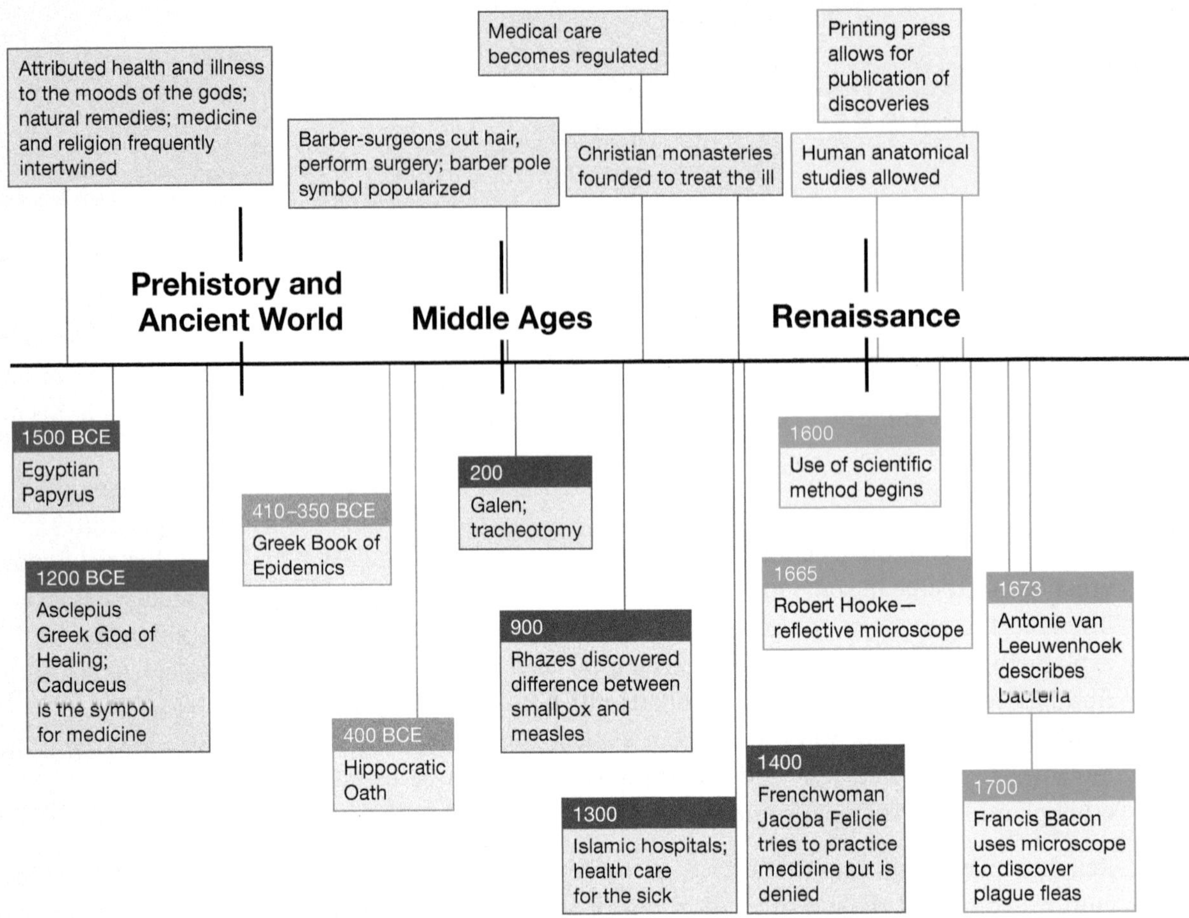

Fig. 2.2 Timeline The timeline highlights of the history of healthcare. *When was the scientific method first used?*

In ancient times, few people could read, and travel was difficult. Nevertheless, the writings of an educated few contributed to the advancement of medicine. Stone tablets showing physicians treating Egyptian nobility and recording treatments for diseases have been found. In later eras, monks spent long hours copying manuscripts, some of which contained vital medical information. In the years before the invention of the printing press, these handmade books were rare and treasured. They increased access to precious information, although their audience was limited.

The Egyptians trained many physicians, among them a Greek man named Galen. Appointed as physician to the gladiators during the second century, he used his skills as a surgeon to treat the injured. Galen documented the importance of the spinal cord to the movement of limbs. He described how to cure breathing difficulties by performing a tracheotomy, a surgical opening of the trachea, or windpipe. He based much of his practice on the teachings of Hippocrates. Galen's manuscripts were hand-copied and used in physician training for centuries — until the Renaissance, which began during the fourteenth century.

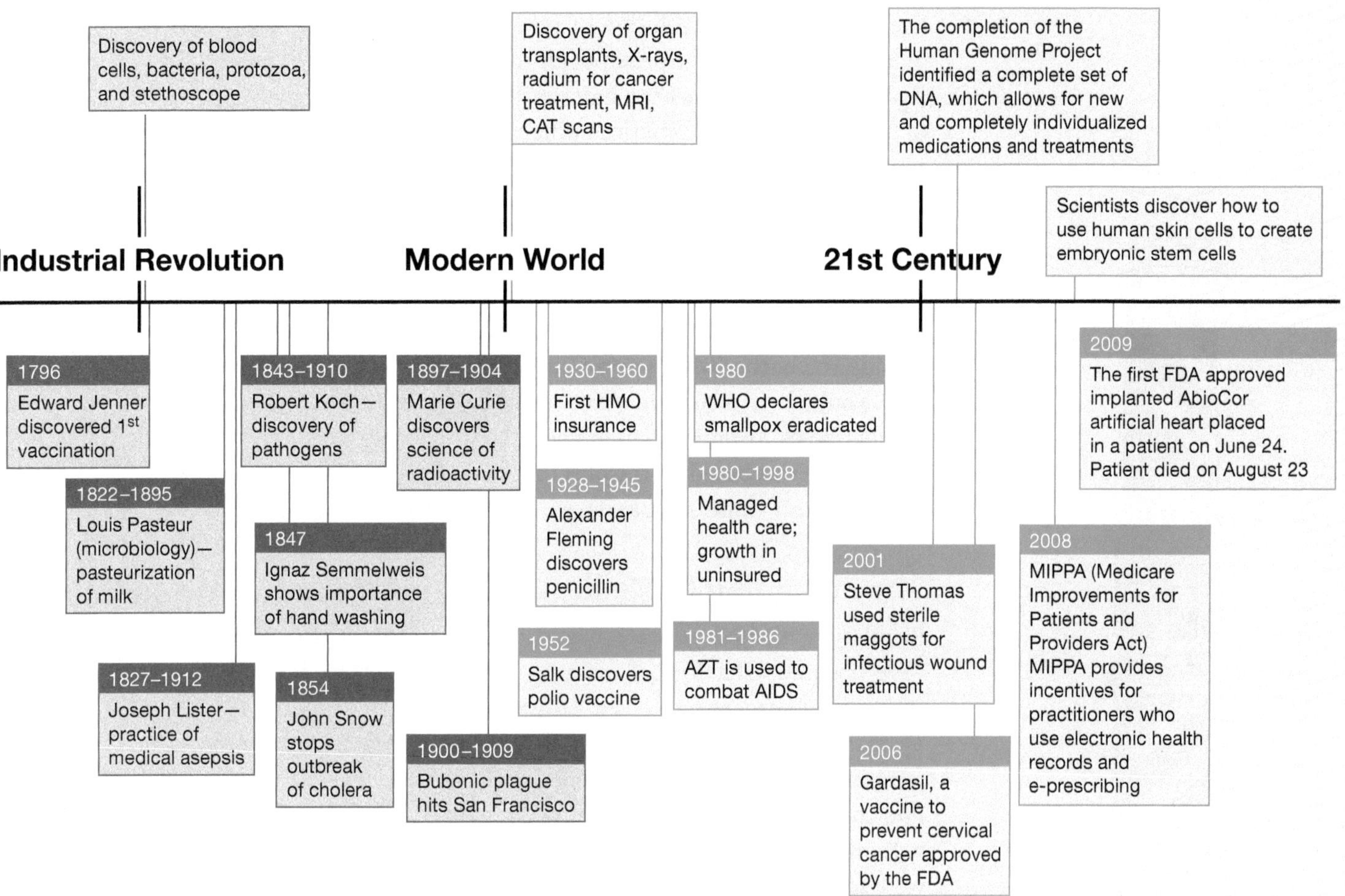
Discovery of blood cells, bacteria, protozoa, and stethoscope
Discovery of organ transplants, X-rays, radium for cancer treatment, MRI, CAT scans
The completion of the Human Genome Project identified a complete set of DNA, which allows for new and completely individualized medications and treatments
Scientists discover how to use human skin cells to create embryonic stem cells
Industrial Revolution
Modern World
21st Century
1796 Edward Jenner discovered 1st vaccination
1822–1895 Louis Pasteur (microbiology)—pasteurization of milk
1827–1912 Joseph Lister—practice of medical asepsis
1843–1910 Robert Koch—discovery of pathogens
1847 Ignaz Semmelweis shows importance of hand washing
1854 John Snow stops outbreak of cholera
1897–1904 Marie Curie discovers science of radioactivity
1900–1909 Bubonic plague hits San Francisco
1930–1960 First HMO insurance
1928–1945 Alexander Fleming discovers penicillin
1952 Salk discovers polio vaccine
1980 WHO declares smallpox eradicated
1980–1998 Managed health care; growth in uninsured
1981–1986 AZT is used to combat AIDS
2001 Steve Thomas used sterile maggots for infectious wound treatment
2006 Gardasil, a vaccine to prevent cervical cancer approved by the FDA
2008 MIPPA (Medicare Improvements for Patients and Providers Act) MIPPA provides incentives for practitioners who use electronic health records and e-prescribing
2009 The first FDA approved implanted AbioCor artificial heart placed in a patient on June 24. Patient died on August 23

READING CHECK

Recall what is stated in the Hippocratic Oath.

The Middle Ages

What was the most important change in medical care in the Middle Ages?

The period in history known as the Middle Ages began around CE 500 and lasted until around CE 1500. During those years, science and reason began to replace people's beliefs in spiritual or superstitious causes for illnesses.

Doctors began to keep careful notes on their cases. A Persian doctor named Rhazes discovered the difference between smallpox and measles. He wrote about his findings around CE 900. His works were used until the 1800s. Like Galen, Rhazes played a role in the development of medicine as a science by building on the ideas of Hippocrates.

The Barber-Surgeon

Even with the slow evolution of medicine into a science, there were practices that would surprise people today. For example, in the Middle Ages barbers cut more than hair. Barber-surgeons performed surgery to treat cataracts and practiced phlebotomy (bloodletting). They also served with the military and treated injuries sustained in battle. They amputated limbs and burned the stumps to seal the blood vessels.

The striped pole we see in front of a barbershop is a symbol left over from the time when barbers were also surgeons. After an operation, the bandages would be hung on a staff or pole and sometimes placed outside the barber's shop as an advertisement. Twirled by the wind, they would form a red and white spiral pattern that was later used on painted poles. A more popular theory of the origin of the colors of a barber pole was based on the idea that red represented the blood, blue, the veins, and white, the bandages. **Figure 2.3** shows a barber pole.

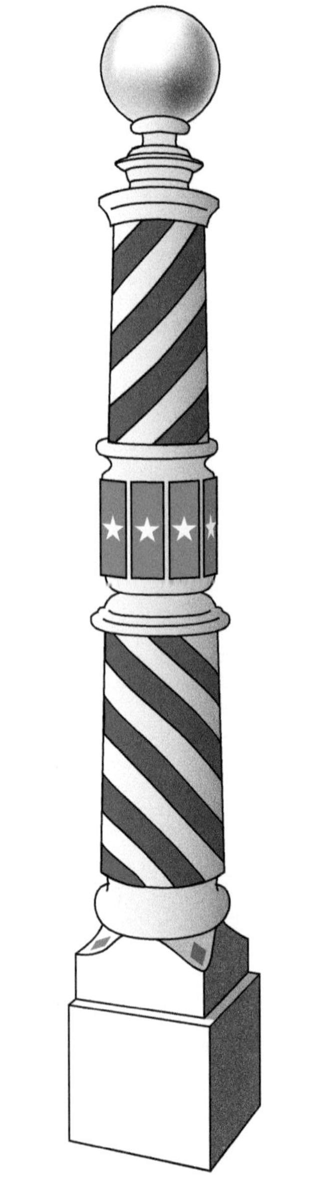

Fig. 2.3 Barber-Surgeons The striped barber pole is a symbol left over from the time when barbers were also surgeons. *How would you feel about your barber or hair stylist drawing your blood or pulling your teeth?*

The Beginning of Medical Care Regulation

Regulation of medical care began in the Middle Ages. Physicians were licensed after formal training with experienced doctors. Physicians and surgeons received different training. Physicians learned by reading books and training with experienced doctors. Women were not allowed to practice medicine. In the fourteenth century, a Frenchwoman named Jacoba Felicie was tried for practicing medicine without a license. She defended herself by explaining that women were sometimes embarrassed to go to a male physician for treatment. The judge did not find in her favor, and she was forbidden to practice medicine.

Religion and Medicine

Religion continued to play a significant role in healthcare. Both Christian and Muslim teachings encourage the care of those in need. By the thirteenth century there were scores of hospitals in the Muslim world. Religious instruction based on the Qur'an (Koran) taught followers social responsibilities, such as the rich providing for the poor and the healthy caring for the sick. These principles led to the founding of many Islamic hospitals. Each hospital had separate wards for different illnesses, employed trained nurses, and maintained stocks of medication.

The teachings of the Christian church also encouraged followers to help the sick and needy. Many monasteries were founded specifically to treat the sick. Local healers, who were often women, served at the monasteries. Otherwise, the treatment consisted of prayer and rest.

READING CHECK

Compare Christian and Muslim teachings about healthcare in the Middle Ages.

The Renaissance

How did the invention of the printing press advance the practice of medicine?

Medical practice went through many changes during the Renaissance, which began during the fourteenth century and lasted until the seventeenth.

In the fifteenth century, the invention of the printing press made it possible to publish books faster. Information about new discoveries could be spread quickly.

During the sixteenth century, the scientific method came into use in Europe. This was a major change in the way people thought about medicine and research. The scientific method is a process used to acquire new knowledge. Instead of using guesswork or the supernatural to explain events and diseases, people began to look for the real causes of what they saw around them. The scientific method was based on observation and taking careful notes. This method was not common practice during the Middle Ages.

The developments that took place during this time were made possible by inventions such as the microscope, which allowed much more accurate observation of patients and symptoms. Doctors could propose an explanation of disease and test it by experimentation and observation. Robert Hooke (1635–1703) built one of the first reflecting microscopes. **Figure 2.4** shows an example of an early microscope.

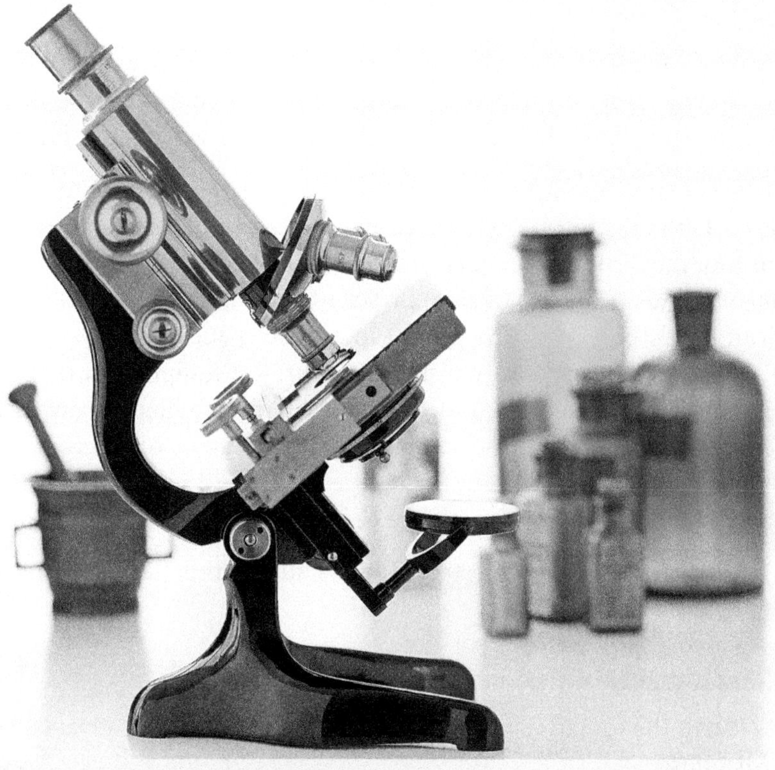

Photo: Tetra Images/CORBIS

Fig. 2.4 Microscope Robert Hooke built one of the first reflecting microscopes. *How did the invention of the microscope change healthcare?*

During the Age of Enlightenment, a philosophical movement of the 1700s, studies of the human anatomy took place. These investigations, which had been forbidden by the church in the past, helped correct many beliefs.

READING CHECK

Identify the sixteenth-century development that brought major change to how people thought about medicine and research.

The Industrial Revolution

What did Edward Jenner discover that led to the practice of vaccination?

During the **Industrial Revolution** of the late eighteenth and early nineteenth centuries, great changes were caused by the introduction of machines. Along with important economic changes, progress was also made in medicine. New diagnostic tools such as the stethoscope were invented. Blood cells, bacteria, and protozoa could now be seen with a microscope. Doctors knew that blood was carried through the body by large vessels, but they did not know how blood circulated throughout the body. This was explained by the discovery of capillaries.

A connection was made between health and the environment . Edward Jenner (1749–1823), an English doctor, discovered that milkmaids exposed to cowpox did not get smallpox. Around 1796 he began inoculating people with the fluid from cowpox blisters, thus beginning the practice of vaccination.

Modern medical practice is based on the discoveries and developments of the nineteenth century. Once the connection between the structure and the function of an organism was made, further discoveries followed.

Louis Pasteur (1822–1895) carried out experiments that became the basis for modern microbiology. Joseph Lister (1827–1912) was ridiculed for insisting on the use of carbolic soap to disinfect instruments and clean hands before doctors moved to another patient. Today we call his practice—the practice of disinfecting surgical equipment and hand washing as a way to prevent the spread of infection—**medical asepsis.** Robert Koch (1843–1910) discovered that **pathogens,** or disease-producing microorganisms, are the source of some diseases and proved that Lister was correct. This was the beginning of modern bacteriology.

The use of ether as an anesthetic began during this period. It made painless surgery possible.

READING CHECK

Name the tool developed in the late 18th century that advanced diagnosis.

Modern Times

What new developments show the most promise for transforming healthcare?

The twentieth century saw rapid growth in healthcare. Discoveries in electronics and computer science changed clinical medicine dramatically. Advances in engineering, chemistry, and physics have contributed to current medical practice. Antibiotics were invented. Radium, used for cancer treatment, was discovered. The use of X-rays gained importance in noninvasive diagnoses. The development of computed axial tomography (CT scan), magnetic resonance imaging (MRI),

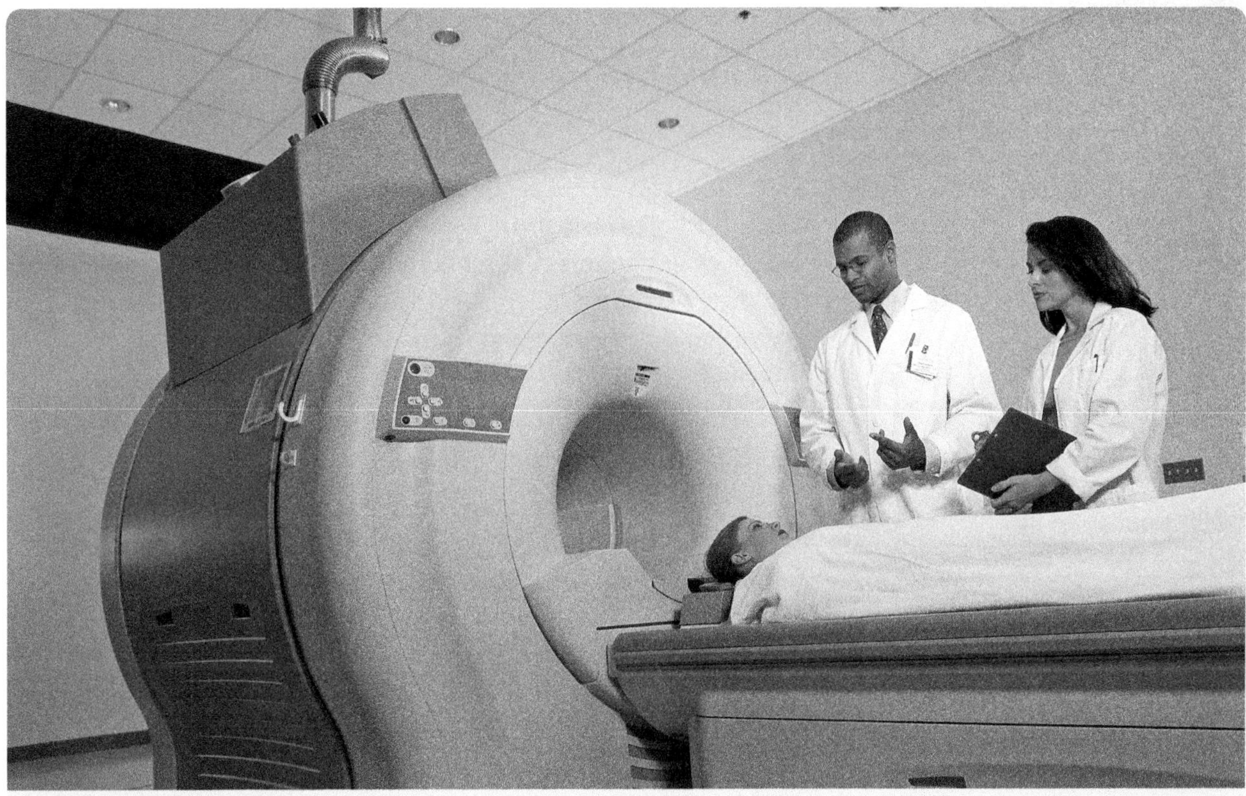

Fig. 2.5 MRI Technology can improve care techniques. *How did the invention of the MRI affect the treatment of clients?*

and ultrasound or sonographic imaging has improved diagnosis and treatment for many diseases. **Figure 2.5** shows an MRI machine. Organ transplants are now common, and are safer and more succcessful than ever before. The development of artificial organs is progressing. In vitro fertilization allows many infertile couples to have children. Research, technology, and improved care techniques are extending the horizon for healthcare.

21st Century

The rapid progress in science and technology is expected to continue through the twenty-first century and bring many more changes and challenges to healthcare professionals. **Electronic health records** and

Photo: CORBIS

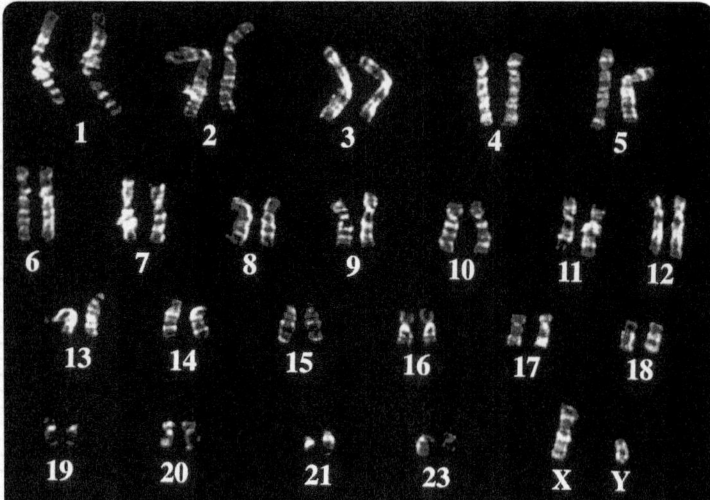

Fig. 2.6 The Human Genome Project The Human Genome Project identified all of the 20,000–25,000 genes in human DNA. This knowledge has been crucial in the development of many new and individualized drugs and treatments. *How can the study of human DNA help people with genetic disorders?*

electronic communication provide instant transmission of information. Physicians and patients need not be in the same room or even the same country to give and receive advice and treatment. Surgeries are performed with intricate computerized equipment. People in many areas of the world are living longer and healthier lives because of vaccines, clean water, and better nutrition. The completion of the Human Genome Project (HGP) and the use of stem cells has opened doors to new types of individualized drugs and treatments (see **Figure 2.6**). Diagnostic screening and preventive care are improving wellness and increasing life expectancy.

Today's healthcare professional needs to be able to think critically and use flexible approaches to problem solving. Learning and adapting to change are necessary to maintain competency in the high-tech environment of modern healthcare. The only certainty in healthcare is change.

READING CHECK

Name three important medical advancements of the twentieth century.

SECTION 2.1 History of Healthcare Review

AFTER YOU READ

1. **Analyze** the effect Hippocrates had on the ethical practice of medicine.
2. **Describe** the history of the caduceus and the striped barber pole.
3. **Identify** a contribution of Persia to the development of medicine as science.
4. **Contrast** thirteenth-century Islamic and Christian healthcare systems.
5. **Indicate** the ways in which Lister contributed to the current practice of medical asepsis.
6. **Examine** the effect that modern science is having on the healthcare professional.

Technology ONLINE EXPLORATIONS

Healthcare Discoveries

So many advancements and discoveries in healthcare have occurred throughout history that they are too numerous to mention in this chapter. Choose one of the time periods discussed in Section 2.1 of this chapter. Research online or in other sources for at least one additional discovery or advancement in healthcare. Write a summary of your findings to present to your class or turn in to your teacher.

SECTION
2.2 Trends in Healthcare

You should be familiar with these trends in modern-day healthcare:

- Technology
- Preventive Medicine and Wellness
- An Aging Population
- Healthcare Reform
- Outpatient Care
- Emergency Preparedness

These trends are discussed in the this section.

Vocabulary

Content Vocabulary

You will learn these content vocabulary terms in this section.

- **baby boom**
- **healthcare reform**
- **geographic information system (GIS)**

Academic Vocabulary

You will see this word in your reading and on your tests. Find its meaning in the Glossary in the back of the book.

- **access**

Technology

What new technology do you see in healthcare?

Over the last decade, the advancement of technology has affected all aspects of our life. This is also true in the field of healthcare.

Healthcare has always been affected by science and technology. In the twenty-first century, however, we could say that the development of technology has been "explosive." For example, during the 1970s mobile telephones seemed to be just science fiction. Prototypes for early mobile phones were described as being as small as a briefcase! Today a nurse may carry a smart phone in a pocket and stay in constant touch with patients, physicians, and other members of the healthcare team. Miniaturization allows physicians to put a tiny camera as well as instruments into the body to perform surgery through small incisions. A physician in a remote area can send digital images across the country or around the world in an instant to consult with a specialist.

Paper charts are becoming a thing of the past. The use of electronic health records (EHR) is gaining momentum and must be accomplished by the year 2014. More and more physicians are joining larger healthcare facilities that already have EHR in place. EHR allows all of a patient's data to be accessible in one location. An electronic chart provides quick access and helps to prevent mistakes with medication and other medical errors. As shown in **Figure 2.7,** patient records are available at any time, and anywhere, to healthcare professionals.

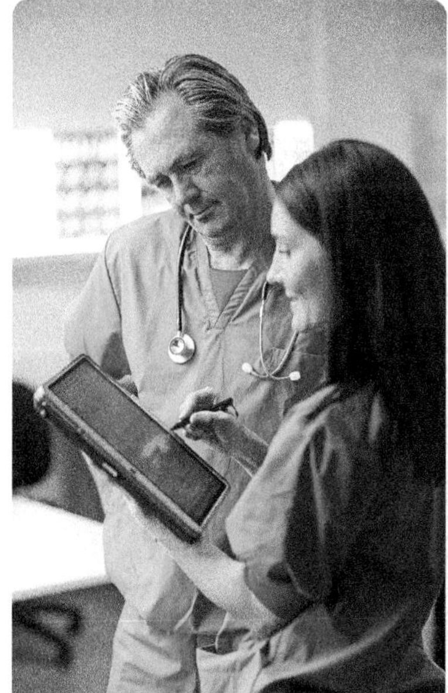

Fig. 2.7 EHR This device makes it possible to gain quick access to a client's medical history from a remote location. *How does this ensure better client care?*

READING CHECK

List two ways in which smaller electronic devices have helped healthcare.

Photo: Thomas Tolstrup/Stone/Getty Images

Preventive Medicine and Wellness

Do you consider your personal wellness when you select activities to do or things to eat?

The words "preventive medicine and wellness" can bring to mind anything from massage therapy to whole foods. The idea of wellness led to the fitness movement, which started in the 1980s. Fitness centers for healthy clients may include aerobic exercise, weight training, and fitness machines. **Figure 2.8** shows a fitness center.

The link between exercise, diet, and good health is strong. Screening tests and drugs to prevent disease are common. A healthy lifestyle goes a long way toward improving your quality of life. Aging baby boomers, physicians, insurance companies, and fitness experts all recognize the value of good health.

Hospital Wellness Centers

The link between wellness and illness is addressed by hospital or medical wellness centers. Hospital or medical wellness centers are different from other fitness centers because they offer programs that focus on older populations and their therapeutic needs. Clinical services are an important component of hospital wellness centers, which offer services such as:

- Cardiac rehabilitation
- Pulmonary rehabilitation
- Occupational medicine
- Sports medicine
- Clinical weight management
- Physical therapy

Personal Responsibility for Wellness

Individuals, and that means you, too, are responsible for promoting their own wellness and choosing their own care.

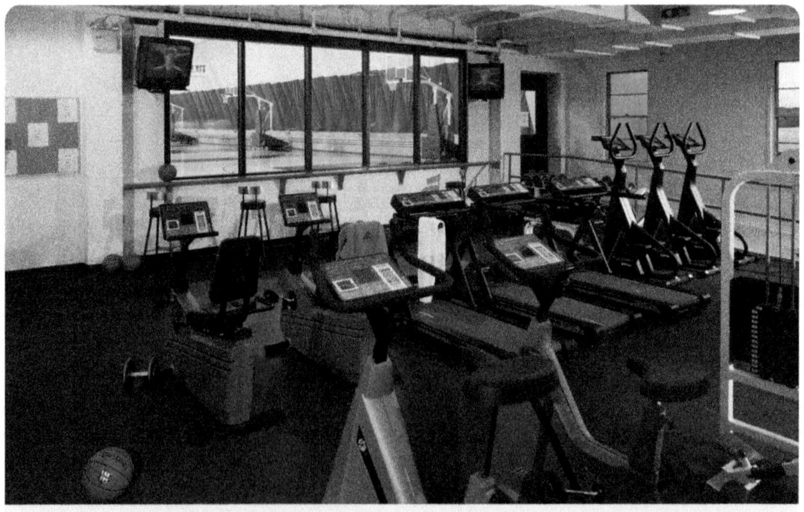

Fig. 2.8 Wellness Exercise and fitness is one part of maintaining wellness. *How do hospital fitness centers differ from commercial fitness centers?*

Photo: Daniel Mirer/CORBIS

Some factors related to wellness are:

- Fitness — including fitness during pregnancy and fitness to prevent heart disease, high blood pressure, and lower back pain
- Preventive care — including immunizations and healthcare screening tests
- Spiritual health — believing in a higher authority, observing religious practices, and living according to a set of values, standards, and morals to help find direction and purpose in life
- Safety — learning life-saving tips to prevent injuries and accidents, how to deliver CPR, and how to be prepared for emergencies
- Nutrition — learning how to eat right, to guard against diseases such as osteoporosis and cancer, to recognize how certain nutrients affect the body, and to know in which foods these nutrients are found
- Tackling tobacco addiction — making a personal plan for quitting or reducing tobacco intake
- Stress management — using techniques to help manage stress and cope with everyday problems

21ST CENTURY SKILLS

Considering Culture

As a healthcare professional, you will be responsible for choosing your own healthcare practices and managing your own wellness. Practicing preventive care and wellness is essential to health and longevity. But you will also encounter clients whose beliefs or healthcare choices are different from your own. Your responsibility will be to help the client make good choices through education. However, the choices are the client's to make, and the client's decisions should be respected, never criticized.

READING CHECK

Identify five factors related to wellness.

An Aging Population

Do you know how the average age of our population is trending?

After World War II, the United States economy boomed. There were plenty of jobs, and people could afford to have large families. This resulted in a phenomenon known as the **baby boom,** which occurred from 1946 to 1964. During this time the average age of the U.S. population decreased because of the large number of births. Many baby boomers are now in retirement age. In 2011 the first boomers began to receive Medicare, our national health insurance for the elderly.

This affects our society because older adults require more healthcare services. The healthcare system and each professional must be prepared to meet the needs of an aging population. Government agencies, healthcare providers, businesses, and families are just a few of the institutions that must adapt to an aging population. Baby boomers can expect to live longer, healthier lives by practicing preventive care. **Figure 2.9** shows active, healthy senior citizens.

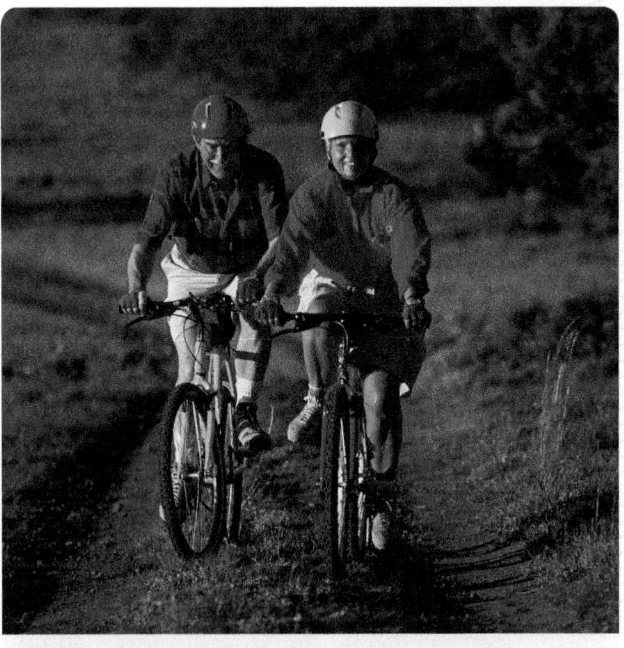

Fig. 2.9 Baby Boomers People are living longer and remaining active later in life than they have in previous generations. *How is the age of our population going to change between now and the year 2015?*

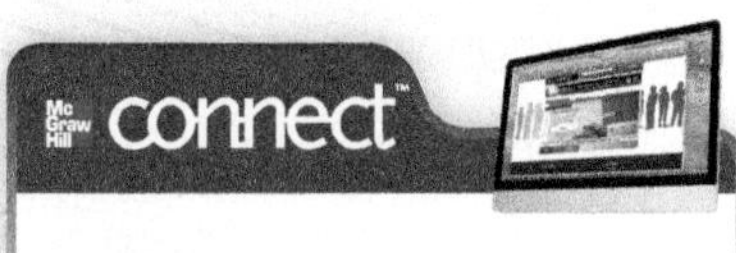

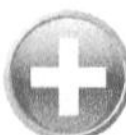

STEM CONNECTION

Medical Math

Calculating the Average Age of a Population
To calculate the average, or mean, age of a population, you must know the number of people in the population and the age of each person. Since the population of the United States is more than 300 million people, assembling this information would be difficult.

Go to connect to calculate the changing average age of a family.

Healthcare Reform

Healthcare costs are increasing in the United States because of growing demand and more costly procedures. Uninsured or underinsured individuals also cause the cost of healthcare to rise.

Where can someone without health insurance go when he or she needs care? Hospitals that are partly supported by taxes provide care to uninsured people with low incomes. Hospitals or healthcare providers often pass on these costs to patients who have insurance or can afford to pay full price. This raises the prices charged by providers and insurance companies. The Affordable Care Act addresses some of these issues over time. **Healthcare reform** is needed to

- increase the number of people with coverage through public sector insurance programs or private sector insurance companies.
- expand the number of providers that a patient may choose from.
- improve access to healthcare specialists.
- improve the quality of healthcare.
- decrease the cost of healthcare.

READING CHECK

Describe how people with no health insurance can get care when they need it.

Outpatient Care

Have you or has someone you know had outpatient surgery?

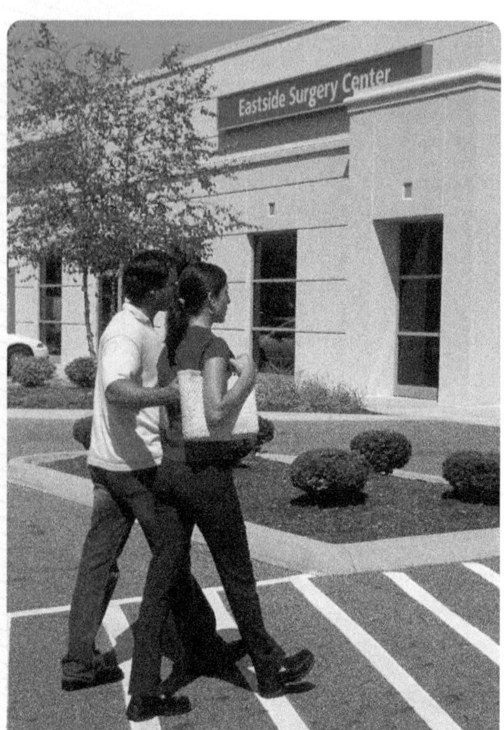

Fig. 2.10 Outpatient Care Outpatient care facilities are increasing in numbers. *How has the increase in outpatient care helped our healthcare system?*

When Medicare and insurance companies reduced the reimbursement paid to inpatient facilities, outpatient care gained popularity.

Many procedures, from diagnosis to treatment, are done on an outpatient basis. A patient may walk into a clinic in the morning, have tests or surgery, and go home in the afternoon (see **Figure 2.10**). Procedures that once required hospitalization now are done in outpatient centers.

If a patient does require time in the hospital, it can be reduced by home healthcare. Patients who once would have spent five days in a hospital may now go home in three days. A skilled professional visits the home to assess the patient's condition and to provide treatment and education. Because of this, much of the care has shifted to families. Patients and families self-administer treatments or perform procedures done by nurses or therapists in the past. In addition to being a healthcare provider, the healthcare professional is now also a teacher and coach.

Photo: Doug Martin

Home health services have many benefits. A patient in his or her home is exposed to fewer pathogens or disease germs. Stress and anxiety are also minimized at home. Nurses and therapists provide assessment, treatment, and education. Unlicensed workers assist with personal care. Many frail or elderly people can remain at home with services including meal delivery, shopping help, transportation, and so on. **Figure 2.11** shows a caregiver in a patient's home.

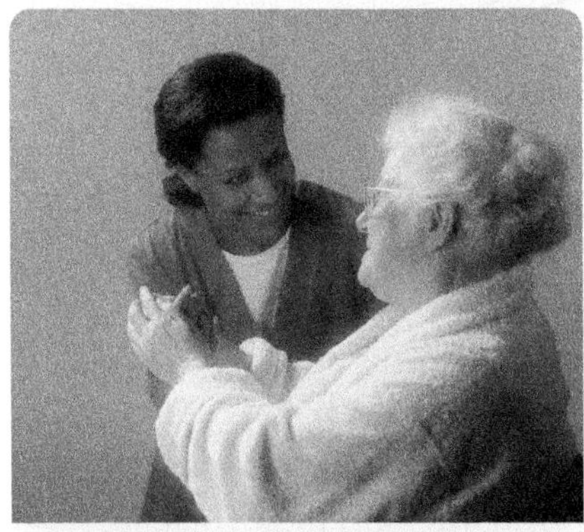

Fig. 2.11 Home Healthcare Shortened hospital stays and outpatient services have expanded the need for home healthcare. *How has the increased use of home healthcare changed the role of healthcare providers?*

READING CHECK

Identify two benefits that home health services have compared with hospitalization.

Emergency Preparedness

Are you concerned about major public health emergencies?

Healthcare professionals respond to all types of emergencies. Bioterrorist threats and pandemic outbreaks require organizations and public health officials to respond to public health emergencies.

A **geographic information system (GIS)** integrates hardware, software, and data for capturing, managing, analyzing, and displaying all forms of geographically referenced information. GIS technologies plan for emergencies and track outbreak patterns. Healthcare professionals at healthcare facilities report suspected or definite outbreaks. Then that data is analyzed so that an appropriate response can be prepared.

READING CHECK

Explain why it is important for public health officials to be able to track outbreak patterns.

SECTION 2.2 Trends in Healthcare Review

AFTER YOU READ

1. **Demonstrate** how each of the following contributes to the rising cost of healthcare:
   a. Technology
   b. An aging population
2. **Analyze** how each of the following helps contain the costs of healthcare:
   a. Home healthcare
   b. Preventive care and wellness
3. **Explain** why all healthcare professionals must be prepared for emergencies.

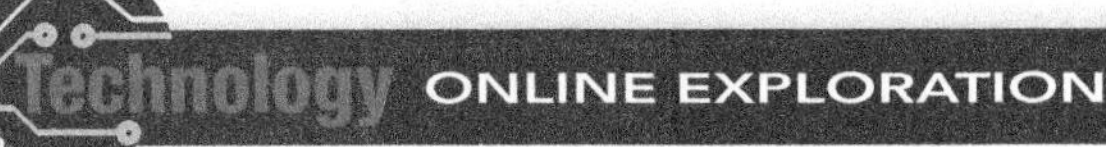

A Wellness Plan

Search the Internet using the keyword "wellness" and find a site that offers a free health or wellness assessment. Participate in the assessment. Then identify behaviors you can change to improve your own wellness. Create a wellness plan that includes three practices you can use to improve your state of wellness.

2.3 Healthcare Facilities

SECTION

Vocabulary

Content Vocabulary

You will learn these content vocabulary terms in this section.

- **residents**
- **assisted-living center**
- **activities of daily living (ADL)**

Healthcare Facilities

Healthcare facilities are places that provide care or make it possible for some type of care to be delivered to patients. Care provided ranges from short appointments to long-term residential care. Some facilities provide care for patients wherever the patient is located. For example, home health services provide care in the home, and emergency care services provide care at the scene of an accident or illness. The facilities and services discussed in this section are:

- Hospitals (inpatient facilities)
- Long-term care facilities
- Practitioners' offices and clinics
- Laboratories
- Emergency medical services
- Home healthcare
- Rehabilitation centers
- Hospices

Hospitals (Inpatient Facilities)

What companies or organizations own and operate the hospitals in your area?

Hospitals provide inpatient care and vary in ownership and operation. They may be

- run by religious organizations.
- private.
- nonprofit.
- run by government organizations.
- specialized.

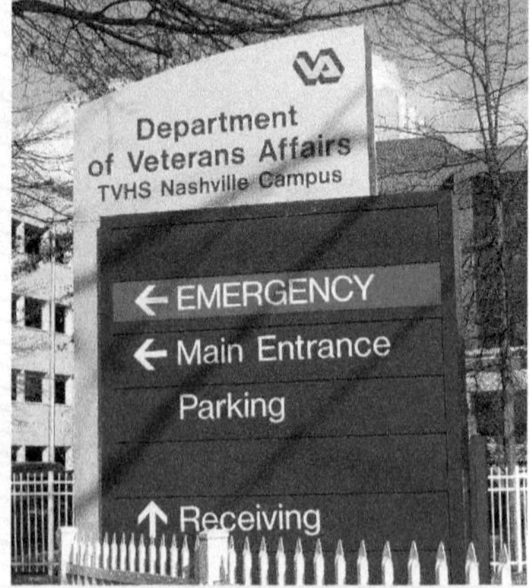

Fig. 2.12 Government Hospital Clients who have little or no money may receive care at these facilities. *What type of client receives care at this facility?*

Photo: Todd Bannor/Alamy

Hospitals Run by Religious Organizations

The beliefs of many religions involve helping people who are sick or needy. Therefore, many churches or religious groups set up hospitals that provide care to the public. A person need not be a member of a certain religion to receive care. However, the care is given in accordance with religious beliefs. For example, a Catholic hospital may not provide birth control, abortions, or other treatments that do not meet with the beliefs of the Roman Catholic Church.

Private Hospitals

A private hospital has shareholders, who invest money in the facility and expect a profit or return on their investment. Often a group of doctors or business professionals own stock in a private hospital.

Nonprofit Hospitals

Nonprofit hospitals do not have shareholders. The goal of these hospitals is not to produce a profit for shareholders; any profit is used to pay for improvements, equipment updates, or expansion of services. These hospitals may be sponsored by a religious or charitable organization.

Hospitals Run by Government Organizations

Some government hospitals provide care for military personnel and their dependents as well as for veterans, as shown in **Figure 2.12.** Military hospitals are funded by federal taxes, while state and county taxes fund state or county hospitals. Patients who have little or no money may receive healthcare free or at a reduced cost in these facilities.

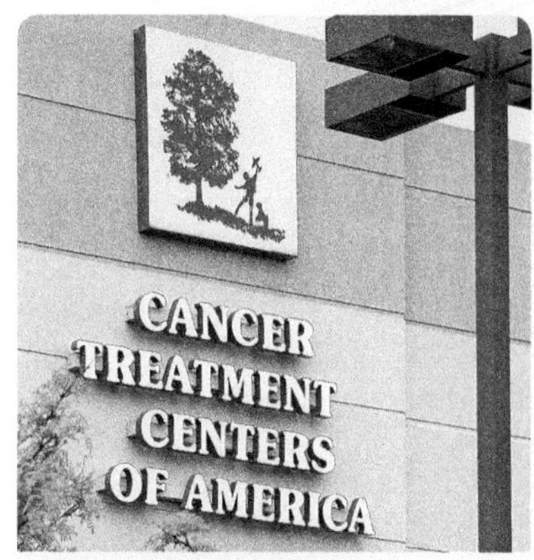

Fig. 2.13 Specialized Hospitals Some hospitals specialize in treating cancer, the number two cause of death in the United States. *Is there a specialized hospital near you?*

Specialized Hospitals

Hospitals may provide care to the general population, or they may specialize in certain types of care or age groups. In specialty hospitals, the physicians, nurses, and other staff are highly trained to meet the needs of these groups. Children's hospitals specialize in the needs of children from birth to young adulthood. Other hospitals specialize in a specific disease or treatment. For example, some hospitals treat diseases of the heart and lungs, some treat cancer, and some specialize in rehabilitation. **Figure 2.13** shows a specialized cancer treatment facility.

READING CHECK

List five types of hospitals and explain what makes each unique.

Long-Term Care Facilities

Have you ever known someone who required long-term care?

Long-term care centers provide care to people who need nursing or other professional healthcare services on a regular basis. These patients may not need round-the-clock nursing services. However, it may be unsafe for them to live alone, or they may have needs their family cannot meet. Many residents in long-term care facilities are frail or elderly. They may also be handicapped or disabled.

In a hospital, a physician usually sees a patient every day. In a long-term facility, a physician usually reviews the care being provided to the patient and sees the patient on a monthly basis. The patient may receive therapy to maintain or increase mobility and independence in dressing, personal hygiene, or eating. A patient may also be admitted for physical rehabilitation following surgery, injury, or serious illness. After regaining strength and mobility, the patient is often able to return home. Others may live there for the rest of their lives. These people may be called **residents** instead of patients. Long-term care facilities may be private, nonprofit, or funded by state and local taxes.

Photo: Stan Gregg/Alamy

With the growth of the aging population, long-term care has developed at various levels. Some patients may choose an **assisted-living center** that offers them separate living quarters while providing meals, housekeeping, and medical supervision. These patients are able to perform many of their own **activities of daily living (ADL).** Other places provide various levels of care, including skilled nursing facilities that offer 24-hour nursing services for patients who are unable to take care of themselves.

READING CHECK

Name two widespread uses of long-term care other than to care for the elderly.

Practitioners' Offices and Clinics

Do you most often get your primary healthcare at a practitioner's office or a clinic?

Healthcare providers such as physicians, nurse practitioners, and physician assistants provide examination and diagnosis for both acute and sudden illnesses as well as chronic or long-term illnesses. They also provide wellness exams, counseling, and treatment for their patients. Many offer some testing and minor surgery. As shown in **Figure 2.14,** dentists and dental hygienists are included in this group. Healthcare providers may have an individual practice or may work with other practitioners in a group practice.

Various practitioners may share office space and support staff in a clinic. Each has his or her own patients. The members of the group share the billing, reception, and recordkeeping staff. A clinic may specialize in cardiology, dentistry, or neurology, for example. Some clinics offer a variety of services. In some clinics there are practitioners with different specialties, so the patient can be treated at the clinic for almost any type of problem. These types of clinics are often privately owned but can also be affiliated with a hospital.

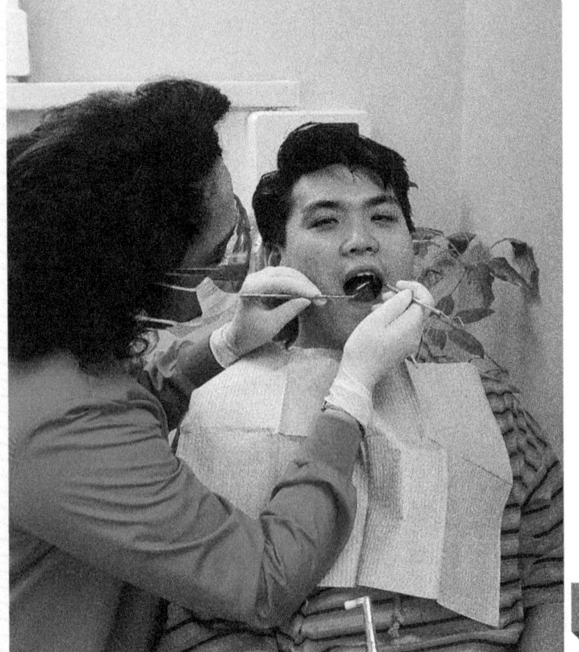

Fig. 2.14 At the Office Most dental offices perform exams and minor surgery. *How often should you see your dentist?*

The word "clinic" may also refer to a type of care or consultation provided on a specific day. Such clinics might last for one day in one location and then move on to another facility. Examples are flu clinics, sexually transmitted disease (STD) clinics, and cardiac clinics. These clinics are often supported by public healthcare funds.

READING CHECK

Describe the level of care that a client can expect to receive at a practitioner's office.

Laboratories

Have you ever visited a medical laboratory?

Laboratories perform tests on blood and other body fluids to assist physicians or other practitioners in making a diagnosis. Labs also examine tissue to determine the presence of disease, to identify infections, and to determine appropriate treatments for infections. A laboratory may be part of a hospital or clinic, or it may be independent. It may also be supported by public funds.

READING CHECK

Explain the purpose of medical laboratories.

Emergency Medical Services

Have you or a loved one ever had to call on emergency medical services?

Emergency medical services (EMS) extend medical care from the emergency room of a hospital into the community. The EMS system is designed to provide care to ill and injured people as quickly as possible.

When a person calls for help with an injury or illness, EMS often responds. Most areas have a 911 telephone system for reporting. A dispatcher answers a call, takes information, and alerts EMS. The caller's address may be automatically identified. The dispatcher is trained to give instructions for handling the emergency before an ambulance arrives.

Many people provide EMS service. In urban areas, police officers, firefighters, and ambulance staff are most likely to provide this type of care. In rural and wilderness areas, volunteers, park rangers, or ski patrol staff may provide it. EMS courses on topics such as first responder, basic first aid, and cardiopulmonary resuscitation (CPR) are offered to the public in many places.

READING CHECK

List five professions that might deliver EMS service.

Home Healthcare

What types of ailments do home healthcare workers most often treat?

Home healthcare, which was discussed in Section 2 of this chapter, is another type of healthcare service. Care is provided in the home for short periods after hospitalizations or for longer periods for patients who have chronic diseases or disabilities.

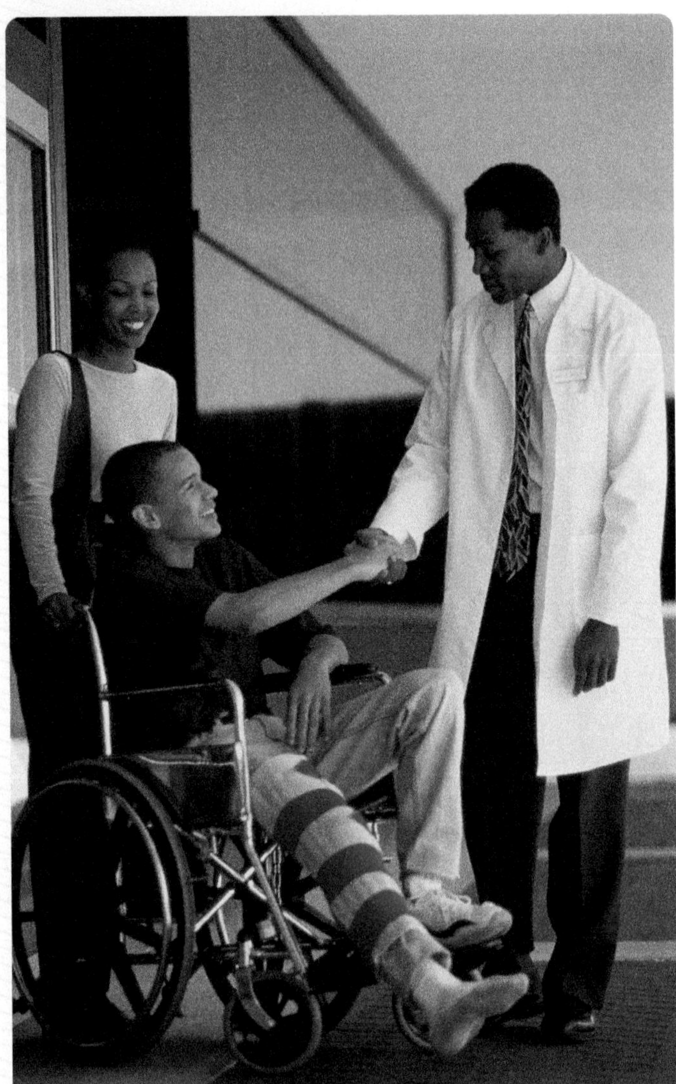
Fig. 2.15 **Rehabilitation Centers** These centers help clients regain physical or mental capacities. *Is there a rehab center in your area?*

Photo: Ron Chapple/Taxi/Getty Images

Rehabilitation Centers

Rehabilitation centers help patients regain physical or mental abilities or teach them how to live with disabilities. Rehabilitation focuses on physical, occupational (job), mental or psychological, and behavior modification therapies. These centers can be part of a hospital or clinic, or privately owned. Their main goal is to help patients regain function, independence, and, as much as possible, the ability to take care of themselves. **Figure 2.15** shows a patient in a rehabilitation center.

READING CHECK

Identify four possible focuses for rehabilitation.

Hospices

What is the goal of hospice care?

Hospice is a special form of care for patients who have terminal illnesses. The goal is to give support to patients who are near death. Hospice care focuses on the ill person and the family, not the disease.

Hospice is usually offered only to patients who are thought to have fewer than six months to live. An example of a hospice patient is a person who has terminal cancer. Anyone who has a terminal condition is eligible for this type of care.

Terminal diseases are allowed to run their natural course. The goal of hospice care is to reduce pain and other symptoms, as well as to give spiritual and emotional support. Hospices often provide care in the patient's home. Hospice centers are also available in many areas.

Hospice care includes treatment from doctors, nurses, therapists, dieticians, social workers, clergy, and volunteers. Therapy is designed to

- improve the quality of life.
- use pain medications effectively.
- relieve symptoms.
- prepare the person and his or her family for death.

Nothing is done to speed death. Instead, death is allowed to occur naturally. Hospice care has been shown to increase patient comfort,

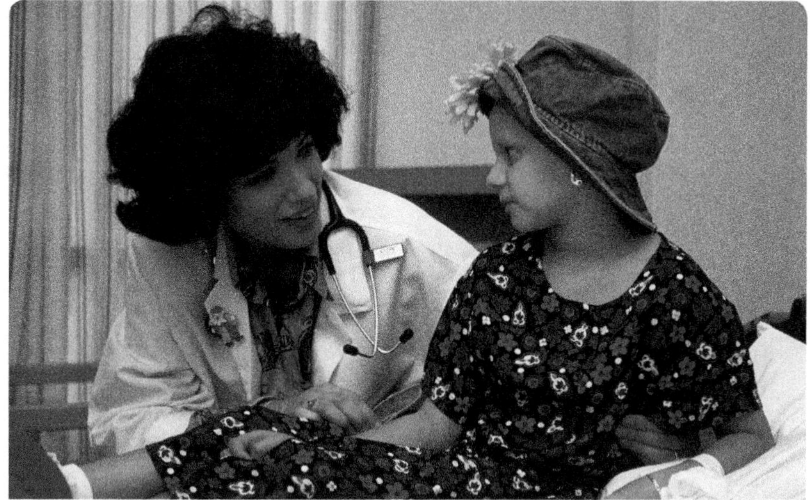

Fig. 2.16 Hospice Care for clients who have a terminal illness is provided by hospice. *What is the focus of hospice care?*

ease family anxiety, and reduce costs. The end of life is a difficult time for patients and their families. For some patients, this time may be better spent at home than in a hospital. For many patients who have terminal diseases, hospice offers a more peaceful way to die. But it is not for everyone. Patients facing death should be allowed to decide for themselves what kind of care is best for them. **Figure 2.16** shows a typical hospice setting.

READING CHECK

Summarize two benefits of hospice care.

SECTION 2.3 Healthcare Facilities Review

AFTER YOU READ

1. **Distinguish** among private, specialty, non-profit, and government hospitals.
2. **Identify** five services provided in practitioners' offices.
3. **Contrast** practitioners' offices and clinics.
4. **Indicate** services provided by laboratories.
5. **Identify** the services that emergency medical services provide.
6. **Compare** rehabilitation to home healthcare.
7. **Explain** the goal of hospice care.

Technology ONLINE EXPLORATIONS

Local Healthcare Facilities

Search the Internet to find the name and phone number of one of each type of healthcare facility discussed in this section. Each facility should be in your local area or state. Call or visit one facility and obtain information about the services it provides. Write a report based on your interview and share it with the class. Include information on the goals of the facility, methods of payment to the facility, availability of federal and/or state funding, and the hours or length of time the facility's services are available.

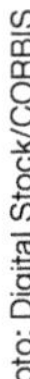
Photo: Digital Stock/CORBIS

SECTION
2.4 Healthcare Agencies

Vocabulary

Content Vocabulary

You will learn these content vocabulary terms in this section.

- **U.S. Department of Health and Human Services (DHHS)**
- **Centers for Disease Control and Prevention (CDC)**
- **Food and Drug Administration (FDA)**
- **National Institutes of Health (NIH)**
- **World Health Organization (WHO)**

Academic Vocabulary

You will see this word in your reading and on your tests. Find its meaning in the Glossary in the back of the book.

- **individuals**

Government Agencies

Have you considered a career with a government agency?

While individuals receive healthcare from hospitals, laboratories, physicians, dentists, and therapists, groups of people also need healthcare services. Cities, counties, states, our nation, and people around the world receive healthcare support from government and nonprofit agencies. Government health services are paid for by taxes. Nonprofit agencies are supported by private contributions or fund raisers.

Government agencies may provide care, but mainly they conduct research, oversee programs providing care to the elderly and children, and establish healthcare policies. Examples of government agencies are:

- Local health departments
- U.S. Department of Health and Human Services
- World Health Organization

Local Health Departments

Local health departments provide immunizations, inspect restaurants, and oversee the protection of the environment. They collect statistics on communicable diseases and share that information with state and national agencies. Local health departments may also provide health education and other health-related services to the community. State, county, or city governments administer local health departments.

U.S. Department of Health and Human Services

The **U.S. Department of Health and Human Services (DHHS)** is the national agency that deals with health in the United States. The President appoints the Secretary of Health and Human Services, who advises on health and welfare plans, policies, and federal government programs. Many departments come under the supervision of the Secretary of Health and Human Services. Some administer programs that provide services to needy children and families. Others support a nationwide network that provides at-home services to the elderly like "meals on wheels." The Agency for Healthcare Research and Quality supports research designed to decrease medical errors, reduce medical costs, and improve healthcare quality.

An important agency in the DHHS is the **Centers for Disease Control and Prevention (CDC).** The CDC has established a system that monitors and prevents disease outbreaks using the GIS. It also guards against international disease transmission, maintains health statistics, provides immunization services, supports disease and injury prevention research, and promotes healthy behaviors and environments. State health departments and other agencies collaborate with the CDC to ensure the health and safety of the nation.

Other agencies within the DHHS are the **Food and Drug Administration (FDA)** and the **National Institutes of Health (NIH).** The role of the FDA is to ensure that food and cosmetics are safe and that medication and medical devices are safe and useful. The NIH, the world's premier medical research organization, supports research projects working to end diseases such as cancer, Alzheimer's, diabetes, arthritis, heart ailments, and AIDS.

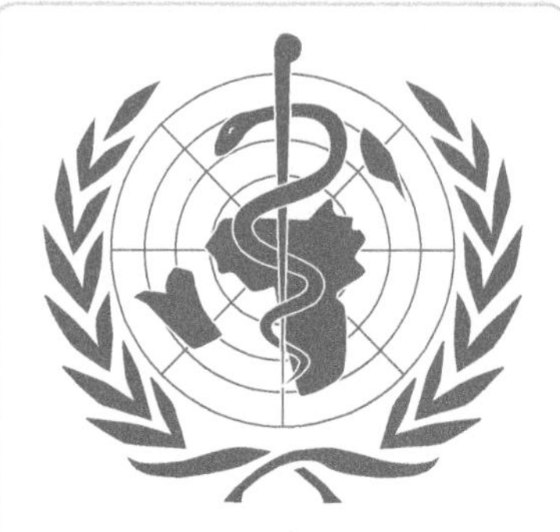

Fig. 2.17 WHO The World Health Organization defines health as a state of complete physical, mental, and social well-being, not merely the absence of disease or infirmity. *What is the primary goal of WHO?*

World Health Organization

The **World Health Organization (WHO)** is an international agency sponsored by the United Nations and is the directing and coordinating authority on international health (see **Figure 2.17**). A goal of WHO is to help people attain the highest possible levels of health. WHO also compiles health statistics and information on disease, and publishes health information. WHO also trains medical personnel in techniques to improve general health or combat specific diseases.

READING CHECK

Describe three functions of local health departments.

Volunteer and Nonprofit Health Agencies

Can you think of a nonprofit health agency that is concerned with a particular disease or group of diseases?

Healthcare services are also provided by nonprofit agencies at the state, local, or national level. Many deal with a specific disease or group of diseases. They provide funding for research and promote education based on information learned through research. They may also provide special services to victims of disease by purchasing equipment or providing treatment centers. Sometimes they act as referral centers.

Volunteer nonprofit organizations make great contributions to the health of those they serve. In addition, they have influenced laws, created standards of care for infants, and educated doctors and other health professionals in new techniques.

The next time you read a pamphlet on smoking cessation, immunization, or cancer prevention, check the name of the publisher. Chances are that a nonprofit organization is the publisher.

Here are two examples of the hundreds of volunteer agencies that promote healthcare-related causes worldwide. You can find more through an Internet search.

American Lung Association Founded in 1904 to fight tuberculosis, the American Lung Association (ALA) is the oldest voluntary health organization in the United States. Today the ALA fights lung disease with an emphasis on asthma, tobacco control, and environmental health. The ALA's advocacy programs lobby for laws and regulations related to lung health at the national, state, and local levels. The ALA played a major role in the passage of the landmark federal Clean Air Act, as well as the law prohibiting smoking on domestic passenger airline flights. Contributions from the public and gifts and grants from corporations and foundations fund the ALA.

March of Dimes The March of Dimes was founded in 1938 by President Franklin D. Roosevelt, himself a victim of paralytic poliomyelitis. The initial goals of the March of Dimes were to provide care for the victims of polio and to develop a vaccine. Before vaccines were developed, an estimated 50,000 people in the United States were paralyzed or died each year from polio. As a result of efforts by the March of Dimes, all babies now receive a vaccine to prevent polio. Having accomplished this goal, the foundation moved on to improving the health of babies, working to prevent birth defects, and reducing infant mortality.

READING CHECK

Explain how nonprofit health agencies that deal with a disease or group of diseases are effective.

SECTION 2.4 Healthcare Agencies Review

AFTER YOU READ

1. **Examine** the role of the U.S. Department of Health and Human Services (DHHS).
2. **Identify** three agencies in the DHHS and their functions.
3. **Indicate** a primary goal of the World Health Organization (WHO).
4. **Explain** how nonprofit and volunteer organizations influence laws.
5. **Illustrate** three ways volunteer and nonprofit organizations contribute to health and healthcare.

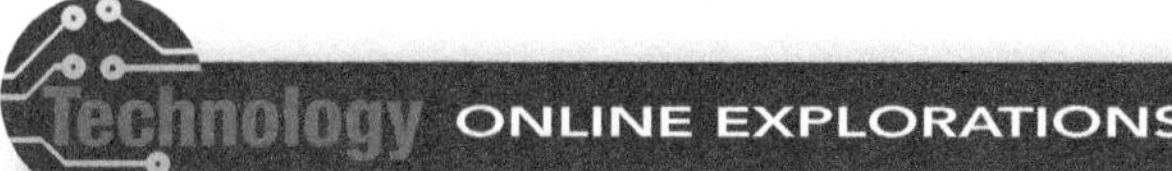

Agency Funding

Use the Internet to find a government or nonprofit agency that is not discussed in this section. Contact the agency and ask how the agency is funded, who works for the agency, and what services the agency provides. Compile your information into a booklet with other students to create a healthcare resource guide for your class.

SECTION
2.5 Health Insurance

Paying for Healthcare

What kind of health insurance do you have, if any?

Most people rely on health insurance to pay for healthcare. A subscriber pays a **premium** to an insurance company. The subscriber is often an employer, but subscribers can also be individuals.

The insurance company decides what services will be covered. If the service is covered, the insurance company pays for that service. The amount paid and type of service covered vary. Many plans limit the amount they will pay for a service and also set deductibles, or the amount an insured person must pay before the insurance company begins to pay. After the deductible is paid, a copayment often applies.

Employers often offer insurance coverage to employees. This is **group insurance.** The employer may pay part or all of the premium as an employment benefit. People without a group policy may buy individual policies. Individual policies often cost more than group policies.

In 2010, President Barack Obama signed the Patient Protection and Affordable Care Act, extending coverage to 32 million previously uninsured Americans. The law also bans lifetime limits on coverage, exclusions for preexisting conditions, and policy cancellations when a person becomes ill. Parents may also keep their children on a family policy until age 26.

Healthcare is also paid for by methods such as Medicare, Medicaid, Managed care (Health Maintenance Organizations and Preferred Provider Organizations), Workers' compensation, and Military healthcare.

Medicare and Medicaid

When were Medicare and Medicaid established?

In 1965 the federal government passed legislation to give certain people better access to healthcare. The legislation targeted people who lacked access to quality care, such as the elderly, infants, children, and the disabled. The programs were Medicare and Medicaid.

Medicare

Medicare provides insurance to people who are 65 and older, disabled, or have permanent kidney failure. There are four parts to Medicare.

Vocabulary

Content Vocabulary

You will learn these content vocabulary terms in this section.

- premium
- group insurance
- managed care
- Health Maintenance Organization (HMO)
- Preferred Provider Organization (PPO)
- workers' compensation

Academic Vocabulary

You will see this word in your reading and on your tests. Find its meaning in the Glossary in the back of the book.

- policy

Part A provides for hospital care. It helps pay for inpatient services, skilled nursing facility services, home health services, and hospice care. Part B helps pay for physicians, outpatient services, and other services. The insured pays a premium for Part B and may have a deductible or purchase other private insurance.

Part C may be called Medicare Advantage or MA. These plans, offered by private companies approved by Medicare, are similar to HMOs or PPOs. A Part C plan provides all of the Part A and Part B coverage and may also offer coverage for vision, hearing, dental, and health and wellness programs, and may also include Part D coverage. Part D is prescription insurance from a private company approved by Medicare.

Medicaid

Medicaid provides insurance for low-income families with children. In many states, dental coverage for children is also included. The aged, the blind, disabled people on Supplemental Security Income, certain low-income pregnant women, and certain people with very high medical bills may also be covered by Medicaid. The states and the federal government run this program and provide funding for it.

There is no co-payment or deductible for Medicaid. The states must cover basic services. They have authority to decide who is eligible, how it is paid, and what is covered. Services considered basic are inpatient and outpatient services in hospitals, laboratory, and X-ray services. Skilled nursing and home health services, doctors' services, family planning, health checks, and diagnosis and treatment for children are also basic. **Figure 2.18** shows a Medicaid identification card.

READING CHECK

Recall which three groups of people are eligible for Medicare.

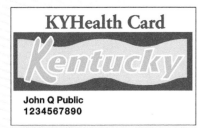

Fig. 2.18 Medicaid Card This is an example of a Medicaid card. *Who uses this identification card?*

Managed Care

Can you name one type of managed care organization?

Managed care plans are designed specifically to control costs. Managed care organizations manage, negotiate, and contract for healthcare with the primary goal of keeping healthcare costs down.

Health Maintenance Organizations

The focus of **Health Maintenance Organizations (HMOs)** is prevention and wellness care. Illness prevention is more cost-effective than treating disease. To belong to an HMO, premiums are paid to the HMO instead of to an insurance company. Because HMOs focus on prevention, wellness care not normally covered by traditional insurance programs is covered. Subscribers can only see providers hired by the HMO. Tests and surgeries are monitored to ensure they are necessary.

Table 2.1

HEALTH MAINTENANCE ORGANIZATION (HMO)	PREFERRED PROVIDER ORGANIZATION (PPO)
you can only use the providers in the network	you can go out of the network but will pay more if you do
pay a copayment	pay an annual deductible; copay possible
you do not have to file any claim forms	if you use services outside the network, you must file a claim form for reimbursement
you need a referral if you want to a see a specialist or anyone other than your primary doctor	you do not usually need a referral to see a specialist

Preferred Provider Organizations

A **Preferred Provider Organization (PPO),** also known as a participating provider organization or preferred provider option is made up of medical doctors, hospitals, and other healthcare providers who have contracted with an insurer or administrator to provide healthcare at reduced rates. PPOs and HMOs are compared in **Table 2.1.**

Workers' Compensation

What is covered by workers' compensation?

Workers' compensation covers accidents, injuries, or diseases that occur in the workplace. Federal law requires employers to purchase and maintain workers' compensation insurance for their employees.

Workers' compensation covers services such as basic medical treatment for inpatient and outpatient care, payments to employees for temporary or permanent disabilities, death benefits, and rehabilitation costs.

READING CHECK

Describe three benefits that are provided through workers' compensation to workers who are injured on the job.

Military Healthcare

Can you identify a military healthcare facility?

The U.S. government provides healthcare benefits for families of current military personnel and veterans through the CHAMPUS/TRICARE program. CHAMPUS stands for Civilian Health and Medical Program of the Uniformed Services. It is a healthcare benefit for members of the uniformed services, including the Army, Navy, Marines, Air Force, Coast Guard, Public Health Service, NASA, and their families.

READING CHECK

Recall Who is eligible for military health services?

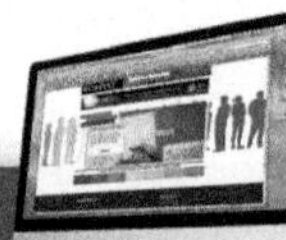

Mc Graw Hill connect™ ONLINE PROCEDURES

PROCEDURE 2-1

Recognizing Historic Events in Healthcare

For as long as human beings have been on the planet, we have practiced medicine. The historic events of medicine have shaped healthcare today.

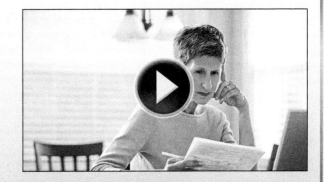

PROCEDURE 2-2

Identifying Healthcare Facilities

Healthcare facilities are places that provide care or make it possible for some type of care to be delivered to patients. Care can be provided on a short- or long-term basis. Knowledge of healthcare facilities will let you chose the correct location to receive care.

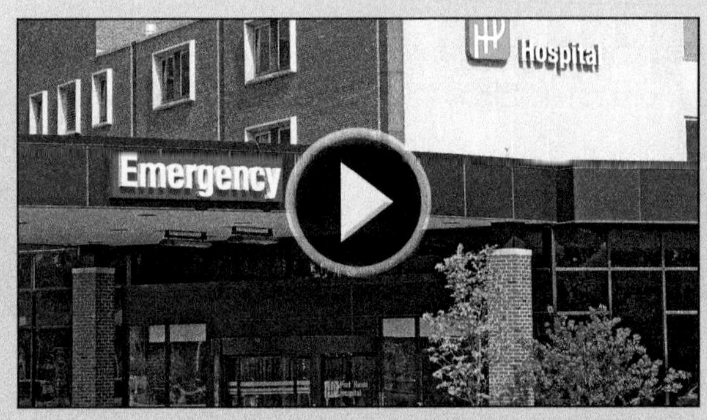

SECTION 2.5 Health Insurance Review

AFTER YOU READ

1. **Discuss** the differences between group and private health insurance.
2. **Indicate** populations who are eligible for federally supported health insurance.
3. **Identify** the groups of people who are eligible for Medicare.
4. **Identify** the groups of people who are eligible for Medicaid.
5. **Indicate** at least five services that must be covered by each state through Medicaid.
6. **Describe** the purpose of managed care.
7. **Compare and Contrast** health maintenance organizations and preferred provider organizations.
8. **Explain** the value of workers' compensation.

Technology ONLINE EXPLORATIONS

Insurance

Visit www.healthcare.gov. Click on the Find Insurance Options link to learn about the policies you may obtain. What type of policy interests you the most? What are the copayments and deductibles? What services are provided?

CHAPTER 2 Review

Chapter Summary

SECTION 2.1

- Numerous inventions and discoveries have had significant effects on healthcare: the printing press, the microscope, the stethoscope, medical asepsis, and the regulation of practicing physicians, to name just a few. **(pg. 24)**
- Healthcare in ancient times was based on tradition, superstition, and religion. As documentation, classification, and reasoning replaced these practices, patterns could be established and the effectiveness of treatment could be documented. **(pg. 25)**
- The practices of healthful living—such as exercise, rest, and good food and water—were encouraged in ancient times as they are now. **(pg. 30)**

SECTION 2.2

- Advances in technology, the growth of the aging population, and increases in the number of uninsured and underinsured people have caused the cost of healthcare to rise. The current trends of wellness and preventive care, outpatient care, and healthcare reform help to control and contain healthcare costs. Emergency preparedness is necessary for all healthcare professionals. **(pg. 31**)

SECTION 2.3

- Healthcare facilities such as hospitals, long-term care facilities, practitioners' offices, clinics, laboratories, emergency medical services, home health, rehabilitation centers, and hospices provide care or allow some types of care to be delivered to patients. **(pg. 36)**

SECTION 2.4

- Cities, counties, states, our nation, and people around the world receive healthcare from government agencies that are supported by taxes. Volunteer agencies provide funding for research and distribution of information gained from research. **(pg. 42)**

SECTION 2.5

- Medicare provides health insurance to people who are at least 65 years old, or are disabled, or have permanent kidney failure. Medicaid provides health coverage to certain low-income families with children, the aged, the blind, disabled people on Supplemental Security Income, certain low-income pregnant women and children, and people with very high medical bills. **(pg. 45)**
- Health maintenance organizations (HMOs) focus on prevention and wellness care and were developed in response to the rising cost of healthcare. **(pg. 46)**
- Workers' compensation is paid for by an employer and covers employee accidents, injuries, or diseases that occur in the workplace. **(pg. 47)**

CHAPTER 2 Assessment

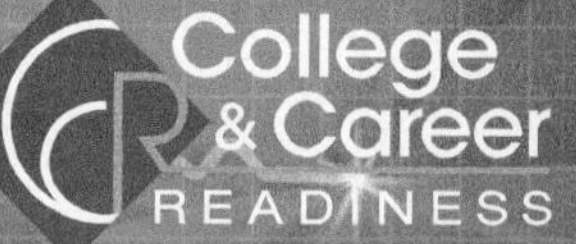

Critical Thinking/Problem Solving

1. Your friend received a bad burn on her arm while at work. The burn is red, blistered, and swollen. She wants to go to a doctor, but her parents do not have health insurance. What would you tell your friend to do?

2. Your best friend's grandmother, who is 66 years old, has just been diagnosed with breast cancer and is said to have less than six months to live. What type of facilities, services, and insurance would she need and be eligible for? Explain your answer.

3. There have been several cases of H1N1 influenza in your city. What should be done to track the potential for a worsening outbreak?

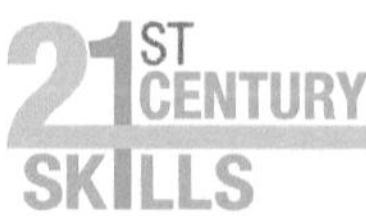

4. **Teamwork** An insurance claim form must be completed before an insurer will pay for medical expenses. A common and standard claim form is the CMS 1500. Download a copy of this form from a trusted website. Complete the form, working with a partner and basing your information on a recent visit to a physician. If you do not have the necessary information, make something up

5. **Communication** Identify an event in the history of healthcare and write down the key details about that event. As a class or as smaller groups, form a human timeline in front of the class. Once the timeline is formed, each student should explain the event he or she has chosen.

6. **Information Literacy** The National Institutes of Health (NIH) consists of a number of institutes that perform research on various diseases and disorders. Search the NIH website and find an institute that you would like to learn more about. Discover the purpose of the institute you have chosen and share this information with your class.

Mc Graw Hill connect™ ONLINE ACTIVITIES

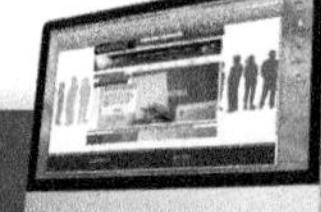

Complete our HST online activities for Chapter 2, which include Concept Check review questions, Reference Flash Cards, and Online Procedures assessment sheets.

- **Concept Check** review questions
- **Reference Flash Cards** medical terminology practice
- **Online Procedures** assessment sheets

CHAPTER 3 Safety and Infection Control Practices

Essential Question:

What can you do to promote the safety of the healthcare workplace?

"Safety" means freedom from danger, risks, and injury. Quality healthcare begins with the safety of the patient and the healthcare professional. Healthcare professionals are responsible for their own safety as well as that of their patients. Their attitude and knowledge are important to ensure safety. When employed in healthcare, you are required to be aware of potential safety risks. You should report any unsafe practices that you observe in a facility to a charge nurse or other supervisor. You should also know how to respond if an emergency occurs. The slogan "safety first" always applies.

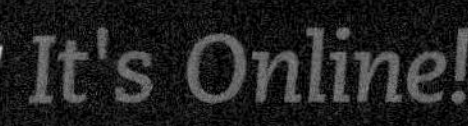

- Online Procedures
- STEM Connection
- Medical Science
- Medical Terms
- Medical Math
- Ethics in Action
- Virtual Lab

READING GUIDE

OBJECTIVES

After completing this chapter, you will be able to:

- **Demonstrate** how safety practices relate to patients.
- **Explain** the importance of body mechanics to workers.
- **Indicate** the five factors that affect microbial growth.
- **Examine** methods used to destroy microorganisms.
- **Distinguish** the parts of a microscope.
- **Discuss** biological agents used for bioterrorism.
- **Analyze** the chain of infection.
- **Compare** common signs and symptoms of infection.
- **Compare** standard and transmission-based precaution guidelines.
- **Demonstrate** four safety procedures.
- **Explain** the cough etiquette standard.

BEFORE YOU READ

Connect Have you ever been in a medical emergency situation? If so, how do you suppose the healthcare personnel involved were able to avoid chaos?

Main Idea

Standardized procedures are used to control infection and establish a safer and more predictable environment.

Note-Taking Activity

Draw this table. Write key terms and phrases under **Cues**. Write main ideas under **Note Taking**. Summarize the section under **Summary**.

Cues	Note Taking
○	○
○	○
Summary	

Graphic Organizer

Before you read the chapter, draw a diagram like the one below. As you read, write the main safety and infection control practices covered in this chapter into the diagram.

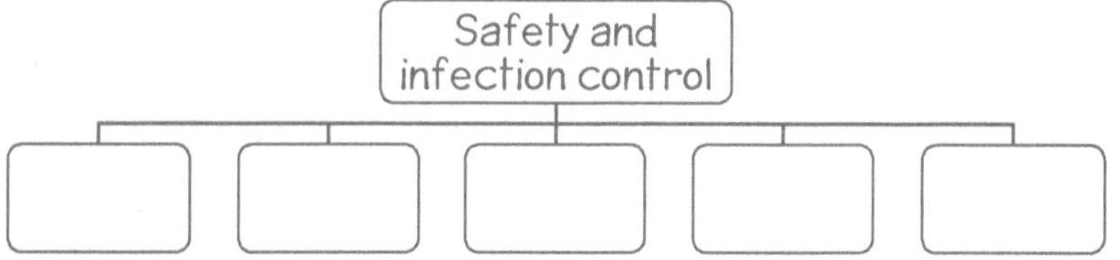

connect
Downloadable graphic organizers can be accessed online.

STANDARDS

HEALTH SCIENCE

NCHSE 1.13 Analyze the basic structure and function of the human body.

NCHSE 1.21 Describe common diseases and disorders of each body system (prevention, pathology, diagnosis, and treatment).

SCIENCE

NSES 1 Develop an understanding of science unifying concepts and processes: systems, order, and organization; evidence, models, and explanation; change, constancy, and measurement; evolution and equilibrium; and form and function.

NCHSE *National Consortium for Health Science Education*

NSES *National Science Education Standards*

COMMON CORE STATE STANDARDS

MATHEMATICS

Geometry

Geometric Measurement and Dimension G-GMD Visualize relationships between two- and three-dimensional objects.

ENGLISH LANGUAGE ARTS

Reading

Range of Reading and Level of Text Complexity R-10 Read and comprehend science/technical texts in the grades 11–CCR text complexity band independently and proficiently.

Speaking and Listening

Comprehension and Collaboration SL-2 Integrate multiple sources of information presented in diverse media or formats evaluating the credibility and accuracy of each source.

SECTION 3.1 Accidents and Injuries

Governing Agencies

What government agencies oversee safety in the workplace?

The Occupational Safety and Health Act of 1970 requires the **Occupational Safety and Health Administration (OSHA)** to oversee workplace **safety.** OSHA enacts and enforces safety and health standards intended to prevent workplace injuries and illnesses.

For example, the Occupational Exposure to Hazardous Chemicals Standard states that employees must be told about all hazards and chemicals in the workplace. OSHA requires that **Material Safety Data Sheets (MSDS)** be kept on all chemicals at a facility (see **Figure 3.2** on page 54). Manufacturers must provide a copy of MSDS for all of the products they sell. The appropriate MSDS should be available to all employees.

The MSDS must contain all of the following information:

- Manufacturer's name and address
- Safety exposure limits
- Chemical name
- Health hazards
- Flammability level
- Reactivity level
- Personal protective equipment (PPE) and other control measures required when handling the chemical
- Hazard rating for the chemical (based on a scale of 0 to 4, with 0 indicating no hazard and 4 indicating extreme hazard)

In addition to maintaining the MSDS, a facility must properly label all hazardous materials. If a label is not readable or is missing, it must be replaced. Healthcare facilities must comply with regulations related to MSDS and chemicals. Failure to comply may result in large fines.

A safety officer may be chosen to oversee safety education. He or she is responsible for preventing accidents and injuries through employee training as seen in **Figure 3.1,** for regular equipment and facility inspections, and for accident investigations. The safety officer is responsible for compliance with OSHA regulations. However, it is the duty of all healthcare employees to follow OSHA guidelines and be actively involved in safety training.

Vocabulary

Content Vocabulary

You will learn these content vocabulary terms in this section.

- **Occupational Safety and Health Administration (OSHA)**
- **safety**
- **Material Safety Data Sheets (MSDS)**
- **National Institute for Occupational Safety and Health (NIOSH)**

Academic Vocabulary

You will see this word in your reading and on your tests. Find its meaning in the Glossary in the back of the book.

- **investigations**

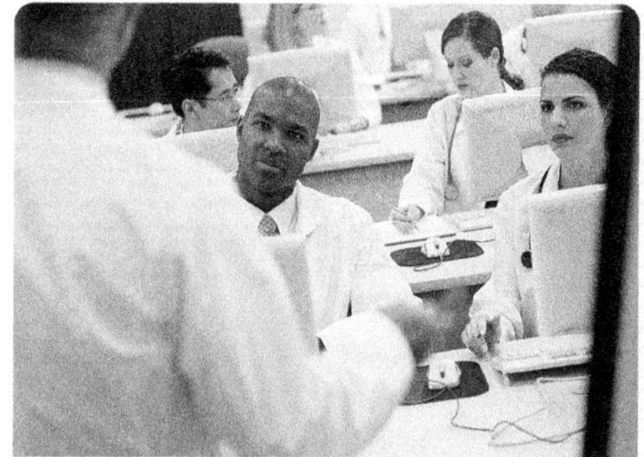

Fig. 3.1 Employee Training Regular in-service training on safety is provided to employees. *What should an employee do if he or she notices unsafe procedures or situations in the healthcare facility?*

The Centers for Disease Control and Prevention (CDC) plays a role in accident and injury prevention. The CDC has developed standard precautions to avoid transmission of disease. OSHA enforces these precautions. These procedures are discussed in Section 3.5.

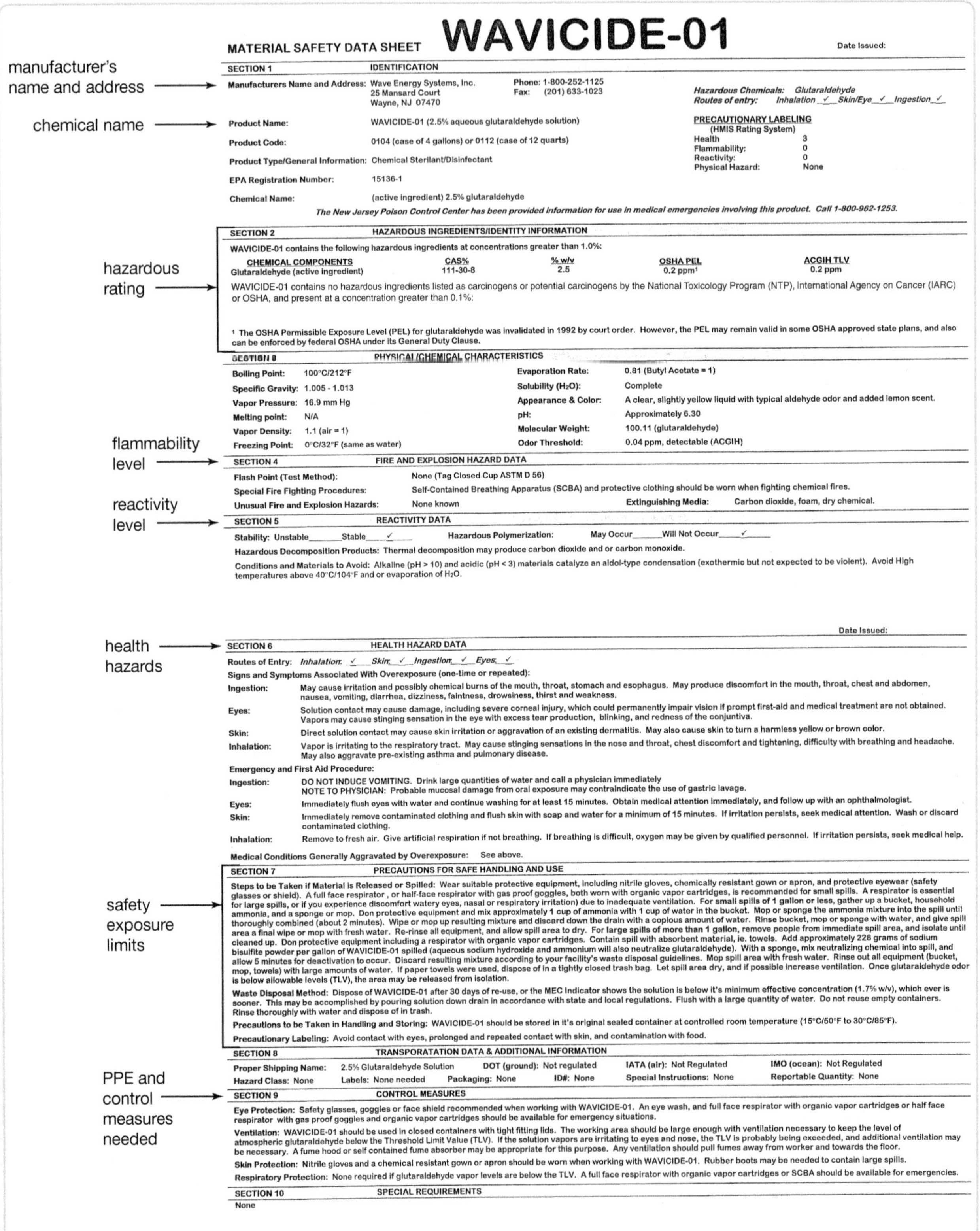

MATERIAL SAFETY DATA SHEET **WAVICIDE-01**

Date Issued:

SECTION 1 IDENTIFICATION

Manufacturers Name and Address: Wave Energy Systems, Inc.
25 Mansard Court
Wayne, NJ 07470

Phone: 1-800-252-1125
Fax: (201) 633-1023

Hazardous Chemicals: *Glutaraldehyde*
Routes of entry: *Inhalation* ✓ *Skin/Eye* ✓ *Ingestion* ✓

Product Name: WAVICIDE-01 (2.5% aqueous glutaraldehyde solution)

Product Code: 0104 (case of 4 gallons) or 0112 (case of 12 quarts)

Product Type/General Information: Chemical Sterilant/Disinfectant

EPA Registration Number: 15136-1

Chemical Name: (active ingredient) 2.5% glutaraldehyde

PRECAUTIONARY LABELING
(HMIS Rating System)

Health	3
Flammability:	0
Reactivity:	0
Physical Hazard:	None

The New Jersey Poison Control Center has been provided information for use in medical emergencies involving this product. Call 1-800-962-1253.

SECTION 2 HAZARDOUS INGREDIENTS/IDENTITY INFORMATION

WAVICIDE-01 contains the following hazardous ingredients at concentrations greater than 1.0%:

CHEMICAL COMPONENTS	CAS%	% w/v	OSHA PEL	ACGIH TLV
Glutaraldehyde (active ingredient)	111-30-8	2.5	0.2 ppm[1]	0.2 ppm

WAVICIDE-01 contains no hazardous ingredients listed as carcinogens or potential carcinogens by the National Toxicology Program (NTP), International Agency on Cancer (IARC) or OSHA, and present at a concentration greater than 0.1%:

[1] The OSHA Permissible Exposure Level (PEL) for glutaraldehyde was invalidated in 1992 by court order. However, the PEL may remain valid in some OSHA approved state plans, and also can be enforced by federal OSHA under its General Duty Clause.

SECTION 3 PHYSICAL/CHEMICAL CHARACTERISTICS

Boiling Point:	100°C/212°F	**Evaporation Rate:**	0.81 (Butyl Acetate = 1)
Specific Gravity:	1.005 - 1.013	**Solubility (H_2O):**	Complete
Vapor Pressure:	16.9 mm Hg	**Appearance & Color:**	A clear, slightly yellow liquid with typical aldehyde odor and added lemon scent.
Melting point:	N/A	**pH:**	Approximately 6.30
Vapor Density:	1.1 (air = 1)	**Molecular Weight:**	100.11 (glutaraldehyde)
Freezing Point:	0°C/32°F (same as water)	**Odor Threshold:**	0.04 ppm, detectable (ACGIH)

SECTION 4 FIRE AND EXPLOSION HAZARD DATA

Flash Point (Test Method): None (Tag Closed Cup ASTM D 56)

Special Fire Fighting Procedures: Self-Contained Breathing Apparatus (SCBA) and protective clothing should be worn when fighting chemical fires.

Unusual Fire and Explosion Hazards: None known **Extinguishing Media:** Carbon dioxide, foam, dry chemical.

SECTION 5 REACTIVITY DATA

Stability: Unstable_____ Stable ✓ **Hazardous Polymerization:** May Occur_____ Will Not Occur ✓

Hazardous Decomposition Products: Thermal decomposition may produce carbon dioxide and or carbon monoxide.

Conditions and Materials to Avoid: Alkaline (pH > 10) and acidic (pH < 3) materials catalyze an aldol-type condensation (exothermic but not expected to be violent). Avoid High temperatures above 40°C/104°F and or evaporation of H_2O.

Date Issued:

SECTION 6 HEALTH HAZARD DATA

Routes of Entry: *Inhalation* ✓ *Skin* ✓ *Ingestion* ✓ *Eyes* ✓

Signs and Symptoms Associated With Overexposure (one-time or repeated):

Ingestion: May cause irritation and possibly chemical burns of the mouth, throat, stomach and esophagus. May produce discomfort in the mouth, throat, chest and abdomen, nausea, vomiting, diarrhea, dizziness, faintness, drowsiness, thirst and weakness.

Eyes: Solution contact may cause damage, including severe corneal injury, which could permanently impair vision if prompt first-aid and medical treatment are not obtained. Vapors may cause stinging sensation in the eye with excess tear production, blinking, and redness of the conjuntiva.

Skin: Direct solution contact may cause skin irritation or aggravation of an existing dermatitis. May also cause skin to turn a harmless yellow or brown color.

Inhalation: Vapor is irritating to the respiratory tract. May cause stinging sensations in the nose and throat, chest discomfort and tightening, difficulty with breathing and headache. May also aggravate pre-existing asthma and pulmonary disease.

Emergency and First Aid Procedure:

Ingestion: DO NOT INDUCE VOMITING. Drink large quantities of water and call a physician immediately
NOTE TO PHYSICIAN: Probable mucosal damage from oral exposure may contraindicate the use of gastric lavage.

Eyes: Immediately flush eyes with water and continue washing for at least 15 minutes. Obtain medical attention immediately, and follow up with an ophthalmologist.

Skin: Immediately remove contaminated clothing and flush skin with soap and water for a minimum of 15 minutes. If irritation persists, seek medical attention. Wash or discard contaminated clothing.

Inhalation: Remove to fresh air. Give artificial respiration if not breathing. If breathing is difficult, oxygen may be given by qualified personnel. If irritation persists, seek medical help.

Medical Conditions Generally Aggravated by Overexposure: See above.

SECTION 7 PRECAUTIONS FOR SAFE HANDLING AND USE

Steps to be Taken if Material is Released or Spilled: Wear suitable protective equipment, including nitrile gloves, chemically resistant gown or apron, and protective eyewear (safety glasses or shield). A full face respirator , or half-face respirator with gas proof goggles, both worn with organic vapor cartridges, is recommended for small spills. A respirator is essential for large spills, or if you experience discomfort watery eyes, nasal or respiratory irritation) due to inadequate ventilation. For **small spills of 1 gallon or less**, gather up a bucket, household ammonia, and a sponge or mop. Don protective equipment and mix approximately 1 cup of ammonia with 1 cup of water in the bucket. Mop or sponge the ammonia mixture into the spill until thoroughly combined (about 2 minutes). Wipe or mop up resulting mixture and discard down the drain with a copious amount of water. Rinse bucket, mop or sponge with water, and give spill area a final wipe or mop with fresh water. Re-rinse all equipment, and allow spill area to dry. For **large spills of more than 1 gallon**, remove people from immediate spill area, and isolate until cleaned up. Don protective equipment including a respirator with organic vapor cartridges. Contain spill with absorbent material, ie. towels. Add approximately 228 grams of sodium bisulfite powder per gallon of WAVICIDE-01 spilled (aqueous sodium hydroxide and ammonium will also neutralize glutaraldehyde). With a sponge, mix neutralizing chemical into spill, and allow 5 minutes for deactivation to occur. Discard resulting mixture according to your facility's waste disposal guidelines. Mop spill area with fresh water. Rinse out all equipment (bucket, mop, towels) with large amounts of water. If paper towels were used, dispose of in a tightly closed trash bag. Let spill area dry, and if possible increase ventilation. Once glutaraldehyde odor is below allowable levels (TLV), the area may be released from isolation.

Waste Disposal Method: Dispose of WAVICIDE-01 after 30 days of re-use, or the MEC Indicator shows the solution is below it's minimum effective concentration (1.7% w/v), which ever is sooner. This may be accomplished by pouring solution down drain in accordance with state and local regulations. Flush with a large quantity of water. Do not reuse empty containers. Rinse thoroughly with water and dispose of in trash.

Precautions to be Taken in Handling and Storing: WAVICIDE-01 should be stored in it's original sealed container at controlled room temperature (15°C/50°F to 30°C/85°F).

Precautionary Labeling: Avoid contact with eyes, prolonged and repeated contact with skin, and contamination with food.

SECTION 8 TRANSPORATATION DATA & ADDITIONAL INFORMATION

Proper Shipping Name: 2.5% Glutaraldehyde Solution	**DOT (ground):** Not regulated	**IATA (air):** Not Regulated	**IMO (ocean):** Not Regulated
Hazard Class: None **Labels:** None needed	**Packaging:** None **ID#:** None	**Special Instructions:** None	**Reportable Quantity:** None

SECTION 9 CONTROL MEASURES

Eye Protection: Safety glasses, goggles or face shield recommended when working with WAVICIDE-01. An eye wash, and full face respirator with organic vapor cartridges or half face respirator with gas proof goggles and organic vapor cartridges should be available for emergency situations.

Ventilation: WAVICIDE-01 should be used in closed containers with tight fitting lids. The working area should be large enough with ventilation necessary to keep the level of atmospheric glutaraldehyde below the Threshold Limit Value (TLV). If the solution vapors are irritating to eyes and nose, the TLV is probably being exceeded, and additional ventilation may be necessary. A fume hood or self contained fume absorber may be appropriate for this purpose. Any ventilation should pull fumes away from worker and towards the floor.

Skin Protection: Nitrile gloves and a chemical resistant gown or apron should be worn when working with WAVICIDE-01. Rubber boots may be needed to contain large spills.

Respiratory Protection: None required if glutaraldehyde vapor levels are below the TLV. A full face respirator with organic vapor cartridges or SCBA should be available for emergencies.

SECTION 10 SPECIAL REQUIREMENTS

None

Fig. 3.2 MSDS Shown are key parts of the MSDS. *Who is responsible for completing the MSDS for chemicals used in a healthcare facility? Where will you find the safety measures you should use when handling this product?*

The **National Institute for Occupational Safety and Health (NIOSH)** conducts research and makes recommendations for the prevention of work-related disease and injury. The Institute is part of the CDC.

Other health and safety agencies are the health departments of the states, the U.S. Department of Health and Human Services (DHHS), the Food and Drug Administration (FDA), and the Environmental Protection Agency (EPA). State and federal departments of health provide education, immunization, and other health services. The FDA regulates food, drug, cosmetics, and medical devices. The EPA regulates waste disposal, including needles and other instruments. It also regulates cleaning products used in healthcare facilities.

READING CHECK

Recall which government agency is concerned with disease prevention.

Preventing Accidents

What are the three general types of accidents?

Every workplace accident should be documented and reviewed to help prevent future accidents. Poor judgment, physical limitations, and lack of training are just a few of the causes of accidents.

The Physical Environment

Knowing your surroundings will help you prevent emergencies. You should always consider the following guidelines:

- Be familiar with the environment. Locate exits, stairs, fire alarms and extinguishers, as shown in **Figure 3.3**; understand call signals, paging systems, and emergency lights.
- Know the safety policies and procedures of your facility.
- Operate only the equipment you are trained to use. Read the operating instructions carefully. Ask for help when you need it.
- Report accidents, spills, and damaged equipment immediately.
- Do not use frayed or damaged electrical cords. Do not plug in a piece of equipment that does not have a third grounding prong.
- Stay on the right side of a hallway when you accompany or transport clients and equipment. Stop at intersections.
- Allow others to exit stairs, doors, and elevators before you enter.

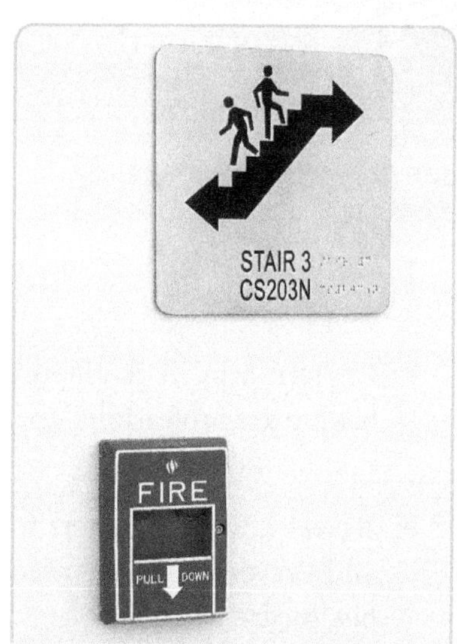

Fig. 3.3 Safety You should know the safety policies and procedures of your environment. *What items should you locate and understand the functions of when starting work at a new facility?*

Photo: PhotoAlto Agency RF Collections/Getty Images

Chemical Safety

Follow the guidelines for handling hazardous or unknown chemicals:

- Never use any product that does not have a readable label.
- Read all labels at least three times before using a product.
- Read the MSDS for any product you use to know potential hazards.
- Wear protective equipment when handling chemicals.

- Never mix solutions or chemicals.
- Know how to report an accident or obtain emergency assistance.

Patient Care

Patient care requires close attention to detail for accident prevention. Follow these guidelines for patient safety:

- Be sure patients know the bathroom location and how to use call signals, emergency call lights, handrails, and safety rails.
- Identify the patient and explain a procedure before you begin.
- Provide privacy. Knock, and ask for permission before opening doors or going behind curtains. Maintain privacy in procedures.
- Perform only procedures you are trained to perform.
- Report safety hazards such as spilled liquids, loose rugs that can cause falls, and extremely hot food or drinks.
- Observe your patient at all times. Report changes, complaints, or problems immediately. Be alert to changes the patient may not report.
- Ensure patient safety and comfort always. For example, if the patient is in bed, the bed should be lowered and the wheels locked. If appropriate, give the patient the call light and raise the side-rails.

READING CHECK

List what you should wear to protect yourself from hazardous or unknown chemicals.

SECTION 3.1 Accidents and Injuries Review

AFTER YOU READ

1. **Define** OSHA. How does it affect the healthcare professional?
2. **Explain** why it is important for you as a healthcare professional to know the information on an MSDS.
3. **Assess** how the Centers for Disease Control and Prevention is involved in the safety of a healthcare worker.
4. **Discuss** three safety practices related to healthcare equipment and the healthcare environment.
5. **Examine** three safety practices related to patient care.

Technology ONLINE EXPLORATIONS

A Cleaning Tool

Download a copy of an MSDS for sodium hypochlorite (bleach) from the Internet. Review the MSDS information and list all the components on a sheet of paper. Explain why sodium hypochlorite is an important cleaning tool in the healthcare field. Using water as a substitute for the bleach, demonstrate how to handle bleach safely.

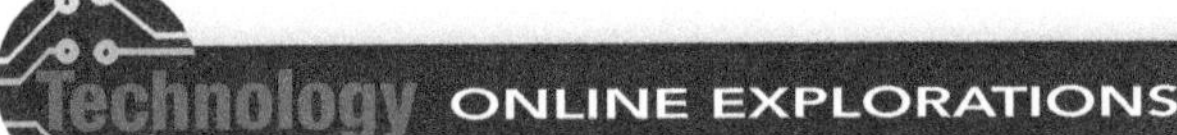

SECTION 3.2 Body Mechanics

Principles of Body Mechanics

What is proper standing posture?

Body mechanics may be defined as positions and movements used to maintain proper posture and avoid muscle and bone injuries. Performing daily activities using correct body mechanics helps prevent physical strains to the human body, especially to the back. Back injury is the number one injury experienced by healthcare professionals.

As a healthcare professional, you will often need to move, lift, and carry objects. You may also lift, transfer, and position patients. Using proper body mechanics is necessary to save energy and to prevent muscle strain and stress to the various parts of your body.

For example, a paramedic who lifts stretchers or equipment bags must practice good body mechanics if he or she plans to continue working in emergency medical services. A nurse who must lift and transfer patients must practice body mechanics to protect his or her back.

Body alignment refers to the correct relationship or position of the head, back, and limbs. If your body is in correct alignment, unnecessary pressure is not placed on the natural curves of your back. Proper body alignment also protects the ligaments and muscles of the back. This is important in preventing muscle strain and spinal disc injury.

Maintain proper standing posture. Place your feet flat on the floor, about 6 to 10 inches apart. This is your **base of support.** Keep your back straight and flex your knees slightly (see **Figure 3.4**).

READING CHECK

Identify which body parts must be correctly aligned.

Body Mechanics Failure

What is elasticity?

All muscles stretch to some extent. Elasticity is a measure of how far a muscle will stretch without injury. When the back muscles are stretched too far, a strain or even disc herniation may occur.

Failure to use proper body mechanics can cause back problems such as acute strains and sprains, disc strain and bulge, disc herniation, and fatigue.

Vocabulary

Content Vocabulary

You will learn these content vocabulary terms in this section.

- **body mechanics**
- **body alignment**
- **base of support**

Academic Vocabulary

You will see this word in your reading and on your tests. Find its meaning in the Glossary in the back of the book.

- **statistics**

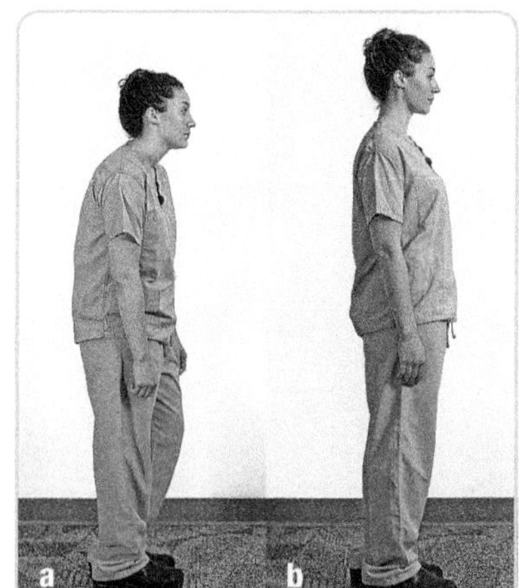

Fig. 3.4 Posture Proper posture is important. *In which photo is this healthcare professional demonstrating proper posture?*

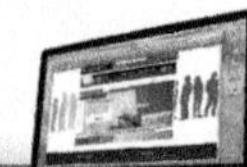

connect

STEM CONNECTION

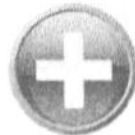

Medical Science

Center of Gravity The earth exerts an attracting force on every object. This is called gravity. The weight of an object is the total amount of this force acting through a single point called the center of gravity. In human beings, the center of gravity is just below the navel or belly button. This center of gravity shifts when a person bends, moves, or carries an object (see **Figure 3.7**).

For an object to be stable, its center of gravity must be directly over its base of support. The base of support for human beings is the feet.

Go to connect to complete the Center of Gravity activity and worksheet.

The best "cure" for back pain is to prevent it. Once you have it, back pain is difficult to treat and recurrence is common. Exercise, proper support for the back, a healthy diet and weight, and good body mechanics are the only ways to avoid back injury. Employees who do daily lifting of patients may be required to wear a specially designed back support. An example of a back support is shown in **Figure 3.5.**

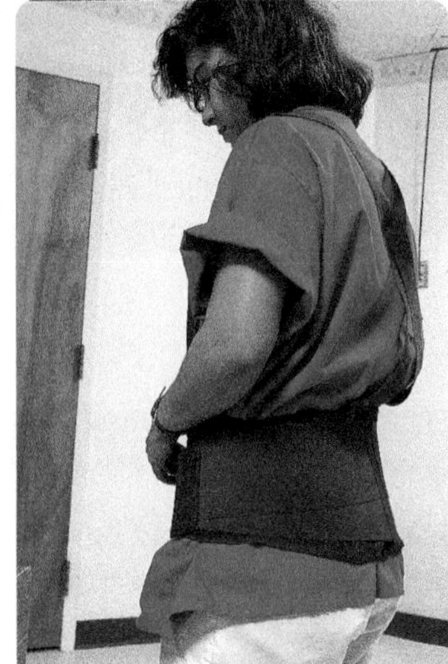

Fig. 3.5 Prevention This is a type of back support *Why should you wear a back support when you lift and move patients?*

READING CHECK

Describe how back pain can be prevented.

Key Components of Body Mechanics

How can posture help protect your back?

Remember these basic guidelines on body mechanics to help maintain the good health of your back and avoid injury:

- Have a good base of support. Keep your feet about shoulder-width apart.
- Always use both hands when moving someone or something.
- Face the way you want to move. Never use a twisting movement.
- Avoid unnecessary reaching.
- Keep your chin up and look straight ahead.
- Keep your shoulders back.
- Bend at the hips and knees (see **Figure 3.6**) instead of bending your back.
- Torque is a force that produces a twisting motion. Since too much torque on the back can result in severe injury, avoid twisting your back.
- Keep the object you are lifting close to your body.
- Exhale when lifting or exerting force.
- Keep your abdominal muscles tight in order to help support your back.
- Lift with your legs, not with your back. Using the stronger leg muscles to lift heavy objects can help you avoid injury to the more delicate back muscles.
- Push, pull, or slide heavy items whenever possible, instead of lifting.

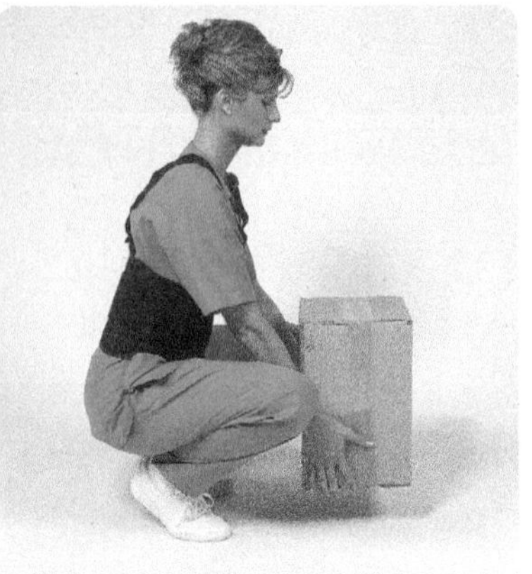

Fig. 3.6 Body Mechanics Always bend from your hips and knees. *Why is it important not to twist your back?*

Photos: (t)Lou Bopp/Lou Bopp Photography, (b)Aaron Haupt Photography

- Pushing is the best technique for moving something large.
- Use the weight of your body to help you push or pull.
- Always ask for help whenever needed.
- When moving or positioning a patient, tell the patient what you are going to do and ask for the patient's help.

Eight of every ten Americans suffer a back injury some time in their lives. Don't become one of those statistics. Plan ahead. A good rule of thumb is to move the object twice: Move it once in your head—the plan. Then actually move it—the action.

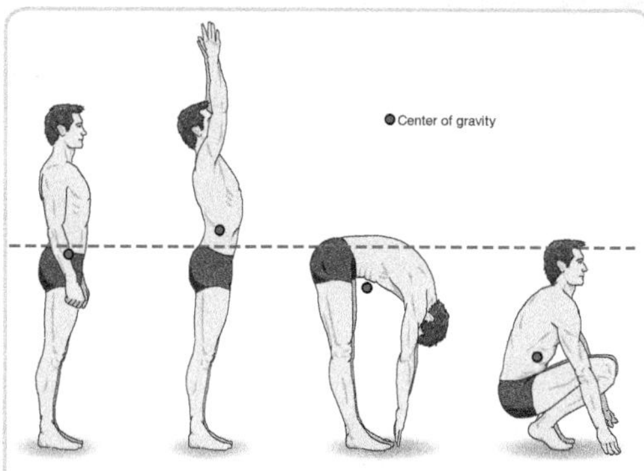

Fig. 3.7 Center of Gravity The center of gravity moves as the body moves. *Why should you keep your center of gravity over the base of support when working?*

READING CHECK

Recall the percentage of Americans that suffers at least one back injury.

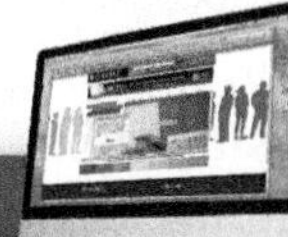

connect ONLINE PROCEDURES

PROCEDURE 3-1

Practicing Proper Body Mechanics

When you practice proper body mechanics, follow the step-by-step guide in the following sections. See the animation in connect that illustrates a worker demonstrating poor body mechanics. After you have viewed the animated procedure and answered the related questions, practice what you have learned with a partner and record the results in your Connect Procedures Recording Log.

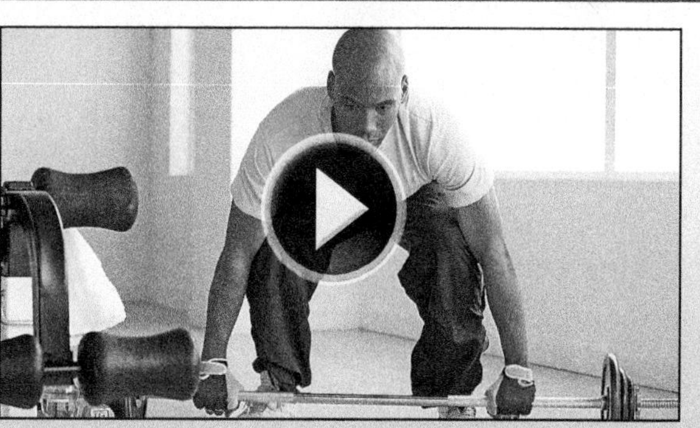

SECTION 3.2 Body Mechanics Review

AFTER YOU READ

1. **Define** the term "body mechanics."
2. **Indicate** at least five guidelines to follow when using good body mechanics.
3. **Explain** three complications resulting from poor body mechanics.
4. **Discuss** some ways to prevent back injury.
5. **Illustrate** how you would place a large suitcase or box into the trunk of your car. Include all the steps of proper body mechanics in your description.

Technology ONLINE EXPLORATIONS

Back Injuries

Research information online about back injuries experienced by healthcare employees. Discuss the severity of the problem and the various ways you can prevent a back injury.

SECTION **3.3** # Basic Microbiology

Vocabulary

Content Vocabulary

You will learn these content vocabulary terms in this section.

- **microbiology**
- **aerobic microbe**
- **anaerobic microbe**
- **antiseptics**
- **disinfection**
- **sterilization**
- **bioterrorism**
- **biological agents**
- **tuberculosis**
- **hepatitis B**

Academic Vocabulary

You will see this word in your reading and on your tests. Find its meaning in the Glossary in the back of the book.

- **environment**

Microorganisms

What are some benefits of microorganisms?

Microbiology is the science that studies living organisms that cannot be seen with the naked eye. A microscope is the only way to view the millions of tiny creatures, known as microorganisms, that live in our environment. Microorganisms are found almost everywhere on this planet. They are on our skin, in the air we breathe, on every surface we touch, and even inside our bodies.

Microorganisms are also referred to as "microbes" or more commonly as "germs," especially by people who do not have a science background. Only a small number of microorganisms, called pathogens, actually cause disease. Most are harmless. In fact, they sometimes benefit humans and the environment. These microbes are referred to as nonpathogens.

However, we usually do not notice or think about microorganisms until they cause some form of physical illness. And we do not often remember that certain microbes play a beneficial role in human health.

The benefits of having these tiny living creatures inhabit our environment are far greater than the problems they may create, as **Table 3.1** demonstrates. As with most organisms, the determining factors for "good" or "bad" effects of microorganisms are based on their individual characteristics and the environment.

Table 3.1 Microorganisms in Our World

PROBLEMS CAUSED BY MICROORGANISMS	BENEFITS OF MICROORGANISMS
• Cause various infections in human beings and animals	• A normal part of our body • Prevent exposure to other harmful microorganisms • Support production of bread, cheese, yogurt, beer, and several other foods and beverages • Contribute to health of soil for farming • Aid in purifying waste water

Some microbes may be pathogenic in certain situations and not in others. One example is the *Escherichia coli (E. coli)* bacterium. Normally it inhabits the intestinal tract. It breaks down waste products and takes part in the synthesis of vitamin K, which helps control bleeding.

However, some varieties of *E. coli* can cause diarrhea. If *E. coli* moves to another part of the body, major problems can result. For example, if *E. coli* traveled to the urinary tract, it would likely cause an infection there.

READING CHECK

Identify how the *E. coli* bacterium can be harmful.

Factors That Influence Microbial Growth

What do microbes need to survive?

Just like human beings, microorganisms need certain conditions to survive and thrive as shown in **Table 3.2.** These conditions include:

- A suitable temperature
- pH, or the values used in chemistry to express the degrees of acidity or alkalinity of a substance
- Food
- Moisture
- Oxygen (but not for all bacteria)

Since these conditions vary all over the human body, certain microorganisms live only in specific areas of the body.

All microbes need food and moisture to survive. Most pathogens prefer a warm, dark environment. Only a few can tolerate an acidic environment (low pH). Some microbes can live only in the presence of oxygen. They are called **aerobic microbes.** Others grow best in the absence of oxygen. They are called **anaerobic microbes.**

Some consume only living matter or tissues. Others prefer dead matter. Removing one or more favorable conditions will decrease or prevent their growth. Altering the preferred living environment of microbes is one way to decrease or eliminate them, but other methods can be used.

READING CHECK

Explain why certain microorganisms are found only on specific body parts.

Table 3.2 Conditions promote the growth of microorganisms.

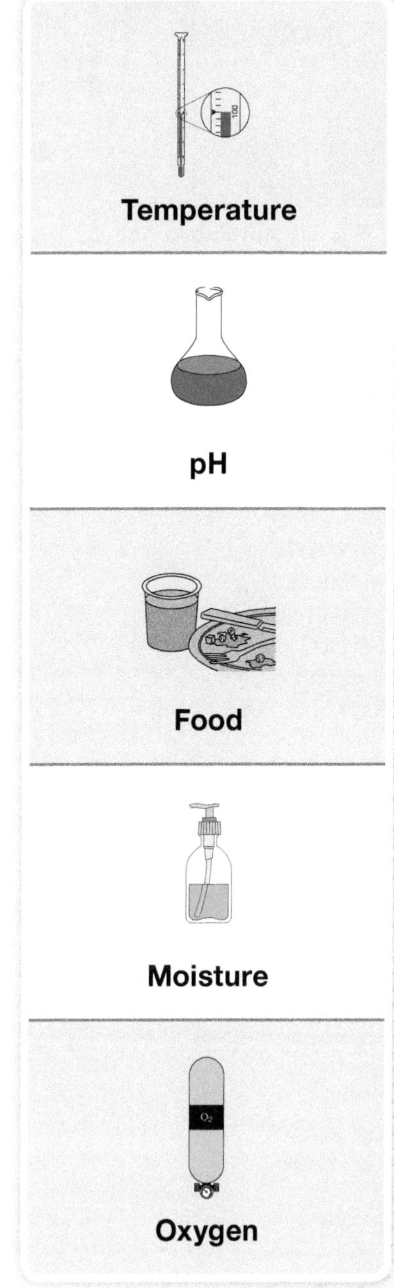

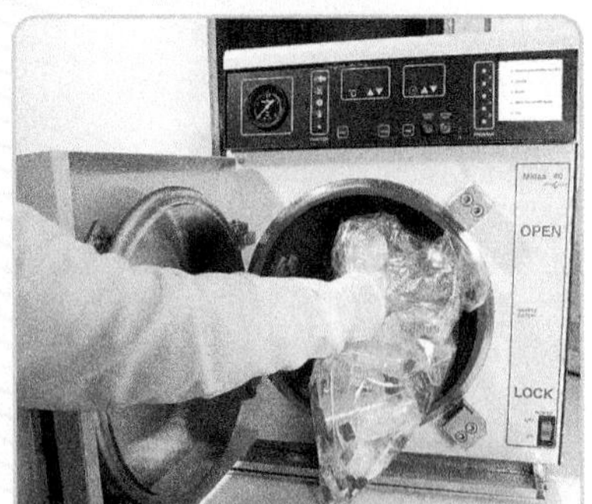

Fig. 3.8 Autoclave The autoclave destroys all microbes and their spores. *How does the autoclave do this?*

Methods That Destroy Microorganisms

How are microorganisms controlled and killed?

Three common practices are used to prevent the growth and spread of microorganisms:

- Antiseptics
- Disinfection
- Sterilization

Antiseptics are solutions that are applied directly to the skin. They prevent or slow the growth of pathogens. Alcohol, betadine, and chlorhexidine gluconate are often used to clean the skin before certain medical procedures. Antiseptics are not useful against all microorganisms.

Disinfection uses strong chemicals such as bleach solution and zephirin to kill many pathogens. These are used mainly on objects and not on the skin because they may cause skin irritation and trauma.

Although many microbes can be eliminated by disinfecting procedures, disinfectants and antiseptics have limited effects against microbe spores. Spores are cells produced by bacteria either to reproduce or to increase their resistance to a harsh environment.

Sterilization is the best way to kill microbes and their spores. For example, an autoclave is used to sterilize medical instruments. It uses steam under pressure. **Figure 3.8** shows an autoclave. Other sterilization methods include the use of chemicals, radiation, and gas.

READING CHECK

Recall which practice kills all microbes and their spores.

Types of Microorganisms

What is the smallest type of microorganism?

Microorganisms are tiny living plants or animals. The five major types are listed below. They are discussed below, and common diseases caused by these organisms are summarized in **Table 3.3:**

- Bacteria
- Fungi
- Protozoa
- Viruses
- Rickettsiae (parasites)

Bacteria

Bacteria are normally found on humans and commonly infect humans. They are one-celled plants classified by their shape and arrangement. Diseases such as strep throat and pneumonia are caused by a form of bacteria. Some are round and are called cocci. Some are rod-shaped and are called bacilli. Others are spiral- or corkscrew-shaped and are called spirochetes or spirilla.

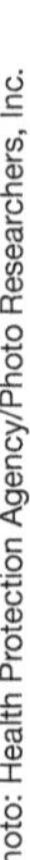

Table 3.3 Disease Causes and Descriptions

DISEASE	MICROBE TYPE	DESCRIPTION
Acquired immune deficiency syndrome (AIDS)	**[VIRUS]**	Syndrome caused by HIV (human immunodeficiency virus), resulting in decreased resistance to infections. Transmitted by blood and body fluids.
Amebic dysentery	**[PROTOZOON]**	Condition characterized by loose stools caused by inflammation of the intestines.
Athlete's foot	**[FUNGUS]**	Known as *Tinea pedis*. This same microorganism can affect the body (*T. corporis*) and the scalp (*T. capitis*).
Boils	**[BACTERIUM]**	Localized skin infection usually caused by the staphylococcus bacterium.
Giardiasis	**[PARASITE]**	Transmitted by the oral-fecal route and through untreated water. Causes diarrhea.
Gonorrhea	**[BACTERIUM]**	Highly contagious condition transmitted by sexual intercourse and caused by gonococcus bacterium.
Hepatitis	**[VIRUS]**	Types A, B, C, D, and E are all caused by a virus. It affects the liver and causes mild symptoms to chronic illness or death. Workers should vaccinated for Hepatitis B.
Lyme Disease	**[BACTERIUM]**	Transmitted by a tick infected with the spirochete Borrelia burgdorferi.
Malaria	**[PROTOZOON]**	Disease transmitted to humans by the bite of infected anopheles mosquitoes. Protozoan parasites invade red blood cells. Symptoms include fever and chills.
Pertussis	**[BACTERIUM]**	Also called whooping cough. Caused by bacillus bacteria.
Pneumonia	**[BACTERIUM, FUNGUS, CHEMICALS]**	Respiratory condition in which lung tissue is inflamed. Can include difficulty breathing and cough.
Rheumatic fever	**[BACTERIUM]**	Febrile (characterized by fever) disease, usually occurring after a streptococcal infection.
Rocky Mountain spotted fever	**[PARASITE]**	Transmitted by a tick infected with Rickettsia. Fever, rash, and headache are common symptoms.
SARS (severe acute respiratory syndrome)	**[VIRUS]**	Highly contagious disease that causes severe flu-like symptoms.
Strep throat	**[BACTERIUM]**	Inflammation and infection of the throat caused by the streptococcus bacterium.
Syphilis	**[BACTERIUM]**	Infectious venereal disease, usually transmitted by sexual contact. Caused by a spirochete bacterium.
Tetanus	**[BACTERIUM]**	Infectious disease produced by the toxins from the tetanus bacillus. The first sign is stiffness of the jaw, hence the common name "lockjaw."
Varicella	**[VIRUS]**	Highly contagious disease caused by the varicella-zoster virus. Also called "chickenpox," or "shingles," it is characterized by the presence of skin lesions.

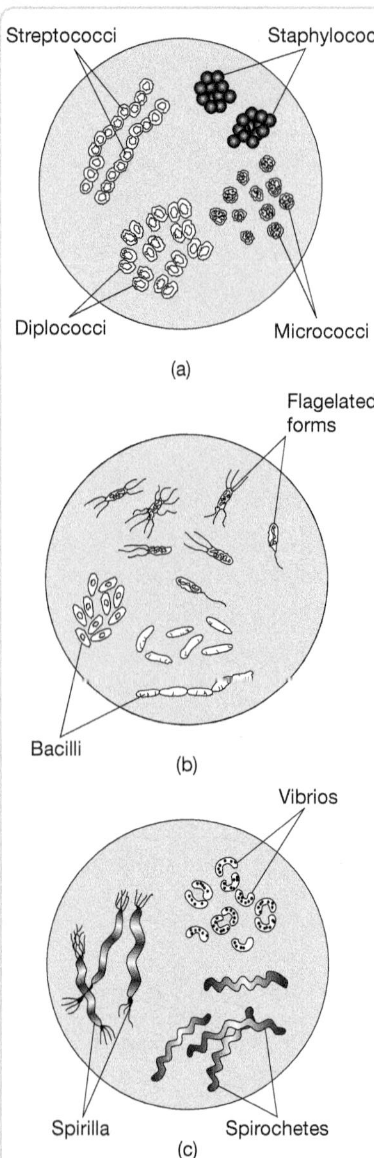

Fig. 3.9 Morphology of Bacteria (a) cocci bacteria, (b) bacilli bacteria, (c) spirilla/ spirochete bacteria. *Why are bacteria arranged in these groups?*

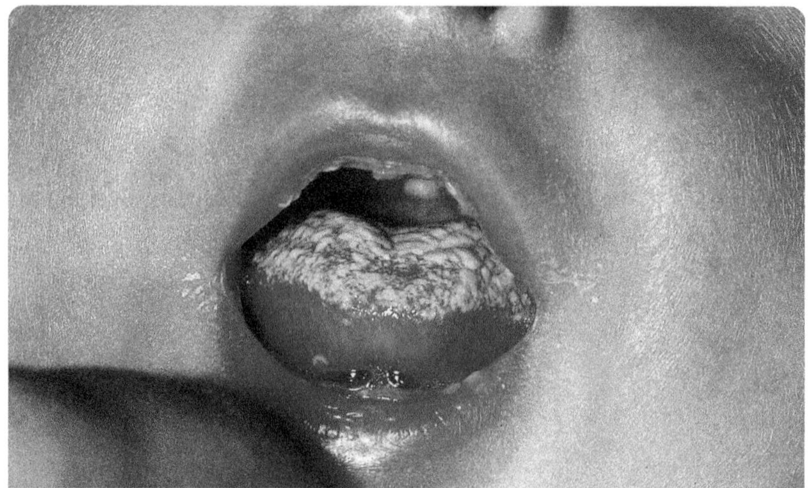

Fig. 3.10 Thrush *(Candida albicans)* This is a yeast infection caused by a fungus, which causes white patches like cheese to appear on the tongue. *Can you name another disease caused by a fungus?*

Bacteria can be categorized according to how they are arranged. The arrangement is a way to identify the exact species. The shape as well as an overview of each type of bacterium and examples of diseases they cause are shown in **Figure 3.9** and **Table 3.4.** Some bacteria are capable of producing spores. Spores are environmentally resistant forms of the bacterium that help it reproduce. The spores go dormant until conditions are again favorable for growth.

Fungi

Fungi also contribute to illness. A fungus is a plantlike organism that lives on dead matter. Fungi are responsible for conditions such as ringworm, athlete's foot, and yeast infections. They also cause thrush, or candida, as shown in **Figure 3.10.**

Table 3.4 Bacteria

TYPE	ARRANGEMENT	COMMON DISEASE CAUSED
Diplococci	• In pairs	• Gonorrhea • Pneumonia
Staphylococci	• In groups or clusters	• Boils • Wound infections
Streptococci	• In chains	• Strep throat • Rheumatic fever
Bacilli	• Rod-shaped in pairs, single, or in chains	• Tuberculosis
Spirilla/ Spirochete	• Corkscrew or spiral	• Tetanus • Syphilis • Bacterial diarrhea

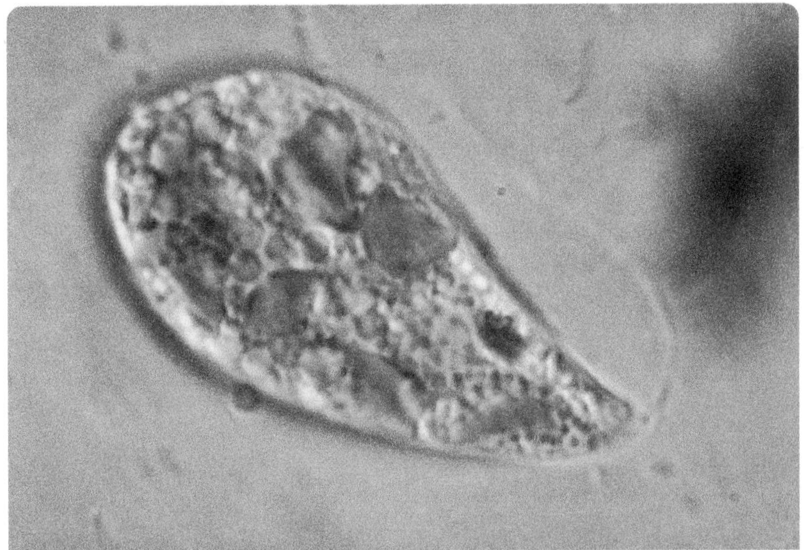

Fig. 3.11 Protozoa Protozoa are found in contaminated water supplies. *What are two diseases caused by protozoa?*

Protozoa/Helminth

Protozoa are tiny animals found in contaminated water supplies, as shown in **Figure 3.11,** and in decayed materials. Helminth are parasites commonly called worms or flukes. Humans can ingest the eggs, larvae, or worms in contaminated food, and some worms can enter the body through the skin. Diseases caused by helminths include pinworms and tapeworms. These microorganisms cause diseases such as malaria, trichomoniasis, and amebic dysentery.

Rickettsiae

Rickettsiae are parasites that must live inside the cells of other living organisms. Diseases caused by these microorganisms are transmitted to human beings by the animal the parasite inhabits, such as mosquitoes, fleas, lice, and ticks. Human beings bitten by an infected tick may contract a disease such as Rocky Mountain spotted fever.

Viruses

The smallest of all the microorganisms is the virus. It can be seen only with the help of a powerful electron microscope. Viruses are difficult to destroy. They can grow and reproduce only inside other living cells. Human beings are infected by viruses from contact with the blood or body fluids of other living beings. Diseases associated with viruses are the common cold, chickenpox, herpes, hepatitis (all types A to E), and acquired immune deficiency syndrome (AIDS), to name a few. Healthcare workers are at great risk of being exposed to the blood and body fluids of patients. Therefore, they must take extra preventive measures.

READING CHECK

Name the type of microorganism that lives on dead matter.

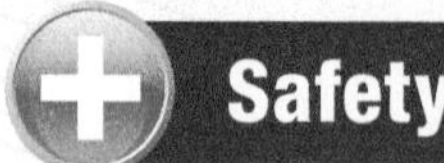

Safety

Immunization and Tests for Healthcare Personnel

For you as a healthcare professional, preventing transmission of disease is crucial. Here are some recommended immunizations and tests for people employed in the healthcare area. These will protect you from disease.

- Tuberculosis (TB) skin test: This is an injection given on the inside of the forearm to test for exposure to tuberculosis. **Tuberculosis** is a highly contagious disease caused by a bacterium. It can be transmitted through the air. A positive test does not mean that you have TB, but it does mean that you have been exposed. If your TB test is positive, you will need to have an X-ray and further evaluation.
- Hepatitis B vaccine: **Hepatitis B** is one of the most serious types of hepatitis and can cause death. The vaccine is given in three injections over a six-month period. It is given to infants as part of their immunization series.
- Influenza vaccine: Influenza ("flu") is easily passed from person to person. The virus is spread by coughing and sneezing or by contact with contaminated skin or other surfaces. The elderly and patients who have chronic medical conditions are at risk for developing severe complications from the flu. Healthcare personnel should get flu shots so that they do not get the flu and pass it on to those at high risk.

Table 3.5 Categories of Biological Agents

CATEGORY	DESCRIPTION	EXAMPLES
A	-highest risk -easily transmitted from person to person -high mortality rates	-Anthrax -Botulism -Smallpox -Tularemia -Viral hemorrhagic fevers
B	-lower risk, because they result in moderate illness and a low death rate -less easily transmitted	-Brucellosis -Salmonella or Escherichia coli in food supplies -Viral encephalitis
C	-emerging pathogens that could be engineered for mass dissemination in the future	-Nipah virus -Hantavirus

Bioterrorism and Biological Agents

Bioterrorism is the use of microorganisms as weapons. A bioterrorism attack is the deliberate release of viruses, bacteria, or other agents to harm others. These **biological agents** cause illness or death in people, animals, or plants. Biological agents can be spread through the air or water, or in food.

Bioterrorism or biological agents can be separated into three categories, depending on how easily they can be spread and the severity of illness or death they cause. **Table 3.5** shows some examples of biological agents. Healthcare professionals should be prepared to respond to a bioterrorism attack. This will be discussed in Chapter 4, Emergency Preparedness.

Microscopes

What are the parts of a microscope?

Body cells and microorganisms are not visible to the naked human eye, but they can be seen with a microscope. Specimens are magnified by a microscope. This enables a skilled person to identify a given microorganism.

A monocular microscope has one eyepiece for viewing. The binocular microscope has two. The triocular microscope has three. The compound Brightfield microscope is often used in laboratories. **Table 3.6** describes some of the more common microscopes.

Table 3.6 Microscopes and Their Characteristics

TYPE	CHARACTERISTICS
Brightfield microscope	• Most commonly used in laboratories • Has visible light source and two lenses • Enables light to pass through the specimen • Used to view microorganism morphology (structure)
Darkfield microscope	• Directs light from the side of the specimen • Causes microorganism to appear very light on a dark background
Fluorescence microscope	• Has an ultraviolet (UV) light source • Used to detect microorganisms in specimens, cells, and tissues
Phase-contrast microscope	• Used for living microorganisms. The specimen does not need to be stained. • Used to identify dense structures in living microorganisms
Electron microscope	• Uses an electron beam instead of light • Uses magnets instead of standard lenses • Has the highest magnification capability • Enables visualization of tiny microorganisms such as viruses

Parts of a Microscope

Figure 3.12 shows the parts of the microscope. Located in the eyepiece, or ocular, the lens magnifies objects. Objectives are on the revolving nosepiece. Each has a different magnifying capability as marked on the objective. Most microscopes have three or four objectives. The objectives are described below:

- The shortest objective is the lowest power of magnification, marked 10 ×.
- The medium-length objective is the high-power magnification, marked 40 ×.
- The longest objective is the oil immersion objective (a layer of oil is located between the specimen and the objective). It provides the greatest power of magnification, marked 100 ×.

The base of the microscope contains the light source and supports the microscope. Specimen slides are held in place by a platform called the stage. Light is controlled by the iris diaphragm, located in the condenser under the stage. Once the slide is in place, use the coarse adjustment knob to bring the specimen into view. Then use the fine adjustment knob to provide a clearer focus of the specimen.

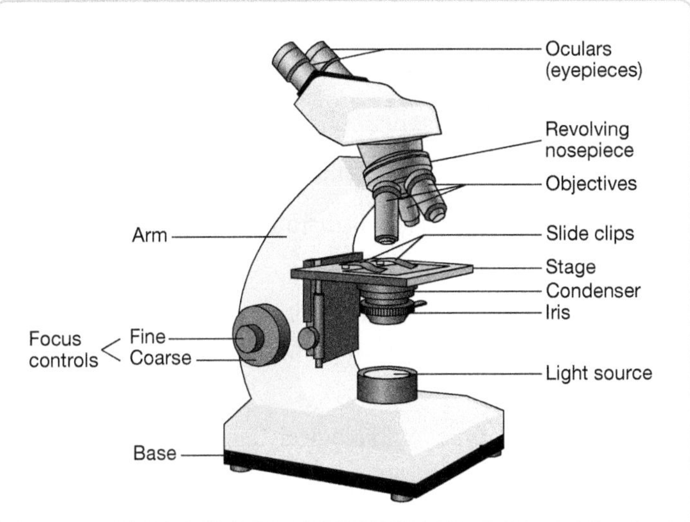

Fig. 3.12 Microscope Labeled are parts of a microscope. *What is the function of this instrument?*

Care of the Microscope

A microscope must be meticulously cared for in order to extend the life of the equipment. Use special lens-cleaning paper to clean the objectives and eyepieces. Clean the oil immersion objective immediately after its use to prevent oil buildup. Then cover the microscope and store it in a safe location with the shortest (low-power) objective in the lowest position. Proper handling, cleaning, and storing will help ensure that this delicate instrument will remain fully functional for many years.

READING CHECK

Name the type of microscope that has the highest magnification capability.

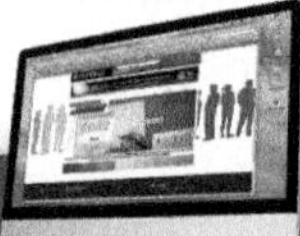

connect ONLINE PROCEDURES

PROCEDURE 3-2

Operating a Microscope

When you practice operating a microscope, follow the step-by-step guide given in this animation. After you have viewed the animated procedure and answered the related questions, practice what you have learned with a partner and record the results in your Connect Procedures Recording Log.

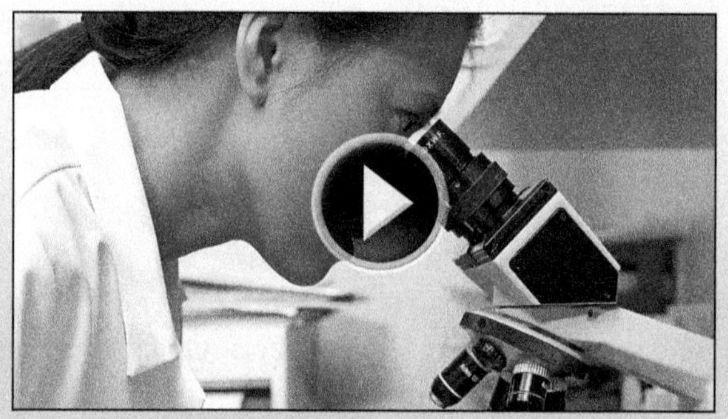

SECTION 3.3 Basic Microbiology Review

AFTER YOU READ

1. **Define** "microorganisms."
2. **Examine** five factors of microbial growth.
3. **Differentiate** between disinfection and sterilization.
4. **Identify** the type of microorganism that can survive only by living on other living creatures.
5. **Assess** the type of biological agent that concerns you the most. Justify your answer.
6. **Indicate** the two main parts of the microscope that must be carefully maintained.

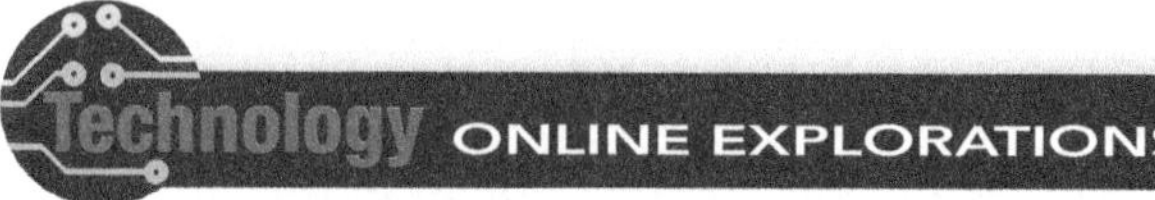

Biological Agents

Research the Internet to learn about biological agents. Select one biological agent that is considered a threat. Write a summary of what you found out about the agent. How would it be used? What problems would occur if the agent is used? What symptoms would it cause? How can the use of this agent be prevented?

Photo: ERproductions Ltd/Blend Images LLC

SECTION

3.4 Principles of Infection

Infection

How is infection transmitted?

The presence of microorganisms does not automatically mean that an infection will result. Infection results only if pathogens increase in number and alter the functioning of normal tissues. Some infections are **contagious,** which means that they can be spread to other people.

The Chain of Infection

Six factors must be present for an infection to result. This is known as the **chain of infection,** which is shown in **Figure 3.13**. If the chain of infection is broken, infection will not occur. The factors are:

- Infectious agent
- Reservoir
- Portal of exit
- Mode of transmission
- Portal of entry
- Susceptible host

Infectious Agent

Many microorganisms cause disease when humans are exposed to them. Others live harmlessly but cause disease if they multiply. These microorganisms are the infectious agent or the first link in the chain.

Reservoir

Humans, insects, food, and water all serve as **reservoirs** for microorganisms, providing food and a place to multiply. Nonliving materials can also house microorganisms. These objects are referred to as **fomites.** Pathogens reside in or on these reservoirs until they can escape.

Portal of Exit

A variety of escape routes, referred to as **portals of exit,** are present in human beings. Common portals of exit are:

- Respiratory tract
- Skin
- Blood or other body fluids
- Food
- Gastrointestinal tract
- Mucous membranes

These sites allow the microorganism to leave the existing reservoir once a mode of transmission becomes available.

Mode of Transmission

The **mode of transmission,** or the way a disease is transmitted, varies. A disease can be spread in many ways. For example, the varicella, or chickenpox, virus is transmitted by contact and airborne droplets.

Vocabulary

Content Vocabulary

You will learn these content vocabulary terms in this section.

- **contagious**
- **chain of infection**
- **reservoirs**
- **fomites**
- **portals of exit**
- **mode of transmission**
- **portal of entry**
- **host**
- **immunity**
- **healthcare-associated infection (HSI)**
- **surgical asepsis**

Academic Vocabulary

You will see this word in your reading and on your tests. Find its meaning in the Glossary in the back of the book.

- **exposed**

The Chain of Infection

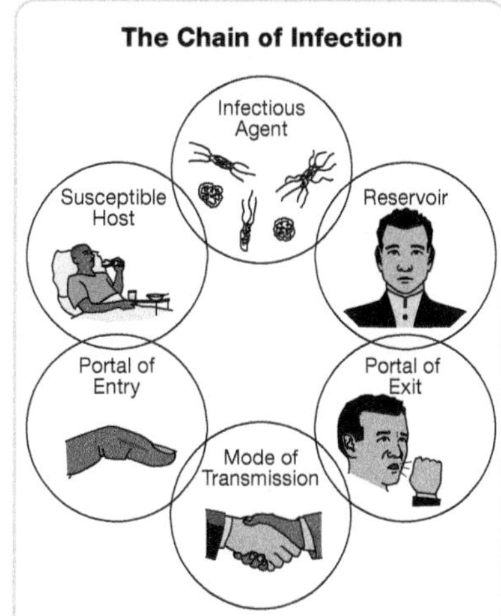

Fig. 3.13 Infection This is the chain of infection. *What happens if one of the links in the chain of infection is broken?*

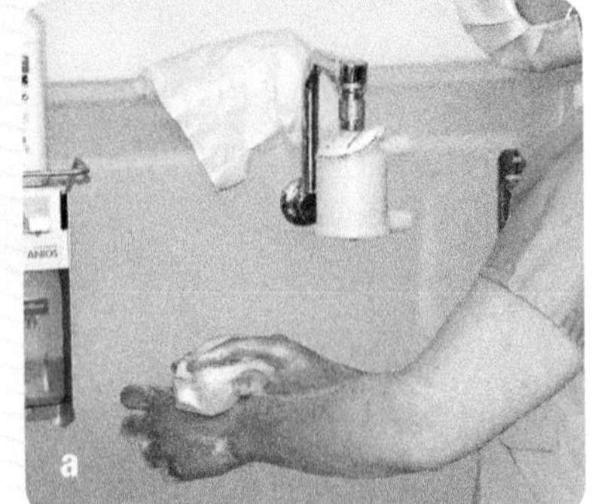

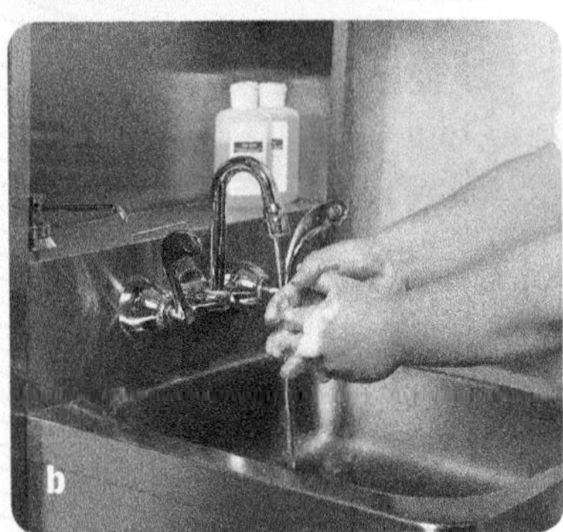

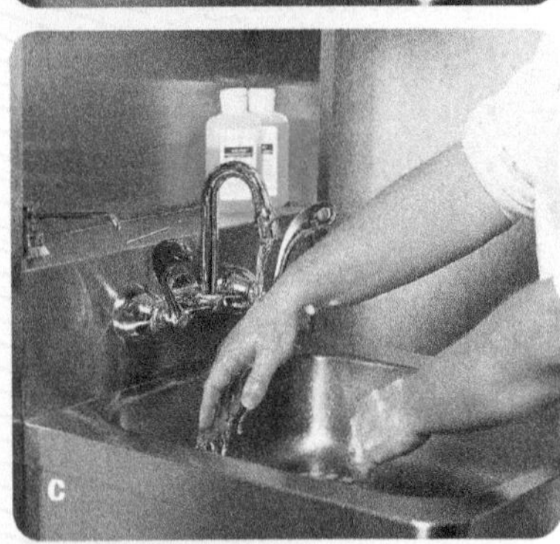

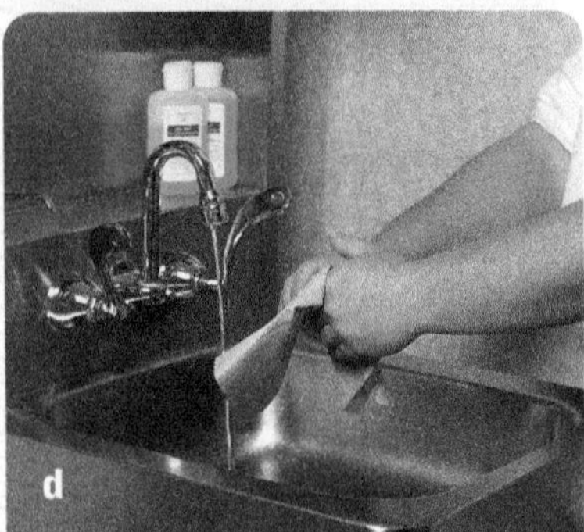

Fig. 3.14 Prevention Steps to follow in hand washing:
(a) Wet hands thoroughly and work up a good lather.
(b) Interlace fingers using friction to cleanse the hands.
(c) Rinse hands thoroughly with fingers pointing downward.
(d) Dry hands completely.

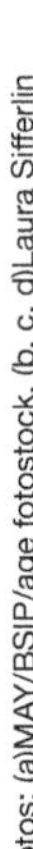

Healthcare professionals can stop the chain of infection by preventing the spread of pathogens. Handwashing, as shown in **Figure 3.14,** is one of the best practices to prevent such transmissions.

Portal of Entry

Transmission of pathogens requires a **portal of entry** into the host or environment. Portals of entry include the respiratory tract, mucous membranes, and the gastrointestinal tract.

Susceptible Host

A susceptible **host** is capable of becoming infected. Individuals develop **immunity** to specific pathogens from natural events, like exposure to the disease or pathogen, or artificial events, like immunization. Having immunity means they are not susceptible to the pathogen.

READING CHECK

Identify the portals of exit for microorganisms that exist in humans.

Signs and Symptoms of Infection

What causes most local infections?

Signs and symptoms of infection can occur when enough pathogens invade a susceptible host. Infection may be present at a site of injury or may be throughout the body. Common signs of local infection include:

- Redness
- Swelling
- Tenderness
- Warmth
- Drainage

Local infections usually result from trauma or injury to the skin. General infections are systemic responses. Treatment for both is aimed at patient comfort and eliminating the cause of the infection.

READING CHECK

List some signs of a local infection.

Asepsis

What is the difference between clean and sterile?

When in a healthcare facility, a patient can get infections unrelated to their illness. These are known as **healthcare-associated infections (HSIs),** or nonsocomial infections. Healthcare professionals care for many patients, so there is risk of transmitting pathogens. Handwashing helps to prevent these infections. Waterless hand cleansers can also be acceptable to prevent HSIs if there is no visible skin contamination.

Aseptic practices can keep an area free of disease-producing microorganisms. Aseptic practices include maintaining cleanliness and preventing or eliminating contamination. Healthcare professionals practice two types of aseptic techniques:

- Medical asepsis
- Surgical asepsis

Medical Asepsis

The purpose of medical asepsis, or "clean technique" is to reduce the number of microorganisms. Medical aseptic practices include hand-washing, using personal protective barriers, and routine cleaning.

Surgical Asepsis

Surgical asepsis is called "sterile technique." For a sterile item to remain sterile, it may only contact sterile items. If a non-sterile object touches a sterile area, the area is contaminated. If in doubt about the sterility of an object or area, consider it contaminated. Sterile technique is covered in Chapter 16, The Clinical Office.

READING CHECK

Recall what type of environment requires a sterile field.

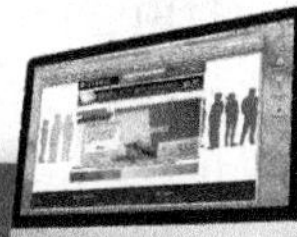

Connect ONLINE PROCEDURES

PROCEDURE 3-3

Hand Hygiene

You should wash your hands for 10 to 15 seconds following patient contact. If your hands are heavily soiled, you should wash them for at least one minute. See the animation that illustrates proper handwashing technique. After you have viewed the animated procedure and answered the related questions, practice what you have learned until you have mastered the skill. Follow your teacher's guidelines for completion of hands-on testing.

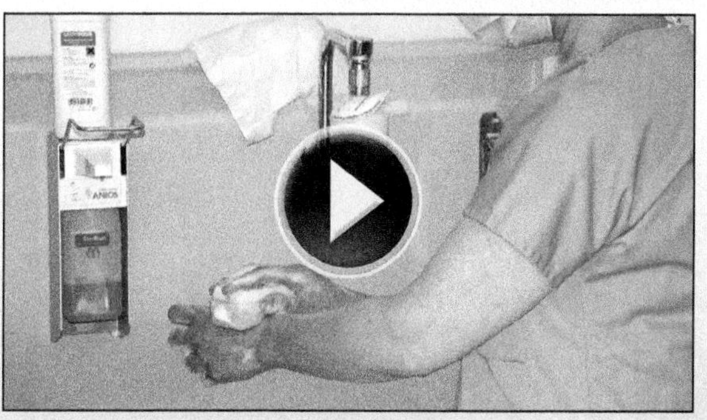

SECTION 3.4 Principles of Infection Review

AFTER YOU READ

1. **Examine** the six links in the chain of infection.
2. **Indicate** two signs of local infection.
3. **Define** nosocomial infection
4. **Compare** the signs of local infection with those of general infection.
5. **Differentiate** between medical and surgical asepsis.

Technology ONLINE EXPLORATIONS

Infection

Using the Internet, go to the Centers for Disease Control and Prevention, or other federal agency site to determine the number of nosocomial infections that occurred last year. Write a brief summary including the number and what types of infections most commonly occur.

SECTION
3.5 Standard and Transmission-Based Precautions

Vocabulary

Content Vocabulary

You will learn these content vocabulary terms in this section.

- **standard precautions**
- **personal protective equipment (PPE)**
- **transmission-based precautions**
- **high-efficiency particulate air (HEPA) filter**

Academic Vocabulary

You will see this word in your reading and on your tests. Find its meaning in the Glossary in the back of the book.

- **minimize**

Standard Precautions

How are infectious diseases spread?

Infectious diseases may be spread by contact with infected blood or body fluids as well as by airborne droplets. Hepatitis B (HBV, inflammation of the liver) and the human immunodeficiency virus (HIV, the virus that causes AIDS) are two blood-borne diseases of great concern. Tuberculosis (TB, caused by a bacterial infection) is an airborne disease that requires meticulous measures to prevent its spread. The Centers for Disease Control and Prevention (CDC) has developed guidelines to minimize the spread of such diseases. These guidelines are called **standard precautions.**

According to standard precautions, all blood and body fluid are considered contaminated. The guidelines for standard precautions are given in **Figure 3.16.** OSHA has established blood-borne pathogen standards that must be followed by all healthcare facilities. Handwashing is vital. Healthcare workers must wear **personal protective equipment (PPE)** when they may be exposed to blood and body fluids. As shown in **Figure 3.15,** gloves, gowns, masks, and face shields are examples of PPE. The equipment used depends on the disease and how it is spread.

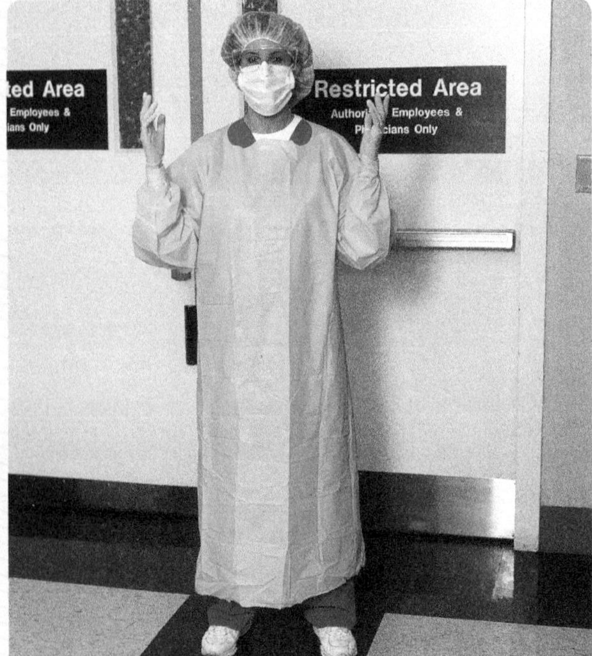

Fig. 3.15 PPE This person is wearing personal protective equipment (PPE). *What PPE is commonly used by healthcare professionals?*

Respiratory Hygiene and Cough Etiquette

Because of the potential for an outbreak of respiratory illness, especially certain types of flu, the CDC has created another set of guidelines for this. The respiratory hygiene/cough etiquette standard applies to everyone and is added to standard precautions for healthcare settings. Individuals should cover their cough or sneeze, use the "flu salute" (coughing or sneezing into the crook of the elbow), and clean their hands frequently. These standards are shown in **Figure 3.17.**

READING CHECK

Describe the precautions that guard against the transmission of respiratory illness.

Photo: Geoff Butler

STANDARD PRECAUTIONS

FOR INFECTION CONTROL

Assume that every person is potentially infected or colonized with an organism that could be transmitted in the healthcare setting.

Hand Hygiene

Avoid unnecessary touching of surfaces in close proximity to the patient.

When hands are visibly dirty, contaminated with proteinaceous material, or visibly soiled with blood or body fluids, wash hands with soap and water.

If hands are not visibly soiled, or after removing visible material with soap and water, decontaminate hands with an alcohol-based hand rub. Alternatively, hands may be washed with an antimicrobial soap and water.

Perform hand hygiene:

Before having direct contact with patients.
After contact with blood, body fluids or excretions, mucous membranes, nonintact skin, or wound dressings.
After contact with a patient's intact skin (e.g., when taking a pulse or blood pressure or lifting a patient).
If hands will be moving from a contaminated body site to a clean body site during patient care.
After contact with inanimate objects (including medical equipment) in the immediate vicinity of the patient.
After removing gloves.

Personal protective equipment (PPE)

Wear PPE when the nature of the anticipated patient interaction indicates that contact with blood or body fluids may occur.

Before leaving the patient's room or cubicle, remove and discard PPE.

Gloves

Wear gloves when contact with blood or other potentially infectious materials, mucous membranes, nonintact skin, or potentially contaminated intact skin (e.g., of a patient incontinent of stool or urine) could occur.

Remove gloves after contact with a patient and/or the surrounding environment using proper technique to prevent hand contamination. Do not wear the same pair of gloves for the care of more than one patient.

Change gloves during patient care if the hands will move from a contaminated body site (e.g., perineal area) to a clean body site (e.g., face).

Gowns

Wear a gown to protect skin and prevent soiling or contamination of clothing during procedures and patient-care activities when contact with blood, body fluids, secretions, or excretions is anticipated.

Wear a gown for direct patient contact if the patient has uncontained secretions or excretions.

Remove gown and perform hand hygiene before leaving patient's environment.

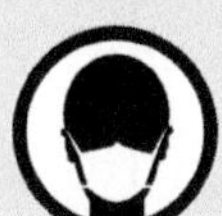

Mouth, nose, eye protection

Use PPE to protect the mucous membranes of the eyes, nose and mouth during procedures and patient-care activities that are likely to generate splashes or sprays of blood, body fluids, secretions and excretions.

During aerosol-generating procedures wear one of the following: a face shield that fully covers the front and sides of the face, a mask with attached shield, or a mask and goggles.

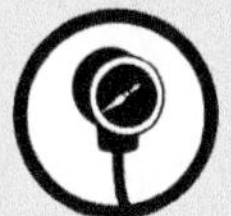

Respiratory Hygiene/Cough Etiquette

Educate healthcare personnel to contain respiratory secretions to prevent droplet and fomite transmission of respiratory pathogens, especially during seasonal outbreaks of viral respiratory tract infections.

Offer masks to coughing patients and other symptomatic persons (e.g., persons who accompany ill patients) upon entry into the facility.

Patient-Care equipment and instruments/devices

Wear PPE (e.g., gloves, gown), according to the level of anticipated contamination, when handling patient-care equipment and instruments/devices that are visibly soiled or may have been in contact with blood or body fluids.

Care of the environment

Include multi-use electronic equipment in policies and procedures for preventing contamination and for cleaning and disinfection, especially those items that are used by patients, those used during delivery of patient care, and mobile devices that are moved in and out of patient rooms frequently (e.g., daily).

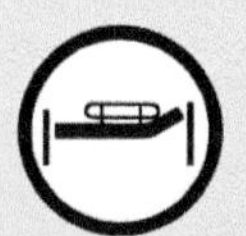

Textiles and laundry

Handle used textiles and fabrics with minimum agitation to avoid contamination of air, surfaces and persons.

Fig. 3.16 Standard Precautions Here are guidelines for standard precautions. *How do standard precautions help break the links in the chain of infection?*

Photo: Brevis Corporation

Stop the spread of germs that make you and others sick!
Cover your Cough

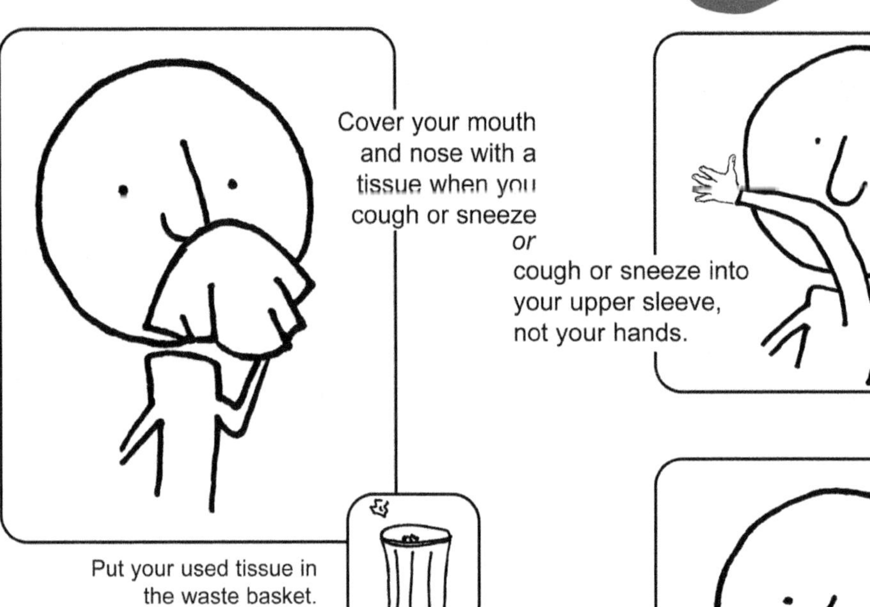
Cover your mouth and nose with a tissue when you cough or sneeze
or
cough or sneeze into your upper sleeve, not your hands.
Put your used tissue in the waste basket.
You may be asked to put on a surgical mask to protect others.

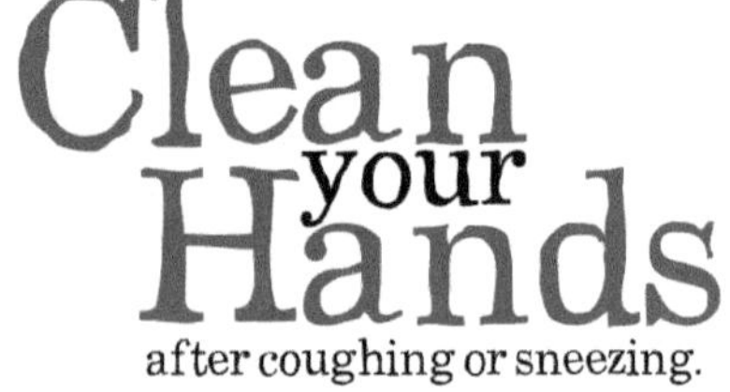
Clean your Hands
after coughing or sneezing.

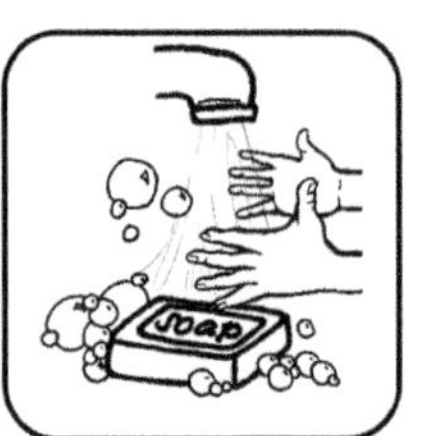
soap

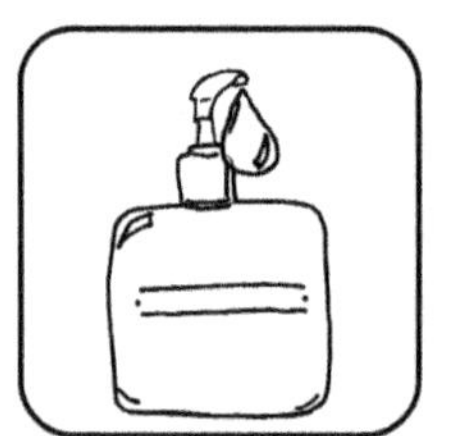

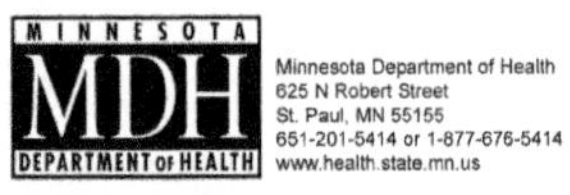
MINNESOTA
MDH
DEPARTMENT OF HEALTH
Minnesota Department of Health
625 N Robert Street
St. Paul, MN 55155
651-201-5414 or 1-877-676-5414
www.health.state.mn.us

Fig. 3.17 Flu Salute This is a Cover Your Cough poster. *Why is it important to sneeze into your sleeve rather than your hands?*

Photo: Courtesy of the Minnesota Department of Health

Transmission-Based Precautions

How is disease spread through the air?

For patients who have highly infectious diseases, other precautions are needed. **Transmission-based precautions** are aimed at preventing the spread of highly infectious agents. The three types of transmission-based precautions are:

- Airborne
- Droplet
- Contact

Airborne Precautions

Diseases such as tuberculosis can be spread by tiny airborne droplets. The droplets can remain suspended in the air for long periods of time because of their small size. Air currents can then transport these infectious agents. Patients who are believed to have tuberculosis require special isolation procedures. Anyone who enters the patient's room must wear a **high-efficiency particulate air (HEPA) filter** or mask. Also, negative pressure must be used to keep the air in the room from being drawn into other areas. The patient's room door must remain closed.

Droplet Precautions

Droplet precautions are required for patients who may have conditions such as pertussis (whooping cough) and other diseases that can be spread when the patient coughs or sneezes. A person who comes in close contact with the patient should wear a mask.

Contact Precautions

Patients who have skin or wound infections that could be transmitted by direct or indirect contact also require special precautions to prevent transmission. With direct contact, this type of infection is transmitted from skin to skin. With indirect contact, the infection can be transmitted from articles of clothing or surfaces in the patient's environment such as linens.

Antibiotic Resistant Bacteria

Antibiotic resistant bacteria cannot be controlled or killed by antibiotics. These include:

- MRSA (methicillin-resistant staphylococcus aureus)
- VRE (vancomycin-resistant enterococcus)
- MDR-TB (multi drug resistant Myobacterium tuberculosis)

These infections are difficult to treat and easy to spread. They are prevented by minimizing the use of antibiotics. To prevent their transmission, good hygiene and standard precautions are used. In a healthcare facility, additional contact precautions must be applied.

Healthcare professionals may need to don a gown and gloves before they enter the room of a patient who may have one of these infections. It is important to perform careful handwashing after removing gloves to prevent the spread of these highly transmissible diseases.

READING CHECK

List precautions that can be taken to reduce the risks posed by antibiotic resistant bacteria.

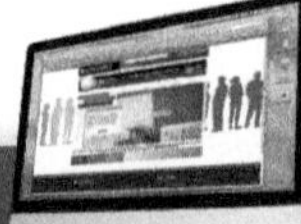

connect ONLINE PROCEDURES

PROCEDURE 3-4

Donning and Removing Personal Protective Equipment

"Donning" personal protective equipment (PPE) simply means to put it on. Personal protective equipment prevents the spread of microorganisms and infection. Different articles are worn depending upon the disease and/or the procedure performed. Refer again to **Figure 3.15** on page 72 for an illustration of personal protective equipment. Removing personal protective equipment must be done carefully, because it is contaminated.

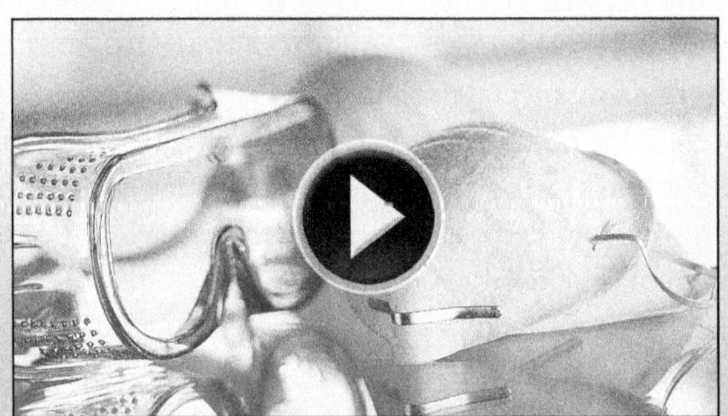

SECTION 3.5 Standard and Transmission-Based Precautions Review

AFTER YOU READ

1. **Discuss** standard precautions.
2. **Choose** two examples of personal protective equipment.
3. **Demonstrate** three parts of the respiratory hygiene/cough etiquette standard.
4. **Differentiate** between droplet precautions and airborne precautions.
5. **Explain** what extra precautions antibiotic-resistant bacteria require.

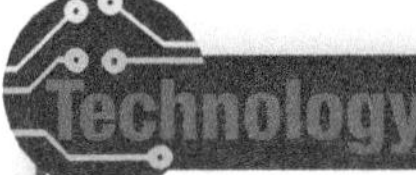

ONLINE EXPLORATIONS

Infection Control

Preventing infection in healthcare as well as the community is essential to wellness. Research the Internet, including OSHA, and review the latest infection control standards. Then create an educational poster, bulletin board, brochure, or presentation.

Photo: Geoff Butler

CHAPTER 3 Review

Chapter Summary

SECTION 3.1

- Education is the way to prevent accidents and injuries in the healthcare setting. **(pg. 53)**
- Governmental agencies such as OSHA, the CDC, and the FDA create rules and regulations to protect healthcare workers from injury and disease. **(pg. 53)**
- Material safety data sheets (MSDS) provide information about chemicals used in healthcare facilities. **(pg. 54)**
- Basic safety guidelines should be followed so that both the environment and equipment are safe for patients and healthcare professionals. **(pg. 55)**

SECTION 3.2

- A healthy diet, good posture, and good body mechanics help prevent back injuries in the healthcare workplace. **(pg. 57)**
- Body mechanics involves lifting, moving, and transferring patients and equipment in a manner that keeps the body in alignment with the center of gravity over the base of support. **(pg. 58)**

SECTION 3.3

- Microorganisms are tiny life forms that can be seen only through the lens of a microscope. Microorganisms may be pathogens or nonpathogens. **(pg. 60)**
- Specific environmental conditions are needed to support the growth and reproduction of microorganisms. The process of sterilization kills all microorganisms and their spores. **(pg. 61)**
- Biological agents are used in bioterrorism, which is the use of microorganisms as weapons. **(pg. 66)**

SECTION 3.4

- The chain of infection is a cyclical pattern describing how infections occur. **(pg. 69)**
- Handwashing is the most important practice in the prevention of the spread of disease. **(pg. 70)**
- The term "medical asepsis" refers to clean technique, and "surgical asepsis" refers to sterile technique. **(pg. 71)**

SECTION 3.5

- According to standard precaution guidelines, all blood and body fluids are considered contaminated. **(pg. 72)**
- Certain microorganisms such as MRSA, VRE, and MDR-TB are resistant to normal antibiotic therapy, so extra precautions must be taken. **(pg. 75)**

CHAPTER 3 Assessment

Critical Thinking/Problem Solving

1. A hospitalized patient has been diagnosed with tuberculosis. According to a physician's order, the patient is to be taken to radiology for a chest X-ray. Your supervisor tells you to take the patient to radiology and to follow all precautions during the transport. How should you do this?

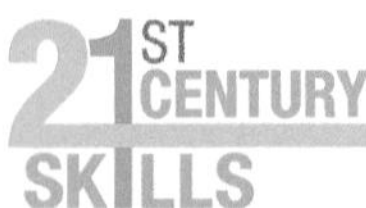

2. **Problem Solving** Obtain a cafeteria tray and a thick textbook. Perform the following procedures and answer the questions:

   a. Stand with your feet apart. Place the book on the tray and hold the tray with both hands at arm's length in front of you. Pull the tray toward you. Stop halfway and note the weight of the tray. Was the tray heavier or lighter at arm's length? Is the tray heavier or lighter halfway toward your body?

   b. Bring the tray close to your body. Is the tray heavier or lighter than it was at arm's length? What is the most comfortable position for holding the tray?

   c. Repeat steps a and b, this time placing your feet together. How does it feel to hold the tray at arm's length with your feet together? Now try with your feet apart again. Record how heavy or light the tray feels away from your body and close to your body.

   d. Place the cafeteria tray with the book on it on the floor. Using correct body mechanics, pick up the tray and book and carry them across the room. Describe exactly how you do this.

3. **Information Literacy** Research drug resistant bacteria on the Internet. The Centers for Disease Control is a good place to start (www.cdc.gov). Create a one- to two-page brochure about how drug resistant bacterial infections can be prevented.

connect ONLINE ACTIVITIES

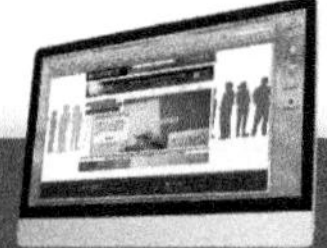

Complete our HST online activities for Chapter 3, which include Concept Check review questions, Reference Flash Cards, and Online Procedures assessment sheets.

- **Concept Check** review questions
- **Reference Flash Cards** medical terminology practice
- **Online Procedures** assessment sheets

CHAPTER 4 Emergency Preparedness

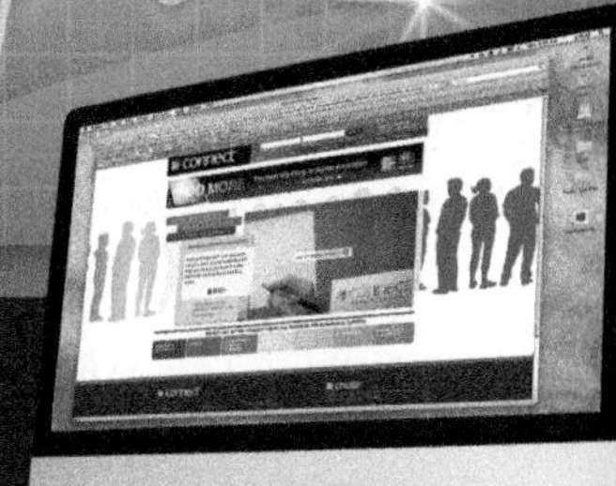

Essential Question:

How do you think you would respond to an emergency in a public place?

Emergencies of all types can occur when you are working in the field of healthcare. No matter where you are, people may have an acute illness or an injury. An appropriate response will be needed, and you may be the one who must respond. You could even experience a disaster—anything from a simple fire to a bomb threat or bioterrorism. As a healthcare professional, you should be prepared to determine the urgency of such a situation and respond properly. No matter what type of emergency occurs, remember to stay calm and think through each situation in order to create the best outcome.

McGraw-Hill connect™

It's Online!

- Online Procedures
- STEM Connection
- Medical Science
- Medical Terms
- Medical Math
- Ethics in Action
- Virtual Lab

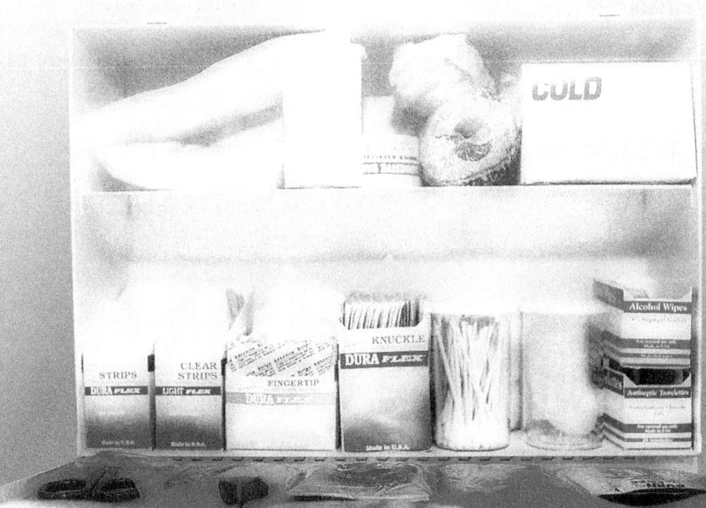

READING GUIDE

OBJECTIVES

After completing this chapter, you will be able to:

- **Identify** causes of emergencies.
- **Distinguish** safety and emergency signs, codes, and symbols.
- **Summarize** how to respond to various disasters.
- **Summarize** fire prevention and fire safety practices.
- **Demonstrate** the appropriate response to an emergency fire situation.
- **Assess** what is wrong with an injured or sick patient.
- **Apply** knowledge to an initial assessment and a focused exam.
- **Demonstrate** cardiopulmonary resuscitation (CPR) for the one-rescuer adult, child, and infant and the two-rescuer adult.
- **Practice** responsive and unresponsive foreign body airway obstruction (FBAO) for adult, child, and infant.
- **Demonstrate** first-aid and CPR procedures.

BEFORE YOU READ

Connect What is the first thing you should do in a medical emergency?

Main Idea

Healthcare professionals must learn how to recognize medical emergencies, analyze them correctly, and act accordingly.

Note-Taking Activity

Draw this table. Write key terms and phrases under **Cues**. Write main ideas under **Note Taking**. Summarize the section under **Summary**.

Cues	Note Taking
o o	o o
Summary	

Graphic Organizer

Before you read the chapter, draw a diagram like the one below. As you read, write the main points covered in the chapter into the diagram.

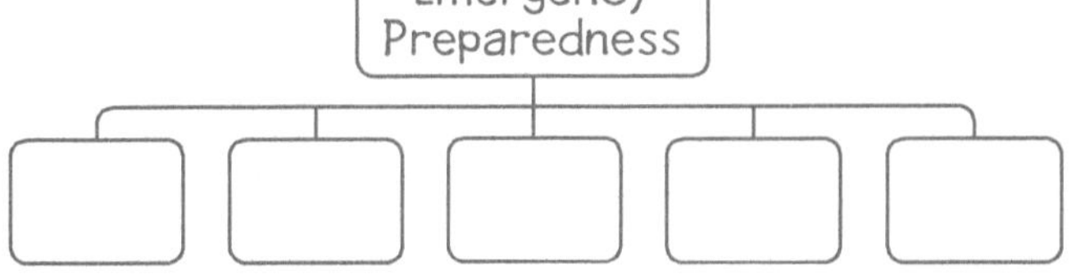

connect
Downloadable graphic organizers can be accessed online.

STANDARDS

HEALTH SCIENCE

NCHSE 1.22 Recognize emerging diseases and disorders.

NCHSE 7.52 Apply principles of basic emergency response in natural disasters and other emergencies.

SCIENCE

NSES A Develop abilities necessary to do scientific inquiry, understandings about scientific inquiry.

NCHSE *National Consortium for Health Science Education*

NSES *National Science Education Standards*

COMMON CORE STATE STANDARDS

MATHEMATICS

Statistics and Probability

Interpreting Categorical and Quantitative Data S-ID Summarize, represent, and interpret data on a single count or measurement variable.

ENGLISH LANGUAGE ARTS

Speaking and Listening

Comprehension and Collaboration SL-2 Integrate multiple sources of information presented in diverse media or formats (e.g., visually, quantitatively, orally) evaluating the credibility and accuracy of each source.

Language

Knowledge of Language L-3 Apply knowledge of language to understand how language functions in different contexts, to make effective choices for meaning or style, and to comprehend more fully when reading or listening.

SECTION

4.1 Emergency Readiness

Medical Emergencies

What are some medical emergencies?

A medical emergency is any situation in which a person suddenly becomes ill or sustains an injury that requires immediate help by a healthcare professional. Some emergencies are not life threatening.

First Aid

Do you know any of the basics of first aid?

First aid is the initial help given to a sick or injured person. It may include dialing 911 for help or providing **cardiopulmonary resuscitation (CPR).** CPR is a series of ventilations (breaths) and chest compressions used on a person who has stopped breathing or whose heart has stopped. First aid provides medical support until expert help arrives.

READING CHECK

Describe the goal of first aid.

Contacting EMS

When should EMS be contacted?

Contacting the Emergency Medical Services (EMS) system is the first step during an emergency. When you call 911, which activates the EMS system for medical assistance and transport, speak clearly and calmly to the dispatcher. Provide all important information, including the location. Do not hang up until the dispatcher gives you permission.

Vocabulary

Content Vocabulary

You will learn these content vocabulary words in this section.

- **first aid**
- **cardiopulmonary resuscitation (CPR)**
- **shelter-in-place**

Academic Vocabulary

You will see this word in your reading and on your tests. Find its meaning in the Glossary in the back of the book.

- **community**

Mc Graw Hill connect™ ONLINE PROCEDURES

PROCEDURE 4-1

Contacting Emergency Medical Services System

Being able to contact emergency medical services quickly and efficiently when an emergency occurs is an essential part of emergency preparedness. Keep emergency numbers posted near your telephone or stored in your cell phone.

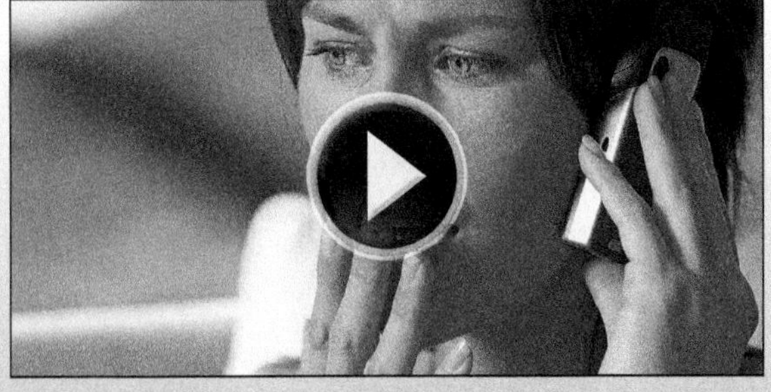

Photo: CORBIS

Safety and Emergency Signs

Which organizations work with safety sign standards?

To maintain safety and be prepared for an emergency, it is essential to recognize safety insignia. These labels, signs, and symbols are required by the Occupational Safety and Health Administration (OSHA). The International Standards Organization (ISO), the National Fire Protection Association (NFPA), and the American National Standards Institute (ANSI) are involved in safety sign standardization and compliance. Common signs and labels are shown in **Table 4.1**. Most healthcare facilities also use emergency codes that are defined by color. **Table 4.2** shows these colors and emergency codes.

READING CHECK

Explain the meaning of "code yellow" in a healthcare facility.

Table 4.1 Safety and Emergency Signs Symbols and Labels

TITLE, SIGN, SYMBOL, OR LABEL	MEANING
Biohazard CAUTION BIOHAZARD SHARPS DISPOSAL ONLY	Indicates the actual or potential presence of a biohazard, including equipment, containers, rooms, and materials that present a risk or potential risk. The biohazard symbol is usually black. The background is typically fluorescent orange, orange-red or other contrasting color.
Fire Safety IN CASE OF FIRE DO NOT USE ELEVATORS USE EXIT STAIRWAYS	A fire extinguisher sign is placed at the location of the extinguisher. An exit sign like this one indicates the appropriate method of exit in case of a fire. Elevators and escalators are not typically in use during an emergency.
First Aid and Automated External Defibrillator (AED) FIRST AID AED	The sign would indicate that a first aid kit and an automated external defibrillator is available for use. These are placed at the location of the equipment.
Wash Your Hands NOTICE STOP WASH YOUR HANDS	Hands should be washed frequently. This is a reminder placed in locations where contamination to hands can occur and available handwashing equipment is nearby.
Handicap	This symbol indicates the route a handicapped person should take. Consider this for patients who are unable to walk or need to avoid steps for any reason.
General Safety Signs EMERGENCY EYE WASH STATION	Provide notices of general practice and rules relating to health, first aid, medical equipment, sanitation, housekeeping, and suggestions relative to general safety measures. For example, an eye wash station is used when chemicals, blood, or other foreign items get in the eye.

Table 4.2 Emergency Codes

CODES	EMERGENCY CODE DEFINITIONS
FIRE	RED—Follow procedures to protect patients, staff, visitors, self, and property from a confirmed or suspected fire.
MEDICAL EMERGENCY	BLUE—Facilitate the arrival of equipment and specialized personnel to the location of an adult medical emergency. Provide life support and emergency care.
INFANT/CHILD ABDUCTION	PINK—Activate response to protect infants and children from removal by unauthorized persons, and descrbe someone attempting to take an infant from the facility.
COMBATIVE ASSAULT PERSON	GRAY—Activate response when staff members are confronted by an assaultive person.
BOMB THREAT	GREEN—Activate response to a bomb threat or discovery of a suspicious package.
PERSON WITH WEAPONS OR HOSTAGE	SILVER—Activate facility and staff response to event in which staff members are confronted by persons with weapons or who have taken hostages in the facility.
HAZARDOUS MATERIAL SPILL	YELLOW—Identify conditions, evacuate an area, and protect others from exposure due to a hazardous materials spill. Perform procedures for a minor or major spill.
INTERNAL DISASTER	TRIAGE INTERNAL—Activate response to incidents that require or may require significant support from several departments in order to continue patient care.
EXTERNAL DISASTER	TRIAGE EXTERNAL—Activate response to external emergencies that may require significant support from several departments in order to continue patient care.
POWER BLACK OUT	CODE EDISON—Activate response to a rolling power failure.

Bioterrorism and Disasters

Have you participated in any community disaster drills?

Bioterrorism is the intentional release of a biologic agent with the intent to cause harm. Bioterrorism requires public health readiness.

A healthcare professional's skills are of great value to the community. You must also be familiar with the steps for responding to disasters, as shown in **Table 4.3** on page 84. Participating in community fire drills or other disaster drills is an excellent way to be prepared.

Evacuation and Shelter-in-Place Plans

A healthcare facility should have evacuation and shelter-in-place plans. **Shelter-in-place** refers to a room in the facility with few or no windows, in which to take refuge when evacuation is too dangerous.

Evacuation plans should include means of communication to employees during and after the emergency. Maps of the facility with escape routes clearly marked should be posted.

READING CHECK

Describe shelter-in-place and its purpose in a healthcare facility.

Table 4.3 Assisting in Disasters

TYPE OF DISASTER	ACTION TO TAKE
Weather disaster, such as a flood or hurricane	• Report to the community command post; have your credentials with you. • Receive an identifying tag or vest; accept only an appropriate assignment. • Document what medical care each victim receives on each person's disaster tag.
Indoor fire	• Activate the alarm system. • Use a fire extinguisher if the fire is confined to a small container. • Turn off oxygen and shut windows and doors; seal doors with wet cloths. • If evacuation is necessary, proceed quietly and calmly. Direct ambulatory patients and family members to the exit. Assist patients who need help leaving.
Bioterrorist attack	• Be alert for a rapidly increasing incidence of disease in a healthy population. • Take appropriate isolation precautions. • Use standard precautions when decontaminating rooms and equipment. • Inform local health departments of suspected bioterrorism agent.
Chemical emergency	• Don appropriate personal protective equipment to avoid secondary contamination. • Identify the chemical and report to the local authorities. • Assist with patient decontamination. • Monitor patient's CABs of CPR and vital signs if indicated. (See section 4.4.) • Document what medical care each victim receives. • Arrange for patient transport if possible.
Mass casualities	• Assess the situation for safety. • If there is an explosion, do not move toward the explosion. • Report to the community command post. • Triage victims as necessary and render first aid as required. • Document what medical care each victim receives.

SECTION 4.1 Emergency Readiness Review

AFTER YOU READ

1. **Indicate** at least five types of emergencies.
2. **Differentiate** between first aid and CPR.
3. **Describe** a shelter-in-place.
4. **Create** a bulletin board, collage, or poster of emergency signs, labels, symbols and codes and their meanings.

Technology ONLINE EXPLORATIONS

The CDC and Bioterrorism

The CDC maintains an Internet site with information about identified biological agents at www.bt.cdc.gov. Create a list of the newest biological agent and five other biological agents used for bioterrorism.

SECTION

4.2 Fire Safety

The Fire Triangle

Can you recognize situations that present a fire risk?

Fire is one of the dangers faced by healthcare providers. Healthcare professionals must recognize and respond to fire risk situations. Caution and a clear head are needed to protect the patient, healthcare professionals, and yourself. If healthcare professionals do not know the steps to take for safety during a fire risk situation, the loss of life in a large healthcare facility could be great. All healthcare professionals should be trained in fire prevention and first response to a fire hazard.

Fire can occur in any setting when three elements are present. The elements necessary for a fire risk to occur are fuel (something that will burn), heat (a temperature high enough to allow the fuel to burn), and oxygen (to feed the fire).

These three elements create the **fire triangle** (see **Figure 4.1**). If one element is missing from the triangle, a fire will not occur. Successful removal of one or more elements will stop a fire that has begun. Fire extinguishers are key to breaking the fire triangle.

READING CHECK

Identify the three elements that are needed for a fire to occur.

Vocabulary

Content Vocabulary

You will learn this content vocabulary word in this section.

- **fire triangle**

Academic Vocabulary

You will see this word in your reading and on your tests. Find its meaning in the Glossary in the back of the book.

- **appropriate**

Types of Extinguishers

Have you ever used a fire extinguisher?

Fire extinguishers are divided into five categories based on different types of fires (see **Table 4.4** on page 86). The most common type is the ABC fire extinguisher. This type is capable of putting out all types of fires except combustible metal fires and cooking-oil fires.

When a Fire Emergency Occurs

What would you do in a fire emergency?

If a fire occurs, you should use the acronym RACE to help keep patients and coworkers safe and to stop the fire from spreading. (An acronym is an abbreviation formed from the first letter of each word in a term or phrase.) The acronym RACE stands for

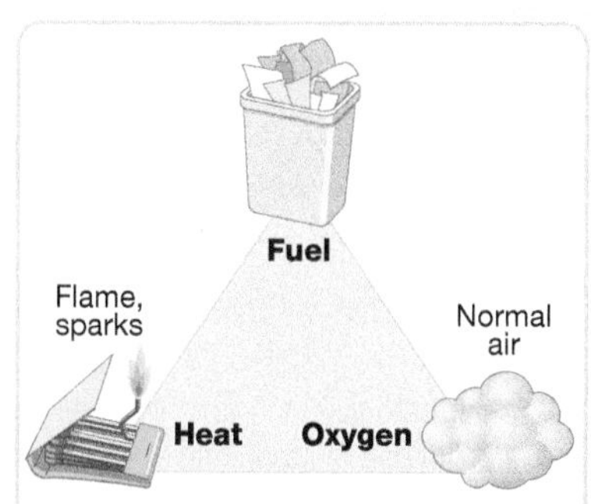

Fig. 4.1 Fire Triangle Shown are the factors needed for fire. *How can you stop a fire once it has started?*

Table 4.4 Fire Types

CLASSES, TYPES OF FIRES	PICTURE SYMBOL
A Wood, paper, cloth, trash, and other ordinary materials	
B Gasoline, oil, paint, and other flammable liquids	
C May be used on fires involving live electrical equipment without danger to the operator	
D Combustible metals and combustible metal alloys	D
K Cooking media (vegetable or animal oils and fats)	

R = Rescue. Once a fire is seen everyone not involved in the fire extinguishing process must leave the scene.

A = Alarm. Assign someone to pull an alarm or pull the alarm yourself. If an alarm is not close by, call a facility phone operator or 911.

C = Contain. Close windows and doors. You can also contain a fire with blankets, pillows, or other things that will help smother it.

E = Evacuate. When fire and smoke are a threat, move everyone, including yourself, out of immediate danger. Smoke and heat can cause great damage to the mucous membranes of the respiratory system. Once damaged, the membranes swell and close off the airway passages. This can be fatal!

You can also think of the E in RACE as standing for "Extinguish." You should only attempt to extinguish a fire that is small and confined. In this case, you may be able to put the fire out with a nearby fire extinguisher. Determine the cause of the fire and check your extinguisher to be sure that it can handle the fire type. Follow the PASS procedure discussed in Procedure 4-2 to extinguish the fire.

READING CHECK

Identify the meaning of the letters in the acronym RACE.

Emergency Fire Rules

Do you know what you would do if there were a fire at your workplace?

Knowing what to do will help you assist patients and yourself. You should also follow these rules. When you do, lives will be saved!

- Be prepared. Know your responsibilities in a fire situation.
- Know when and how to evacuate your location. (**Figure 4.2** shows an evacuation route.)
- Know where fire alarms are located and how to activate them.

Mc Graw Hill connect™ ONLINE PROCEDURES

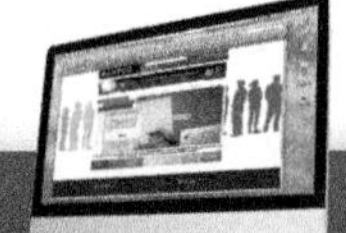

PROCEDURE 4-2

How to Use a Fire Extinguisher

The best way to fight a fire is to practice the strategies required to eliminate the fire emergency. The PASS practice, explained in this procedure, will prepare you to extinguish a small fire and prevent a tragedy in the workplace.

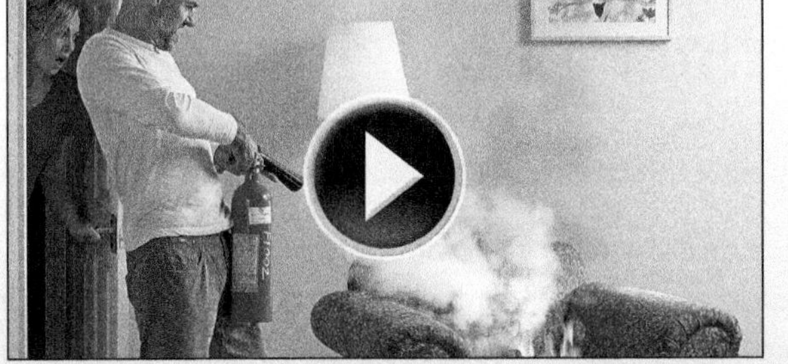

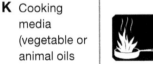

Photo: Michael Blann/Digital Vision/Getty Images

- Keep fire extinguishers in plain view. Make sure there are no obstructions that block access to fire extinguishers.
- Keep areas uncluttered and free of debris.
- Evacuate ambulatory clients first, then the wheelchair-bound, and finally the bed-bound.
- If possible, never leave a client alone during a fire emergency.
- Never use an elevator in a fire situation.
- Never open windows. Open windows allow oxygen to feed the fire.
- Always feel a door if you think fire is in the area behind the door. If the door is hot, never open the door!

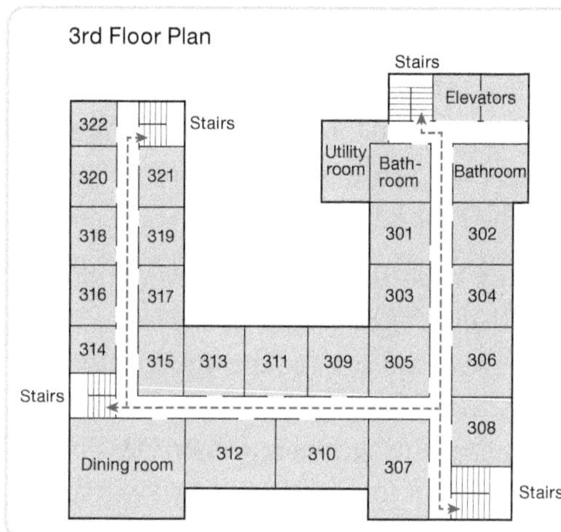

Fig. 4.2 Evacuation Route Diagram Know the evacuation route at the facility where you are employed. *In what order should clients be evacuated?*

READING CHECK

Explain what you would do if you came to a closed door as you were escaping a workplace fire.

21ST CENTURY SKILLS

Problem Solving

No matter the emergency, you must be able to respond calmly. Knowing your responsibilities and emergency procedures will help you be prepared. Act quickly and efficiently. When giving directions, use short sentences. Pay attention to details. Be prepared to do whatever is **appropriate.**

In addition to smoke, panic kills more people than fire itself. Healthcare facilities have a plan in place for fire emergencies. Yearly training and review are provided to employees to remind them of fire and other emergency procedures. Some facilities conduct periodic fire drills for all shifts and in all areas. Everyone must know how to respond to a fire. The safety committee reviews employees' response to the fire drill. The safety committee also makes recommendations. Practice will prevent deaths if a fire occurs.

SECTION 4.2 Fire Safety Review

AFTER YOU READ

1. **Assess** how, in a fire emergency, you would decide whether you should enter a room. For example, if a door were hot, would you enter?
2. **Choose** the order in which you would evacuate the following:
   - **a.** Patient A, who uses a walker.
   - **b.** Patient B, who is in a wheelchair.
   - **c.** A visitor of patient A, who is ambulatory.
   - **d.** Patient C, who is in a coma.
3. **Indicate** the three elements of the fire triangle.
4. **Explain** why each element of the fire triangle is necessary to produce a fire.
5. **Define** the acronyms PASS and RACE.

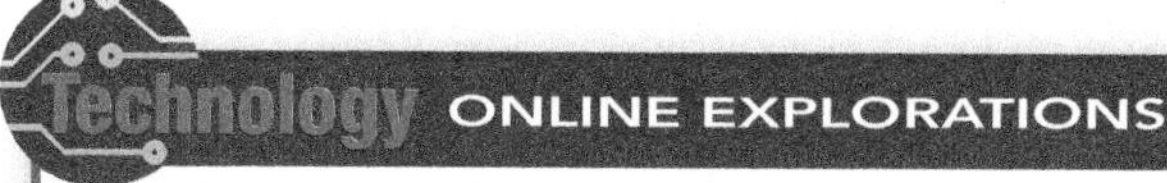

Fire Prevention

Research online to determine the most common cause of fires as well as ways to prevent fires. Create a list of the causes and a set of rules to prevent fires.

SECTION
4.3 Basics of First Aid

Vocabulary

Content Vocabulary

You will learn these content vocabulary words in this section.

- **conscious**
- **unconscious**
- **primary assessment**
- **abdominal thrusts**
- **secondary assessment**

Academic Vocabulary

You will see this word in your reading and on your tests. Find its meaning in the Glossary in the back of the book.

- **aware**

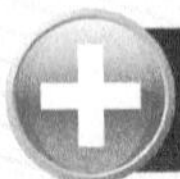

Safety

Protection from Blood-Borne Pathogens

While providing first aid, you may encounter blood and other body fluids. These are potential hazards to your health. Take precautions to avoid direct contact with such fluids. Ideally, you should wear vinyl gloves and follow standard precautions. If gloves are unavailable, improvise by using plastic wrap, plastic grocery bags, shopping bags, thick towels, or any other material as a protective barrier between you and the blood or body fluid. Be careful especially to protect your eyes, mouth, and nose from coughed or sneezed blood or other body fluids.

Consent

What must you do before administering first aid?

Providers of first aid must be able to recognize medical emergencies. They must then seek professional medical help and offer basic emergency care. When properly given, first aid can be the difference between temporary and permanent disability. It can even mean the difference between life and death.

Before giving first aid, you must have the patient's permission, or consent. Obtain verbal consent from all **conscious** adults of legal age capable of making a sound decision. Consent for the **unconscious** or unresponsive patient is implied. This means that it is assumed that consent to emergency assistance would be given. When possible, a child's parent or guardian gives consent for a child to receive first aid. Never withhold first aid from a child by spending unnecessary time obtaining parental or guardian permission. Keep in mind that a conscious, competent adult patient has the right to refuse your help. However, if, in your opinion, a patient really needs help, call 911 regardless of what the patient says.

READING CHECK

Describe the concept of implied consent.

Responsibilities of First-Aid Providers

Have you ever needed to provide first aid to a stranger?

First-aid providers are a vital link between an injured or sick patient and the activation of Emergency Medical Services (EMS). It is essential for the person providing first aid to do the following:

- Recognize that an emergency exists based upon the patient's appearance, behavior, or surroundings.
- Make a decision to help. The decision to help someone is important. This decision must take into account your own personal safety if you provide first aid.
- Call EMS if the situation requires you to do so. See **Procedure 4-1.**

- Safely gain access to the patient and determine what is wrong.
- Provide first aid.
- Stay with the patient until EMS arrives.

Evaluating the Scene

Before offering help, it is important to survey the scene of the incident:

- Determine whether there are threats to your own safety or to the safety of the patient or bystanders. At the scene of an automobile accident, hazards may include downed power lines, spilled gasoline or other fluids, broken glass, metal, fire, blood, or a vehicle running in gear.
- At the scene of a home incident, hazards may include angry or violent family members, hazardous household chemicals, blood or other body fluids. If you believe that the scene is too dangerous, do not offer assistance. Call 911 and wait in a safe place until help arrives.
- Determine the nature or cause of the illness or injury. Determine the basis of the patient's medical complaint or the cause of the accident.
- Determine the number of sick or injured patients involved. Call EMS, if necessary, and report your findings.

The Primary Assessment

If the patient is responsive, introduce yourself and state that you know first aid. (See **Figure 4.3.**) Ask the patient if you can help. How the patient responds to your questions will provide essential information regarding the status of his or her airway, ability to breathe, and circulatory status. It will also tell you whether the patient wants your help. The first part of the **primary assessment** consists of evaluating the patient's responsiveness through his or her answers to your questions. If the client can talk, you can assume that the patient's airway is open.

Ask the patient to tell you his or her name, explain what has happened, and tell you how you can help. If the patient knows his or her name and what has happened, you can assume that he or she is alert and aware of the surroundings. Pay close attention to how the patient speaks. If the patient speaks in short, choppy phrases or cannot speak or cough, he or she might be having breathing problems. Ask yourself:

- How does the patient look?
- How is the patient behaving?
- Does the patient appear to be in distress or pain?
- Is the patient bleeding?
- What color is the patient? Pale, blue-gray, or grayish skin tones can indicate serious problems with breathing or circulation.

If you detect conditions that compromise the patient's breathing and circulation, correct them immediately. For example, if a foreign body is obstructing an adult patient's airway, perform **abdominal thrusts.** If the patient cannot breathe, perform rescue breathing. If he or she has severe bleeding, control the bleeding using direct pressure to the site. First aid for foreign body airway obstruction and bleeding, rescue breathing, and other skills are discussed later in this chapter.

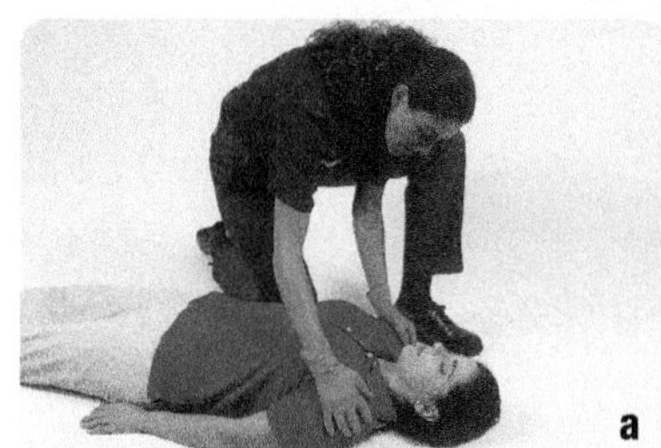
a

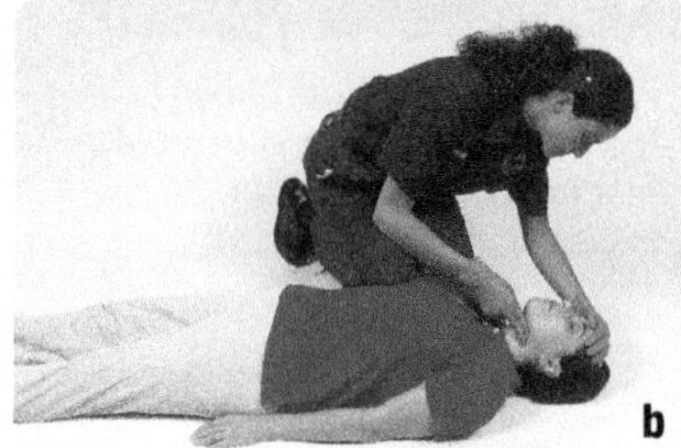
b

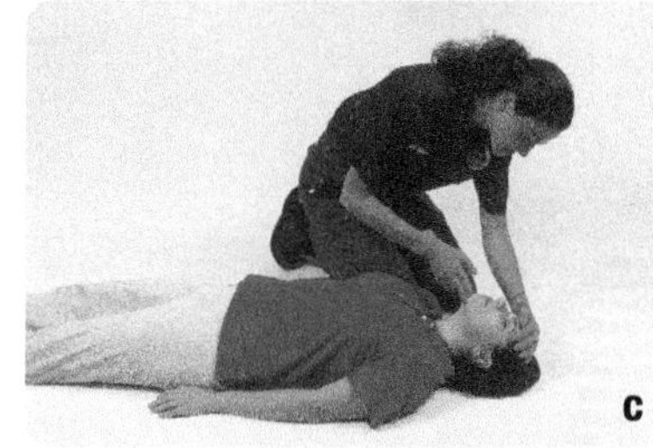
c

Fig 4.3 First Aid (a) Primary assessment: Unresponsive patient: check for hazards. If the scene is not safe, leave immediately. If it is safe, check the patient for responsiveness. If responsive say "My name is ___________, and I know first aid. May I help you?" If you get no response, assume the patient is unresponsive. If there is no possibility of injury to the head, neck or back, position the patient on his or her back, then use the CABs. **(b) Compressions:** Check for breathing. If the patient is not breathing or breathing is not normal (i.e. gasping), quickly check the carotid pulse in the neck for no longer than 10 seconds. If the pulse is absent or you are not sure, perform 30 chest compressions. If breathing is normal, open the airway and continue with the assessment. **(c) Airway:** Open and check airway using the head tilt-chin lift method or the jaw thrust maneuver. **Breathing:** Give 2 rescue breaths that make the chest rise. Return to chest and perform continuous cycles of 30 compressions to 2 breaths. Stop about every 2 minutes, for no longer than 10 seconds, to check for a pulse and breathing.

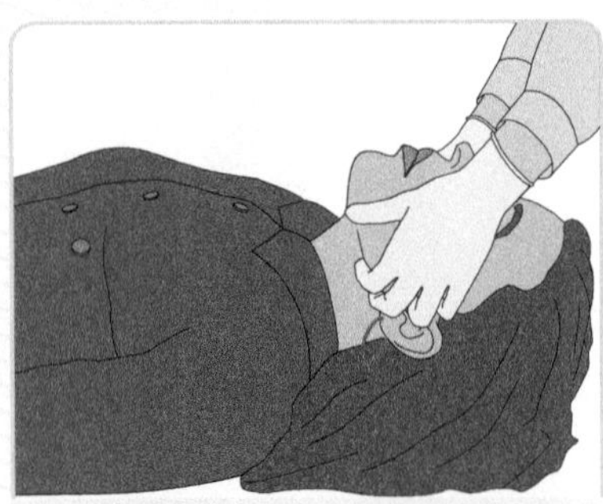

Fig. 4.4 Jaw Thrust Open the airway using the jaw thrust maneuver. *When should the jaw thrust maneuver be used?*

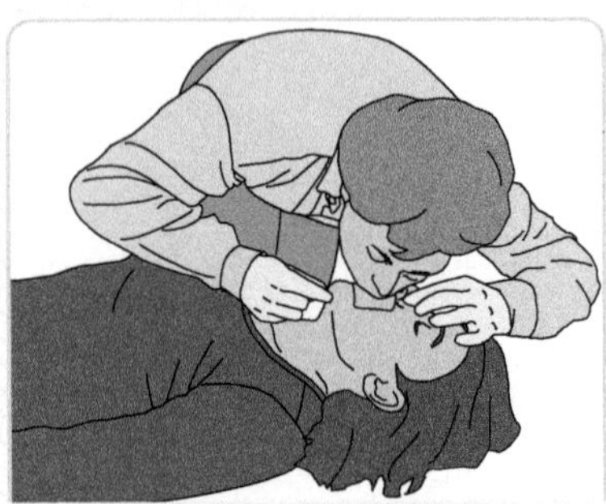

Fig. 4.5 Open the Airway Use the head tilt-chin lift method to open the airway. *What should you do after opening the airway?*

Unresponsive Patient

For a patient who is not breathing or is gasping for breath, you will begin CABs. C = check circulation, A = Airway, B = Breathing. Follow these steps as illustrated in **Figure 4.3** on page 89.

1. If there is no possibility of injury to the neck or back, position the patient on his or her back.
2. Check for responsiveness by tapping the patient on the shoulder and saying "Are you okay? Can you hear me? My name is ____, and I know first aid." If the patient is unresponsive follow the CABs as shown in steps 3, 4, and 5.
3. **C (circulation):** Check for signs of circulation. This includes feeling for a pulse, observing breathing, coughing, and movement, noting skin color and temperature, and looking for major bleeding. Feel for a pulse at the carotid artery on an unresponsive patient or the radial pulse on a responsive patient. Signs of normal circulation are natural skin color and temperature, and spontaneous movement, coughing, and breathing. Check for major bleeding by scanning the body from head to toe. Control any significant bleeding with direct pressure while avoiding direct contact with the patient's blood. Check for signs of shock, which will be discussed later. If there are no signs of shock, begin cardiopulmonary resuscitation (CPR), discussed in Section 4.4 of this chapter.
4. **A (airway):** If you suspect a neck or back injury, open the airway using the jaw thrust maneuver (see **Figure 4.4**). If you have help, direct the helper to hold the patient's head motionless to protect the neck. If there is no possibility of a neck or back injury, open the patient's airway using head-tilt, chin lift (see **Figure 4.5**).
5. **B (breathing):** Check for breathing. Place your ear over the patient's mouth and watch the patient's chest. Do this for at least 10 seconds. If the client is breathing, you should see the chest rise and fall, and you will hear and feel air exiting the mouth. If you hear snoring, wheezing, gurgling, or groaning, the patient is experiencing breathing difficulties and may require EMS services. If the patient is not breathing, provide rescue breaths to the patient. Rescue breathing is discussed in Section 4.4.

Secondary Assessment

If the patient's injury or illness does not need an immediate first-aid measure, conduct a **secondary assessment**. This includes checking the patient's head, neck, chest, abdomen, pelvis, legs, arms, and portions of the back that are reachable without moving the patient. Perform this assessment on patients who are unconscious or unresponsive and on those who have sustained significant trauma. Remember, if a patient is not breathing, has no pulse, or has major bleeding, correct these before performing the secondary assessment. NEVER move a patient when you think that the patient has a neck or back injury.

If it is not already being done, ask someone to hold the patient's head still as you check it. Begin your secondary assessment by starting at the head and performing the following steps. **Figure 4.6** illustrates these steps.

1. **Head:** Begin by looking at and feeling the patient's head for deformities, bruises, open wounds, tenderness, depressions, and swelling. Check the ears and nose for blood as well as for clear fluid. Check the mouth for bleeding, loose teeth, or foreign bodies.
2. **Eyes:** Gently open the patient's eyes and compare the pupils. They should be the same size and should react equally to light.
3. **Neck:** Look and feel for deformities, bruises, depressions, open wounds, tenderness, and swelling. Check for a medical-alert necklace.
4. **Chest:** Look and feel for deformities, bruises, open wounds, tenderness, depressions, and swelling.
5. **Abdomen:** Look and feel for deformities, bruises, open wounds, tenderness, depressions, and swelling.
6. **Pelvis:** Look and feel for deformities, bruises, open wounds, tenderness, depressions, and swelling. Gently press downward on the pelvis to check for pain. Gently grasp the upper thighs and press inward to check for pain.
7. **Legs:** Look and feel for deformities, bruises, open wounds, depressions, tenderness, and swelling. Compare the skin color, temperature, condition (for example, dry or moist), and size of both legs. If the injury does not keep you from doing so, check for movement and sensation. Have the patient wiggle his or her toes. Touch the patient's toe and have him or her identify the toe. If the patient can wiggle his or her toes as well as identify which toe is being touched, assume that the nerve pathways to that extremity are intact and not damaged.
8. **Arms:** Look and feel for deformities, bruises, open wounds, depressions, tenderness, and swelling. Compare the skin color, temperature, and size of both arms. If the injury does not keep you from doing so, check for movement and sensation. Have the patient wiggle his or her fingers. Touch a finger and ask the patient to identify the finger you have touched. Check for a medical-alert bracelet.
9. **Back:** Slide your hand under the back as far as it will go without moving the patient. Look and feel for bleeding, deformities, bruises, open wounds, depressions, tenderness, and swelling.

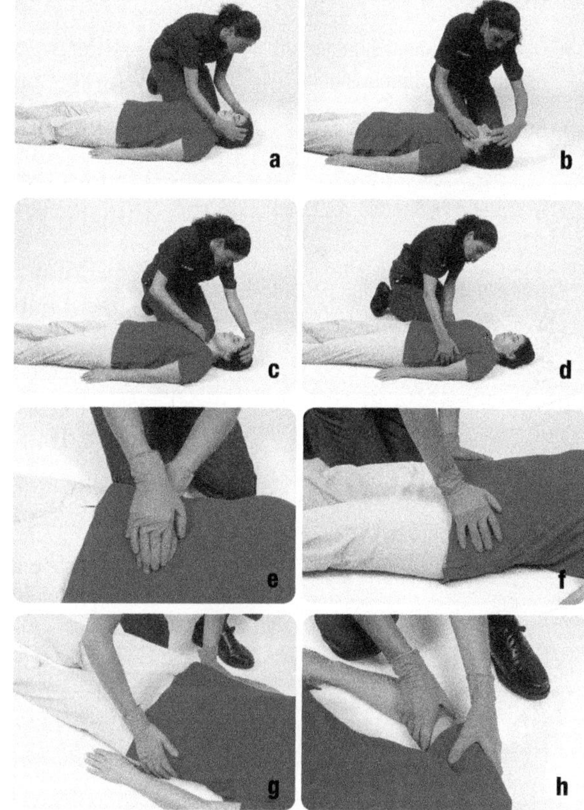

Fig. 4.6 Secondary Assessment (a) Head: Check the skull and scalp. **(b)** Gently open both eyes and compare the pupils—they should be the same size. **(c) Neck:** Check for a medical-alert necklace. **(d) Chest:** Gently squeeze the chest for rib pain. **(e) Abdomen:** Gently press the four abdominal quadrants. **(f) Pelvis:** Gently press downward on the tops of the hips for pain. **(g) Pelvis:** Gently press towards each other for pain. **(h) Extremities:** Check the full length of both arms and legs. *If a patient is not breathing, what should you do before performing a focused exam?*

Photos: Aaron Haupt Photography

21ST CENTURY SKILLS

Communication

When providing first aid to a sick or injured patient, incorporate these communication skills:

- Identify yourself and state that you know first aid.
- Obtain the patient's name and use it when communicating.
- Speak slowly and use your normal tone of voice.
- Maintain eye contact with the patient.
- Calm and reassure the patient.

Obtaining Information from a Patient

Use the memory aid SAMPLE to gather information relating to the patient's symptoms and medical history.

S = Signs and Symptoms: "What seems to be bothering you today?" or "What is wrong?"

A = Allergies: "Are you allergic to any medications?" "What are they?"

M = Medications: "What prescription or over-the-counter medications, vitamins, or herbal remedies are you taking?"

P = Pertinent Past Medical History: "Have you ever had this problem before?" "What was it?" "What other medical problems or conditions do you have?"

L = Last Oral Intake: "When was the last time you ate or drank something?" "What was it?"

E = Event preceding: "What were you doing when this happened?" "How did it happen?"

If possible, write down the findings of your primary and secondary assessments and history. Give this to the EMS providers when they arrive. If this is not possible, provide EMS with a brief oral report.

READING CHECK

List the nine body parts checked in a focused examination.

SECTION 4.3 Basics Of First Aid Review

AFTER YOU READ

1. **Describe** first aid.
2. **Identify** the three conditions a first-aid provider should evaluate during a survey of an incident.
3. **Describe** three potential hazards that might exist at the scene of an automobile accident.
4. **Explain** what you could use as a protective barrier to prevent being exposed to blood if a patient is bleeding and you do not have gloves.
5. **Illustrate** some ways in which to appraise an injured or sick patient's condition without asking questions.
6. **Describe** appropriate first aid for an unconscious or unresponsive patient without a pulse.
7. **Recall** the appropriate first aid for an unconscious and unresponsive patient with a pulse.
8. **Explain** the purpose of doing a secondary assessment on an injured patient.

Technology ONLINE EXPLORATIONS

Primary and Secondary Assessment

Assessing a patient requires attention to detail. Visit the American Heart Association's Internet site to review the steps of the Primary and Secondary Assessment. Create reference cards to help you perform the assessment completely and accurately.

SECTION **4.4**

Cardiopulmonary Resuscitation

The Chain of Survival

Do you know what the chain of survival is?

Cardiopulmonary resuscitation (CPR) is one of the initial first-aid skills you should learn. It can truly save lives.

Cardiovascular disease is the leading cause of death in the United States. Nearly 1 million Americans die each year from **heart attacks** or related causes. Of these, nearly half die from sudden **cardiac arrest.** The most likely cause is an abnormal heart rhythm called **ventricular fibrillation (VF).** This is when the heart stops beating and starts to fibrillate, or quiver. Performing CPR on a client in cardiac arrest can double the chances of survival.

Survival rates also improve dramatically if the chain of survival is started. The American Heart Association's chain of survival guidelines provide five major measures to deal with life-threatening emergencies such as sudden cardiac arrest, heart attack, stroke, or choking. The key features of the five links in the chain of survival are:

- **Early access to EMS.** Early access includes knowing the warning signs of sudden cardiac arrest, heart attack, **stroke,** or choking, and seeking immediate medical assistance.
- **Early CPR with an emphasis on chest compressions.** Start CPR on an unresponsive client without a pulse emphasizing chest compressions of adequate rate and depth, allowing complete chest recoil after each compression, minimizing interruptions in compressions, and avoiding excessive ventilation. These procedures buy clients of cardiac arrest time and improve survival chances.
- **Rapid defibrillation.** Most clients in sudden cardiac arrest are experiencing ventricular fibrillation. Treatment for this condition is **defibrillation** or the restoration of normal heart rhythm. Trained CPR and EMS providers use **automated external defibrillators (AEDs),** devices designed to return normal rhythm to the heart. Access to an AED is crucial. When someone suffers sudden cardiac arrest, survival chances decrease 7 to 10 percent for each minute without defibrillation. Public access defibrillation (PAD) is a program to train people to use AEDs and make them available.
- **Effective Advanced Life Support.** Trained EMS providers, called paramedics, provide the necessary combinations of drugs, airway management, and defibrillation to improve the chances of survival for clients of cardiac arrest, heart attack, stroke, and choking.

Vocabulary

Content Vocabulary

You will learn these content vocabulary words in this section.

- **heart attacks**
- **cardiac arrest**
- **ventricular fibrillation (VF)**
- **stroke**
- **defibrillation**
- **automated external defibrillators (AEDs)**
- **barrier devices**
- **bag-valve mask (BVM)**

Academic Vocabulary

You will see this word in your reading and on your tests. Find its meaning in the Glossary in the back of the book.

- **guidelines**

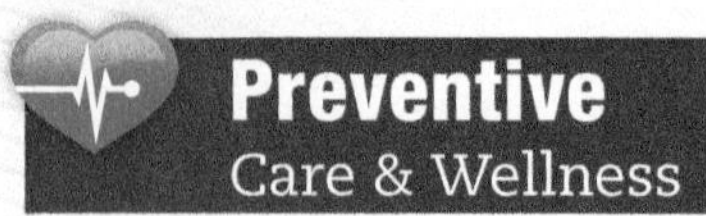

Preventive
Care & Wellness

Healthy Arteries

The arteries of your brain and heart need your help to stay healthy. Habits such as smoking, a diet high in fat and cholesterol, overeating to obesity, and lack of exercise can damage arteries. When this happens, blood clots may cause a stroke, a heart attack, or death. You can reverse the effects of these habits by not smoking, having your blood cholesterol checked periodically, exercising regularly, eating a healthy diet, and monitoring your blood pressure.

21ST CENTURY SKILLS

Problem Solving

Cardiac arrest is when your heart stops beating. Not all people who experience this condition are older. According to the American Heart Association, about 5,900 children age 18 and under suffer cardiac arrest each year due to trauma, cardiovascular disease, and sudden infant death syndrome. The incidence of sudden cardiac arrest in high school athletes in the U.S. is from .28 to 1 death per 100,000 high school athletes annually. Everyone should know what to do when cardiac arrest occurs.

- **Integrated post–cardiac arrest care.** This link emphasizes the importance of hospital based Intensive Care Unit (ICU) post-cardiac arrest care including therapeutic hypothermia in selected cases.

READING CHECK

Summarize the process of defibrillation.

Using Barrier Devices and Face Masks

Can you think of some barrier devices you can use in an emergency?

Before initiating and performing CPR, first-aid providers should follow infection-control procedures. These procedures include using gloves and **barrier devices.** The risk of infection from the human immunodeficiency virus (HIV), the virus that causes AIDS, or any hepatitis virus through mouth-to-mouth rescue breathing is remote. However, the American Heart Association and the American Red Cross recommend the use of barrier devices and bag-valve masks.

Using a Bag-Valve Mask

Have you ever seen a bag-valve mask?

A **bag-valve mask (BVM)** consists of a self-inflating bag and a one-way valve attached to a face mask. EMS and hospital personnel prefer to use this device for giving rescue breaths in CPR. The mask works best when it is used with supplemental oxygen. The proper use of the BVM requires practice. It is most effective when used by two first-aiders (see **Procedure 4-5**) ; however, a single first-aider can also use the BVM (see **Procedure 4-6**).

READING CHECK

Explain why groups such as the American Red Cross recommend using barrier devices and bag-valve masks for rescue breathing.

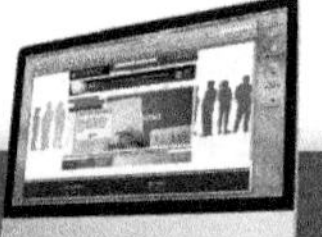

McGraw Hill connect ONLINE PROCEDURES

PROCEDURE 4-3

Using a Face Mask—No Trauma

Face masks are used to reduce the spread of infection. Most face masks are made of plastic and have a rim that creates a seal around the client's nose and mouth.

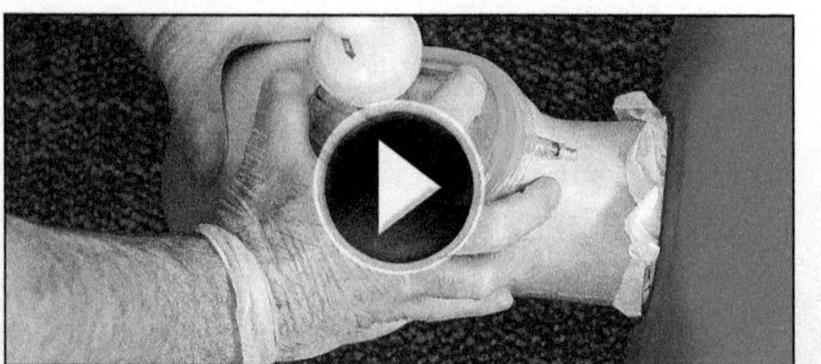

Photo: McGraw-Hill Companies, Inc./Scott Thompson, photographer

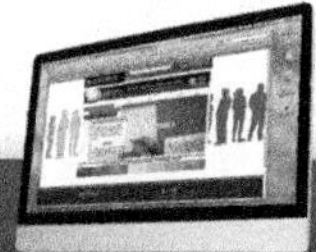

Connect ONLINE PROCEDURES

PROCEDURE 4-4

Using a Face Shield—No Trauma

Place the shield over the client's face and avoid directly touching the client's mouth. Face shields have a center opening to permit the first-aid provider to give rescue breaths.

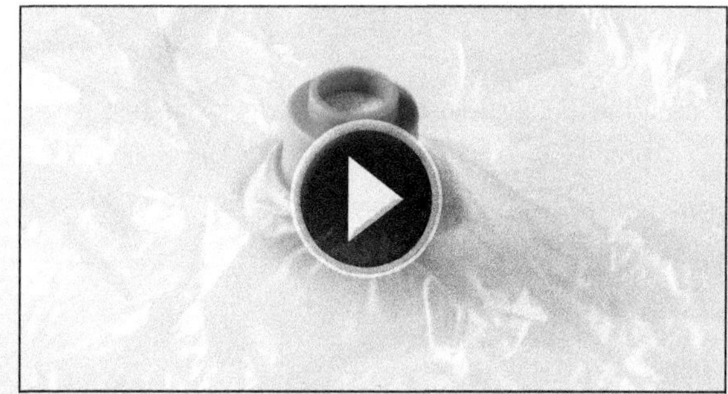

PROCEDURE 4-5

Using a Two-Rescuer Bag-Valve Mask—No Trauma

With two rescuers, the first rescuer uses the thumb and index finger of each hand to provide a complete seal. The other three fingers are used to lift the jaw and open the airway. The second rescuer squeezes the bag.

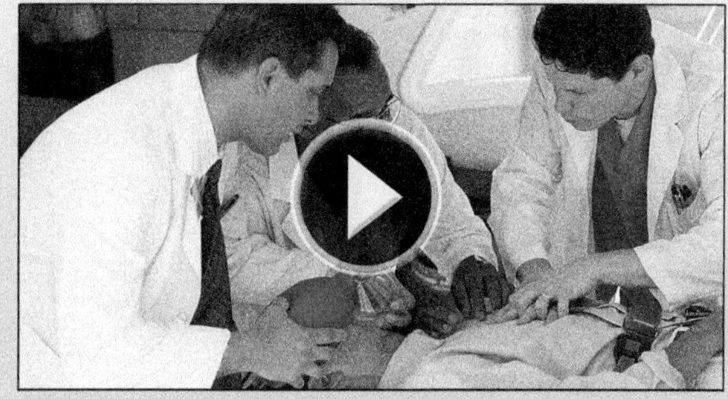

PROCEDURE 4-6

Using a One-Rescuer Bag-Valve Mask—No Trauma

The first aider circles the top edges of the mask with the thumb and index finger, and uses the other three fingers to lift the jaw and open the airway.

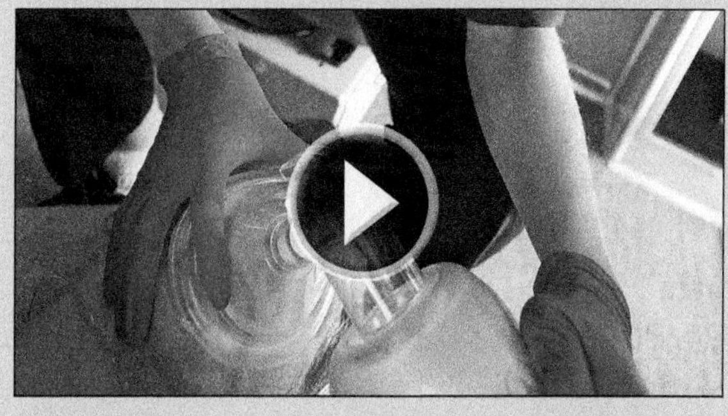

Cardiopulmonary Resuscitation

Have you ever performed CPR?

If sudden cardiac arrest occurs, blood flow stops and the heart, brain, and other vital organs are deprived of oxygen. There are three "red flags" for victims of sudden cardiac arrest:

- No response
- No signs of circulation
- No breathing or inadequate breathing

If there is no response, no sign of circulation, and no breathing or inadequate breathing, begin CPR. Follow CAB guidelines when performing One-Rescuer Cardiopulmonary Resuscitation (see **Figure 4.7**).

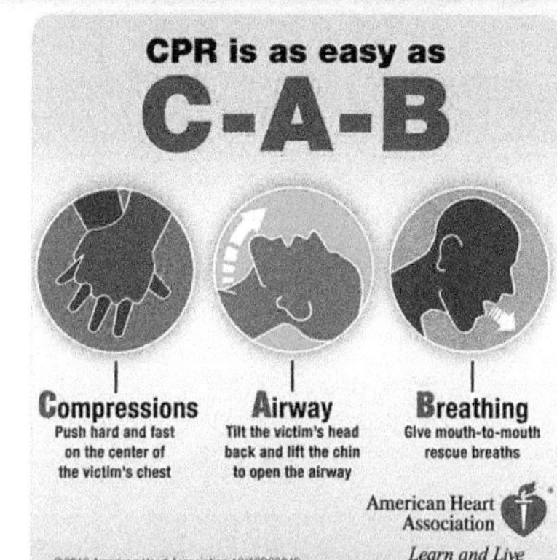

CPR is as easy as
C-A-B
Compressions
Push hard and fast on the center of the victim's chest
Airway
Tilt the victim's head back and lift the chin to open the airway
Breathing
Give mouth-to-mouth rescue breaths
American Heart Association
Learn and Live
©2010 American Heart Association 10/10DS3849

Fig. 4.7 CAB This CPR poster from the American Heart Association promotes the three main elements of CPR. *What do the initials CAB stand for?*

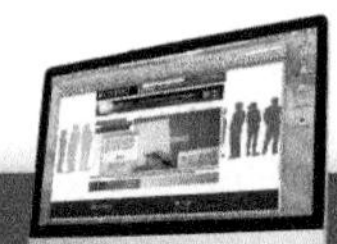

connect ONLINE PROCEDURES

PROCEDURE 4-7

One-Rescuer Cardiopulmonary Resuscitation—Adult

Follow the CAB guidelines when performing one-rescuer CPR. CAB refers to compressions, airway, and breathing.

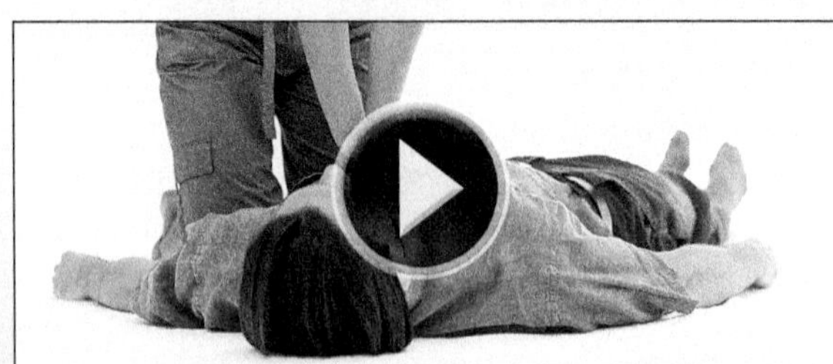

PROCEDURE 4-8

Two-Rescuer Cardiopulmonary Resuscitation—Adult

One person is positioned at the head to open the airway and provide rescue breathing. The second rescuer is positioned at the patient's side to provide chest compressions.

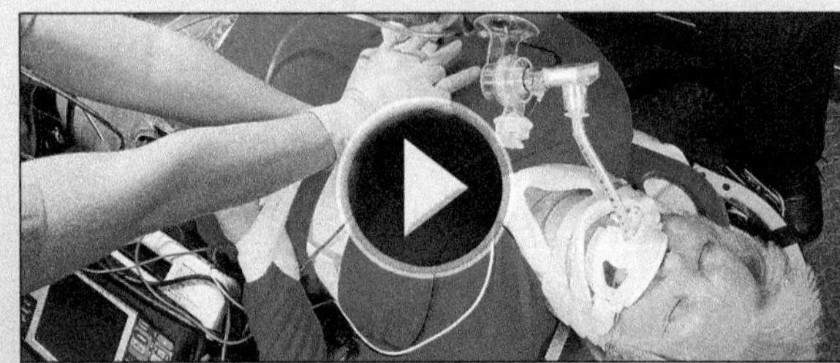

PROCEDURE 4-9

Cardiopulmonary Resuscitation for Infants and Children

According to the American Heart Association, an infant is a person from birth to one year of age, and a child is a person between age one and the onset of puberty. The usual cause for cardiac arrest in infants or children is a lack of oxygen to the brain, heart, and other vital organs.

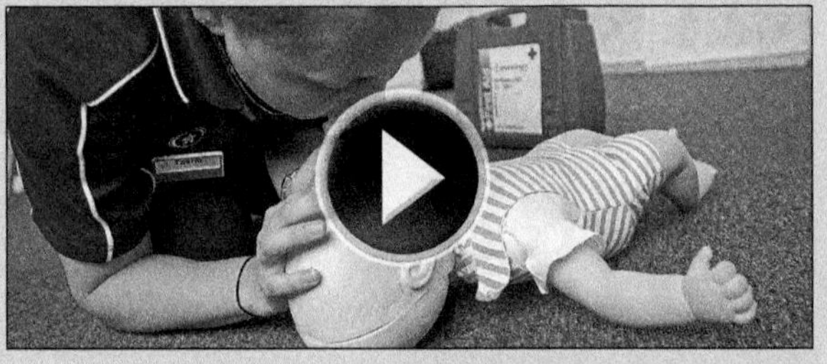

PROCEDURE 4-10

Foreign Body Airway Obstruction in a Responsive Adult or Child

In adults, an FBAO is common in situations involving alcohol and food. A patient may choke while eating and talking. Infants and children are more likely to choke on small objects.

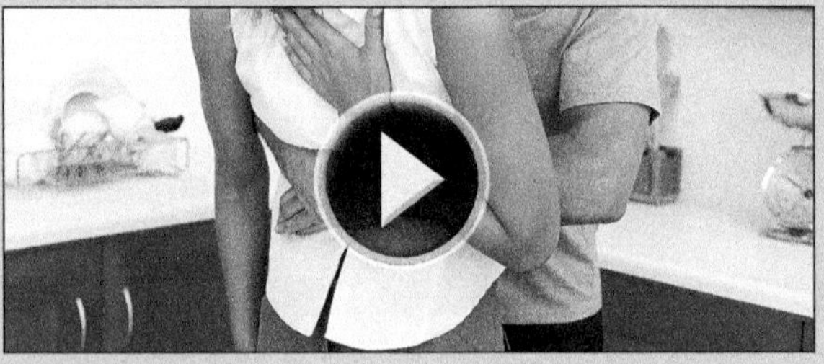

Photos: (t-b)Stockbyte Platinum/Alamy, Ocean/CORBIS, Ian Miles-Flashpoint Pictures/Alamy, Stockbyte/George Doyle/Getty Images

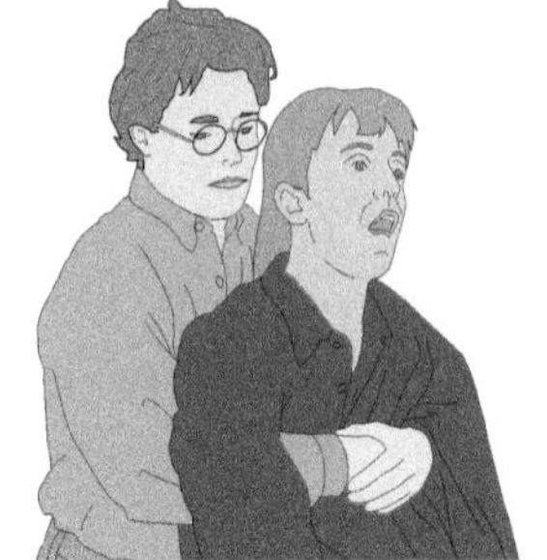

Fig. 4.8 Choking Aid *When would you perform a chest thrust rather than an abdominal thrust?*

Foreign Body Airway Obstruction

What could you do if you saw someone choking in a restaurant?

Foreign body airway obstruction (FBAO), or choking, can occur in patients of all ages. In adults, an FBAO is common in situations involving a combination of alcohol and food. Often, a patient chokes on a piece of food while eating and talking at the same time. Infants and children more frequently choke on small objects such as toys.

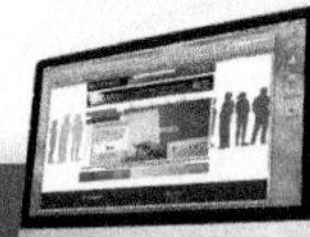

Mc Graw Hill connect™ ONLINE PROCEDURES

PROCEDURE 4-11

Foreign Body Airway Obstruction in an Unresponsive Adult or Child

When you come to the aid of an adult or child who has an FBAO and is unresponsive, call 911 or a local emergency number. Check for obstructions in the patient's airway, then perform CPR. Check for obstructions each time the airway is opened during CPR.

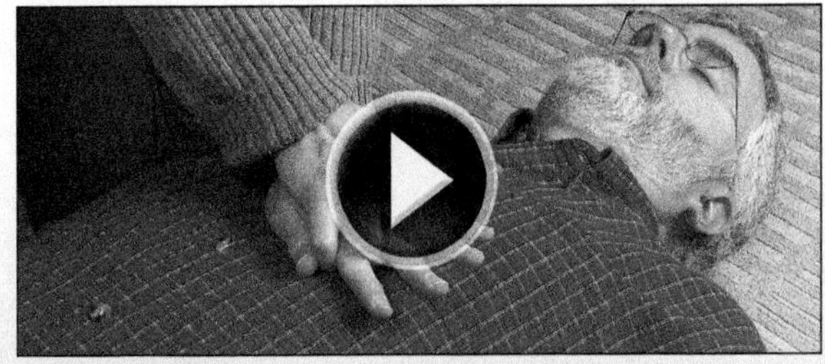

PROCEDURE 4-12

Foreign Body Airway Obstruction in a Responsive Infant

When you aid an infant who has an FBAO and is responsive, position the infant as described and alternate back blows and chest thrusts until the object is expelled or the infant becomes unresponsive.

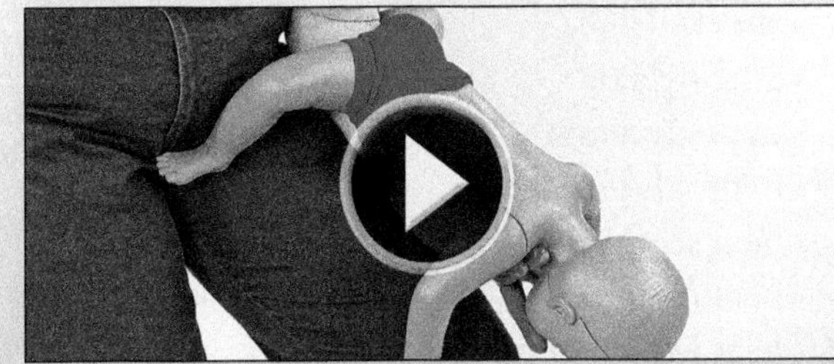

PROCEDURE 4-13

Foreign Body Airway Obstruction in an Unresponsive Infant

When you aid an unresponsive infant who has an FBAO, check for breathing and open the airway. Perform rescue breaths and CPR if necessary.

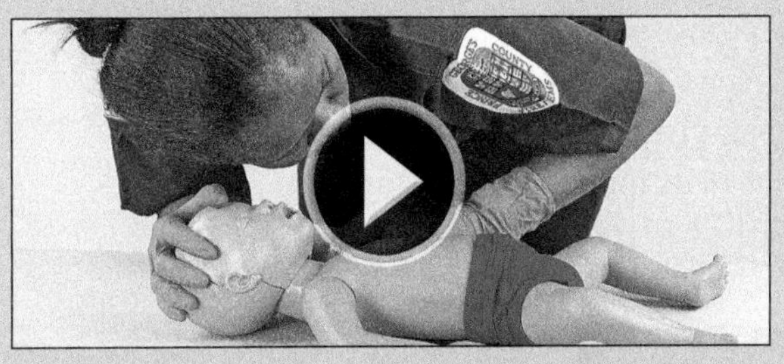

Photos: (t)The McGraw-Hill Companies, Inc./Photo by Chris Hammond, (c b)The McGraw-Hill Companies, Inc./Rick Brady, photographer

SECTION 4.4 Cardiopulmonary Resuscitation Review

AFTER YOU READ

1. **Assess** what you should do if you discover a patient lying unresponsive on the floor.
2. **Indicate** what you should do if a woman sitting next to you during lunch begins coughing, clutches her throat, and becomes silent.
3. **Analyze** what you should look for to determine whether rescue breaths are effective.
4. **Describe** the signs of circulation.
5. **Name** your first action if you enter a room to find a middle-aged man collapsed on the floor.
6. **Explain** what you should do if an infant has choked on a grape and becomes unresponsive after you are unable to dislodge the grape.
7. **Arrange** the steps to take if a 3-year-old child near you suddenly becomes limp.
8. **Explain** what to do if a pregnant woman clutches her throat and cannot cough or speak.

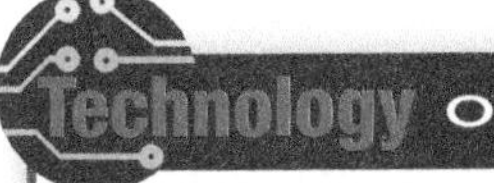

Technology ONLINE EXPLORATIONS

CPR Reference

Using items found on the Internet, develop a visual tool to help assist someone in providing CPR. Make the bulletin board or presentation as visual as possible with graphics, pictures, and photos.

SECTION

4.5 First Aid for Specific Emergencies

Vocabulary

Content Vocabulary

You will learn these content vocabulary words in this section.

- **shock**
- **anaphylaxis**
- **hypoglycemia**
- **hyperglycemia**
- **heat stroke**
- **heat cramps**
- **heat exhaustion**
- **hypothermia**

Academic Vocabulary

You will see this word in your reading and on your tests. Find its meaning in the Glossary in the back of the book.

- **constant**

Medical Emergencies

What kinds of medical emergencies have you encountered?

As a first-aid provider, you will need to respond to a variety of emergency situations. This section explains how to deal with the most common types of emergencies and gives guidelines that you can apply when the unexpected occurs.

Procedures covered in this section address a number of different emergencies that you may encounter. These include recognizing and administering first aid for a heart attack and a stroke, as well as minor wound care, stopping or controlling external and internal bleeding, and treatment for shock. Also covered in this section are first aid procedures for burns, ingestion of (or exposure to) poisons, heat emergencies, cold-related emergencies, muscle and bone injuries, diabetic emergencies, and seizures.

McGraw Hill connect™ ONLINE PROCEDURES

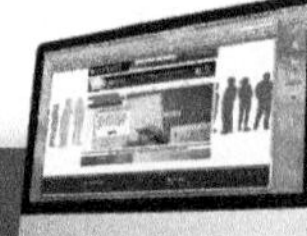

PROCEDURE 4-14

First Aid for Heart Attack

A heart attack occurs when the heart muscle is deprived of oxygen-rich blood and nutrients. The arteries that supply blood to the heart can become narrow because of an accumulation of plaque and cholesterol. The artery becomes blocked and no oxygen nourishes the cardiac muscle. Without oxygen, the heart muscle starts to die.

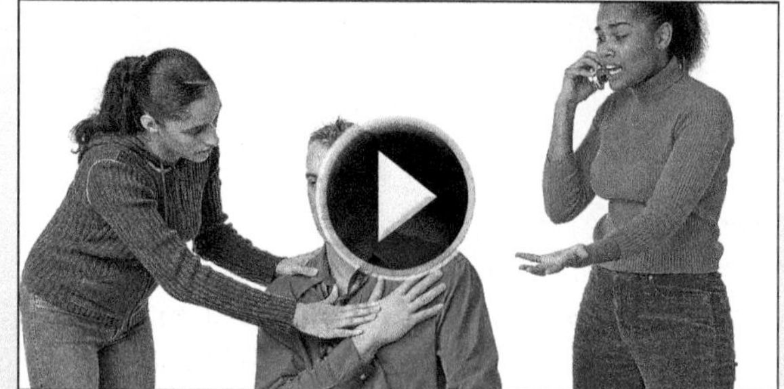

PROCEDURE 4-15

First Aid for Stroke

A stroke involves the brain. The cause of a stroke is similar to that of a heart attack. An artery supplying blood to the brain becomes blocked, cutting off oxygen and nutrients. A stroke can also occur when a blood vessel in the brain ruptures and bleeds into the brain. Strokes are the third leading cause of death in the United States.

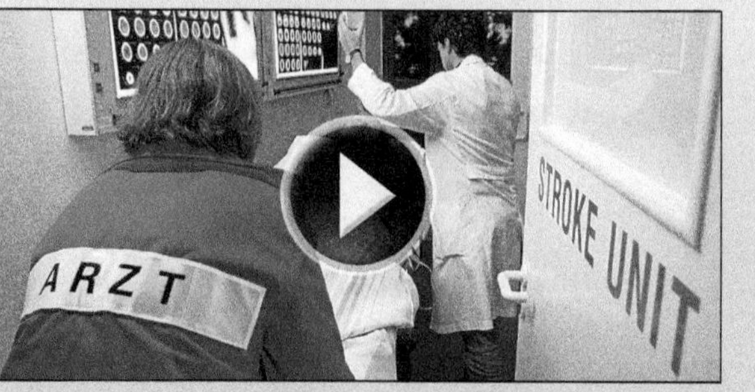

Photos: (t)Ken Karp for MMH, (b)Norbert Michalke/imagebroker/Alamy

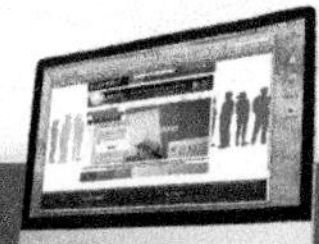

connect ONLINE PROCEDURES

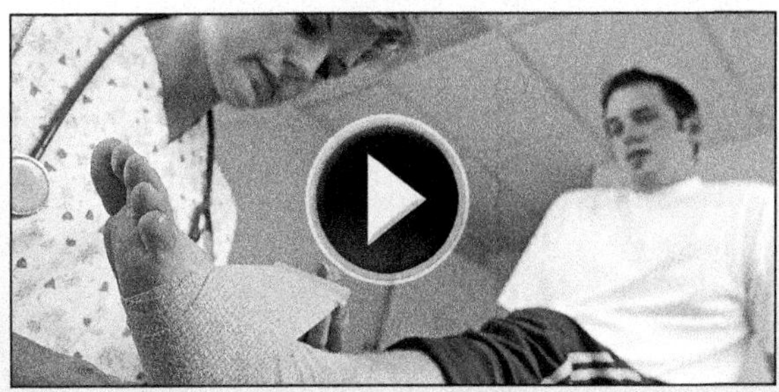

PROCEDURE 4-16

Minor Wound Care

Wash minor wounds with soap and water to help prevent infection. Keep in mind that wound cleaning generally restarts bleeding. If the wound is shallow, continue with washing anyway. On the other hand, if the wound is deep, postpone washing and seek immediate medical assistance. A physician should remove matter embedded in the skin.

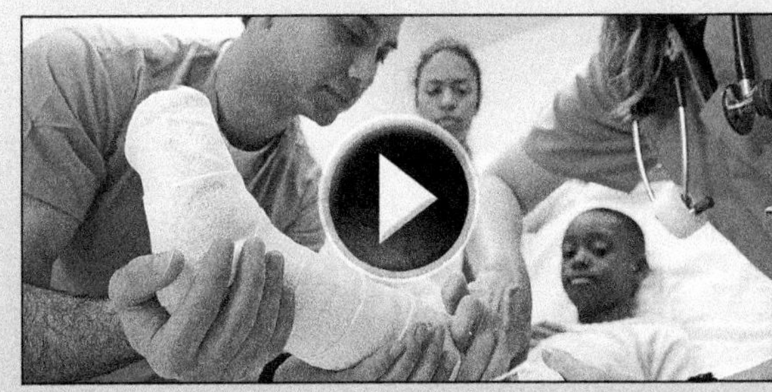

PROCEDURE 4-17

Controlling External Bleeding

External bleeding occurs when an object penetrates, tears, avulses (tears away), severs, or scrapes the outer protective layer of skin. These injuries are open wounds or soft tissue injuries. Controlling bleeding is the first priority in taking care of an open wound. Left alone, significant external bleeding can lead to severe blood loss and shock. Regardless of the bleeding or wound type, the first aid for external bleeding is the same: control the bleeding.

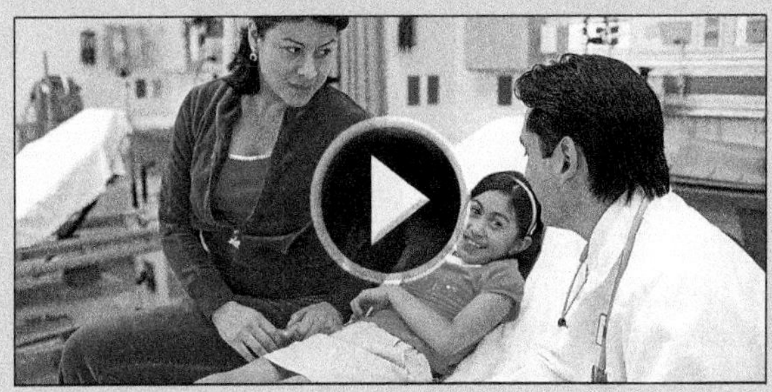

PROCEDURE 4-18

Internal Bleeding

Internal bleeding occurs when a blunt or penetrating force is applied to the skin, resulting in trauma to one or more internal organs, such as the liver, spleen, or kidneys. Internal bleeding can also result from non-traumatic conditions such as a stomach ulcer. Internal bleeding is difficult to recognize.

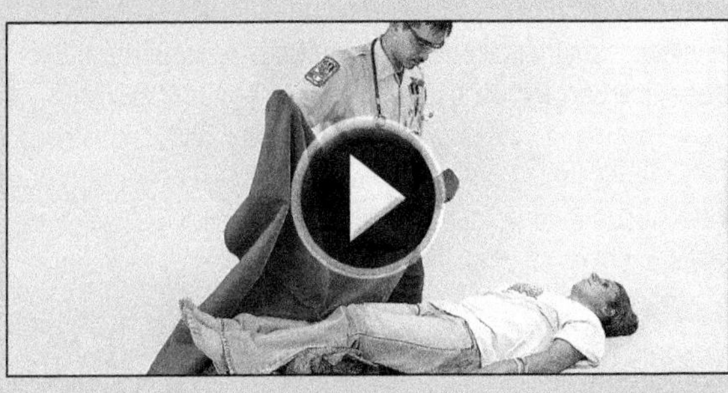

PROCEDURE 4-19

Shock

Shock refers to a condition that occurs when too little oxygen and nutrients reach the body's cells, tissues, and organs. Oxygen and nutrients travel to these structures by way of the circulatory system. Because every injury and some medical conditions affect the circulatory system to some degree, providers of first aid should treat all injured or sick patients for shock even though they may not exhibit the signs of shock.

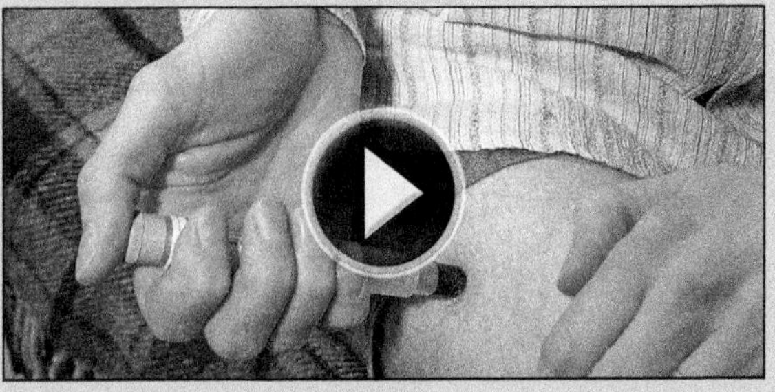

PROCEDURE 4-20

Anaphylaxis

Anaphylaxis is a type of shock that occurs quickly, even in minutes, with severe life-threatening consequences. Exposure to a substance to which the patient is severely allergic causes anaphylaxis. Exposure to this substance, called an allergen, occurs by contact, injection, or ingestion. Common allergens are bee stings, strawberries, shrimp, peanuts, aspirin, and penicillin. Anaphylaxis is a true medical emergency, and immediate assistance from EMS is essential.

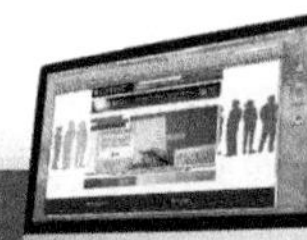

Mc Graw Hill connect ONLINE PROCEDURES

PROCEDURE 4-21

Burns

When the outer protective layer of the body, the skin, encounters thermal energy (heat), chemicals, or electricity, burns occur.

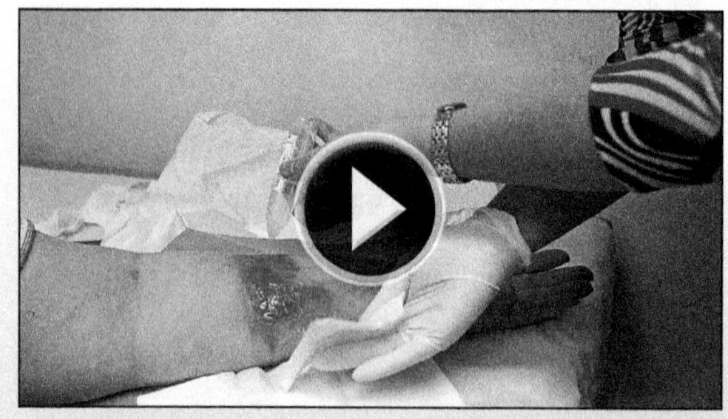

PROCEDURE 4-22

Injuries to Bones, Joints, and Muscles

Injuries to bones, joints, and muscles commonly result from motor vehicle or sporting accidents and falls. The four common injuries to bones, joints, and muscles are fractures, dislocations, sprains, and strains. Unless there is an apparent deformity, it may be impossible or even unimportant for a first-aid provider to decide whether a patient has a fracture, dislocation, sprain, or strain. In general, the first aid for each is the same.

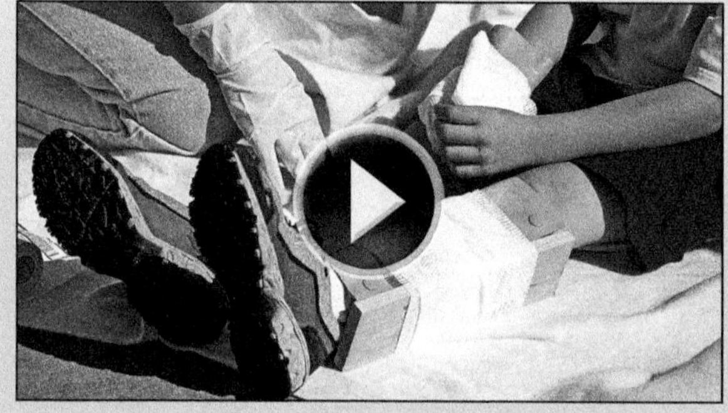

PROCEDURE 4-23

Diabetic Emergencies

Diabetes is a condition in which the pancreas, the organ that produces insulin, no longer produces enough insulin, or the insulin it produces is ineffective. Insulin, a hormone, helps the body use carbohydrates or sugar to produce energy. Insulin moves sugar from the bloodstream to the cells. The cells use sugar to produce energy. Diabetics may suffer from two diabetic emergencies: **hypoglycemia** or **hyperglycemia.**

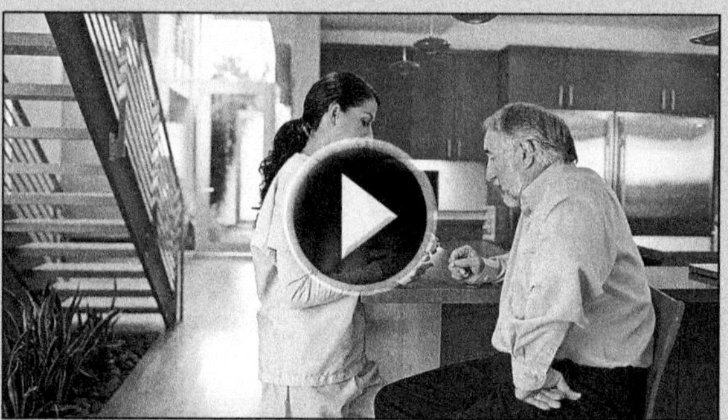

PROCEDURE 4-24

Seizures

A seizure or convulsion may be an unexpected, intense, unmanageable contraction of a group of muscles. In other cases a seizure may be subtle, consisting of only a brief "loss of awareness" or a few moments of what appears to be daydreaming. Seizures are caused by abnormal bursts of electrical activity in the brain. Grand mal seizures, or tonic-clonic seizures, involve the entire body.

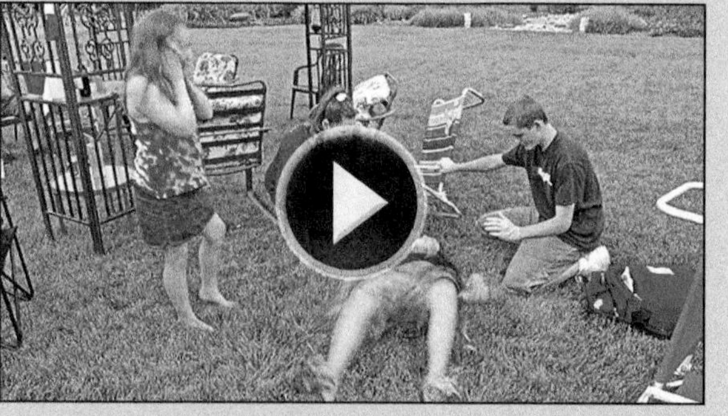

Photos: (t)Crispin Hughes/Photofusion Picture Library/Alamy, (c)Brand X Pictures/Getty Images, Hello Lovely/Corbis, (b)The McGraw-Hill Companies, Inc./Rick Brady, photographer

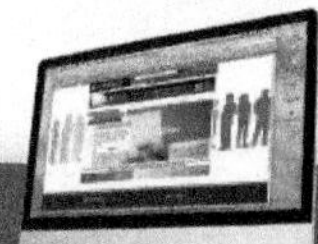

McGraw Hill **connect**™ ONLINE PROCEDURES

PROCEDURE 4-25

Heat Emergencies

Our body constantly works to rid itself of the heat it produces. If the body is exposed to excessive heat, the struggle to maintain a constant internal temperature of 98.6°F intensifies. This can result in heat-related illnesses such as **heat stroke, heat cramps,** and **heat exhaustion.**

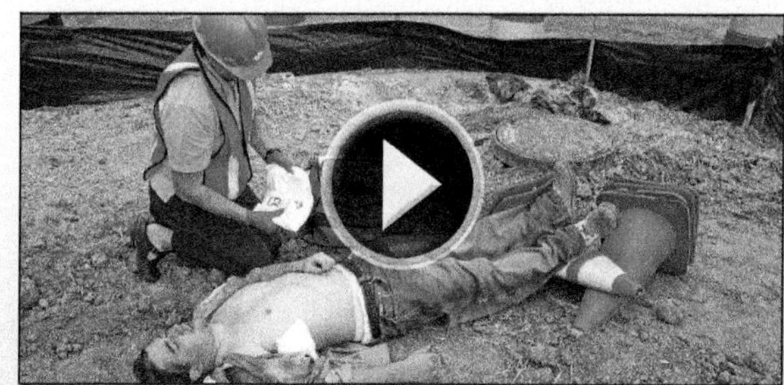

PROCEDURE 4-26

Cold-Related Emergencies

Exposure to cold can affect the entire body or the individual parts of the body. **Hypothermia** is when a patient's entire body is affected. Excessive exposure of the skin to cold can cause freezing of the skin and tissues under the skin.

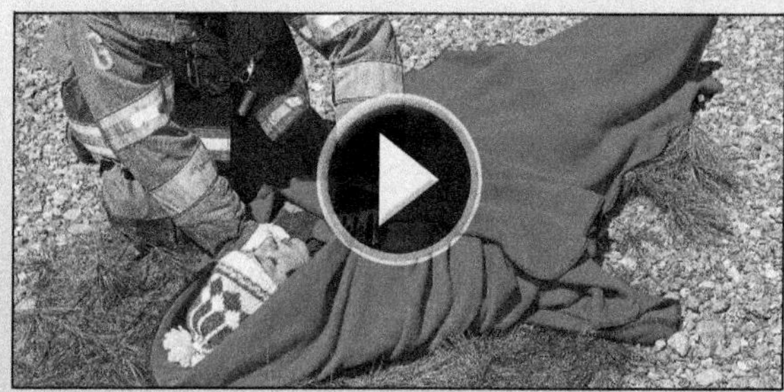

PROCEDURE 4-27

Poisons

Poisons are substances that produce harmful effects after being ingested, inhaled, or absorbed through the skin. Most poisonings occur in children under the age of 5. Ingested poisons include household chemicals, medications, petroleum products, and insect and weed control products.

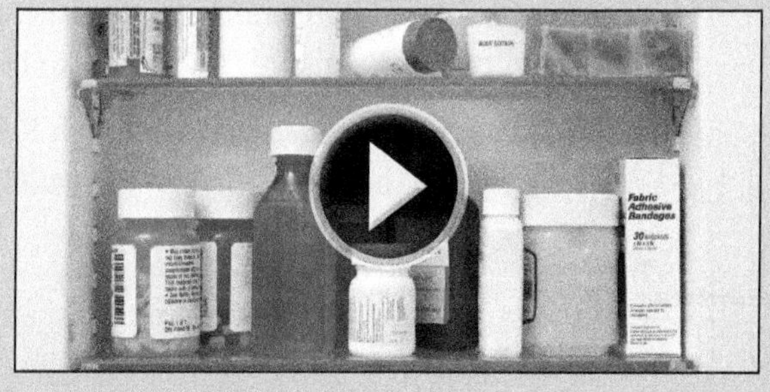

SECTION 4.5 First Aid For Specific Emergencies Review

AFTER YOU READ

1. **Recognize** the appearance and behavior of a patient who is having a heart attack.
2. **Explain** the action you should take when blood is flowing freely from a wound.
3. **Indicate** the information that should be obtained for cases of ingested poisons.
4. **Explain** how to determine whether a patient is having a low or high blood sugar episode.

Technology ONLINE EXPLORATIONS

CPR Training

The American Health Association and National Safety Council provide courses to become certified in first aid and/or CPR. Look online to find a course being taught in your local area.

CHAPTER 4 Review

Chapter Summary

SECTION 4.1

- Emergency care may be needed for medical emergencies, fire emergencies, bioterrorism, or other disasters. First aid is the initial help and care provided to a sick or injured person. **(pg. 81)**
- First aid is the essential link between the injured or sick person and the activation of EMS. **(pg. 81)**
- Recognizing safety and emergency signs, labels, and codes is necessary to be prepared for an emergency. **(pg. 82)**
- Healthcare professionals must be prepared to respond to any type of disaster. **(pg. 83)**

SECTION 4.2

- Fires can occur when there is a supply of fuel, heat, and oxygen. **(pg. 85)**
- Fire drills are important in the healthcare setting. Lives can be saved when the healthcare professionals know how to handle the emergency. **(pg. 86)**
- When a fire occurs, use the acronym RACE to respond to the fire and the acronym PASS to use the fire extinguisher. **(pg. 86)**

SECTION 4.3

- Before offering first aid, survey the scene of the incident to determine threats to your own safety or to the safety of the patient or bystanders, to determine the nature or cause of the illness or injury, and to determine the number of patients involved. **(pg. 89)**
- Before providing first aid, identify yourself, say you know first aid, obtain the patient's name, and use the patient's name when communicating with him or her. **(pg. 89)**

SECTION 4.4

- Always perform an primary assessment to determine whether there are problems with the patient's circulation, airway, or breathing (the CABs). Correct these problems immediately. **(pg. 95)**

SECTION 4.5

- Cardiovascular disease is the leading cause of death in the United States. Therefore, it is important for first-aid providers to recognize the signs and symptoms of heart attack and stroke and to perform CPR when required. **(pg. 98)**
- Controlling bleeding is the first priority in treating an open wound. First-aid providers may need to perform procedures for internal and/or external bleeding. **(pg. 99)**
- To perform first aid safely and correctly, you must first recognize the signs and symptoms of shock; burns; bone, muscle, and joint injuries; poisonings; heat and cold emergencies; seizures; and diabetic emergencies. **(pgs. 99-101)**

CHAPTER **4 Assessment**

Critical Thinking/Problem Solving

1. You are working the evening shift in the laboratory. As you approach the urinalysis department, you smell smoke. The door is closed, and smoke is coming from under it. There are two other technologists at the other end of the laboratory. Explain what you should you do. Use the acronyms RACE and PASS if applicable.
2. You just witnessed an automobile accident. What must you consider before offering your assistance? What should you tell the emergency dispatcher? If you choose to assist any of the injured patients, what should you do?
3. Your neighbor has disturbed a nest of yellow jackets and has been stung numerous times. He is short of breath and complains of severe itching. You notice that his legs and face are becoming puffy. What should you do?
4. Your father is busy remodeling your basement. He accidentally drives a nail through his right hand with a nail gun. What should you do?

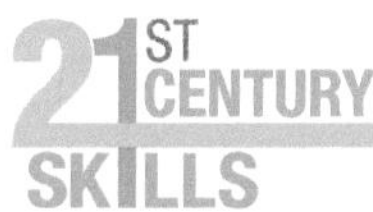

5. **Communication** Role-play various emergencies. Describe your symptoms and have a partner or the class identify your illness or injury. Take turns and find out how many emergency situations you can determine when you are told the symptoms.
6. **Teamwork** Obtain a bag-valve mask. Practice using it correctly on a mannequin.
7. **Information Literacy** Search the Internet for organizations that issue certification in first aid and CPR. Look for the American Heart Association, the American Red Cross, or the National Safety Council. Find out the requirements for enrolling in a course in first aid or CPR and the location of a course in your area.

connect™ ONLINE ACTIVITIES

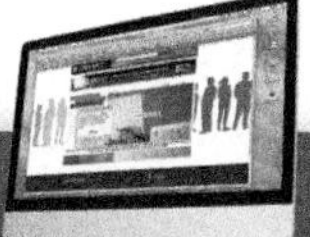

Complete our HST online activities for Chapter 4, which include Concept Check review questions, Reference Flash Cards, and Online Procedures assessment sheets.

- **Concept Check** review questions
- **Reference Flash Cards** medical terminology practice
- **Online Procedures** assessment sheets

CHAPTER 5

Medical Terminology

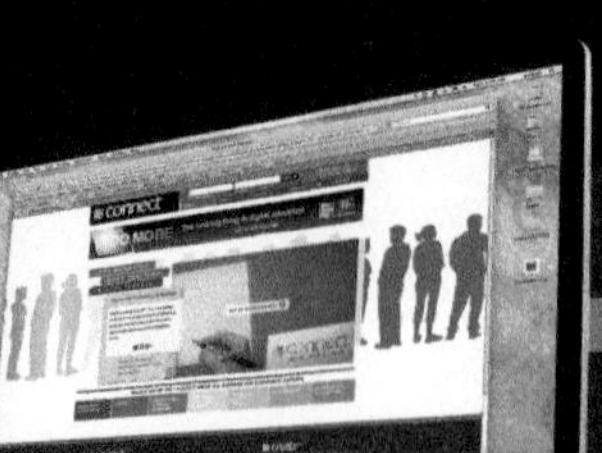

McGraw-Hill connect™

It's Online!

- Online Procedures
- STEM Connection
- Medical Science
- Medical Terms
- Medical Math
- Ethics in Action
- Virtual Lab

Essential Question:

How can you tell if the medical terminology used on a TV show or in a movie is accurate?

You may have heard many medical terms used, for example, in TV programs. Have you ever thought about what they mean or how they were **created**? Medical terminology has been formed mainly from Greek and Latin words, so it often looks like a foreign language. One medical term can mean a complete phrase in English. To learn medical terminology, you need to understand the basic word parts and be able to build and decode the terms in order to read them. In this chapter, the word "read" sometimes means "understand," "analyze," or "decode." A sound knowledge of medical terminology is important for a successful career in healthcare.

READING GUIDE

OBJECTIVES

After completing this chapter, you will be able to:

- **Identify** the four medical terminology word parts.
- **Define** and recall key medical terminology.
- **Apply** the common medical terminology and abbreviations for each body system.
- **Distinguish** common medical abbreviations.
- **Recognize** and correctly use abbreviations.

BEFORE YOU READ

Connect What do you need to know in order to be able to determine the meaning of a medical word that you may never have seen before?

Main Idea

To be able to learn medical terminology, you will need to understand the basic word parts and be able to build the terms in order to "read" them.

Note-Taking Activity

Draw this table. Write key terms and phrases under **Cues.** Write main ideas under **Note Taking.** Summarize the section under **Summary.**

Cues	Note Taking
o	o
o	o
Summary	

Graphic Organizer

Before you read the chapter, draw a diagram like the one below. As you read, write the medical terminology word parts covered by the chapter into the diagram.

Understanding Medical Terms

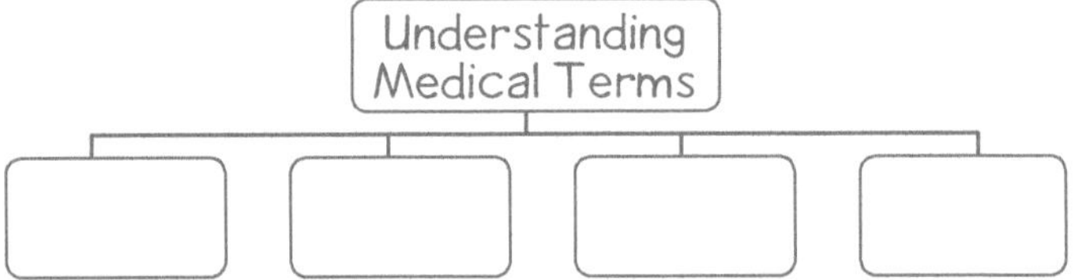

connect

Downloadable graphic organizers can be accessed online.

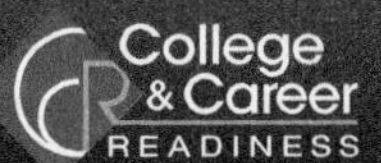

STANDARDS

HEALTH SCIENCE

NCHSE 2.21 Use roots, prefixes, and suffixes to communicate information.

NCHSE 2.22 Use medical abbreviations to communicate information.

SCIENCE

NSES 1 Develop an understanding of science unifying concepts and processes: systems, order, and organization; evidence, models, and explanation; change, constancy, and measurement; evolution and equilibrium; and form and function.

NCHSE *National Consortium for Health Science Education*

NSES *National Science Education Standards*

COMMON CORE STATE STANDARDS

MATHEMATICS

Quantities N-Q Reason quantitatively and use units to solve problems.

ENGLISH LANGUAGE ARTS

Reading

Key Ideas and Details R-2 Determine the central ideas or conclusions of a text; trace the text's explanation or depiction of a complex process, phenomenon, or concept; provide an accurate summary of the text.

Language

Knowledge of Language L-3 Apply knowledge of language to understand how language functions in different contexts, to make effective choices for meaning or style, and to comprehend more fully when reading or listening.

SECTION
5.1 Understanding Medical Terminology

Vocabulary

Content Vocabulary

You will learn these content vocabulary terms in this section.

- word root
- combining form
- prefix
- suffix

Academic Vocabulary

You will see this word in your reading and on your texts. Find its meaning in the Glossary in the back of the book.

- create

Using Word Parts to Understand Medical Terminology

Can you tell what a medical term means by examining its word parts?

Medical words are divided into parts. To understand the word, each part is identified. Then the basic meaning of the word is defined. We use common rules to break the word apart and "read" it as a sentence. Four word parts make up a medical term:

- Word root
- Combining form
- Prefix
- Suffix

Let's look at each of these word parts individually:

1. **Word root (WR)** is the basic meaning of the medical term. In medical terminology, a **word root** normally indicates a body part. If a medical term contains more than one word root, it is a compound word, which you will learn about in Section 5.2. All medical terms must have one or more word roots. Examples of word roots are:

Root	Meaning
neur	nerve
cost	rib

For example, the word ***perineuritis*** means "inflammation around the nerve." *Neur* is the word root.

2. **Combining form (CF)** is a word root plus a vowel that is used to help pronounce certain medical terms. The most common vowel added to a word root is the letter *O*. A **combining form** is used between word roots in a compound word or when a suffix (word ending) starts with a consonant. Medical terms with multiple word roots, or word roots combined with a suffix that starts with a consonant, will use combining forms. Examples of combining forms are:

Combining Form	Meaning
neur/o	nerve
cost/o	rib

For example, the word ***neurobiology*** means study of the life of nerves. *Neuro* is the combining form.

3. **Suffix (S)** is the word ending. To change the meaning of a term, frequently we change the **suffix.** When connected to the word root, the suffix will make the word a noun (N), an adjective (A), or a verb (V). An example of a noun suffix is *-logist,* "a specialist

in the study of" (for example, psychologist or anesthesiologist). All medical terms have suffixes. Examples of suffixes are:

Suffix	Meaning
-ectomy	excision or surgical removal (N)
-al	pertaining to (A)

Use the combining form of the word root when the suffix begins with a consonant. For example: neuropathy = *neur* + *o* + *pathy.* The suffix *-pathy* begins with a consonant, so the letter *o* must be added to the word root *neur.* When the suffix begins with a vowel, do not use the combining form of the word root. For example: neuritis = *neur* + *itis.* The suffix *-itis* begins with a vowel, so the combining form is not needed.

4. **Prefix (P)** is used at the beginning of a medical term. A **prefix** describes, modifies, or limits the term. Not all medical terms have prefixes. Examples of prefixes are:

Prefix	Meaning
trans-	across, through
intra-	in, within
sub-	less than, under

For example, in the term ***subcutaneous,*** which relates to anything that is or goes under the skin, *sub* means "under," while the term ***cutaneous*** just means "pertaining to the skin."

READING CHECK

Identify the four parts of a medical term.

Understanding Medical Terms

Do you look at medical term parts in a certain order?

"Reading" a medical term is a step-by-step process. This process will help you understand terminology. To read, or decode, medical terms, follow these steps:

1. Start with the suffix (the word's ending) and define the suffix.
2. Go to the prefix (the word's beginning) and define the prefix.
3. Go to the middle of the word; define the word root, combining form, or both if both exist in the same word.
4. Combine the definitions to decode the complete medical term or phrase **(see Figure 5.1).**

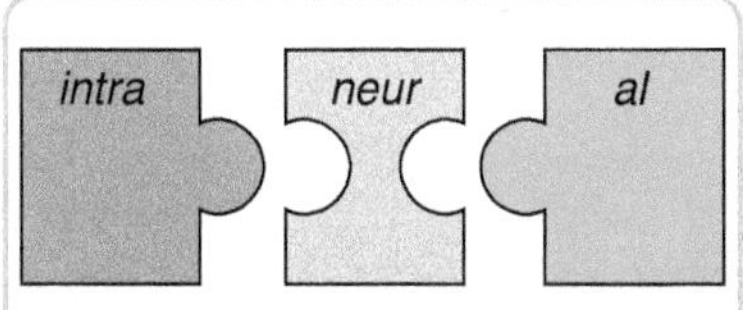

Fig. 5.1 Word Parts Reading the term "intraneural." *In what order should you define the parts of a medical term?*

Some terms can be used as a prefix, combining form, or a suffix. The placement of the word part will be the key to its usage. For example *mega-* and *megal/o-* mean "large" or "great" and *megaly* means "large," "great," "extreme," or "an enlargement of."

READING CHECK

Recall the recommended order in which medical terms can be decoded.

PART USAGE		
WORD PART	MEDICAL TERM	MEANING
Mega — prefix	megadose	many times greater than recommended dose
megal(o) — combining form	megalocephalic	pertaining to an abnormally large head
megaly — suffix	cardiomegaly	enlargement of the heart

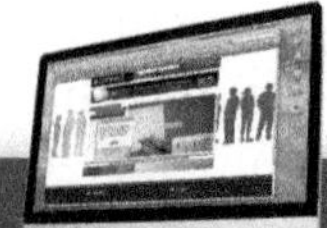

connect ONLINE PROCEDURES

PROCEDURE 5-1

Reading Medical Terms

Medical words are divided into parts. Each part is identified. Then, the basic meaning of the word is defined. We use common rules to break the word apart and "read" it as a sentence. Four word parts make up a medical term: word root, combining form, prefix, and suffix.

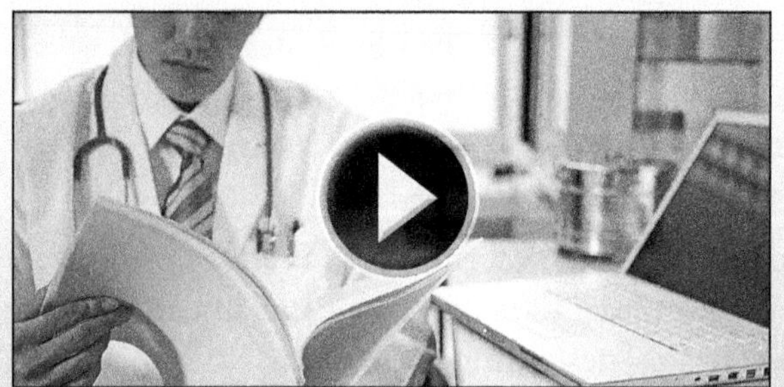

PROCEDURE 5-2

Building Medical Terms

"Reading" a medical term is a step-by-step process. This process will help you become adept in understanding terminology. To read, or decode, medical terms, start with the suffix; go to the prefix; then, go to the word root, combining form, or both; finally, combine the definitions to decode the complete medical term or phrase.

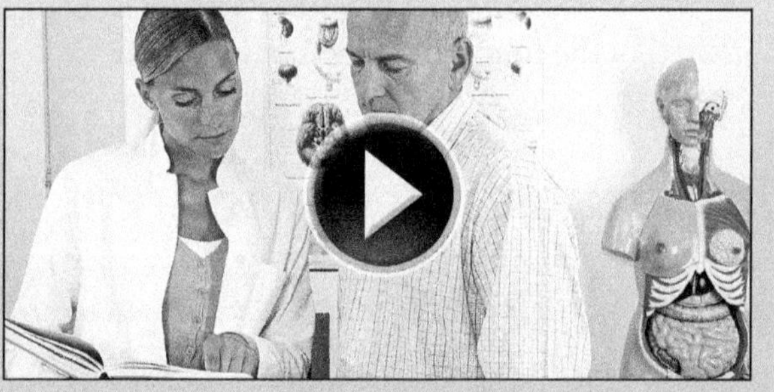

Photos: (t)Michael Hitosh/Digital Vision/Getty Images, (b)Alessandra Schellnegger/zefa/CORBIS

SECTION 5.1 Understanding Medical Terminology Review

AFTER YOU READ

1. **Identify** the 4 word parts used in medical terminology.
2. **Indicate** which vowel is most often used in a combining form.
3. **Set up** the steps used to "read" a medical term
4. **List** 3 words that end with the suffix *-ologist.*
5. **Name** 3 words that include the word root *neur/o.*

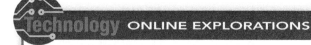

Technology ONLINE EXPLORATIONS

Decoding Terms

Go online to find five medical terms. Identify the word parts contained in each word and try to decode the terms.

SECTION **5.2** # Building Medical Terms

Using Word Parts to Build Medical Terminology

Can you build a medical term by constructing it from various word parts?

Once you have "read" a medical term, you can then construct, or build, other medical terms by using word parts. First let's read some terms.

Read ***neurectomy***

Word root *neur* + suffix *-ectomy* =

1. Start with the suffix: *-ectomy* means "excision (of)"
2. Go to the beginning of the word: *neur* means "nerve"

The medical term ***neurectomy*** means "excision (of) (a) nerve."

Read ***neural***

Word root *neur-* + suffix *-al* =

1. Suffix: *-al* means "pertaining to"
2. Word root: *neur* means "nerve"

The medical term ***neural*** means "pertaining to (a) nerve."

Read ***costectomy***

Word root *cost* + suffix *-ectomy* =

1. Suffix: *-ectomy* means "excision (of)"
2. Word root: *cost* means "rib"

The medical term ***costectomy*** means "excision (of) (a) rib."

Read ***costal***

Word root *cost* + suffix *-al* =

1. Suffix: *-al* means "pertaining to"
2. Word root: *cost* means "rib"

The medical term ***costal*** means "pertaining to (a) rib."

Read ***transcostal***

Prefix *trans-* + word root *-cost* + suffix *-al* =

1. Suffix: *-al* means "pertaining to"
2. Prefix: *trans-* means "across" or "through"
3. Word root: *cost* means "rib"

Vocabulary

Academic Vocabulary

You will see these words in your reading and on your tests. Find their meanings in the Glossary in the back of the book.

- **construct**
- **compound**

The medical term ***transcostal*** means "pertaining to something going across or through (the) rib."

Read ***intracostal***

Prefix *intra-* + word root *cost* + suffix *-al* =

1. Suffix: *-al* means "pertaining to"
2. Prefix: *intra-* means "in," "within," or "between"
3. Word root: *cost* means "rib"

The medical term ***intracostal*** means "pertaining to something that is in, within, or between (the) rib/s."

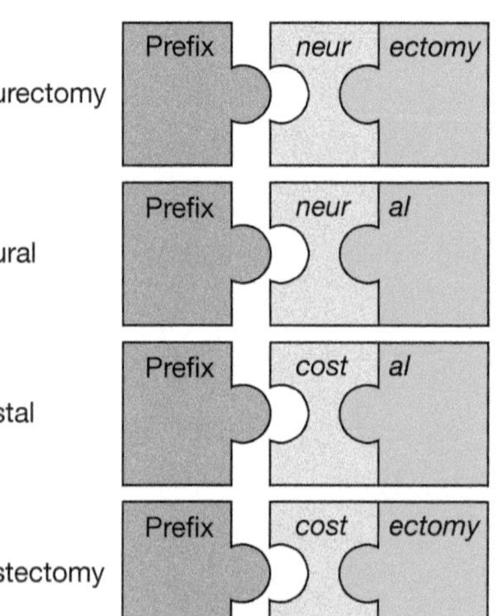

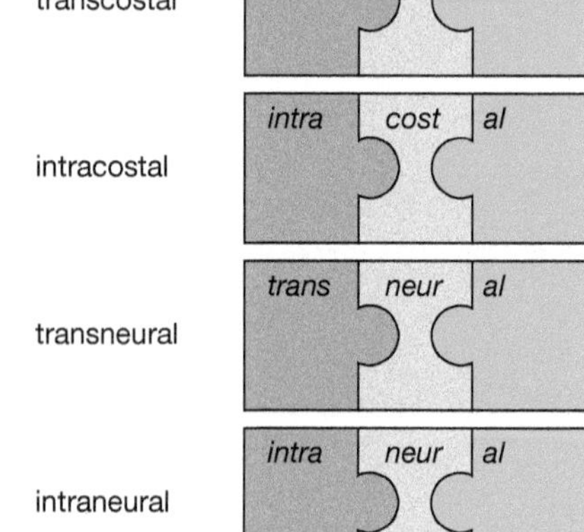

Fig. 5.2 Building Medical Terms. The prefix, word root, and suffix provide clues to the word's meaning. *What is the key to understanding medical terms?*

Read ***transneural***

Prefix *-trans* + word root *neur* + suffix *-al* =

1. Suffix: *-al* means "pertaining to"
2. Prefix: *trans-* means "across" or "through"
3. Word root: *neur* means "nerve"

The medical term ***transneural*** means "pertaining to something that goes across or through (a) nerve."

Read ***intraneural***

Prefix *intra-* + word root *neur* + suffix *-al* =

1. Suffix: *-al* means "pertaining to"
2. Prefix: *intra-* means "in" or "within"
3. Word root: *neur* means "nerve"

The medical term ***intraneural*** means "pertaining to something that is in or within (a) nerve."

Compound Words

How do you build compound words?

When you are building compound words, you should always remember that combining forms are used between word roots. For example:

Read ***transneurocostal***

1. Start with the suffix *-al,* pertaining to
2. Then the prefix *trans-*, across
3. Next, the combining form *neur/o,* nerve
4. Finally, the word root *cost,* rib

Once you have learned to break apart and read medical terms, it is easy to build them. All you need to do is place a prefix, word root (combining form) and suffix in the correct order to build a term. **Figure 5.2** shows some medical terms built in this manner. Following are some more common word parts:

Prefixes

sub- = less than, under
poly- = many

Word Root (Combining Form)

cutane/o = skin
hemat = blood
ling/u = tongue
rhin/o = nose

Suffixes

-rrhea = flow, discharge
-ology = study of
-ous = pertaining to

READING CHECK

Recall the type of forms used between word roots and compound words.

SECTION 5.2 Building Medical Terms Review

AFTER YOU READ

1. **"Read"** the following medical terms.
   - sublingual
   - subcutaneous
   - transneurocostal
2. **Use** the steps you have learned in this section to read the following compound words.
   - transpolyrhinal
   - subpolylingual
   - transdermal

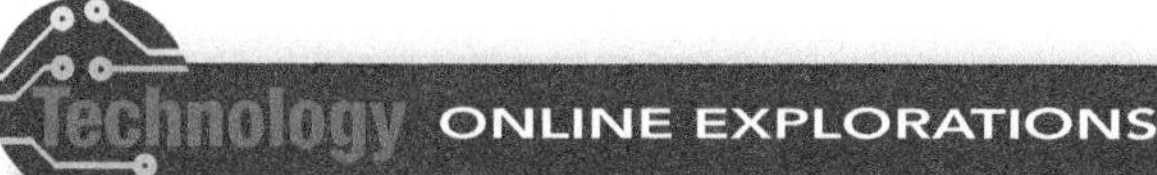

Expand Your Vocabulary

In an online medical dictionary, look up five unfamiliar terms. Listen to the pronunciations.

SECTION

5.3 Frequently Used Word Parts

Frequently Used Suffixes

Are you familiar with the frequently-used suffixes and prefixes?

In addition to the word parts in Section 5.2, there are many other frequently used word parts. Suffixes, prefixes, plural forms, roots, descriptive terms, directional terms, and word parts relating to colors and numbers are all included.

SUFFIX	MEANING	SUFFIX	MEANING
-al, -eal, -iac, -ic, -ical, -ior	pertaining to	*-ian*	specialist
-algia	pain	*-ism*	condition, method, process
-asis, -esis, -iasis	condition of	*-itis*	inflammation
-blast	germ, embryonic cell	*-logy*	study of
-cele	swelling, tumor, cavity, hernia	*-oid*	like, resembling
-centesis	surgical puncture to remove fluid	*-oma*	tumor
-cide	causing death	*-pathy*	disease condition
-ectomy	excision, surgical removal	*-scope*	instrument to visually examine
-gram	record	*-scopy*	process of visually examining
-graph	instrument to record	*-tomy*	process of cutting, incision
-ia	condition of		

Frequently Used Prefixes

PREFIX	MEANING	PREFIX	MEANING
a-, an-	no, not, without	*hyper-*	excessive, above
anti-, contra-	against	*hypo-*	deficient, below
auto-	self	*micro-*	small
dia-	through, complete	*peri-*	around, surrounding
dys-	abnormal, painful, difficult	*post-*	after
endo-	within	*pre-*	before
epi-	above, upon	*pro-*	before
ex-	out	*re-*	back, again
fore-	in front of	*ultra-*	beyond, excess

READING CHECK

Recall a suffix that means "the study of" and a prefix that means "self."

Plural Forms

Sometimes, the spelling of the term will change when used in the plural. For example:

SINGULAR	PLURAL	SINGULAR	PLURAL
bacterium	bacteria	phalanx	phalanges
cavity	cavities	vertebra	vertebrae

When a singular word ends in **y,** the plural is often made by changing **y** to **i** and adding **es.** When a singular word ends in **a,** add **e** to form the plural. If a singular word ends in **um,** change **um** to **a** to form the plural.

Commonly Used Word Roots

How many commonly used medical word roots can you list?

WORD ROOT	MEANING	WORD ROOT	MEANING	WORD ROOT	MEANING	WORD ROOT	MEANING
abdomin/o	abdomen	*crani/o*	skull	*hist/o*	tissue	*phleb/o*	vein
aden/o	gland	*cutane/o, derm/o, dermat/o*	skin	*kary/o, nucle/o*	nucleus	*psych/o*	mind
arthr/o	joint	*cyt/o*	cell	*nephr/o, ren/o*	kidney	*rhin/o*	nose
cardi/o	heart	*dors/o*	the back	*neur/o*	nerve	*spin/o*	spine, backbone
cephal/o	head	*gastro/o*	stomach	*oste/o*	bone	*thorac/o*	chest
cervic/o	neck	*hemat/o, hem/o*	blood	*ot/o*	ear	*vertebr/o*	vertebrae, backbones
chondr/o	cartilage	*hepat/o*	liver	*pelv/o, pelvi/o*	hip, pelvic cavity		

Descriptive Terms

TERM	MEANING	TERM	MEANING	TERM	MEANING	TERM	MEANING
algia, dynia	pain	*cry/o*	cold	*eu*	good, normal	*megaly*	enlargement
ankyl/o	bent, crooked	*cyan/o*	blue	*itis*	inflammation	*melan/o*	black, dark
brachy	short	*dys*	difficult, abnormal	*leuk/o*	white	*quadra, quadri*	four
chrom/o	color	*erythr/o*	red	*malacia*	softening	*tachy*	*fast*

READING CHECK

Name the word roots for "heart" and "skin" and the descriptive term for "pain."

Directional Prefixes

Do you know how to use word parts that indicate direction?

PREFIX	MEANING	PREFIX	MEANING	PREFIX	MEANING	PREFIX	MEANING
ab-	away from	*circum-*	around	*ex/o*	out of, away from	*later/o-*	side
ad-	toward	*dist-*	far, distant	*hemi-*	half, one side	*medi/o-, mes/o-*	middle
ante-	before	*end/o-*	within	*inter-*	between	*poster/o-*	back
anter/o-	front						

Color and Number Prefixes

PREFIX	MEANING	PREFIX	MEANING	PREFIX	MEANING	PREFIX	MEANING
bi(s)-	twice, double, both	*deca- or deci-*	ten	*leuk/o-*	white	*poly-*	many
cent-	one hundred	*di-*	double, twice	*melan/o-*	black, dark	*uni-*	one
chrom/o-	color stain	*erythr/o-*	red	*quad- or tetra-*	four	*xanth/o-*	yellow
cyan/o-	blue	*hemi- or semi-*	half				

READING CHECK

Classify the following prefixes as indicating either numbers or colors: cent-, melan-, uni-, erythr-, bi-.

SECTION 5.3 Frequently Used Word Parts Review

AFTER YOU READ

1. **Identify** the word part that contains the suffix.
2. **Identify** the word part that contains the prefix.
3. **Explain** the meaning of the following terms: distal, melanoma, neuropathy, phlebotomy.
4. **Describe** how you would change the singular form of a medical term to the plural.
5. **Choose** three word prefixes for direction.

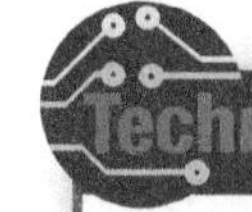

ONLINE EXPLORATIONS

Word Construction

Build at least five medical terms that you do not already know. Using an online dictionary, find the new terms that you have created and listen to their pronunciation. Review the definition. Is it the same as the definition for the term that you built?

SECTION 5.4 Organ Systems

Integumentary System

Do you know what parts of the body are included in the integumentary system?

Many word parts represent each of the major organ systems. These word parts are used to describe diseases and conditions related to each system. In this section, we will review each system and its associated word parts, and also look at abbreviations pertaining to those systems. In Chapters 6 and 7 we will learn more about the organ systems.

The skin (*derm/o, dermat/o, cutane/o*) and its structures, such as hair (*trich/o*), glands (*aden/o*), and nails (*onych/o, ungu/o*), make up the integumentary system (see **Figure 5.3**). The function of this system is to protect the body against infection, dehydration, and injury. The skin also regulates body temperature and helps in sensory perception.

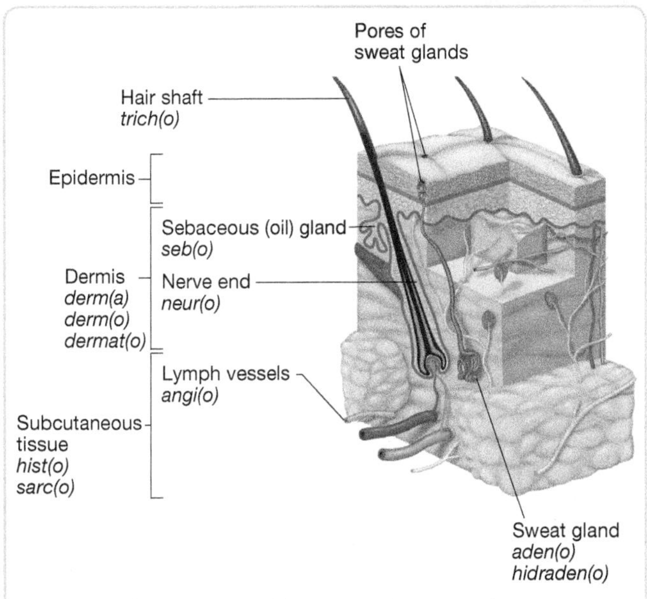

Fig. 5.3 The Integumentary System. This figure shows parts of the integumentary system. *What are the functions of the integumentary system?*

Integumentary System Terms

WORD ROOT	MEDICAL TERM	DEFINITION
derm/o, dermat/o	dermatology	study of skin and its diseases
cutane/o	subcutaneous	under the skin
hidr/o	hidradenitis	inflammation of a sweat gland
lip/o	lipocyte	fat cell
myc/o	mycosis	condition caused by fungus
trich/o	trichogenic	producing hair
ungu/o, onych/o	subungual	under a nail

Vocabulary

Academic Vocabulary

You will see these words in your reading and on your tests. Find their meanings in the Glossary in the back of the book.

- **internal**
- **external**
- **transport**

READING CHECK

Name the part of the integumentary system indicated by the word root *trich*.

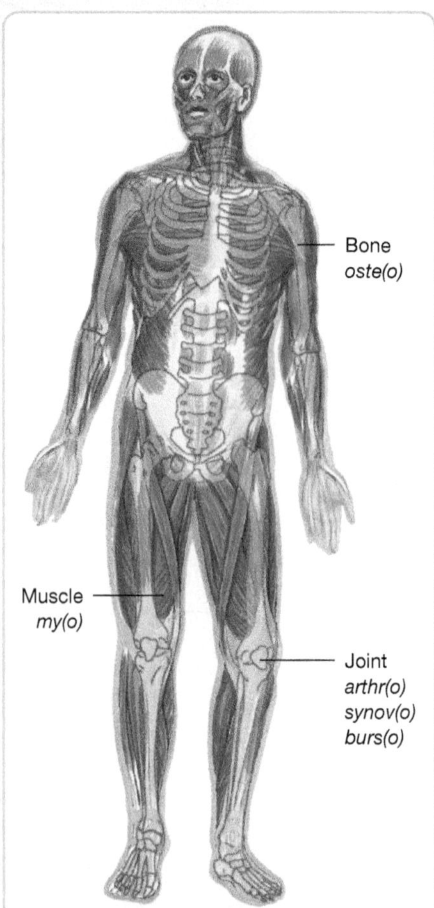

Fig. 5.4 The Musculoskeletal System. *What are two word roots used in the name of this system?*

Musculoskeletal System

What is the primary function of the muscular system?

Muscle (*my/o, muscul/o*) tissue (*hist/o, histi/o*) will contract or shorten to move parts of the skeleton, vessels (*angi/o, vas/o, vascul/o*), or internal organs (*viscer/o*). Some muscles stay partially contracted to maintain posture. The muscles also generate heat for the body. Muscles receive direction from the nervous system to contract or relax. The muscular system includes the muscles and connective tissue (*sarc/o*).

The skeleton supports and protects the body (see **Figure 5.4**). The bones of the body also function as a storage area for excess calcium (*calc/i*). This system includes bonés (*oste/o*), cartilage (*chondr/o*), and joints (*arthr/o, articul/o*). The tables below show abbreviations and terms associated with the musculoskeletal system.

READING CHECK

Name the part of the muscular system indicated by the word root *my*.

Musculoskeletal System

ABBREVIATION	MEANING
ACL	anterior cruciate ligament
Ca	calcium
CT	computed tomography
EMG	electromyography
IM	intramuscular
MRI	magnetic resonance imaging
Ortho	orthopedics
RA	rheumatoid arthritis
ROM	range of motion
TMJ	temporomandibular joint

Musculoskeletal System Terms

WORD ROOT	MEDICAL TERM	DEFINITION
arthr/o	arthrogram	X-ray of a joint
cervic/o	cervicodynia	neck pain
chondr/o	chondroplasty	surgical repair of cartilage
crani/o	craniotomy	incision, or surgical cutting, of the skull
kinesi/o	dyskinesia	difficulty or abnormality of movement
my/o	myositis	inflammation of muscle
oste/o	osteoporosis	decrease in bone density
physis	symphysis	growing together
tend/o, ten/o	tenorrhaphy	suture of a tendon
troph/o	atrophy	decrease in size of organ or tissue

Nervous System

What is the function of the nervous system?

The nervous system is responsible for conscious and unconscious actions (see **Figure 5.5**). The two major divisions are the central nervous system (CNS) and the peripheral nervous system (PNS). The CNS consists of the brain (*encephal/o*) and the spinal cord (*myel/o*). The cranial (*crani/o*) nerves (*neur/o, neur/i*) and the spinal nerves make up the PNS. The nervous system functions by electrical impulses. Neurons, or nerve cells, make up the conducting tissue of the nervous system. The connective tissue that supports and protects the nervous tissue is the neuroglia ("nerve glue"). This system includes the brain, spinal cord, and peripheral nerves.

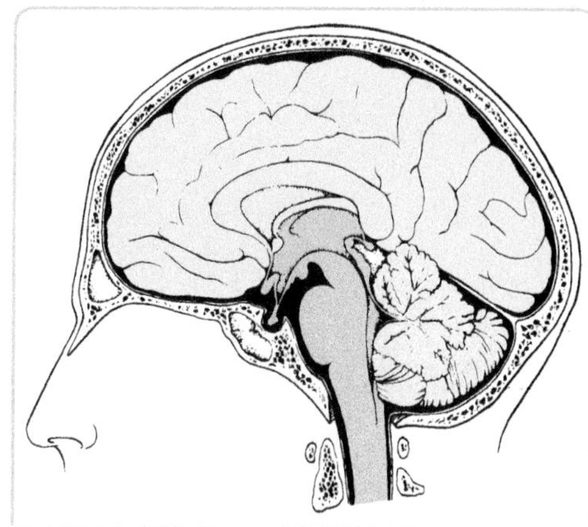

Fig. 5.5 The Nervous System The nervous system has two major divisions, the central nervous system and the peripheral nervous system. *What is the medical term that describes nerve pain?*

READING CHECK

Identify the two major divisions of the nervous system.

Nervous System Terms

WORD ROOT	MEDICAL TERM	DEFINITION
cerebell/o	cerebellum	posterior part of the brain
cerebr/o	cerebral	pertaining to the brain
cervic/o	cervical	pertaining to the neck
crani/o	craniomalacia	softness of the skull
mening/o, meningi/o	meningitis	inflammation of the meninges
myel/o	myelogram	X-ray of the spinal cord
neur(i), neur/o	neuralgia	nerve pain
neur(i), neur/o	neuron	a nerve cell
vertebr/o	vertebral	pertaining to the vertebrae (bones of the spine)

Nervous System

ABBREVIATION	MEANING	ABBREVIATION	MEANING
CNS	central nervous system	EEG	electroencephalogram
CSF	cerebrospinal fluid	MS	multiple sclerosis
CVA	cerebrovascular accident (known as stroke)	TIA	transient ischemic attack
CVD	cerebrovascular disease		

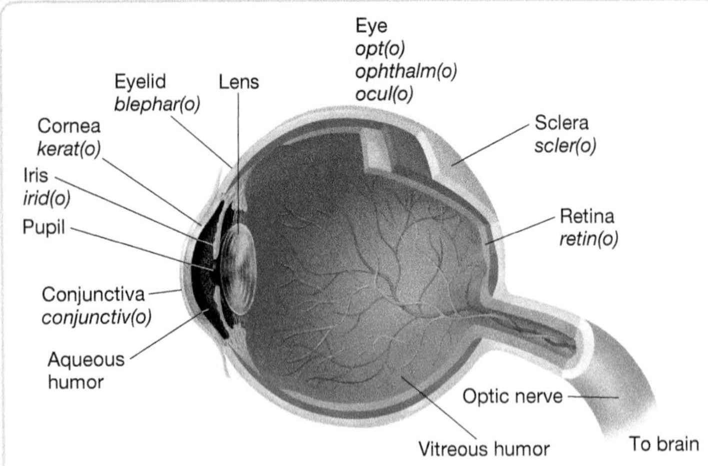

Fig. 5.6(a) The Eye This illustration shows the parts of the eye. *What are two word roots referring to the eye?*

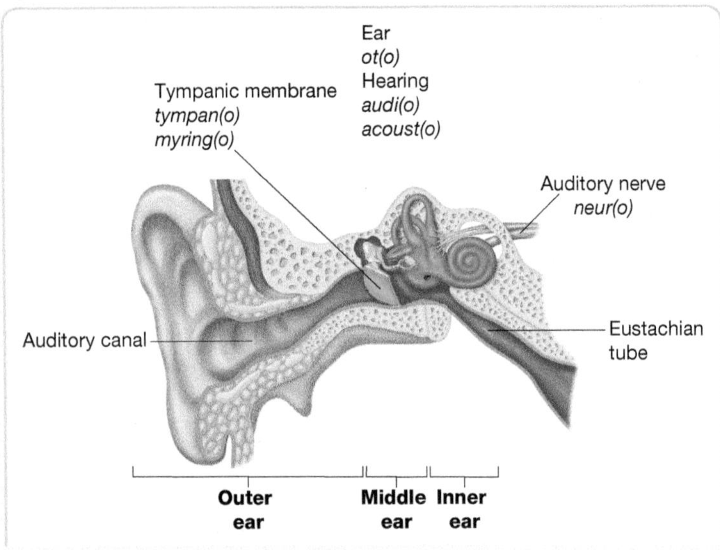

Fig. 5.6(b) The Ear This illustration shows the parts of the ear. *What is a word root referring to the ear?*

Sensory System

Do you know how the sensory system works?

The senses detect stimuli from the external and the internal environment. The eyes respond to stimuli by sending nerve impulses along sensory neurons that lead to the brain. The ears are essential not only to both hearing, but also to balance. The eyes (*ocul/o, ophthalm/o, opt/o, -opia*), the ears (*ot/o*), and parts of other systems make up the sense organs. The parts of the eye and the ear are shown in **Figures 5.6(a)** and **5.6(b)**. Abbreviations and medical terms associated with the sensory system are shown in the tables at the bottom of the page.

READING CHECK

Name the part of the sensory system that's indicated by word root *ocul.*

Sensory System

ABBREVIATION	MEANING
EENT	eyes, ears, nose, and throat
ENT	ears, nose, and throat
OD	*oculus dexter*; right eye
OM	*otitis media*, infection of the middle ear
OS	*oculus sinister*; left eye
PERRLA	pupils equal, round, reactive to light accommodation

Sensory System Terms

WORD ROOT	MEDICAL TERM	DEFINITION
audi/o	audiometer	instrument to measure hearing
conjunctiv/o	conjunctivitis	inflammation of the conjunctiva (pinkeye)
esthes/o	anesthesia	without sensation
myring/o	myringotomy	incision of an eardrum
ocul/o	intraocular	within the eye
ot/o	otoscopy	visual examination of the ear
retin/o	retinitis	inflammation of the retina

The Circulatory System

What parts of the body does the circulatory system include?

The survival of the body (*somat/o*), the cells (*cyt/o, cyte*), and the tissues (*hist/o, histi/o*), are all controlled by the circulatory system (**Figure 5.7**). This system includes the heart (*cardi/o*) and the blood vessels. Blood vessels include arteries, veins, and capillaries. Blood (*hem/o, hemat/o*) travels through the these vessels (*angi/o, vas/o, vascul/o*) to bring oxygen (*ox/o, -oxia*) and food to all cells. Blood also carries away the waste products of metabolism. Medical terms and abbreviations associated with the circulatory system may be found in the tables at the bottom of this page.

READING CHECK

Explain what you learn about a patient when you are told that he or she has cardiomegaly.

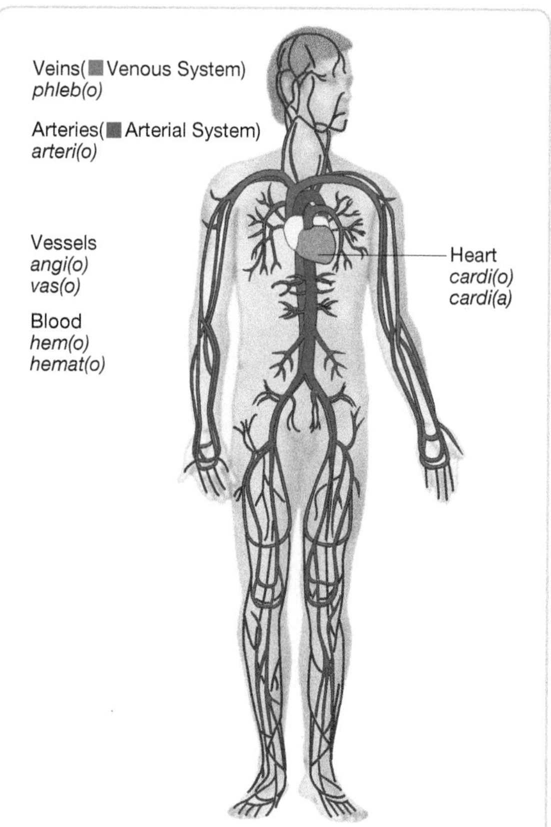

Fig. 5.7 The Circulatory System This system is also called the cardiovascular system. *What are two word roots that make up the word "cardiovascular"?*

Circulatory Terms

WORD ROOT	MEDICAL TERM	DEFINITION
angi/o	angiogram	image or record of a blood vessel
arteri/o	arteriotomy	surgical incision into an artery
cardi/o	cardiomegaly	enlargement of the heart
my/o	cardiomyopathy	disease of the heart muscle
phleb/o	phlebotomy	incision of a vein
thromb/o	thrombolysis	destruction of clots
vas/o	vasoconstriction	narrowing of a blood vessel
ven/o	venous	pertaining to a vein

Circulatory System

ABBREVIATION	MEANING	ABBREVIATION	MEANING
ASHD	arteriosclerotic heart disease	CHF	congestive heart failure
BP	blood pressure	ECG, EKG	electrocardiogram
CABG	coronary artery bypass graft	ECHO	echocardiogram
CCU	coronary care unit	MI	myocardial infarction
CHD	coronary heart disease		

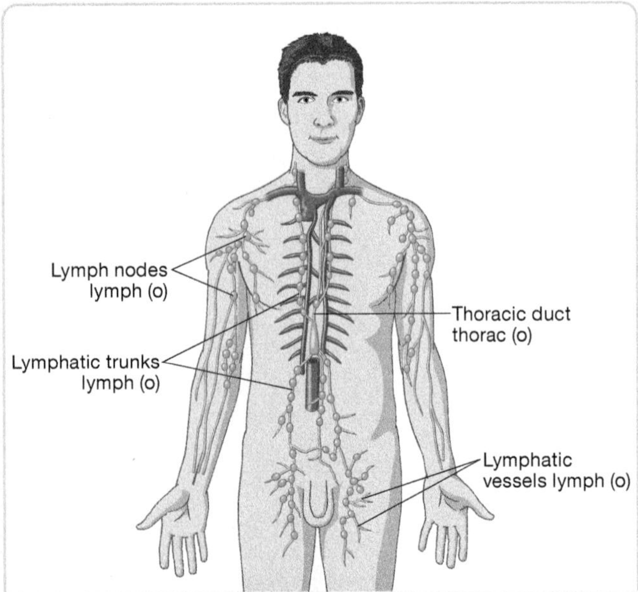

Fig. 5.8 The Lymphatic System. This illustration shows the parts of the lymphatic system. *What two things does the fluid in the lymph nodes do to help the body?*

Lymphatic System

Do you know what the lymphatic system does?

The lymphatic (*lymph/o*) system also travels through vessels (*angi/o, vas/o, vascul/o*). It returns excess fluid and proteins from the tissues to the bloodstream. It also protects the body from bacteria and viruses as part of the immune system. The system includes glands (*aden/o*) and tissues (see **Figure 5.8**). Medical terms and abbreviations associated with the lymphatic system may be found in the tables below.

READING CHECK

Name the part of the lymphatic system indicated by the word root *splen*.

Lymphatic System Terms

WORD ROOT	MEDICAL TERM	DEFINITION
immun/o	immunosuppressor	agent that suppresses the immune response
lymph/o	lymphoid	resembling lymph
path/o	pathogen	disease-causing agent
splen/o	splenomegaly	enlargement of the spleen
thym/o	thymectomy	removal of the thymus
tox/o	toxic	pertaining to poison

Lymphatic System

ABBREVIATION	MEANING
AIDS	acquired immunodeficiency syndrome
CMV	cytomegalovirus
HD	Hodgkin's disease
HIV	human immunodeficiency virus
HSV	herpes simplex virus

Respiratory System

What is the purpose of the respiratory system?

The respiratory (*pneum/o-*, *pneumon/o-*, *pneumat/o-*) system provides oxygen (*ox/o-*, *-oxia*) to body cells and removes carbon dioxide (*-capnia*). Internal and external respiration, or breathing (*pnea*, *spir/o*), is the taking in of oxygen and the giving off of carbon dioxide. Internal respiration refers to the gas exchange between the blood and body cells. External respiration refers to the exchange of air between the body (*pulm/o-*, *pulmon/o-*) and the outside environment. This system includes the lungs and the airways (see **Figure 5.9**). Medical Terms and abbreviations associated with the respiratory system may be found in the tables below.

READING CHECK

Recall what you can determine about a patient if you are told that he or she has adenoiditis.

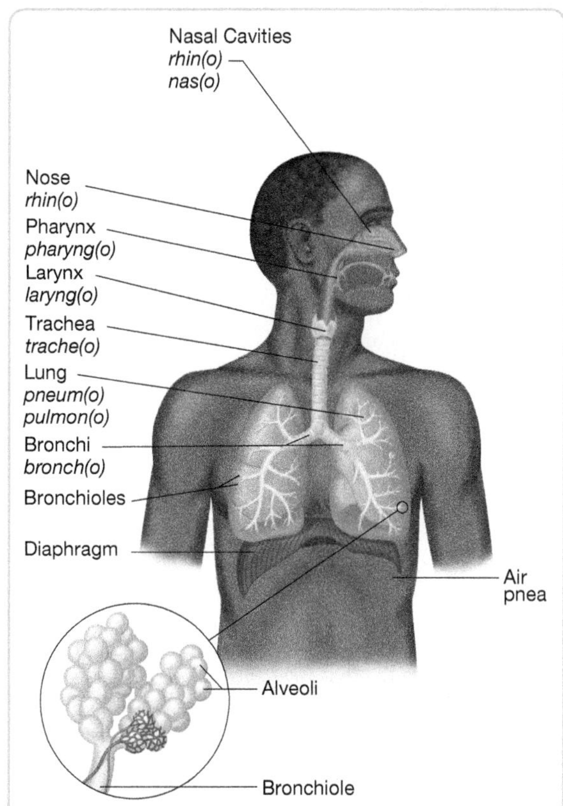

Fig. 5.9 The Respiratory System. This figure shows parts of the respiratory system. *What is the word root that means "respiratory"?*

Respiratory System Terms

WORD ROOT	MEDICAL TERM	DEFINITION
aden/o	adenoidectomy	removal of the adenoids
bronchi/o	bronchitis	inflammation of the bronchi
laryng/o	laryngocentesis	surgical puncture of the larynx
lob(i)-, lob/o	lobectomy	surgical removal of one lobe of the lungs
laryng/o	laryngitis	inflammation of the voice box
rhino/o	rhinitis	inflammation of the nose (nasal cavities)
pneum/o-, pneumon/o	pneumonia	acute infection of the alveoli
nas/o	nasogastric	pertaining to the nose and stomach
sept/o	septoplasty	surgical repair of the nasal septum
tonsill/o	tonsillitis	inflammation of the tonsils

Respiratory System

ABBREVIATION	MEANING	ABBREVIATION	MEANING
ABG	arterial blood gases	ICU	intensive care unit
COPD	chronic obstructive pulmonary disease	TB	tuberculosis
CXR	chest X-ray	URI	upper respiratory infection

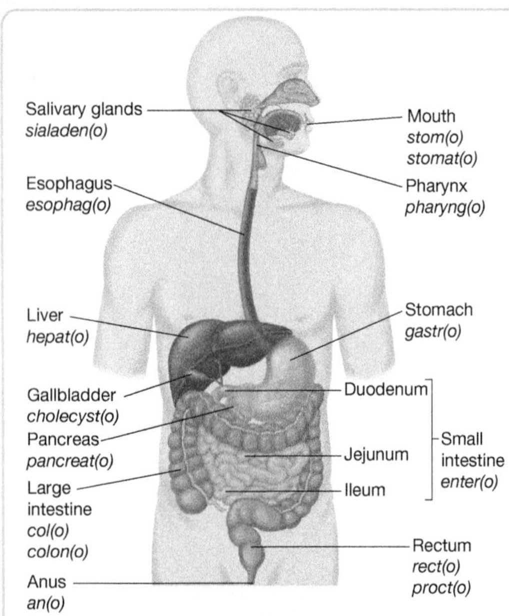

Fig. 5.10 The Digestive System. This figure shows parts of the digestive system. *What functions does the digestive system perform?*

Digestive System

What parts of the body are included in the digestive system?

This system is responsible for the intake of food, digestion of food, absorption of nutrients, and removal of solid waste. Digestion (*pepsia*) starts when food enters the mouth (*or/o*). Food must be broken down until it can be absorbed and the waste products removed. The tongue (*gloss/o*), mouth (*stom/o, stomat/o*) and teeth (*odont/o, dent*) are part of this process. This system includes all the organs of digestion and manages the excretion of waste (see **Figure 5.10**). Medical terms and abbreviations associated with the digestive system may be found in the tables below.

READING CHECK

Identify the part of the digestive system indicated by the word root *col*.

Digestive System Terms

WORD ROOT	MEDICAL TERM	DEFINITION
amyl/o	amylase	enzyme that digests starch
append/o	appendicitis	inflammation of the appendix
cholecyst/o	cholecystectomy	removal of the gall bladder
col/o	colitis	inflammation of the colon
dont/o	orthodontist	specialist in straightening teeth
enter/o	enteritis	inflammation of the small intestine
enzym/o	enzyme	chemical that speeds up a reaction between substances
esopha/o	esophageal	pertaining to the esophagus
gastr/o	epigastric	pertaining to the area above the stomach
hepat/o	hepatopathy	broad term for liver disease
lingu/o	sublingual	under the tongue
pancreat/o	pancreatitis	inflammation of the pancreas
pharyng/o	pharyngitis	inflammation of the pharynx
proct/o	proctoscopy	visual exam of the rectum and anus

Digestive System

ABBREVIATION	MEANING	ABBREVIATION	MEANING
EGD	esophagogastroduodenoscopy	NPO	nothing by mouth
GI	gastrointestinal	TPN	total parenteral nutrition
NG	nasogastric		

Urinary System

What is the purpose of the urinary system?

The urinary (*ur/o-, -uria*) system is responsible for removing the liquid waste from the blood, maintaining the proper balance of water (*hydro*), salts, and acids in the body fluids, and removing excess fluids from the body. The urinary system includes the kidneys (*nephr/o, ren/o*), ureter (*ureter/o*), bladder (*cyst/o, vesic/o*), and urethra (*urethr/o*) (see **Figure 5.11**). Medical terms and abbreiviations associated with the urinary system may be found in the tables below.

READING CHECK

Indicate the part of the urinary system indicated by the word root *ren*.

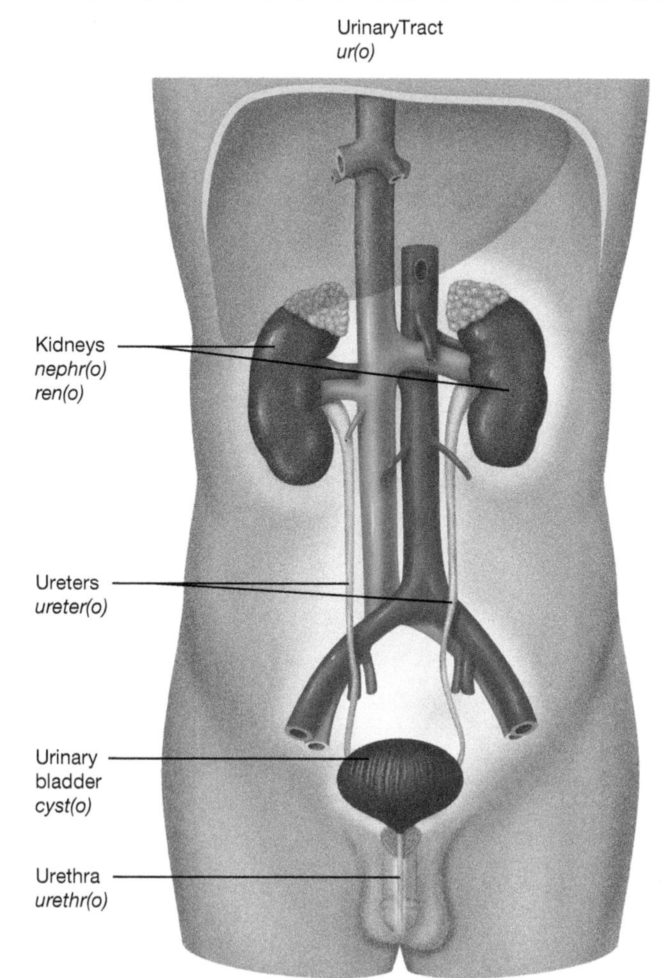

Fig. 5.11 The Urinary System. This figure shows parts of the urinary system. *What functions does the urinary system perform?*

Urinary System Terms

WORD ROOT	MEDICAL TERM	DEFINITION
arteri/o	arteriole	small artery
cyst/o	cystopexy	surgical fixation of the bladder
urin/o	urinoma	a cyst or tumor containing urine
nephr/o	nephropathy	kidney disease
ren/o	renomegaly	enlargement of the kidney
peritone/o	retroperitoneal	posterior to, or behind, the peritoneum

Urinary System

ABBREVIATION	MEANING
ADH	antidiuretic hormone
BPH	benign prostatic hypertrophy
BUN	blood urea nitrogen
IVP	intravenous pyelogram
PKU	phenylketonuria
PSA	prostate-specific antigen
TURP	transurethral resection of the prostate
UA	urinalysis
UTI	urinary tract infection

Endocrine System

Do you know the purpose of the endocrine system?

The endocrine system is made up of a number of glands (see **Figure 5.12**). These glands affect body functions by releasing hormones directly into the bloodstream. *End/o* means "in" or "within" and *crine* means "secrete." The endocrine system influences body tissue by secreting hormones that react with receptors located within the various tissues.

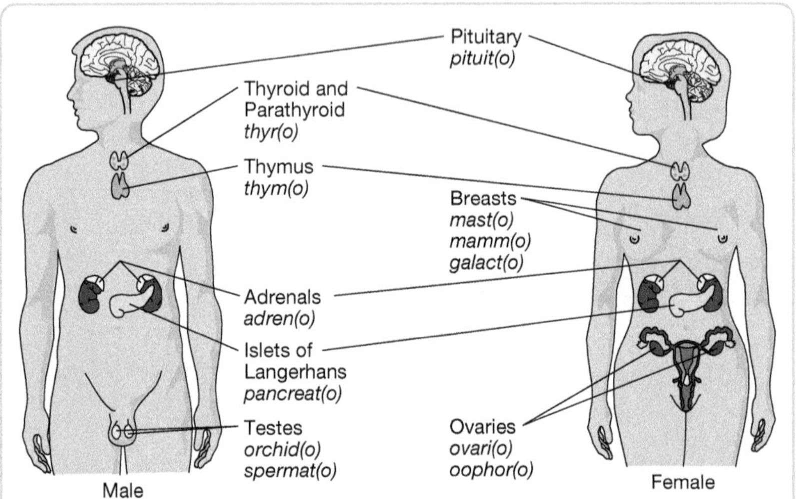

Fig. 5.12 The Endocrine System This illustration shows parts of the endocrine system. *What are two word roots associated with the endocrine system?*

READING CHECK

Name the part of the endocrine system indicated by the word root *adren.*

Endocrine System Terms

WORD ROOT	MEDICAL TERM	DEFINITION
adren/o	adrenopathy	disease of a the adrenal glands
calci/o	hypocalcemia	deficient calcium in the blood
crin/o	endocrinologist	one who studies endocrine diseases
gluc/o	glucogenesis	production of glucose
pancreat/o	pancreatectomy	removal of the pancreas
thyroid/o	thyroiditis	inflammation of the thyroid gland

Endocrine System

ABBREVIATION	MEANING
ACTH	adrenocorticotropic hormone
BMR	basal metabolic rate
DM	diabetes mellitus
FBS	fasting blood sugar
GTT	glucose tolerance test
IDDM	insulin-dependent diabetes mellitus, known as type 1 diabetes
TSH	thyroid-stimulating hormone

Reproductive Systems

Do you know what is included in the reproductive system?

The organs of the reproductive system are shown in **Figures 5.13(a)** and **5.13(b)**. The female reproductive system controls the production and movement of female sex cells (ova) to a site of fertilization. If an ovum, or egg, is fertilized by a male sex cell (sperm), the female system normally nurtures the fertilized ovum until birth. In the male, several organs are parts of both the reproductive and the urinary systems. The male reproductive system produces and transports sperm.

READING CHECK

Name the part of the reproductive system indicated by the word root *cervic.*

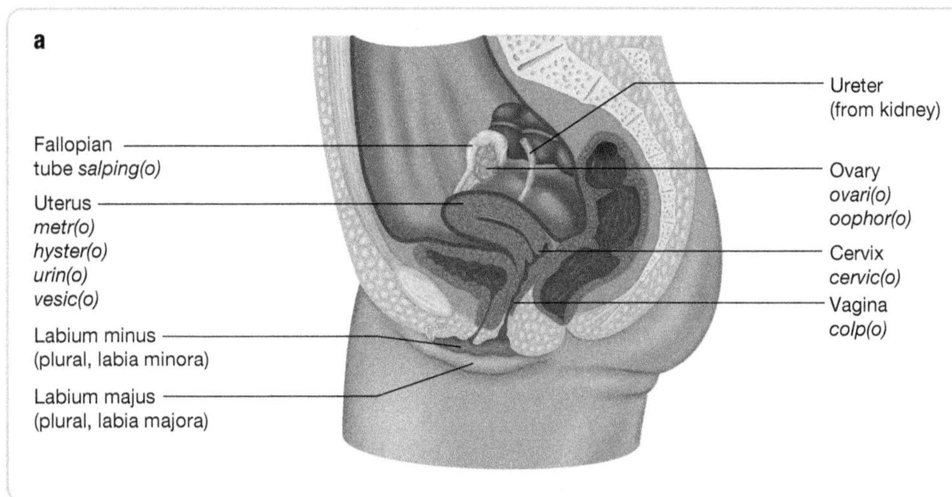

Fig. 5.13(a) The Female Reproductive System. This figure shows parts of the female reproductive system. *What are two word roots referring to the female reproductive system?*

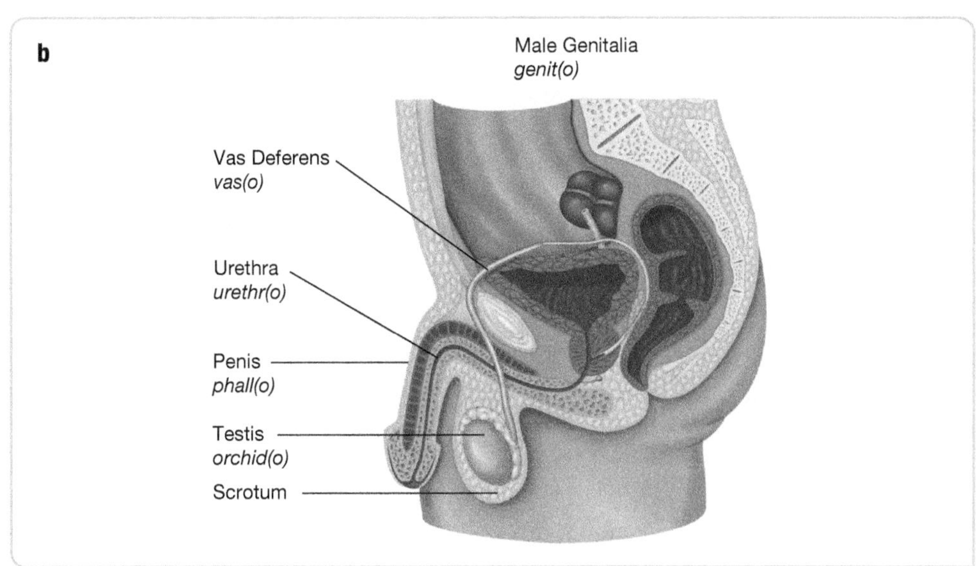

Fig. 5.13(b) The Male Reproductive System. This figure shows parts of the male reproductive system. *What word root refers to the male reproductive system?*

Reproductive System Terms

WORD ROOT	MEDICAL TERM	DEFINITION
andr/o	android	resembling a (male) human
cervic/o	cervicitis	inflammation of the cervix
galact/o	galactorrhea	abnormal discharge of milk
hyster/o	hysterectomy	removal of the uterus
men/o	dysmenorrhea	painful menstruation
nat/i	neonatal	pertaining to newborn

Reproductive System

ABBREVIATION	MEANING
AB	abortion
AFP	alpha-fetoprotein
BSE	breast self-exam
C-section, CS	cesarean section
D&C	dilation and curettage
EDC	expected date of confinement (birth)
GU	genitourinary
GYN	gynecology
LMP	last menstrual period
STD	sexually transmitted-disease

SECTION 5.4 Organ Systems Review

AFTER YOU READ

1. **Choose** and define one medical term from each organ system.
2. **Create** one new medical term for each of the organ systems.
3. **Identify** one medical abbreviation related to each system.
4. **Indicate** which parts of the body are affected by the following disorders: appendicitis, cervicitis, colitis, and tonsillitis.
5. **Identify** which part of the body is the root of the word *glossary*.

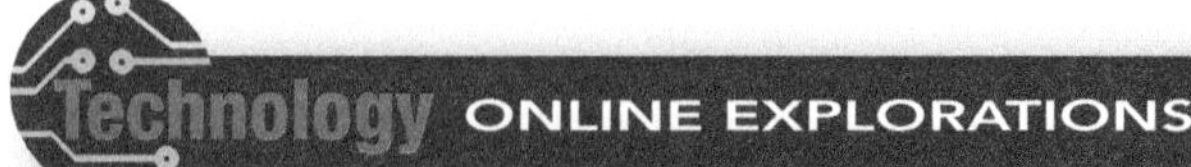

Explore a System

Select a system of the body to explore further. Go online to find two new abbreviations and two new medical terms used to describe the system you selected.

SECTION 5.5 Medical Abbreviations

Medical Abbreviations

What are some of the other medical abbreviations used in healthcare?

Many abbreviations are used in healthcare that are not directly related to the systems of the body. They are part of the physician's orders, a medication prescription, or a patient's chart. Abbreviations may be letters of the words they represent. Sometimes medical abbreviations are derived from Latin or Greek terms.

For example:

tsp. = **tea**s**p**oon

q.d. = every day (Latin: ***q**uaque* ***d**ie*)

Be careful when using abbreviations. If carelessly handwritten, they can result in errors, especially medication errors. For this reason, The Joint Commission (TJC) and the Institute for Safe Medication Practice (ISMP) have identified frequently misinterpreted abbreviations and symbols that have contributed to harmful medication errors. TJC and ISMP are two healthcare organizations whose mission includes promotion of patient safety. An example of an error-prone abbreviation is U (for unit). When handwritten, U can be mistaken for a zero, potentially leading to a drug overdose. See **Table 5.1** below and in Appendix B for examples of abbreviations.

Vocabulary

Academic Vocabulary

You will see this word in your reading and on your tests. Find its meaning in the Glossary in the back of the book.

- **derive**

21ST CENTURY SKILLS

Communication

Electronic Health Records

Electronic health records (EHRs) help to reduce the chance of medication and other medical errors. The risk of misinterpreting a medical term or abbreviation is reduced because all of the terms are entered electronically or selected from a predetermined list within the healthcare records. Although they are not to be handwritten, in some cases you may see "do not use" or "error prone" abbreviations that are preprinted or used in EHRs.

Table 5.1 Commonly Used Medical Abbreviations

ABBREVIATION	MEANING	ABBREVIATION	MEANING
@	at	BE	barium enema
AA	Alcoholics Anonymous	BID, b.i.d., bid	twice a day
a.c.	before meals, usually one-half hour preceding meals	BM	bowel movement
abd	abdomen, abdominal	BMI	body mass index
ACLS	Advanced cardiac life support	BP	blood pressure
ad lib	freely, as often as desired	BR	bed rest
am, AM	morning	BRP	bathroom privileges
amb.	ambulate, ambulatory	Bx, Bx	biopsy
Ax	axillary (armpit)		

ABB	MEANING	ABB	MEANING	ABB	MEANING
CA, Ca	carcinoma (cancer)	Fx, fx	fracture	K+, K	potassium
cap.	capsule	g, gm	gram	mcg	microgram
CC	chief complaint	gt, gtt	drop, drops	mg	milligram
cc	cubic centimeter	h	hour	N&V	nausea and vomiting
disc, DC, d.c.	discontinue	H_2O	water	Na, Na+	sodium
DNR	Do not resuscitate.	HBV	hepatitis B virus	NC	nasal cannula
drg, drsg, dsg	dressing	HIPAA	Health Insurance Portability and Accountability ACT	NA	Narcotics Anonymous
Dx, dx	diagnosis	h.s.	hour of sleep (at bedtime)	NPO	nothing by mouth
ED	emergency department	Ht., ht	height	NPO p MN	nothing by mouth past midnight
EHR	electronic health records	inj.	injection	oint., ung	ointment
ER	emergency room	I and O, I/O	intake and output	OOB	out of bed
Fvo	fever unknown origin	IV	intravenous (through a vein)	OTC	over the counter

For additional medical abbreviations and commonly-used medical symbols, see Appendix B.

SECTION 5.5 Medical Abbreviations Review

AFTER YOU READ

1. **Write** the following sentences in long form, eliminating all the abbreviations:
   a) The patient had **COPD** and was taking a **Rx bid.** He was having his **VS** done **q4h.** He will have a **CXR** done **stat** if he develops **SOB.**
   b) After the patient had an **ECG** it was discovered he needed a **CABG** done and was placed in the **CCU** to have his **BP** and **TPR** monitored **q.h.**
   c) The patient had an incomplete **AB** and required a **D&C.** After that she had difficulty having a **BM** and was **Dx** with **CA.**
2. **Identify** three places where medical abbreviations might be used.
3. **Examine** the possible consequences of using carelessly written medical abbreviations.
4. **Assess** the greatest benefit of using electronic health records (EHRs).
5. **Indicate** the meaning of "DNR" on a patient's medical chart.

Technology ONLINE EXPLORATIONS

ISMP and TJC Research

Visit the website of The Joint Commission (www.jointcommission.org) or the Institute for Safe Medication Practices (www.ismp.org) and find the latest list of Do Not Use or Error-Prone Abbreviations. Use this list as a reference while working in the healthcare profession.

CHAPTER 5 Review

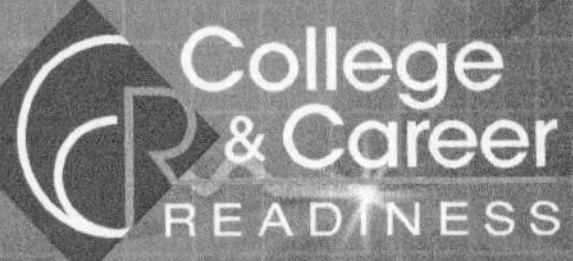

Chapter Summary

SECTION 5.1

- Medical terminology consists of word roots that are the basic meaning of the medical term. When a word root ends in a vowel, it is a combining form. Prefixes and suffixes modify the word root. **(p. 106)**
- In order to create and define medical terminology, you must break each term into its parts and define each part. "Read" each medical term using these steps:
  1. Start with the suffix (the word ending); define the suffix.
  2. Go to the prefix (the beginning of the word); define the prefix.
  3. Go to the middle of the word; define the word root, combining form, or both, if both exist in the same word.
  4. Combine the definitions of the word parts to decode the complete medical term or phrase. **(p. 107)**

SECTION 5.2

- When you are building compound words, you should always remember that combining forms are used between word roots. **(p. 110)**
- To build medical terms, all you need to do is place a prefix, root word (combining form) and suffix in the correct order to build the term. **(p. 111)**

SECTION 5.3

- Other frequently used word parts include suffixes, prefixes, plural forms, roots, descriptive terms, directional terms, and word parts relating to colors and numbers. **(p. 112)**
- Word parts are often combined to represent the major organ systems. When using medical abbreviations related to body systems remember "When in doubt, spell it out." **(p. 113)**

SECTION 5.4

- The body is made up of several major organ systems. There are a number of word parts that represent each of those systems and the organs and components in those systems. These word parts are used to describe diseases and conditions related to each system. **(p. 115)**
- Each body system has a number of related abbreviations pertaining to that system. **(p. 115)**

SECTION 5.5

- Medical abbreviations are derived from the letters of the word they represent or from the Greek or Latin form of the word. **(p. 127)**

CHAPTER **5 Assessment**

Critical Thinking/Problem Solving

1. You have read a diagnostic medical term in a client's chart and have knowledge regarding the client's condition. How will you respond if the client asks you the meaning of the medical term?

2. Your best friend's mother just had a mammogram and was diagnosed with fibrocystic disease. After the examination she became upset and developed rhinitis. The next week she had a Bx and the M.D. told her to do a BSE. Can you tell your friend what happened to her mother in simpler terms?

21ST CENTURY SKILLS

3. **Teamwork** Obtain copies of the "Review of Systems" portion of a client's chart. Make sure that the names are removed before you begin. With a partner or in a group, write the "Review of Systems" section in simple terms, defining all of the medical terms and abbreviations.

4. **Communication** Select two prefixes, two suffixes, and four word roots, and with a partner or group build as many medical terms as you can. Write each word on the front of a card and its definition on the back. Use these cards as a class review for a test or to play word-building games in a game-show format, such as *Jeopardy!*.

5. **Information literacy** Explore the National Health Information Center's (NHIC) website. Look for references to diseases in the new items posted at the site. You may also use your local newspaper or a magazine. See if you can recognize word roots, combining forms, prefixes, and suffixes within the information. Relate the information that you find about diseases to specific body systems. Share your results with the class.

connect™ ONLINE ACTIVITIES

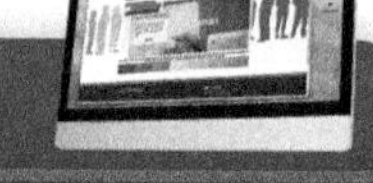

Complete our HST online activities for Chapter 5, which include Concept Check review questions, Reference Flash Cards, and Online Procedures assessment sheets.

- **Concept Check** review questions
- **Reference Flash Cards** medical terminology practice
- **Online Procedures** assessment sheets

CHAPTER 6

Human Structure and Function

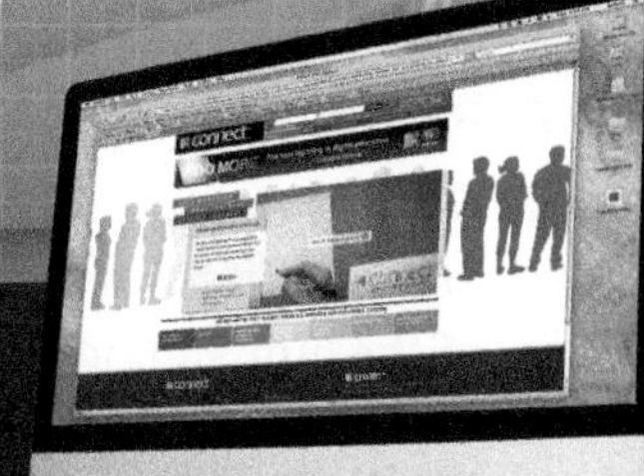

Essential Question:

How do the organs and systems in my body work together?

To understand how the human body works, it is necessary to understand its systems. The smallest element of the body is the cell; a group of cells makes tissue; various tissues make organs; and a group of organs makes a system. This chapter introduces thirteen systems: integumentary, skeletal, muscular, nervous, sensory (or special senses), circulatory, lymphatic, immune, respiratory, digestive, urinary, endocrine, and reproductive.

McGraw Hill connect™

It's Online!

- Online Procedures
- Anatomy Activities
- STEM Connection
- Medical Science
- Medical Terms
- Medical Math
- Ethics in Action
- Virtual Lab

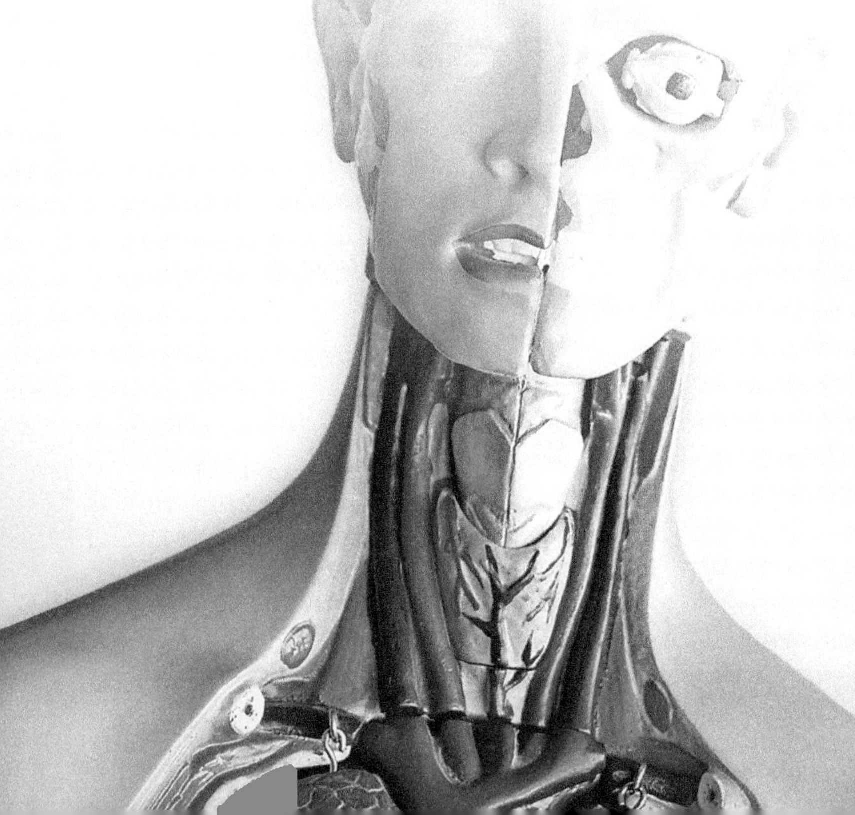

READING GUIDE

OBJECTIVES

After completing this chapter, you will be able to:

- **Categorize** the structural and functional organization of the human body.
- **Identify** body planes, directional terms, quadrants, and cavities.
- **Describe** the organs of the integumentary, skeletal, muscular, nervous, special senses, circulatory, lymphatic, immunue, respiratory, digestive, urinary, endocrine, and reproductive systems.
- **Indicate** the functions of the integumentary, skeletal, muscular, nervous, special senses, circulatory, lymphatic, immune, respiratory, digestive, urinary, endocrine, and reproductive systems.
- **Distinguish** the structure and functions of the body systems.

BEFORE YOU READ

Connect Can you describe how the human body is structured and the systems it includes?

Main Idea

Students will understand the structural and functional organization and identify the major organs and systems of the human body.

Note-Taking Activity

Draw this table. Write key terms and phrases under **Cues.** Write main ideas under **Note Taking**. Summarize the section under **Summary**.

Cues	Note Taking
o	o
o	o
Summary	

Graphic Organizer

Before you read the chapter, draw a diagram like the one below. As you read, write the human body systems covered by the chapter into the diagram.

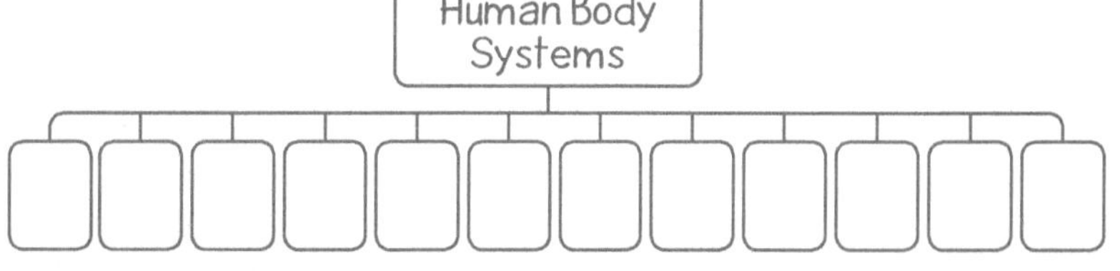

connect

Downloadable graphic organizers can be accessed online.

STANDARDS

HEALTH SCIENCE

NCHSE 1.11 Classify the basic structural and functional organization of the human body (tissue, organ, and system).

NCHSE 1.12 Recognize body planes, directional terms, quadrants, and cavities.

SCIENCE

NSES C Develop understanding of the cell; molecular basis of heredity; biological evolution; interdependence of organisms; matter, energy, and organization in living systems; and behavior of organisms.

NCHSE *National Consortium for Health Science Education*

NSES *National Science Education Standards*

COMMON CORE STATE STANDARDS

MATHEMATICS

Number and Quantity

Quantities N-Q3 Choose a level of accuracy appropriate to limitations on measurement when reporting quantities.

ENGLISH LANGUAGE ARTS

Language

Vocabulary Acquisition and Use L-5 Demonstrate understanding of figurative language, word relationships, and nuances in word meanings.

Reading

Range of Reading and Level of Text Complexity R-10 By the end of grade 12, read and comprehend science/technical texts in the grades 11–CCR text complexity band independently and proficiently.

SECTION
6.1 Understanding the Human Body

Overview

How is your body organized?

Our bodies are amazingly complex! This chapter explains how our bodies' many systems work together.

The organization, as shown in **Figure 6.1,** begins with the smallest element, the cell, and extends to a collection of systems. In other words, the organization starts out with the simple and proceeds to the complex:

- Cells are made up of chemicals that combine to form tissue.
- Tissues are specialized cells that function together to form organs.
- Organs work cooperatively to form systems.
- Systems work together to make up the human body.

Vocabulary

Content Vocabulary

You will learn this content vocabulary term in this section.

- **respiration**

Academic Vocabulary

You will see these words in your reading and on your tests. Find their meanings in the Glossary in the back of this book.

- **function**
- **structures**
- **regions**

Cells

What substance performs the work of the cell?

The body is made up of cells that vary in size, shape, and function. All cells need food, water, and oxygen to live and function. The basic structures of cells are the cell membrane, nucleus, and cytoplasm:

- The membrane is the outer covering of the cell. It holds the cell together and helps to maintain cell shape.
- The nucleus is the central portion of the cell. It directs cell activities and contains chromosomes, which are the bearers of genes. Genes determine traits such as eye color, height, hereditary diseases, and gender. Chromosomes are made of deoxyribonucleic acid (DNA), which contains the genetic information. **Figure 6.2** on page 134 shows a cell with its chromosomes.
- All cells have a nucleus, with the exception of the red blood cells (RBC). Those cells are enucleated, which means they do not have a nucleus.
- The cytoplasm surrounds the nucleus. The cytoplasm is the substance that performs the work of the cell, such as reproduction and movement.

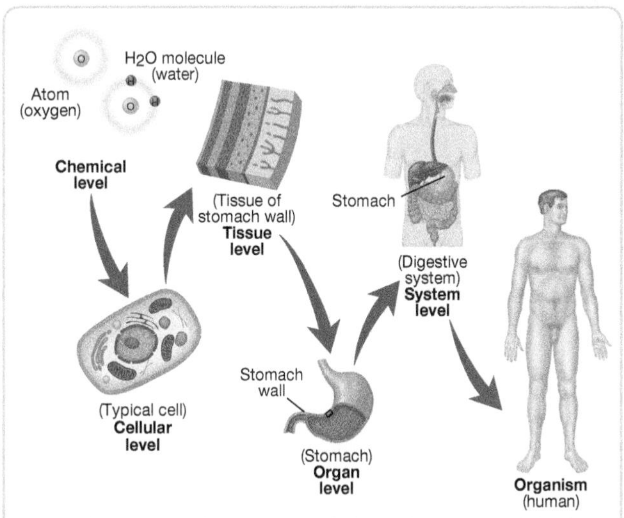

Fig. 6.1 Organization The body's many systems all work together. *What is unique about each system of the body?*

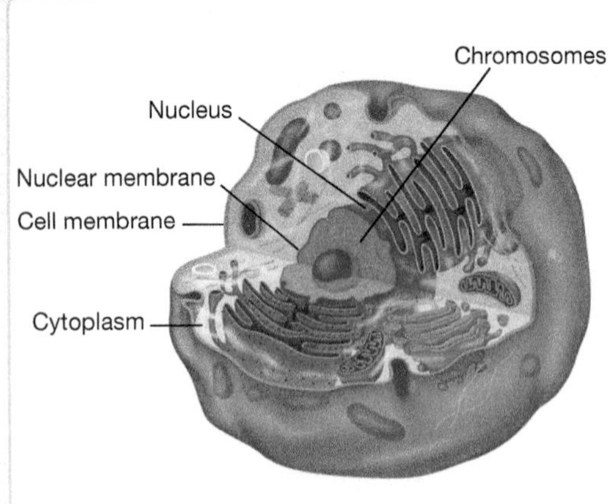

Fig. 6.2 Cell Structure This is the composition of a cell. *What is the function of the chromosomes found in the cell?*

Cell Types

All cells have special functions, which are influenced by their shape. There are several different cell types, whose shape and function are adapted to meet a specific need, for example:

- Nerve cells usually have long, thin extensions that can transmit nerve impulses over a distance.
- Epithelial cells are thin, flat, and tightly packed, forming a protective layer over underlying cells.
- Muscle cells are slender rods that attach at the ends of the structures they move.

READING CHECK

List what cells need to live and function.

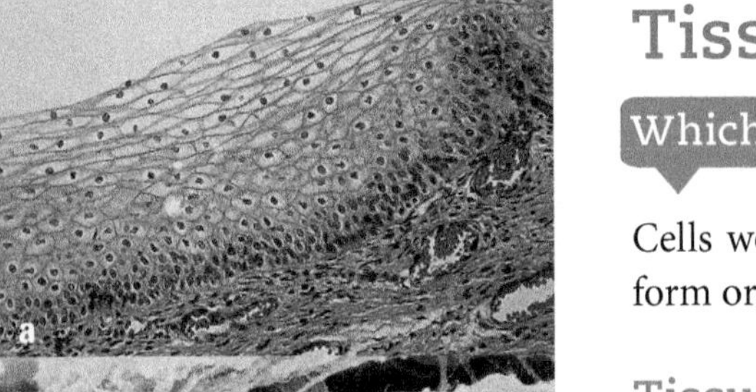

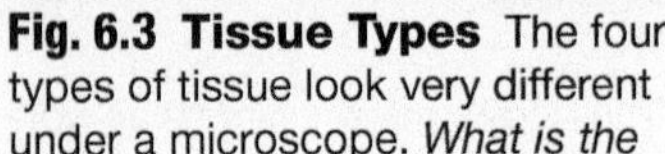

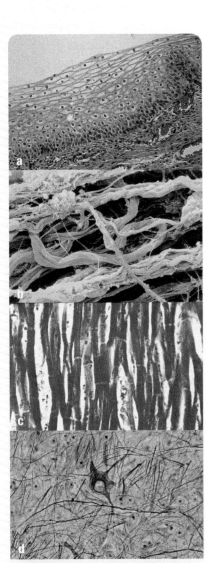

Fig. 6.3 Tissue Types The four types of tissue look very different under a microscope. *What is the function of epithelial tissue?*

Tissues and Organs

Which type of tissue expands and contracts?

Cells work together to become tissues, and tissues work together to form organs.

Tissues

Groups of cells that work together to perform the same task are called tissue. As shown, the body has four types of tissue:

- Connective tissue (see **Figure 6.3a**) holds body parts such as bones, ligaments, and tendons together and connects them.
- Epithelial tissue (see **Figure 6.3b**) covers the internal and external body surfaces. The skin and linings of internal organs, such as the intestines, are epithelial tissue.
- Muscle tissue (see **Figure 6.3c**) expands and contracts, allowing the body to move.
- Nervous tissue (see **Figure 6.3d**) carries messages from all parts of the body to and from the brain and spinal cord.

Organs

Groups of tissue that work together to perform a specific function are called organs. Examples include

- the kidneys, which maintain water and salt balance in the blood.
- the stomach, which breaks down food into substances that the circulatory system can transport throughout the body as nourishment for its cells.

READING CHECK

Name the four types of tissue.

Photos: (t to b)Biophoto Associates/Science Source/Photo Researchers, Prof. P. Motta, Dept. of Anatomy, University "La Sapienza," Rome/Science Photo Library/Photo Researchers, Michael Abbey/Photo Researchers, Biophoto Associates/Photo Researchers

Systems

Which system regulates most body activities?

Groups of organs working together to perform one of the body's major functions are called a system. Systems have separate and distinct functions, but they rely on one another to perform their tasks. The systems of the body are:

- The integumentary system consists of the skin and the accessory structures, which are hair, nails, sweat glands, and oil glands. The skin is the largest organ and serves to cover and protect our body.
- The musculoskeletal system supports and protects the body and is the body's framework. It also provides body movement. It consists of bones, muscles, and cartilage. Without bones and muscles, we would not be able to stand or move.
- The nervous system consists of the brain, spinal cord, and peripheral nerves. The nervous system regulates most body activities and sends and receives messages from the sensory organs.
- The special senses system includes the eyes, the ears, and the parts of other systems that are involved in the reactions of the senses. This is also known as the sensory system.
- The circulatory system consists of the heart and blood vessels, which pump and transport blood throughout the body. The blood carries oxygen and nutrients to the tissues and removes waste from the tissues through the circulatory system.
- The lymphatic and immune systems consist of the lymph, the glands of the lymphatic system, the lymphatic vessels, and the nonspecific and specific defenses of the immune system. These systems help protect the body from infection and disease.
- The respiratory system consists of the lungs and the airways, which perform **respiration** to supply the body oxygen.
- The digestive system is all the organs of digestion, absorption of nutrients, and elimination of waste. The digestive system is necessary for the normal intake of food and water into our body.
- The urinary system consists of the kidneys, ureters, bladder, and urethra. It eliminates metabolic waste, helps to maintain the acid-base and water-salt balance, and helps regulate blood pressure.
- The endocrine system consists of the glands that secrete hormones for the regulation of many of the body's activities.
- The reproductive system controls reproduction and heredity. The female reproductive system includes the ovaries, vagina, fallopian tubes, uterus, and mammary glands, or breasts. The male reproductive system includes the testes, penis, prostate gland, vas deferens, and seminal vesicles.

READING CHECK

Describe the main purpose of the circulatory system.

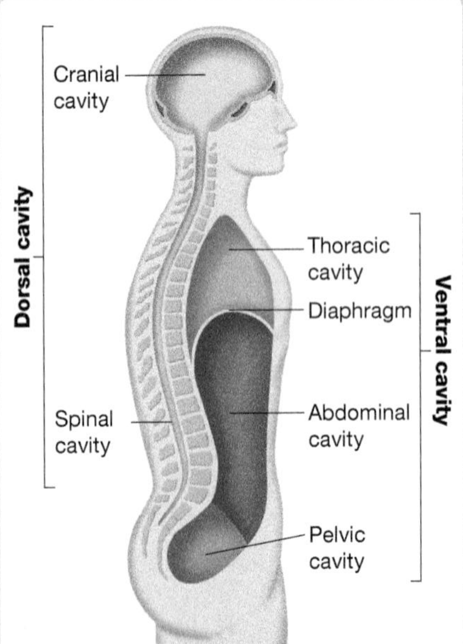

Fig. 6.4 Body Cavities The two main body cavities are the dorsal and the ventral. *Which organs are found within the dorsal cavity?*

Body Cavities

Which organ separates the two parts of the ventral cavity?

Seen in **Figure 6.4,** the body has two main cavities, or spaces:

- The dorsal cavity, on the back side of the body, contains the cranial cavity, which holds the brain, and the spinal cavity, which holds the spinal cord.
- The ventral cavity, on the front side of the body, is divided in two by a muscle called the diaphragm. Above the diaphragm is the thoracic cavity, holding the heart, lungs, and major blood vessels. Below the diaphragm is the abdominal cavity, holding the organs of the digestive and urinary systems. The bottom portion of the abdominal cavity, called the pelvic cavity, contains the reproductive system.

Directions, Planes, Regions

How many planes divide the body?

Special terms are used to identify areas of the body. They are based upon anatomical position, when the body is standing erect, facing forward, with the arms at the sides and the palms facing forward.

Directional terms refer to a path going to or from the body or a path that is related to another part of the body. Body planes are imaginary lines that divide the body into sections. Regions of the body are also identified using special names.

Directional Terms

Directional terms locate a portion of the body or describe a position of the body. **Figure 6.5** illustrates directional terms for the body, including frequently used terms and their definitions:

- Anterior, or ventral: the front side of the body
- Posterior, or dorsal: the back side of the body
- Inferior: below another structure
- Superior: above another structure
- Lateral: to the side. For example, the eyes are lateral to the nose.
- Medial: middle or near the medial plane of the body
- Deep: through the surface, as in a deep cut
- Superficial: on or near the surface, as with a scratch on the skin
- Proximal: near the point of attachment to the trunk
- Distal: away from the point of attachment to the trunk
- Supine: lying on one's spine, facing upward
- Prone: lying on one's stomach, facing downward

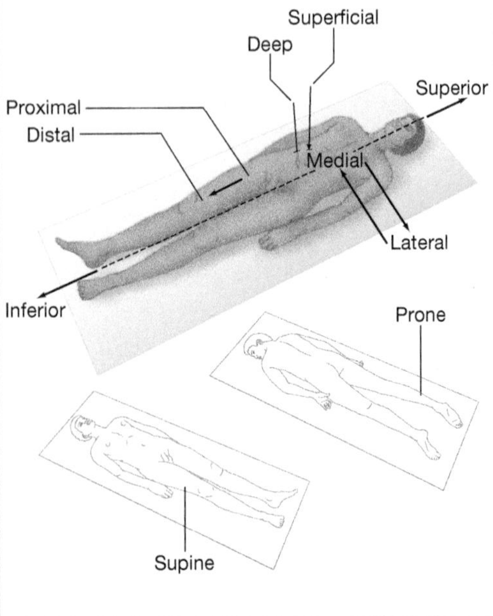

Fig. 6.5 Directional Terms Directional terms refer to locations on or positions of the body. *What is one example of the directional term "superior"? Of the term "inferior"?*

Planes of the Body

In order to visualize the various body structures in relationship to each other, three imaginary planes divide the body. These planes cut through the body in different directions.

- The sagittal plane divides the body into two parts, right and left. If it divides the body into equal right and left parts, as shown in **Figure 6.6,** it is called the midsagittal plane.
- The frontal, or coronal, plane divides the body into anterior and posterior sections.
- The transverse plane divides the body horizontally into a top, or superior, part and a bottom, or inferior, part.

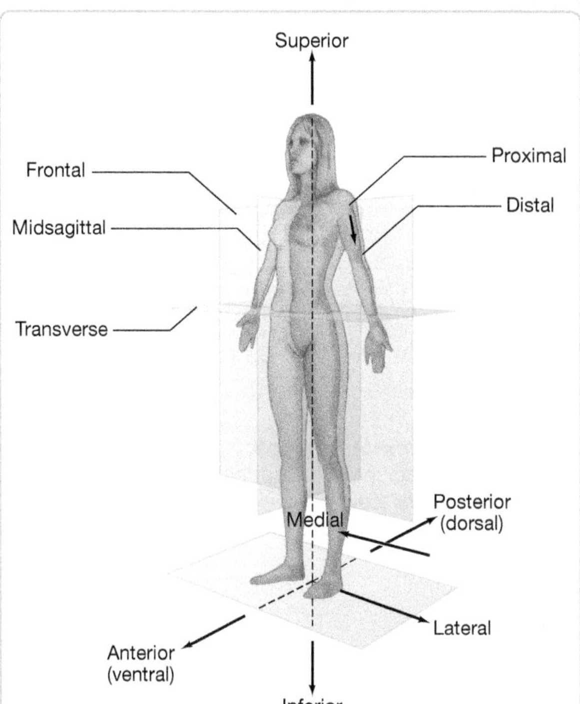

Fig. 6.6 Sagittal Plane The sagittal plane divides the body into two parts. *How does the midsagittal plane divide the body?*

Regions of the Abdominal Cavity

Because the abdominal cavity is so large, it is helpful to divide it into nine regions, as shown in **Figure 6.7** on page 138. This is done for many reasons. For example, regions are used to describe the location of an organ, injury, or pain.

connect ONLINE PROCEDURES

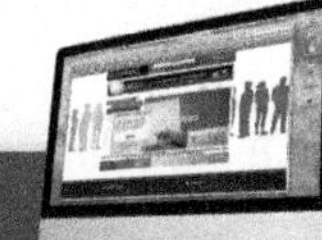

PROCEDURE 6-1

Identifying Organs and Body Quadrants

Because the abdominal cavity is so large it is helpful to divide it into four quadrants. These quadrants are helpful when describing the injury or pain, or the location of an organ.

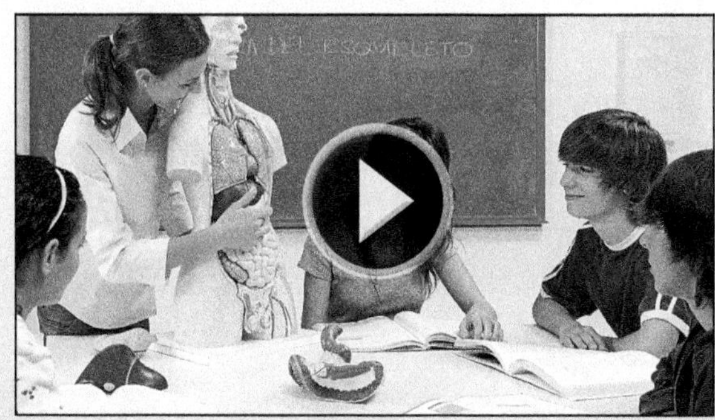

PROCEDURE 6-2

Recognizing Body Systems

Groups of organs working together to perform one of the body's major functions are called a "system." Systems have separate and distinct functions, but they rely on one another to perform their tasks.

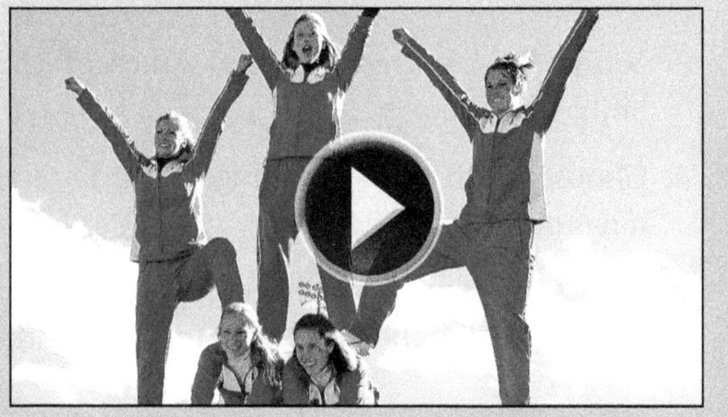

Photos: (t)Image Source/Alamy, (b)U.S. Air Force photo by Danny Meyer

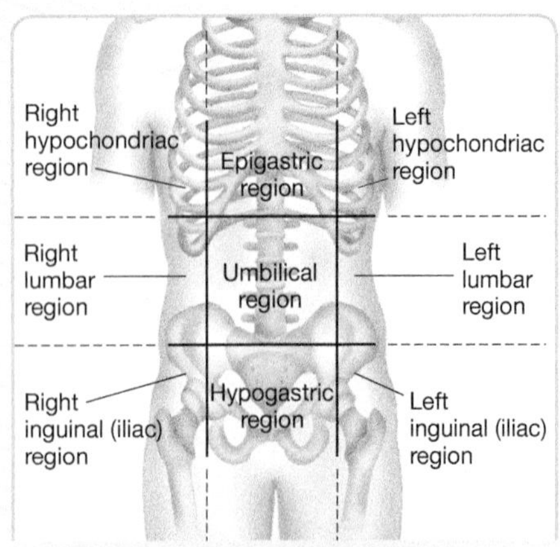

Fig. 6.7 Abdominal Regions These are the regions of the abdominal cavity. *How many ways are there to divide the abdomen for medical purposes?*

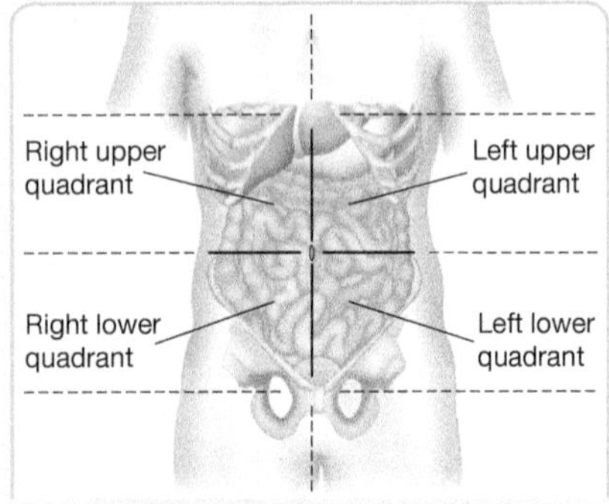

Fig. 6.8 Abdominal Quadrants There are 4 abdominal quadrants. *Name two of the organs found in each quadrant.*

The nine regions of the abdominal cavity are:

- Epigastric region, the area above the stomach
- Hypochondriac regions (left and right), the two regions just below ribs, immediately over the abdomen
- Umbilical region, the region surrounding the umbilicus (navel)
- Lumbar regions (left and right), the two regions near the waist
- Hypogastric region, the area just below the umbilical region
- Iliac, or inguinal, regions (left and right), the two regions near the upper portion of the hipbone

A simpler way to divide the abdominal cavity is into four quadrants, as shown in **Figure 6.8.**

- Right upper quadrant (RUQ), on the right anterior side; contains part of the liver, the gallbladder, and parts of the pancreas and intestinal tract
- Right lower quadrant (RLQ), on the right anterior side; contains the appendix, parts of the intestines, reproductive organs in the female, and urinary tract
- Left upper quadrant (LUQ), on the left anterior side; contains the stomach, spleen, and parts of the liver, pancreas, and intestines
- Left lower quadrant (LLQ), on the left anterior side; contains parts of the intestines, reproductive organs in the female, and urinary tract.

READING CHECK

Identify the region above the stomach.

SECTION 6.1 Understanding the Human Body Review

AFTER YOU READ

1. **Explain** how the human body is organized, starting with the simplest structure.
2. **Name** the cavities and the planes of the body.
3. **Choose** which of the following is superior: the lungs or the intestines.
4. **Choose** which of the following is more distal: the wrist or the shoulder.
5. **Identify** where your stomach is located: abdominal cavity, left upper quadrant, or left hypochondriac region.

Technology ONLINE EXPLORATIONS

Chromosomes

Research online the purpose of chromosomes. Identify three ways in which knowledge of chromosomes is used in medical science.

SECTION

6.2 The Integumentary System

The Skin

What determines the thickness of skin?

An integument is a covering. The integumentary system includes the skin, hair, nails, sweat glands, and oil-producing glands. **Figure 6.9** shows the integumentary system.

The skin is the largest body organ. The average adult has about 21.5 square feet of skin. The skin has the following functions:

- Protects the body from injury
- Protects the body from the intrusion of harmful microorganisms
- Protects the body from the ultraviolet (UV) rays of the sun
- Helps to maintain the proper internal temperature of the body
- Serves as a site for excretion of waste through perspiration
- Serves as an important sensory organ

The skin varies in thickness, depending on the part of the body it covers and its function in covering that part. For example, the skin on the upper back is about ten times thicker than the skin on the eyelid. The eyelid skin must be light, flexible, and movable, so it is thin. The skin on the upper back must cover and move with large muscle groups and bones, so it is thick to provide strength and protection.

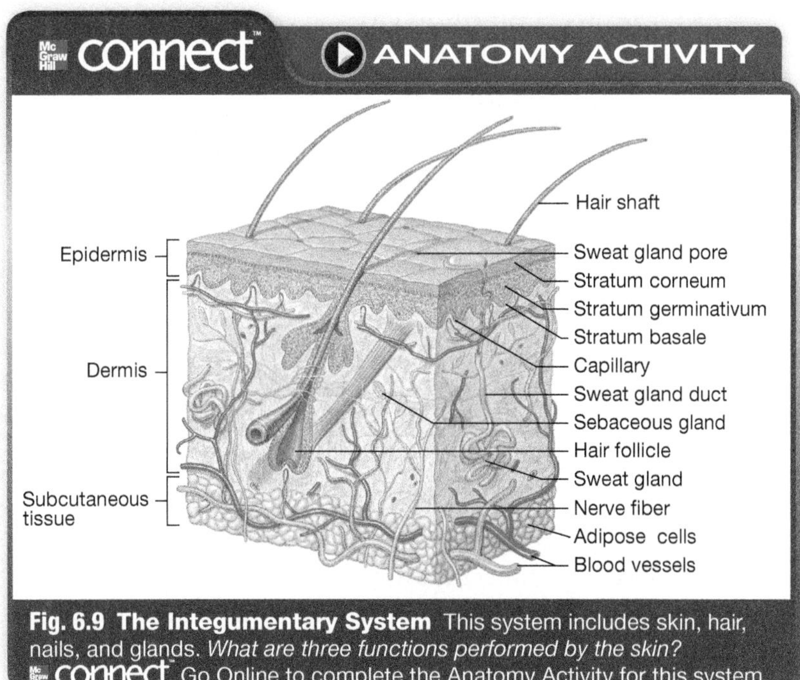

Fig. 6.9 The Integumentary System This system includes skin, hair, nails, and glands. *What are three functions performed by the skin?*
connect Go Online to complete the Anatomy Activity for this system.

Vocabulary

Content Vocabulary

You will learn these content vocabulary terms in this section.

- **epidermis**
- **dermis**
- **subcutaneous layer**

Academic Vocabulary

You will see this word in your reading and on your tests. Find its meaning in the Glossary in the back of this book.

- **flexible**

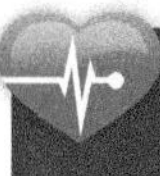

Preventive Care & Wellness

Sun Safety

The incidence of skin cancer is rapidly increasing due to overexposure to the sun. The FDA recommends Seven Steps to Safer Sunning:

- Stay in the shade. Avoid the hottest sun from 10 A.M. to 4 P.M.
- Always use sunscreen products that have a sun protection factor (SPF) on the label of at least 15.
- Wear a brimmed hat that shades the neck, ears, eyes, and head.
- Wear sunglasses with a label indicating that they block 99 to 100 percent of the sun's rays.
- Wear loose, lightweight, long-sleeved shirts and long pants or long skirts.
- Avoid artificial tanning methods.
- Check your skin regularly for signs of skin cancer.

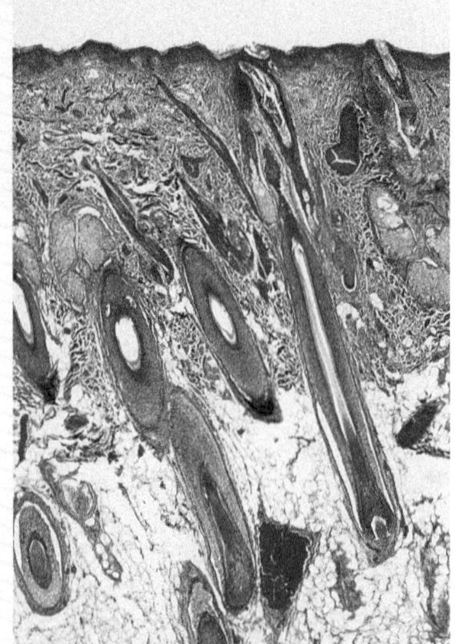

Fig. 6.10 Hair Follicles Tiny muscles called arrector pili attached to this hair follicle contract to cause goose bumps. *What triggers this contraction?*

Parts of the Skin

The skin has three main parts, or layers:

- The **epidermis** is the outer layer of skin and consists of several sublayers. The two main sublayers are the stratum corneum and the stratum germinativum. The stratum corneum is the top sublayer. It consists of a flat layer of dead cells arranged in parallel rows. As new cells are produced, the dead cells are sloughed off. The stratum germinativum is the bottom sublayer of the epidermis. Here, new cells are produced and pushed up to the stratum corneum. Specialized cells in the epidermis produce a pigment called melanin, which helps determine skin and hair color. It is essential in screening out the sun's UV rays, overexposure to which causes skin cancer.
- The **dermis** contains connective tissue that holds many capillaries, lymph cells, nerve endings, sebaceous and sweat glands, and hair follicles. These nourish the epidermis and serve as sensitive touch receptors. The papillary layer, or top layer of the dermis, fits into ridges on the stratum germinativum to form lines that are unique to each individual. On the fingers, these lines are known as fingerprints.
- Skin shade changes based upon the amount of oxygenated blood in the dermis. Oxygen is carried by a pigment in the red blood cells called hemoglobin. Hemoglobin with lots of oxygen will be bright red. Hemoglobin with less oxygen will be a darker red color. When a person has a lot of oxygen in his or her blood, the skin will have a pinkish hue. If the supply of oxygen in the blood is low, the skin will look pale or bluish.
- The **subcutaneous layer** is the layer between the dermis and the body's inner organs. It consists of fatty tissue and some layers of fibrous tissue. Within the subcutaneous layers lie blood vessels and nerves. The layer of fatty tissue serves to protect the inner organs and to maintain the body's temperature.

READING CHECK

Explain the functions of the dermis.

Other Parts of the Integumentary System

What are the sebaceous glands?

Hair

Hair grows from the epidermis to cover various parts of the body. It serves to cushion and protect the areas it covers. Hair has two parts: the shaft (above the skin) and the root (beneath the skin surface). Hair grows upward from the root through the hair follicles (**Figure 6.10**). Most hair follicles have an arrector pili muscle. When you get cold or nervous these muscles contract, causing goose bumps to form.

The shape of the follicle determines the shape of the hair, which can be straight, wavy, or curly. Hair color is determined by the presence of melanin. Gray hair occurs with aging, when we stop producing melanin. These hair characteristics are generally determined by heredity. Baldness, or alopecia, may be caused by heredity, or it may result from disease, injury, or medical treatments such as chemotherapy (see **Figure 6.11**).

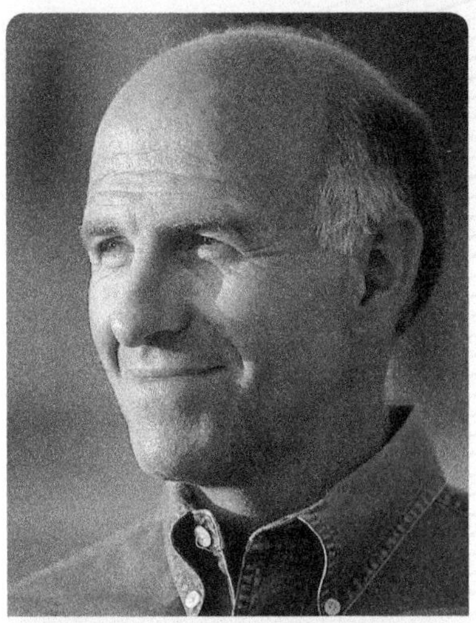

Fig. 6.11 Baldness This is a man with baldness, or alopecia. *What is the usual cause of alopecia?*

READING CHECK

Identify what determines the color of hair.

Nails

Nails are plates made of hard keratin that cover the dorsal surface of the distal bone of the fingers and toes. Nails serve as a protective covering, help us grasp objects, and allow us to scratch. Healthy nails appear pinkish; the whitish half-moon at the base is called the lunula. The cuticle is a narrow band of epidermis that surrounds nails on three sides. **Figure 6.12** shows the parts of a nail.

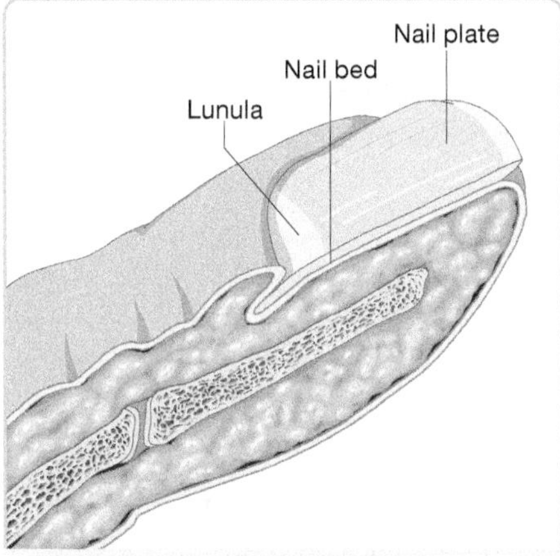

Fig. 6.12 Section of a Nail The lunula is at the base of the nail and looks like a half moon. *What purposes do nails serve?*

Sweat and Sebaceous Glands

Sweat glands are also called sudoriferous glands. They are found almost everywhere on the surface of the body. Sweating provides a means for the body to cool itself. These glands, which secrete outward toward the surface of the body through ducts, are called exocrine glands. The excretion of sweat is called diaphoresis. Secretions exit the body through pores or tiny openings in the skin surface.

Sebaceous glands, located in the dermis, secrete an oily substance called sebum. Sebum is found at the base of the hair follicles. This substance lubricates and protects the skin. Sebum forms a skin barrier against bacteria and fungi and also softens the surface of the skin.

SECTION 6.2 The Integumentary System Review

AFTER YOU READ

1. **Name** the organs that make up the integumentary system.
2. **Compare** the three layers of the skin.
3. **List** the functions of the skin.
4. **Identify** some of the ways an individual can avoid getting skin cancer.
5. **Explain** what might cause an individual to have dark brown, curly hair.

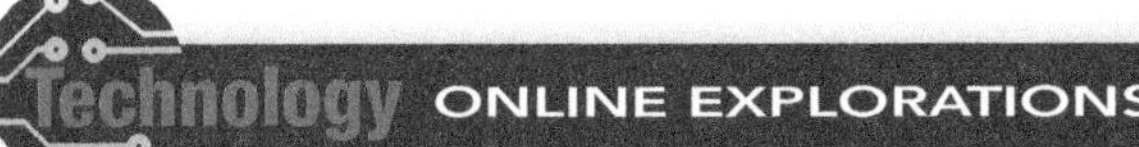

Sizing Up the Skin

The skin is considered our largest organ. Research online to learn more about the size of the skin and its size compared to other organs in the body.

Photo: Frank Siteman/Stock Boston

SECTION

6.3 The Skeletal System

Vocabulary

Content Vocabulary

You will learn these content vocabulary terms in this section.

- **osteocytes**
- **ossification**

Academic Vocabulary

You will see this word in your reading and on your tests. Find its meaning in the Glossary in the back of this book.

- **framework**

Overview of the Skeletal System

What nutrient is stored by the bones?

A newborn baby has over 300 bones. Some of these bones fuse later, leaving the mature adult with only 206 bones in his or her skeleton. **Figure 6.13** shows the bones of the skeleton. The skeletal system consists of bones and joints, which serve the following purposes:

- Provide a framework for the body
- Protect vital organs like the brain and spinal cord
- Serve as levers, when muscles are attached, to help us lift and move

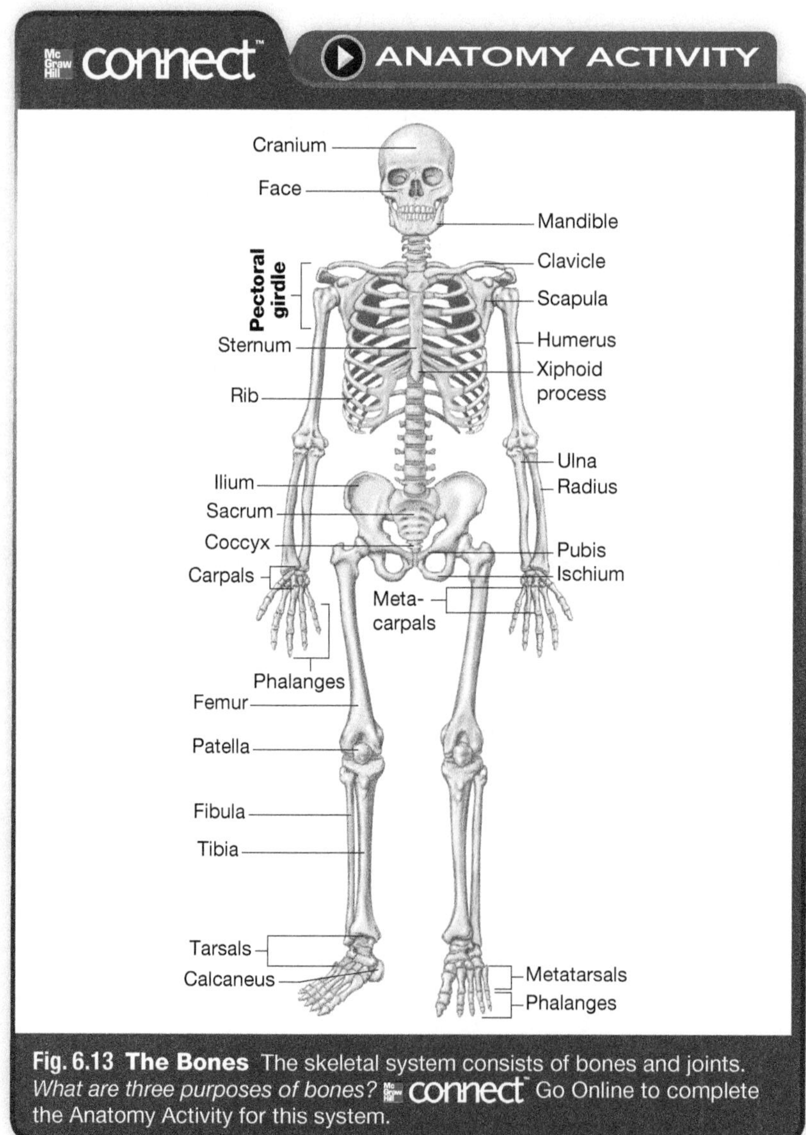

Fig. 6.13 The Bones The skeletal system consists of bones and joints. *What are three purposes of bones?* connect Go Online to complete the Anatomy Activity for this system.

- Store calcium, which may be reabsorbed into the blood if there is not enough calcium in the diet
- Produce blood cells in the red bone marrow

READING CHECK

Explain why a baby has more bones than an adult.

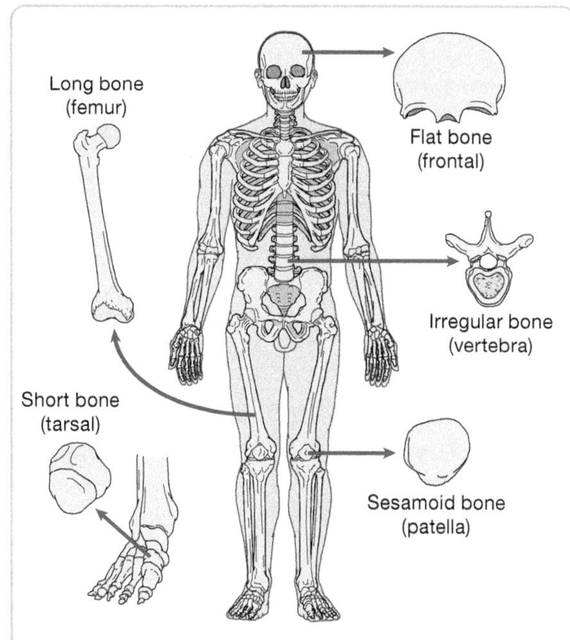

Fig. 6.14 Classification of Bone by Shape Five different classes of bone are recognized according to shape – long, short, flat, irregular, and sesamoid. *What type of bone are the bones of the face?*

Types of Bones

What purposes do flat bones serve?

As shown in **Figure 6.14,** the five most common categories of bones are long, short, flat, irregular, and sesamoid.

Long Bones

Long bones form legs and arms. As shown in **Figure 6.15,** they include the humerus and femur. The shaft is the longest part of long bones. The outer part is compact bone. It is solid and does not bend easily. Oxygen and nutrients come from the bloodstream to compact bone.

Another name for the shaft is diaphysis. Each end of the shaft, or epiphysis, is shaped to connect to other bones by ligaments and muscles. The epiphysis is covered by cartilage to protect the bone at movable points.

Inside the compact bone is spongy bone that covers the space in which marrow is stored. There is also spongy bone in the epiphyses. The medullary cavity has a lining called the endosteum. A fibrous membrane called the periosteum covers the outside of the bone.

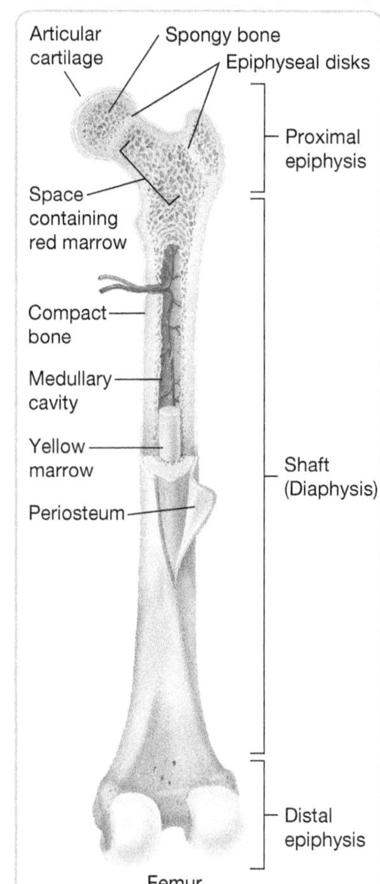

Fig. 6.15 The Femur The femur is a long bone in the leg. *What is the epiphysis?*

Short Bones

Short bones are the small, cube-shaped bones of the wrists, ankles, and toes. Short bones consist of an outer layer of compact bone with an inner layer of cancellous bone, or bone with a latticework structure.

Flat Bones

Flat bones usually have large, rather flat surfaces that cover organs or provide a surface for large areas of muscle. The shoulder blades, pelvis, and skull have flat bones.

Irregular Bones

Irregular bones are specialized bones with specific shapes. The bones of the ears, vertebrae, and face are irregular bones.

Sesamoid Bones

Sesamoid bones are located in a tendon near joints. The patella, or kneecap, is a sesamoid bone. These bones are also in hands and feet.

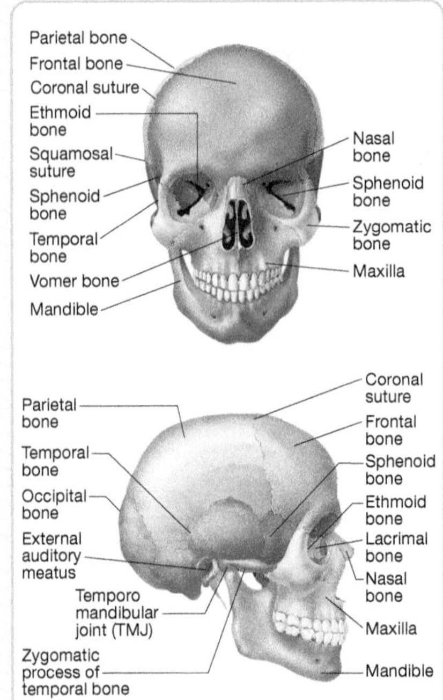

Fig. 6.16 The Bones of the Head The head bones are irregular. *What is the only movable bone in the head?*

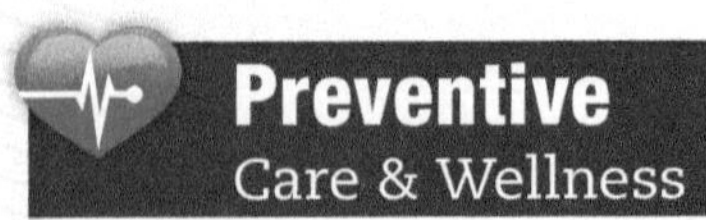

Preventive Care & Wellness

Bone Health

After the age of 35, the bones begin to lose their volume and become porous, in a condition known as osteoporosis. For this reason, you need to build up bone mass before you reach 35 years of age and maintain your bone mass later in life. To prevent osteoporosis, you should have an adequate intake of calcium and vitamin D, engage in regular exercise, and avoid alcohol and cigarettes.

Bone Extensions and Depressions

Bones have extensions and depressions where muscles and tendons attach. For example, the greater trochanter is a bony extension near the upper end of the femur.

Inside the Bone

Marrow is soft connective tissue. It is important in the production of blood cells. Red bone marrow is where red blood cells start to develop. Yellow bone marrow, found in most adult bones, is filled with fat.

READING CHECK

Recall some locations where sesamoid bones are found.

Categories of Bones

What bones are found within the spinal column?

The human body contains five areas of bones. These areas are the head, the spinal column, the chest, the pelvis, and the extremities.

Bones of the Head

Cranial bones (the bones of the head; see **Figure 6.16**) form the skull, which protects the brain and the structures inside the skull. The skull, or cranial, bones join at points called sutures. These bones include:

- Frontal bone: the forehead and roof of the eye sockets
- Ethmoid bone: the nasal cavity and the orbits of the eyes
- Parietal bone: top and upper parts of the sides of the skull
- Temporal bone: lower part of the skull and the lower sides, including the openings for the ears
- Occipital bone: back and base of the skull, with an opening in the foramen magnum through which the spinal cord passes
- Sphenoid bone: the base of the cranium; holds together the frontal, occipital, and ethmoid bones

The temporomandibular joint (TMJ) is the connection of the temporal bone and the mandible, or lower jawbone. It can be a site of pain or aches while chewing, or TMJ syndrome. This syndrome can cause a clicking sound while chewing, ringing in the ears, and deafness.

The mandible is the only movable bone in the face. It contains sockets for the lower teeth. Maxillary bones form the upper jawbone and contain the sockets for the upper teeth.

The Spinal Column

The spinal, or vertebral, column consists of five sets of vertebrae. Each vertebra is a bone segment separated from other vertebrae by a thick disc of cartilage. The discs cushion vertebrae and help the movement and flexibility of the spinal column. The spinal cord passes between the vertebral body and the back of the vertebra. As **Figure 6.17** shows, the five sections of the spinal column are

- cervical vertebrae, the seven vertebrae of the neck.
- thoracic vertebrae, the twelve vertebrae that connect to the ribs.
- lumbar vertebrae, the five bones of the middle back.
- sacrum, the curved bone of the lower back, consisting at birth of five separate bones that fuse in early childhood.
- coccyx, the tailbone, formed from four fused bones.

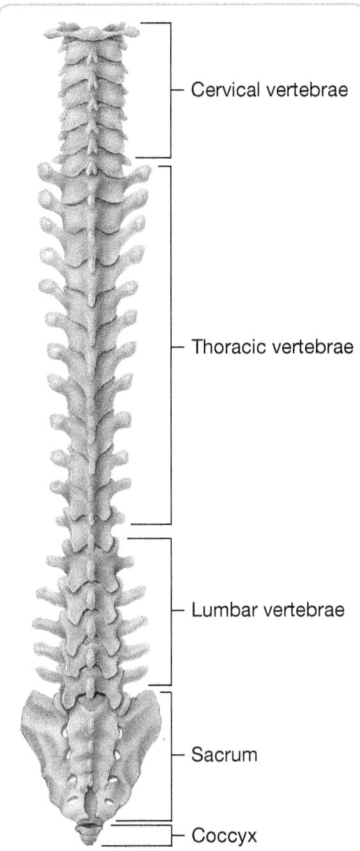

Fig. 6.17 Spinal Column The Spinal Column has five sections. *Describe the purpose of discs.*

Bones of the Chest

The clavicle, and the scapula are at the top of the chest cavity. The sternum, or breastbone, extends down the middle of the chest. Extending from the sternum are twelve rib pairs. The first seven pairs, called true ribs, are joined to the vertebral column and to the sternum. The next three pairs, called false ribs, are attached to the vertebral column and the seventh rib. The last two ribs are also false ribs. They are known as floating ribs and do not attach to the sternum or to other ribs.

Bones of the Pelvis

The pelvic girdle is a large bone that forms the hips and supports the trunk of the body. Composed of three fused bones—the ilium, ischium, and pubis—it is the point of attachment for the legs. Inside the pelvic girdle is the pelvic cavity. The area where the two pubic bones are connected by cartilage is called the pubic symphysis.

Bones of the Extremities

The following are the bones of the extremities:

- The upper arm bone, the humerus, attaches to the scapula and clavicle. The two lower arm bones are the ulna and the radius, which attach to the eight carpals or wrist bones.
- The metacarpals are the five bones of the palm that radiate out to the finger bones, the phalanges.
- The femur, in the thigh, is the longest bone in the body. It meets the two bones of the lower leg, the tibia, or shin, and fibula, at the kneecap, or patella.
- The tarsals form the ankle. The largest tarsal is the calcaneus, or heel. Metatarsals in the foot connect to the phalanges of the toes.

Bone Growth and Joints

How are bones connected?

The cells of the bone, called **osteocytes,** are part of a dense network of connective tissue. The hardening and development process of the osteocytes is called **ossification.** Ossification depends upon calcium, phosphorus, and vitamin D. Bones grow in length as long as there is cartilage within the bone known as the epiphyseal disk, or growth plate. This growth process stops between the ages of 18 and 25 years.

Bone mass, or the density of the bone, increases through ossification. Bone density peaks at about 35 years of age. Osteoblasts are bone-forming cells that turn membrane into bone. They use excess blood calcium to build new bone. Osteoclasts are known as bone-dissolving cells. When bone is dissolved, calcium is released into the bloodstream.

Even after bone length growth stops, osteoclasts and osteoblasts continually remodel bone tissue. Throughout life, osteoclasts break down bone when the body needs more calcium in the blood, while osteoblasts replace the bone when there is excess calcium in the blood.

Joints

Joints are points where bones connect. Bones are connected to other bones with ligaments, which are bands of fibrous tissue. The movement at a particular joint varies depending on the body's needs.

- Diarthroses are joints that move freely, such as the knee joint.
- Amphiarthroses are cartilaginous joints that move slightly, such as the joints between vertebrae.
- Synarthroses do not move. Examples are the fibrous joints between the skull bones.
- Symphyses are cartilaginous joints that unite two bones firmly. An example is the pubic symphysis.
- Synovial joints are covered with a membrane that secretes a fluid lubricant and helps the joint move easily. The hip joint is an example of a synovial joint.

READING CHECK

Identify when bones stop growing.

SECTION 6.3 The Skeletal System Review

AFTER YOU READ

1. **State** the five purposes of bones.
2. **Identify** the five types of bones, and name one bone of each type.
3. **Name** the divisions of the spinal column, and recall how many vertebrae are in each part.
4. **List** and describe the types of joints.
5. **Name** the longest bone in the human body.
6. **Identify** what cells are involved in ossification.

Technology ONLINE EXPLORATIONS

Bones

Go online to find images of the human skeleton. Practice naming the bones of the body alone and with a partner. How many bones can each of you name without looking at reference materials?

SECTION

6.4 The Muscular System

Functions of Muscles

What is the main function of muscles?

The muscular system is made up of more than 600 individual muscles, accounting for about 40 percent of the total adult body weight. Its main function is movement. Walking, waving, and making facial expressions are all controlled by muscles. Smooth muscles in your stomach and intestines help you digest food. Cardiac muscle in the heart pumps blood throughout your body.

In addition to movement, muscles provide stability. Tiny muscles in your spine hold bones together. Some muscles for openings, called sphincters, control the movement of substances. For example, the urinary sphincter prevents urination until relaxed. When muscles contract, they release heat which helps the body maintain a normal temperature. That is why moving your body can help warm you up.

READING CHECK

Recall how many muscles make up the muscular system.

Types of Muscles

How are skeletal muscles attached to bones?

- Involuntary muscles govern movement that is not controlled by will, such as respiration and digestion. Involuntary muscles that move the internal organs and systems are called smooth muscles.
- Cardiac muscle controls the contractions of the heart. Cardiac muscle is also an involuntary muscle.
- Voluntary muscles can be contracted at will. These muscles, called skeletal muscles, are responsible for the movement of all bones.

In addition to providing movement, skeletal muscles help maintain posture, protect internal organs, and produce heat and energy for the body. Muscles attach to a stationary bone at a point called the origin. They attach to a movable bone at a point called the insertion. Some spaces between tendons and joints have a bursa, a sac lined with a synovial membrane that helps the movement of joints. The **tendons**, or bands of fibrous tissue, connect muscles to bone. Movement takes place at the joints and uses the muscles, ligaments, and tendons. Remember that **ligaments** attach bone to bone.

Vocabulary

Content Vocabulary

You will learn these content vocabulary terms in this section.

- **tendons**
- **ligaments**
- **range of motion**

Academic Vocabulary

You will see this word in your reading and on your tests. Find its meaning in the Glossary in the back of this book.

- **voluntary**

Table 6.1 Muscles

NAME	LOCATION	FUNCTION
Orbicularis oculi	Circles eyelids	Closes eyelid
Masseter	Mandible	Closes jaw
Sternocleidomastoid	From sternum and clavicle to temporal bone	Flexes and rotates head
Trapezius	From occipital bone to scapulae	Raises shoulder and pulls shoulder back
Pectoralis major	Chest	Flexes and adducts anteriorly
Deltoid	Shoulder	Abducts arm; injection site
Biceps brachii	Front of upper forearm	Flexes forearm
Triceps brachii	Back of upper forearm	Extends forearm
Intercostals	Between ribs	Moves ribs to permit breathing
Diaphragm	Floor of thoracic cavity	Increases vertical diameter of thoracic cavity for breathing
Rectus abdominus	From symphysis pubis to sternum	Flexes and rotates vertebral column
Gluteus medius (dorsogluteal)	Upper buttocks	Abducts femur; injection site
Vastus lateralis	Upper outer thigh	Extends knee; injection site
Hamstrings	Posterior aspect of the thigh	Flexes lower leg
Quadriceps femoris	Anterior aspect of thigh	Extends lower leg
Tibialis anterior	Front of lower leg	Flexes foot
Gastrocnemius	Prominent muscle of the calf	Adducts foot, allows plantar flexions

As seen in **Figures 6.18**, skeletal muscles provide movement. Some movements provided by skeletal muscles include:

- Flexion; bending. Flexing your arm muscles bends your elbow.
- Extension: straightening. You "extend your hand" to shake someone's hand by straightening your elbow.

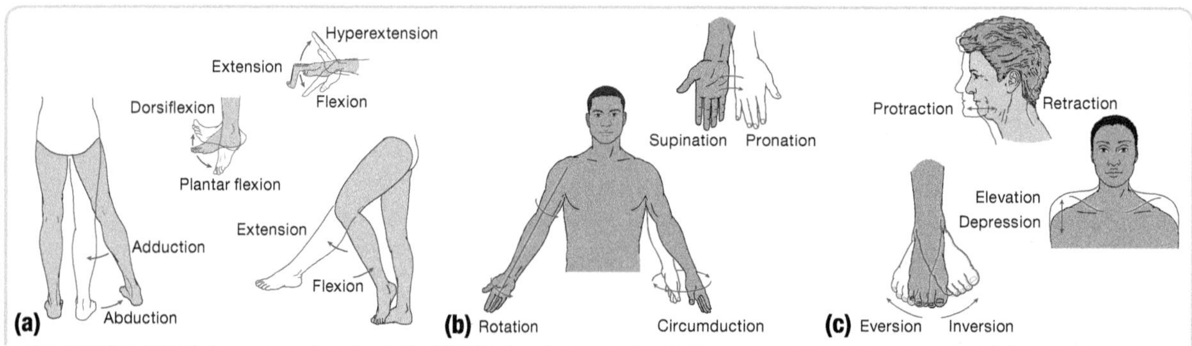

Fig. 6.18 Muscle Movements (a) Adduction, Abduction, Dorsiflexion, Plantar Flexion, Hyperextension, Extension, and Flexion. (b) Rotation, Circumduction, Supination, and Pronation. (c) Eversion, Inversion, Protraction, Retraction, Elevation, and Depression. *Which type of movement goes toward the body?*

- Abduction: moving something away from the body. To abduct your arm or leg, you move it away from your body.
- Adduction: moving toward or adding something to the body. When you adduct your arm, you move it toward your body.
- Rotation: moving something around an axis. A ballet dancer rotates his or her leg from the hip.

Understanding the movement of muscles and the **range of motion** of muscles and joints is important for nurses, physical therapists, athletic trainers, and many other healthcare personnel. In addition, certain muscles of the body must be located to give an intramuscular (IM) injection into that muscle. **Table 6.1** and **Figure 6.19** show some of the important skeletal muscles and their locations and functions.

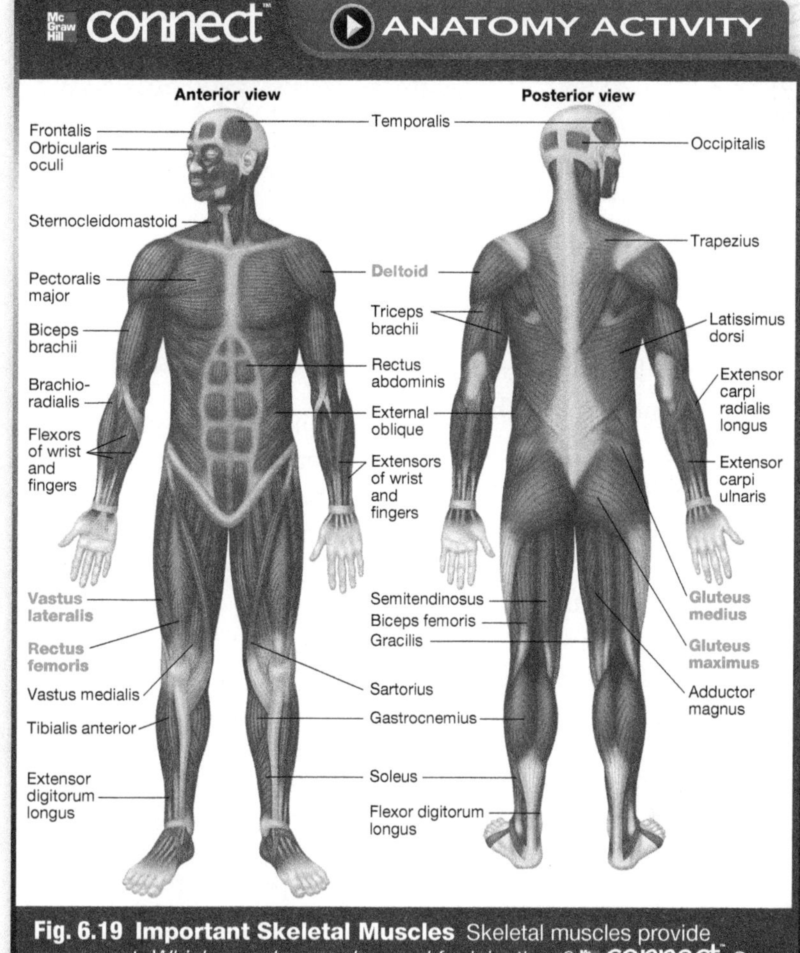

Fig. 6.19 Important Skeletal Muscles Skeletal muscles provide movement. *Which muscles may be used for injections?* connect Go online to complete the Anatomy Activity based on this system.

READING CHECK

Contrast the functions of involuntary and voluntary muscles.

SECTION 6.4 The Muscular System Review

AFTER YOU READ

1. **Name** the three types of muscle tissue and their main functions.
2. **Differentiate** between the origin and the insertion of a muscle.
3. **Compare** a ligament and a tendon.
4. **Predict** what might happen if you exercise on a hot day.
5. **Name** and **demonstrate** three skeletal muscle movements.

Technology ONLINE EXPLORATIONS

Joint Movements

Research online the types of movements that are specific to each of the types of joints of your body. Practice these movements and state the name of each movement as you perform it. Make a list of all of the joints and all of the movements that you are able to perform.

SECTION

6.5 The Nervous System

Vocabulary

Content Vocabulary

You will learn these content vocabulary terms in this section.

- **neurons**
- **synapse**
- **homeostasis**

Academic Vocabulary

You will see this word in your reading and on your tests. Find its meaning in the Glossary in the back of this book.

- **process**

Overview

How does the nervous system control your body?

The nervous system directs the functions of all the human body systems. Every activity, voluntary or involuntary, is controlled by some of the more than 100 billion nerve cells in the body. The brain and spinal cord—the central nervous system—act as a control center. Nerves—the peripheral nervous system—carry messages to and from this center.

Neurons

What are nerve impulses?

Nerve cells, or **neurons,** are the basic element of the nervous system. Neurons are highly specialized types of cells that vary greatly in function, shape, and size. **Figure 6.20** shows a neuron. All neurons have three parts:

- The cell body, which includes branches or fibers that reach out to send or receive impulses
- Dendrites, which are thin branching extensions of the cell body. They conduct nerve impulses toward the cell body.
- The axon, which conducts nerve impulses away from the cell body. It is a branch covered by tissue called the myelin sheath. At the end of the axon are fibers through which the impulses leaving the neuron pass. The impulse then jumps between neurons over a space called a **synapse,** after being stimulated to do so by a neurotransmitter, a tiny sac at the end of nerve fibers.

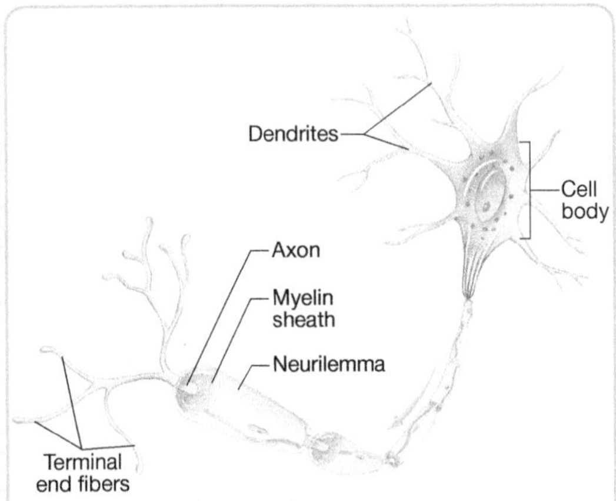

Fig. 6.20 Nerve Cells Neurons are composed of three parts. *What stimulates a nerve impulse to jump from one nerve to another?*

All neurons have two basic properties:

- Excitability, the ability to respond to a stimulus
- Conductivity, the ability to transmit a signal

There are three types of neurons:

- Efferent, or motor, neurons, which convey information to the muscles and glands from the central nervous system
- Afferent, or sensory, neurons, carrying information from sensory receptors to the central nervous system
- Interneurons, which carry and process sensory information

Neurons form bundles called nerves that bear electrical messages to the body's organs and muscles. Some nerves contain two or more types of neurons. The cells in the body contain stored electrical energy that is released when they receive outside stimuli or when internal chemicals stimulate the cells. The released energy passes through the nerve cell, causing a nerve impulse. The impulses are received or transmitted by tissues or organs called receptors and are then transmitted to other receptors throughout the body.

connect ANATOMY ACTIVITY

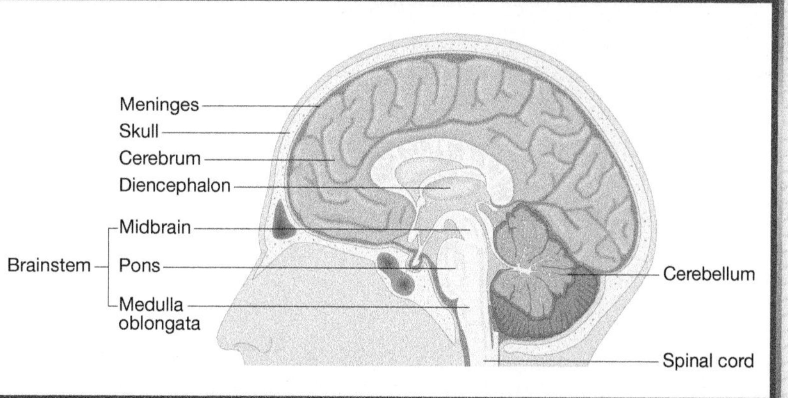

Fig. 6.21 Divisions of the Brain The brain is divided into several parts. *In which division of the nervous system is the brain located?*

connect Go Online to complete the Anatomy Activity for this system.

Neuroglias

In addition to nerve cells, other cells in the nervous system support, connect, protect, and remove debris from the system. These cells, called neuroglias, do not transmit impulses. Certain neuroglias, along with the almost solid walls of the brain's capillaries, form what is known as the blood-brain barrier. This barrier permits some chemical substances to reach the brain's neurons but blocks most others.

READING CHECK

Name the three parts of a neuron.

The Central Nervous System

What part of the brain makes decisions?

The central nervous system consists of the brain and the spinal cord. This is the center of control. It receives and interprets all stimuli and sends nerve impulses to instruct muscles and glands to act or to respond to certain actions. These actions include both voluntary and involuntary movement, seeing, hearing, thinking, secreting of hormones, remembering, and responding to outside stimuli. As shown in **Figure 6.21,** the brain has four major parts:

- The brainstem is made up of the midbrain, the pons, and the medulla oblongata. The midbrain is concerned with visual reflexes. The pons controls certain respiratory functions. The medulla oblongata contains centers that regulate heart and lung functions, swallowing, vomiting, coughing, and sneezing.
- The cerebellum is the area that coordinates musculoskeletal movement to maintain posture, balance, and muscle tone.
- The cerebrum lies above the cerebellum. The cerebrum has left and right hemispheres and an outer portion called the cerebral cortex. The cerebral cortex is the area of conscious decision making. The left and right lobes of the cerebrum are each divided into four parts or lobes. The frontal lobe controls voluntary motor movements,

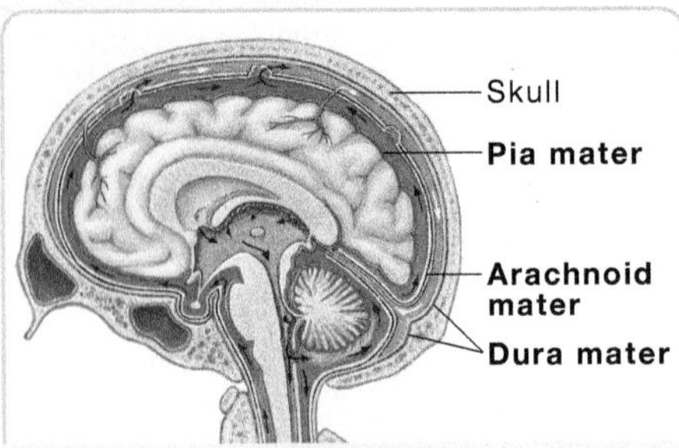

Fig. 6.22 The Meninges The meninges have three layers. *What is the function of the meninges?*

expression, and moral behavior. The parietal lobe controls and interprets the senses and taste. The temporal lobe controls memory, equilibrium, emotion, and hearing. The occipital lobe controls vision and various forms of expression.

- The diencephalon is the deep portion of the brain containing the thalamus and the hypothalamus. The diencephalon serves as a relay center for sensations. It integrates with the autonomic nervous system to control heart rate, blood pressure, temperature regulation, water and electrolyte balance, digestive functions, behavioral responses, and glandular activities.

The area between the brain and the cranium is filled with cerebrospinal fluid (CSF). CSF is a watery fluid that contains various compounds and flows throughout the brain and around the spinal cord. This watery fluid cradles and cushions the brain. Ventricles or cavities in the brain also contain this fluid. The meninges, which are described below, also protect the brain.

The spinal cord extends from the base of the brain to near the first lumbar vertebra in the lower back. The spinal cord is contained within the vertebral column in a space called the vertebral canal. The spinal cord is protected by the bony structure of the vertebral column, by the cerebrospinal fluid that surrounds it, and by the spinal meninges. Extending out from the spinal cord are the nerves of the peripheral nervous system.

The meninges, which are shown in **Figure 6.22,** are three layers of membranes that cover the brain and spinal cord:

- The outer layer, the dura mater, is a tough, fibrous membrane that covers the entire length of the spinal cord and contains channels for blood to enter brain tissue.
- The middle layer, a weblike structure called the arachnoid membrane, runs across the space containing cerebrospinal fluid.
- The pia mater, the innermost layer of the meninges, is a thin membrane containing blood vessels that nourish the spinal cord. The space between the dura mater and the bones of the spinal cord is called the epidural space. Containing blood vessels and fat, it is the space into which medication may be injected to dull pain. An epidural may be given during childbirth and for some pelvic operations. **Figure 6.23** illustrates the epidural space.

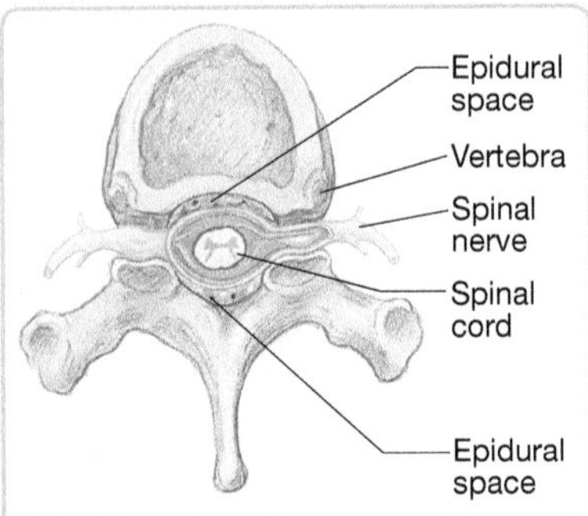

Fig. 6.23 The Epidural Space The epidural space is the space between the dura mater and the bones of the spinal cord. *What might a physician inject into the epidural space?*

READING CHECK

Identify the role of cerebrospinal fluid.

The Peripheral Nervous System

Which part of the peripheral nervous system processes sensory information?

The peripheral nervous system includes 12 pairs of cranial nerves that carry impulses to and from the brain **(see Figure 6.24)** and 31 pairs of spinal nerves that carry messages to and from the spinal cord. The spinal nerves are grouped with the segments of the spinal cord from which they extend.

The peripheral nervous system has two subsystems. These are divided according to their function.

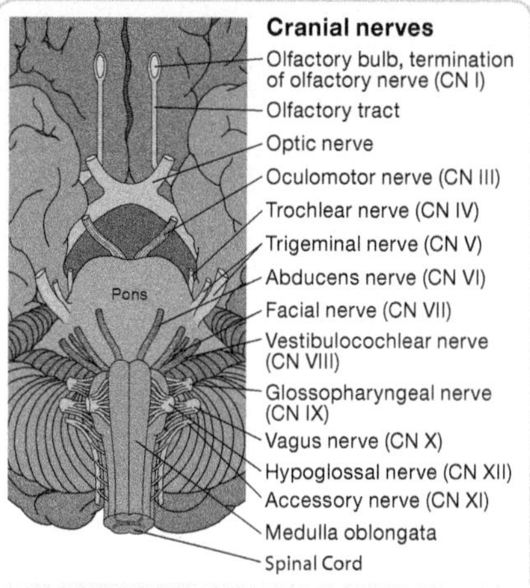

Fig. 6.24 The Cranial Nerves
Cranial nerves carry impulses to and from the brain. *What other group of nerves is part of the peripheral nervous system?*

The Somatic Nervous System

The nerves of the somatic nervous system receive and process sensory input from the skin, muscles, tendons, joints, eyes, tongue, nose, and ears. They also excite the voluntary contraction of skeletal muscles. The somatic nervous system is voluntary. For example, it allows you to pull away if you touch something hot.

The Autonomic Nervous System

The nerves of the autonomic nervous system carry impulses from the central nervous system to glands, various involuntary muscles, cardiac muscle, and various membranes. The autonomic nervous system stimulates organs, glands, and senses by stimulating secretions of substances.

The autonomic nerves are further divided into the sympathetic and the parasympathetic divisions. The two divisions play opposite roles. The sympathetic division operates when the body is under stress. It helps to activate responses necessary to react in dangerous or abnormal situations. The parasympathetic division, on the other hand, operates to keep the body in **homeostasis,** or balance, under normal conditions.

READING CHECK

Explain how the peripheral nervous system stimulates organs.

SECTION 6.5 The Nervous System Review

AFTER YOU READ

1. **Explain** the two properties that allow nerves to respond to a stimulus and transmit a signal.
2. **Research** what would happen if a client lacked a functioning myelin sheath.
3. **Name** the part of the nervous system that would activate if someone held a gun to your head.
4. **Recall** the part of the brain that is responsible for conscious decision making.
5. **Name** and **describe** the three parts of a neuron.

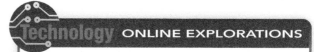

Technology ONLINE EXPLORATIONS

Cranial Nerves

There are 12 pairs of cranial nerves that have important functions. Research online to determine the function of each pair of cranial nerves. Then review with a partner each nerve pair and its function.

SECTION

6.6 The Sensory System

Vocabulary

Content Vocabulary

You will learn these content vocabulary terms in this section.

- **pinna**
- **olfactory**

Academic Vocabulary

You will see this word in your reading and on your tests. Find its meaning in the Glossary in the back of this book.

- **react**

Overview

How can the body receive stimuli other than through the five basic senses?

The sensory system, also known as the special senses, includes any organ or part that perceives or receives stimuli from the outside world and from within our bodies. **Figure 6.25** shows the sensory system.

You probably know the five basic senses. They are sight, touch, hearing, smell, and taste. However, there are other ways in which our bodies "sense" and react to stimuli. For example, the islets of Langherhans sense high blood sugar levels and are stimulated to release insulin. As another example, the muscles, joints, and semicircular canals of the ears provide a sense of position and balance.

The major parts of the sensory system are related specifically to the organs of the five senses and to the senses experienced by those organs:

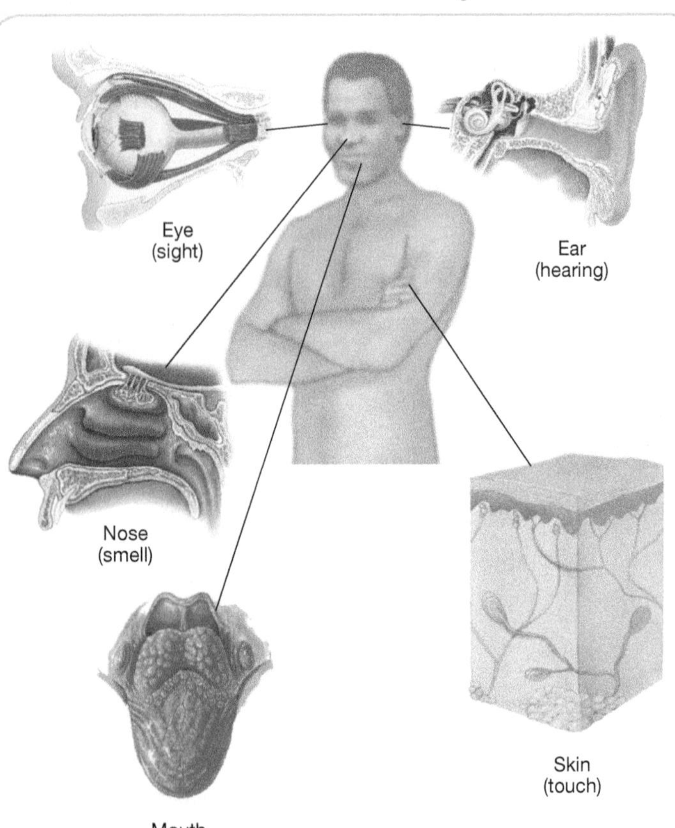

Fig. 6.25 The Sensory System The sensory system includes organs of the five basic senses. *In addition to the basic senses, what is one way in which the body "senses"?*

- Sight—the eye
- Touch—the skin
- Hearing—the ears
- Smell—the nose
- Taste—the mouth

Sight—the Eye

What is vision?

Each eye is a sphere consisting of an outer layer, a middle layer, and an inner layer. The eyelid covers the outer layer. The anterior surface of the eye and the posterior surface of the eyelid are lined with a mucous membrane called the conjunctiva.

The Parts of the Eye

As shown in **Figure 6.26,** the parts of the eye are as follows:

- The smooth, firm, white posterior section of the outer layer, called the sclera, is made up of a thick, tough membrane. The sclera supports the eyeball. The cornea is the transparent, anterior section, which is the first place where light is bent, or refracted, as it enters the eye. The sclera is white and has blood vessels that nourish the cornea. The cornea is transparent, has no blood vessels, and refracts light rays.

- The middle layer is a layer of blood vessels consisting of a thin posterior membrane called the choroid. In the front are the ciliary muscles, used for focusing the eyes.
- The interior layer of the eye contains a light-sensitive membrane called the retina. The retina decodes light waves and sends the information on to the brain, which interprets what we see. The retina consists of specialized nerve receptor cells called rods, which are sensors of black and white shades, and cones, which are sensors of color and the brightest light. The region where the retina connects to the optic nerve is called the optic disk. The optic disk is known as the blind spot because it has no rods or cones to receive images.

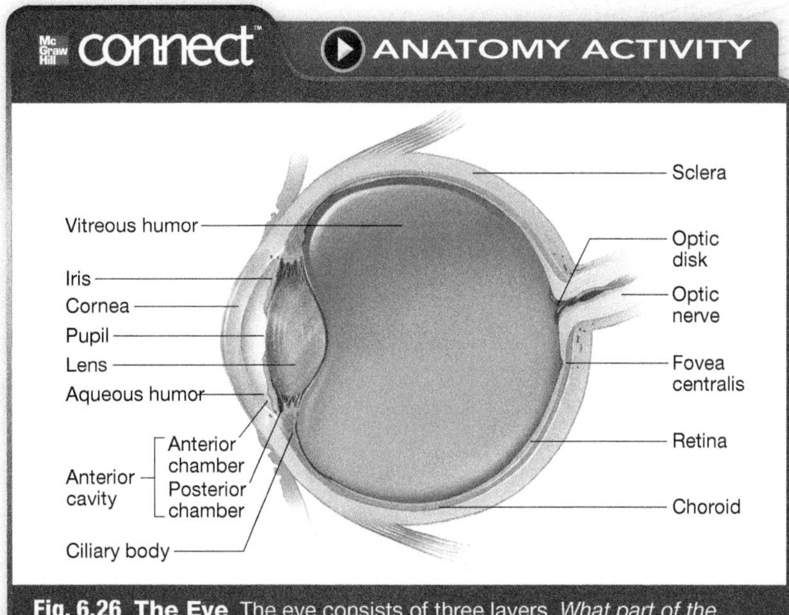

Fig. 6.26 The Eye The eye consists of three layers. *What part of the eye helps maintain the shape?* connect Go Online to complete the Anatomy Activity for this system

Vision

Vision is the process that begins when light is refracted as it hits the cornea and again when it hits the retina. Light passes through the pupil, the black circular center of the eye. It next passes through the lens, which is a colorless, flexible, transparent body behind the iris. The iris is the colored part of the eye that expands and contracts in response to light, thereby opening and closing the pupil.

The Eyeball

The eyeball is divided into three cavities called chambers. The anterior chamber lies between the cornea and iris. The posterior chamber lies between the iris and the lens. Both the anterior and the posterior chambers are filled with aqueous humor, a thin, watery liquid that provides nourishment to the lens and cornea. It also maintains a constant pressure within the eyeball. The vitreous chamber occupies about 80 percent of the space in the eyeball. It is filled with vitreous humor, a gelatinous substance that nourishes parts of the eye and maintains a supportive structure to keep the eye from collapsing.

Other Eye Structures

Several other structures are important to the eye. The eyelids close to protect the eyes and to allow rest and sleep. The eyebrows and eyelashes help keep foreign particles from entering the eye. The lachrymal glands secrete moisture into the tear ducts. The resulting tears moisten the eyes, wash foreign particles off the eye, and distribute water and nutrients to parts of the eye. Tears may be secreted more heavily than necessary as a reaction to eye irritations, allergies, infections, or emotional upset.

READING CHECK

Explain how the retina functions.

Hearing and Equilibrium—the Ear

How does the ear regulate equilibrium?

The ear is the organ of hearing and equilibrium, or balance. The three major divisions of the ear are the external ear, the middle ear, and the inner ear (see **Figure 6.27**).

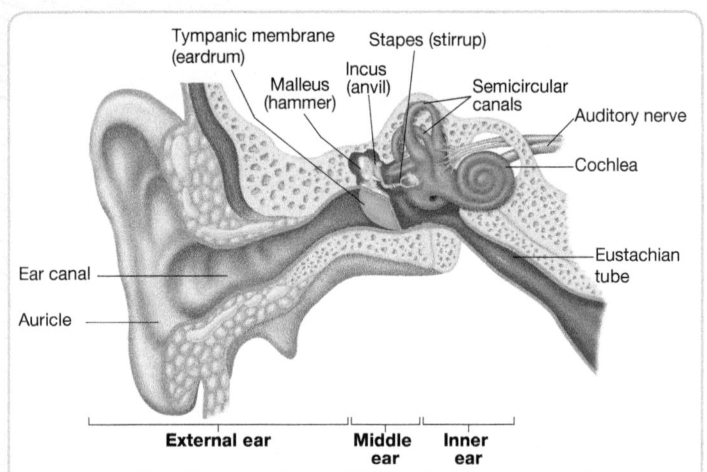

Fig. 6.27 The Ear The ear has three major divisions: the external, the middle, and the inner ear. *What are the functions of the inner ear?*

- The external ear, or **pinna,** is on the outside of the body. The external auditory meatus contains glands that secrete earwax.
- The middle ear includes the eardrum, or tympanic membrane, and three small bones called the ossicles. The eardrum is an oval, semitransparent membrane with skin on its outer surface and a mucous membrane on the inside. The three ossicles are the malleus (hammer), incus (anvil), and stapes (stirrup). Sound waves cause the ossicles to vibrate and produce sound. The middle ear is connected to the pharynx through the eustachian tube. This tube helps equalize air pressure on both sides of the eardrum.
- The inner ear is complex. It contains three semicircular canals and the cochlea. The semicircular canals are important to hearing. The cochlea is a snail-shaped structure important to equilibrium. Inside the cochlea are hairlike cells that make up the organ of Corti. The hairs move back and forth in response to sound waves and eventually send messages to the brain to interpret sound.

Touch, Pain, and Temperature—the Skin

How does the skin sense different types of touch?

The skin's layers sense different intensities of touch. Light touch is felt in the top layer of skin, whereas touch with harder pressure is felt in the middle or bottom layer. The skin's receptors can sense touch, pressure, pain, and hot and cold temperatures. The skin also has pain receptors that sense any injury to skin tissue.

Smell—the Nose

How does the sense of smell change with time?

The sense of smell is activated by receptors located at the top of the nasal cavity. The receptors are nerve cells covered with hairlike cilia that send messages about smell to the brain. **Figure 6.28** shows the **olfactory** area. The term "olfactory" relates to the sense of smell. The receptors in the nose that give us our sense of smell can only be stimulated for a short amount of time. This is why when you enter a room the smell seems strong, but in time you stop noticing it. The sense of smell is closely related to the sense of taste.

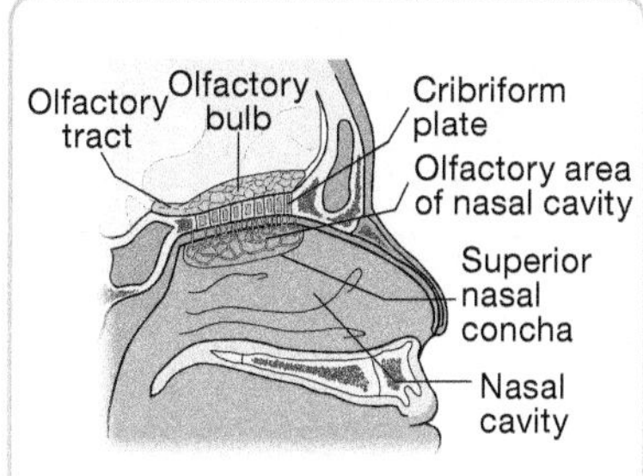

Fig. 6.28 The Sense of Smell The olfactory area that allows us to have a sense of smell is in the upper part of the nasal cavity. *How is the sense of smell affected if you have a cold or a dry nose?*

Taste—the Tongue and Oral Cavity

What activates the taste buds?

Taste buds sense the taste of food (see **Figure 6.29**). Most taste buds are on the surface of the tongue in small raised structures called papillae. Some taste buds line the roof of the mouth and the walls of the pharynx. The taste buds are activated when the item being tasted dissolves in the watery fluid around them (secreted by the salivary glands). There are four main types of taste buds to match the primary taste sensations: sweet, sour, salty, and bitter. Different parts of the tongue contain concentrations of receptors for each of those sensations. Some receptors sense the texture, odor, and temperature of food. In the case of food that is too hot, spicy, or cold, pain receptors are activated.

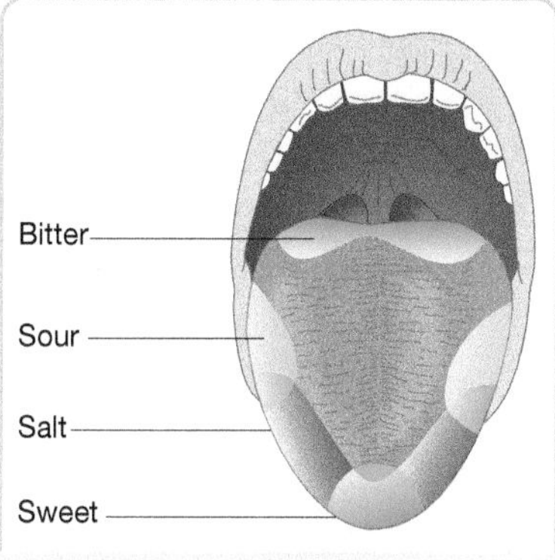

Fig. 6.29 The Tongue The tongue is the location of taste buds, or papillae. *How are the taste buds activated?*

READING CHECK

Name the types of taste buds.

SECTION 6.6 The Sensory System Review

AFTER YOU READ

1. **Name** the five basic senses.
2. **Name** at least one other way the body senses and reacts to stimuli.
3. **Explain** this scenario: when you got to chemistry class, the room smelled like smoke, but after a while you did not notice the smell.
4. **Describe** what the skin can sense.
5. **Explain** the function of the retina.

Technology ONLINE EXPLORATIONS

ESP

The term ESP (extrasensory perception) is used to describe a sixth sense. Do some online research about ESP. Write a summary of what you find. In your summary, answer this question: "Is ESP truly one of the special senses?"

6.7 The Circulatory System

Vocabulary

Content Vocabulary

You will learn these content vocabulary terms in this section.

- **circulation**
- **arteries**
- **veins**
- **coronary**
- **pulmonary**
- **systemic**

Academic Vocabulary

You will see this word in your reading and on your tests. Find its meaning in the Glossary in the back of this book.

- **stable**

The Heart

What parts of the heart control blood flow?

The circulatory system is the body's delivery service. The heart pumps blood through the blood vessels to the entire body. This process is known as **circulation.**

The average adult heart is about the size of your fist and lies in the thoracic cavity between the lungs. Two thirds of the heart lies to the left of the sternum, or breastbone. It is an amazingly powerful muscular pump that beats an average of 72 times a minute, 100,000 times a day, and 3,000 million times (three trillion times!) in an average lifetime. **Figure 6.30** shows how blood flows through the heart.

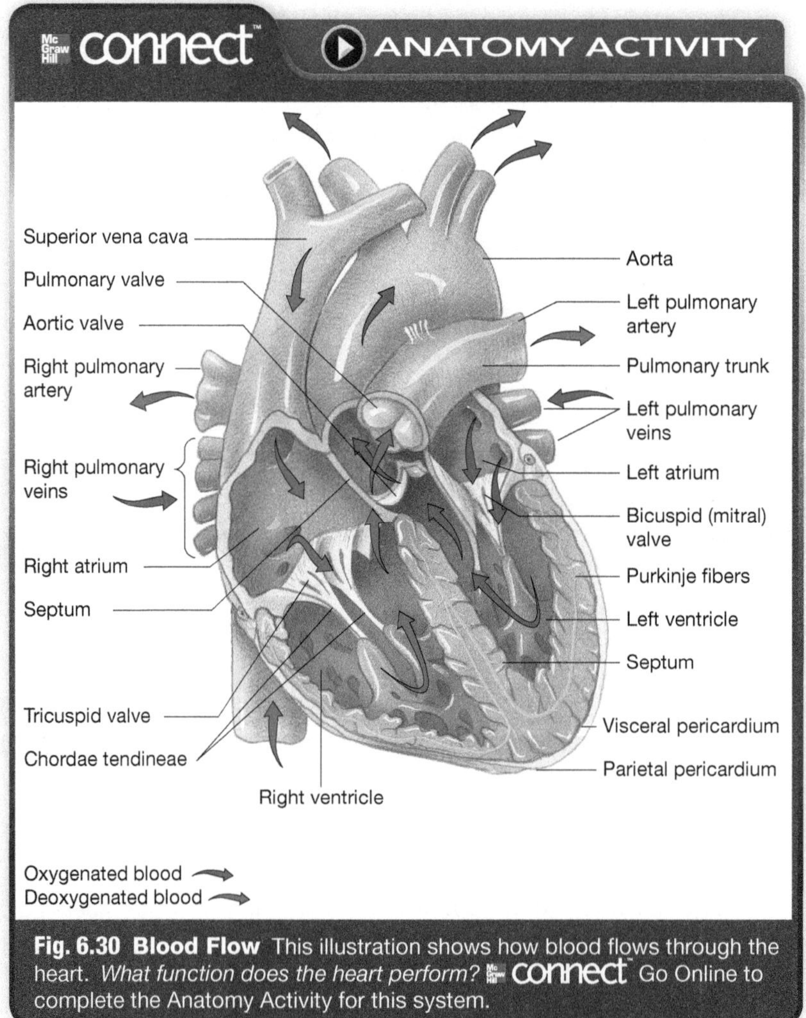

Fig. 6.30 Blood Flow This illustration shows how blood flows through the heart. *What function does the heart perform?* connect Go Online to complete the Anatomy Activity for this system.

The Pericardium

The heart is covered by the pericardium, a protective sac. The pericardium has two layers: the visceral pericardium, which is the inner layer next to the heart, and the parietal pericardium, which is the outer portion of the pericardium.

Inside the pericardium, the heart has three layers of tissue. The outermost layer is the epicardium. The middle layer is the myocardium, a layer of muscular tissue. The inner layer, the endocardium, forms a membranous lining for the chambers and valves of the heart.

Parts of the Heart

The heart is divided into right and left sides. Each side has two chambers. The right atrium (upper chamber) and right ventricle (lower chamber) on the right side are separated from the left atrium and left ventricle on the left side by a partition called a septum.

Blood Flow

Blood flows through the chambers of the heart in only one direction, with the flow regulated by valves. The blood is pumped through the system of arteries and veins. **Arteries** carry blood away from the heart. **Veins** carry blood toward the heart. The arteries carry blood rich in oxygen, except for the pulmonary artery, which brings blood low in oxygen from the heart to the lungs. The veins carry blood low in oxygen except for the pulmonary vein, which returns blood rich in oxygen from the lungs.

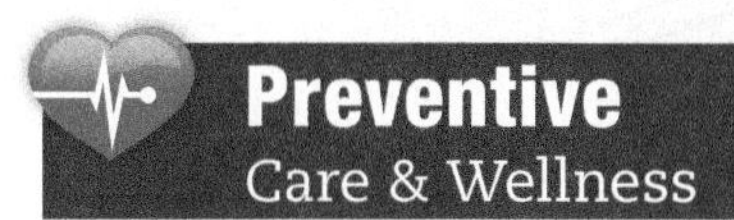

Preventive Care & Wellness

A Healthy Heart

Circulatory diseases are the number one cause of death in the United States. Many of these deaths could be prevented by a healthy diet and lifestyle. The following are some guidelines provided by the American Heart Association.

- Use up at least as many calories as you take in. If you eat more, exercise more.
- Exercise 30 minutes a day most days of the week.
- Eat a variety of nutritious foods from all the food groups (fruit, vegetables, whole grains, and lean meat such as fish and poultry).
- Eat less of the nutrient-poor foods. Reduce your intake of fats, trans fat, sugary foods and beverages.
- Do not smoke tobacco, and stay away from tobacco smoke.

Valves of the Heart

The valves of the heart control the blood flow to and from the heart. The valve between the left atrium and left ventricle is the bicuspid, or mitral, valve. The valve between the right atrium and right ventricle is the tricuspid valve. These valves control the flow of blood within the heart between the atria and ventricles. The pulmonary and aortic valves stop the backflow of blood into the heart. **Figure 6.31** shows the valves of the heart.

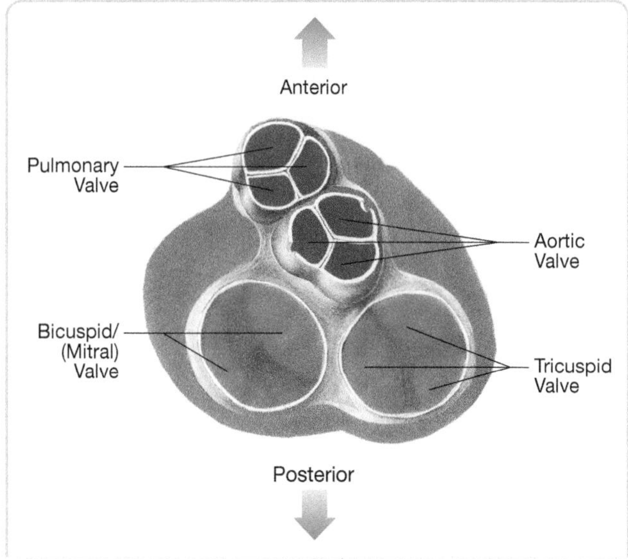

Fig. 6.31 Valves This illustration shows the valves of the heart. *Which valves prevent the backflow of blood into the heart?*

The Cardiac Conduction System

The cardiac conduction system controls the electrical impulses that cause the heart to contract. It is contained in special heart tissue called conductive tissue. This system is discussed in more detail in Chapter 26, "Medical Testing."

READING CHECK

Explain why blood flows in one direction only.

Circulation

Why does the heart need a continuous supply of oxygen?

The arteries and veins are the vessels that carry blood to and from the heart and lungs and to and from the heart and the rest of the body. This is the main function of the circulatory system.

There are three types of circulation:

- coronary
- pulmonary
- systemic

Figure 6.32 illustrates the pulmonary and systemic circulation system.

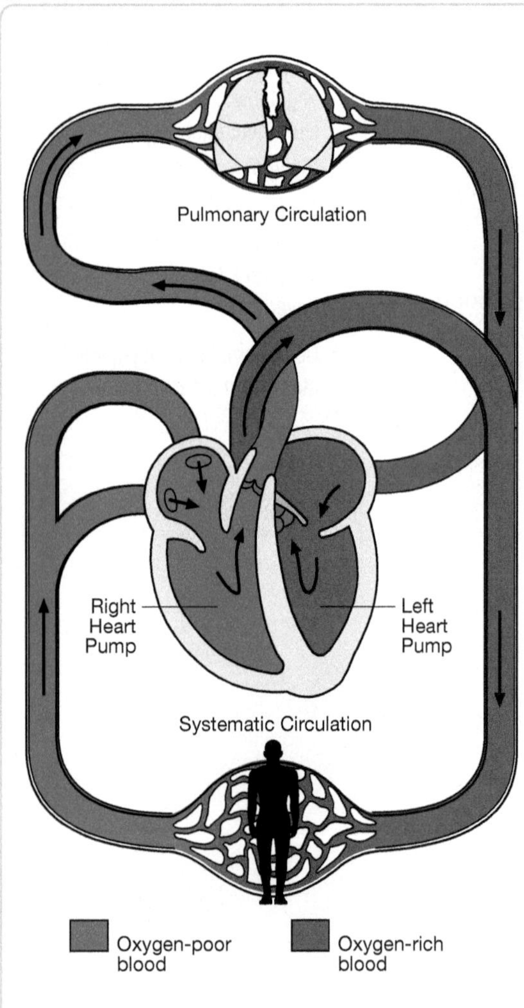

Fig. 6.32 Pulmonary and Systemic Circulation This illustration shows the basic flow of the circulatory system. *What is the major difference between the pulmonary and the systemic circulation?*

Coronary Circulation

Coronary circulation is the circulation of blood within the heart. The coronary arteries branch off the aorta to supply blood to the heart muscle. The aorta is the main artery through which blood exits the heart. The heart needs more oxygen than any other organ except the brain. About 100 gallons of blood per day is pumped to the heart through the coronary arteries.

Pulmonary Circulation

Pulmonary circulation is the flow of blood between the heart and lungs. The pulmonary arteries carry blood that is low in oxygen from the right ventricle of the heart to the lungs to pick up more oxygen. Blood that is rich in oxygen flows from the lungs to the left atrium of the heart through the pulmonary veins.

Systemic Circulation

Systemic circulation is the flow of blood between the heart and the cells of the body. The heart contracts to pump blood through the arteries to the cells of the body. The blood that goes from the heart to the cells of the body is rich in oxygen. Specialized arteries carry this blood to other areas of the body.

For example, the carotid artery supplies blood to the head and neck, and the femoral artery supplies the thigh. The arteries divide into smaller vessels called arterioles, which then divide into very narrow vessels called capillaries. The capillaries provide the cells they serve with essential nutrients. The capillaries also remove waste products and carbon dioxide from the cells.

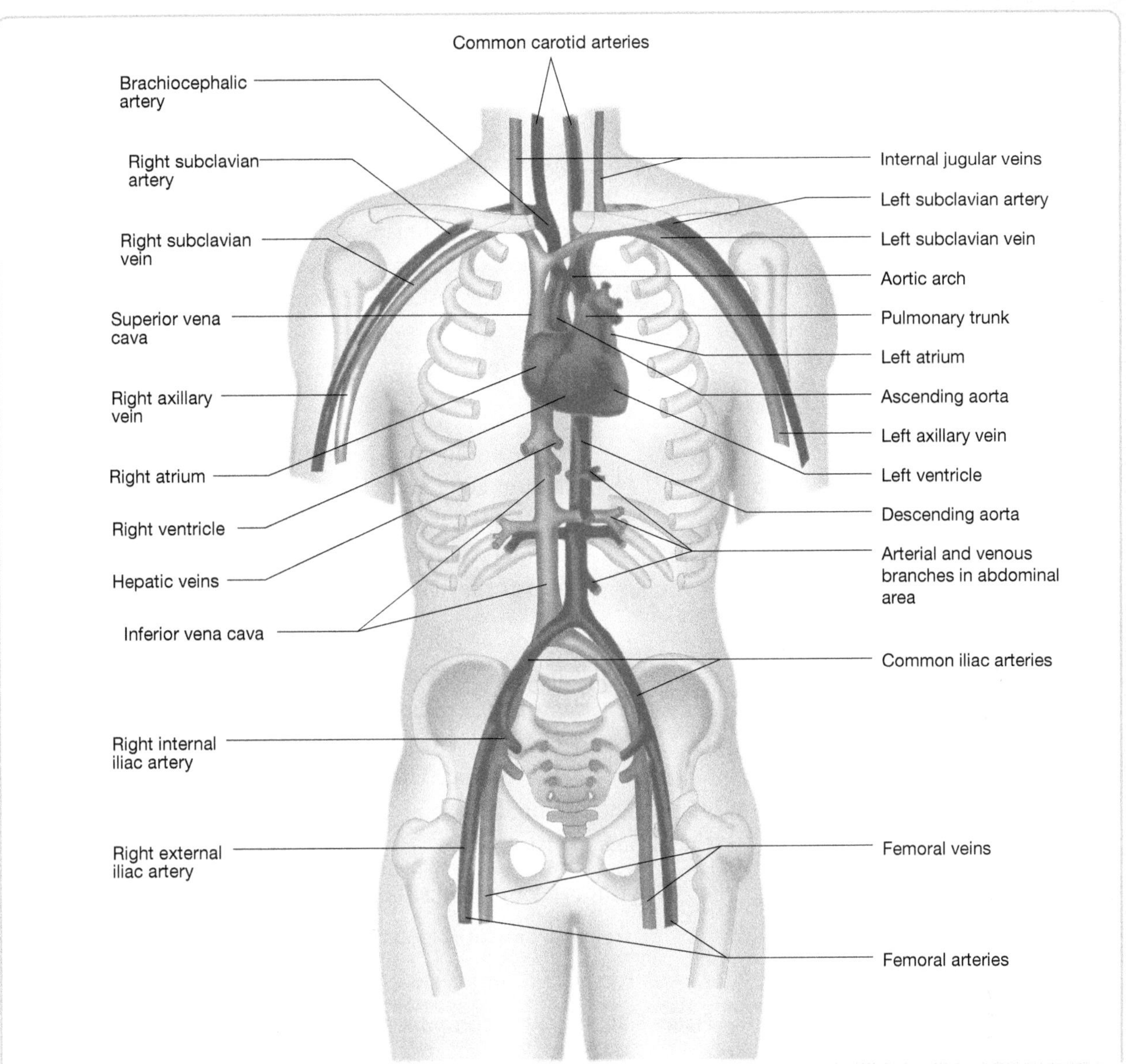

Fig. 6.33 Arteries and Veins This illustration shows the major arteries and veins of the body. *How is blood collected from the upper part of the body and carried to the heart?*

The blood travels back to the heart through the venules, which are small branches of veins. The veins take the blood low in oxygen back to the heart. The blood from the upper part of the body is collected and carried to the heart through a large vein called the superior vena cava. The blood from the lower part of the body goes to the other large vein, the inferior vena cava. Both of these large veins bring the blood to the right atrium of the heart.

Figure 6.33 shows the major arteries and veins of the body.

READING CHECK

Define the three types of circulation.

Blood

How do red blood cells transport oxygen?

Blood is a complex mixture of cells, water, and various proteins and sugars. It sends life-sustaining nutrients, oxygen, and hormones to all parts of the body. It also removes waste products from cells of the body to prevent toxic buildup. It helps keep the fluid volume that exists within body tissues stable and helps regulate body temperature. Human life is not possible without blood.

There are about five liters of blood circulating within the average adult body. If a person loses blood, either through bleeding or by donating blood, the body replaces most of the blood within 24 hours. If bleeding is extensive, blood transfusions may be needed.

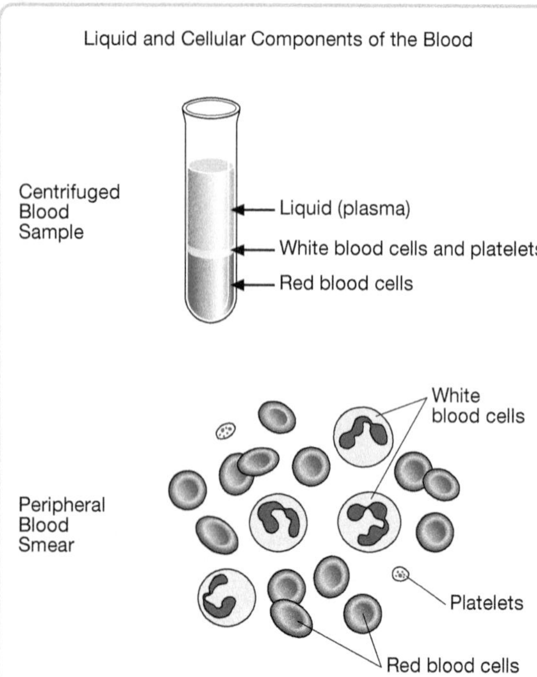

Fig. 6.34 Components of the Blood
Blood contains both liquids and solids. *What is in the liquid and solid portion of the blood?*

Blood is a thick liquid made up of a fluid part, called plasma, and a solid part. Plasma consists of water, proteins, salts, nutrients, vitamins, and hormones. Plasma, which is about 55 percent of the blood, is a clear liquid. The cells or solids of blood make up about 45 percent of blood. The solid part of blood, which is suspended in the plasma, consists of:

- Erythrocytes, or red blood cells (RBCs)
- Leukocytes, or white blood cells (WBCs)
- Thrombocytes, or platelets

Figure 6.34 shows the components of blood.

The measurement of the percentage of packed red blood cells is known as the hematocrit. Chapter 25 discusses how to take this measurement on a blood sample. Red blood cells, which are produced in the bone marrow, circulate in the body for about 120 days. Hemoglobin, a protein within red blood cells, aids in the transport of oxygen to the cells of the body.

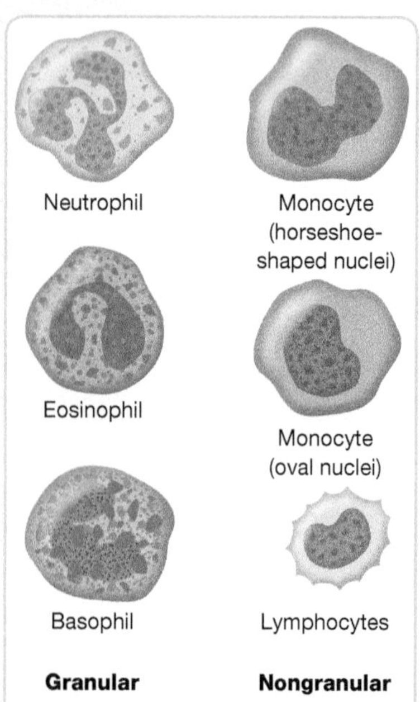

Fig. 6.35 White Blood Cells
White blood cells perform a variety of functions. *What are two types of white blood cells and their functions?*

Leukocytes, or white blood cells (see **Figure 6.35**), protect against disease in many ways. Leukocytes are transported in the bloodstream to the site of an infection to help fight that infection. The five types of leukocytes and their functions are:

- basophils, which release heparin to stop clotting, produce histamine to cause the blood vessels to dilate, help control inflammation, and kill parasites.
- eosinophils, which kill parasites and help control inflammation and allergic reactions.

- monocytes, which destroy large unwanted particles in the bloodstream.
- neutrophils, which remove small unwanted particles and materials from the blood.
- lymphocytes, which are essential to the immune system and protect the body against the formation of cancer cells.

Platelets, or thrombocytes, are fragments that break off from large cells in the red bone marrow. Platelets live for about ten days and help in blood clotting. When an injury occurs, platelets stick to damaged tissue and to each other, to control blood loss from a blood vessel.

Blood Types

When blood is needed for transfusion, the blood being donated is tested and categorized into one of four human blood types, or groups. Donated blood must be tested because, if the donor and the recipient have incompatible blood types, adverse reactions might result. Common blood types are O, A, B, and AB.

In addition to the four human blood types, there is a positive or negative element in the blood, known as the Rh factor. It was first found in rhesus monkeys. Rh-positive blood contains this factor, and Rh-negative blood does not. The Rh factor is a type of antigen, or substance that causes the body to produce antibodies. Testing for blood types is described in Chapter 25.

READING CHECK

Summarize how blood makes human life possible.

connect

VIRTUAL LAB: The Cardiac Cycle

The cardiac cycle is the heart's well-choreographed process of relaxation and contraction. For a basic understanding behind the cardiac cycle's role in the circulation system, watch this animation to see the heart's choreography in action.

connect Go online to view the animation of the cardiac cycle and complete the related questions.

SECTION 6.7 The Circulatory System Review

AFTER YOU READ

1. **Illustrate** the purpose of each the following:
   a. Valves
   b. Pericardium
   c. Arteries
   d. Veins
2. **Explain** the difference between coronary, pulmonary, and systemic circulation.
3. **Name** the components of blood and what they contain.

Technology ONLINE EXPLORATIONS

How Blood Travels

Demonstrate how blood travels through the circulatory and respiratory systems. Go online to find diagrams of several organs or body parts that show how blood enters and leaves each structure. On cards or sheets of paper, print the name of the structure, and give one card to each student in your class. With your classmates, line up in order of how the blood travels, starting with the right atrium.

SECTION 6.8

The Lymphatic and Immune Systems

Vocabulary

Content Vocabulary

You will learn these content vocabulary terms in this section.

- lymph
- antibodies

Academic Vocabulary

You will see this word in your reading and on your tests. Find its meaning in the Glossary in the back of this book.

- network

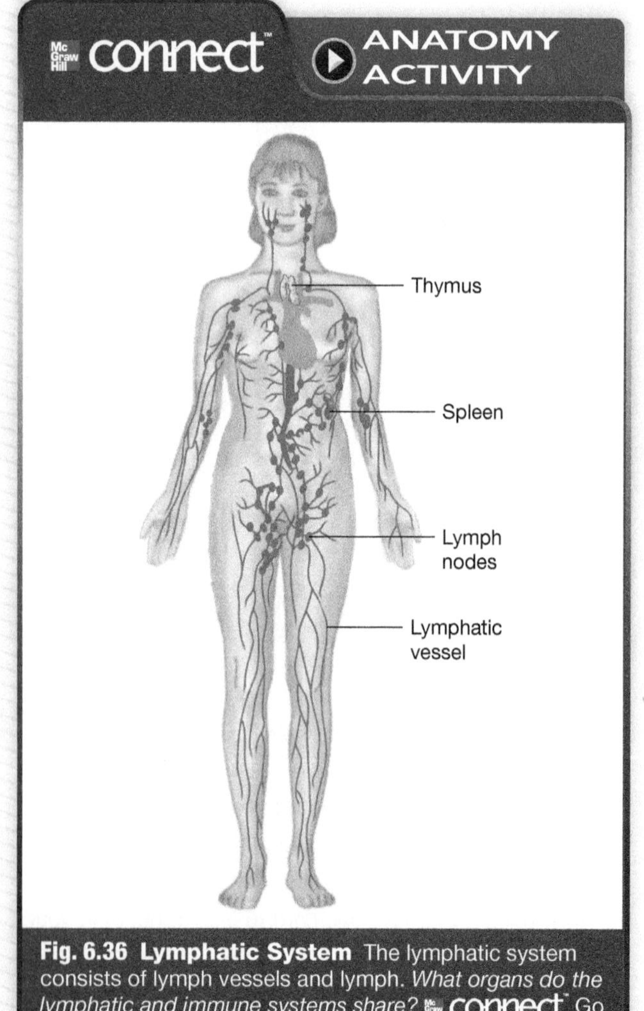

Fig. 6.36 Lymphatic System The lymphatic system consists of lymph vessels and lymph. *What organs do the lymphatic and immune systems share?* connect Go online to complete the Anatomy Activity for this system.

Lymphatic Organs and Structures

How does the lymphatic system resemble the circulatory system in function?

The lymphatic and immune systems share some of the same structures and functions, as shown in **Figure 6.36.** Both systems contain the lymph nodes, spleen, and thymus gland, and both systems produce some of the disease-fighting immune cells. The lymphatic system contains lymph vessels and the lymph itself. The immune system regulates all the types of immunity, either natural or acquired by the body.

The lymphatic system is also similar to the circulatory system. A network of lymphatic vessels transports lymph fluid to and from the bloodstream. Lymph, like blood, transports various substances around the body. Unlike blood, lymph does not contain either red blood cells or platelets. Like blood, it contains white blood cells. It carries less protein than blood but about the same amount of water, salts, sugar, and waste material.

Microscopic lymphatic capillaries are the smallest parts of the lymphatic system. The capillaries have thin walls that allow the fluid in tissues to flow between the capillaries and the tissues. The fluid in the spaces between tissues is called interstitial fluid. When this fluid flows into the lymphatic capillaries, it is called **lymph.**

The capillaries merge to form larger pathways, which are the lymphatic vessels. These vessels bring lymph to the lymph nodes. **Figure 6.38** illustrates a lymph node. Lymph nodes are specialized organs that produce lymph cells and filter harmful substances from the tissues. Lymph nodes contain special cells that devour foreign substances. These cells are known as macrophages. Lymph nodes become swollen with lymph cells and macrophages.

Lymphocytes are white blood cells that produce antibodies. **Antibodies** are specialized proteins that fight disease. Substances called antigens also fight disease by provoking an immune response in other cells.

The lymph vessels also gather fluid and substances that have leaked from the blood capillaries into the tissues and transport them back to the bloodstream, where they are needed. In addition, they bring lipids or fats from the small intestine to the bloodstream where parts of the lipids are used. Lymph travels in only one direction, toward the thoracic cavity where it empties into the right lymphatic duct and the thoracic duct. The two ducts carry the lymph into veins in the neck and then into the heart. The heart circulates the blood to the body's tissues, where the process of fluid and substances leaking into the lymphatic capillaries begins again.

Lymph nodes are located everywhere in the body except in the central nervous system. The tonsils and adenoids are lymph tissue. Other major groups of lymph nodes are found in the neck, armpit, chest, and groin.

The Spleen and the Thymus Gland

Two organs of the lymph system are the spleen and the thymus gland:

- The larger organ, the spleen, is shown in **Figure 6.37.** It is located in the upper left portion of the abdominal cavity. The function of the spleen is to filter foreign material from the blood, to store blood, to destroy old red

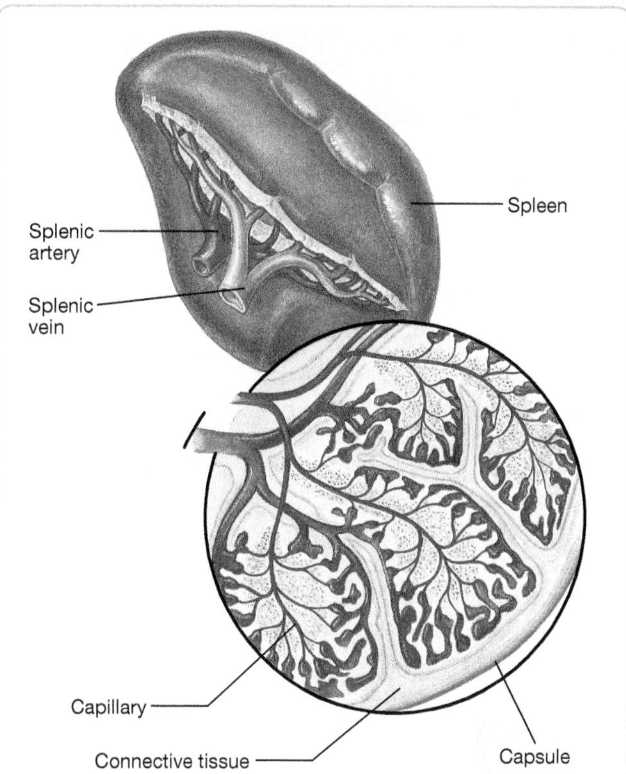

Fig. 6.37 Spleen The Spleen is the larger of two organs in the lymph system. *What can happen if the spleen is injured? What is the treatment?*

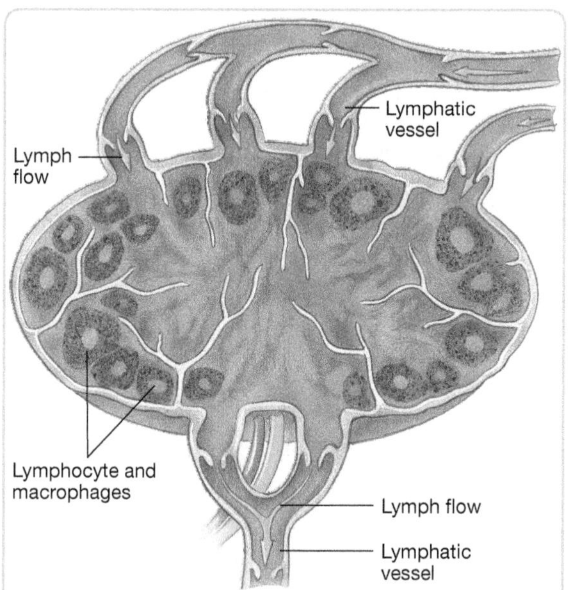

Fig. 6.38 Lymph Nodes Lymph nodes are located throughout the body. *How does the lymph fluid get back into the bloodstream?*

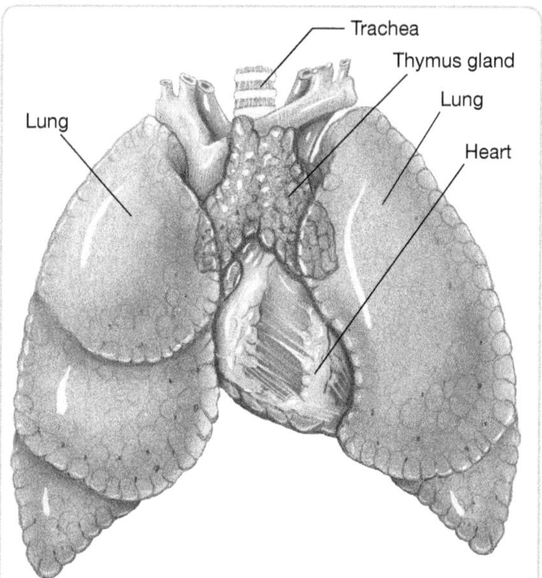

Fig. 6.39 Thymus Gland The thymus gland is located between the lungs. *Why does the thymus gland shrink as we reach adulthood?*

blood cells, and to activate lymphocytes. If ruptured by an injury, the spleen must be repaired or removed. If it is removed, its functions are taken over by the lymph nodes, liver, and bone marrow.

- The thymus gland, shown in **Figure 6.39,** is a soft gland with two lobes. It is large during infancy and early childhood when immunity is most crucial, but it gradually shrinks until it is often quite small in adulthood. By adulthood, our bodies have natural immunities, and we do not need the thymus gland. The thymus gland contains certain important cells that mature into T cells, which provide immunity after they leave the thymus.

READING CHECK

Identify where the lymph nodes are located.

The Immune System

What types of barriers make up the immune system?

The immune system consists of a series of defenses against intruders, such as viruses and bacteria. The lymph nodes, spleen, and thymus gland serve as defense mechanisms that protect the body. Parts of other systems, such as the skin, also play an important role in protecting the body from disease.

The human body has a number of mechanical, chemical, and other defenses against disease. When disease-causing agents, called pathogens, try to enter the body, the skin often stops them. Mechanical barriers include the cilia in the nostrils and other mucous membranes. If pathogens get past the mechanical barriers, chemical barriers, such as gastric juices in the stomach, may stop them. Specialized cells, called macrophages, ingest and destroy pathogens in the bloodstream. In addition, human beings are naturally resistant to some diseases that affect other animals. On the other hand, some pathogens prefer the environment of the human body as opposed to that of other animals.

Types of Immunity

The specific defenses of the immune system provide immunity, which is resistance to particular pathogens. There are three major types of immunity:

- Natural immunity is the human body's natural resistance to certain diseases. This natural resistance varies from one individual to the next. Natural resistance depends on the individual's genetic characteristics and on some of his or her natural chemical defenses.

21ST CENTURY SKILLS

Emerging Technology about Immunity

The human body is continually under assault. There is a multitude of viruses, bacteria, fungi, and parasites, which all have different modes of attack. Confronting these attacks is the amazing human immune system. The immune system is complex, and scientists are challenged to understand it. These scientists want to know how we respond to pathogens, so that new vaccines and drugs can be designed to prevent and treat infections. They are also striving to understand why the immune system sometimes works incorrectly, as in allergies and in autoimmune diseases such as rheumatoid arthritis or type-1 diabetes.

The sequencing of the human genome is helping scientists answer these questions. The human genome contains the genes that encode the entire immune defense system. Scientists already know of 765 proteins that resemble antibodies and are thought to play a role in immunity, but the task of deciphering the genome is large. There are 30 – 40,000 genes that must be studied to determine which of them produce molecules that are involved in immunity. It is even more important to know how the genes and molecules work together to keep us healthy.

- Acquired active immunity is acquired either by having a disease and producing natural antibodies to it or by being vaccinated against the disease. Vaccination, sometimes called immunization, provides immunity by introducing into the body an antigen from a different organism that causes active immunity. Acquired active immunity is divided into two types. One type is immunity provided by plasma cells, which produce antibodies called immunoglobulins. The other type of acquired active immunity, cell-mediated immunity, is provided by the action of T cells. The T cells respond to antigens by multiplying rapidly and producing proteins that have antiviral properties.
- Acquired passive immunity is immunity provided in the form of antibodies or antitoxins that have been developed in another person or another species. Acquired passive immunity is necessary in cases such as snakebites, when a dose of antitoxin often must be given immediately. Passive immunity may also be administered to lessen the chance of catching a disease or to lessen the severity of the course of the disease. Gamma globulin is a preparation of collected antibodies given to prevent or lessen the effects of certain diseases, such as hepatitis A, varicella, and rabies.

READING CHECK

Explain how vaccination provides immunity.

SECTION 6.8 The Lymphatic and Immune Systems Review

AFTER YOU READ

1. **Compare** blood and lymph.
2. **Name** the organs that are shared by the lymphatic and immune systems.
3. **Describe** what type of immunity you receive from a vaccine.
4. **Suggest** the most likely reason for your doctor to recommend an injection of a gamma globulin.
5. **Compare** acquired active immunity to acquired passive immunity.

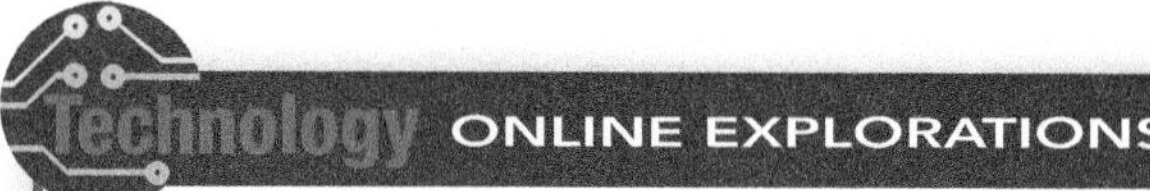

ONLINE EXPLORATIONS

Lymphatic Fluid

Imagine that you are a drop of lymphatic fluid. Write a paragraph explaining what your job is and how you would get into the heart. Go online to research the pathway of lymphatic fluid.

SECTION 6.9 The Respiratory System

Vocabulary

Content Vocabulary

You will learn these content vocabulary terms in this section.

- **pleura**
- **inhalation**
- **exhalation**
- **cilia**
- **aspiration**

Academic Vocabulary

You will see this word in your reading and on your tests. Find its meaning in the Glossary in the back of this book.

- **relaxes**

Overview

Can the body function without both lungs?

The cells of our bodies must have oxygen in order to live. The respiratory system supplies oxygen. It is carried in the blood to the cells by the circulatory system. As shown in **Figure 6.40,** the respiratory system consists of the following parts.

- The lungs are the main organ of the respiratory system, and provide the body with oxygen and eliminate carbon dioxide from the blood. The outside of the lungs is a moist, double layer of membrane called the **pleura.** (The plural of *pleura* is *pleurae.*). The outer layer of this membrane is the parietal pleura. The inner layer is the visceral pleura. Both layers make lung movement in the thoracic cavity easier by protecting the lungs and providing the moisture that allows movement. The space between the two pleurae is called the pleural cavity. The right, larger lung is divided into three lobes. The left lung is divided into two lobes. Human beings can function with one or more lobes removed or even when an entire lung has been removed, as is necessary in some cases of lung cancer.
- The respiratory tract is the system of passageways through which air moves in and out of the lungs.
- Muscles move air into and out of the lungs.

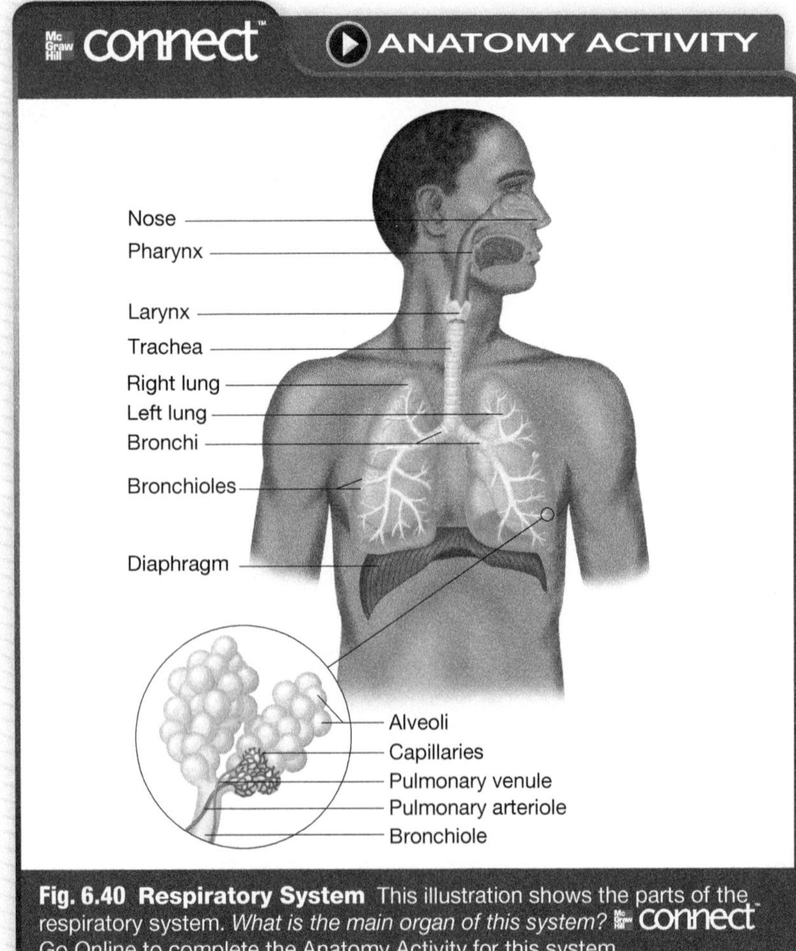

Fig. 6.40 Respiratory System This illustration shows the parts of the respiratory system. *What is the main organ of this system?* connect Go Online to complete the Anatomy Activity for this system.

The respiratory system performs two major tasks:

- External respiration, or breathing, is the exchange of air between the body and the outside environment (see **Figure 6.41**).
- Internal respiration is the process of bringing oxygen to the cells and removing carbon dioxide from them (see **Figure 6.42**).

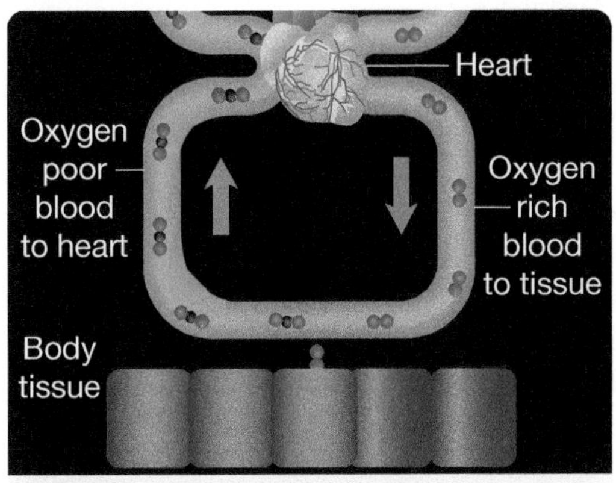

Fig. 6.41 External Respiration The air between the body and the outside environment is exchanged. *What is another term for external respiration?*

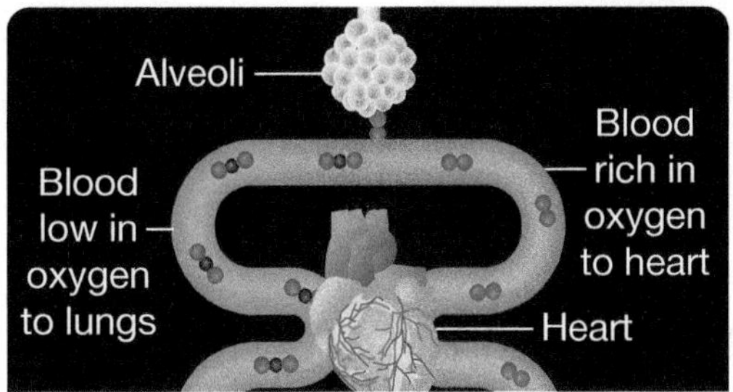

Fig. 6.42 Internal Respiration Oxygen is carried to and from the cells. *What is removed from the cells?*

Breathing (external respiration) involves two actions: **inhalation** (breathing in) and **exhalation** (breathing out). We breathe in air that is about 21% oxygen. When we inhale (breathe in), the diaphragm contracts by flattening and the intercostal muscles raise the ribs. These actions increase the space in the thoracic cavity and air rushes in. When we exhale (breathe out), the diaphragm relaxes and the ribs lower, causing air to rush out. **Figure 6.43** shows the events of inhalation and exhalation.

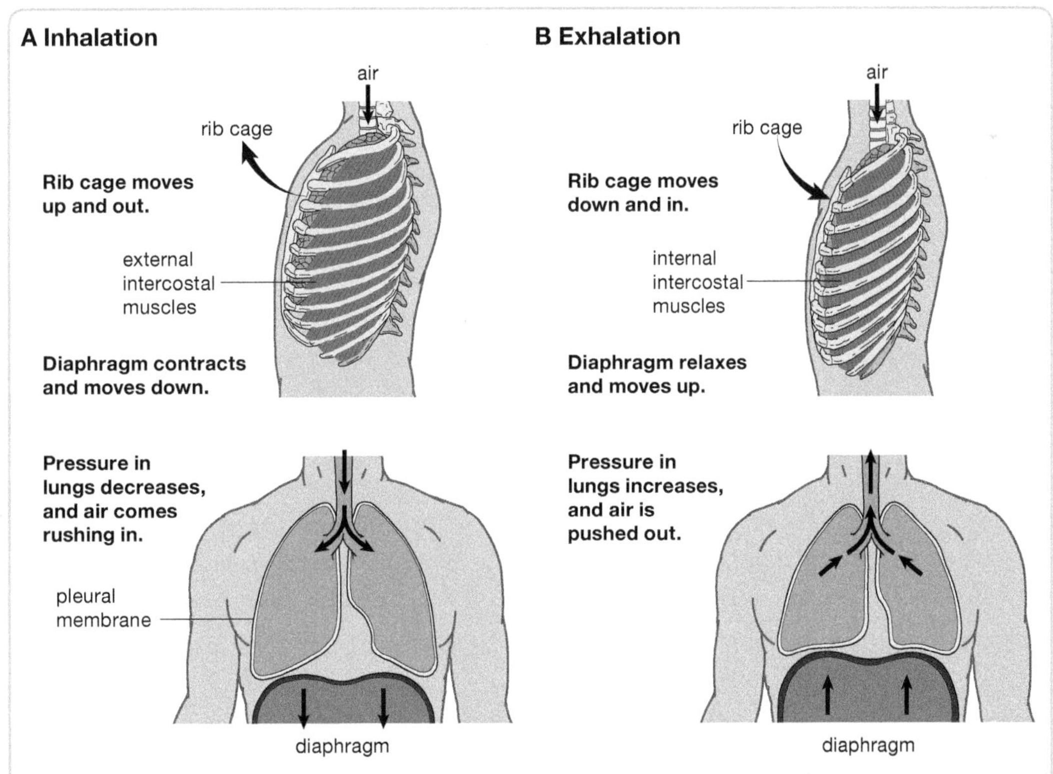

Fig. 6.43. Breathing Inhalation and Exhalation (a) Events of inhalation; (b) Events of exhalation. *Which muscles raise the ribs for inhalation?*

READING CHECK

Recall the number of lobes in each lung.

External Respiration

What prevents food from entering the larynx?

Inhalation, also called inspiration, brings air into the mouth or nose. The nose is divided into two nasal cavities by a piece of cartilage called the nasal septum. As air passes through the nasal cavity and the paranasal sinuses, it is warmed by blood in the mucous membranes that line these areas. Small hairs, called **cilia,** are present in the nasal cavity. They filter out foreign bodies. **Figure 6.44** shows the upper respiratory system.

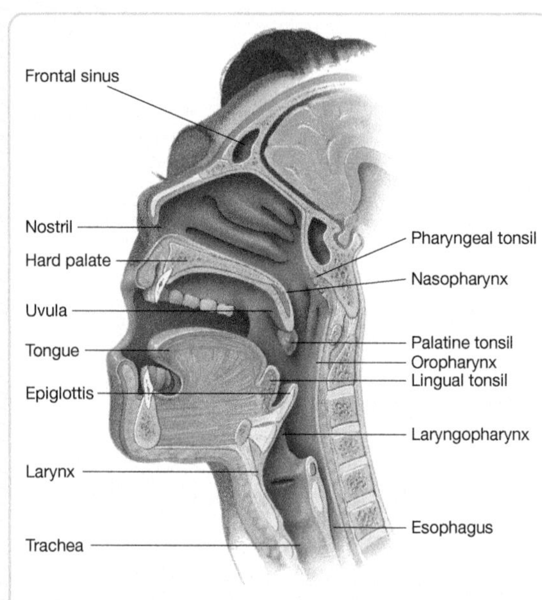

Fig. 6.44 The Upper Respiratory System These are the major structures of the upper respiratory system. *What is the function of the cilia?*

The Throat

The air next reaches the throat, or pharynx, a passageway for both air and food. It is divided into three sections:

- The nasopharynx lies above the soft palate. The soft palate is a flexible, muscular sheet that separates the nasopharynx from the rest of the pharynx. The nasopharynx contains the pharyngeal tonsils, more commonly known as the adenoids. The adenoids aid in the body's immune defense.
- The oropharynx, or the back portion of the mouth, contains the palatine tonsils. They are made up of lymphatic tissue that works as part of the immune system. The oropharynx is part of the mechanism of the mouth that triggers swallowing.
- The bottom section of the pharynx is the laryngopharynx. It is at this point that the respiratory tract divides into the esophagus and larynx.

The Esophagus

The esophagus is the passageway for food and is part of the digestive system. Every time you swallow, food is prevented from going into the larynx by the epiglottis. The epiglottis is a movable flap of cartilage that covers the opening to the larynx, which is called the glottis.

Occasionally, a person may swallow and inhale at the same time. This causes some food to be pulled into the larynx and is known as **aspiration.** Usually, a strong cough forces out the food, but sometimes an individual may choke. If this occurs, the food must be dislodged using the Heimlich maneuver, which you learned about in Chapter 4.

The Larynx

The larynx, or voice box, is the place from which air passes to the trachea, or windpipe. Air goes into the larynx, which is the area where the sounds of speech and singing are produced. The larynx contains vocal cords. The size and thickness of the cords determine the pitch of sound. The male's thicker and longer vocal cords produce a lower pitch than do the shorter and thinner vocal cords of most women and children. The larynx is supported by various structures, one of which consists of two disks joined at an angle to form the thyroid cartilage, or Adam's apple.

The Trachea

The trachea, or windpipe, is a tube that connects the larynx to the right and left bronchi. Both bronchi contain cartilage and mucous glands. Bronchi are the passageways through which air enters the right and left lungs. These passageways divide and get smaller and smaller until they reach their smallest size, which are the bronchioles. During exhalation, which is also called expiration, air that is pushed out of the lungs travels up through the respiratory structures and is expelled into the environment.

connect

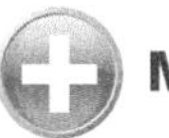

STEM CONNECTION

Medical Science

Boyle's Law and Breathing
Boyle's law explains how breathing works. According to Boyle's law, if volume decreases, pressure increases, and if volume increases, pressure decreases.

connect Go online to learn how Boyle's Law applies to the functioning of your lungs.

Internal Respiration

What two structures exchange oxygen and carbon dioxide inside the lungs?

The structures inside the lungs resemble an upside-down tree, with smaller parts branching off. At the end of each bronchiole is a cluster of air sacs known as alveoli. The one-celled, thin-walled alveoli connect to small blood vessels, known as capillaries, in the lungs. Oxygen is exchanged between the alveoli and the capillaries. Carbon dioxide is sent from the capillaries into the alveoli. Oxygen is then delivered to the body's other cells during this phase of respiration. Carbon dioxide is expelled back up through the respiratory tract during exhalation.

READING CHECK

Name the organ in which the sound of speech is produced.

SECTION 6.9 The Respiratory System Review

AFTER YOU READ

1. **Describe** the two actions that make up the act of breathing.
2. **Identify** the sections of the throat and their purposes.
3. **Explain** the function of the epiglottis.
4. **Compare** external and internal respiration.
5. **Explain** what causes differences in vocal pitch.

Technology ONLINE EXPLORATIONS

Respiratory Research
The website of the National Heart, Lung, and Blood Institute, part of the National Institutes of Health, includes a summary of the respiratory system, "How the Lungs Work." Click on "clinical trials" to learn more about current research related to the respiratory system. Write a brief summary of one of the studies currently being conducted.

SECTION 6.10 The Digestive System

Vocabulary

Content Vocabulary

You will learn these content vocabulary terms in this section.

- **peristalsis**
- **enzymes**
- **mastication**

Academic Vocabulary

You will see this word in your reading and on your tests. Find its meaning in the Glossary in the back of this book.

- **eliminate**

Digestion

How does the digestive system move food through the gastrointestinal tract?

Every cell in the body needs a constant supply of food to provide energy and the building blocks to manufacture body substances. This food is called intake. Once the body breaks down the food, it must eliminate the waste. The digestive system is responsible for the intake of food and elimination.

Digestion is the process of breaking down foods into nutrients that can be absorbed by cells. The digestive system consists of the digestive tract or gastrointestinal (GI) tract and several accessory organs, which are:

- mouth
- pharynx
- esophagus
- stomach
- small intestine
- large intestine
- liver
- gallbladder
- pancreas

CONNECT ANATOMY ACTIVITY

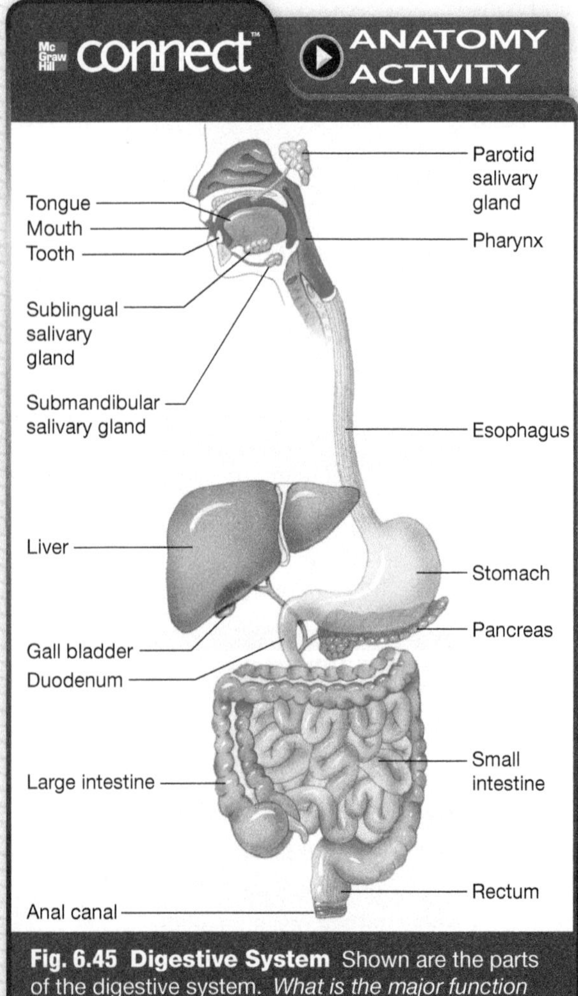

Fig. 6.45 Digestive System Shown are the parts of the digestive system. *What is the major function of the digestive system?* connect *Go Online to complete the Anatomy Activity for this system.*

The GI tract and the accessory organs are discussed in the following sections. **Figure 6.45** shows the components of the digestive system.

The GI tract is sometimes referred to as the alimentary canal. It is a tube that extends from the mouth to the anus. The wall of the GI tract has four layers that aid in the digestion of the food that passes through it:

- The outer covering is a serous layer of tissue, which is a layer of tissue that contains a serum or serumlike substance. It protects the canal and lubricates the outer surface. This covering allows the organs within the abdominal cavity to slide freely and not get lodged next to the abdominal cavity.
- The next layer is the muscle layer, which contracts and expands in wavelike motions, called **peristalsis,** to move food along the canal.
- The third layer is made of loose connective tissue containing various vessels, glands, and nerves that both nourish the surrounding tissue and carry waste away from it.
- The innermost layer is a mucous membrane that secretes mucus and digestive **enzymes** while protecting the tissues within the canal. Digestive

enzymes convert complex proteins, sugars, and fat molecules into simpler substances that can be used by the body.

READING CHECK

Name the substances that help the body break down food into nutrients and waste.

Organs of the Digestive System

How does the liver assist in digestion?

The digestive system consists of the mouth, the pharynx, the esophagus, the stomach, the small and large intestines, the liver the gall bladder, and the pancreas.

The Mouth

Food is taken into the oral cavity, or mouth. The lips sense the temperature and texture of the food and protect the mouth from food that is too hot or too rough on the surface. Once in the mouth, food is chewed by the teeth in a process called **mastication,** which uses the muscles of the cheeks and the tongue. Deglutition is the process of swallowing. At the back of the tongue, lingual tonsils form two mounds of rounded tissue that play an important role in the immune system.

The roof of the mouth is formed by the hard palate and the soft palate. At the back of the soft palate is a downward-pointing, cone-shaped projection called the uvula. On either side of the back of the mouth are rounded masses of lymphatic tissue called the palatine tonsils. The mouth also contains the gums, which hold the teeth.

Digestion of food begins in the mouth with mastication. Also, three sets of salivary glands surrounding the oral cavity secrete saliva. This fluid contains enzymes that begin the digestion of carbohydrates and aid in breaking down food. Each salivary gland has ducts through which the saliva travels to the mouth. As **Figure 6.46** shows, the three pairs of salivary glands are the parotid glands, the submandibular glands, and the sublingual glands.

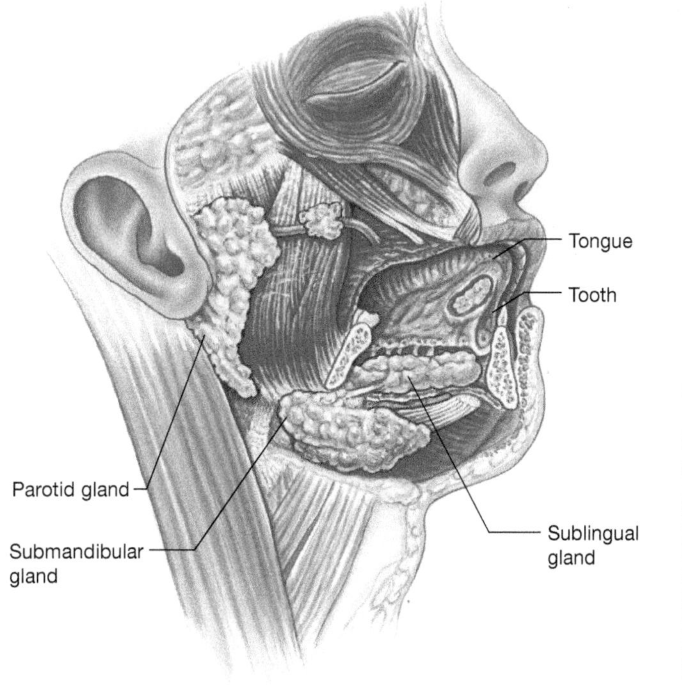

Fig. 6.46 Salivary Glands There are three pairs of salivary glands. *What do the salivary glands do in the process of digestion?*

The Pharynx

From the mouth, food goes through the throat, or pharynx. Food and air share this passageway. The pharynx is a muscular tube that moves food into the esophagus. When food is swallowed, the epiglottis, a flap of tissue, covers the trachea until the food is moved into the esophagus.

The Esophagus

The esophagus is a muscular tube that connects the throat with the stomach. When you eat, the esophagus contracts rhythmically to push food toward the stomach. At the bottom of the esophagus, just above the stomach, is a group of thickened muscles in the esophageal wall called the cardiac sphincter. This group of muscles contracts and closes the entrance to the stomach when food is present to prevent backflow or vomiting. Every time more food comes through the esophagus to the stomach, the muscles relax and allow the food to pass through.

The Stomach

The stomach is a pouch-like organ in the left hypochondriac region of the abdominal cavity. The stomach receives food from the esophagus and mixes it with gastric juice. Gastric juice contains hydrochloric acid and enzymes. Pepsin, an enzyme in the gastric juice, begins protein digestion.

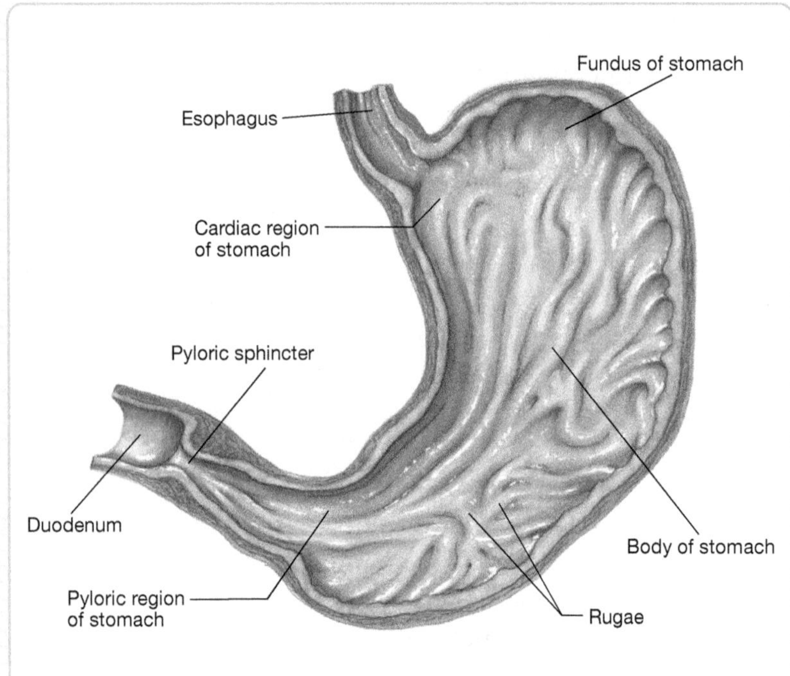

Fig. 6.47 Stomach The stomach has four regions. *What is the function of the stomach?*

The lining of the stomach is relatively thick and has many folds of mucous tissue called rugae. As the stomach fills up, the wall distends, and the folds disappear. The size of the stomach is similar to that of the human fist.

As shown in **Figure 6.47,** the stomach has four regions:

- Cardiac region: the region closest to the heart
- Fundus: the upper, rounded portion
- Body: the middle portion
- Pylorus: the narrowed bottom part

The pylorus has a powerful circular muscle at its base, the pyloric sphincter. This sphincter controls the emptying of the stomach's contents into the small intestine.

After a meal, the muscles of the stomach move. The food is then mixed with gastric juice to form a semifluid mass called chyme. Chyme may consist of food that has been in the stomach for several hours, or it may contain food that has been broken down in as little as one hour. The type of food and the amounts eaten determine how long it takes the stomach to release the chyme.

The stomach muscles release the chyme in small batches at regular intervals into the small intestine, where further digestion takes place.

Small Intestine

The small intestine receives chyme from the stomach, bile from the liver, and pancreatic juice from the pancreas. Bile is a substance secreted by the liver that ranges in color from yellow-brown to green.

The small intestine has three parts:

- The duodenum is only about 10 inches long. Here the chyme mixes with bile, pancreatic juice, and intestinal juice. Bile aids in fat digestion. Pancreatic juice aids in digestion of starch, proteins, and fat. Intestinal juice aids in digesting sugars such as glucose. Secretions from mucous glands lubricate the entire small intestine. The small intestine is lined with villi, which are tiny, one-cell-thick finger-like projections with capillaries through which digested nutrients are absorbed into the bloodstream and lymphatic system.
- The jejunum is a section of the small intestine that is eight feet long. It continues the digestive process.
- The ileum, the third section, connects the small intestine to the large intestine. The food is released from here into the large intestine.

Chyme takes from one to six hours to travel through the small intestine. The length of time for digestion varies depending on the food being digested and the health of the digestive system. Absorption, which begins in the small intestine, is the passage of material through the walls of the GI tract to the bloodstream. The small intestine is about 20 feet long from the stomach to the large intestine.

Large Intestine

The large intestine is about five feet long and forms a rectangle around the tightly packed small intestine. Waste products from digestion usually remain in the large intestine from 12 to 24 hours.

The large intestine has four parts:

- The cecum is the first part and has three openings: one from the ileum into the cecum, one from the cecum into the colon, and one from the cecum into the appendix, a worm-like pouch on the side. The appendix is filled with lymphatic tissue and is considered an accessory part of the body because it has no function or role in the digestive process. The appendix can, however, become inflamed and may require surgical removal. Within the cecum, the process of turning waste material into feces (stool) begins when water and certain necessary substances are absorbed back into the bloodstream. As the water is removed, the semisolid mass known as feces is formed and moved into the colon.
- The colon is divided into three parts that form a horseshoe shape in the abdominal cavity. The ascending colon extends upward. The transverse colon extends across. The descending colon extends downward, to where it connects to the sigmoid colon.
- The sigmoid colon is an S-shaped body that goes across the pelvis to the middle of the sacrum, where it connects to the rectum.

- The rectum attaches to the anal canal. The sphincter muscles at the mouth of the anus open during the release of feces from the body. This release is known as defecation.

The Liver

The liver is an important digestive organ located in the upper right quadrant of the abdominal cavity. Although it is not within the GI tract, it performs many digestive functions. The liver is a relatively large organ weighing about three pounds in the average adult. The hepatic portal system is the group of blood vessels that transports blood and other substances to and from the liver. The liver helps change food nutrients into usable substances. It secretes bile, a yellow-brown to green substance, which is stored in the gallbladder. It stores glucose and certain vitamins for release when the body needs them. The liver also secretes bilirubin, a bile pigment that is combined with bile and excreted into the duodenum.

The Gallbladder

The bile released from the liver goes into the gallbladder. The gallbladder stores bile until it is needed for digestion. Then it is forced out into the duodenum, where it aids in the breaking down of fats.

The Pancreas

The pancreas is five to six inches long and lies across the posterior side of the stomach. It is part of the digestive system because it secretes pancreatic juice into the small intestine through its system of ducts. Pancreatic juice contains various enzymes such as amylase and lipase. The pancreas is also an endocrine gland.

READING CHECK

List the substances that the body adds to food during digestion.

SECTION 6.10 The Digestive System Review

AFTER YOU READ

1. **List** the organs of digestion and the accessory organs of the digestive system.
2. **Identify** the purpose of intake.
3. **Illustrate** the path of a bite of food from your mouth to its exit from your body.
4. **Explain** the functions performed by the liver.
5. **Discuss** the function of the gallbladder.

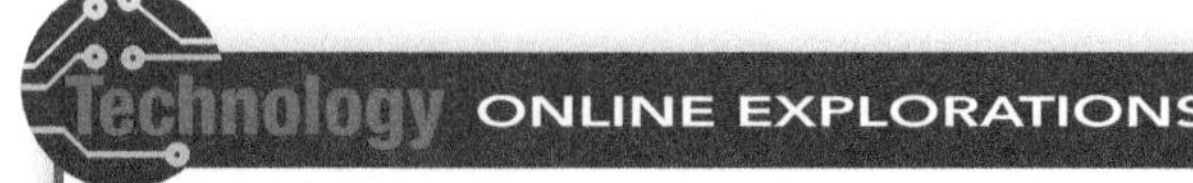

The Right Weight

Using the Internet or a reliable weight chart, determine your ideal body weight. Use this number to determine the weight at which you would be considered overweight, obese, and morbidly obese.

SECTION

6.11 The Urinary System

The Kidneys and Their Functions

How does urine move to the urinary bladder?

The urinary, or renal, system regulates water in the body, removes waste from blood, and stimulates red bone marrow to create red blood cells and regulate blood pressure. The system consists of the kidneys, ureters, urinary bladder, and the **urethra** (see **Figure 6.48**).

The kidneys form urine for excretion and retain substances the body needs. Urine begins forming with the filtration of water, salts, sugar, urea, and other waste from the blood. Average adult kidneys filter about 1,700 quarts of blood daily and create about 1.5 quarts of urine.

Kidneys have an outer protective part (cortex) and an inner soft part (medulla). On the concave side is the hilum, through which blood vessels, nerves, and ureters enter and exit. Nephrons perform the kidney's functions. Because kidneys have more nephrons than needed, people can live with one kidney or a part of a kidney.

Blood enters each kidney through the renal artery and exits through the renal vein. In the kidney, the renal artery branches into smaller arteries, or arterioles. Each arteriole leads into a nephron. A nephron is a group of capillaries called a glomerulus, which filters fluid from the blood. This is the first place urine is formed. Each nephron also contains a renal tubule to carry urine to ducts in the cortex. Surrounding each glomerulus is the Bowman's capsule, where fluid collects and then passes into a renal tubule. **Figure 6.49** on page 178 shows the formation of urine in the kidney.

Capillaries surround the renal tubule which allows most water, sugars, and some salts to reabsorb into the bloodstream. The remaining fluid is now urine. It travels to the renal pelvis, a collecting area in the center of the kidney.

Other Urinary Organs

What creates the urge to urinate?

In addition to the kidneys, the urinary system includes the ureters, the urinary bladder, and the urethra.

Vocabulary

Content Vocabulary

You will learn these content vocabulary terms in this section.

- **urethra**
- **voiding**
- **micturition**

Academic Vocabulary

You will see this word in your reading and on your tests. Find its meaning in the Glossary in the back of this book.

- **consists**

connect ANATOMY ACTIVITY

UrinaryTract

Kidneys

Ureters

Urinary bladder

Urethra

Fig. 6.48 The Urinary System
The urinary system is also known as the renal or excretory system. *What are the functions of the urinary system?* connect Go Online to complete the Anatomy Activity for this system.

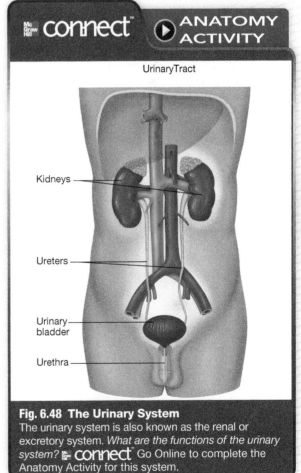

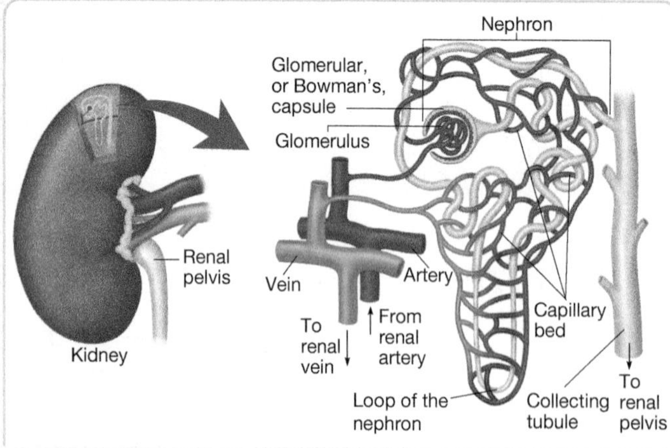

Fig. 6.49 Urine Formation The kidneys form urine for excretion. *What are the functions of the nephron?*

connect

VIRTUAL LAB: **Nephron**

The nephron is the basic functional unit of the kidney. Its main purpose is to control the concentration of water and substances such as salt by filtering blood—reabsorbing what the body needs and eliminating the rest as urine. The animation shows how the nephron works.

connect Go online to view the animation of the Nephron and complete the related questions.

The Ureters

Attached to each kidney is a ureter, a tube about six inches long that takes urine from the renal pelvis to the urinary bladder. Rhythmic contraction of the smooth muscle in the ureters moves urine to the urinary bladder. It travels in waves in a process similar to the progression of digested food through the intestines.

The Urinary Bladder

The urinary bladder is a hollow, muscular organ that stores urine until it is excreted from the body. Urine is pumped into the bladder every few seconds. The bladder can hold 300–400 milliliters (about $1\frac{1}{2}$ to 2 cups) of urine. The bladder walls contain epithelial tissue that can stretch to allow the bladder to hold twice as much as it does when normally full. When the bladder is stretched, nerve endings that create the urge to urinate are stimulated. The walls also contain three layers of muscle that help in the emptying process.

The Urethra

Urine is excreted through the urethra, a tube of smooth muscle with a mucous lining. The female urethra, about 1.5 inches long, opens through the meatus, located at the distal end of the urethra. The male urethra, about eight inches long, extends through three different regions before exiting through the meatus on the distal end of the penis. Excreting urine is called **voiding** or **micturition.**

READING CHECK

Recall how much urine the average adult produces in one day.

SECTION 6.11 The Urinary System Review

AFTER YOU READ

1. **Identify** another name for the urinary system.
2. **Recall** how much blood is filtered by the kidneys each day.
3. **Explain** the process of urine formation.
4. **Describe** how urine is transferred from the kidney to the urinary bladder.
5. **Analyze** what is happening in your body when you feel the urge to urinate.

Technology ONLINE EXPLORATIONS

Urine Contents

What is in our urine can reveal a lot about our health. Research the Internet with a partner to determine what is normally in urine and what is not. Create a table of your results.

SECTION

6.12 The Endocrine System

Endocrine Functions and Organs

What gland regulates the secretion of essential hormones from other glands?

The endocrine system is made up of glands that act as the body's master regulator. **Figure 6.50** shows the parts of the system, which acts by means of chemical stimuli only. Unlike the nervous system, which has immediate and short-term effects on the muscles and glands, the endocrine system has widespread, slower, and longer-lasting effects. The endocrine system affects growth, metabolism, and reproduction.

The glands and other tissues of the endocrine system secrete special chemicals, or **hormones**, into the bloodstream. Hormones work in specific target cells. Glands that secrete hormones are ductless glands because the hormones are not secreted into ducts.

Vocabulary

Content Vocabulary

You will learn this content vocabulary term in this section.

- **hormones**

Academic Vocabulary

You will see this word in your reading and on your tests. Find its meaning in the Glossary in the back of this book.

- **factor**

Organs and Glands that Secrete Hormones

The following organs and glands secrete hormones:

- The hypothalamus, which is part of the nervous system, also serves as an endocrine gland because it releases hormones that regulate pituitary hormones. Hormones released by the hypothalamus have either a releasing or an inhibiting factor. A releasing factor allows secretion of other hormones to take place. An inhibiting factor prevents the secretion.
- The pineal gland is located superior and posterior to the pituitary gland. It releases melatonin, a hormone believed to affect sleep.
- The pituitary gland is the body's master gland to regulate the secretion of hormones.
- The thyroid gland releases secretions that control metabolism and blood calcium. Two of the hormones secreted, thyroxine (T4) and triiodothyronine (T3), are produced in the thyroid gland using iodine from blood. T4 and T3 circulate throughout the bloodstream, helping to stimulate and control various bodily functions, such as regulating the metabolism of carbohydrates, lipids, and proteins. Iodine is necessary for proper thyroid functioning.

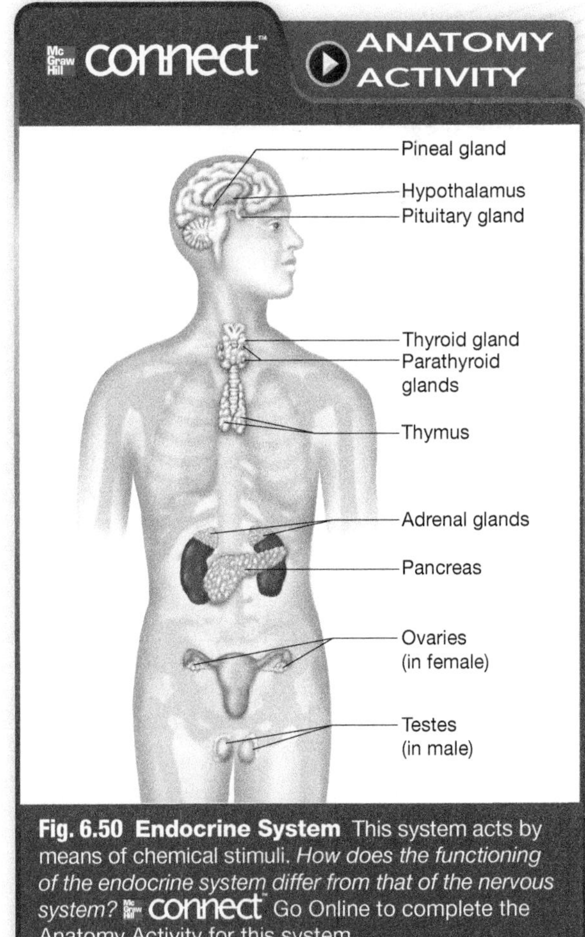

Fig. 6.50 Endocrine System This system acts by means of chemical stimuli. *How does the functioning of the endocrine system differ from that of the nervous system?* connect Go Online to complete the Anatomy Activity for this system

- The parathyroid glands help regulate the levels of calcium and phosphate, two elements necessary to maintain homeostasis (balance), or normal functioning, of the body.
- The thymus gland is considered to be part of the endocrine system because it secretes a hormone and is ductless. However, it is also part of the immune system. The hormone it releases stimulates the production of T cells and B cells, which are important to the development of an immune response.
- The adrenal glands are a pair of glands. Each gland sits atop a kidney, and each consists of two parts: the adrenal cortex, which

Table 6.2 Hormones

GLAND OR ORGAN	HORMONE	FUNCTION
Hypothalamus	Pituitary-regulating hormone	Stimulates or inhibits pituitary secretions
Pineal gland	Melatonin	Affects sexual function and wake-sleep cycle
Pituitary, anterior	Growth hormone (GH) and somato-tropic hormone (STH)	Stimulate bone and muscle growth; regulate some metabolic functions
Pituitary, anterior	Thyroid-stimulating hormone (TSH)	Stimulates thyroid gland to secrete hormones
Pituitary, anterior	Adrenocorticotropic hormone (ACTH)	Stimulates secretion of adrenal cortex hormones
Pituitary, anterior	Follicle-stimulating hormone (FSH) and luteinizing hormone (LH)	Stimulate development of ova and production of female hormones
Pituitary, anterior	Prolactin	Stimulates breast development and milk production
Pituitary, posterior	Antidiuretic hormone (ADH), also known as vasopressin	Increases water reabsorption
Pituitary, posterior	Oxytocin	Stimulates uterine contractions and lactation
Pituitary, posterior	Melanocyte-stimulating hormone	Stimulates production of melanin
Thyroid	T3, T4	Regulate metabolism and stimulate growth
Parathyroid	Parathyroid hormone	Increases blood calcium as necessary to maintain homeostasis
Thymus	Thymosin, thymic humoral factor (THF), serum thymic factor (STF)	Aid in development of T cells and some B cells; function not well understood
Adrenal, medulla	Epinephrine (adrenaline) and norepinephrine	Work with the sympathetic nervous system to regulate the reaction to stress
Adrenal, cortex	Glucocorticoids, mineralocorticoids, and gonadocorticoids	Affect metabolism and growth, and aid in electrolyte and fluid balance
Pancreas	Insulin and glucagon	Maintain normal level of blood glucose concentration
Ovaries	Estrogen and progesterone	Promote development of female sex characteristics, menstrual cycle, reproductive functions
Testes	Testosterone	Promotes development of male sex characteristics and sperm production

is the outer portion, and the adrenal medulla, which is the inner portion. The adrenal glands regulate electrolytes, or essential mineral salts, in the body. The mineral salts affect metabolism and blood pressure. They also secrete hormones in response to stress.

- The pancreas helps in maintaining a proper level of blood glucose. Within the pancreas, specialized hormone-producing cells, known as the islets of Langerhans, secrete insulin when blood sugar levels are high and glucagon when blood sugar levels are low. When insulin is released in response to high blood sugar levels, it stimulates the sending of glucose to the body's cells for use as energy. When glucagon is released in response to low blood sugar levels, it stimulates stored glycogen to be transformed into glucose again. The islets of Langerhans serve the pancreas's endocrine functions, and the remaining cells are part of the digestive system.
- The ovaries produce the female sex hormones, estrogen and progesterone. They are also part of the female reproductive system.
- The testes produce a male sex hormone called testosterone. The testes are also part of the male reproductive system.

Too much or too little of a hormone in the body creates an imbalance and, often, a disorder or disease. Most endocrine illnesses are the result of a hormonal imbalance. Understanding hormones will help you understand what happens when an imbalance occurs. **Table 6.2** lists the organs that produce hormones and their names and functions.

READING CHECK

Identify which part of the endocrine system is also part of the immune system.

SECTION 6.12 The Endocrine System Review

AFTER YOU READ

1. **Compare** the nervous and endocrine systems. How are they alike? How are they different?
2. **Name** the organ that is part of both the endocrine system and the digestive system. What does it do for each system?
3. **Identify** the organ that secretes factors that control the release of hormones but is part of the nervous system. What factors does it release?
4. **Recall** which gland has two parts. What are the functions of these parts?
5. **Explain** how the pancreas helps to regulate blood glucose.

Technology ONLINE EXPLORATIONS

Your Internal Thermostat

The endocrine system works like an automatic thermostat. When the room gets hot, the air conditioner turns on; when it is cold, the heater turns on. When we need fuel, hormones are released to stimulate feelings of hunger. When we are threatened, a hormone prepares our muscles for action. Keep a 24-hour record of your level of energy, how sleepy you feel, your temperature, and hunger. Compare your record with those of other students. Research online to help establish what organ or gland and hormone caused your results.

SECTION

6.13 The Reproductive System

Vocabulary

Content Vocabulary

You will learn these content vocabulary terms in this section.

- **germ cells**
- **menstruation**
- **menarche**
- **menopause**

Academic Vocabulary

You will see this word in your reading and on your tests. Find its meaning in the Glossary in the back of this book.

- **layers**

Overview

What role is played by the accessory reproductive organs?

Human reproduction requires specialized sex cells from a male and a female. These are **germ cells,** or gametes. The male cells are spermatozoa or sperm. The female cells are ova. Germ cells have half as many chromosomes as other cells in the body. Those other cells have 23 chromosome pairs or 46 chromosomes. Sperm and the ova each contain 23, one of each pair. When they unite, a new life begins.

Although the reproductive systems of males and females are different, the reproductive organs of both sexes may be divided into two groups:

- The primary organs are the gonads, or sex glands. These produce the germ cells and make hormones. Female gonads are ovaries and male gonads are testes.
- Accessory organs, which are glands and ducts, transport and protect germ cells.

Female Reproductive System

What events signal the beginning and end of a woman's childbearing years?

The female reproductive system is shown in **Figure 6.51.** The ovaries release an egg as part of the ovarian cycle. A fertilized egg is transported via one of the fallopian tubes to the uterus, where it develops into an embryo and then into a fetus. At the end of gestation, the infant is born through the vagina in a routine delivery or surgically through the abdomen in a Caesarean delivery.

The ovaries lie on either side of the uterus and usually release only one mature ovum during each monthly cycle. This is called ovulation. In rare cases, more eggs are released.

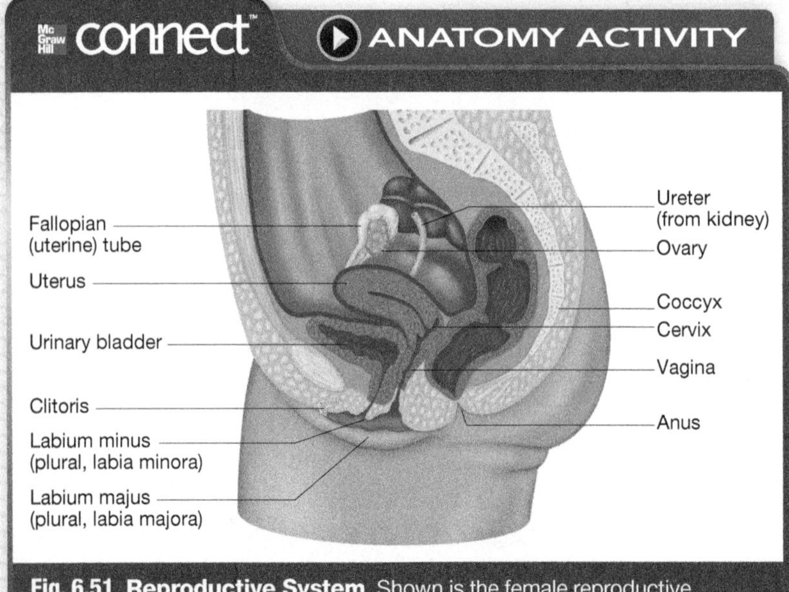

Fig. 6.51 Reproductive System Shown is the female reproductive system. *What is the primary organ of reproduction in females?*
connect Go Online to complete the Anatomy Activity for this system.

At birth, most females have from 200,000 to 400,000 immature ova in each ovary. Many of these disintegrate before the female reaches puberty and the first **menstruation,** called **menarche. Menopause** is the end of the menstruation cycle and of the child-bearing years.

As shown in **Figure 6.52,** when an ovum (oocyte) is released, it enters the fallopian tubes, which have hair-like ends called fimbriae. Fimbriae sweep the ovum into one of the fallopian tubes, where it may be fertilized by a sperm. Fertilized or not, the ovum moves by contractions of the tube to the uterus. The uterus is about three inches long. Once inside the uterus, a fertilized ovum attaches to the uterine wall, where it will be nourished for about 40 weeks of development called gestation. The upper portion of the uterus, the fundus, is the place where the placenta grows into the uterine wall. An ovum that has not been fertilized is released along with the lining of the uterus during menstruation.

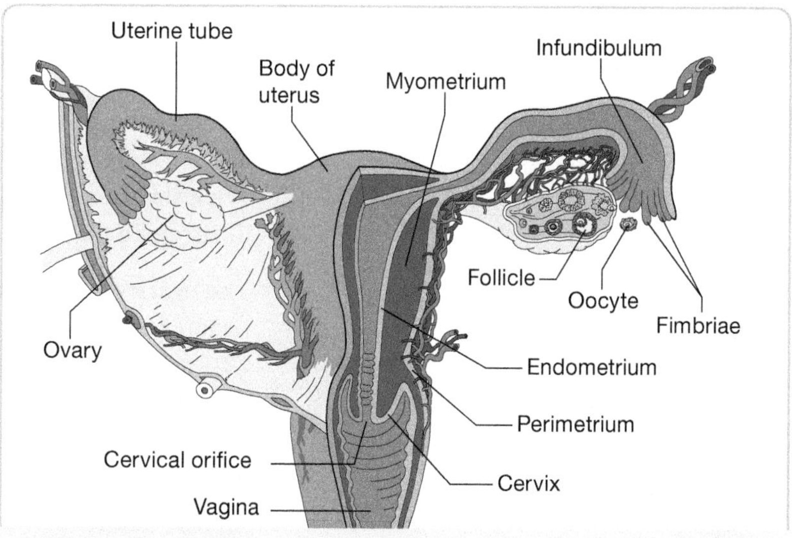

Fig. 6.52 Female Reproductive Organs This is an anterior view of the female reproductive organs. *Which organ releases the ovum?*

The cervix is a protective body with glands that secrete mucous substances into the vagina. The vagina can expand to accommodate the passage of a baby during childbirth.

The uterus is made up of three layers of tissue. The outer layer, the perimetrium, is a protective layer of membranous tissue. The myometrium, which is the middle layer, has three layers of smooth muscle. This middle layer stretches during pregnancy and provides muscle contractions during labor to push the infant out of the uterus.

The inner mucous layer, the endometrium, is deep and velvety, and has an abundant supply of blood vessels and glands. Each month it is built up in expectation of the arrival of a fertilized ovum. Without a fertilized egg, the endometrium is broken down and becomes the blood and mucus of the menstruation cycle.

The external female genitalia are collectively known as the vulva. The vulva consists of the mons pubis, the labia majora, and the labia minora. The space between the labia minora contains Bartholin's glands, which secrete fluid into the vagina, and the openings for the vagina and urethra. The space between the bottom of the labia majora and the anus is called the perineum. **Figure 6.53** shows the external female genitalia.

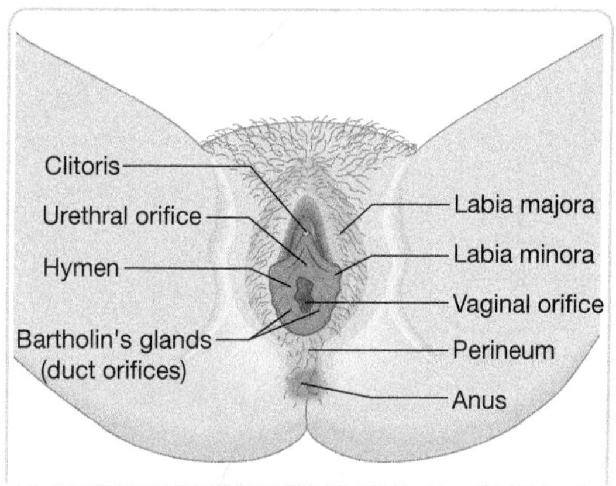

Fig. 6.53 Genitalia Two hormones play an important role in the development of mature genitalia in women. *What are those hormones?*

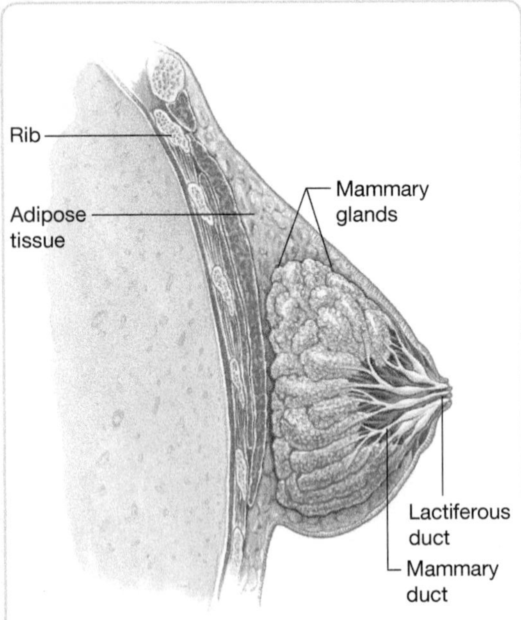

Fig. 6.54 Mammary Glands The breasts are full of glandular tissue that responds to the cycles of menstruation and birth. *What is lactation?*

The female breast, or mammary gland, is an accessory organ, providing milk to nurse the infant after birth. The breasts are full of glandular tissue that is stimulated by hormones after puberty to grow and respond to the cycles of menstruation and birth.

During pregnancy, hormones stimulate the milk-producing ducts and sinuses that transport milk to the nipple. The dark-pigmented area surrounding the nipple is called the areola. After birth, the mammary glands experience a "let-down" reflex, which allows milk to flow through the nipples when the infant suckles. This is called lactation. **Figure 6.54** illustrates a mammary gland and its milk-producing ducts.

The ovaries secrete estrogen and progesterone, the primary female hormones. In the stages before and during puberty, estrogen and progesterone play an important role in the development of mature genitalia and of secondary sex characteristics, such as pubic hair and breasts. Other hormones help in childbirth and milk production.

READING CHECK

Recall how many ova are present in the ovaries of a newborn girl.

Male Reproductive System

How many sperm are needed to fertilize an ovum?

The male reproductive system is shown in **Figure 6.55.** The spermatozoa, or sperm, are produced in the testes. The testes also produce testosterone, the most important male hormone. The testes are contained within the scrotum, a sac outside the body, where the temperature is lower than it is inside the body. The lower temperature is necessary for the safe development of sperm.

Sperm cells are contained in seminiferous tubules.. At the top part of each testis is the epididymis. In the epididymis the sperm develop to maturity and become able to move. They leave the epididymis and enter a narrow tube called the vas deferens. The sperm then travel to the

connect ANATOMY ACTIVITY

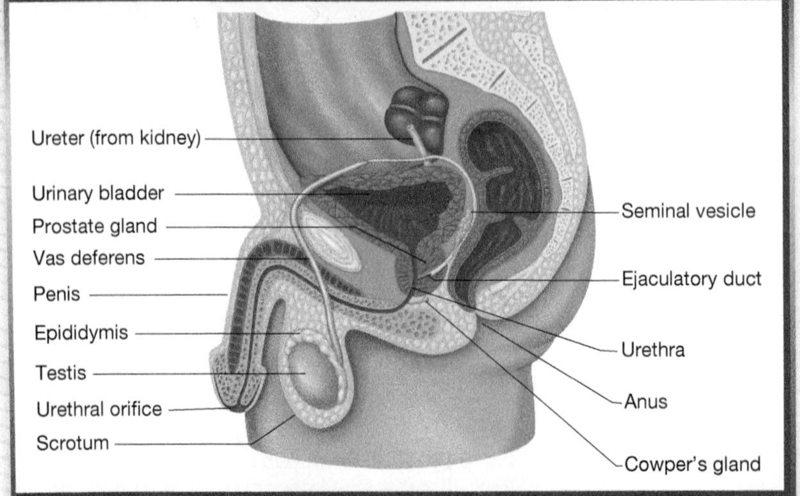

Fig. 6.55 Male Reproductive System Shown is the male reproductive system. *What are the accessory organs of the male reproductive system?*
connect *Go Online to complete the Anatomy Activity for this system*

seminal vesicles. The seminal vesicles secrete fluid to help the sperm move.

Next the sperm pass through the ejaculatory duct leading to the prostate gland and the urethra. The prostate gland also secretes a fluid that helps the sperm move. The gland then contracts its muscle tissue during ejaculation to help the sperm exit the body.

Just below the prostate are the two bulbourethral glands, or Cowper's glands, which also secrete a fluid that lubricates the inside of the urethra to help the semen move easily. The urethra passes through the penis to the outside of the body. The tip of the penis is called the glans penis, a sensitive area that is covered at birth by the foreskin.

The spermatozoon is a microscopic cell, much smaller than an ovum. It has a head region that carries genetic material. It has a tail called the flagellum that propels the sperm forward. During ejaculation, hundreds of millions of sperm are released.

Usually only one sperm can fertilize a single ovum. In some cases, two or more ova are fertilized at a single time, resulting in multiple births such as twins or triplets. Identical twins are the result of the splitting of one ovum after a single sperm has fertilized it. Fraternal twins are the result of two sperm fertilizing two ova.

READING CHECK

Recall how identical twins are created.

SECTION 6.13 The Reproductive System Review

AFTER YOU READ

1. **Compare** the male and female reproductive systems.
2. **Describe** the difference between primary and accessory organs of reproduction.
3. **Explain** what happens when an ovum (egg) is not fertilized.
4. **Trace** the path of sperm. What organs does it travel through? How does it become part of semen?
5. **Compare** how identical twins are created as opposed to fraternal twins.

Technology ONLINE EXPLORATIONS

The Hormonal Cycle

There are four hormones involved in the 28-day menstrual cycle. Go online to research these hormones and draw a map or diagram of how they work to create the menstrual cycle.

CHAPTER **6 Review**

Chapter Summary

SECTION 6.1

- The body's smallest element is the cell; grouped cells make tissue; various tissues make organs; and a group of organs makes a system. Body cavities separate organs. **(pg. 133)**

SECTION 6.2

- The integumentary system consists of the skin, hair, nails, sweat glands, and oil-producing glands. **(pg. 139)**

SECTION 6.3

- The skeletal system, the body's framework, consists of bones and joints. **(pg. 142)**

SECTION 6.4

- The muscular system allows us to move, keeps our heart beating, and helps us digest food. It also provides stability. **(pg. 147)**

SECTION 6.5

- The nervous system works through electrical and chemical stimuli. **(pg. 150)**

SECTION 6.6

- The sensory system includes five senses: sight, hearing, touch, taste, and smell. **(pg. 154)**

SECTION 6.7

- The circulatory system includes the heart, blood, and blood vessels. **(pg. 158)**

SECTION 6.8

- The lymphatic system contains vessels that transport lymph fluid to and from the bloodstream. **(pg. 164)**
- The immune system provides defenses against diseases and disorders. **(pg. 166)**

SECTION 6.9

- The respiratory system includes the lungs and other structures that provide oxygen to all of the body's cells. **(pg. 168)**

SECTION 6.10

- The digestive system provides intake and elimination through the gastrointestinal tract and accessory organs. **(pg. 172)**

SECTION 6.11

- The urinary system removes waste products from the blood and eliminates them from the body. **(pg. 177)**

SECTION 6.12

- The endocrine system works through chemical stimuli called hormones. **(pg. 179)**

SECTION 6.13

- The male and female reproductive systems contain primary organs and accessory organs. **(pg. 182)**

CHAPTER 6 Assessment

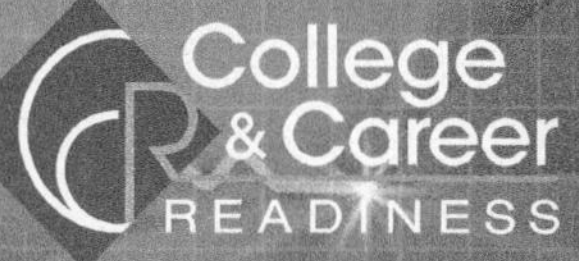

Critical Thinking/Problem Solving

1. Although all healthcare professionals need to know anatomy and physiology, certain professionals specialize in (or exercise special knowledge about) one or more particular body systems. Review the healthcare professions below and determine the body system that is most closely matched to each. Explain why you chose that system.

- Esthetician
- Urologist
- Massage Therapist
- Dietician
- Athletic Trainer
- Radiologic Technologist
- Mental Health Nurse
- Optometrist
- Respiratory Therapist
- Obstetrician

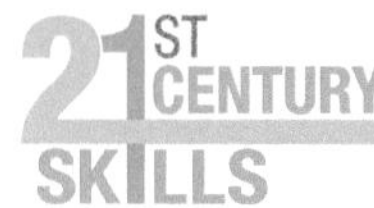

2. **Teamwork** With a partner as a client, count the number of times in one minute that he or she breathes. Make a note of the number. Then have your partner count your own respiration rate. Compare the results.

3. **Communication** Working with a partner, perform range of motion tests on joints, fingers, elbows, shoulders, and head. Record each movement for each joint listed.

4. **Information Literacy** Go online to find five diseases or disorders related to a system presented in this chapter. Create a "What Went Wrong" chart showing the cause of each disease.

connect™ ONLINE ACTIVITIES

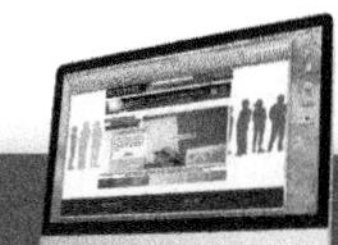

Complete our HST online activities for Chapter 6, which include Body Systems Anatomy animated tutorials, Concept Check review questions, Reference Flash Cards, and Online Procedures assessment sheets.

- **Body Systems Anatomy** animated tutorials with drag-and-drop activities
- **Concept Check** review questions
- **Reference Flash Cards** medical terminology practice
- **Online Procedures** assessment sheets

CHAPTER 7 Diseases and Disorders

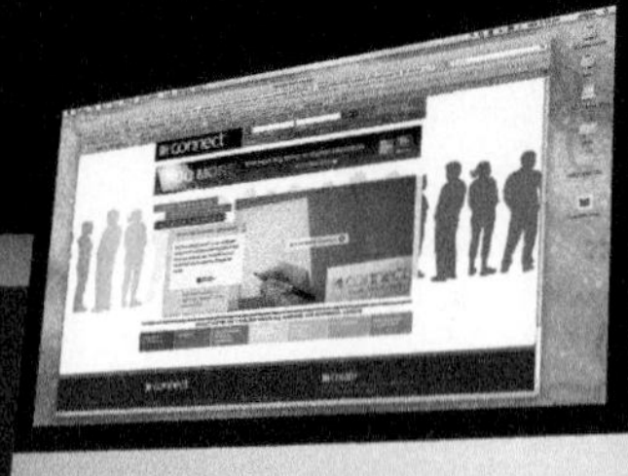

McGraw Hill connect™

It's Online!

- **Online Procedures**
- **STEM Connection**
- **Medical Science**
- **Medical Terms**
- **Medical Math**
- **Ethics in Action**
- **Virtual Lab**

Essential Question:

What are the main types of diseases and disorders?

Diseases and disorders can be caused by many things, including cell injury or death, infection, allergy, autoimmune issues, developmental and genetic anomalies, and change in blood flow. This chapter will discuss the diseases and disorders that affect each of the body's systems and the methods used to treat those conditions.

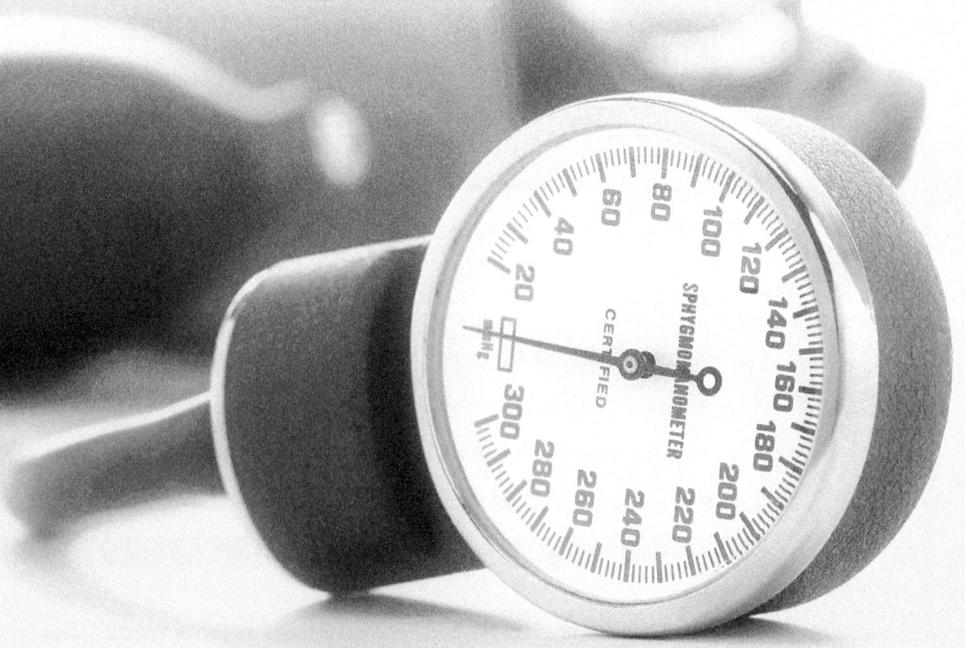

Photo: Dale Wilson/Photographer's Choice RF/Getty Images

READING GUIDE

OBJECTIVES

After completing this chapter, you will be able to:

- **Identify** the sources of diseases and disorders of the body systems.
- **Describe** diseases and disorders of the integumentary, skeletal, muscular, nervous, special senses, circulatory, lymphatic, respiratory, digestive, urinary, endocrine, and reproductive systems.
- **Categorize** diseases and disorders of the integumentary, skeletal, muscular, nervous, special senses, circulatory, lymphatic, respiratory, digestive, urinary, endocrine, and reproductive systems.
- **Recognize** emerging diseases, disorders, and therapies.

BEFORE YOU READ

Connect Can you recognize common ailments of the various body systems?

Main Idea

The ability to recognize and define common diseases and disorders of body systems and to identify appropriate treatments for them is an essential healthcare skill.

Note-Taking Activity

Draw this table. Write key terms and phrases under **Cues**. Write main ideas under **Note Taking**. Summarize the section under **Summary**.

Cues	Note Taking
o o	o o
Summary	

Graphic Organizer

Before you read the chapter, draw a diagram like the one below. As you read, write the diseases and disorders as covered in this chapter into the diagram.

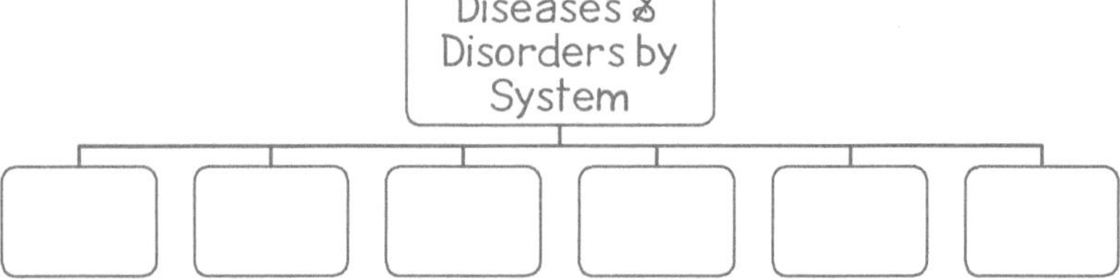

connect
Downloadable graphic organizers can be accessed online.

STANDARDS

HEALTH SCIENCE

NCHSE 1.21 Describe common diseases and disorders of each body system (prevention, pathology, diagnosis, and treatment).

SCIENCE

NSES C Develop understanding of the cell; molecular basis of heredity; biological evolution; interdependence of organisms; matter, energy, and organization in living systems; and behavior of organisms.

NCHSE 1.22 Recognize emerging diseases and disorders.

NCHSE *National Consortium for Health Science Education*

NSES *National Science Education Standards*

COMMON CORE STATE STANDARDS

MATHEMATICS

Number and Quantity

Quantities N-Q 3 Choose a level of accuracy appropriate to limitations on measurement when reporting quantities.

ENGLISH LANGUAGE ARTS

Reading

Key Ideas and Details R-2 Determine the central ideas or conclusions of a text; summarize complex concepts, processes, or information presented in a text by paraphrasing them in simpler but still accurate terms.

Speaking and Listening

Comprehension and Collaboration SL-2 Integrate multiple sources of information presented in diverse media or formats (e.g., visually, quantitatively, orally) evaluating the credibility and accuracy of each source.

SECTION

7.1 Causes of Diseases and Disorders

Vocabulary

Content Vocabulary

You will learn these content vocabulary terms in this section.

- pathology
- cancer
- inflammation
- hemodynamics
- autoimmune
- neoplasm
- malignant
- benign

Academic Vocabulary

You will see this word in your reading and on your tests. Find its meaning in the Glossary in the back of this book.

- involve

connect

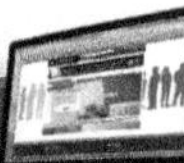

STEM CONNECTION

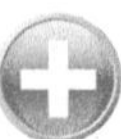

Medical Science

Cancer Cell Growth
Cancer is a group of closely related diseases that can occur in many different tissues and systems. One in three individuals will develop some form of cancer. The most common cancers occur in the lungs, colon, rectum, prostate, breast, and uterus. The term "malignancy" means a cancerous tumor or cancer in the blood or lymph tissue.

Go to connect to complete a brief assignment on cancer.

Pathology: Diseases and Disorders

What is the most common cause of illness and death worldwide?

The term **pathology** comes from *pathos*, "suffering," and *-ology*, "the study of." It is therefore the study of suffering.

More precisely, pathology is the study of disease. Disease is any structural or physiological change that disrupts homeostasis in the body.

Diseases and disorders can be caused by many things, including:

- Cell injury or death. When a cell is injured by toxins, trauma, infection, **cancer,** or other agents, it may adapt or die.
- **Inflammation** is a vascular response of tissue to an injury, infection, allergy, or autoimmune disease. Inflammation is normally a protective response intended to destroy or limit both the injurious agent and the damaged tissue. At times it can go out of control and cause even more damage. Inflammation can be classified as acute (short term) or chronic (long term), based on how long the inflammation lasts.
- Developmental and genetic diseases are those that are passed on from our parents. There are over 250,000 birth defects in newborns in the U.S. each year. Approximately 20 percent of these are due to heredity.
- A change in **hemodynamics** (blood flow) is a cause of disease. These diseases involve the heart and blood vessels. For example, a blood clot causes disruption of the blood flow to the heart, causing a heart attack.
- **Autoimmune** diseases occur when the body's immune system attacks the body. Basically, the body is unable to distinguish between self and non-self. Autoimmune diseases can be very debilitating and even cause death. Autoimmune diseases are more common in women and seem to be on the rise.
- **Neoplasms** ("new growths") are tissues that grow out of control. Neoplasms are categorized as benign or **malignant.** Solid neoplasms are referred to as tumors. If the tumor stays localized in the tissue, it is designated as **benign.** If the tumor has the ability to spread to distant sites, it is referred to as a malignant tumor, or a cancer.

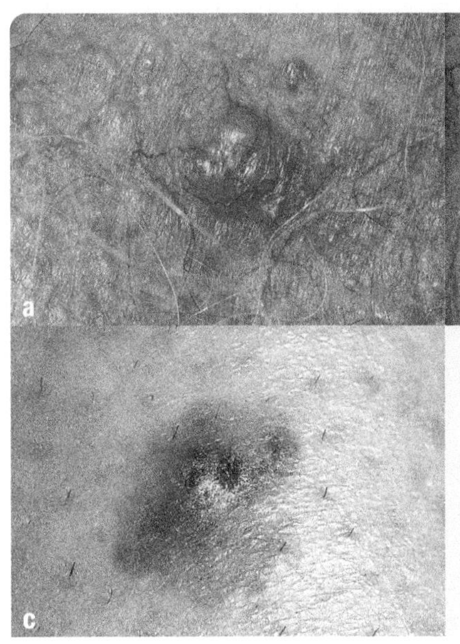

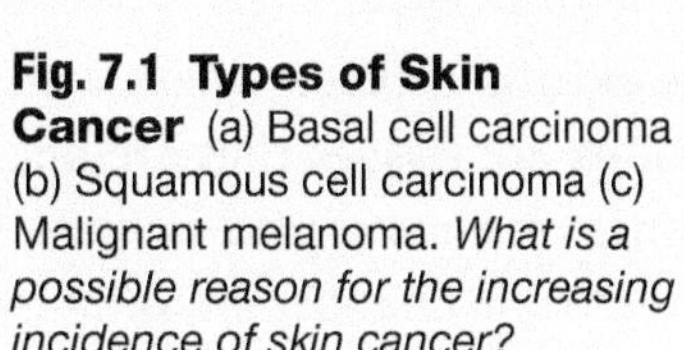

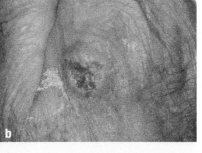

Fig. 7.1 Types of Skin Cancer (a) Basal cell carcinoma (b) Squamous cell carcinoma (c) Malignant melanoma. *What is a possible reason for the increasing incidence of skin cancer?*

Photos: (l-r)Science Photo Library RF/Getty Images, Biophoto Associates/Science Source/Photo Researchers, John Kash M.D./Photo Researchers

- Environmental and nutritional pathology covers all aspects of our environment that cause disease. For example, smoking, alcoholism, poor nutrition, obesity, and drug abuse can all cause disease.
- Infections are the most common cause of illness and death worldwide. Infectious organisms cause tissue damage and death. The study of these organisms is called microbiology, as discussed in Chapter 3.

READING CHECK

Name the types of diseases that often occur due to heredity.

21ST CENTURY SKILLS

Technology and Aging

We are all aware that the life expectancy of Americans has increased dramatically over the last 100 or so years. In 1900, the average life expectancy for men in the U.S. was 43.6 years. In 2005, that had risen to 75.2 years. The average life expectancy for women in 1900 was 48.3 years and 80.4 years by 2005. Factors that have impacted these statistics are women surviving childbirth, fewer infectious diseases, better nutrition, better access to healthcare, safer work environments, and higher awareness of healthy lifestyles. Of course, disease still has a powerful effect on life expectancy, but with new research and genetic engineering, it will not be surprising if life expectancy rises even further in the future.

SECTION 7.1 Causes of Diseases and Disorders Review

AFTER YOU READ

1. **Indicate** at least five causes of disease.
2. **Compare** and **contrast** benign and malignant tumors.
3. **Identify** four causes of inflammation.
4. **Choose** and **discuss** three environmental factors that can cause disease.
5. **Discuss** how a change in hemodynamics can cause disease.

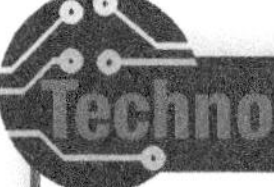

Technology ONLINE EXPLORATIONS

Life Expectancy

Research the Internet for more information about your life expectancy and disease potential. Based upon your age and date of birth, determine your life expectancy. Then determine the top three causes of death for your age and sex.

SECTION 7.2

Diseases and Disorders of the Integumentary System

Vocabulary

Content Vocabulary

You will learn this content vocabulary term in this section.

- lesions

Academic Vocabulary

You will see these words in your reading and on your tests. Find their meanings in the Glossary in the back of this book.

- primary
- annually

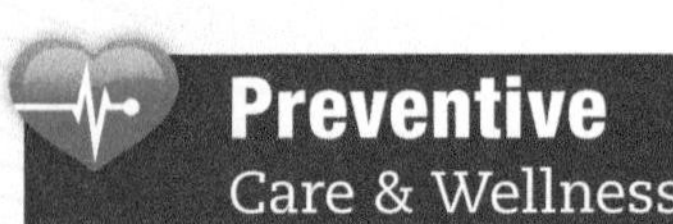

Preventive Care & Wellness

Check Your Moles

Moles should be checked for signs of possible melanoma (skin cancer). The acronym ABCDE is used to remember the possible signs.

A = Asymmetry The mole should look equal in size from side to side.

B = Border The border of the mole should not be irregular; it should be smooth.

C = Color The mole should be even. It should not darken or lighten or contain a mixture of colors.

D = Diameter The mole should not grow larger than 6 mm, about the diameter of a pencil eraser.

E = Evolving The mole should not change in size, shape, color, or appearance, or grow on an area of previously normal skin. The texture of an existing mole should not change and become hard, lumpy, or scaly.

Lesions

What are primary and secondary lesions?

The skin is a place where some internal diseases show symptoms. **Lesions** are tissues that are altered because of a disease or disorder. Primary lesions appear on previously normal skin. Secondary lesions result from changes in primary lesions. Secondary lesions usually involve either loss of skin surface or material that forms on the skin surface. Vascular lesions are blood vessel lesions that show through the skin. Several specific types of lesions are shown in **Figure 7.2.**

Microorganism-Related Diseases

How is shingles related to chickenpox?

Some common diseases are caused by viruses or other microorganisms.

- Rubella, or German measles, poses a threat to an unborn child. If a pregnant woman contracts rubella, severe defects in the fetus can occur. Immunizations should be given to children. Women who have not been immunized should be before getting pregnant.
- Chickenpox is caused by the varicella-zoster virus. It is spread by direct contact or by breathing in germs when someone coughs or sneezes. Chickenpox produces a blister-like rash, itching, tiredness, and fever. It tends to produce more severe symptoms in older clients and can cause birth defects if contracted by a mother during pregnancy. A vaccine is available to prevent this contagious disease.
- Herpes zoster is the virus that causes shingles. A client who has had chickenpox has a 20 percent chance of developing shingles. Shingles is an inflammation that affects the nerves on one side of the body and results in skin blisters. It can be extremely painful. A vaccine is now available for adults to prevent herpes zoster.
- Herpes simplex 1 causes cold sores or fever blisters around the mouth. It is not the same as herpes simplex 2, or genital herpes.
- Impetigo, caused by staphylococci or streptococci, appears as a blistery rash. When the blisters open, they produce a thick, golden-yellow discharge. It is spread through direct contact with discharge from the lesions. It is treated with oral and/or topical antibiotics.
- Tinea, or ringworm, is caused by fungi. On the feet it is called athlete's foot, or tinea pedis. On the scalp it is scalp ringworm, or tinea capitis. Treatment is topical antifungal medication.

READING CHECK

Explain how rubella can complicate pregnancy.

Other Skin Diseases and Disorders

Which skin cancer causes the most deaths?

- Furuncle (or boil) is a localized, pus-producing infection originating in a hair follicle.
- Carbuncle is a pus-producing infection that starts in subcutaneous tissue and usually comes with fever and a general feeling of illness.
- Abscess is a localized infection usually accompanied by pus and inflammation.
- Gangrene, or death of tissue, is due to loss of blood supply.
- Acne, or acne vulgaris, is a skin condition that causes eruptions on the face and upper back, usually starting around puberty.
- Psoriasis is a recurrent skin condition that causes scaly lesions on the trunk, arms, hands, legs, and scalp, often associated with stress.
- Pediculosis is infestation of lice. It can occur on the head or in the genital area. It is very common among school-age children and can be contracted only by coming in contact with a person with lice.
- Scabies is a contagious skin eruption caused by mites that often occurs between fingers, on areas of the trunk, or on male genitalia.

Skin Cancer

There are three types of skin cancer. More than 90 percent of skin cancers are on sun-exposed skin, usually the face, neck, ears, forearms, and hands. A change of color, size, shape, or texture of a mole is a common indicator. A bleeding or itching mole is another indicator.

Basal cell and squamous cell carcinomas can cause serious illness and, if untreated, can cause considerable damage, disfigurement, or even death. Malignant melanoma causes more than 75 percent of all deaths from skin cancer. This disease can spread to other organs, most commonly the lungs and liver.

Burns

The second leading cause of accidental death in the United States, after motor vehicle accidents, is burn injuries. There are more than 200 special burn care centers in the United States. More than 2 million burn injuries are reported each year, and more than 11,000 patients die annually from burn injuries. This year, about 1 million people will suffer a burn injury that causes a significant or permanent disability.

READING CHECK

List the procedures used to treat and prevent pediculosis.

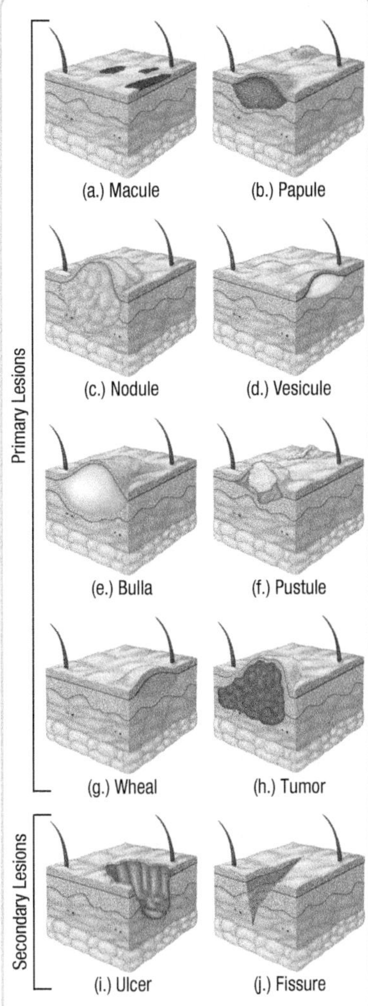

Fig. 7.2 Types of Lesions Lesions are tissues altered because of a disease or disorder. *What are three types of lesions?*

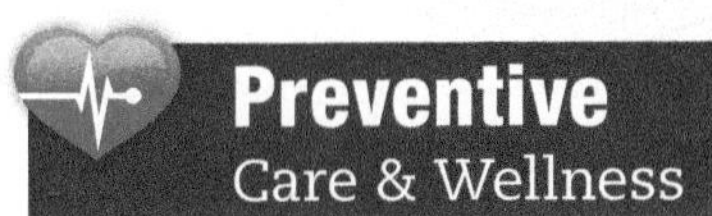

Preventive Care & Wellness

Cancer Warning Signs

Knowing the seven warning signs of cancer can help save lives. Learn the acronym "CAUTION":

- **C**hange in bowel or bladder habits.
- **A** sore that does not heal.
- **U**nusual bleeding or discharge.
- **T**hickening or lump in breast or elsewhere.
- **I**ndigestion or difficulty swallowing.
- **O**bvious change in a wart or mole.
- **N**agging cough or hoarseness.

connect ONLINE PROCEDURES

PROCEDURE 7-1

Identifying Cancer

Cancer can occur in any system of the body and cause a multitude of problems. Knowing how to recognize the warning signs and types of skin cancer is important to helping to prevent it.

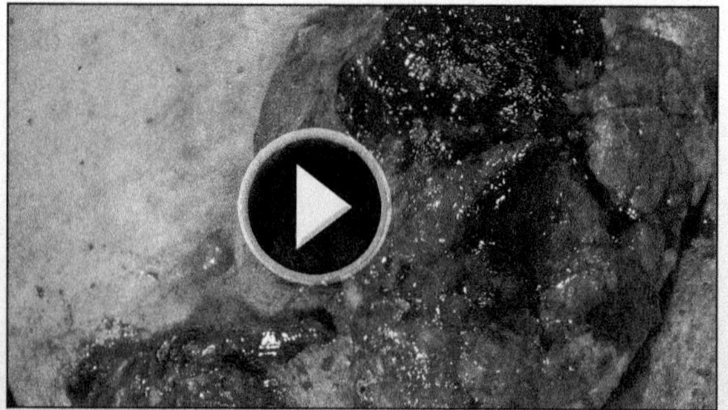

PROCEDURE 7-2

Recognizing Skin Lesions

Skin lesions are caused by a disease or a disorder. They are changes in the skin that come from either an external or internal source. External sources can include contact with a substance such as poison ivy or an injury to the skin. Internal sources include infections such as streptococcus or measles.

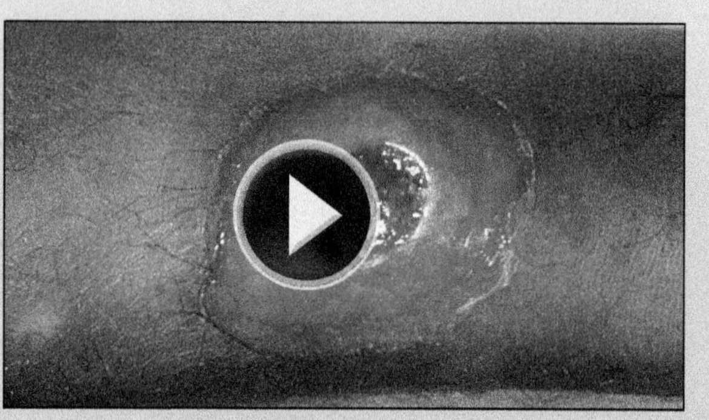

7.2 Diseases and Disorders of the Integumentary System Review

AFTER YOU READ

1. **Discuss** the difference between primary and secondary lesions.
2. **Describe** three diseases caused by micro-organisms that affect the skin.
3. **Compare** the three types of skin cancer.
4. **Explain** the meaning of the acronym ABCDE when checking for the signs of skin cancer.
5. **Suggest** three steps that may help to control acne vulgaris.

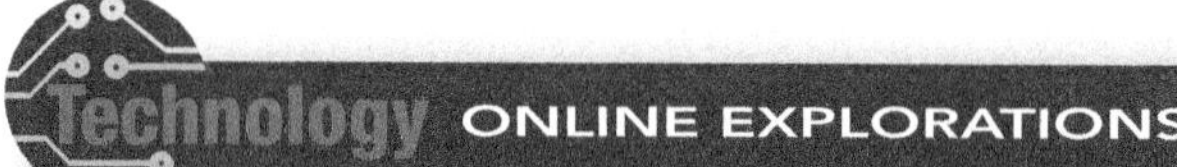

ONLINE EXPLORATIONS

Lesions

Using the Internet and **Figure 7.2** ("Types of Lesions,") select three types of lesions and identify a disease or disorder that would cause each type of lesion. For example, if you have measles, you would have macules.

SECTION
7.3 Diseases and Disorders of the Skeletal and Muscular Systems

Fractures

What are the most serious types of fractures?

Fractures, which are breaks or cracks in bones, are injuries of the skeletal system. **Figure 7.3** and the following list give some examples.

- A closed fracture is a break with no open wound.
- A simple fracture, also known as a hairline fracture, does not move any part of the bone out of place.
- An open fracture, also called a compound fracture, is a break with an open wound.
- A complex fracture is a separation of part of the bone and usually requires surgery to be repaired.
- A greenstick fracture is an incomplete break of a bone. It usually occurs to a child's soft bone and does not go entirely through the bone.
- A comminuted fracture is a break in which the bone is fragmented or shattered.
- A Colles' fracture is a break of the lower end of the radius, in the arm. It is usually caused by falling and landing on an outstretched hand. This type of break results in a bulge at the wrist.
- A complicated fracture involves extensive soft tissue injury.
- An impacted fracture occurs when a fragment from one part of a fracture is driven into the tissue of another part. When this injury occurs to the skull, it is called a depression fracture.
- A compression fracture is a break in one or more vertebrae caused by a compressing or squeezing of the space between the vertebrae.
- A spiral fracture occurs when a bone is broken by a twisting force. This is common in skiing accidents.

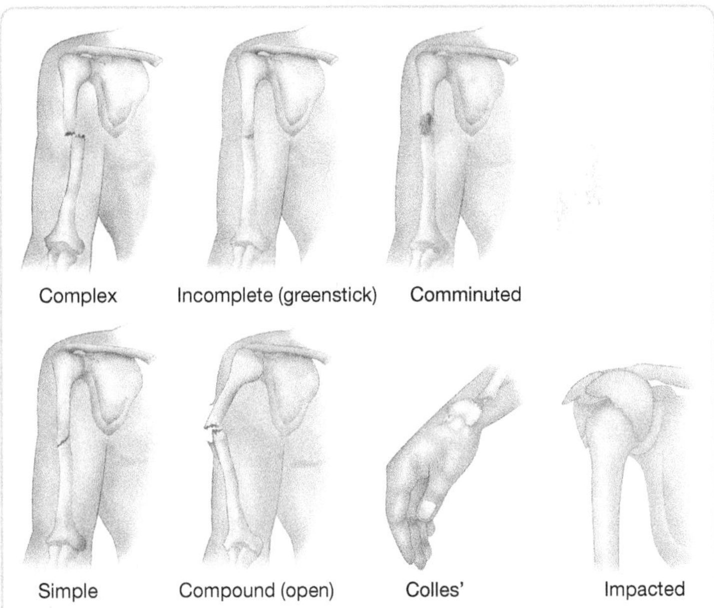

Fig. 7.3 Fractures Shown are several types of fractures. *Which type of fracture is the most severe?*

Vocabulary

Content Vocabulary

You will learn these content vocabulary terms in this section.

- **trauma**
- **RICE**

Academic Vocabulary

You will see this word in your reading and on your tests. Find its meaning in the Glossary in the back of this book.

- **detects**

READING CHECK

Identify the cause of a Colles' fracture.

Skeletal Diseases and Disorders

What is a sprain?

- Osteoporosis is a softening of the bones due to a lack of calcium. More common in women after menopause, this condition results in a loss of bone density and easily broken bones. Treatment is to take calcium and vitamin D and increase the patient's weight-bearing exercise level. A bone density test detects this condition.
- Osteomyelitis is caused by bacteria in the bone tissue. It is an infection in the bone that spreads rapidly. It can cause severe pain at the end of the bone and bone damage if left untreated. Although osteomyelitis is difficult to treat, hospitalization and intravenous (IV) antibiotics are commonly used. Treatment is especially important in children to stop destruction of the developing bone tissue.
- Arthritis is an inflammation of the joints causing pain, stiffness, aching, and limited range of motion. Range of motion measures the degree to which a joint is able to move. Two common types of arthritis are osteoarthritis and rheumatoid arthritis. Osteoarthritis is the degeneration of the joints and erosion of the joint cartilage due to aging. Rheumatoid arthritis is a systemic disease affecting connective tissue (see **Figure 7.4**). It occurs three times more often in females than in males and usually starts between the ages of 35 and 45. Treatment for both types of arthritis includes rest, pain relief, steroids, and anti-inflammatory medications. When severe joint damage occurs, a client may need surgery to replace damaged joints.

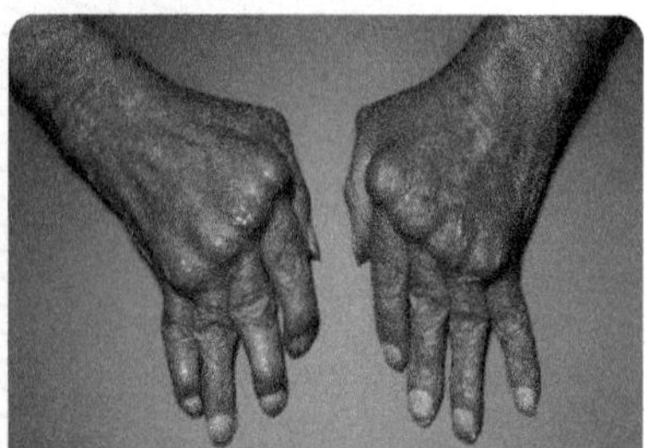

Fig. 7.4 Rheumatoid Arthritis The person pictured here is suffering from rheumatoid arthritis. *Name another type of arthritis.*

Photo: James Stevenson/SPL/Photo Researchers

- A sprain is a joint injury or **trauma** that tears ligaments. A severe sprain is accompanied by pain, swelling, tenderness, and inability to move the joint. Mild sprains are treated with rest, ice, and elevation in the first 24 hours. Most sprains heal within two weeks.
- A herniated disc, sometimes called a slipped or ruptured disc, is when one or more of the spinal discs balloon out from inside the bony parts of the vertebrae. If the bulge is large enough, it may press on a nerve, causing severe pain. Pain from a herniated disc can be relieved with bed rest, muscle relaxants, and anti-inflammatory drugs. Traction and/or surgery may be necessary.
- Carpal tunnel syndrome is caused by overuse of the wrist. It is more common in keyboarders, assembly line workers, and people who play sports like racquetball. Symptoms include weakness and numbness in the hand and pain in the wrist, hand, or elbow. Treatment includes splints, medication, and a change in work habits.

Abnormal Posture Conditions

Some abnormal posture conditions are due to spinal curvature, which may cause pain and/or require surgery. These conditions are:

- Kyphosis is humpback, or rounding at the thoracic vertebrae.
- Lordosis is swayback, or an abnormal inward curvature of the lumbar vertebrae.

- Scoliosis is side-to-side curvature of the spine, as shown in **Figure 7.5.** A simple test for scoliosis is commonly done on children. The child is asked to lean forward, exposing the vertebrae. Scoliosis may first appear at age six but may not be noticeable until adolescence.

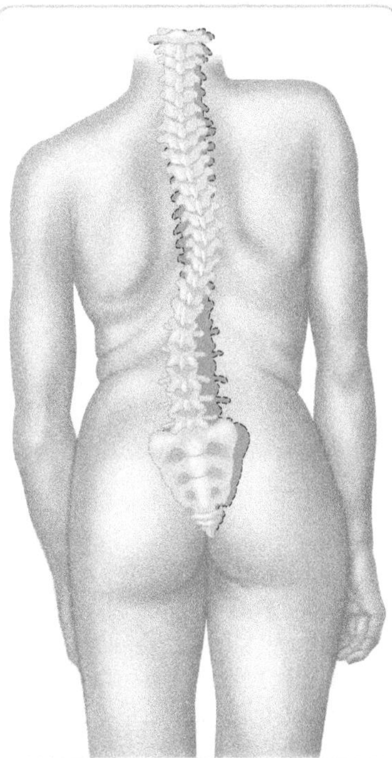

Fig. 7.5 Scoliosis Scoliosis is one type of abnormal posture condition. *What type of abnormal curvature of the spine is found with scoliosis?*

READING CHECK

Recall the causes of carpal tunnel syndrome.

Muscular Diseases and Disorders

What disorders affect the joints?

Muscle diseases and disorders arise from congenital conditions, injury, degenerative disease, or other systemic disorders. Some examples are:

- Strain is the overuse of a muscle and/or tendon. Muscles in the back, arms, and legs are prone to strains. Strains cause pain, swelling, and limited movement. They should be treated immediately with **R**est, **I**ce, **C**ompression, and **E**levation, or **RICE** (see **Figure 7.6**). Depending on the injury and location, hot applications, pain medications, and medication to relax the muscles are also given.
- Fibromyalgia is chronic pain in muscles and in the fibrous tissue that surrounds them. Although the cause is unknown, this disease can also cause numbness, tingling, fatigue, headaches, sleep disturbances, and depression. Clients who have fibromyalgia are treated with pain medication, physical therapy, massage, and muscle relaxants, and are helped to reduce stress.
- Bursitis is inflammation of the bursa surrounding a joint. Inflammation of a tendon in a joint caused by overwork is called tendonitis. Both of these conditions can be very painful, can restrict movement, and can cause swelling. Both are usually treated with rest, pain medication, splinting, and/or steroids.
- Dislocation may result from an injury or from a strenuous, sudden movement. A dislocated joint is characterized by pain, swelling, rapid discoloration of surrounding tissue, inability to move the area, and a misshapen appearance. The joint must be relocated by a physician and then immobilized and splinted to allow for healing.
- Muscular dystrophy is the name of a group of inherited diseases that cause progressive weakness and disability. The muscles atrophy (get smaller). The disease may result in disability and death. No cure is known. However, physical therapy can slow the progress of the disease.
- Botulism is a rare but serious disorder caused by bacteria. If the bacteria get into food, they can cause food poisoning. This disease starts within eight to 40 hours after ingesting the toxin. To prevent

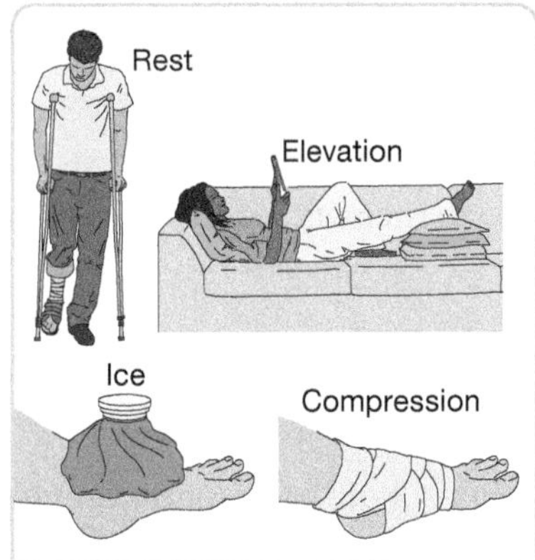

Fig. 7.6 RICE RICE is an acronym for the treatment needed for muscular injuries such as a strain. *Which muscles are most likely to experience strain?*

this disease, never give honey or corn syrup to infants, sterilize home-food containers properly at 250°F for 35 minutes, do not use foods from bent or bulging cans, and cook and store food properly.

READING CHECK

List the symptoms of fibromyalgia.

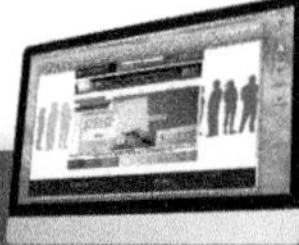

McGraw Hill connect™ ONLINE PROCEDURES

PROCEDURE 7-3

Identifying Types of Fractures

Fractures to bones vary in type depending upon the specific injuries sustained. The type of fracture determines the type of treatment a patient should receive. Most fractures are under the skin, but others result in broken bones that may break through the skin.

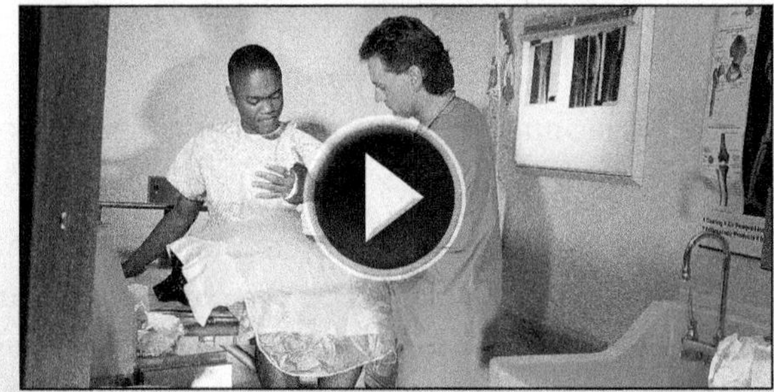

PROCEDURE 7-4

Administering RICE

When someone has an acute injury or overuse of a muscle, joint, or tendon, the appropriate treatment is known by the acronym RICE. These treatment measures reduce pain and swelling and can help improve movement.

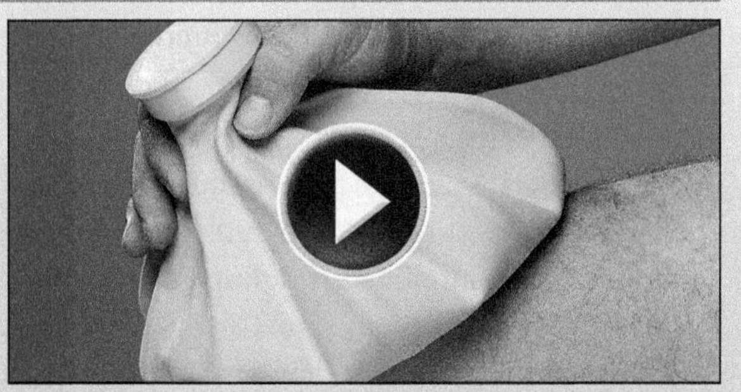

SECTION 7.3 Diseases and Disorders of the Skeletal and Muscular Systems Review

AFTER YOU READ

1. **Identify** which type of fracture would most likely occur to a child.
2. **Compare** two types of arthritis.
3. **Describe** three types of abnormal posture.
4. **Choose** the most common type of treatment for disorders caused by inflammation of a part of the muscular system
5. **Evaluate** which muscular system disease the following patient would most likely have: Sally Samson, a 35-year-old woman with persistent muscle pain, frequent headaches, inability to sleep, and fatigue.
6. **Describe** how you can prevent botulism.

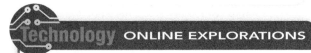

Technology ONLINE EXPLORATIONS

Fracture Causes

Review the types of fractures in this chapter and select one. Go online to learn which types of accidents would most likely result in the fracture that you selected. Then write a short story about such an accident and share it with the class or a partner.

Photos: (t)Photodisc Collection/Getty Images, (b)Royalty-Free/CORBIS

SECTION 7.4
Diseases and Disorders of the Nervous System

Traumatic Disorders of the Brain

What is the difference between a concussion and a contusion?

There are many types of diseases and disorders of the nervous system. The brain is part of the central nervous system.

The following kinds of trauma (injury) can occur to the brain.

- Concussion is an injury to the brain caused by an impact with an object. Cerebral concussions usually clear up within 24 hours. A severe concussion can lead to coma, which is abnormally deep sleep with little or no response to stimuli. Coma may also result from other causes, such as a stroke.
- Brain contusion is a bruising of the surface of the brain without penetration into the brain. Traumatic injury, such as that which might occur during a car accident, may cause the brain to hit the skull and then to rebound to the other side of the skull. An injury of this type is called a "closed-head trauma," because there is no penetration of the skull.

Vocabulary

Content Vocabulary

You will learn these content vocabulary terms in this section.

- **degenerative**
- **paralysis**

Academic Vocabulary

You will see this word in your reading and on your tests. Find its meaning in the Glossary in the back of this book.

- **response**

Congenital Diseases

What is a congenital disease?

Congenital diseases (conditions present at birth) of the central nervous system can be devastating and nearly always have some impact on the client's activities of daily living (ADL). Some examples are:

- Spina bifida is a defect in the spinal column in which the spinal cord and/or its covering protrudes outside the vertebrae. Mild cases are visible only by X-ray. However, with severe cases the protrusion is clearly visible. The condition causes varying degrees of paralysis or lack of feeling and movement below the site of the protrusion. Since it can be diagnosed in a fetus during pregnancy, it is sometimes possible to perform corrective surgery on the fetus. **Figure 7.7** shows an example of spina bifida.

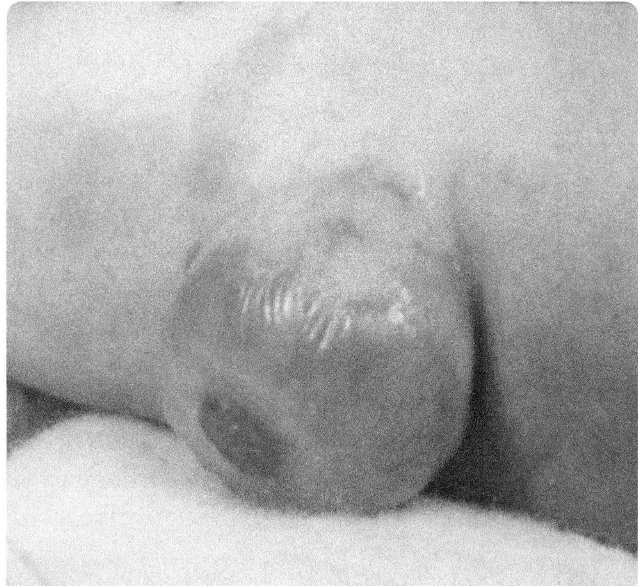

Fig. 7.7 Spina Bifida This image shows a severe case of spina bifida. *What may be contained in this sac on an infant's back?*

Photo: Biophoto Associates/Science Source/Photo Researchers

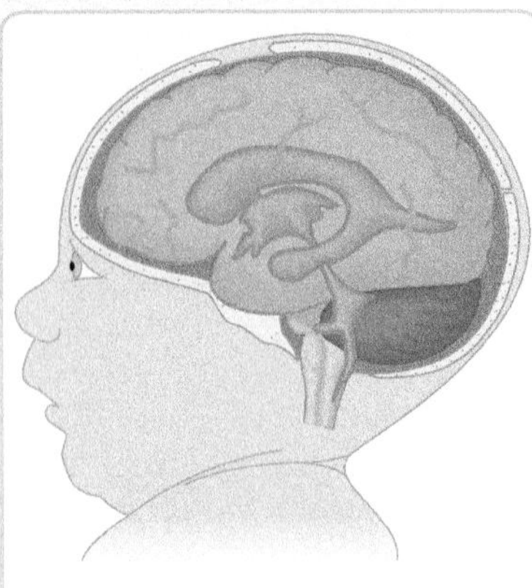

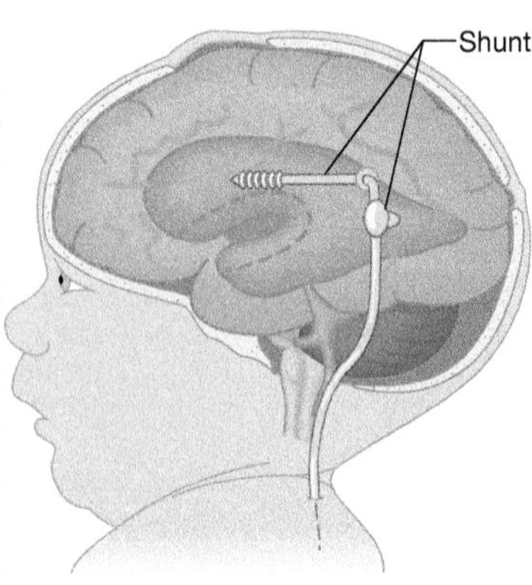

Fig. 7.8 Hydrocephalus Shown is a treatment of hydrocephalus. *Why is a shunt used for this treatment?*

- Hydrocephalus is an overproduction of cerebrospinal fluid in the brain. It usually occurs at birth, although it may be prenatal and can also occur in adults as the result of infections or tumors. Hydrocephalus is treated by draining the cerebrospinal fluid. **Figure 7.8** illustrates a shunt used to treat hydrocephalus.
- Cerebral palsy is caused by cerebral damage during gestation or birth and results in lack of motor coordination and other neurological deficiencies.

READING CHECK

Summarize the potential effects of spina bifida on the patient's activities of daily living.

Degenerative Diseases

How does myasthenia gravis weaken muscles?

Diseases of the nervous system can affect almost any part of the body. These diseases are called **degenerative** because they cause tissue or organs to worsen, or degenerate, over time. Some examples are:

- Alzheimer's disease is a progressive degeneration of neurons in the brain. It eventually leads to death. Mental capacity worsens over time. Symptoms that worsen as Alzheimer's disease progresses are loss of memory, inability to properly use familiar objects, and inability to receive and understand outside stimuli. This condition occurs in people as early as the age of 40 but is most common around 60 years of age.
- Amyotrophic lateral sclerosis (ALS) is a degenerative disease of the motor neurons leading to loss of muscle control and death. It is also known as Lou Gehrig's disease.
- Multiple sclerosis (MS) destroys the myelin sheath and causes muscle weakness, unsteady walking, paresthesia (tingling), extreme fatigue, and some paralysis.
- Myasthenia gravis is a disease causing muscle weakness. An overproduction of antibodies prevents neurotransmitters from sending proper nerve impulses to skeletal muscles. Muscles become very tired very quickly. There is no cure, but medication can help. A client suffering from myasthenia gravis may need to make some lifestyle changes in order to cope with the disease.
- Parkinson's disease is a degeneration of nerves in the brain, which causes tremors, muscle weakness, and difficulty in walking. It is treated with drugs that increase the levels of dopamine in the brain. Treatment helps relieve symptoms but cannot cure the disease.

READING CHECK

Name the chief symptoms of Alzheimer's disease.

Other Disorders of the Nervous System

What are the three common types of paralysis?

- Epilepsy is a chronic, recurrent seizure activity. Epilepsy has been known since ancient times when victims were thought to be under the influence of outside, and even supernatural, forces. Now it is understood that epilepsy is caused by abnormal conditions in the brain that trigger sudden, excessive electrical activity. The seizures caused by this activity can be preceded by an aura, a collection of symptoms felt just before the actual seizure. Seizures may be mild or intense. Petit mal seizures are mild and usually involve only a momentary disorientation. Grand mal, or tonic-clonic, seizures are more severe and include loss of consciousness, convulsions, and twitching of limbs.
- Tourette's syndrome is a neurological disorder that causes a client to make sounds and twitch uncontrollably. Some drugs are helpful in controlling symptoms to allow sufferers to lead normal lives.
- Meningitis is an inflammation of the meninges. When caused by bacteria, it is called bacterial meningitis and involves symptoms such as fever, headache, and stiff neck. It is usually treated with antibiotics. In some severe cases, it can be fatal. Viruses cause viral meningitis. Viral meningitis has the same symptoms as bacterial meningitis, but it is not treated with antibiotics. Medications are given to relieve some of the more uncomfortable symptoms such as fever and headache.
- Guillain-Barré syndrome occurs when the body's immune system attacks the peripheral nerves. It comes on quickly, causing weakness and progressing to difficulty breathing or paralysis. Supportive treatment, including a respirator, may be required. With time and a correct diagnosis and treatment, the disease runs its course and is usually not fatal.
- Encephalitis is an inflammation of the brain that results from a viral infection or from the spread of an infection to the brain. This infection can originate from measles, mumps, chickenpox, or some other illnesses. Clients have a variety of symptoms including fever, headache, seizures, weakness, visual disturbances, vomiting, stiff neck and back, and disorientation. When the infection is severe, the client can suffer from paralysis and coma. The severity of the infection and the chances for recovery depend upon the virus and the client's response. One serious form of encephalitis, caused by the herpes simplex (Type I) virus, can be fatal. The use of antiviral medications has decreased the number of deaths from encephalitis.

Types of Paralysis

Paralysis is the loss of movement and sensation in a part of the body. It is a type of physical disability, which means that it is a condition that

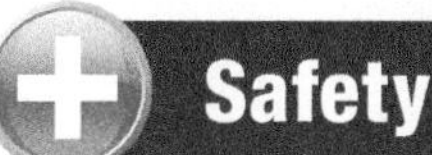

Safety

Clients Who Have Dementia

Dementia is the loss of mental functioning characterized by a decrease in intellectual ability, loss of memory, impaired judgment, personality change, and disorientation. There are many causes of dementia, and it can occur in varying degrees. Alzheimer's is one type of dementia. Regardless of the cause or the type of dementia, clients should be kept safe and secure. These are some techniques to ensure client safety:

- Keep dangerous objects or substances out of reach or locked away. Some examples of dangerous objects or substances are drugs, poisons, scissors, knives, cleaning solutions, matches, and lighters.
- If a client tends to wander, maintain a secure area or provide the client with a sensor that will alert others if he or she has left a particular area.
- Keep the environment calm. Avoid loud noises and crowds, because they can disorient the client.
- Provide simple activities that last for short periods of time.
- Keep pictures, clocks, and calendars where the client can see them.

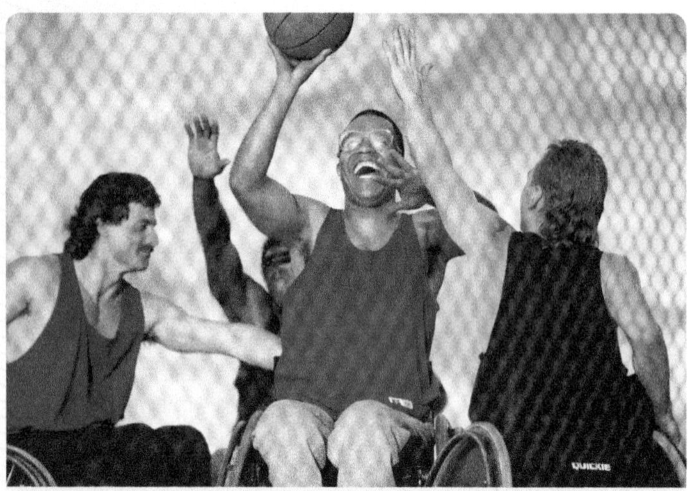

Fig. 7.9 **Paraplegia** Clients with paraplegia and quadriplegia are frequently confined to a wheelchair. *What is the definition of "paralysis"?*

limits a major activity. The clients in **Figure 7.9** have paralysis. Three common types of paralysis are:

- Hemiplegia, paralysis on one side of the body, is usually the result of a stroke. The client is unable to move one side effectively and cannot feel heat, cold, pressure, and pain on that side. The client may also have a drooping eyelid or side of the face. Paralyzed clients are at an increased risk for choking because of the effect of the stroke on the mouth and throat. They are also at risk for burns on the affected side.
- Paraplegia, paralysis from the waist down, is often caused by a motorcycle or car accident, fall, gunshot or stab wound, or sports injury. These clients are prone to pressure sores on their buttocks from using a wheelchair and may need assistance with urinary and bowel functions.
- Quadriplegia, paralysis from the neck down, is usually the result of an injury below the fourth cervical vertebra. Clients may have some use of their upper arms, depending on the location of the injury. They frequently need complete care and are prone to respiratory and urinary tract infections and pressure sores.

READING CHECK

Identify the cause of epilepsy.

SECTION 7.4 Diseases and Disorders of the Nervous System Review

AFTER YOU READ

1. **Explain** the difference between a degenerative and a congenital disease of the nervous system.
2. **Analyze** the following situation: A patient arrives at the hospital with head trauma. The physician calls the injury a closed-head trauma. What does that mean?
3. **Identify** two disorders of the nervous system that are types of inflammation.
4. **Compare** the different types of epileptic seizures.
5. **Indicate** some of the diseases that can lead to encephalitis.

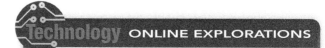

Technology ONLINE EXPLORATIONS

Nervous System Disease

Research one disease of the nervous system that you would like to know more about. Write a brief summary of its cause, signs and symptoms, and treatment.

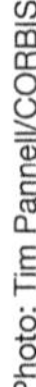

SECTION 7.5

Diseases and Disorders of the Sensory System

Eye Diseases and Disorders

What is the most common cause of vision loss in the United States?

Most common eye disorders involve defects in the curvature of the cornea and/or lens or defects in the refractive ability of the eye due to an abnormally short or long eyeball. Some of these disorders, which will be discussed in more detail in Chapter 28, Ophthalmic Care are:

- Astigmatism is a distortion of sight. It is caused by an abnormal shaped cornea or lens.
- Hyperopia, farsightedness (Vision is better at a distance.)
- Myopia, nearsightedness (Vision is better for nearby objects.)
- Presbyopia, loss of close vision due to a loss of ability to focus and accommodate (a common disorder after age 40)
- Cataracts, cloudy vision caused by cloudiness of the lens of the eye. This is usually a result of aging, but may also be congenital or the result of a disease or injury (see **Figures 7.10 a and b**).

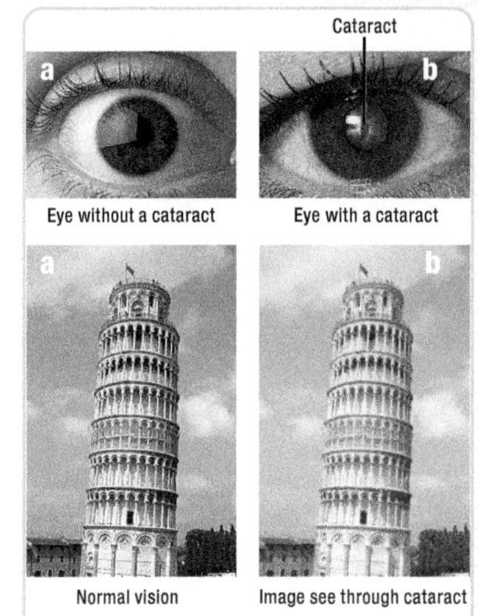

Fig. 7.10 (a) and (b) Cataracts Shown is the same view as seen normally and by a person with a cataract. *How do cataracts distort vision?*

There are a number of other diseases and disorders of the eye:

- Asthenopia, also known as eyestrain, is a condition in which the eyes tire easily. Symptoms may include pain in or around the eyes, headache, dimness of vision, dizziness, and slight nausea. It can occur when the eyes are focused on objects 12 to 18 inches away for long periods of time.
- Diplopia, or double vision, may be the result of a disease or injury.
- Photophobia, or light sensitivity, is sometimes the result of disease.
- Glaucoma is any disease caused by abnormally high pressure within the eye. It can be treated in most cases by using medication or surgery to relieve the pressure. If not treated, it can lead to blindness.
- Macular degeneration, also called low vision, is a breakdown of macular tissue. It leads to the loss of central vision, which is the vision we use for reading and driving. It is the most common cause of vision loss in the United States.
- Conjunctivitis, also known as pinkeye, is a highly infectious inflammation of the conjunctiva. The eyes become red and irritated and have a burning feeling. Sometimes pus is visible in the eyes. Antibiotic eye drops or ointments are used for treatment.

READING CHECK

Name eye diseases and disorders that are typical to older adults.

Ear Diseases and Disorders

What causes tinnitus?

Common diseases and disorders of the ears are:

- Deafness, or partial or total hearing loss. Diminished or lessened hearing can be caused by various conditions. Lessening of vibrations in the ear causes conductive hearing loss. This can be caused by abnormal wax buildup, hardening of the bone of the ear, infection, or foreign body obstruction. Lesions or dysfunction of parts of the ear can cause a condition called sensory hearing loss.
- Tinnitus is a constant ringing or buzzing in the ear. It can be the result of conditions such as high blood pressure.
- Otitis media is inflammation and/or infection of the middle ear. It may result in blockage of the eustachian tube by fluid. It causes pain and temporary hearing loss. Treatment includes antibiotics, nasal decongestants, and antihistamines.
- Otitis externa, also known as "swimmer's ear," is inflammation of the external ear canal. The ear becomes itchy, painful, and may swell. It is treated with steroid and antibiotic eardrops. No water should be allowed to enter the ear canal during the healing process.
- Ménière's disease is fluid pressure within the cochlea. It causes disturbances of equilibrium, hearing loss, and vertigo or dizziness. A low-sodium diet and reduction of nicotine and caffeine can help symptoms. It is also treated with medication and surgery.

READING CHECK

Explain why otitis externa is often called "swimmer's ear."

SECTION 7.5 Diseases and Disorders of the Sensory System Review

AFTER YOU READ

1. **Identify** the eye disorder a patient has when he or she cannot see things at a distance.
2. **Analyze** what eye disease you most likely have if your left eye is red and itchy, and when you woke up this morning, there was some pus in the corner of that eye.
3. **Explain** what you should do to treat and prevent the case described in question 2 above.
4. **Compare** otitis media and otitis externa.
5. **Describe** some of the treatments for Ménière's disease.

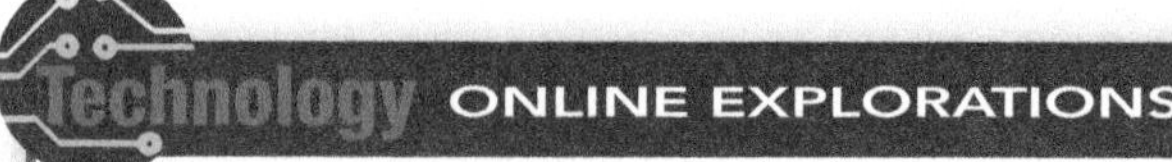

Cataract Surgery

Your grandmother needs to have cataract surgery and has asked you to tell her what to expect. Research the surgery on the Internet and provide the information your grandmother needs, including how the surgery is done, how long it will take to recover, and what your grandmother can expect during and after the surgery.

SECTION

7.6 Diseases and Disorders of the Circulatory System

Diseases and Disorders of the Heart and Blood Vessels

What are the two causes of strokes?

Diseases and disorders of the heart, blood vessels, and blood include the following:

- **Hypertension** is high blood pressure. Blood pressure is the force of the blood against the walls of the arteries. It is affected by lifestyle factors. Overeating leading to excessive weight, smoking, lack of exercise, and stress are factors that affect blood pressure. Medication can help control blood pressure. Untreated hypertension can damage the liver, blood vessels, and kidneys, or it may lead to a cerebrovascular accident (CVA), or stroke.
- A stroke can occur when a blood clot blocks the flow of blood in a vessel, or when a blood vessel bursts in the brain. As blockage increases, the client may experience symptoms before a stroke. These short incidents are known as transient ischemic attacks (TIAs). If a clot travels from somewhere in the body to the brain, or if a blood vessel ruptures in the brain, a sudden stroke can occur. A client can recover completely from a mild stroke. However, damage may be permanent in a severe stroke. Common damage caused by strokes includes thought disorders, loss of or difficulty with speech, loss of muscle control, some paralysis, and disorientation.
- Arteriosclerosis is hardening of the arteries. Arteries lose their elasticity and ability to contract. Arteriosclerosis commonly occurs as a result of aging and can lead to high blood pressure and other cardiovascular diseases. Atherosclerosis is a type of arteriosclerosis caused by the build up of fats, called plaque, in the arteries.
- An aneurysm occurs when the wall of an artery is weakened as a result of a disease or a defect present at birth, or trauma. An aneurysm is a ballooning out or a saclike formation on an artery wall. It may cause pain and pressure, but often there are no symptoms. If found, most aneurysms must be surgically removed.
- Coronary artery disease (CAD) is the narrowing of the coronary arteries that supply blood to the heart. It is usually caused by atherosclerosis, which is a build up of fatty plaque inside the blood vessels of the heart. CAD can lead to angina or myocardial infarction. As seen in **Figure 7.11** on page 206, CAD may be treated by placing a stent inside the blocked blood vessels in the heart.

Vocabulary

Content Vocabulary

You will learn these content vocabulary terms in this section.

- **hypertension**
- **myocardial infarction (MI)**
- **remissions**
- **relapses**

Academic Vocabulary

You will see this word in your reading and on your tests. Find its meaning in the Glossary in the back of this book.

- **recover**

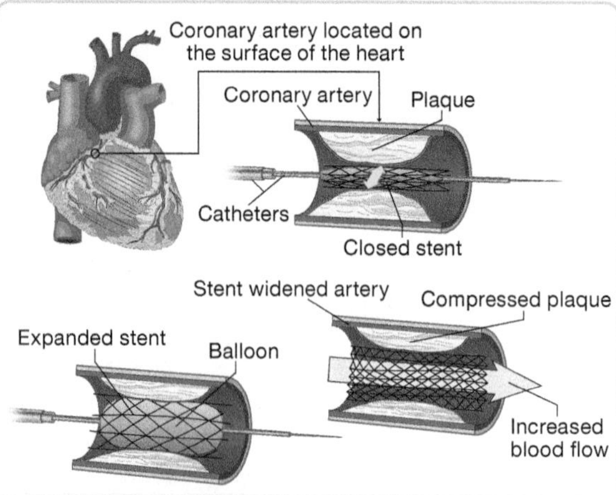

Fig. 7.11 Coronary Angioplasty Coronary angioplasty involves placing a stent in the heart. *What disease is treated with this procedure?*

- **Myocardial infarction (MI),** or heart attack, is when blood flow to the heart is cut off. This can result in permanent damage to the heart tissue. Without a fresh supply of blood, the deprived heart tissues begin to die. Angina is a temporary lack of blood in the heart muscle, which can cause symptoms similar to a heart attack.
- Congestive heart failure (CHF) occurs when the heart cannot pump at its usual capacity. When this happens, the vital organs do not receive enough blood. CHF may occur from atherosclerosis and/or myocardial infarction. If the heart is weakened and cannot pump with its usual force, blood backs up into the heart and lungs, causing congestion.
- Arrhythmias occur when the heart beats abnormally. They can be caused by a genetic disorder, CAD, or medication. Symptoms vary from none to shortness of breath or even death.

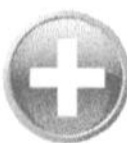
connect

STEM CONNECTION

Medical Science

Shock and Circulation

To understand why shock occurs, we need to examine the three basic components of the circulatory system. These are the pump (heart), fluid (blood), and pipes to carry blood (blood vessels). A failure of any one of these three components leads to shock.

- **Pump failure.** Any significant damage to the pump affects its ability to move blood. This can occur when the heart is damaged, as in a heart attack.
- **Fluid loss.** A significant loss of blood or body fluid can result in shock. Usually excessive external or internal bleeding, excessive vomiting, diarrhea, sweating, and burns can cause this loss.
- **Pipe failure.** When blood vessels suddenly become enlarged, there is not sufficient fluid volume to fill them. This can occur when there is an injury to the nervous system such as a spinal injury.

READING CHECK

Name some causes of congestive heart failure.

Table 7.1 Anemia

TYPE	CAUSE	TREATMENT
Iron-deficiency anemia	Insufficient iron in the blood affecting the production of hemoglobin	Iron supplements and increased intake of green leafy vegetables
Aplastic anemia	Failure of the bone marrow to produce enough red blood cells	Bone marrow transplant, immuno-suppressive drugs.
Pernicious anemia	Change in the shape and number of the red blood cells due to a lack of sufficient vitamin B_{12}	Vitamin B_{12} injections
Sickle cell anemia	Hereditary condition, most commonly seen in persons of African-American ancestry, characterized by sickle-shaped red blood cells and a breakdown in the membranes of red blood cells	Transfusion of packed red blood cells and supportive therapy
Posthemorrhagic anemia	Sudden, dramatic loss of blood	Blood transfusions

Blood Diseases and Disorders

In what two systems can leukemia occur?

- Anemia is a condition in which the red blood cells do not send enough oxygen to the tissues. It is caused by a low volume of either red blood cells or hemoglobin. Symptoms are pallor, fatigue, difficulty breathing, and rapid heart rate. **Table 7.1** lists the types of anemia. Blood transfusion is common (see **Figure 7.12**).
- Hemophilia is a blood disorder that involves excessive bleeding. Hemophiliacs can be treated with medications and transfusions.
- Leukemia involves an abnormal increase in white blood cells in bone marrow and the bloodstream. People with leukemia may experience **remissions,** during which the disease disappears. **Relapses** are recurrences of the disease. Symptoms include fever, pallor, anemia, bleeding gums, excessive bruising, and joint pain. Treatment may include chemotherapy, radiation, and/or bone marrow transplant.

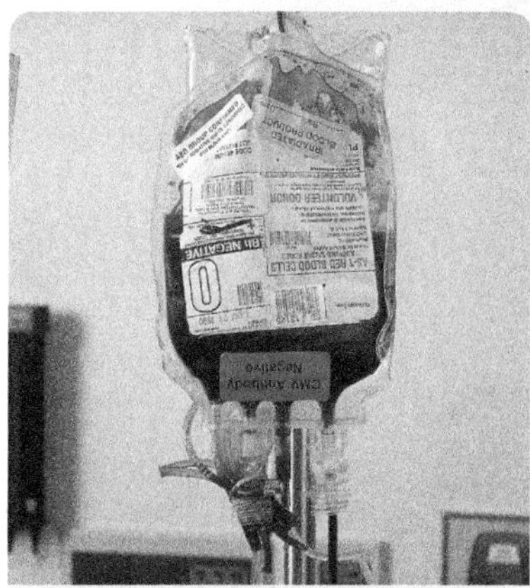

Fig. 7.12 Blood Transfusion This donor unit is being used in a blood transfusion. *What is a condition that requires treatment with transfusions?*

READING CHECK

Explain how hemophilia is treated.

connect ONLINE PROCEDURES

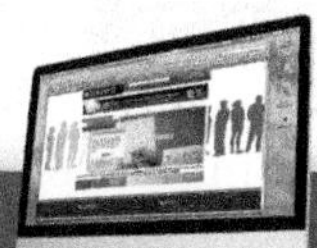

PROCEDURE 7-5

Recognizing how Coronary Angioplasty is Performed

Coronary angioplasty, or the repair of the coronary arteries, is done by inserting a device known as a stent. This procedure opens the arteries and allows improved blood flow to the heart.

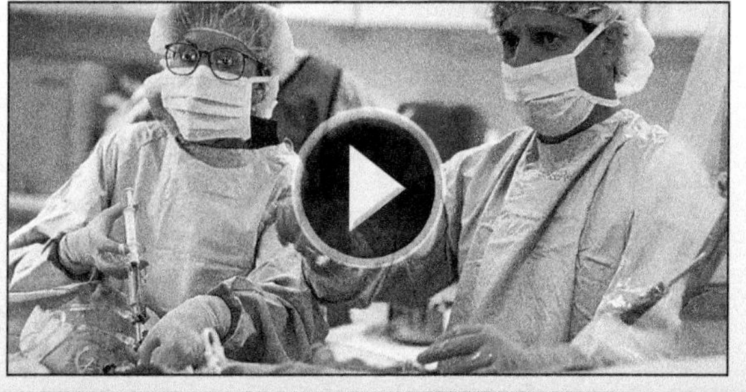

SECTION 7.6 Diseases and Disorders of the Circulatory System Review

AFTER YOU READ

1. **Compare** two disorders of the cardiovascular system that affect the heart.
2. **Describe** two disorders of the blood.
3. **Identify** which type of anemia is caused by heredity.
4. **Explain** the procedure of coronary angioplasty.

Technology ONLINE EXPLORATIONS

Cardiovascular Disease

The diagnosis and treatment of cardiovascular disease keeps progressing. Search online for one of the following terms and write a brief summary of that term: thrombolytic or fibrinolytic, cardiac catheterization, enhanced external counter pulsation (EECP) therapy, coronary artery bypass graft, and Coumadin.

Photos: (t)Doug Martin, (b)Rob Crandall/SCPhotos/Alamy

SECTION 7.7

Diseases and Disorders of the Lymphatic and Immune Systems

Vocabulary

Content Vocabulary

You will learn these content vocabulary terms in this section.

- **Acquired immunodeficiency syndrome (AIDS)**
- **Human immunodeficiency virus (HIV)**
- **opportunistic**
- **mononucleosis**

Academic Vocabulary

You will see this word in your reading and on your tests. Find its meaning in the Glossary in the back of this book.

- **affect**

Conditions Related to Immunity and to the Lymph Nodes

What is an autoimmune disease?

Some diseases and disorders of the lymphatic and immune systems are:

- **Acquired immunodeficiency syndrome (AIDS),** AIDS, is caused by the **human immunodeficiency virus (HIV),** a virus spread by sexual contact, exchange of bodily fluids, receipt of tainted blood, or use of intravenous drugs. AIDS clients are subject to a number of infections that take hold because of the lowered immune response. These are known as **opportunistic** infections and may be present in a number of body systems. These infections may affect the entire body with diseases, such as herpes, candidiasis, skin cancer in the form of Kaposi's sarcoma, and pneumonia. AIDS is considered to be a sexually transmitted disease; however, it can also be transmitted at birth, or through blood and IV drugs. Advancements in research have made it possible to manage the disease and prolong the life of many AIDS victims. Death from AIDS and related illnesses has greatly declined in the United States since the 1990s largely due to antiretroviral therapy and screening, while education about prevention methods has reduced the incidence of HIV infection. In developing nations where advanced treatment is not available, however, HIV infection and death from AIDS continue to be problems of alarming proportions.
- Lymphoma is cancer of the lymph nodes. It is a relatively common cancer with high cure rates. Two of the most common types of lymphoma are Hodgkin's disease and non-Hodgkin's lymphoma. Hodgkin's disease is a type of lymph cancer of uncertain origin that generally appears in early adulthood. Non-Hodgkin's lymphoma is a cancer of the lymph nodes, with a severe overgrowth of cells that spread in a diffuse pattern. It usually appears in midlife. Depending on how far the disease has spread, both types of lymphoma can usually be arrested with chemotherapy and radiation. Surgery in the form of a bone marrow transplant is also useful in Hodgkin's disease.
- Infectious **mononucleosis,** sometimes called "mono," is a highly contagious disease common in teenagers and young adults. It is associated with the Epstein-Barr virus. Symptoms include fatigue, weakness, sore throat, fever, weight loss, enlarged lymph nodes,

and an enlarged spleen. It is treated with plenty of rest, fluids, and pain medication. Infectious mononucleosis is often called the "kissing disease" because it is usually transmitted through mouth-to-mouth contact when kissing, sharing drinks, or through eating utensils.

- Allergies, which are a problem of the immune system, affect millions of people. The incidence and severity of allergies varies depending on the time of year, amount of exposure to various allergens, or allergy-causing substances, and other problems. Common substances that cause allergies are dust mites, cat dander, and pollens. Many people have serious allergic reactions to certain types of foods or medicines. Allergic problems include asthma, nasal and sinus allergies, hives, and even severe anaphylactic reactions that can be fatal.
- Autoimmune diseases occur when the immune system turns against its own healthy tissue. An autoimmune response is the result of T cells attacking one's healthy cells. Examples include rheumatoid arthritis and Guillain-Barré syndrome, which were discussed in Section 7.4. Another example is lupus, which can cause severe joint and muscle pain, extreme exhaustion, fevers, and skin rashes. It can also lead to organ failure and death. The exact cause of lupus remains unclear, and there is no cure. Diagnosis is difficult, because the symptoms mimic those of other illnesses and there is no specific diagnostic test.

READING CHECK

Identify the type of cancer that affects the immune system.

SECTION 7.7 Diseases and Disorders of the Lymphatic and Immune Systems Review

AFTER YOU READ

1. **Explain** why the rate of death caused by HIV has decreased in the United States since the 1990s.
2. **Indicate** the infections that can result when a patient has AIDS (acquired immunodeficiency syndrome).
3. **Compare** two autoimmune diseases.
4. **Describe** what you can do to reduce the chances you will get mono if your best friend has it.

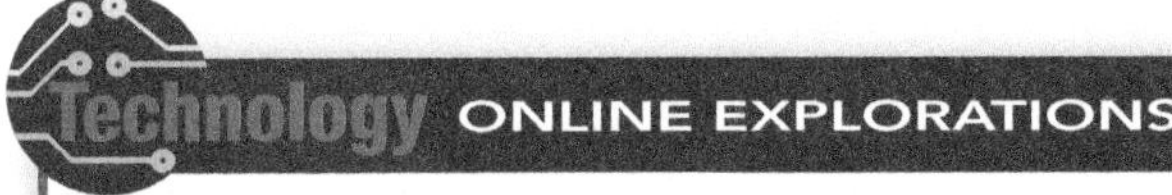

Autoimmune Diseases

Many diseases are autoimmune. Use the Internet to determine why a disease is called autoimmune and explain what happens in the body.

SECTION **7.8** # Diseases and Disorders of the Respiratory System

Vocabulary

Content Vocabulary

You will learn these content vocabulary terms in this section.

- asthma

Academic Vocabulary

You will see this word in your reading and on your tests. Find its meaning in the Glossary in the back of this book.

- occur

Diseases and Disorders

What are the symptoms of asthma?

The respiratory system is the site of many inflammations (swelling, pain, and/or dysfunction in a body part), disorders, and infections. This system must contend with foreign material coming into the body from outside, as well as internal problems that may affect any of its parts. When a part of the respiratory system becomes inflamed, the suffix *-itis* may be placed at the end of the word. For example, an inflammation of the bronchi is called bronchitis.

Examples of diseases and disorders of the respiratory system are:

- Bronchitis is an inflammation of the bronchi. It causes increased secretions from the mucous membranes of the bronchi, obstructing breathing. Allergies, dust, infections, and pollution can cause bronchitis.
- **Asthma,** which also occurs in the bronchi, is a condition of bronchial airway obstruction causing sudden breathing difficulty accompanied by wheezing and coughing. An asthma attack may be caused by allergy, infection, or anxiety.
- Emphysema is a disease that often affects the elderly, especially those who smoke heavily or have asthma or chronic bronchitis. A client with emphysema is unable to exhale all air from the lungs, causing carbon dioxide buildup and damage to the alveoli. As the disease progresses, the client's breathing becomes more difficult.
- Chronic obstructive pulmonary disease (COPD) is a term for any disease that causes chronic obstruction of the bronchial tubes and lungs. Chronic bronchitis and emphysema are two COPD processes.
- Hemoptysis is the coughing up of blood from the lungs or bronchial tubes. This serious condition can occur with chronic lung diseases, tuberculosis, lung cancer, or trauma.
- Lung cancer is caused by exposure to carcinogens, such as cigarette smoke or other cancer-causing substances. Symptoms appear in later stages; the client may have hemoptysis (bloody sputum), dyspnea (shortness of breath), weight loss, and chest pain.
- Upper respiratory infection (URI) is a viral infection of all or part of the upper respiratory tract that is more commonly known as the common cold. A URI is highly contagious. Symptoms include sneezing, watery eyes, sore throat, and cough. There is no cure. However, clients should get plenty of rest and treat the symptoms with pain relievers and other cold medicines.

- Epistaxis, or nosebleed, results from a trauma, or a rupture of a blood vessel in the nose. To treat a nosebleed, lean the patient's head forward. Pinch the nostril(s) toward the midline. Apply a cold compress to the bridge of the nose.
- Pneumonia is an inflammation and infection of the lungs. Pneumonia often affects bedridden, elderly, and frail people.
- Tuberculosis is an infectious disease caused by bacilli, bacteria that invade the lungs and cause small swellings and inflammation.
- Anthracosis, or black lung, is caused by coal dust in the lungs.
- Pleurisy is an inflammation of the pleurae, or membranes around the lungs. It causes a sharp pain while breathing, dyspnea, fever, and grating sounds, or crepitation, in the lungs when breathing.
- Influenza, or flu, occurs suddenly and is caused by a virus. Symptoms include fever, chills, body aches, sore throat, and fatigue.

Changes in Breathing

Diseases and disorders of the respiratory system may affect normal breathing and can change normal breathing to any of the following:

- Bradypnea, slow breathing
- Tachypnea, rapid breathing
- Hypopnea, shallow breathing
- Hyperpnea, abnormally deep breathing
- Dyspnea, difficult breathing
- Apnea, inability to breathe
- Orthopnea, difficulty in breathing, especially while lying down
- Cheyne-Stokes respiration, a period of apnea followed by deep, labored breathing that becomes shallow and then returns to apnea. Cheyne-Stokes respiration can indicate impending death.

READING CHECK

List some conditions that could lead to coughing up blood.

SECTION 7.8 Diseases and Disorders of the Respiratory System Review

AFTER YOU READ

1. **Describe** two diseases of the respiratory system that cause inflammation.
2. **Compare** a cold and the flu.
3. **Determine** which disease of the respiratory system you are least likely to contract.
4. **Choose** three different respiratory diseases and describe their causes.

Technology ONLINE EXPLORATIONS

Respiratory Diseases

Do you know anyone with asthma? Imagine that you need to teach a classmate about how to care for his or her asthma. Go to the National Heart Lung and Blood Institute website. In the Health Professionals section about lung diseases, review the materials about asthma. Create a brief lesson or handout to use to teach a classmate about the disease.

SECTION 7.9

Diseases and Disorders of the Digestive and Urinary Systems

Vocabulary

Content Vocabulary

You will learn these content vocabulary terms in this section.

- **symptoms**
- **jaundice**
- **urinary tract infection (UTI)**

Academic Vocabulary

You will see this word in your reading and on your tests. Find its meaning in the Glossary in the back of this book.

- **widespread**

Eating Disorders

What are the three classifications of obesity?

Digestive system diseases and disorders can be classified into eating disorders, digestive diseases, and disorders that are **symptoms** (problems a patient has that can be seen or measured) of other diseases.

Eating disorders are at the top of the list of problems associated with the digestive system. These are discussed in more detail in Chapter 8.

- Clients who have anorexia nervosa refuse to eat because they want to be thin. Anorexia nervosa occurs most often in adolescents and young adults. It can produce many health problems.
- Bulimia nervosa is a disorder involving bingeing on food and then purposely purging or vomiting in a quest for weight loss. Like anorexia nervosa, it occurs in adolescents and young adults and can produce many health problems.
- Obesity is often the result of overeating but may also be hereditary. It can be a factor in many health problems, such as heart disease and diabetes. Obesity is classified in three levels: (1) an overweight client is less than 20 percent over his or her ideal body weight, (2) an obese client is 20 percent over his or her ideal body weight, and (3) a morbidly obese client is 100 pounds over his or her ideal body weight. Morbid obesity is a severe threat to health and life.

READING CHECK

Identify the age groups that are most associated with anorexia nervosa and bulimia nervosa.

Digestive Diseases

How can gastroenteritis be prevented?

The diseases of the digestive system include:

- Esophageal varices is twisted veins in the esophagus that can hemorrhage and ulcerate. This is a very serious condition that can cause fatal bleeding. It is frequently related to a disease of the liver known as cirrhosis.
- Gastroenteritis is an inflammation of both the stomach and the small intestine, which is also known as stomach flu. This condition is usually caused by a virus and may produce nausea, vomiting,

diarrhea, abdominal pain, cramping, and fever. Recovery is usually rapid, within one or two days. Clients should increase their fluid intake, especially clear fluids, and reduce their solid food intake during recovery. Gastroenteritis may be prevented by good hygiene, hand washing, not sharing eating or drinking utensils, and other measures of infection control. In addition, not eating unwashed raw fruits and vegetables or uncooked foods is important to prevention.

- Nausea is a sick feeling in the stomach caused by illness or the ingestion of spoiled food. Nausea may also be felt in certain situations such as early pregnancy or when repetitive motion causes discomfort, as in car sickness or seasickness.
- Gastrointestinal (GI) ulcers are also known as peptic or stomach ulcers. These are sores on the mucous membrane of any part of the GI tract. Symptoms include a gnawing pain or burning sensation that is relieved by drinking milk or taking antacids. Medication is commonly used to treat ulcers, but recurring ulcers may require surgery. Duodenal ulcers are another type of peptic ulcer. They are caused by the Helicobacter pylori bacterium (see **Figure 7.13**). The discovery of this bacterium has led to the widespread use of antibiotics to treat many types of ulcers.
- Hiatal hernia is a protrusion of the stomach through an opening in the diaphragm. Stomach acids flowing back into the esophagus cause pain and burning in the stomach and chest. Certain eating habits and practices make the condition worse. The client should not bend over or lie down after eating and should not drink carbonated beverages, talk while eating, or chew gum. Losing weight (if a client is obese), eating small, frequent meals, and taking antacids are treatments. Surgery may be indicated but is very infrequently performed.
- Cirrhosis is a chronic liver disease usually caused by chronic hepatitis, poor nutrition, or excessive alcohol consumption.
- Cholecystitis is an acute or chronic inflammation of the gallbladder. It is most commonly caused by hardened masses known as gallstones, in the ducts of the gallbladder. Treatment may include weight loss, a low-fat diet, medication, or surgery.
- Appendicitis is inflammation of the appendix caused when gastric substances leak into it from the duodenum. Symptoms include abdominal pain, constipation, fever, and an elevated white blood cell count. Surgery is required to prevent the appendix from bursting.
- Inflammatory bowel diseases include ulcerative colitis and Crohn's disease. Ulcerative colitis is a chronic type of inflammatory bowel disease with recurring ulcers and inflammation of the large intestine. Other symptoms may include cramping, abdominal pain, and diarrhea. Crohn's disease is similar to ulcerative colitis. It sometimes includes the production of abnormal openings in tissue walls. Crohn's disease affects both the small and the large intestine. Both diseases are often associated with stress and are usually treated with medication.

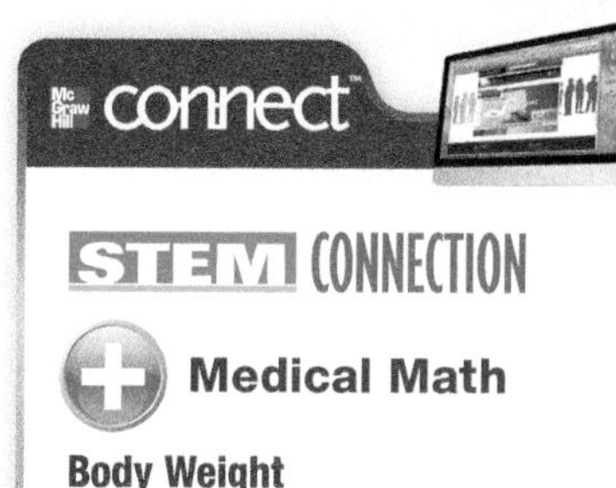

STEM CONNECTION

Medical Math

Body Weight
The client's ideal body weight is 150 lbs. Using the guidelines, determine at what weight he would be overweight (<20 percent), obese (>20 percent over to 99 lbs. over) and morbidly obese (>100 lbs. over). connect Go online to read more about calculating ideal body weight, and complete the activity.

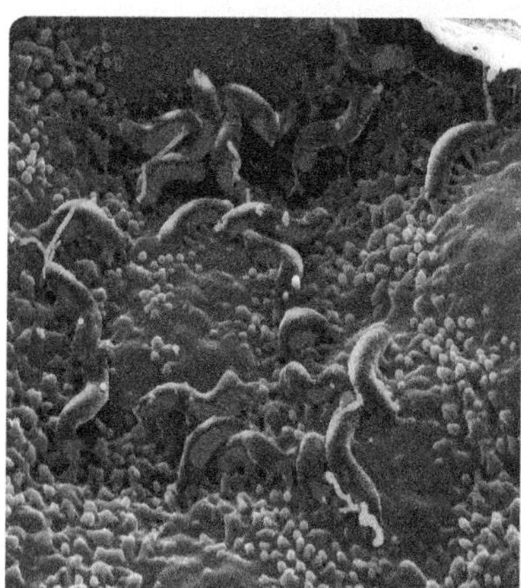

Fig. 7.13 Heliobacter Pylori This bacterium has been found to cause stomach ulcers and gastritis. *What is the definition of an ulcer?*

Photo: Eye of Science/Science/Source/Photo Researchers

- Diverticulitis is an inflammation of the small pouches in the intestinal wall caused by trapped food or bacteria. This condition causes pain and fever. Treatment includes bed rest, antibiotics, liquid diet, or low-fiber diet. Once the inflammation subsides, clients should increase their fiber consumption and avoid nuts, popcorn, raisins, and food with seeds that can lodge in the pouches of the colon.

READING CHECK

List the types of inflammation that occur in the digestive system.

Disorders That Can Be Symptoms

What causes halitosis?

Certain disorders can also be symptoms of another disease or problem.

- Constipation is infrequent or difficult release of bowel movements. It is sometimes the result of insufficient moisture to soften and move stools.
- Diarrhea is loose, watery stools that may be caused by insufficient roughage in the diet or by an internal disorder. An analysis of stool for blood, bacteria, and other elements can provide a clue to the cause.
- Hemorrhoids are swollen, twisted veins that can cause great discomfort in and around the anal area. Medication to soothe the pain and itching is available. Maintaining soft stool with plenty of bran in the diet and warm baths may help prevent recurrence.
- Halitosis is foul mouth odor, or bad breath. It may be caused by poor dental hygiene or by lung or intestinal disorders.
- Flatulence is accumulation of gas in the stomach or intestines. Flatus is the release of gas through the anus.
- Eructation, which is belching or burping, is the release of gas from the stomach through the mouth.

Both belching and flatulence are normal bodily functions unless they are excessive or associated with a disorder.

- **Jaundice** is excessive bilirubin in the blood that causes a yellow discoloration of the skin. The white part of the eye, or the sclera, frequently turns yellow as well, as shown in **Figure 7.14.** Jaundice may be a result of liver disease. Newborn jaundice, a common condition, is discussed in Chapter 8.

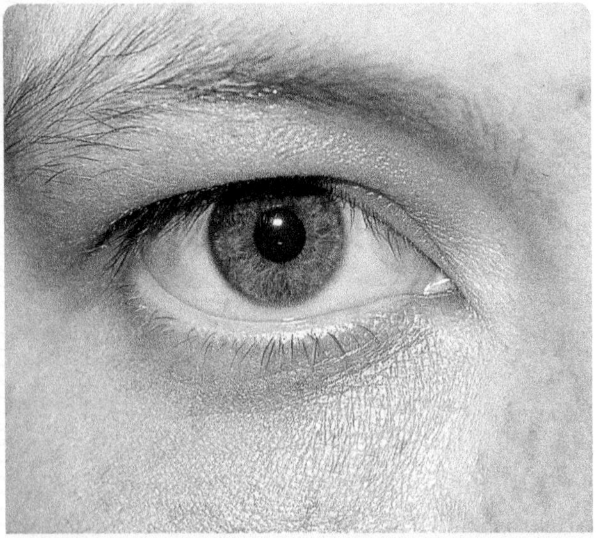

Figure 7.14 Jaundice Jaundice, which is yellow discoloration of the skin, can also affect the sclera, or white part, of the eye. *What disease can cause jaundice?*

Photo: Garry Watson/Science Photo Library/Photo Researchers

READING CHECK

Name the substance that causes jaundice.

Urinary Diseases and Disorders

Why are women at greater risk than men for contracting a urinary tract infection?

A **urinary tract infection (UTI)** can occur anywhere in the urinary tract, most commonly in the bladder or urethra. Urinary tract infections are much more common in women than in men because the distance from the meatus to the bladder in women is much shorter. Examples of UTIs and other urinary diseases and disorders are:

- Cystitis is an inflammation of the bladder. Symptoms include painful and frequent urination and discomfort. Treatment generally includes antibiotics and plenty of liquids. If more than three infections occur in a year, surgery may be required.
- Incontinence is the involuntary discharge of urine or feces. It is usually a symptom of another disease or disorder and is more common in certain disabled or elderly clients.
- Kidney stones, or renal calculi, are hardened lumps of matter that tend to form in the kidneys and other parts of the urinary system. If possible, the stones are allowed to pass from the body in the urine.
- Glomerulonephritis refers to a kidney inflammation located in the glomerulus. This inflammation can be acute or chronic; if chronic, high blood pressure, kidney failure, and other conditions can result.
- Pyelonephritis is a bacterial infection in the renal pelvis. It can be acute or chronic, and is manifested by shaking chills, fever, and joint and muscle pain. Chronic pyelonephritis can lead to kidney failure.
- Kidney or renal failure is a loss of kidney function. Causes may be by diabetes or infection. Treatment is dialysis and medication.

READING CHECK

Identify the treatment for a patient with a kidney stone.

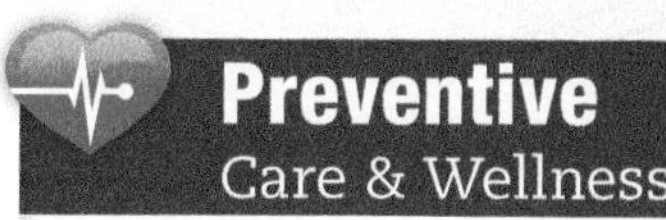

Preventing Urinary Cystitis

In females, the openings for the digestive, urinary, and reproductive systems are all very close. Because of this and a shorter urethra, women are more likely than men to suffer from cystitis, which is more commonly known as a bladder infection.

Here are some prevention tips.

- Always urinate when the urge occurs. Otherwise, urine stays in the bladder and the upper urethra, allowing bacteria to grow.
- Drink lots of clear fluids. The more clear liquids (especially water) one drinks, the more urine created, ensuring that the system is flushed on a regular basis. Cranberry juice or cranberry tablets are often recommended as a preventive measure.
- Wipe front to back. This is especially important after a bowel movement. Doing so prevents contamination of both the vagina and urethra by gastrointestinal (GI) bacteria (E. coli).
- Urinate after intercourse. If sexually active, females should urinate immediately following intercourse, to flush away any contamination.

SECTION 7.9 Diseases and Disorders of the Digestive and Urinary Systems Review

AFTER YOU READ

1. **Describe** the treatment for diverticulitis.
2. **Name** and describe two disorders of the digestive system that you have experienced.
3. **Discuss** possible solutions for this scenario: When visiting your grandfather in a long-term care facility, you notice the odor of urine and feces upon entering. How can the severity of the odor be reduced?.
4. **Compare** the three urinary diseases that are caused by inflammation.

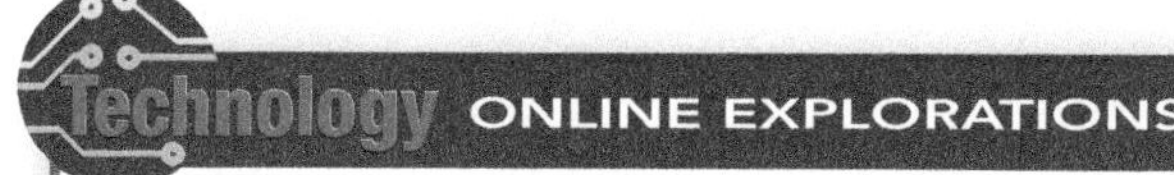

Dialysis

Dialysis is a treatment for renal or kidney failure. Go online to discover how this common treatment helps. Write a summary of the treatment, what it does, how it is done, and any problems that result.

SECTION **7.10**

Diseases and Disorders of the Endocrine System

Vocabulary

Content Vocabulary

You will learn these content vocabulary terms in this section.

- **oversecretion**
- **undersecretion**

Academic Vocabulary

You will see this word in your reading and on your tests. Find its meaning in the Glossary in the back of this book.

- **supplements**

Diseases and Disorders

Which organ produces insulin?

Too much or too little of a hormone creates an imbalance and, often, a disorder or disease. Most endocrine illnesses are the result of **oversecretion** or **undersecretion** of hormones. Understanding hormones will help you to understand what happens when an imbalance occurs.

Disorders of the Pituitary Gland

Imbalances in hormones produced in the pituitary gland can cause disorders such as those listed here.

- Acromegaly, an enlargement of features after childhood, is caused by an oversecretion of growth hormone (see **Figure 7.15**). Oversecretion can also result in gigantism (see **Figure 7.16**).
- Dwarfism, or stunted growth, caused by undersecretion of growth hormone by the pituitary gland results in a person being small but having normally proportioned features (see **Figure 7.17**). Dwarfism with disproportionate features is usually caused by the congenital absence of the thyroid gland or by another genetic defect.
- Diabetes insipidus is caused by undersecretion of the antidiuretic hormone (ADH). It is characterized by excessive amounts of water

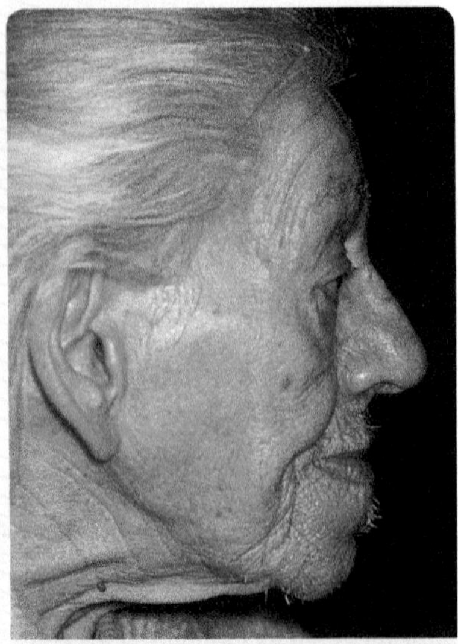

Fig. 7.15 Acromegaly Excess growth hormone in an adult causes enlarged face and hands. *Which gland produces this growth hormone?*

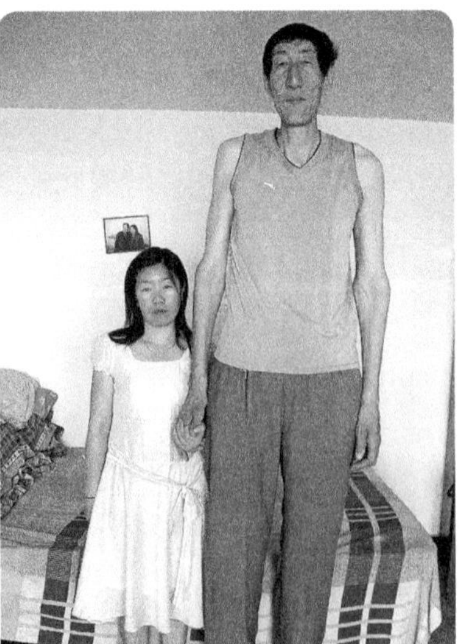

Fig. 7.16 Gigantism Gigantism is caused by oversecretion of growth hormone. *What condition is caused by undersecretion of the same hormone?*

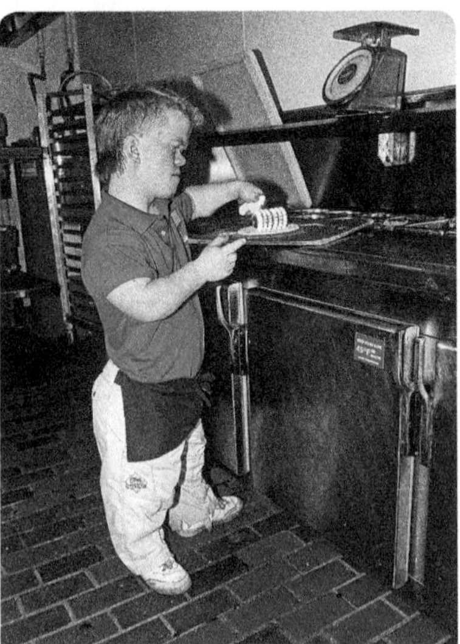

Fig. 7.17 Pituitary Dwarfism A person with pituitary dwarfism is small but has normally proportioned features. *What causes this condition?*

being secreted in the urine and excessive and constant thirst. It can be treated with an antidiuretic medication.

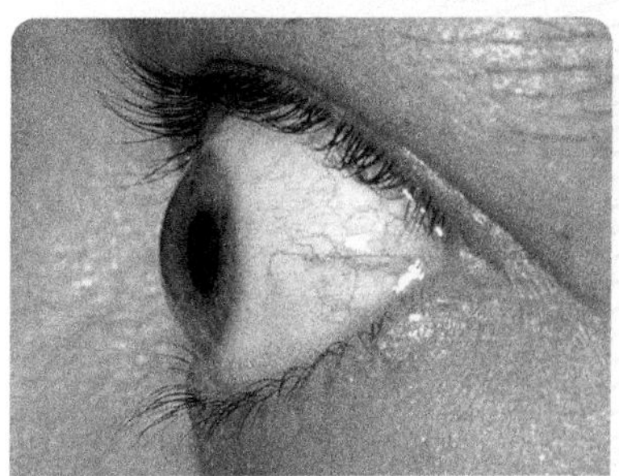

Fig. 7.18 Exophthalmos Bulging of the eyeball is due to an excess of T3 and/or T4. *What endocrine gland is responsible for this disorder?*

Disorders of the Thyroid Gland

Some diseases and disorders associated with the thyroid gland are:

- Hyperthyroidism, also known as Graves' disease, is caused by an overactive thyroid gland. Hyperthyroidism is characterized by bulging of the eyes. Oversecretion of thyroid hormones, a tumor, or a lack of iodine in the diet can cause a goiter, which is an expansion of the thyroid gland that develops into a large growth in the neck. **Figure 7.18** shows one symptom of hyperthyroidism, which is exophthalmos, or bulging eyes.
- Hypothyroidism is caused by underactivity of the thyroid gland and results in sluggishness, slow pulse, and often obesity. Myxedema is a specific type of hypothyroidism in adults. It has a range of symptoms, including puffiness in the extremities, slow muscular response, and dry skin. Hypothyroidism can be treated with synthetic hormones.

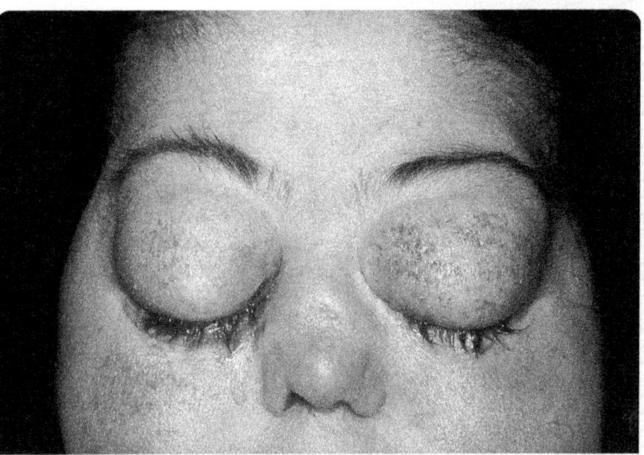

Fig. 7.19 Cushing's Syndrome Symptoms of Cushing's syndrome are a round and red face, an obese trunk of the body, and wasted limbs. *What three conditions can lead to this syndrome?*

Disorders of the Parathyroid Gland

Overactivity of the parathyroid gland is usually caused by a tumor in the parathyroid gland. It often results in many clinical symptoms from bone loss to severe cases of kidney failure.

Underactivity of the parathyroid gland results in low blood calcium levels, causing many symptoms such as bone loss and some muscle paralysis. Medications and supplements that increase calcium absorption may be prescribed.

Disorders of the Adrenal Glands

Some diseases and disorders associated with the adrenal glands are:

- Cushing's syndrome results from an oversecretion of glucocorticoids, an adrenal tumor, or an oversecretion of ACTH from the pituitary gland. If Cushing's syndrome is caused by a tumor, it is usually cured by removal of the tumor. Some symptoms of Cushing's syndrome are a round and red face, an obese trunk of the body, and wasted limbs (see **Figure 7.19**).
- Addison's disease is caused by underactivity of the adrenal gland. It may result in anemia, abnormal skin pigment, and general malaise. It can be controlled with cortisone.

Disorders of the Pancreas

Diseases and disorders associated with the pancreas are:

- Hypoglycemia is a lowering of blood sugar levels that deprives the body of needed glucose and is caused by oversecretion of insulin.

connect

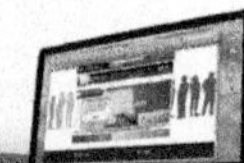

VIRTUAL LAB:
The Digestive and Endocrine Systems

Your digestive system is affected by what you put into it. In this virtual lab, you will create a daily menu, and track the nutritional contents of the choices you make.

connect Complete the Virtual lab online for this chapter,

- Diabetes mellitus is a widespread disease that affects about 4 percent of the U.S. population and is caused by undersecretion of insulin.

  Diabetes occurs either as Type I, which is insulin-dependent diabetes, or as Type II, which is noninsulin-dependent diabetes. Type I occurs in childhood or in adulthood and is the result of underproduction of insulin by the pancreas. Type I diabetes can be treated with controlled doses of insulin. Type II diabetes occurs in adulthood, usually in overweight people whose responsiveness to insulin is abnormally low. Mild Type II diabetes is controllable by exercise and diet. More severe cases need medication that helps lower the blood glucose level. Oral medications or insulin, which is given by injection, are common. If either type of diabetes is left uncontrolled, the client will suffer from excess glucose in the blood that spills into the urine, and excessive thirst, hunger, and urination. Complications of diabetes involve a wide range of ailments from circulatory problems to infections. Clients can suffer from kidney disease and failure, loss of sensation in the extremities, and visual loss leading to blindness.

READING CHECK

Identify the organ that is the source of gigantism and dwarfism.

connect ONLINE PROCEDURES

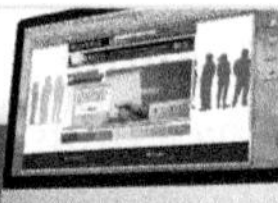

PROCEDURE 7-6

Identifying Endocrine Disorders

Endocrine disorders are usually caused by too much or not enough of a hormone. Knowing the hormones and their function will help you understand and recognize endocrine disorders.

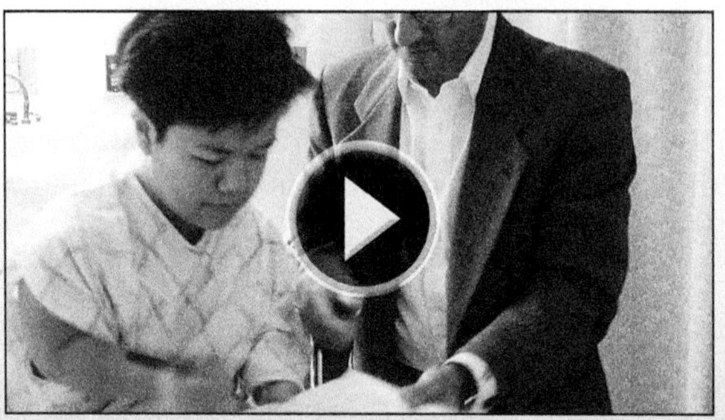

SECTION 7.10 Diseases and Disorders of the Endocrine System Review

AFTER YOU READ

1. **Describe** the symptoms you would expect a client with hypothyroidism to exhibit.
2. **List** the symptoms of diabetes mellitus.
3. **Explain** how diabetes mellitus is treated.
4. **Identify** some complications of diabetes mellitus.

Technology ONLINE EXPLORATIONS

Obesity

Obesity is a common cause of disease. Research the topic online, and then create a mini-brochure or presentation to help educate patients in at least five ways to prevent obesity.

Photo: DY Riess MD/Alamy

SECTION 7.11
Diseases and Disorders of the Reproductive System

Female Reproductive System Disorders

What is the difference between PMS and PMDD?

Both female and male reproductive systems may be the site of various diseases and disorders. Some disorders of the female reproductive system are:

- Pelvic inflammatory disease (PID) is a bacterial infection that can occur anywhere in the female reproductive system. Women with PID are at risk of chronic pelvic pain, ectopic pregnancy, and tubal infertility. Symptoms are lower abdomen pain, fever, and vaginal discharge. Treatment is antibiotics, rest, and an increase in fluids.
- **Premenstrual syndrome (PMS)** is a group of symptoms that appear 3 to 14 days before the onset of menstruation. The exact cause is not known. However, PMS is linked to hormone or chemical imbalance, poor nutrition, and stress. Women with PMS may experience physical symptoms such as breast swelling and tenderness, abdominal bloating, headache, backache, and constipation. **Premenstrual dysphoric disorder (PMDD)** is similar to PMS. However, PMDD includes more severe mental and emotional symptoms. These include nervousness, irritability, tension, and depression. Treatment targets the symptoms and includes medication, stress reduction, changes in diet, and exercise.

Abnormal Growths

Growths in the female reproductive system may be either benign or malignant. They can cause pain, abnormal bleeding, infertility, and pregnancy complications. Some abnormal growths are:

- Endometriosis is a condition in which uterine wall or endometrial tissue is found in the pelvis or on the abdominal wall. It can cause pain, irregular bleeding, and can result in infertility. Treatment includes pain medication, hormonal therapy, and surgery.
- Cervical cancer is a disease that can be detected early with a pelvic exam and Pap smear. Symptoms include abnormal vaginal bleeding and discharge and/or an enlarged uterus. Treatment involves hysterectomy, chemotherapy, and/or radiation.
- Ovarian cancer is difficult to diagnose in its earliest stages because there are few noticeable symptoms or the symptoms are thought to be something else. It often spreads before it is detected.

Vocabulary

Content Vocabulary

You will learn these content vocabulary terms in this section.

- **premenstrual syndrome (PMS)**
- **premenstrual dysphoric disorder (PMDD)**
- **sexually transmitted diseases (STD)**

Academic Vocabulary

You will see this word in your reading and on your tests. Find its meaning in the Glossary in the back of this book.

- **cultures**

- Breast tumors are tissue with dense, irregular, and bumpy "cobblestone" consistency. This is called fibrocystic breast change. The client may have discomfort, premenstrual tenderness and swelling, and nipple sensation or itching. This may be improved by decreasing caffeine and fat. It is sometimes normal variation in breast tissue. Whenever a woman finds a change in her breast, she should consult a practitioner to check for breast cancer.
- Breast cancer is a malignant tumor that may be found in one site. If it has spread to the lymph nodes, extensive treatment may be required. Depending upon the severity, one or more of these treatments may be used: hormone therapy, lumpectomy, mastectomy, radical mastectomy, radiation, and chemotherapy.

Pregnancy is considered to be a normal process. However, some pregnancies are in themselves not normal and end in abortion. Abortion is the premature end of a pregnancy. This end can be spontaneous, by miscarriage, or can be surgically performed. An ectopic pregnancy occurs when the fertilized egg is implanted outside the uterus. If implantation occurs in the fallopian tube, this is called a tubal pregnancy. An ectopic pregnancy usually requires surgery to remove the fetus. It will die because of lack of nourishment, or it may rupture the fallopian tube as it grows.

READING CHECK

List three possible treatments for breast cancer.

Male Reproductive System Disorders

What is the common age range for men to develop testicular cancer?

Here are some diseases and disorders of the male reproductive system.

- Epididymitis is inflammation of the epididymis. The cause may be gonococcus, streptococcus, or staphylococcus. Symptoms are pain and swollen testes. Treatment is antibiotics and pain medication.
- Benign prostatic hypertrophy (BPH) is an enlargement of the prostate gland not involving cancer but causing obstruction of the urinary tract. Symptoms include a slowed, weak, or delayed start of the urinary stream, frequent urination, pain and/or blood during urination, a sudden urge to void, and incontinence. Treatment depends upon severity of symptoms. Until symptoms impact lifestyle, surgery may be withheld. Medications include antibiotics.
- Prostate cancer is not related to BPH. However, it is an enlargement of the prostate gland due to a cancerous tumor. Symptoms include delayed or slowed start of urinary stream; urinary dribbling, especially immediately after urinating; urinary retention; pain with urination, bowel movement, or ejaculation; and lower back pain. Treatment may include any or all of the following: surgical

removal, chemotherapy, radiation, and hormonal therapy aimed at reducing the amount of testosterone in the body.

- Testicular cancer is an abnormal, rapid, and invasive growth of malignant cells in the testicles. There may be no symptoms, or the client may experience enlargement of a testicle or a change in the way it feels; a lump or swelling in either testicle; a dull ache in the back or lower abdomen; testicular discomfort; or a feeling of heaviness in the scrotum. Surgery, chemotherapy, radiation, or a bone marrow transplant may be used as treatment.

READING CHECK

Summarize the symptoms of prostate cancer.

Sexually Transmitted Diseases

What is the most common sexually transmitted disease?

Sexually transmitted diseases (STDs) are diseases that are transmitted primarily through sexual contact and exchange of body fluids. In most cases of STDs, both sexual partners should be treated. Sexually active individuals are at risk. Individuals who have multiple partners are at a higher risk for the following diseases.

- Chlamydia is the most common sexually transmitted disease in the United States. Untreated chlamydia can lead to pelvic infection and infertility in females. In men, chlamydia may produce symptoms such as discharge from the penis or rectum or a burning sensation on urination or defecation. It can also cause epididymitis and orchitis. However, up to 25 percent of infected men may have no symptoms at all. Only approximately 30 percent of women have symptoms due to chlamydia. Women who do have symptoms may note vaginal discharge, burning on urination, or abdominal pain. Antibiotics are used for treatment.
- Gonorrhea is a highly contagious infection caused by a bacterium. It is one of the most common infectious bacterial diseases. In women, the gonorrhea bacterium can cause sore throat or vaginitis and may lead to PID. Men may experience pain and/or discharge from the urethra. The first aspect of treatment is to use antibiotics to cure the affected person. The second is to locate and test all sexual contacts and to treat them to prevent further spread of the disease.
- Syphilis is an acute disease treatable with antibiotics. It has three stages. During the primary stage, a painless chancre or sore appears on the penis or vulva. This may go unnoticed. The secondary stage occurs if the primary stage is not treated and is more noticeable. The client experiences fever, swollen glands, sore throat, and a non-itching rash. The third stage comes more than a year later, when major organs may be involved, and can include permanent damage such as mental disorder, paralysis, deafness, or blindness.

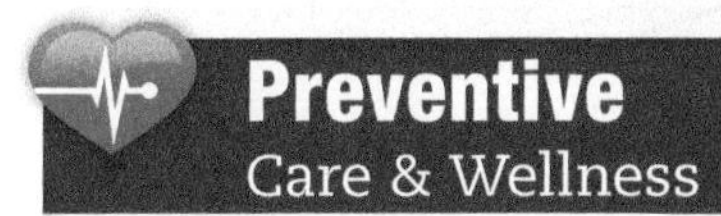

Preventive Care & Wellness

Screening for Reproductive System Cancer

Reproductive cancers can be prevented, but early detection is essential. The American Cancer Society has made the following general recommendations.

Breast cancer:

- Monthly self-examinations
- Periodic examinations by a healthcare professional
- Periodic mammograms

Cervical cancer:

- Pap tests
- Pelvic examinations

Testicular cancer:

- Monthly self-examinations

Prostate cancer:

- Prostate-specific antigen (PSA) test

21ST CENTURY SKILLS

Cultural Diversity in Illness and Treatments

Different cultures have different ideas about the body and how it works. For example, people in some cultures believe that there are forces in the body that must be in balance. In addition, some cultures may refuse certain treatments or may have their own cultural practices. For example, some clients may believe that illness is the will of God or that illness is a punishment for sins. Some religions and cultures do not believe in transfusions or amputations. In addition, some cultural or religious groups practice spiritual healing. The roles of men and women and the role of the family can differ widely from culture to culture. As a healthcare provider, you must be understanding and accepting of these differences. It is important that you treat all individuals with respect and not make judgments about clients who have beliefs different from yours.

- Trichomoniasis is caused by a parasite. The symptoms are different in men than they are in women. In men, the infection often produces no symptoms and clears spontaneously in a few weeks. Symptomatic men may experience a mild urethral itching or discharge or a mild burning after urination or ejaculation. Women develop a frothy, foul-smelling, green-white or yellowish vaginal discharge. The volume of discharge may be large. Itching may occur on the labia and inner thighs, and the labia may appear swollen. The treatment is with antibiotics.
- Herpes simplex 2 is known as genital herpes, because it affects the genital area. This virus has no cure. When painful genital blisters appear, the symptoms are treated. The virus lives in the nervous system waiting to strike again when the immune system is weakened. Medications are available to reduce the severity of the symptoms and may help prevent its spread.
- Condyloma is a growth on the outside of the genitalia that may be a result of a disease such as human papilloma virus, or genital warts. Women who have human papilloma virus are at risk for cervical cancer and should have a pelvic exam and Pap smear up to every six months. The growth, which is sometimes not noticeable, may be the only symptom. The warts can be removed. A vaccine that provides immunity to many types of HPV viruses is available.
- Hepatitis B is caused by a virus and is also considered a sexually transmitted disease. It was discussed in Chapter 3, Safety and Infection Control Practices.
- Human immunodeficiency virus (HIV) is the cause of AIDS, as discussed in Section 7.7.

READING CHECK

Compare and contrast the symptoms of trichomoniasis in men and in women.

SECTION 7.11 Diseases and Disorders of the Reproductive System Review

AFTER YOU READ

1. **Identify** what all sexually transmitted diseases have in common.
2. **Explain** how reproductive system cancers can be prevented and detected.
3. **Describe** the stages of syphilis.

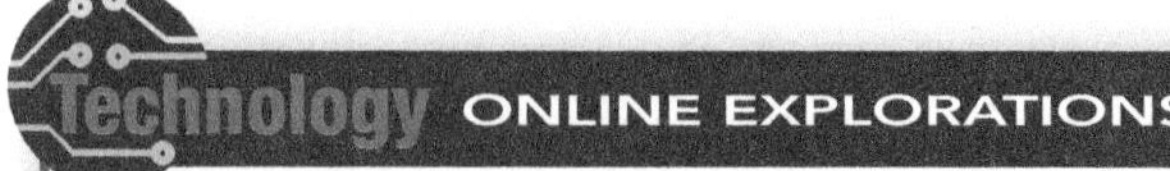

Self-Exams

Go to the American Cancer Society's website to learn the procedure for a breast or testicular self-exam. Once you are familiar with the procedure, teach/explain it to a classmate as if he or she were one of your patients, or write a list of the steps you would use to explain a self-examination to a client.

CHAPTER
7 Review

Chapter Summary

SECTION 7.1

- Diseases and disorder causes include inflammation, genetics, hemodynamic changes, autoimmunity, neoplasms, environment, and infection. **(pg. 190)**

SECTION 7.2

- Diseases and disorders of the integumentary system include various lesions that may be symptoms of other disorders. **(pg. 192)**

SECTION 7.3

- Fractures are often a disorder of the skeletal system. Skeletal system diseases include osteoporosis, arthritis, osteomyelitis, herniated disc, and spine curvatures. **(pg. 195)**
- Muscular system disorders include strain, dislocation, and fibromyalgia. **(pg. 197)**

SECTION 7.4

- Diseases and disorders of the nervous system may be caused by traumatic injury, or they may be congenital. **(pg. 199)**

SECTION 7.5

- Diseases and disorders of the sensory system usually result from age-related disorders or age-related wear and tear on the senses. **(pg. 203)**

SECTION 7.6

- Diseases may occur when the red blood cells do not transport enough oxygen to the tissues, or when the white blood cell levels are increased. **(pg. 205)**

SECTION 7.7

- AIDS is a disease of the lymphatic and immune system. **(pg. 208)**

SECTION 7.8

- Diseases of the respiratory system range from mild inflammations and infections to chronic problems that block the airways and reduce oxygen exchange. **(pg. 210)**

SECTION 7.9

- Obesity can affect long-term health and cause diseases in other systems. **(pg. 212)**
- Infections and inflammations are the most common urinary system disorders. **(pg. 215)**

SECTION 7.10

- Most endocrine system diseases are caused by hormone over- or underproduction. **(pg. 216)**

SECTION 7.11

- Reproductive system cancer screening should be done in males and females. **(pg. 221)**
- AIDS is also a sexually transmitted disease related to the reproductive system. **(pg. 222)**

CHAPTER 7 Assessment

Critical Thinking/Problem Solving

1. While running, you turn your ankle. In great pain, you limp home. What is the name of what you have done? How would you treat the injury?
2. Your client has Alzheimer's disease. How would you explain the disease to the family? What advice would you provide to the family about how to keep their loved one safe?
3. A client is concerned about the prevalence of Type II diabetes and wants to know how to prevent her child from developing this condition. What advice and recommendations would you provide?
4. A client complains about a sore spot on his arm. What criteria would you use to decide if this spot could be cancerous?

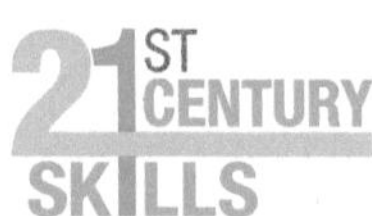

5. **Teamwork** Role-play various diseases presented in this chapter by "acting out" the symptoms of each disease. See if your partner or the class can identify the disease being portrayed.
6. **Information Literacy** Choose a disease or disorder described in this chapter that you would like to learn more about. Research online for more information about the disease. Compile a document that includes its name, definition, causes, prevention, symptoms, treatments, complications, and prognosis.

McGraw Hill connect ONLINE ACTIVITIES

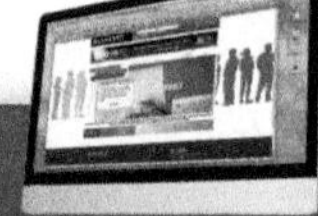

Complete our HST online activities for Chapter 7, which include Concept Check review questions, Reference Flash Cards, and Online Procedures assessment sheets.

- **Concept Check** review questions
- **Reference Flash Cards** medical terminology practice
- **Online Procedures** assessment sheets

CHAPTER 8

Human Growth and Development

Essential Question:

At what age do people undergo the most dramatic changes?

Every individual is unique. However, as we grow and mature, all of us pass a series of developmental milestones. From fetal development to mature adulthood, there are specific aspects of physical, intellectual, emotional, and social development associated with each stage of life. Familiarity with these stages and their characteristics will benefit healthcare professionals, whether they specialize in working with one or all age groups.

McGraw Hill connect™

It's Online!

- Online Procedures
- STEM Connection
- Medical Science
- Medical Terms
- Medical Math
- Ethics in Action
- Virtual Lab

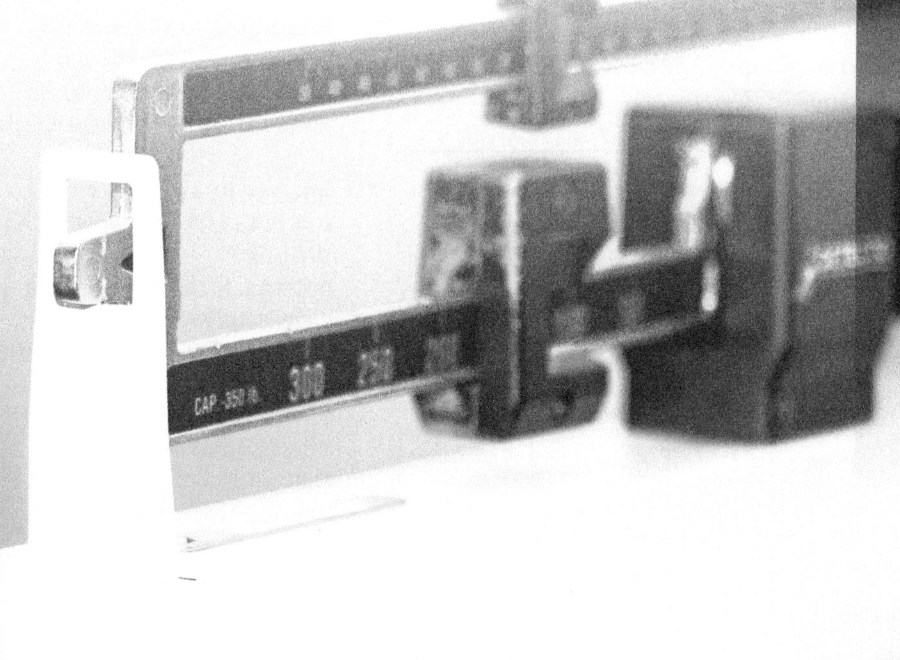

Photo: The McGraw-Hill Companies Inc.

READING GUIDE

OBJECTIVES

After completing this chapter, you will be able to:

- **Identify** four developmental milestones.
- **Identify** two human growth and development principles.
- **Describe** the development of the embryo and fetus.
- **Recognize** the appearance of a healthy full-term newborn.
- **Illustrate** the development of an infant.
- **Compare** toddler and preschooler development.
- **Discuss** two developmental tasks of elementary and middle-school children.
- **Propose** reasons for three major health-related issues with which teenagers may have to cope.
- **Select** one major health-related issue with each age level of adults.
- **Demonstrate** four development procedures.

BEFORE YOU READ

Connect Can you identify some stages of human development?

Main Idea

Healthcare workers should recognize the changes and challenges that humans experience, including various stages of development and important milestones, as they grow from conception through old age.

Note-Taking Activity

Draw this table. Write key terms and phrases under **Cues**. Write main ideas under **Note Taking**. Summarize the section under **Summary**.

Cues	Note Taking
∘	∘
∘	∘
Summary	

Graphic Organizer

Before you read the chapter, draw a diagram like the one to the right. As you read, write the developmental stages covered in this chapter into the diagram.

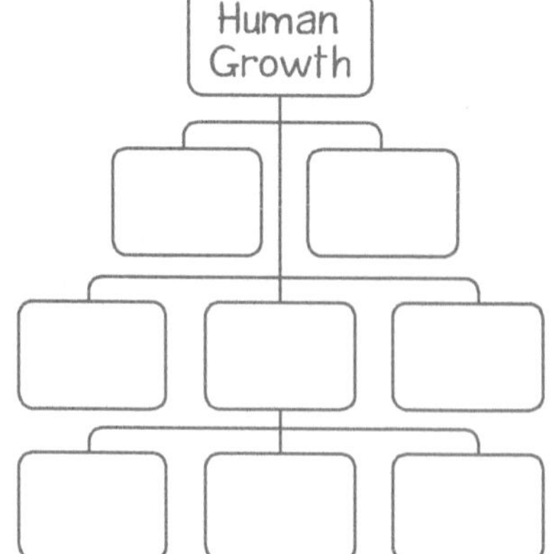

connect

Downloadable graphic organizers can be accessed online.

STANDARDS

HEALTH SCIENCE

NCHSE 1.11 Classify the basic structural and functional organization of the human body (tissue, organ, and system).

NCHSE 1.32 Analyze diagrams, charts, graphs, and tables to interpret healthcare results.

SCIENCE

NSES 1 Develop an understanding of science unifying concepts and processes: systems, order, and organization; evidence, models, and explanation; change, constancy, and measurement; evolution and equilibrium; and form and function.

NCHSE *National Consortium for Health Science Education*

NSES *National Science Education Standards*

COMMON CORE STATE STANDARDS

MATHEMATICS

Geometry

Geometric Measurement and Dimension G-GMD Visualize relationships between two-dimensional and three-dimensional objects.

ENGLISH LANGUAGE ARTS

Writing

Research to Build and Present Knowledge W-8 Gather relevant information from multiple authoritative print and digital sources, using advanced searches effectively; assess the usefulness of each source in answering the research question; integrate information into the text selectively to maintain the flow of ideas, avoiding plagiarism and following a standard format for citation.

SECTION

8.1 Growth and Development

Developmental Milestones

How is wellness related to development?

Different periods of life present different changes and challenges. The **wellness** of individuals depends partly on their stage of growth and development.

This chapter describes the different stages in the life of a human being from conception to mature adult. Understanding growth and development will improve your abilities as a healthcare professional.

During each stage of growth, **developmental milestones** occur.

- Physical development refers to the actual bodily changes observed in a client during a particular period of growth.
- Intellectual-cognitive development refers to the thinking skills a client develops.
- Psycho-emotional development refers to the changes in feelings a client experiences during a particular period.
- Social development involves the way that a person relates to others.

For each stage of development described in this chapter, look for the heading *Aspects of Care* to find a description of the special health needs for that particular stage.

READING CHECK

Define social development.

Vocabulary

Content Vocabulary

You will learn these content vocabulary terms in this section.

- **wellness**
- **developmental milestones**
- **cephalocaudal development**
- **embryo**
- **fetus**
- **gene**

Academic Vocabulary

You will see this word in your reading and on your tests. Find its meaning in the Glossary in the back of this book.

- **mature**

Principles of Growth and Development

What body system is the first to begin developing in the embryo?

In the uterus, the embryo and fetus develop in a head-to-tail manner known as **cephalocaudal development.** The brain and an elementary nervous system begin to develop first. Then development progresses downward. The word **embryo** refers to a human being growing in the uterus from conception to about the eighth week. The word **fetus** refers to a human being growing in the uterus from the eighth week until birth. Children learn gross motor skills, such as walking, first. Then a child learns fine motor skills, such as using a crayon.

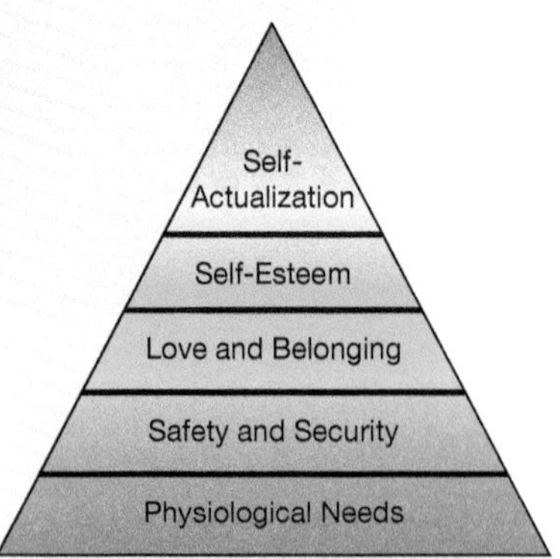

Fig. 8.1 Maslow's Hierarchy The five levels of human needs. *Using Maslow's Hierarchy, put the following in order from lowest (most basic) to highest (most complex): house, significant other, dinner, ability to drive a car, charity work.*

Human Needs

Sociologist and psychologist Abraham Maslow proposed five levels of human needs. According to his theory, all people have needs, but some are more important. Thus, needs can be placed in a hierarchy according to their importance to human life (see **Figure 8.1**).

There are five levels of needs. The first four are called Deficit Needs. If these needs are not met, there is a deficit. If they are met, there is balance, or homeostasis. The fifth level is Being Needs. When they are met, people reach their highest potential. These are the five levels:

- Physiological needs, which are the most basic, include the need for air, food, water, heat, activity, rest, pain avoidance, and sex.
- Safety and security needs are second in the hierarchy. They include the need for stability, protection, structure, order, and limits.
- Love and belonging needs involve the need for friends, spouses, children, and community.
- Esteem needs are more complex. Lower-level esteem needs include the need to be respected by others. Higher-level esteem needs include the need for confidence and independence.
- The highest-ranked needs involve self-actualization, or the continuous need to fulfill one's potential.

Genes and the Environment

Genes and environment influence development in many ways. **Genes** are units of hereditary material contained in a person's cells. The environment is also a powerful factor in development. There has been much discussion about whether people are a product of heredity or of environment. It can be argued that both play equally important roles.

READING CHECK

Recall when an embryo becomes a fetus.

SECTION 8.1 Growth and Development Review

AFTER YOU READ

1. **Explain** the four categories of human development.
2. **Identify** two factors that influence human growth and development.
3. **Using** Maslow's hierarchy, **compare** the need for water to the need for a fulfilling career.
4. **Describe** cephalocaudal development.
5. **Examine** which human need, if met, helps people to achieve their highest potential.

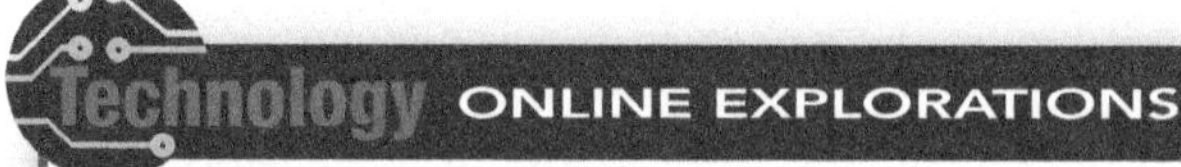

Milestones

Research online the topic of growth and development. Determine the stage you are in and the developmental milestones that you have already passed through.

SECTION 8.2 From Conception through the Teenage Years

Conception to Full Term

When does a fetus's heart begin to beat?

The stages of human development from the time of conception through the teen years, though few in number, bring about enormous changes.

Pregnancy lasts ten lunar months, or 40 weeks. This is about nine calendar months, or 266 to 280 days. Pregnancy is divided into three trimesters during which growth and development inside the uterus occur. (A trimester is about three months.) **Table 8.1** lists the stages of growth and development that take place during each trimester.

Table 8.1 Growth and Development During Each Trimester

TRIMESTER	LENGTH OF TIME	GROWTH AND DEVELOPMENT
First trimester	Conception through third month	Development of major organ systems
Second trimester	Fourth through sixth month	Refinement of organ systems
Third trimester	Seventh through ninth month	Weight gain and maturation to prepare for life outside uterus

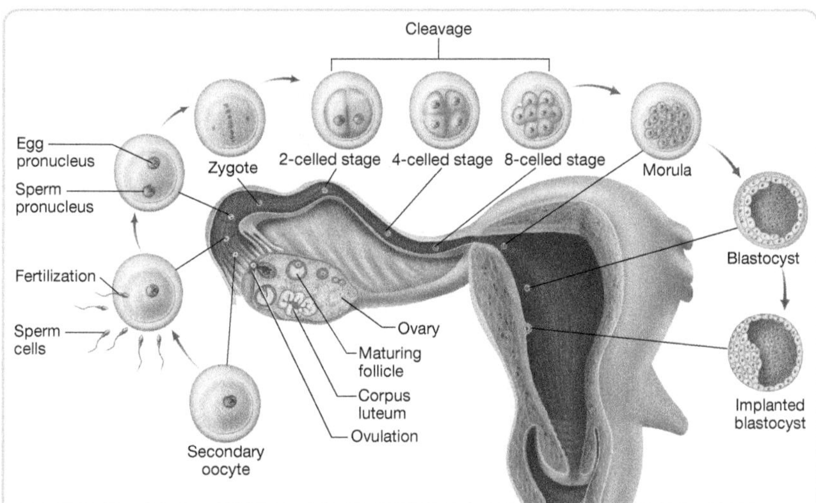

Fig. 8.2 Progress of the Zygote The fertilized ovum (egg) takes 3 to 5 days to travel through the fallopian tube. *How does implantation occur?*

Vocabulary

Content Vocabulary

You will learn these content vocabulary terms in this section.

- conception
- fallopian tube
- fertilization
- zygote
- morula
- implantation
- chorion
- amniotic sac
- circumcision
- puberty

Academic Vocabulary

You will see these words in your reading and on your tests. Find their meanings in the Glossary in the back of this book.

- physical
- maintained
- proportion
- normal

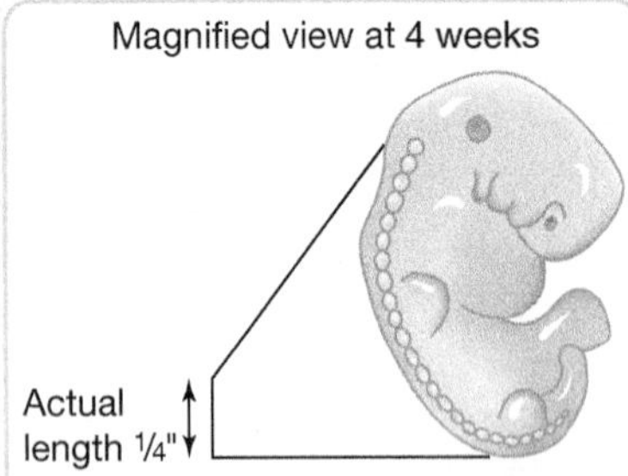

Fig. 8.3. Embryo at 4 Weeks This is a magnified view of the embryo at four weeks. *Can you describe the growth and development in this four-week-old embryo?*

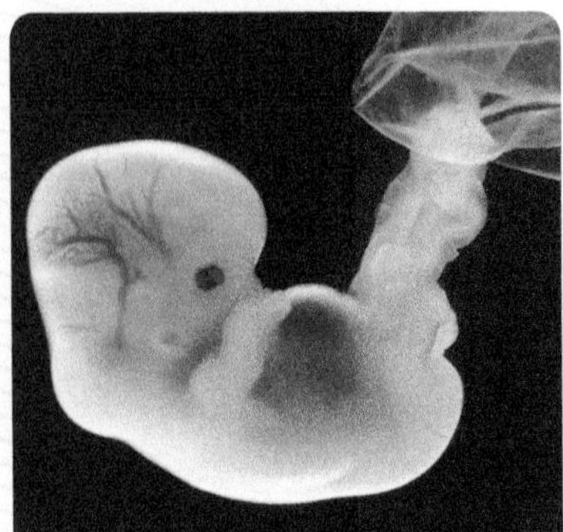

Fig. 8.4 Embryo at 6 Weeks Here, a six-week-old embryo is magnified to more than six times its actual size. *What is the average length of a six-week-old embryo?*

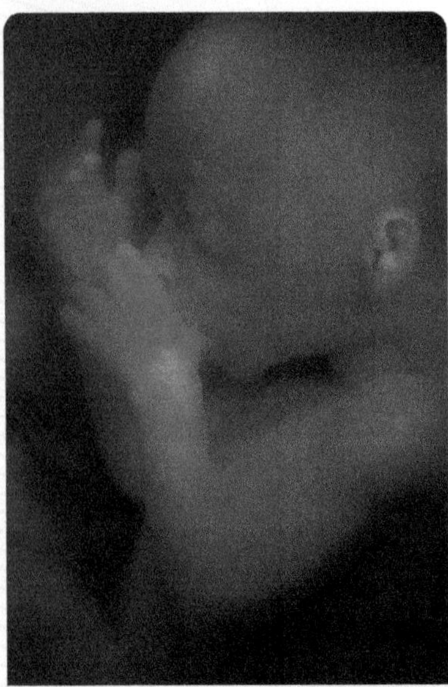

Fig. 8.5 Second Trimester While in the uterus, the fetus may suck its thumb. *When does hair begin to appear?*

First Trimester

Conception occurs when a sperm penetrates the ovum in the outer third of the **fallopian tube,** the tube that extends from the uterus to the ovary. This is called **fertilization**. The fertilized ovum is called a **zygote** (see **Figure 8.2**). The zygote travels through the fallopian tube toward the uterus. It divides into two cells, then four cells, and so on.

The journey through the fallopian tube takes three to five days. The cells, or **morula,** now look like a cluster of grapes. At the back of the cluster is a rootlike projection that will become the placenta, which is the organ that links the blood supplies of the mother and baby. This group of cells becomes implanted into the upper rear wall of the uterus. During implantation, the rootlike projection penetrates an increasing number of blood vessels. The cells facing away from the uterine wall become the outer fetal membrane, or **chorion.**

The **amniotic sac,** a fluid-filled membrane that surrounds the fetus, begins to develop over these cells. The outer cells start to develop a head and a tail. An intestine and a circulatory system start to form. By 21 to 25 days after conception, a rudimentary heart is beating and the nervous system begins to develop. Development continues as follows.

- At four weeks (see **Figure 8.3**), the embryo is about ¼ inch long. There are arm buds on each side. The embryo now has a head, body, tail, eyes, and ears.
- At five weeks, a nose can be seen.
- At six weeks (see **Figure 8.4**), the embryo is a little less than ½ inch long and is floating in the amniotic sac. The leg buds are present.
- At seven weeks, the embryo is about ¾ inch long and can move its hands. The fingers are defined, the internal organs are now visible, and the skull bones are growing at the crown.
- At eight weeks, the embryo is almost an inch long, the liver is very large, the bones are beginning to form, and testes and ovaries are distinguishable. The developing infant is now called a fetus.
- At ten weeks, the fetus is about 1½ to two inches long, the kidneys are making urine, and lower trunk muscles are developing.

Second Trimester

Some development highlights in the second trimester are:

- At 12 weeks, the head of the fetus is about one-third the size of its outstretched length and ribs can be seen. Hair begins to appear.
- At 16 weeks the fetus is about 4½ inches long and weighs about three to four ounces. The face looks human, blood cells form in the spleen, the cerebrum lies over other brain parts, and the testicles of males are in position for descent. The mother feels fetal movements. The heartbeat can be heard with special instruments.
- At 20 to 24 weeks the fetus is about 12 inches long. Major systems continue to develop and bones continue to form. The fetus may move its thumb into its mouth (see **Figure 8.5**). The eyes are sealed closed. If the fetus were born now, survival would be unlikely.

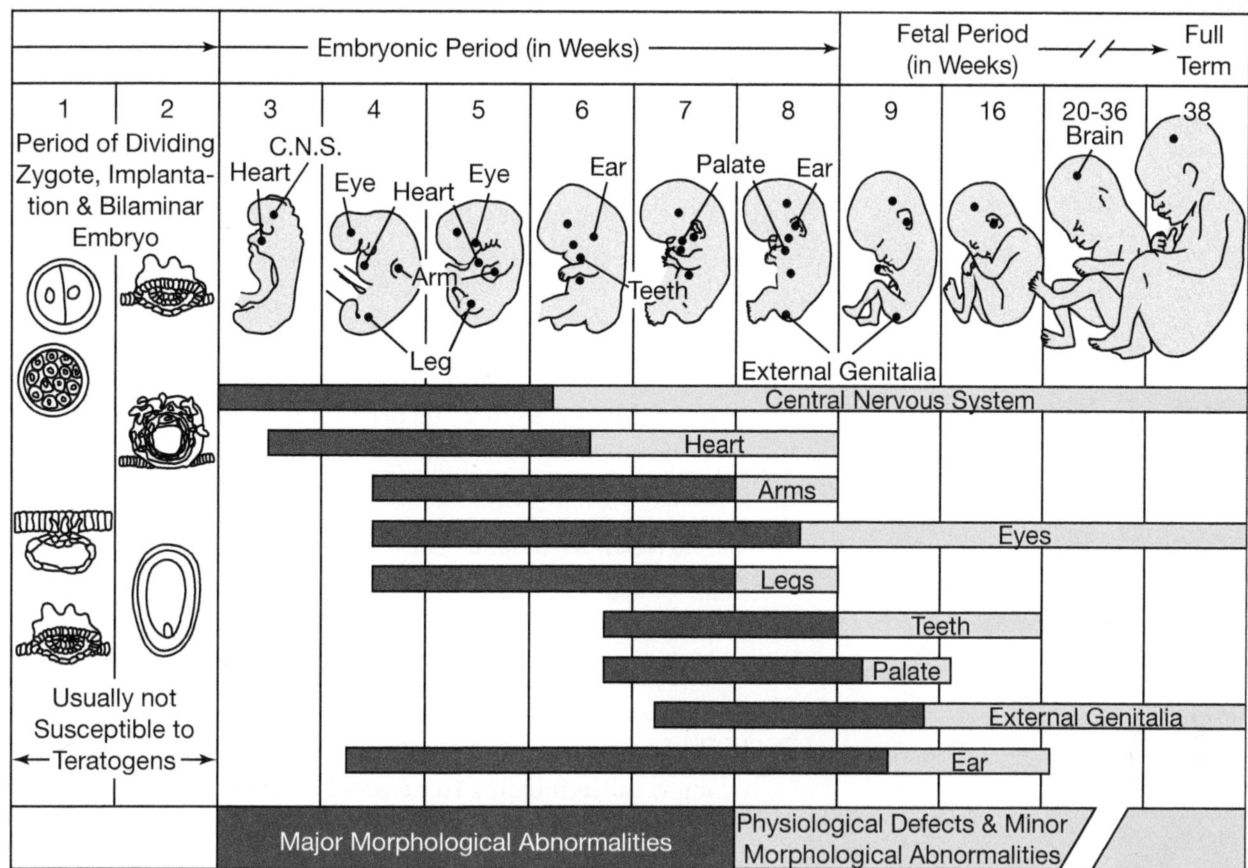

Fig. 8.6 Prenatal Development This chart shows the order of prenatal development. *When does the heart begin to develop?*

Third Trimester

After 26 weeks, the pregnancy enters the third trimester. At 28 weeks, the fetus is about 14 inches long and weighs about 2½ pounds. If the fetus were born at this time, it could survive outside the uterus but would face major threats from infection and immaturity.

The key developments in the third trimester are weight gain, growth in length, and maturation of organs in preparation for survival outside of the uterus. Until the fetus reaches term, the best place for growth and development is in the uterus. At about 38 to 40 weeks of pregnancy, the now full-term infant is ready for birth and labor begins.

During pregnancy, the developing embryo and fetus are influenced by what the mother consumes. Some substances, such as alcohol, drugs, and tobacco, can harm the growing infant even when taken in very small amounts.

See **Figure 8.6** for an overview of prenatal development. Prenatal refers to the time before birth. Can you tell from this chart of prenatal development when the major sensory organs begin to develop?

READING CHECK

Name the point at which the fetus will be able to survive outside the uterus.

The Neonate: Birth to One Month

Why are the bones of a newborn's head not permanently joined?

An infant is called a neonate from birth to one month of age. Many changes take place in this short time.

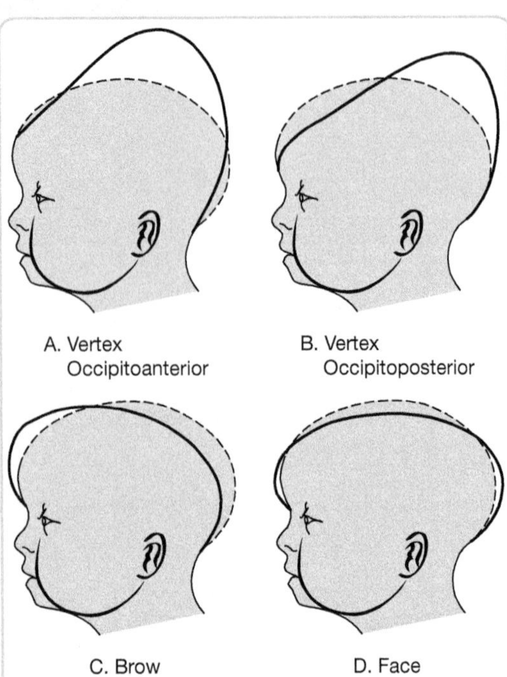

Fig. 8.7 Molding Molding varies depending upon the position of the infant in the birth canal. *What allows the shape of the head to change?*

Physical Development

The full-term infant usually weighs between seven and nine pounds and is 18 to 22 inches in length. Many factors, such as heredity and maternal nutrition, affect the weight and length of the baby.

The Newborn's Head The head of the newborn infant seems to be large in comparison to the rest of her body. In fact, the head is one-fourth of the infant's entire length.

The bones of the newborn's head are not firmly fixed at birth. This allows the plates of the skull to slide over one another during a normal delivery through the birth canal. This sliding is called molding (see **Figure 8.7**). Molding may cause an infant's head to look pointy or like a cone at birth. This rapidly disappears, and the head of the newborn becomes more rounded.

An infant's head has two soft spots, or fontanels, which are tough cartilage. The fontanels are shown in **Figure 8.8.** The anterior, or front, fontanel is diamond-shaped. The baby's pulse can sometimes be seen here. This fontanel closes between the first and second birthdays.

The posterior, or back, fontanel is triangular in shape and can be felt at the crown of the head. It is smaller than the anterior fontanel and usually closes by the third month of life.

The infant can move her head from side to side. However, the neck muscles are not strong enough to hold the head up. The person holding the infant must provide support.

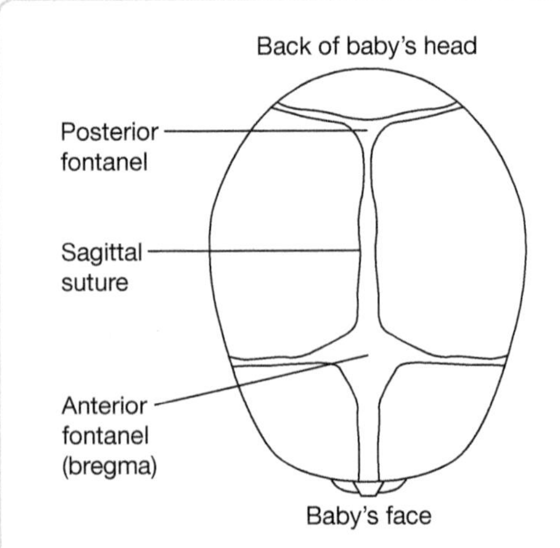

Fig. 8.8 The Back of a Baby's Head The anterior fontanel usually closes by the third month of life, and the posterior fontanel closes between the first and second birthdays. *Would it be dangerous to apply pressure to the fontanels of an infant? Why or why not?*

The Skin of the Newborn The skin of the newborn baby is usually loose, wrinkled, and somewhat red in appearance. At birth, the hands and feet may be bluish, or cyanotic, but usually turn pink after the baby takes its first few deep breaths. The skin color of newborns may vary during the first few days of life because of activity, temperature, and circulatory changes that are occurring.

During the first week of life, the newborn's skin may start to peel. This is not harmful, and nothing needs to be done about it.

Vernix caseosa is the white waxy substance that protected the skin in the uterus may still be in the folds of the skin. Vernix may be patted dry. It is not necessary to wipe it off. Babies may also have some lanugo (soft, downy hair) covering the body, especially around the shoulders. Babies sometimes develop little white bumps around the nose and chin. These are called milia and go away naturally.

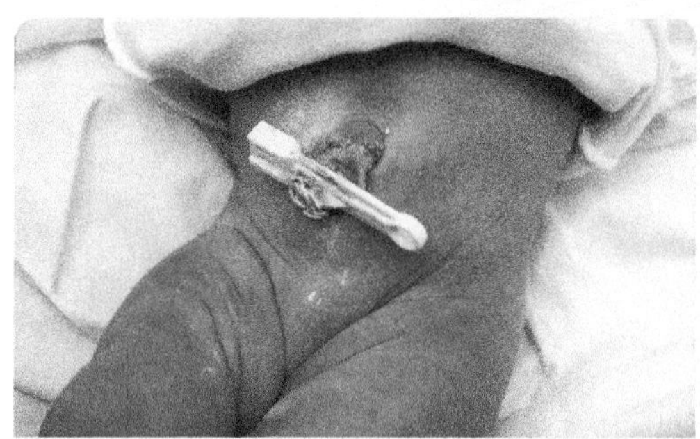

Fig. 8.9 The Clamped Umbilical Cord The umbilical cord is clamped after it is cut. *At what age would you expect the umbilical stump to fall off?*

The part of the umbilical cord still attached to the baby's body is a "stump" about one to 1½ inches in length. It has a white, waxy appearance. It usually falls off around the tenth day of life. The umbilical cord is shown in **Figure 8.9.**

Sometimes infants develop neonatal jaundice, a yellowish color of the skin, in the first few days of life. This is caused by an accumulation of bilirubin, the waste product from the normal breakdown of the red blood cells. Babies have large numbers of red blood cells at birth. Their immature liver is unable to handle the breakdown of these cells. The waste product accumulates, giving the skin a yellowish tint. The whites of the eyes may also appear yellow, and the urine and feces may have a dark yellow color.

Other Physical Characteristics of the Newborn The eyes of the newborn may have a puffy appearance. This is caused by the passage through the birth canal. Some infants have sucking blisters on their lips from thumb sucking while in the uterus. Breast tissue and genitalia may also appear swollen. This swelling may be due to hormonal influences from the mother. Any swelling or puffiness will quickly go away.

Infants' fists are tightly closed. Infants tend to assume the fetal position, which is the position they were in while in the uterus.

Certain reflexes can be observed in the newborn. Some are protective. For example, blinking is a reflex that protects the eye. Everyone, including newborns, has this reflex. Other reflexes are due to the immature nervous system of an infant. These reflexes stop at a certain age and are considered normal until the infant reaches that age. **Table 8.2** on page 234 shows reflexes that are seen in the newborn.

Newborns cry for many different reasons, not just from hunger. Within about three weeks, most parents have learned the different cries of their child and can respond appropriately. In the first few weeks, newborns eat about seven or eight times per day.

Infants can see objects within eight inches of their eyes. They probably detect brightness rather than color. Their eyes tend to turn outward initially. In terms of sound, infants seem to prefer high-pitched tones.

Intellectual-Cognitive Development

Newborns will become calm when picked up and held firmly. They tune out disturbing stimulation by sleeping.

21ST CENTURY SKILLS

Identification and Security of Newborns

Immediately after birth, identification bands are placed on one wrist and one leg of the newborn. A matching band is placed on the mother's wrist. Footprints of the newborn and thumb prints of the mother are also taken. These measures are used for security purposes. Maternity units have special doors with pass codes and monitors at the entrances and exits. The healthcare provider must follow these necessary precautions when working with newborns.

Photo: Nancy Durrell McKenna/Photo Researchers

Table 8.2 Reflexes in the Newborn

REFLEX	DESCRIPTION
Protective	Yawning, coughing, sneezing, blinking, and withdrawing from pain. These reflexes are present throughout life.
Grasping	When an object, for example, an adult's index finger, is placed in the palm of an infant's hand, the infant grasps tightly. The grasp is strong enough to make it possible to briefly lift the infant.
Rooting	When the infant's cheek is stroked with a finger or a nipple, the infant will turn his head toward that side and open her mouth to suck.
Sucking	When something is placed in the infant's mouth or touches her lips, the infant begins sucking. Sucking is consoling to the infant, even when she is not feeding.
Babinski	This reflex is a fanning or hyperextension of the infant's toes. It is caused by stroking the lateral aspect of the sole from the heel to the toes. In adults, the toes flex.
Tonic neck	This is known as the fencer position. When an infant is placed in the supine position (lying on her back) with her head turned to one side, the extremities on the same side will straighten; on the opposite side, the extremities will flex.
Moro	This is known as the startle reflex. It occurs when sudden sound or movement surprises the newborn. The newborn straightens, with arms and hands outward and knees flexed. Slowly the arms return to the chest. The fingers spread, forming a C, and the infant may cry. This reflex continues for six months after birth.
Stepping	When an infant is held in an upright position and one foot is placed on a flat surface, the infant will put one foot in front of the other.

Photos: (t to b)CORBIS, Spencer Grant/PhotoEdit, Inc., Cathy Melloan/PhotoEdit, Inc., Plush Studios/Brand X Pictures/Jupiterimages, Jennie Woodcock/Reflections Photolibrary/CORBIS, Edward Hattersley/Alamy, Petit Format/Photo Researchers, Inc., Phanie/Photo Researchers, Inc.

Social Development

Early on, infants respond to stimulation and establish an individual activity pattern. Generally, an infant responds to a soft, gentle voice and tries to focus on the voice and face. Newborns can show excitement and distress. An example of distress would be another crying infant in the hospital nursery. It takes just one infant crying to start all of the babies crying!

Aspects of Care: The Newborn

A healthcare provider should be familiar with the following guidelines when caring for newborns.

- Newborns should be kept warm, especially immediately after birth, when their skin is still wet. The body temperature of newborns regulates their respiratory pattern.
- A Vitamin K injection is given to the baby to prevent unnecessary bleeding from the umbilical cord where it was cut and clamped.
- Medicated eye drops are put into the baby's eyes within an hour after birth to prevent infection from gonorrhea, which can cause blindness.
- Daily care of the umbilical cord requires cleaning at the base of the cord with rubbing alcohol and applying a cotton ball soaked in alcohol to the stump.
- After the infant is given a small feeding of water, to be sure that he or she can swallow, and the temperature has stabilized, the infant is taken to the mother's room for feedings. Many parents choose to have their infant "room in." This means that the infant spends most of the time in the mother's room and goes back to the nursery only when necessary.
- Blood is taken from the infant to determine whether he or she has any metabolic disorders. Such disorders are treatable with diet and/or medication.
- Sponge baths with tepid water and limited amounts of mild infant cleansing soap are given until the cord has fallen off. The infant's face should be washed with tepid water. No oil should be rubbed on the baby. Lotions and powders should also be avoided.
- The infant is fed by breast or bottle or a combination of both. If an infant is to be breast-fed, parents are given instruction about frequency of feedings, duration of feedings, and care of the mother and her breasts while breast-feeding (see **Figure 8.10**). If an infant is to be bottle-fed, parents must be given instruction about the type of formula and how to prepare it correctly. **Figure 8.11** on page 236 shows an infant being bottlefed. Parents should also be taught about bowel movements and spitting up.

21ST CENTURY SKILLS

Cultural Diversity and Circumcision

Circumcision is the surgical removal of the foreskin of the penis. Parents are responsible for making the decision to circumcise an infant and must sign a surgical permit. In the United States, the physician does the circumcision when the child is 24 to 48 hours old and is stable.

Some parents have their sons circumcised because of religious beliefs. Jews and Muslims have ritual circumcision performed on the infant male on the eighth day of life. The circumcision is done by a person in the religious community. In the Jewish faith, this person is called the *mohel* and the ceremony is called a *berit mila.* The circumcision, called the *bris,* is an important rite in the religious life of the family and is celebrated with family and friends. Native Americans, Asians, and Hispanics generally do not have their infant males circumcised.

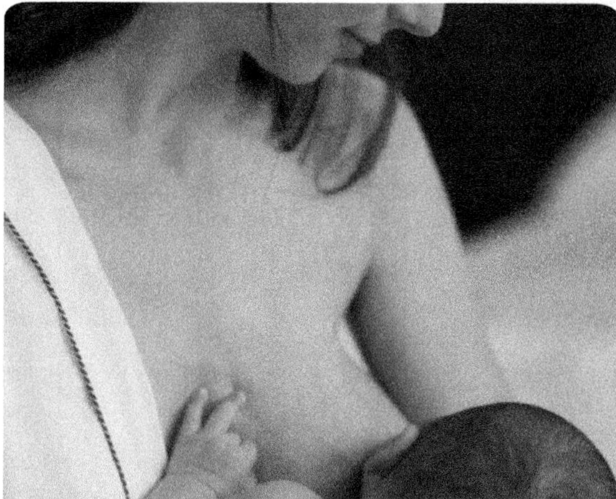

Fig. 8.10 Breastfeeding. Breastfeeding helps in developing a close relationship between mother and infant. *How can the father and any siblings be involved in this process?*

Photo: Lisette Le Bon/Purestock/SuperStock

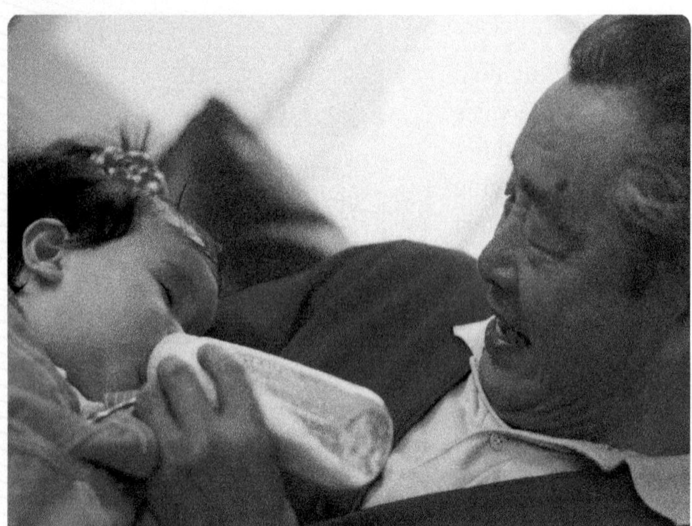

Fig. 8.11 Bottle Feeding The position of the infant during bottle-feeding is important. *Why does position during bottle-feeding matter?*

- The treatment for jaundice in the newborn is keeping the infant well hydrated with breast milk or formula. If necessary, the infant is placed under ultraviolet light, after making sure that the infant's eyes are protected. Blood tests should be performed fairly often to ensure that the bilirubin level does not become dangerously high.
- Follow-up appointments with the infant's healthcare provider should be scheduled.

READING CHECK

List some reasons why newborn babies cry.

The Infant: One Month to One Year

What safety measures should be taken in the home of an infant?

Many changes occur in an infant during the first year. This is why so many parents cherish the wonder of their growing, developing child during this period.

Physical Development

Growth is rapid during the first year of life. Infants triple their birth weight by their first birthday. They develop in a cephalocaudal fashion, first gaining control of the head, neck, and shoulders, and then the arms, torso, and legs. Larger groups of muscles develop before the smaller groups of muscles develop. The nervous system develops rapidly. Changes are seen in reflexes and in the development of coordinated movement and eye-hand coordination.

The following is a brief look at some specific types of physical development in infants.

- By about three weeks of age, infants can focus on objects.
- By about four weeks, infants can follow an object with their eyes and make eye-to-eye contact. The infant can lift his or her head when lying on the stomach.
- At two months, infants can follow objects with their eyes from one side to the other, listen to sounds, bat at objects, and respond to sounds. At this age the infant may string together vowel sounds.
- By three months, an infant may raise the head and shoulders while on the abdomen, and may hold up the head. When the infant is pulled to a sitting position, the head remains in line with the backbone.

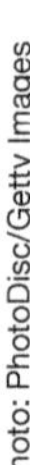

- By four months, the infant may roll from stomach to back and may begin to play with a rattle placed in the hand. Teething may begin.
- By five months, the infant may transfer a rattle from one hand to the other.
- At six months the infant rolls from back to stomach, may be able to sit up briefly, is able to transfer objects from one hand to the other, and can reach to retrieve a dropped object. The two bottom front teeth have probably erupted, or emerged, from the gums.
- At nine months, the infant is able to sit and to creep on hands and knees. The infant is beginning to use the pincer grasp, as illustrated in **Figure 8.12.** The infant can put consonants with vowels and make repetitive sounds such as "mama" and "dada."
- At 12 months the child can hold onto a piece of furniture and move around it, perhaps taking a step or two. With tooth development and the pincer grasp, the infant can pick up and eat small pieces of food.

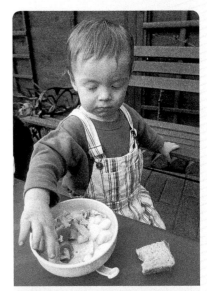

Fig. 8.12 The Pincer Grasp An infant using the pincer grasp picks up finger foods. *When does self-feeding begin?*

Intellectual-Cognitive Development

At birth, an infant can make brief eye contact. By one month of age there is definite eye contact. This progresses to recognition of familiar faces and then to "making faces" at four to five months. Around six months of age, the child is making babbling sounds and by nine months is able to play games such as peek-a-boo. The infant begins to understand cause and effect. If the infant drops a toy and someone retrieves it, the infant will drop it again. This becomes a game. At 12 months, an infant can follow simple directions.

Psycho-Emotional Development

By the time a child is one month old, he or she can smile at another smiling face. By three months, the infant smiles spontaneously and displays pleasure in making sounds. At four months, the infant can vocalize a mood. At six months, there may be abrupt mood changes. At nine months, the infant displays pleasure in playing simple games, and by one year has learned to express many emotions.

For infants to develop physically and emotionally, it is important that their physical needs be addressed quickly and calmly. Physical contact and cuddling is one way to help infants develop a sense of security and trust.

Social Development

Infants become social beings very quickly. By the time infants are one month, they are able to smile. At three months the infant responds to voices. This can be seen when the infant pays attention and coos along with a person speaking in a quiet and gentle manner. At six months the baby "babbles" and is interested in his or her own voice. Imitative play becomes an important part of the infant's interaction with others. At nine months, the first development of words can be observed. This leads to increased interaction with family and others.

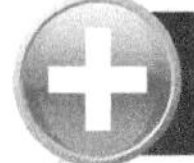

Safety

Sleeping and SIDS

Every year in the United States, about 4,500 apparently healthy babies die in their sleep of sudden infant death syndrome (SIDS), also known as crib death. Usually no cause is found. Most deaths occur in children between two and four months of age. A family history of SIDS seems to put a child at greater risk. These at-risk children are usually closely monitored.

To reduce the risk of SIDS, infants should be placed on the back to sleep, rather than on the stomach. There should be no fluffy pillows, blankets, or other soft items in the infant's crib. The risk of SIDS may also be reduced if adults avoid smoking around the infant and if he or she is given a pacifier.

Photo: Bob Watkins/Photofusion Picture Library/Alamy

Aspects of Care: One Month to One Year

- Regular health checkups and immunizations should be followed according to the healthcare provider's recommendations.
- Infants need tactile stimulation for growth and development. Physical contact and cuddling, as well as prompt attention to their needs, help infants develop a sense of security and trust, which is necessary for them to thrive.
- In the first six months, the mother's breast milk or infant formula meets the needs of the growing infant. The healthcare provider can offer guidance about the introduction of solid foods to the diet.

Safety issues must be considered at all times. The following list contains some essential safety measures.

- Keep emergency phone numbers close to the phone for family and babysitter.
- Make sure the crib meets federal safety standards.
- Never hold the infant on your lap in a car. Use an approved car seat placed in the back of the vehicle. Understand the current recommendations on forward-facing or rear-facing infants.
- Never leave the child unattended in the car.
- Do not put pillows, comforters, or plush toys in the crib.
- Prevent falls. Place the baby on a low surface and use correctly installed gates across stairs.
- Prevent choking. Check toys for small objects that might come loose. Be sure that clothing does not have cords around the neck.
- Do not leave hanging toys in the crib once the child begins to reach, pull, and roll over.
- Keep all cords on window blinds, lamps, and electrical equipment out of reach.
- Although many people are willing to offer advice, the child's healthcare provider is the best resource on healthcare issues.

READING CHECK

Recall how much weight a baby usually gains by his or her first birthday.

The Toddler: One to Three Years

How does a toddler's speech develop by age three?

Children from the age of one to three years need constant attention from parents and others. They also grow less rapidly during this period than they did in the first year; however, growth is still fast, and their communication skills begin to take shape in their use of language.

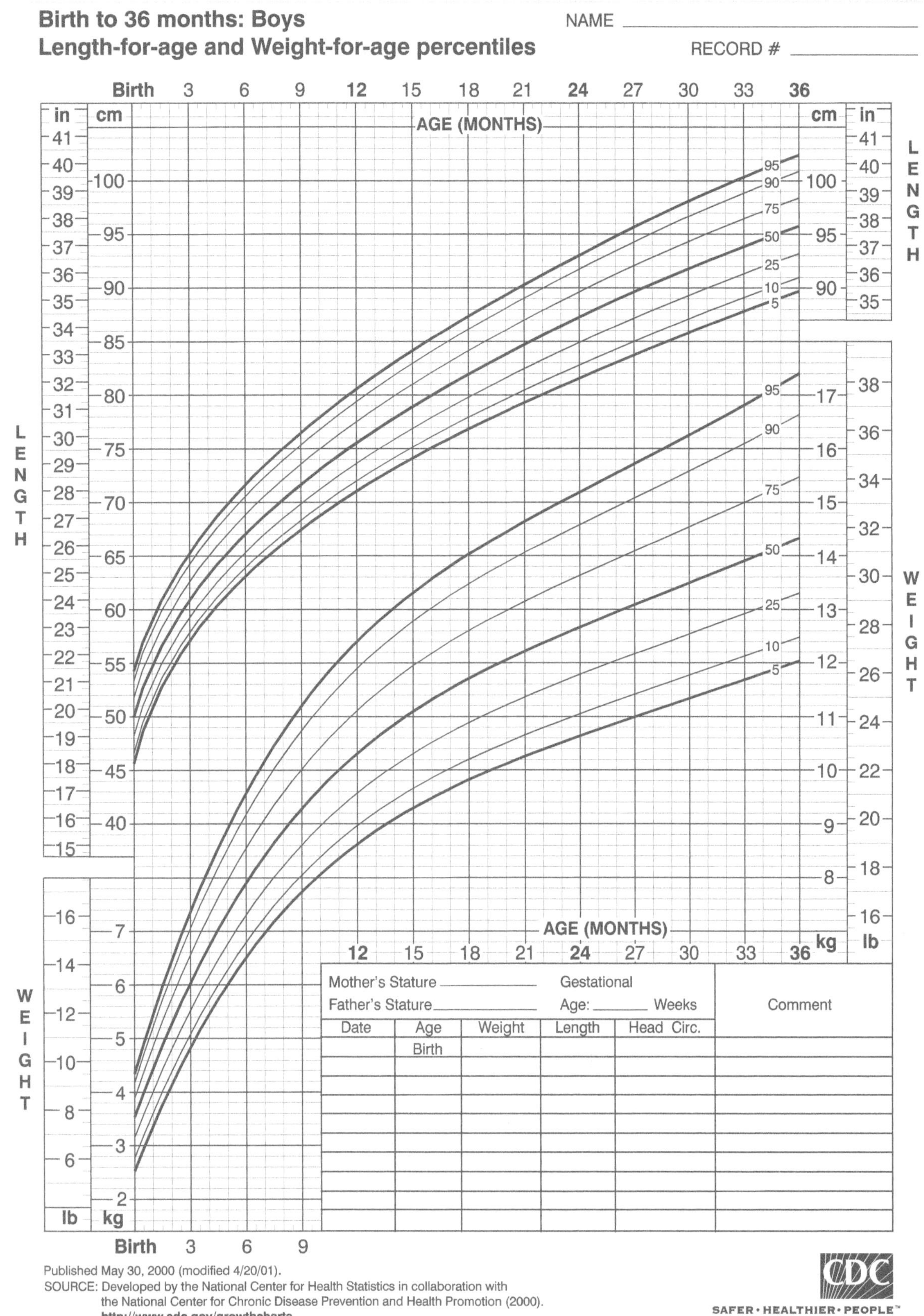

Fig. 8.13 Growth Chart A young child's physical growth and development should be measured and recorded. This chart is used for boys from birth to 36 months. *Which gender grows more quickly?*

Photo: National Center for Health Statistics in Collaboration with CDC

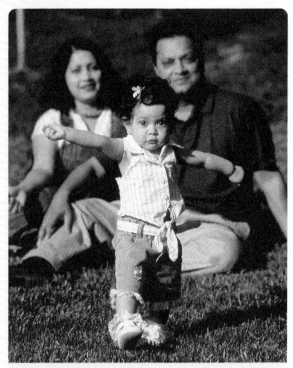

Fig. 8.14 The First Steps This toddler is taking her first steps. *How old would you think she is?*

Physical Development

Weight gain between one and two years is not as rapid as it was earlier. The arms and legs grow more than the trunk and head, and now seem to be in proportion to the overall size of the child. Girls usually reach half of their adult height between 1½ and two years of age; boys reach half of their expected adult height between two and 2½ years. **Figure 8.13** on page 239 shows a growth chart that healthcare providers will use to determine a child's growth in relation to average rates.

Most toddlers will walk independently by 15 months of age. **Figure 8.14** shows a toddler taking her first steps. At 18 months, a toddler can squat to reach for a toy, kneel and remain upright, and precisely perform the pincer grasp. The toddler may use a spoon for self-feeding. By two years of age, the child can run, throw a ball, and scribble with a pencil. The child may want to feed herself or himself.

At three years, the child is very active. Children of this age can dress themselves, ride a tricycle, throw a ball, draw simple shapes, and use a pair of child's scissors. Many children are toilet-trained between two and three years of age.

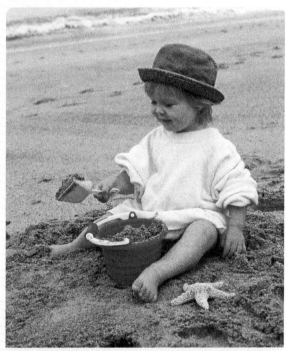

Fig. 8.15 Early Learning The toddler learns by imitation and independent play. *What development purposes does play serve?*

Intellectual-Cognitive Development

During the toddler years, the child begins to learn about the world through play. Children enjoy imitating sweeping, raking, and making things they have seen adults make. **Figure 8.15** shows a toddler at play.

A major task for the toddler is to develop independence. Toddlers are curious about their world, and their play may involve experimenting. Safety must be uppermost in the minds of parents and child care providers, particularly at this stage.

The toddler progresses with speech in the following ways:

- Speaks a few single words at 12 to 15 months
- Makes sentences containing six to 20 words in the second year
- Repeats nursery rhymes at three years.

At 15 months, the child enjoys looking at books. Between two and three years of age, the toddler seems to be constantly asking "Why?"

By three years, the child may participate in the retelling of familiar stories, and can draw and recognize simple shapes. During the toddler years, the child also enjoys playing with blocks.

Psycho-Emotional Development

At one year of age, children are able to express many emotions. As children move from one year to three years, they gain some control over ways of expressing their feelings. Temper tantrums may become a problem between 18 months and two to 2½ years of age. A child of 15 months may respond to "no," but by the time the toddler approaches 18 to 21 months, he or she is resisting authority and is the one who is saying "No!" Children of this age need consistent limits.

If the child learns that a certain behavior will gain nothing, the behavior will stop fairly soon. As toddlers approach three years of age, they become sensitive to the feelings of others and may be characterized as affectionate.

Social Development

Between one and two years the toddler is unlikely to be able to truly play with another child. Play may involve taking toys from another child rather than sharing. Between two and three years children become able to share and play with others. Adult guidance is necessary for the toddler to develop an awareness of what is appropriate when playing with other children.

Aspects of Care: One to Three Years

People who care for toddlers should be aware of the following.

- Toddlers need opportunities to work on their fine motor skills, such as those used in writing with crayons.
- Toddlers are developing their language skills, so simple explanations provide a positive environment for development.
- Healthcare monitoring and vaccinations that are needed.
- When considering toilet training, notice what signs of readiness a child is displaying.

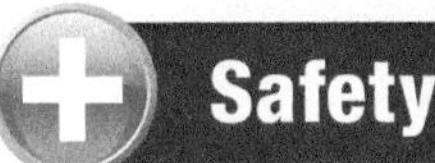

Safety

The Toddler's Environment

During the toddler years, it is very important to allow a child to increase independence in a safe environment. Setting limits helps the child to develop boundaries in relationships and behavior. At the same time, the environment should not be one in which the child is constantly told "No." With these points in mind, observe the following safety measures when caring for a toddler:

- Never leave a child who is unattended around, near, or in any kind of water including the water in toilets, mop buckets, or pools.
- Set the water temperature of the household hot water tank at 120°F.
- Turn pot handles inward, away from the edge of the stove, while cooking.
- Cover electrical outlets.
- Keep medicines and chemicals, including household cleaners, out of reach or in locked cabinets.
- Post the phone number of the local poison control center in an clearly visible location.

The Preschooler: Three to Five Years

How large is the vocabulary of a five-year-old?

The child of three to five years is preparing to go out into the world.

Physical Development

Individual differences such as heredity account for differences in height and weight among children between the ages of three and five years. During this time, the legs and trunk are getting longer. By the time the child is six years old, the trunk and the legs are about equal in length. Girls progress more rapidly toward their adult height and weight than do boys. At this stage, the head grows less rapidly, and the chin and jaw get longer. The respiratory rate and the heart rate are beginning to slow down and coming closer to the adult range.

Bones begin to ossify, or harden, between two and seven years of age. During these years, it is important for children to be active in their play. They also need adequate calcium intake for the development of strong bones.

Most children will have achieved nighttime bowel and bladder control by the time they are three or four years of age. If lack of bowel and/or bladder control persists beyond four or five years, this should be discussed with the child's healthcare provider.

Large muscle development and coordination is seen in a child of three years. This development and coordination is noticed by the child's ability to go up and down stairs, using an alternating step approach, and the ability to ride a tricycle.

At four years of age, the child can skip, hop on one foot, and throw a ball overhand. The four-year-old child is very active. By five years of age, children are coordinated enough to engage in some team sports, such as soccer. They may not understand exactly what the goal of the game is, but they take great pleasure in participating in the activity of the sport. **Figure 8.16** shows a group of children playing together.

Fine motor skills will also improve. By the end of the first year, children usually demonstrate a preference for one hand over the other. Girls are usually about a year ahead of boys in small muscle coordination and fine motor skills. A child of three can draw simple shapes and use a pencil to imitate the way an adult writes. At four, the child can draw a simple human figure and can cut with blunt scissors, though not well at this age. A child of five can reproduce some shapes, letters, and numbers. By the age of five, some children may also have learned how to tie their shoes.

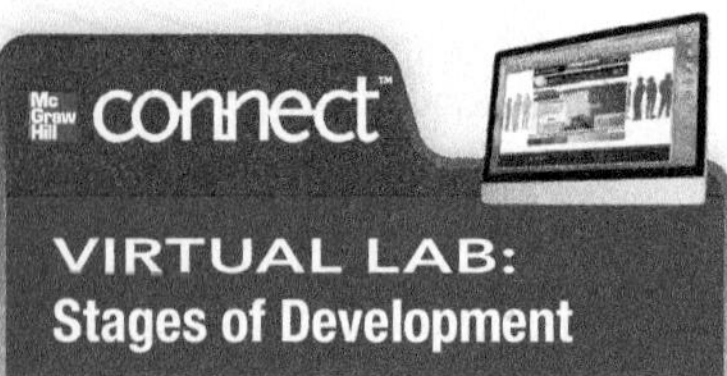

VIRTUAL LAB: Stages of Development

A nine-month human pregnancy has three main stages, known as trimesters. It all starts when a fertilized female egg (ovum) implants itself into the wall of the uterus. The resulting embryo goes through radical development and by the end of the first trimester is considered a fetus. Along the way its major body organs develop, its heart begins to beat, and its gender becomes discernable. The fetus continues to grow and develop during the second and third trimesters. At the end of the nine months, the cervix dilates and the uterus begins contracting to force the fetus out. A baby is born!

This lab will take you through a virtual pregnancy. You'll see just how quickly a baby can develop.

connect Complete the Virtual Lab online for this chapter.

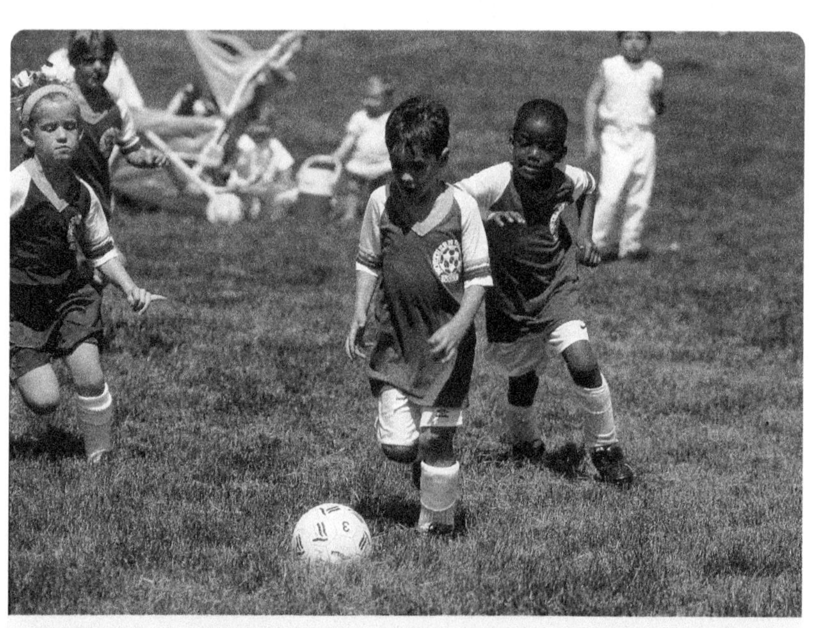

Fig. 8.16 Group Play Group play is an important part of the development of a five-year-old. *What characteristics make a five-year-old more likely to enjoy organized play than a four-year-old?*

Photo: Mark C. Burnett/Photo Researchers

Intellectual-Cognitive Development

As the child's nervous system continues to mature, the child's ability to engage in skillful play and to perform finer and more complicated tasks improves. Language grows by leaps and bounds during these years. The imaginative child of three years has a vocabulary of about 900 words, forms simple sentences, and can tell simple stories that may be very "I"-oriented.

At four years of age, the child's vocabulary is about 1600 words, sentences are complete, and the favorite question is "Why?" Parents need to give very simple answers such as "Because it will keep you safe right now." The child's vocabulary at age five exceeds 2000 words, and the stories the child tells involve more detail. At this age, the child has learned the difference between telling stories and lying.

Psycho-Emotional Development

The three-year-old child is very easy and pleasant. Overall, the child is willing to go along with change. Children of this age usually enjoy music. A child at this age has an increasing sense of self. But imagination may lead the child to have unfounded worries and fears, especially at night.

At four years of age, negativity may increase. Parents hear more of the "No's" that they heard when the child was two years old. The four-year-old child is testing limits and needs guided opportunities for freedom.

Once a child reaches five years, life settles down a little. The child is more self-assured, well-adjusted, and home-centered. At this age, the child likes to follow the rules, may want to "play by the rules," and is capable of accepting some responsibility.

Social Development

Three-year-old children know what gender they are. Children at three years have a keen interest in playing "doctor." The child knows how to take turns and may enjoy brief activities in a group with other children. A three-year-old child likes to "help."

Four-year-old children are very social and enjoy playing simple group games, such as tag and hide and seek.

At five years, the child continues to be very social, enjoys playing with other children, and likes games in which the "rules" are observed.

Aspects of Care: Three to Five Years

Parents and caregivers should be acquainted with the healthcare needs of a three- to five-year-old. Some important needs are listed below.

- Regular checkups should be maintained. The child of five years should receive a complete preschool developmental assessment and physical that includes an evaluation of hearing and vision.

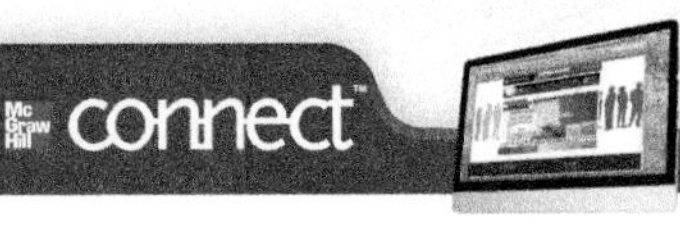

STEM CONNECTION

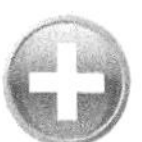

Medical Math

Converting to Feet and Inches
Quickly converting lengths from inches to feet and inches is a useful skill for medical professionals.

Go to connect to learn how to perform this conversion.

Using a Tape Measure
When you record height, weight, and head circumference measurements, you need to determine the number of inches or centimeters and the fraction of inches or centimeters.

Go to connect to learn about working with these measurements.

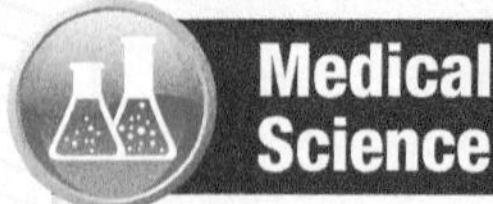

Emerging Diseases and Immunization

Because of the vaccine discoveries of the 20th century, parents and healthcare providers of the 21st century have seen little of diseases such as polio, smallpox, or measles. Debate surrounding vaccine safety has clouded the success of these life-saving vaccines.

Go to connect to read and review a chart of recommended immunizations.

- Immunizations must be up to date when the child enters kindergarten.
- Children of about three years may have night terrors. If these are persistent, parents should discuss them with the healthcare provider. Children may use delaying tactics at bedtime and may need to be shown repeatedly that there is nothing in the closet or under the bed. A night light is useful.
- Nighttime routines are important in helping a child feel secure.

READING CHECK

Recall some ways in which preschool-aged girls develop more quickly than boys.

The Elementary School Child: Six to Ten Years

When does the influence of peers begin to rival the influence of a child's parent?

The following describes the stages of development of the six- to ten-year-old child.

Physical Development

During childhood, girls may be taller and heavier than boys. Bones continue to ossify. Facial proportions verge on those of adulthood. Permanent teeth replace "baby teeth." Muscles continue to develop. Regular exercise is needed to encourage strength and coordination. Postural habits are established.

The fine motor skills become increasingly complex. The nervous system continues to develop. At nine and ten years of age, the reproductive system will also be developing.

Intellectual-Cognitive Development

Knowledge explosion happens once a child enters school. On entering school, the six-year-old child has a brief attention span. By ten years old, she or he is able to focus for longer periods of time. Children move from recognizing simple numbers to doing math. Written language moves from reading and writing in printed letters to cursive writing.

Most children of this age like to talk. They may use more expressive vocabulary when interacting with peers than they do at home. As children approach nine and ten years of age, they can handle concepts relative to time, such as the past and the future. As children move from five or six years of age toward nine and ten years, they are better able to separate fantasy from reality. They develop a sense of what is right and wrong, of honesty and fairness.

Psycho-Emotional Development

When children enter the first grade, parents and other adults are still central in their lives. In the early school years, children like to abide by the rules and to please adults who are important to them. Parental influences and standards of behavior established in the home are still stronger than peer influences.

When children approach ten years of age, they may be more influenced by their peers than by their parents. During these years, children are beginning to develop a sense of self and also learn gender-related roles. Children are very expressive and move quickly from one feeling to another. Children of six to eight years of age may have trouble thinking about disasters that they hear about. Their concern centers on how the event will affect them. Parents need to reassure children that they are safe and will be cared for.

As children approach ten years of age, they are better able to grasp concepts of time and distance. A nine- to ten-year-old child may want to do something to help others. School-age children may be very sensitive to criticism and to what they see as failure.

Social Development

School is central to the life of a child between six and ten years of age. Young school-age children enjoy playing together and exploring new activities. Children enjoy "sleep-overs," organized sports, and video games. **Figure 8.17** shows children of this age engaged in a team sport. Parents need to avoid having the child become overwhelmed with too many organized activities at this time, though. Children also need time to be quiet and alone. Outdoor activities help to use up some of the child's energy. Appropriate social behaviors are learned during this time stage.

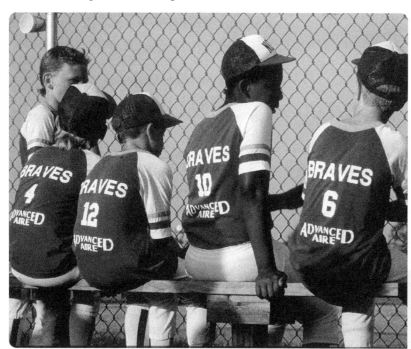

Photo: Aaron Haupt Photography

Fig. 8.17 Sports Organized sports give the nine- and ten-year-old a chance to be noisy and expressive. *How does this help meet other needs of children at this age?*

Aspects of Care: Six to Ten Years

Some important healthcare issues for the six- to ten-year-old child are:

- Structure and a schedule help to maintain order and discipline.
- Monitoring of physical activities to prevent injury. The American Academy of Pediatrics advises against elementary school-age children participating in contact sports.
- Consistency in daily activities and in discipline to help the child to develop intellectually, emotionally, and socially.
- Regular healthcare and dental care to help maintain a child's health. School-age children tend to catch numerous communicable diseases.
- Immunization schedules be maintained.

READING CHECK

List why group activities are important for children between six and ten years of age.

The Middle-School Child: Eleven to Thirteen Years

Why do school grades often slip for 11- to 13-year-old children?

The following sections will give you some insight into the stages of development of the 11- to 13-year-old child.

Physical Development

Girls tend to mature more rapidly than boys. In the United States and in most Western cultures, the onset of **puberty** occurs in females around 12 or 13 years of age, but some may experience changes as early as nine. By the time a girl reaches middle school, a significant occurrence may be the onset of menstruation. It is important for everyone to remember that even though her body may be maturing, she is still only between nine and 12 years old. Males tend to go through the changes of puberty later than females (see **Figure 8.18**). The average age for males to experience these changes is around 14 years.

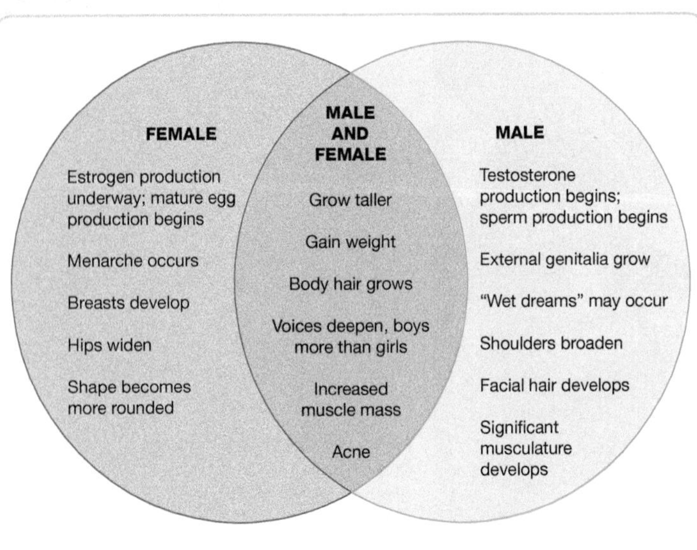

Fig. 8.18 Physical Development Puberty brings significant changes. *What physical changes are expected in both males and females during puberty?*

Bones continue to grow and fuse during early adolescence. Adequate calcium intake and weight-bearing exercise are necessary for strong bones to develop. Girls may begin to take on a more curvy shape. Parents may note an increase in appetite. Hormonal changes may contribute to development of skin problems and acne.

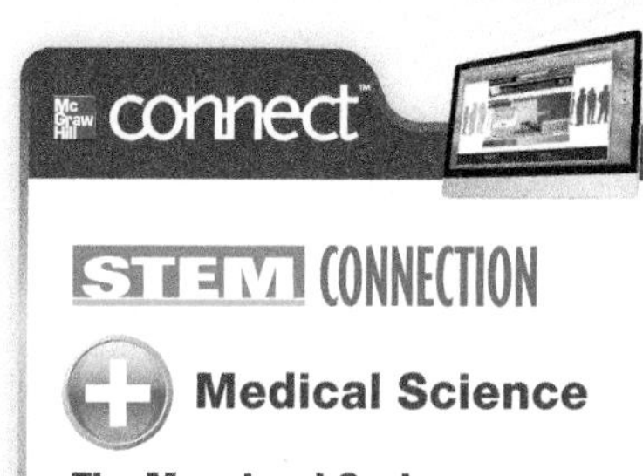

STEM CONNECTION

Medical Science

The Menstrual Cycle
From menarche to the end of menopause, females have cyclic changes to their uterus, ovaries, vagina, and breasts known as the menstrual cycle. This cycle includes a monthly flow of blood known as the menses, more commonly known as the "period." The monthly cycle ranges from 18 to 40+ days.

Go to connect to read and review a table detailing the menstrual cycle.

Intellectual-Cognitive Development

Grades may slip during this time. So much physical growth is taking place and so many physiological changes are occurring that less energy is available to concentrate on academics. In early adolescence, children are developing their ability to think abstractly and critically. This may lead to arguments about academic subjects, world events, and rules imposed in the home and school. The preadolescent may express herself or himself through writing or music or physical activities. Preadolescents may tend to exaggerate and "bend the truth."

Psycho-Emotional Development

Although preadolescents crave independence, they are also very unsure of themselves. They are experiencing a wide range of physical changes and, at the same time, are learning the roles of sexuality. It is very important for preadolescents to receive accurate information about their changing bodies and feelings from appropriate and reliable sources.

Middle-school-age students may not be comfortable asking parents questions about sexuality. Students may be referred to a school nurse or other reliable healthcare provider. Preadolescents should be encouraged to communicate with parents.

Conflict may arise at this time. Parents may find that the preadolescent is easily annoyed and may be temperamental. Frequently, the preadolescent child will take on the behaviors of his or her peer group.

Social Development

Becoming part of a group is often an important part of life for the 11- to 13-year-old. It is usual during the middle-school years for children to have same-sex friends (see **Figure 8.19**). These children are still learning about their own sexual identity and may not be comfortable in heterosexual relationships. Girls express an earlier interest in male-female relationships than do boys. Frequently, peers are the source of support and information for the middle-school child, but children of this age need to be able to turn to an adult with whom they are comfortable, so they can ask personal and intimate questions.

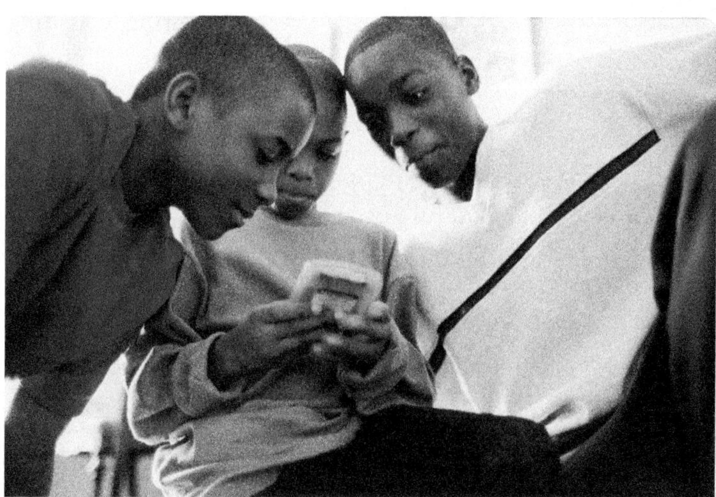

Fig. 8.19 Socialization Friendships are an important part of life for a middle-school child. *Which gender is more comfortable with mixed-gender friendships at this age?*

Photo: CORBIS

Aspects of Care: Eleven to Thirteen Years

Here are some important points to keep in mind.

- The child needs to be assured that he or she is valued and loved.
- Consistency in discipline is very important.
- Parents should not be hypercritical or make too many demands.
- Friendships and associations should be monitored.
- Maintain regular healthcare checkups and immunizations.
- Overscheduling of the child's time should be avoided.

READING CHECK

Summarize the changes that take place at the onset of puberty.

The Adolescent: Fourteen to Nineteen Years

How do teens demonstrate concern for others?

The teen years can be full of excitement for teenagers and their family and friends. They can also be difficult years. Tremendous physiological changes during this time may cause internal conflicts that can turn into external clashes. Parents may feel anxious about their child's quest for independence and about the child's upcoming departure from the home. The teen may experience anxiety about career and school choices. During adolescence teens are:

- Developing their sexual identity
- Establishing increasing independence
- Making career and school choices
- Developing more mature and meaningful relationships
- Preparing to assume their adult roles

Physical Development

During the later teen years, females attain their adult height and weight. Males may continue to grow in height until 25 years of age. Bone structure, genetics, and general health and nutrition all contribute to the overall stature of the individual. Weight control may become an issue. Some health problems of adulthood can be traced back to lifelong habits of poor dietary choices and lack of exercise begun in adolescence. **Figure 8.20** shows an example of appropriate exercise for teens.

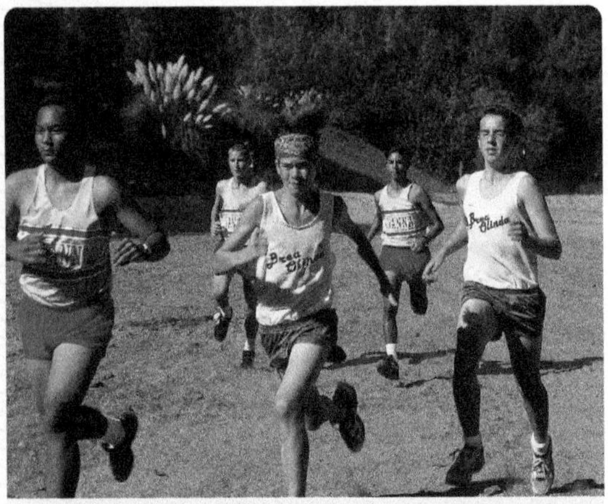

Cardiac, respiratory, and digestive functions are approaching their adult stages. Since teenagers are capable of reproduction, education about sexual behavior provided by trusted, well-informed adults is necessary.

Fig. 8.20 Exercise Group exercise and outdoor activity has long-term benefits. *Why is physical exercise important for adolescents?*

Photo: Tony Freeman/PhotoEdit

Intellectual-Cognitive Development

During the early adolescent years, the child may have taken the word of an adult or a peer without question. Now the teen asks questions and needs to work out answers that fit into his or her values. Reasoning and critical thinking are developing. Adolescents often do not see the connection between behavior and consequences. This may lead to experimentation with drugs, alcohol, or sex.

Psycho-Emotional Development

An adolescent knows the socially acceptable and appropriate ways to express feelings. However, the pressures that are felt by adolescents may result in angry outbursts. Anger that is directed inward can be harmful. Anxiety is also part of adolescence. Teens often worry about their appearance and think that "everyone is looking at me." At the same time, they may believe that "I am all alone" and "no one understands me."

Adolescents may think that they are invulnerable, and may engage in risk-taking behavior. Teens often have an "it won't happen to me" attitude.

Social Development

Friendships are very important to adolescents. (see **Figure 8.21).** They are eager to learn effective interpersonal skills. Teens tend to be concerned about the welfare of others and often get involved in community service projects. As teens get older, they become more comfortable with their parents and outgrow the attitude of "not wanting to be seen dead" with their parents.

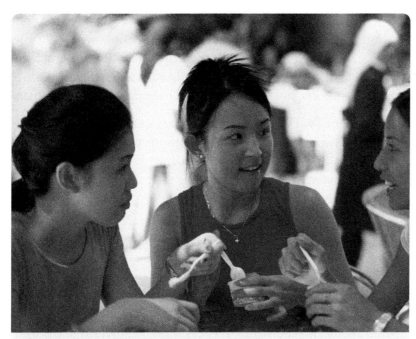

Fig. 8.21 Friendship Classmates and friends are important to the teenager. *What goals can be met through these relationships?*

Photo: Yang Liu/CORBIS

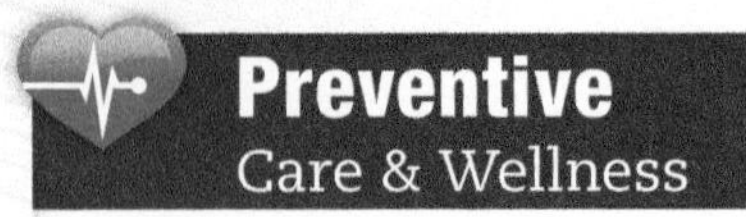

Drug and Alcohol Use

People start using drugs for a variety of reasons.

- They are curious.
- They want relief from problems.
- Their friends are doing it.

Now that you know the usual reasons, you do not have to fall for them. Take time to think. Avoid people who pressure you to take drink or drugs, or offer drugs. Trust your instincts and make your own decisions. Engage in other behaviors that make you feel good. Learn to say "No."

Physical dependence is when your body needs the drug to feel good or normal. When the drug is stopped, your body goes through painful withdrawal.

Mental dependence is even more powerful than physical dependence. With repeated use, you become psychologically "hooked." You may think that you are in control long after you have lost control.

Remember, anyone, at any time, can become hooked on drugs or alcohol!

Problems Faced by Teens

As mentioned earlier, the teen years are wonderful and difficult at the same time. Some of the problems faced by teens are discussed below.

Eating Disorders Adolescents feel pressured to look good. This pressure may lead them to develop abnormal eating behaviors such as anorexia nervosa. Clients who have this disorder starve themselves. Males and females may suffer from anorexia, but it is more often seen in females from a fairly high socioeconomic group. Signs may include

- extreme weight loss.
- intense fear of weight gain due to altered body image. Anorexics, although quite thin, see themselves as being overweight.
- refusal to eat or eating only small amounts of select foods.
- menstrual irregularity or absence of menstruation.

Another eating disorder is bulimia nervosa, a pattern of binge eating and purging. Purging is done by vomiting, taking excessive doses of laxatives, abusing diuretics, or excessive exercise. Signs may include

- overachieving behaviors.
- ritualistic behavior with food.
- binge eating (excessive amounts of food eaten in two hours or less).
- purging or vomiting, usually secretive.
- avoidance of social situations involving food.
- excessive exercise and fasting.
- irregular or absent menstruation.
- changes in the teeth due to acid from vomiting, usually noticed by a dentist during a regular checkup.
- anxiety and/or depression.
- low self-esteem.

A teen suffering from bulimia may still be of normal weight. Regular physicals and dental checkups may help to identify this problem. Males and females may experience this disorder, although females are more frequently diagnosed. Anorexia and bulimia can occur together.

Substance Abuse The use of alcohol, tobacco, club drugs, marijuana, cocaine, and heroin is a concern. The abuse of controlled prescription drugs such as Ritalin or OxyContin is similarly dangerous. Parents, coaches, educators, and friends must be alert for signs of substance abuse, which may include:

- Change in personality
- Withdrawal from activities the teenager once enjoyed
- Change in friends
- Falling school grades
- Change in health habits and appearance

Medical and health counseling services must be provided to the teen who has a substance abuse problem.

Violence Violence takes many forms. Teens of many cultures are exposed to violence in movies, television, video games, and music. Excessive exposure leads to insensitivity toward violence. Teens may also be victims of physical, emotional, psychological, or sexual violence at home.

Bullying, browbeating, or abusing is recognized as a cause of violence at school. Many youths who have carried out homicidal acts of violence were deeply disturbed by repeated bullying experiences such as being teased, taunted, and rejected by peers. Most students are able to tolerate moderate amounts of teasing, but students who are depressed and harbor resentment and anger for a long time may explode in a violent way.

Sexually Transmitted Diseases Teens must be well informed of the risks of contracting a sexually transmitted disease (STD) if they engage in sexual activity. STDs threaten long-term health and well-being. They are spread by blood-borne pathogens and require public education for teens as well as adults. Information and education are available through schools, local and state departments of health, television ad campaigns, the Internet, and the Centers for Disease Control.

Pregnancy Teen pregnancy is associated with many problems. Teen pregnancy prevention is usually a focus of public health education programs for adolescents. Parents should share their philosophies and values with their teenagers to help them make sensible choices. Teaching teens which situations are risky and helping them to avoid those situations gives adolescents some of the guidance they need.

Suicide According to the Centers for Disease Control, suicide is the third leading cause of death for people aged 15 to 24. The suicide rate among young people is greater for males than for females. Females are more likely to attempt suicide than males, but males are more likely to be successful in their first attempt at suicide. Males tend to use firearms to commit suicide. Warning signs include:

- Depression
- Anger that is directed inward, toward the self
- Alcohol and/or other substance abuse
- Changes in habit—carelessness, sloppiness, and a lack of interest in personal appearance
- Giving away personal possessions
- Giving verbal hints about committing suicide

What should you do if you notice these signs or if you hear someone talking about committing suicide? Here are some suggestions.

- Listen
- Take the person seriously
- Get help from a responsible adult
- Do not promise to "keep the secret"
- Never assume that it's "just talk"

21ST CENTURY SKILLS

Cross-Cultural Sensitivity

The Hispanic tradition Quinceañera celebrates a girl's coming of age at 15. **Figure 8.22** shows a typical celebration. In the Hispanic culture, Quinceañera is as important as a woman's wedding day. The girl celebrating her Quinceañera must begin to consider what she plans to do with her life as an adult. The celebration is formal, with the young woman dressed like a bride and accompanied by a court of honor and their escorts. A religious service usually takes place first, followed by an elegant formal reception. Parents may plan the celebration for years.

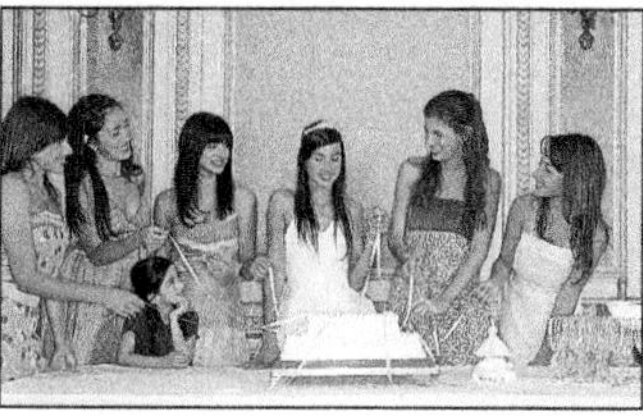

Fig 8.22 Celebrating Quinceañera. *Which culture celebrates this coming-of-age tradition?*

Photo: Image Source Black/Alamy

Aspects of Care: Fourteen to Nineteen Years

People who are responsible for teenagers should know the following important facts about teens.

- Teens need adequate amounts of calcium and weight-bearing exercise for strong bone development.
- Teens should know the risks of early, unplanned pregnancy and sexually transmitted diseases when considering engaging in sexual activity.
- The adolescent needs to spend time enjoying friendships, sporting events, and social events.

People who are caring for teens should do the following:

- Listen
- Give them the facts
- Trust them
- Provide them with firm and friendly discipline
- Be consistent
- Educate them with their independence in mind
- Set limits and stick to them
- Set examples of good behavior and good taste
- Remember how it feels to be an adolescent

READING CHECK

List some signs of eating disorders.

SECTION 8.2 From Conception Through the Teenage Years Review

AFTER YOU READ

1. **Describe** the appearance of a healthy, full-term newborn.
2. **Describe** the progression of an infant's development.
3. **Select and describe** two major developmental tasks for each of the following age groups:
   - **a.** Toddler
   - **b.** Preschooler
   - **c.** Elementary school child
   - **d.** Middle-school child
   - **e.** Adolescent
4. **Describe** three problems with which adolescents may have to deal.

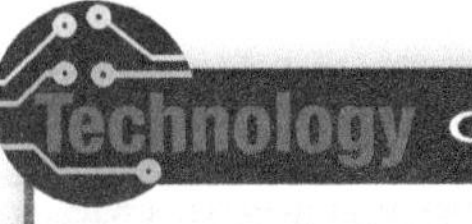

ONLINE EXPLORATIONS

Human Development

Using the Internet, develop a collage of images of human development, from either conception to full term or birth to one year. Find an image that represents each month of life for either of these topics. Present the completed collage to your class.

SECTION

8.3 The Adult Years

The Young Adult: Twenty to Forty Years

When does an adult's vision often begin to weaken?

During this period of life, many people complete their education, start a career, and begin to raise a family.

Physical Development

In the young adult, physical growth generally has stopped as bones have matured. However, adults continue to need a steady source of calcium and regular weight-bearing exercise. Muscle strength is at its peak.

Regular exercise is necessary to maintain cardiovascular and respiratory function, as well as flexibility, strength, and agility. Visual acuity may begin to decline, especially depth perception. Around age 40, most people notice that their vision has weakened. They may hold the newspaper farther away to read it. This usually indicates that **presbyopia** has developed. Reading glasses solve the problem. Hearing loss may be noted. This loss may have begun as early as 14 years of age.

Intellectual-Cognitive Development

The young adult gains knowledge at an amazing rate, through formal education or on-the-job training. Critical thinking and reasoning skills are refined with increasing life experience and practice. Intellectual skills continue to develop. Intellectual curiosity stimulates continued mental growth.

Psycho-Emotional Development

The earliest part of the young adult years is characterized by increasing independence. Many young adults complete their education and begin careers. Although this is exciting, it can create some stress and anxiety. The young adult who has learned coping skills, developed self-esteem, and has a vision of who he or she is will proceed with assurance. Establishing relationships with peers and other adults is another aspect of emotional growth. Lifelong relationships based on genuine concern for the well-being of others develop during the young adult years. Positive communication and interpersonal skills help young adults cope with the ups and downs of relationships. **Figure 8.23** shows one of the milestones of a young adult's life.

Vocabulary

Content Vocabulary

You will learn these content vocabulary terms in this section.

- **presbyopia**
- **geriatrics**
- **osteoarthritis**
- **kyphosis**

Academic Vocabulary

You will see this word in your reading and on your tests. Find its meaning in the Glossary in the back of this book.

- **adequate**

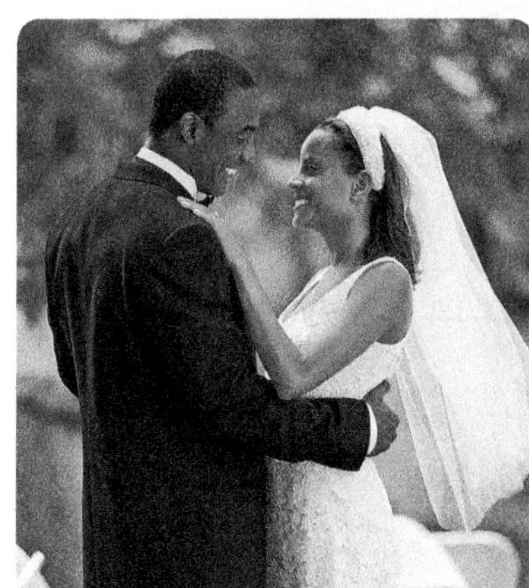

Fig. 8.23 Marriage Choosing a life partner is usually part of the young adult's life. *What are some other milestones that come at this age?*

Social Development

Young adults establish careers, marriages, families, and homes within a community. In the mobile American culture, this may happen miles from family members. Young adults must establish their own values and decide how they wish to interact with others. Social relationships are sometimes based more on common interests than on age. Contributing to the community is another important goal.

Aspects of Care: Twenty to Forty Years

- Regular weight-bearing and aerobic exercise should be continued to prevent or reduce bone loss.
- A balanced nutritional plan should be in place.
- The need for social contact persists throughout adult life. When adults are establishing careers and families, there are many opportunities for social contact, including church, school, and community activities.
- Stress management techniques are essential for the adult who is juggling a full-time job and family life. Regular exercise is a great "stress buster." Some people turn to yoga, meditation, and prayer.
- Regular health checkups provide preventive maintenance. Monitoring weight, blood pressure, cholesterol, and glucose is important. Annual pap smears for women, along with breast examinations and self-examinations, are a necessary part of health maintenance. Men need to perform regular testicular self-exams.
- Regular dental care is necessary. The American Dental Association recommends cleaning and dental checkups twice a year.

READING CHECK

List skills that young adults can use to handle the stress of education and careers.

The Middle-Aged Adult: Forty to Sixty-Five Years

When does the brain begin to shrink?

During these years, people are active and productive but begin to notice signs of aging.

Physical Development

In a female, bone density loss may begin as early as age 35, while men may not experience bone loss until age 65. Regular weight-bearing exercise, combined with a proper diet, helps to maintain bone density. Muscle strength and endurance may begin to decline during these years, particularly if there is no regular exercise regimen. In addition, weight gain may be noticed.

Women in Western cultures experience menopause (end of menstruation) around the ages of 45 to 50. However, menopause is not a single, momentous event, but a process that occurs over a number of years. Research suggests that hormone levels may begin to change in the female as early as the mid- to late thirties. Males experience some changes in testosterone levels at this stage, though they normally continue to produce testosterone well into old age.

During these years, hair may begin to turn gray and become thinner. Wrinkles may appear on the skin, particularly if there had been extensive, unprotected exposure to the sun in earlier years or if the individual is or was a smoker. Chronic health problems such as hypertension (high blood pressure), heart disease, and diabetes may begin to surface during the middle adult years.

Intellectual-Cognitive Development

Around age 50, the brain begins to decrease in size, mostly because of water loss. Starting in middle age, information processing probably begins to slow. Although there may be changes going on in the brain, the middle-aged adult is still capable of multitasking, learning new information, and retrieving old information (see **Figure 8.24**).

Psycho-Emotional Development

Many middle-aged adults feel a sense of pride and accomplishment in career and family. A stable marital relationship contributes to a sense of security. At the same time, there may be a sense of loss as children move out of the home, this is known as the "empty nest" syndrome. Adults who have continued to grow and develop as individuals have more resources to deal with changes in the home situation and may even look forward to having more free time to pursue other interests.

Sometimes people find their life situation difficult. They may lack financial security if careers have taken multiple turns or have suddenly collapsed. Marriages may begin to disintegrate as the family structure and dynamics change. The parents of the middle-aged adult may become increasingly dependent on their adult child as their own health begins to decline.

During the middle adult years, people gain an increasing awareness that life does not last forever and they often reflect on their own mortality.

Social Development

The same events that cause emotional stress may also play a role in the social relationships of middle-aged adults. Careers, growing children, and aging parents may affect many of their activities. Relationships with young adult children may change for the better; on the other hand,

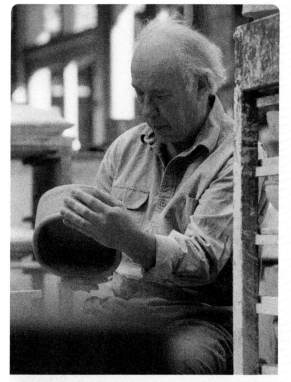

Fig. 8.24 Middle Age The brain becomes smaller after age 50. *What can middle-aged and older adults do to reduce the chances of mental decline?*

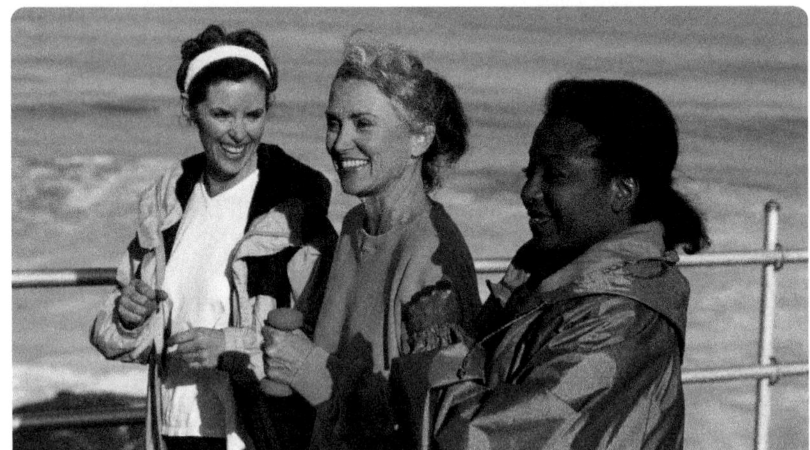

Fig. 8.25 Strength in Relationships Enduring friendships lasting into middle age provide support and strength. *What might these friends have in common?*

conflicts can continue. Aging parents whose needs are increasing may make great demands on the time and energy of middle-aged adults. Healthy adults should seek creative, social, and enjoyable outlets to meet their needs for personal growth. **Figure 8.25** shows the importance of social relationships in the middle years.

Aspects of Care: Forty to Sixty-Five Years

- Regular weight-bearing and aerobic exercise should be continued to prevent or reduce bone loss.
- A balanced nutritional plan should be in place. If there are complicating medical conditions, such as cardiovascular disease or diabetes, the development of a nutrition plan may need to be discussed with a healthcare practitioner.
- Adequate rest helps an individual to be alert and better able to perform the tasks of the day. Disturbances in sleep or excessive fatigue should be reported to a physician.
- The need for social contact throughout the working years and years of raising children remains fairly constant. Social contacts may be established and maintained through church and club affiliations.
- Applying stress management techniques is essential for the adult juggling a full-time job and family life. Stress-management techniques should be continued throughout the middle adult years.
- Regular health and dental checkups help an individual to practice preventive maintenance. Weight and blood pressure, as well as cholesterol and glucose, must be monitored. Women should continue to get annual Pap smears and should begin having mammograms if they have not done so from early adulthood. Annual prostate exams for men should begin at 40 years of age.

READING CHECK

Describe the “empty nest” syndrome.

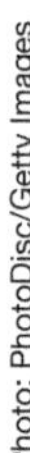

The Mature Adult Years: Sixty-Five Years and Older

Why do many mature adults experience memory loss?

Mature adults may retire from jobs and careers. Retirement has both advantages and disadvantages.

Physical Development

During these years all body systems begin to show signs of aging. Not all people experience all changes. Increasing numbers of individuals are living longer, healthier lives. Many live well into their 90s and beyond.

Geriatrics is the field of medicine concerned with the problems of aging. This field is growing because of increases in the normal life span.

Some of the physical signs of aging are listed below.

Integumentary System

- Thinning and wrinkling skin caused by decreased amounts of collagen and elastin in the dermis
- Atrophy, or degeneration, of the subcutaneous layer of skin, caused by a decrease in adipose tissue
- Decreased number of the cells that produce pigment, or melanocytes, which protect against ultraviolet light
- Graying and thinning hair
- Brittle nails
- Decreasing inflammatory response, resulting in slower healing

Nervous System

- Slower reaction time and thought processing
- Decreased blood flow to the brain caused by arteriosclerosis, a group of disorders that causes thickening of the artery walls
- Shortened attention span and difficulty handling several tasks at one time, caused by decreased frontal lobe size
- Shrinkage of temporal lobes, leading to weaker signals to the brain for processing
- Impairment of fine motor activities such as writing, caused by shrinkage of the substantia nigra, a layer of gray matter in the brain
- Memory loss caused by changes in the part of the brain called the hippocampus and a lack of acetylcholine, a chemical that transmits messages between nerve cells or between nerve cells and muscle cells
- Impaired vision and hearing

Musculoskeletal System

- Osteoporosis or decreased bone density, leading to increased incidence of fracture, particularly fractures of the hip
- **Osteoarthritis** or joint disease
- Decreased numbers of musculoskeletal fibers

Cardiovascular System

- Decreased cardiac output, especially during exercise
- Arteriosclerosis
- Postural hypotension or loss of blood pressure when standing or sitting up abruptly
- Increased risk of heart disease

Respiratory System

- Some loss of elasticity of the lungs
- Calcification of the intercostal cartilage, located between the ribs, and the development of **kyphosis** (curvature of the spine), making it difficult for the lungs to expand properly
- Increased shortness of breath, caused by the physical changes listed above

Immune System

- General decline, giving rise to susceptibility to infectious diseases and autoimmune diseases such as cancer and rheumatoid arthritis

Digestive System

- Constipation, caused by lack of exercise and poor diet
- Fecal incontinence, caused by lack of muscle tone

Genitourinary System

- Decreased number of nephrons, the functional units of the kidney
- Reduced tolerance for stress, so the kidneys may respond to disease in other parts of the body
- Loss of voluntary control of urination

Endocrine System

- Decreased thyroid function
- Loss of estrogen production in postmenopausal females
- Decreasing levels of aldosterone, a hormone that has a role in regulating blood pressure
- Increase in the time it takes for levels of the hormone cortisol to return to normal after stressful events
- Deficiencies in response to insulin by various organs

Intellectual-Cognitive Development

Mature adults may take longer to process information. However, they can and do continue to learn. Long-term memory seems to remain intact. Short-term memory may be less acute. If they do not have a disease such as Alzheimer's, they can continue to perform the same functions as they always have. Their accumulated wealth of information and life experiences make mature adults great teachers.

Psycho-Emotional Development

Many changes may occur in the life of the mature adult. In Western cultures, people retire when they are about 65 to 70 years of age. This is a major change that may have benefits or may cause difficulties. For example, people who no longer have a career may feel a sense of loss and grief. Those who have developed interests outside of their careers may make a smoother transition to retirement. The death of a spouse and of friends are life events with which the mature adult must deal. In addition, mature adults face the reality of their own eventual death. Physical ailments and infirmities can lead to increasing dependence on other family members, frequently middle-aged children.

Grieving, Death, and Dying

While researching death and dying, psychiatrist and author Dr. Elisabeth Kübler-Ross identified five stages of grieving. These stages apply to many situations in life. For example, if a patient has surgery for breast cancer, she will experience grief over the loss of an important part of her body.

There is no defined order in which the stages occur. Clients may move from one stage to another before coming to the stage of acceptance.

- **Denial.** In this stage, the client says, "No, not me!" or "I don't believe it!" She or he may refuse to discuss the illness or refuse to believe the situation. The healthcare professional should offer support and allow the client to express his or her feelings.
- **Anger.** This stage usually occurs when the client can no longer deny the diagnosis or situation. Frequently, the client will say, "Why me?" or "Why did this happen?" Clients who are experiencing loss may be hostile to those around them. Healthcare professionals need to recognize that the client is responding to the situation or illness and not to any particular individual. Good listening skills are essential here. This stage ends when the anger is exhausted and concern for others begins to take over.
- **Bargaining.** This stage occurs when the client tries to make deals. The client acknowledges the inevitability of the diagnosis but wants, or needs, more time. Clients may turn to religion and faith. Also, the client fights to achieve goals that he or she has set. For example, a dying client may want to live until a child graduates. The healthcare professional needs to be a good listener, to be supportive, and to help the client achieve goals whenever it is possible.
- **Depression.** At this stage the client realizes the inevitability of the situation or diagnosis. The client may withdraw, becoming quiet and overcome with sadness and despair. The role of the healthcare professional is again to be a good listener and to provide support.
- **Acceptance.** At this stage the client accepts the inevitability of the diagnosis or situation and may even help others to deal with the circumstances. The healthcare professional can provide physical and emotional support and comfort. For the client who is dying, physical touch from others is a simple way to offer comfort.

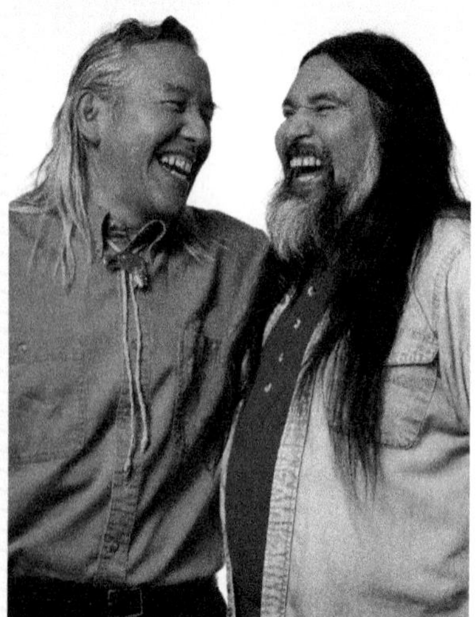
Fig. 8.26 **Maturity** These brothers have remained close through their mature adulthood. *How old do you think they are?*

Social Development

Mature adults may experience increased spirituality. Individuals who are able may prefer to remain in their own home and neighborhood. Still others choose to move to their dream retirement home. Most mature adults in the United States live independently, contributing numerous volunteer hours to their communities. Relationships with grandchildren or other family members can be a source of great pleasure (see **Figure 8.26**).

Aspects of Care: Sixty-Five Years and Older

- Weight-bearing and aerobic exercise should be continued to prevent or reduce bone loss.
- A balanced nutritional plan should be maintained. This may need to be discussed with a healthcare practitioner, particularly if there are complicating medical conditions, such as cardiovascular disease or diabetes.
- As adults reach maturity, periods of extended sleep may decrease, but short periods of rest may help. Sleep disturbances or fatigue should be reported to a healthcare practitioner.
- As an adult matures, retires from work, and maybe even loses a spouse, opportunities for socialization may decrease. It is essential that an individual stay in touch with other members of the community, perhaps through volunteer activities.
- Regular health and dental checkups, and breast and prostate exams should continue.
- Keeping the brain active is necessary to prevent loss of function. Studies have shown that individuals who have active interests maintain mental function better than individuals who do not.

READING CHECK

Name some positive and negative effects of retirement.

SECTION 8.3 The Adult Years Review

AFTER YOU READ

1. **Examine** one major developmental task that the young adult is expected to accomplish.
2. **Describe** one developmental task with which the middle-aged adult is faced.
3. **Explain** one challenge that faces the mature adult.
4. **Indicate** at least five physical changes that occur in the mature adult.
5. **Discuss** some of the ways older adults can maintain physical and mental health.

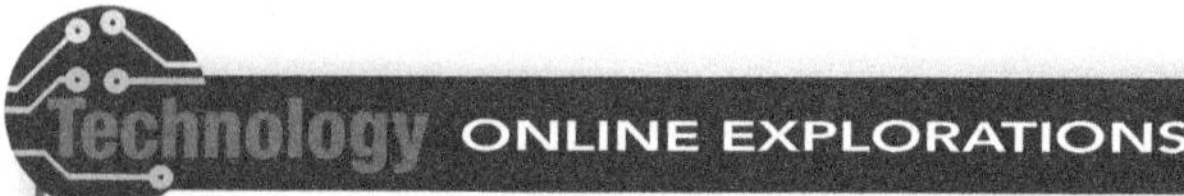

ONLINE EXPLORATIONS

Geriatric Development

Geriatric patients (those over age 65) experience many changes to each of their body systems as they age. Review these changes in the text and then research online to find at least five images that depict some of these changes. Create a summary identifying the system and change seen in each image you have selected.

Photo: PhotoDisc/Getty Images

SECTION
8.4 Procedures for Measuring Weight, Height, and Head

Measuring Weight, Height, and Head Circumference

Why is it important to measure a child's weight, height, and head on a regular basis?

The measurements of weight, height, and head **circumference** are important indicators of physical growth and development, especially in infants and children. These measurements are also used to evaluate health problems, including obesity. In the hospital, daily weighing may be ordered for clients who have conditions that cause **edema** or swelling, such as heart or kidney disease.

Prior to performing the procedures shown in this section, you should become familiar with the **scale, height bar, tape measure,** and other equipment you will be using. Scales measure weight in pounds and/or **kilograms.** Height and head circumference are measured in inches and/or centimeters. Usually, you will record your measurements in one system and will not need to convert your measurements to another system. However, you need to be able to read a tape measure precisely and to convert measurements from inches to feet and inches.

Vocabulary

Content Vocabulary

You will learn these content vocabulary terms in this section.

- circumference
- edema
- scale
- height bar
- tape measure
- kilograms

Academic Vocabulary

You will see this word in your reading and on your tests. Find its meaning in the Glossary in the back of this book.

- convert

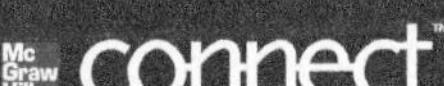

ONLINE PROCEDURES

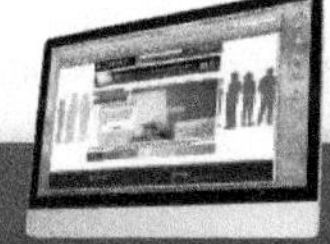

PROCEDURE 8-1

Measuring the Infant

An infant's weight and length are measured frequently. Normal growth is checked and diseases and disorders can be found. When you measure the weight and height of an infant, follow the step-by-step guide provided in this procedure.

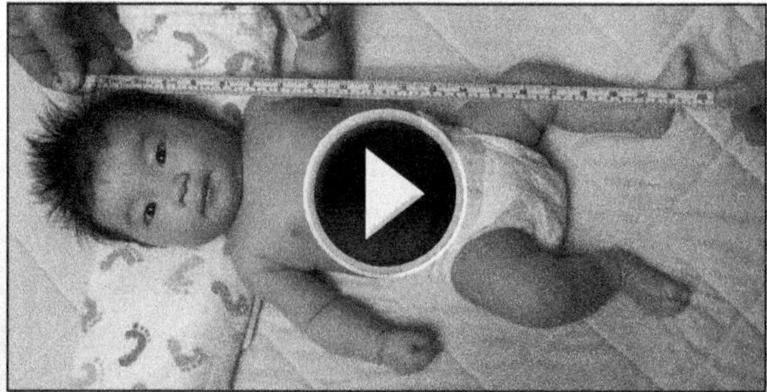

PROCEDURE 8-2

Measuring Head Circumference

The head circumference (HC) of an infant is an important factor in growth and development. Usually a nurse or medical assistant measures head circumference. If there are any preexisting conditions or questions about the head circumference of the infant, the physician may do the measurement or repeat the measurement taken by the staff member.

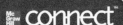

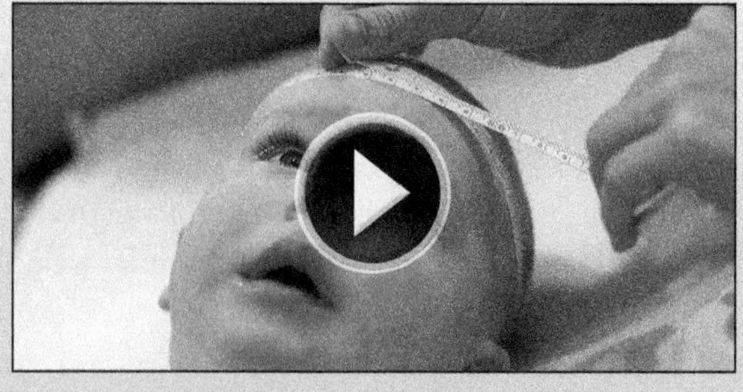

Photos: (t)Roy Hsu/Getty Images, (b)Susan Barr/Workbook Stock/Getty Images

connect ONLINE PROCEDURES

PROCEDURE 8-3

Measuring the Toddler

Infants and children are weighed and measured at every office visit. If toddlers cannot remain still on an adult scale, weight will be measured by measuring the adult holding the toddler and then subtracting the weight of the adult.

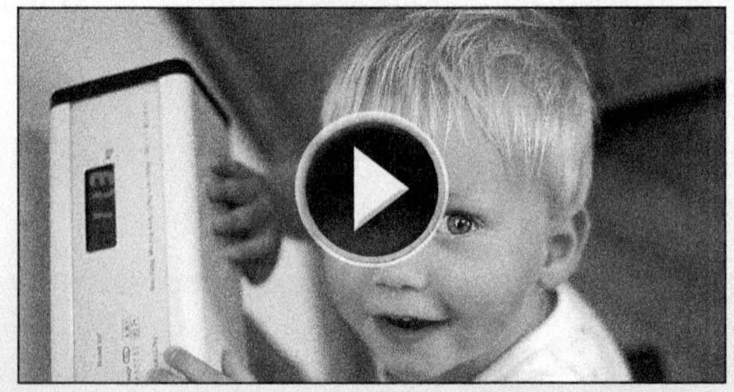

PROCEDURE 8-4

Measuring the Adult

An adult's weight is usually measured at every office visit. It is measured to the nearest quarter of a pound or tenth of a kilogram. Height is measured to the nearest quarter of an inch or centimeter.

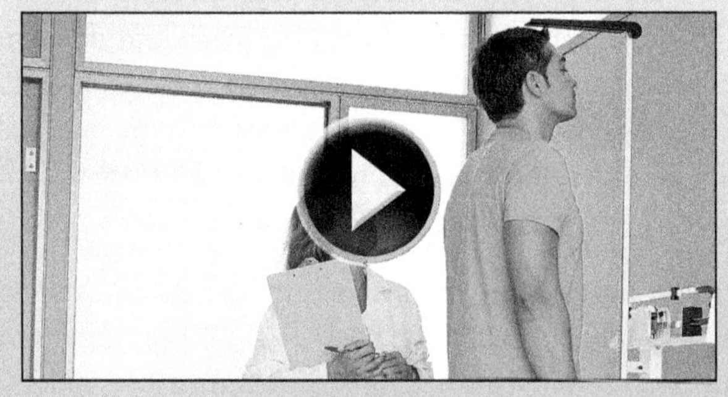

SECTION 8.4 Procedures for Measuring Weight, Height, and Head Circumference Review

AFTER YOU READ

1. **Make** the following calculations:
   a. If the scale balances with the bottom weight marker at the 150 pound mark and the top weight marker balances at 37 pounds, how much does the client weigh?
   b. If the bottom weight marker is at 100 kg and the top weight marker is at 33 kg, what is the client's weight?
   c. The total weight of a parent and child is 158 pounds. When you weigh the parent, she weighs 121 pounds. How much does the child weigh?
   d. The combined weight of a parent and toddler is 139 pounds. The parent weighs 105 pounds. How much does the toddler weigh?
   e. When you measure an infant's head circumference, the 1-inch mark overlaps at the 24½-inch mark on the tape measure. What is the infant's head circumference?

Technology ONLINE EXPLORATIONS

Measurements

Visit the Centers for Disease Control website. For the patient noted below, find and print copies of the following growth charts: Head Circumference for Age, Weight for Length, Length for Age, and Weight for Age. Then chart the measurements provided.

18-month-old girl:
Length—30¼ inches
Weight—23½ lbs.
Head Circumference—18 inches

CHAPTER 8 Review

Chapter Summary

SECTION 8.1

- The major categories of development are physical, intellectual-cognitive, psycho-emotional, and social. **(pg. 227)**
- In children, growth and development proceed in a head-to-tail fashion (cephalocaudal) and from gross motor skills such as running to fine motor skills such as writing. **(pg. 227)**

SECTION 8.2

- The unique combination of genetic material from the egg of the mother and the sperm of the father creates an entirely new and separate person. Cellular division, multiplication, and refinement of function are complete after approximately nine calendar months in the mother's uterus. **(pg. 230)**
- The newborn infant may have cyanotic hands and feet, a pointed head caused by molding, a white cheesy substance on its skin known as vernix caseosa, and soft downy hair called lanugo on the body. The newborn infant is unable even to hold up his or her head. **(pg. 232)**
- In a relatively brief time, infants learn to hold up their head, roll over, sit, crawl, stand, walk, and run. The infant then moves on to gaining increased control over large and small muscles as well, permitting him or her to acquire fine motor skills such as writing and many other skills requiring coordinated eye-hand activity. **(pg. 236)**
- Toddlers explore their environment and gain independence from their parents by learning the word "No." Learning language is one of the key developmental tasks of the preschool child. **(pg. 241)**
- During the early school years, children come under the influence of their peer group. The middle-school child experiences physiological changes, develops complex thought processes, and seeks increasing independence while moving toward stronger peer relationships. **(pg. 245)**
- Teenagers face many health-related problems, including eating disorders, substance abuse, violence, sexually transmitted diseases, pregnancy, and suicide. **(pg. 250)**

SECTION 8.3

- During the early adult years, individuals complete their education and establish themselves in the community. **(pg. 253)**
- The children of middle-aged adults become less dependent, while their parents may become more dependent. **(pg. 255)**
- Mature adults undergo many physical and social challenges. **(pg. 257)**

SECTION 8.4

- Measurements of height, weight, and head circumference are important for monitoring the growth and development of individuals and must be done accurately. **(pg. 261)**

CHAPTER

8 Assessment

Critical Thinking/Problem Solving

1. What would you say to a teenager who tells you that she may be pregnant and has not yet been to a physician?
2. Your client is middle-aged, smokes, is 25 pounds overweight, has a diet low in dairy and calcium-rich foods, and does not exercise. What health-related suggestions can you give your client?
3. Obtain a copy of a growth and development chart for a 2- to 18-year-old female and chart her height and weight using the information shown here.

AGE	HEIGHT (STATURE)	WEIGHT
2 years 6 months	35 in	28 lb
4 years 3 months	41 in	35¼ lb
7 years	48½ in	55 lb

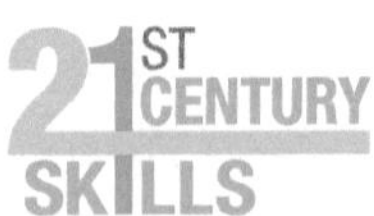

4. **Teamwork** Obtain a partner and a tape measure. Practice measuring your partner's head circumference.
5. **Information Literacy** Using the Internet or another source, research a health issue important to an age group of your choice. Prepare a written report or present the issue and solutions to your classmates in the form of an oral report.

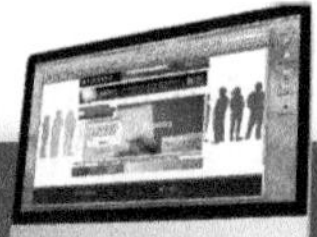

connect ONLINE ACTIVITIES

Complete our HST online activities for Chapter 8, which include Concept Check review questions, Reference Flash Cards, and Online Procedures assessment sheets.

- **Concept Check** review questions
- **Reference Flash Cards** medical terminology practice
- **Online Procedures** assessment sheets

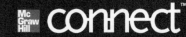

CHAPTER 9 Nutrition

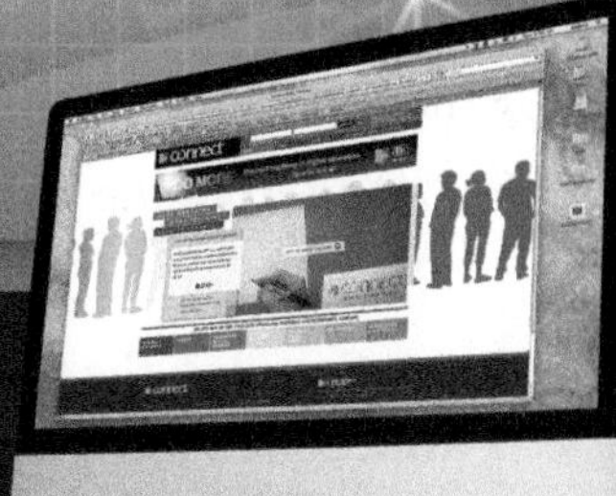

Essential Question:

How healthy is your diet?

What you eat has a direct impact on your health, both today and in your future. In this chapter, you will learn about the six categories of nutrients, where they are found, and the purpose they each serve. You will also learn how to determine how much of each nutrient is needed by different people, in order to be able to understand your patients' and your own needs.

McGraw Hill connect™

It's Online!

- Online Procedures
- STEM Connection
- Medical Science
- Medical Terms
- Medical Math
- Ethics in Action
- Virtual Lab

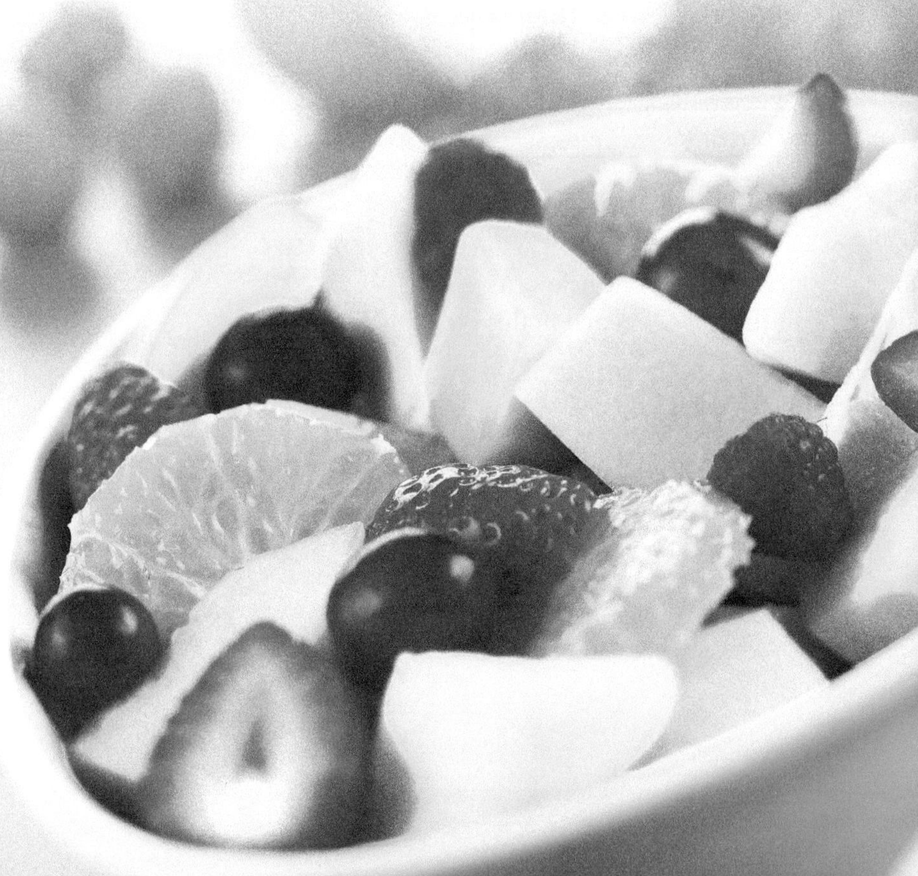

Photo: Foodfolio/the food passionates/CORBIS

READING GUIDE

OBJECTIVES

After completing this chapter, you will be able to:

- **Categorize** the six types of nutrients.
- **Distinguish** the key functions of each nutrient.
- **Illustrate** why each individual's energy needs are different.
- **Discuss** the purpose of the *Dietary Guidelines for Americans.*
- **Identify** the major food groups.
- **Compare** the effects on your health of getting too few or too many nutrients.
- **Demonstrate** one nutrition procedure.

BEFORE YOU READ

Connect Do you know what nutrients the human body needs on a regular basis, and how to get them?

Main Idea

Healthcare workers should recognize nutrition guidelines and be able to explain the recommended nutritional priorities and calorie levels.

Note-Taking Activity

Draw this table. Write key terms and phrases under **Cues**. Write main ideas under **Note Taking**. Summarize the section under **Summary**.

Cues	Note Taking
○ ○	○ ○
Summary	

Graphic Organizer

Before you read the chapter, draw a diagram like the one below. As you read, write the types of nutrients and their uses covered in this chapter into the diagram.

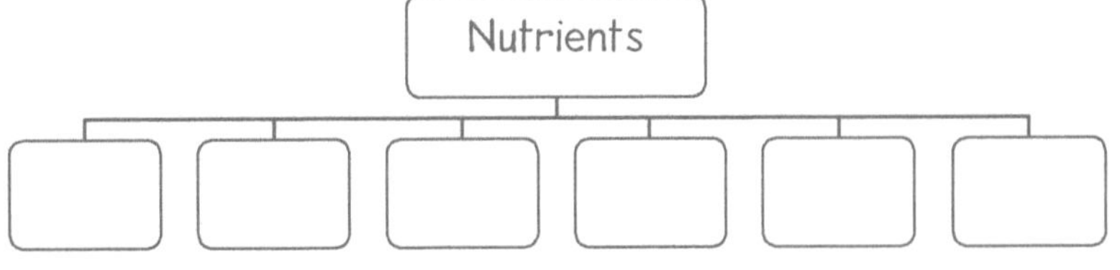

connect

Downloadable graphic organizers can be accessed online.

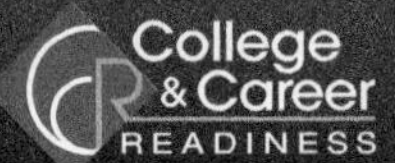

STANDARDS

HEALTH SCIENCE

NCHSE 1.31 Apply mathematical computations related to healthcare procedures (metric and household, conversions and measurements).

NCHSE 9.11 Apply behaviors that promote health and wellness.

SCIENCE

NSES 1 Develop an understanding of science unifying concepts and processes: systems, order, and organization; evidence, models, and explanation; change, constancy, and measurement; evolution and equilibrium; and form and function.

NCHSE *National Consortium for Health Science Education*

NSES *National Science Education Standards*

COMMON CORE STATE STANDARDS

MATHEMATICS

Number and Quantity

Quantities N-Q 3 Choose a level of accuracy appropriate to limitations on measurement when reporting quantities.

ENGLISH LANGUAGE ARTS

Reading

Key Ideas and Details R-2 Determine the central ideas or conclusions of a text; summarize complex concepts, processes, or information presented in a text by paraphrasing them in simpler but still accurate terms.

Speaking and Listening

Comprehension and Collaboration SL-2 Integrate multiple sources of information presented in diverse media or formats (e.g., visually, quantitatively, orally) evaluating the credibility and accuracy of each source.

SECTION 9.1 Essentials of Nutrition

Nutrition and Your Health

How does my diet today affect my health later in life?

Nutrition is the science of how the foods you eat affect your body. Good nutrition is important to sustain life, promote health, and prevent disease. In fact, eating right can make a big difference in how often you are sick, how quickly you recover, and even how long you live.

Nutrition plays an essential role in maintaining general health from the moment a child is born. As a child grows, nutrition influences growth, development, and resistance to disease. Lifelong eating habits are often established in early childhood. Growing children build a foundation for good health by learning healthy eating behaviors and by taking part in regular physical activity at a young age.

As you age, good nutrition continues to be vital to health. What you eat affects how you look, how you feel, and your energy level. Over a lifetime, what you eat affects positively or negatively your chances of developing a **chronic disease,** which is a disease that may progress slowly and not show dramatic change over short periods of time. Chronic diseases include heart disease, cancer, and diabetes.

Nutrients

As **Figure 9.1** on page 268 shows, for overall health, energy, and growth, you need to eat a variety of foods in moderate yet adequate amounts. That is because food supplies **nutrients,** which are substances that nourish your body. Nutrients can be grouped into the six categories of carbohydrates, fats, proteins, vitamins, minerals, and water.

Functions of Nutrients

Nutrients in the foods you eat have important roles in your body.

- Nutrients supply energy. Carbohydrates, proteins, and fats provide you with the energy you need to perform daily activities, such as dressing, brushing your teeth, and walking up and down stairs. These nutrients also supply the energy you need for more active pursuits, such as playing basketball, swimming, or dancing.
- Nutrients build and repair. Proteins are used to promote growth, build new body tissues, and repair worn-out body cells. Proteins can also provide the body with energy when carbohydrates and fats are in short supply. When this happens, however, those proteins are not available for their specialized functions.

Vocabulary

Content Vocabulary

You will learn these content vocabulary terms in this section.

- **nutrition**
- **chronic disease**
- **nutrient**
- **protein**
- **dietary fiber**
- **calorie**
- **saturated fat**
- **unsaturated fat**
- **cholesterol**
- **amino acid**
- **vitamins**
- **antioxidant**
- **osteoporosis**
- **recommended daily allowance (RDA)**
- **basal metabolic rate (BMR)**

Academic Vocabulary

You will see these words in your reading and on your tests. Find their meanings in the Glossary in the back of this book.

- **overall**
- **complex**

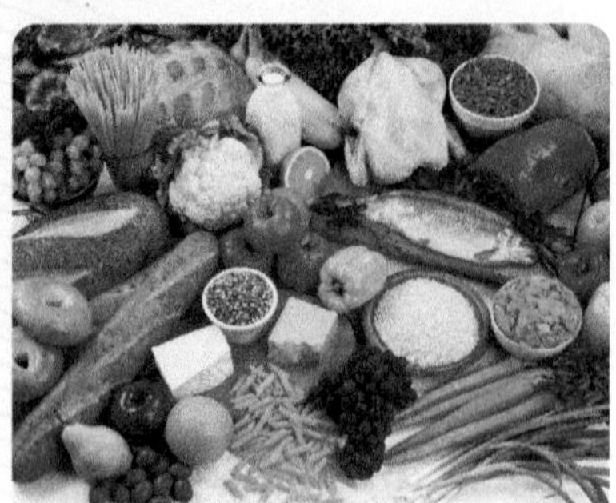

Fig. 9.1 Food Variety For health, energy, and growth, you need to eat a variety of foods in moderate, yet adequate, amounts. *Which food groups can you identify?*

- Nutrients regulate body processes. Vitamins and minerals help regulate many of your body's systems to keep them running smoothly. For example, vitamins and minerals help your body obtain energy from carbohydrates and fats. Vitamins and minerals also work with **proteins** to build body tissues. Water aids in digestion, helps transport nutrients and wastes, regulates body temperature, and much more.

READING CHECK

Name some major life functions and processes that are affected by nutrition.

Nutrients and Their Uses

How can you determine if you are getting all of the nutrients your body needs each day?

Carbohydrates

Carbohydrates are your body's main source of energy. As you can see in **Figure 9.2,** the two categories of carbohydrates are simple and complex.

- Simple carbohydrates, also called sugars, are composed of one or two sugar units. Some foods, such as fruit and milk, contain natural sugar and also contain other important nutrients. Other foods, such as candy, soft drinks, and sweet desserts, are high in added sugar and have few other nutrients.
- Complex carbohydrates, also called starches, are composed of many sugar units. When you eat foods containing carbohydrates, your body breaks down starches into smaller sugar units that are used by your body to produce energy. Among the sources of complex carbohydrates are breads, cereals, rice, pasta, starchy vegetables (potatoes, corn, squash), and legumes (beans, peas, and lentils). Many foods high in complex carbohydrates also supply fiber. **Dietary fiber** is a plant substance that your body cannot digest. It helps your digestive tract work properly and may help protect against heart disease and cancer. **Figure 9.3** shows some examples of dietary fiber.

Your body may run short on energy if you skip meals or limit foods that contain carbohydrates. If you eat more than you need of foods high in carbohydrates, you may get more **calories,** or units of energy derived from food, than your body needs. Over time, eating too many calories from any nutrient source can lead to weight gain.

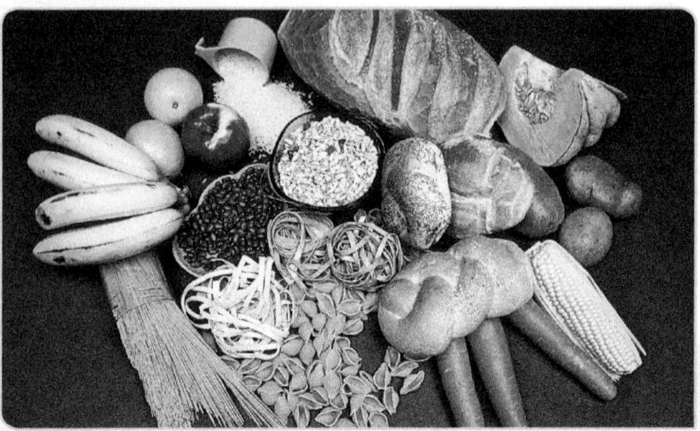

Fig. 9.2 Carbohydrates There are two categories of carbohydrates. *Can you name the two types?*

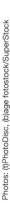

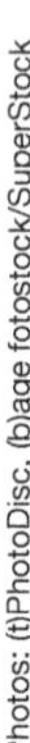

Photos: (t)PhotoDisc, (b)age fotostock/SuperStock

Fats

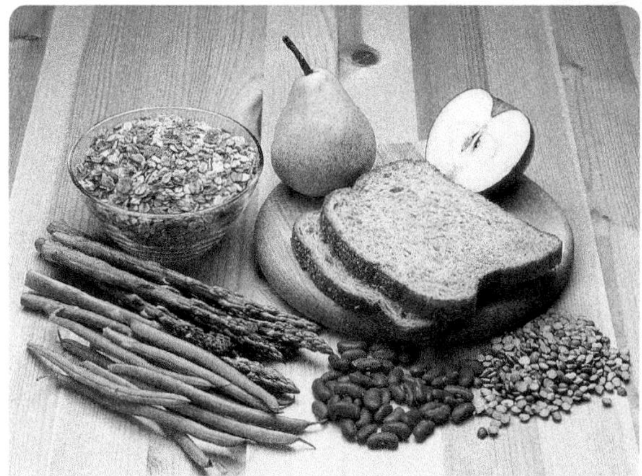
Fig. 9.3 **Dietary Fiber** Dietary fiber is a plant substance that your body can not digest. *Why is it necessary to include dietary fiber in your daily diet?*

Your body needs fat. It is an essential nutrient. It is also a category of food that gives flavor and texture to other foods. As a nutrient, fat promotes healthy skin and normal growth. It also carries certain vitamins to wherever your body needs them. The fat stored in your body acts as insulation against extreme temperatures and helps cushion and protect organs such as the heart and liver.

Fats are a natural part of certain foods such as meat, poultry, fish, dairy products, and nuts. Other foods—for example, vegetable oil, butter, margarine, cream, and mayonnaise—are composed primarily of fats. These sources of fats are often used as ingredients in foods such as salad dressings, gravy, ice cream, cakes, cookies, and many other baked goods. Foods fried in oil absorb some of the fats, which increases their fat content.

There is more than one type of fat. Fats in food may be classified as **saturated fat** or **unsaturated fat,** as shown in **Figure 9.4.** Most fat-containing foods have a mixture of these types of fats. Some foods that contain fats also contain a fatlike substance called **cholesterol.**

- Saturated fats are found in butter, stick margarine, meats, poultry, and some dairy products. These fats are solid at room temperature.
- Unsaturated fats are found in vegetable oils, nuts, olives, and avocados. These fats are typically liquid at room temperature.
- Cholesterol is not a fat. It is a waxy substance that is part of every cell in your body. Cholesterol is found in foods from animal sources, including meat, poultry, fish, egg yolks, and dairy products. Foods from plant sources have no cholesterol. Your body does not need cholesterol from food because it can produce all the cholesterol it needs.

Eating too much cholesterol and fat, especially saturated fats, such as coconut oil or palm kernel oil, can increase your chances for health problems later in life. Saturated fats and cholesterol tend to raise the level of cholesterol in your blood, which increases your risk for heart disease. Eating too many calories from fats can also lead to weight gain.

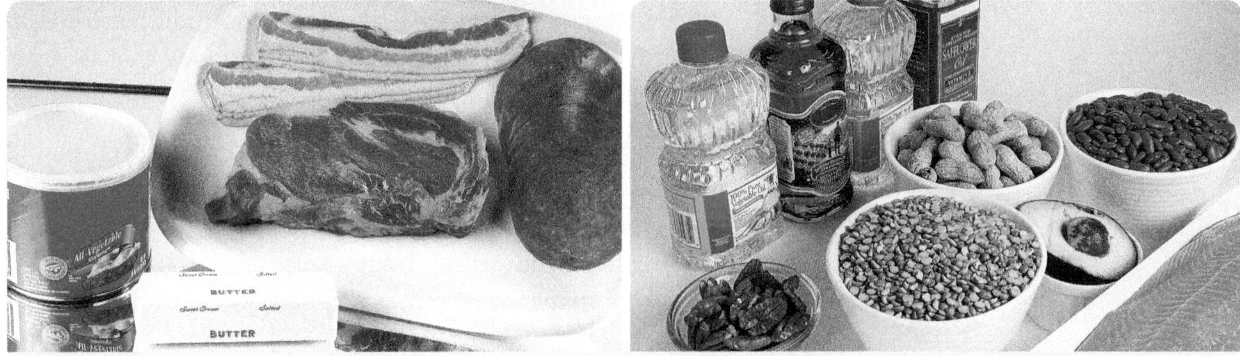

Fig. 9.4 **Fats** One of these images is an assortment of saturated fats, and the other is a an assortment of unsaturated fats. *Which of these are saturated fats and which are unsaturated fats?*

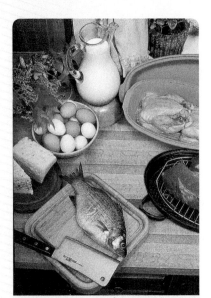

Fig. 9.5 Complete Proteins Proteins are considered the body's building blocks. *How does your body get the essential amino acids you need?*

Proteins

Proteins are considered the body's building blocks because they help your body grow, repair itself, and fight disease. In fact, every part of your body is made up of proteins, including your bones and organs. When necessary, your body can also use proteins for energy.

Proteins are made up of units called **amino acids.** Various amino acids can be arranged in many ways to create various proteins. Your body makes the proteins it needs from the amino acids in the foods you eat. Your body can also make some amino acids. The amino acids your body cannot make, called essential amino acids, must come from the food you eat.

Proteins in food come from both animal and plant sources. Meat, poultry, fish, eggs, and dairy products supply proteins containing all the essential amino acids. For this reason, they are called complete proteins. The foods shown in **Figure 9.5** contain all the essential amino acids.

Some plant sources of proteins are dry beans and peas, nuts, and grain products. Plant sources of protein lack one or more essential amino acids. Therefore, they are considered incomplete proteins. **Figure 9.6** illustrates some foods that supply incomplete proteins. However, eating the right variety of plant-based foods can supply all the essential amino acids you need.

When you eat a variety of foods, it is easy to get the protein you need each day. You do not need to eat extra protein because you are growing, and eating more protein will not build bigger muscles. Only physical activity builds bigger and stronger muscles. When you eat more protein than your body needs, it is stored in your body as fat.

Vitamins

Vitamins are vital nutrients, but you need them only in small amounts. They help other nutrients do their jobs. Vitamins do not provide energy or build body tissues but they do help regulate these processes as well as many others. Vitamins are grouped into two main categories: water-soluble and fat-soluble.

Water-Soluble Vitamins Water-soluble vitamins dissolve in water. Vitamin C and the B vitamins are examples of water-soluble vitamins. Water-soluble vitamins cannot be stored in the body. Therefore it is important that your food choices regularly include these vitamins.

Although your body needs water-soluble vitamins, you should not take large amounts of these vitamins from supplements. This is because your body gets rid of excess water-soluble vitamins through your urine. Taking large amounts of these vitamins from supplements causes your kidneys to work very hard

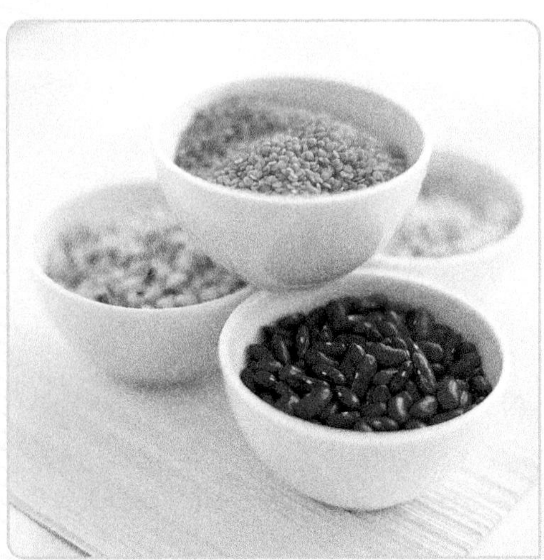

Fig. 9.6 Incomplete Proteins *How can you make sure to get adequate supplies of amino acids with these incomplete proteins?*

Photos: (t)Spangler Studios, (b)David Munns/Photo Researchers, Inc.

to remove the excess, and may cause damage to your kidneys and other organs. **Table 9.1** lists the specific functions of water-soluble vitamins and some food sources for these vitamins.

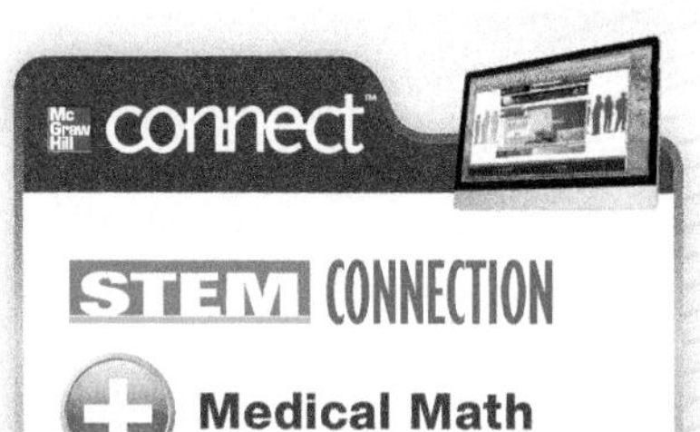

STEM CONNECTION

Medical Math

Determining Your Daily Water Needs

Sufficient water intake is especially important if you are active. It is recommended that each day we drink one-half as many ounces of water as the number of pounds in our body weight. For example, if you weigh 150 lbs, you should drink 75 ounces of water. Go to connect to complete the Water Needs activity.

Table 9.1 Water-Soluble Vitamins

VITAMIN AND FUNCTIONS	FOOD SOURCES
Thiamin (Vitamin B_1) Helps in energy production Maintains healthy nerves, brain, and muscle functions	Enriched and whole-grain breads and cereals; lean pork; dry beans and peas
Riboflavin (Vitamin B_2) Helps in energy production Helps the body resist infection Keeps lining of nose, mouth, and digestive tract healthy	Enriched and whole-grain breads and cereals; milk and dairy products; dry beans and peas; meat; poultry; fish; green, leafy vegetables
Niacin (Vitamin B_3) Helps in energy production Needed for a healthy nervous system	Meat; poultry; fish; liver; enriched and whole-grain breads and cereals; dry beans and peas; peanuts
Vitamin B_6 (Pyridoxine) Helps in energy production Needed for a healthy nervous system Helps protect against infection Helps form red blood cells	Poultry; fish; meat; dry beans and peas; whole wheat products; some fruits and vegetables; liver; eggs
Vitamin B_{12} (Cyanocobalamin) Helps in energy production Helps build red blood cells Needed for a healthy nervous system Helps form genetic material	Meat; poultry; fish; shellfish; eggs; milk and dairy products; some foods, such as breakfast cereals, fortified with vitamin B_{12}
Folate (folic acid) Helps build red blood cells May help protect against heart disease Helps to prevent birth defects	Fruits; whole-grain products; dark green, leafy vegetables; dry beans and peas; liver; bread, cereal, rice, pasta, flour, and other grain products fortified with folic acid
Vitamin C Increases resistance to infection Maintains healthy teeth and gums Helps wounds heal Helps keep blood vessels healthy	Citrus fruits such as oranges and grapefruits; cantaloupes; tomatoes; green peppers; strawberries; kiwi fruit; mangoes; potatoes; broccoli; cabbage

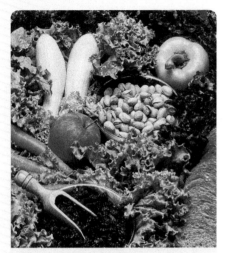

Fig. 9.7 Antioxidants These foods contain antioxidants. *Why are antioxidants important?*

Fat-Soluble Vitamins Fat-soluble vitamins, which include vitamins A, D, E, and K dissolve in fats, both in foods and in your body. Your body stores fat-soluble vitamins in body fat and in your liver. When you need them, your body pulls these vitamins out of storage. Excessive amounts of fat-soluble vitamins can build up to harmful levels in your body. **Table 9.2** lists specific functions and some food sources of fat-soluble vitamins.

Some vitamins have special roles in your body. Vitamins A, C, and E act as **antioxidants,** helping to protect your body cells from damage that can lead to health problems. As shown in **Figure 9.7,** fruits, vegetables, whole-grain breads and cereals, and nuts are good sources of antioxidants.

Minerals

Like vitamins, minerals are "team players." They work as partners with other nutrients to help regulate body processes. Minerals also

Table 9.2 Fat-Soluble Vitamins

VITAMIN AND FUNCTIONS	FOOD SOURCES
Vitamin A An antioxidant Promotes growth and healthy skin and hair Helps eyes adjust to darkness Helps body resist infections	Dairy products; dark green, leafy vegetables such as spinach; deep yellow or orange fruits and vegetables such as carrots, pumpkin, winter squash, cantaloupe, peaches, apricots
Vitamin D Helps build strong bones and teeth Enhances calcium absorption	Fortified milk; egg yolks; fatty fish such as salmon and mackerel; liver. The body can also produce vitamin D itself, when the skin is exposed to sunlight.
Vitamin E An antioxidant Helps form red blood cells and muscles Protects other nutrients from damage	Vegetable oils; whole-grain breads and cereals; dark green, leafy vegetables; dry beans and peas; nuts and seeds
Vitamin K Helps blood to clot	Dark green, leafy vegetables; wheat bran and wheat germ; some fruits; egg yolks; liver

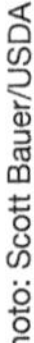

give structure to bones and teeth and provide materials for healthy blood and tissue. **Table 9.3** lists specific functions and food sources of some of the minerals your body needs.

Table 9.3 Minerals

MINERAL AND FUNCTIONS	SOURCES
Calcium Builds and renews bones and teeth Regulates heartbeat, muscles, nerves	Milk; yogurt; cheese; dark green, leafy vegetables; canned fish with edible bones; dry beans; calcium-fortified juices and cereals
Phosphorus Builds and renews bones and teeth Helps in energy production	Milk; yogurt; cheese; meat; poultry; fish; egg yolk; whole-grain breads and cereals
Magnesium Builds and renews bone Helps nerve and muscle function	Whole-grain products; dark green, leafy vegetables; dry beans and peas; nuts and seeds
Sodium, chloride, and potassium Help maintain the body's balance of fluid Help with muscle and nerve actions	Sodium and chloride: salt and foods containing salt; Potassium: fruits such as bananas and oranges; vegetables; meat; poultry; fish; dry beans and peas; dairy products
Iron Helps build and renew hemoglobin to carry oxygen to cells	Meat; poultry; fish; egg yolk; dark green, leafy vegetables; dry beans and peas; enriched grain; dried fruits
Zinc Helps heal wounds and form blood Helps in growth and maintenance of body tissues	Meat; liver; poultry; fish; dairy products; dry beans and peas; whole-grain breads and cereals; eggs
Fluoride Helps prevent tooth decay by strengthening teeth	Small amounts added to the water supply in many communities; toothpaste with fluoride, absorbed when teeth are brushed

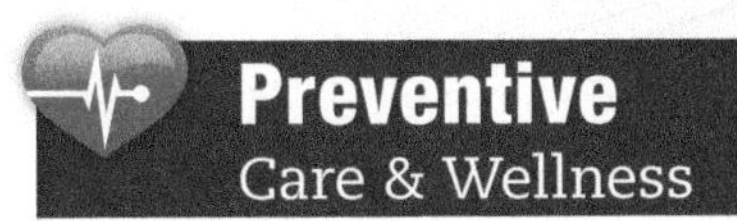

Losing Weight Safely

Your diet and activity level play important roles in determining what you weigh.

Plan meals and snacks that meet your nutritional needs without taking in too many calories. Consider this: To gain one pound, your body needs in excess of about 3500 calories. Likewise, to lose one pound, you need to cut out about 3500 calories. The safest way to do this is to lower your calorie intake from food by about 250 to 500 calories per day and increase your physical activity so that you are burning more calories. This can help promote gradual weight loss of about ½ to 1 pound per week. Losing weight more rapidly than that can be dangerous to your health and may mean that you are losing muscle rather than fat.

Always consult a physician and/or registered dietician before starting a diet.

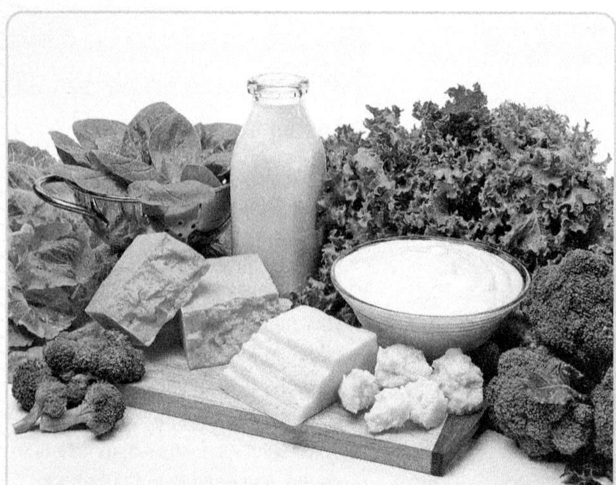

Fig. 9.8 Foods High in Calcium Here are some foods that are high in calcium. *What diseases can an adequate intake of calcium help to prevent?*

Calcium, phosphorus, and magnesium all help build and maintain your bones over your lifetime. Your need for these minerals is highest during your teen years, when bones are growing and becoming more dense. If you do not get enough of these minerals, your body extracts what it needs from your bones. Later in life, **osteoporosis,** a condition in which bones become brittle and break easily, may develop because of a lack of these minerals. **Figure 9.8** shows some foods that are high in calcium.

Iron is very important. It helps red blood cells carry oxygen to all your body's cells. Without enough iron, your blood cannot carry all the oxygen your cells need to produce energy. Over time, this may lead to a condition called anemia, which causes weakness and fatigue. Women are more likely than men to get anemia. Women have a greater need for iron because of the monthly menstrual cycle.

Water

Water is considered a nutrient because it is essential to life. In fact, about two-thirds of your body's weight is made up of water. You need to maintain a regular supply of water to help your body perform its many life-supporting activities. Although it is possible for you to live for many days without food, you can live for only a few days without water.

Water does much more than satisfy your thirst. It helps the body regulate its internal temperature so that it stays constant at around 98.6°F. Water transports nutrients to your body cells and carries waste products away from them. It aids in digestion, moistens body tissues such as your eyes, mouth, and nose, and helps cushion your joints and protect your body organs and tissues. Each day, your body loses about two to three quarts of water. It is important to replace this loss by drinking water and other fluids throughout the day. If you do not drink enough water, you can quickly develop a headache. Choose liquids such as plain water, fruit juices, milk, and soups. Beverages with caffeine, such as coffee, tea, and soda, also count, but caffeine can act as a diuretic, causing your body to lose some water. Many foods also supply your body with water. For example, broccoli, lettuce, tomatoes, and watermelon all contain more than 90 percent water. Even foods such as bread and meat supply small amounts of water. However, water itself is your best source of fluid.

Getting Enough Nutrients

Everyone needs the same nutrients for good health. The amounts of nutrients needed vary according to the individual. How much you need of each nutrient depends on your age, size, how active you are, and whether you are male or female.

Through nutrition research, health experts know approximately how much of each nutrient you need each day to stay healthy. The amounts of specific nutrients—vitamins, minerals, and protein—needed by individuals of all ages are known as the **recommended dietary allowances (RDAs).** These allowances are used mainly by health professionals to evaluate the intake of nutrients by individuals. RDAs for carbohydrates and fats have not been established, because the recommended amounts of these nutrients depend on energy requirements, not on age or gender.

Health experts have determined daily nutrient values, which are included on many food labels. Consumers can use these nutrient levels, based on the RDAs, as a quick reference. These figures do not take age or gender into account, so you may need to adjust the amounts to fit your own daily needs. The inclusion of daily values in food labeling helps consumers understand how a particular food fits into their daily diet. **Figure 9.9** gives an example of nutrition information found on a food label.

Nutrition Facts

Serving Size 8 Crackers (29g)
Servings Per Container about 7

Amount Per Serving

Calories 130	**Calories from Fat** 30
	% Daily Value*
Total Fat 3g	5%
Saturated Fat 1g	5%
Cholesterol 0mg	0%
Sodium 310mg	13%
Total Carbohydrate 22g	7%
Dietary Fiber Less than 1g	3%
Sugars 3g	
Protein 3g	

Vitamin A 2% • Vitamin C 0%
Calcium 0% • Iron 4%

*Percent Daily Values are based on a 2,000 calorie diet. Your daily values may be higher or lower depending on you calorie needs:

	Calories:	2,000	2,500
Total Fat	Less than	65g	80g
Sat Fat	Less than	20g	25g
Cholesterol	Less than	300mg	300mg
Sodium	Less than	2,400mg	2,400mg
Total Carbohydrate		300g	375g
Dietary Fiber		25g	30g

Fig. 9.9 An Example of a Nutrition Facts Label *If you ate this whole container how many calories would you eat? How many grams of fat?*

Energy and Calories

Your body uses the energy it obtains from foods to fuel everything you do—from riding a bike to brushing your teeth to solving a math problem to sleeping. These everyday activities are called voluntary work.

You may not realize that your body also uses energy to power the many processes that are constantly happening inside your body, such as breathing and keeping your heart beating. The rate at which your body uses energy just for maintaining its own tissue, without doing any voluntary work, is called the **basal metabolic rate (BMR).** The units that measure the energy your body obtains from nutrients and the energy your body uses for body processes and activity are called calories.

Carbohydrates, fats, and proteins all supply calories. Carbohydrates and proteins each provide four calories per gram (of carbohydrate or protein). Fats, however, provide nine calories per gram (of fat), which is more than twice the amount that carbohydrates or proteins provide. This explains why high-fat foods tend to be high in calories. Health experts recommend that you make food choices that supply carbohydrates, fats, and proteins in the following proportions (also see **Figure 9.10**).

- Carbohydrates: about 55 percent of your daily calories
- Fats: no more than 30 percent of your daily calories
- Proteins: about 12 to 15 percent of your daily calories

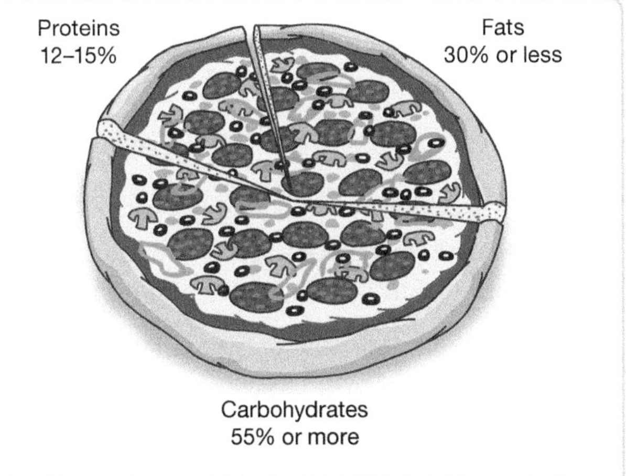

Fig. 9.10 Food Choice Proportions *Does your diet conform to these proportions?*

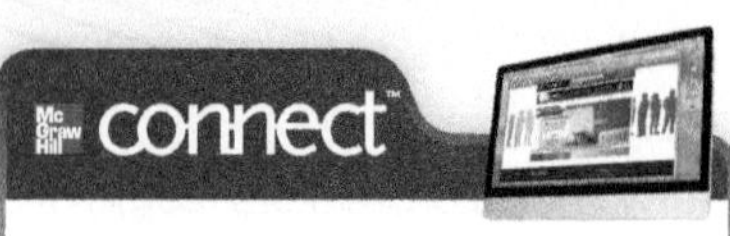

STEM CONNECTION

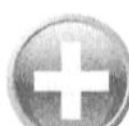

Medical Math

Figuring Your Energy Needs
Nutrition scientists have long been estimating energy requirements for individuals. In 1919, a formula was developed to estimate an individual's basal metabolic rate (BMR). This determines the approximate number of calories an individual needs for basic body functions, considering age, height, and weight.

Go to connect to learn how to calculate a person's energy needs.

Table 9.4 Average Calorie Needs

CATEGORY	APPROXIMATE NUMBER OF CALORIES PER DAY
Women who are not active and some older adults	1,600
Most children, teenage girls, active women, and moderately active men	2,200
Women who are pregnant or breastfeeding	2,200+
Teenage boys, many active men, and some very active women	2,800

Your daily energy, or calorie, needs depend on several factors: age, gender, body size, body's proportion of muscle to fat, genetic makeup, and level of activity. The amount of physical activity is the factor that has the greatest impact on the number of calories your body uses. The longer and more intense your activity, the more calories you burn. As you build more muscle, your body also requires more energy when you are not exercising just to maintain the muscle. **Table 9.4** shows the approximate number of calories you need each day.

READING CHECK

Analyze what would happen if you removed a nutrient category from your diet.

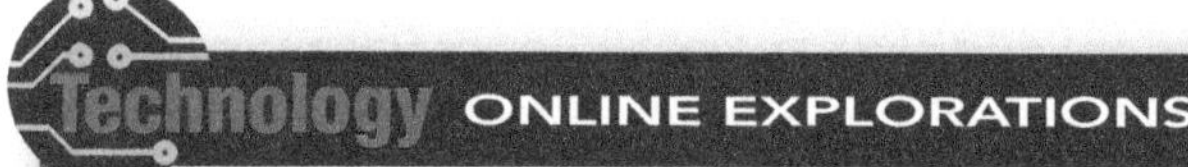

SECTION 9.1 Essentials of Nutrition Review

AFTER YOU READ

1. **Describe** the six nutrients necessary for health.
2. **Examine** the difference between simple and complex carbohydrates.
3. **Compare** saturated and unsaturated fats.
4. **Define** amino acids.
5. **Calculate** what percentages of your diet should consist of fats, carbohydrates, and proteins.
6. **Discuss** the purpose of recommended daily allowances (RDAs).
7. **Identify** the stage of life at which your body most needs minerals.
8. **List** several dietary sources of water.

Technology ONLINE EXPLORATIONS

Water

Water is a key component to life and health. Using the Internet, determine the effects of a low amount of water (fluid) in your body. What is the medical term to describe a body that has a decreased or low level of fluid? What symptoms will you have if you do not consume enough water? How long can you live if you do not have any intake of fluid?

SECTION

9.2 Maintaining Good Nutrition

Dietary Guidelines for Americans

In which food group or groups do beans and nuts fall?

During your teenage years, your body experiences its biggest growth spurt since infancy. By the time this growth spurt is over, you are likely to be 20 percent taller and 50 percent heavier than you were before. Good nutrition is very important to help you reach your growth potential. After you stop growing, good nutrition, along with regular physical activity, helps you stay healthy and fit.

Maintaining good nutrition requires being aware of what you eat, so that you can make the choices that are right for you. Dietary guidelines, a how-to guide for good nutrition, have been established to help Americans make wise food choices. As part of the ***Dietary Guidelines for Americans,*** a new icon, called MyPlate, has been developed to help us understand how to eat healthier. The icon in **Figure 9.11** is based on the dietary guidelines design (see **Figure 9.12**).

These guidelines provide advice about food and lifestyle choices that promote wellness for healthy people two years of age and older. They are based on current knowledge of the effects of nutrition on health. These guidelines can help you meet your nutrient needs, reduce your chances of getting certain diseases, and help you live a healthful, active life.

The guidelines include key recommendations for the general population and for specific groups, such as pregnant women and people over age 50. **Table 9.5** on page 279 provides a summary of the key recommendations. Additional recommendations can be found on the USDA website.

USDA Food Guide

The *Dietary Guidelines* contain technical information that is helpful to policy makers, nutrition educators, and healthcare providers. To help consumers apply the guidelines, various tools, such as brochures and websites, have also been developed. The ***USDA Food Guide*** is one such tool. It puts foods into the following basic groups:

- Fruits. Eat a variety of fruits. Fresh, frozen, canned, and dried fruits generally provide more nutrients than fruit juices.

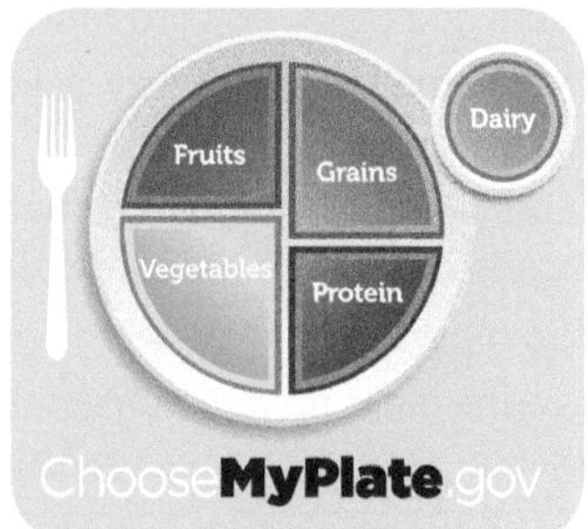

Fig. 9.11 MyPlate The MyPlate icon illustrates the types and quantities of foods a person is recommended to eat. *Is your diet balanced according to the My Plate guidelines?*

Vocabulary

Content Vocabulary

You will learn these content vocabulary terms in this section.

- **Dietary Guidelines for Americans**
- **USDA Food Guide**
- **nutrient-dense**
- **malnutrition**

Academic Vocabulary

You will see these words in your reading and on your tests. Find their meanings in the Glossary in the back of the book.

- **technical**
- **equivalent**

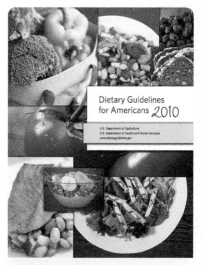

Fig. 9.12 Dietary Guidelines for Americans These guidelines provide advice about food and lifestyle choices that promote wellness for healthy people aged two and older. *How is it beneficial to follow these guidelines?*

Photos: (l)USDA Center for Nutrition Policy and Promotion, (r)U.S. Department of Agriculture, www.dietaryguidelines.gov

- Vegetables. This group includes several subgroups. Dark green vegetables include such foods as broccoli and spinach. Carrots and yams are examples of orange vegetables. Legumes include dried beans and peas as well as soybean products. Legumes can be counted in either the vegetable group or the meat and bean group. When figuring your daily intake, be sure you count the foods you eat in only one group, not both. Starchy vegetables include such foods as green peas, corn, and white potatoes. "Other" vegetables include tomatoes, tomato juice, lettuce, green beans, and onions.

Table 9.5 Some of the Key Recommendations from the *Dietary Guidelines for Americans*

BALANCING CALORIES TO MANAGE WEIGHT	• Promote healthy weight through improved eating and physical activity behaviors. • Control total calorie intake to manage body weight. For people who are overweight or obese, this will mean consuming fewer calories from foods and beverages. • Increase physical activity and reduce time spent in sedentary behaviors. • Maintain appropriate calorie balance during each stage of life: childhood, adolescence, adulthood, pregnancy and breastfeeding, and older age.
FOODS AND FOOD COMPONENTS TO REDUCE	• Reduce daily sodium intake to less than 2,300 milligrams (mg) and further reduce intake to 1,500 mg among persons who are 51 and older and those of any age who are African American, have hypertension, diabetes, or chronic kidney disease. • Consume less than 10 percent of calories from saturated fatty acids by replacing them with monounsaturated and polyunsaturated fatty acids. • Consume less than 300 mg per day of dietary cholesterol. • Keep *trans* fatty acid consumption as low as possible by limiting foods that contain synthetic sources of *trans* fats, and by limiting other solid fats. • Reduce the intake of calories from solid fats and added sugars. • Limit the consumption of foods that contain refined grains, especially refined grain foods that contain solid fats, added sugars, and sodium. • If alcohol is consumed, it should be consumed in moderation (up to one drink per day for women and two drinks per day for men) and only by adults of legal drinking age.
FOOD AND NUTRIENTS TO INCREASE (within calorie needs)	• Increase vegetable and fruit intake. • Eat a variety of vegetables, especially dark green, red-and-orange, beans, and peas. • Consume at least half of all grains as whole grains. • Increase intake of fat-free or low-fat milk and milk products. • Choose a variety of protein foods, which include seafood, lean meat and poultry, eggs, beans and peas, soy products, and unsalted nuts and seeds. • Increase the amount and variety of seafood consumed by choosing seafood in place of some meat and poultry. • Replace protein foods that are higher in solid fats with choices that are lower in solid fats and calories and/or are sources of oils. • Use oils to replace solid fats where possible. • Choose foods that provide more potassium, dietary fiber, calcium, and vitamin D, which are nutrients of concern in American diets.
BUILDING HEALTHY EATING PATTERNS	• Select an eating pattern that meets nutrient needs at an appropriate calorie level. • Monitor foods and beverages consumed, and their fit within a healthy eating pattern. • Follow food safety recommendations when preparing and eating foods.

- Meat, poultry, fish, dry beans and peas, eggs, nuts, and seeds. In this group, choose lean meat and poultry. Vary your choices.
- Milk, yogurt, and cheese. Choose low-fat or fat-free products from this group. These foods are rich in calcium. If you choose not to eat dairy products, look for other foods that supply calcium.

Foods in these groups are **nutrient-dense.** This means that they contribute a significant amount of several nutrients relative to the food energy, or calories, they contain. On the other hand, oils, fats, and sugars have many calories and relatively few nutrients. Use them sparingly.

Table 9.6 shows the recommended daily or weekly amounts for each food group. Note that several calorie levels are given. Recommended daily calories vary with age, gender, level of activity, and physical condition. In general, the following amounts are recommended:

- 2,800 calories for teen males, active men, and very active women.
- 2,200 calories for older children, teen females, active women, and most men. Pregnant or breast-feeding women may need more.
- 1,600 calories for younger children, many women, and older adults.

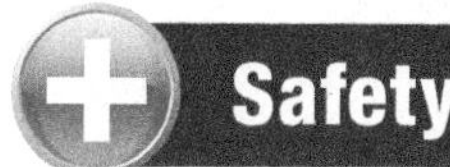

Food Safety

Whatever you eat, always remember to take steps to keep your food safe.

- Wash your hands often, with hot water and hand soap, when preparing food.
- Keep raw meats and ready-to-eat foods separate.
- Cook foods to proper temperature.
- Chill cooked food promptly to below 40° F.
- Avoid unpasteurized juices and dairy products, raw sprouts, and raw or undercooked eggs, meat, and poultry.

Table 9.6 Sample USDA Food Guide

FOOD GROUPS*	CALORIE LEVELS			
	1,600	2,000	2,200	2,800
Fruits	1.5 c (3 srv)	2 c (4 srv)	2 c (4 srv)	2.5 c (5 srv)
Vegetables	2 c (4 srv)	2.5 c (5 srv)	3 c (6 srv)	3.5 c (7 srv)
• Dark green	• 2 c/wk	• 3 c/wk	• 3 c/wk	• 3 c/wk
• Orange	• 1.5 c/wk	• 2 c/wk	• 2 c/wk	• 2.5 c/wk
• Legumes	• 2.5 c/wk	• 3 c/wk	• 3 c/wk	• 3.5 c/wk
• Starchy	• 2.5 c/wk	• 3 c/wk	• 6 c/wk	• 7 c/wk
• Other	• 5.5 c/wk	• 6.5 c/wk	• 7 c/wk	• 8.5 c/wk
Grains	5 oz-eq	6 oz-eq	7 oz-eq	10 oz-eq
• Whole	• 3	• 3	• 3.5	• 5
• Other	• 2	• 3	• 3.5	• 5
Meat, poultry, fish, dry beans and peas, eggs, nuts, and seeds	5 oz-eq	5.5 oz-eq	6 oz-eq	7 oz-eq
Milk, yogurt, and cheese	3 c	3 c	3 c	3 c
Oils	22 g	27 g	29 g	36 g
Discretionary calorie allowance**	132	267	290	426

*Food group amounts are shown in cups (c), cups per week (c/wk), and ounce-equivalents (oz-eq). Where it applies, the number of servings (srv) is given in parentheses. Oils are shown in grams (g).

**This number shows calories that can be eaten in addition to the amounts of nutrient-dense foods in each group. Any solid fats and added sugars in foods are counted here.

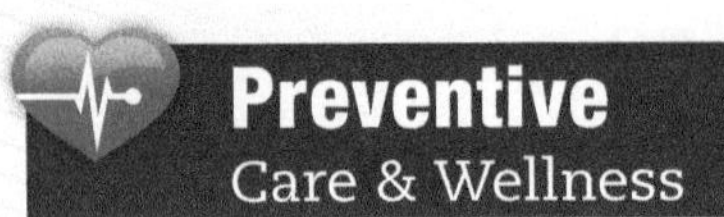

Preventive Care & Wellness

Do You Need a Dietary Supplement?

A dietary supplement provides extra nutrients in the form of pills, capsules, liquid, or powder (see **Figure 9.13**). If you eat a variety of nutritious foods on most days, you are probably getting enough nutrients and do not need a supplement. A doctor or registered dietitian may recommend a dietary supplement for some individuals, such as:

- Young children with many food dislikes
- Older adults
- People taking certain medications
- People recovering from illness
- People following special diets or low-calorie diets
- Women during pregnancy

If you decide on your own to take a dietary supplement, a multivitamin-mineral supplement that provides no more than 100 percent of the daily value of each nutrient is your safest option.

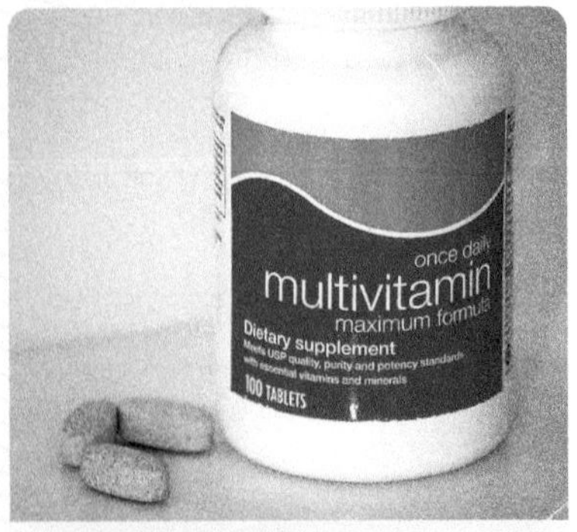

Fig. 9.13 Dietary Supplements Dietary supplements provide extra nutrients in the form of pills, capsules, liquid, or powder *Do you take any dietary supplements?*

Serving Sizes

The Food Guide gives recommended servings in ranges to allow for different energy (calorie) needs. For good health, eat at least the smallest number of servings from each major food group every day. Depending on your daily energy needs, you may need more servings.

Various forms of food may provide various amounts of nutrients. For example, 1/4 cup of dried fruit is equivalent to 1/2 cup of fresh fruit. **Table 9.7** shows the *equivalent* amounts for different food choices in each group.

You need to know the specific amounts of food that make up a serving. Your portions, or helpings, may be different from the Food Guide servings, but that is not a problem. Just compare the size of your helpings to the size of the Food Guide servings. If your helping is bigger, it counts as more than one serving. For example, if you have a hamburger on a bun, it counts as two servings from the grain group.

Table 9.7 Equivalent Amounts

Fruits 1/2 cup equivalent is:	• 1/2 cup fresh, frozen, or canned fruit • 1 medium piece of fruit • 1/4 cup dried fruit • 1/2 cup fruit juice
Vegetables 1/2 cup equivalent is:	• 1/2 cup of cut-up raw or cooked vegetable • 1 cup raw leafy vegetable • 1/2 cup vegetable juice
Grains 1 ounce equivalent is:	• 1 slice bread • 1 cup dry cereal • 1/2 cup cooked rice, pasta, cereal
Meat, poultry, fish, dry beans, eggs, nuts, and seeds 1 ounce equivalent is:	• 1 ounce of cooked lean meat, poultry, fish • 1 egg • 1/4 cup cooked dry beans or tofu • 1 tablespoon peanut butter • 1/2 ounce nuts or seeds
Milk, yogurt, and cheese 1 cup equivalent is:	• 1 cup low-fat or fat-free milk, yogurt • 1 1/2 ounces low-fat or fat-free natural cheese • 2 ounces of low-fat or fat-free processed cheese
Oils 4 grams = 1 teaspoon 1 teaspoon equivalent is:	• 1 teaspoon soft margarine • 1 tablespoon low-fat mayonnaise • 2 tablespoons light salad dressing • 1 teaspoon vegetable oil

Judging food amounts is easier if you compare them to everyday items. For example, three ounces of meat is about the size of a deck of cards (see **Figure 9.14**).

Many foods are mixed, or combination, foods. For instance, pizza, vegetable lasagna, an egg roll, and a chicken burrito all contain foods from more than one food group. To determine Food Guide serving sizes, estimate the amount of each food ingredient from the various food groups. Decide whether each food ingredient provides more, less, or the same amount as one Food Guide serving in that group.

READING CHECK

List some factors that affect your recommended daily calorie amount.

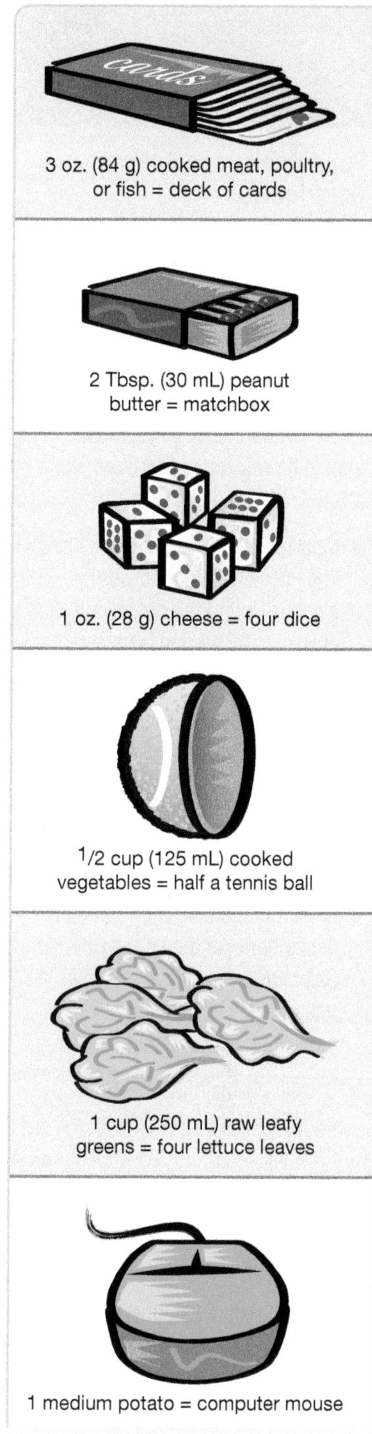

cards
3 oz. (84 g) cooked meat, poultry, or fish = deck of cards
2 Tbsp. (30 mL) peanut butter = matchbox
1 oz. (28 g) cheese = four dice
1/2 cup (125 mL) cooked vegetables = half a tennis ball
1 cup (250 mL) raw leafy greens = four lettuce leaves
1 medium potato = computer mouse

Fig. 9.14 Serving Sizes
Serving sizes for some foods compared with the sizes of everyday non-food items. *How do your normal helpings of food compare with these samples?*

Effects of Poor Nutrition on Health

What common habits have a negative effect on nutrition?

Poor nutrition may result from getting too few or too many nutrients. In either case, your health may be compromised as a result.

Getting Too Few Nutrients

When your food choices do not supply enough of the nutrients you need over a period of time, a nutrient deficiency, or nutrient shortage, may result. Some nutrient deficiencies may not become apparent for many years. For instance, if you do not get enough calcium when you are young, you may develop osteoporosis when you are older.

A continued lack of nutrients may lead to a serious condition called **malnutrition.** Malnutrition may also occur when the body cannot absorb or use nutrients properly.

Malnutrition is most often the result of food shortages that limit an individual's energy and nutrient intake. However, even people who have enough to eat can develop malnutrition if they make poor food choices. Fortunately, nutrient deficiencies and malnutrition can be treated, although some of the health effects may remain. Once a nutrient deficiency or malnutrition is identified, the treatment is to improve food choices or provide extra nutrients as a dietary supplement.

Getting Too Many Nutrients

Poor nutrition may also result from getting more nutrients than you need. For instance, eating too much fat can increase your chances of developing heart disease and other serious health problems. Eating too many calories may lead to weight gain, which can increase your chances of developing diabetes.

Excessive amounts of certain vitamins and minerals, especially fat-soluble vitamins, can also cause harm to your body. For instance, very large amounts of vitamin A from a dietary supplement can cause damage to your liver. Eating too much sodium (from salt) can cause a rise in blood pressure in some individuals. When you take excess vitamins and minerals in the form of pills, capsules, liquids, or powders, you run the risk of getting too many nutrients.

READING CHECK

Identify some causes of malnutrition.

21ST CENTURY SKILLS

Food Habits and Cultural Restrictions

Ethnic background, religious customs, holiday customs, and regional differences affect the way food is grown, cooked, served, and eaten. All diets should be evaluated for the basic food groups. If a diet requires improvement, dietary restrictions should be respected. Here are just a few common examples.

- Muslims avoid pork and shellfish. They usually do not consume alcohol. During the holy month of Ramadan, all-day fasts are required for those who are able.
- Some Buddhists and Hindus do not eat meat.
- Roman Catholics and members of the Greek Orthodox Church may avoid meat at certain times.
- Most members of the Church of Jesus Christ of the Latter-Day Saints (Mormons) avoid coffee, tea, caffeine-containing beverages, and alcoholic beverages.
- Jewish clients may observe certain dietary laws called "kosher."
- Seventh-Day Adventists are encouraged to practice a vegetarian diet.
- Most Christian Scientists do not drink alcohol, coffee, or tea.

Principles of Healthful Eating

Why is it important to eat a variety of foods?

The texture, color, aroma, and flavors of food are what make eating so much fun. No single food or type of food provides all the nutrients you need in the right amounts for a day. That is why the *Dietary Guidelines* recommend choosing many different foods for the nutrients and energy they provide.

The array of food choices available today makes it possible to choose various ways to eat healthfully. Two important things to think about are what and how much you eat. All foods supply nutrients, so all foods can be part of a healthy way of eating. There are no good or bad foods, just good or bad eating patterns. What is important is the total amount and types of foods you eat over several days.

The *USDA Food Guide* shows you how to put the *Dietary Guidelines for Americans* into practice. At the same time, it can help you follow the three basic principles of healthful eating.

- Variety. Eating a variety of foods boosts your chances of getting the many nutrients your body needs to grow strong and stay healthy. Be adventurous and experience variety. Try different and new foods for their great taste.
- Balance. Make your food choices count over several days. This means that you can balance your choices over several days and still get enough of the nutrients you need. If you come up short on servings from the Food Guide one day, just make up for it the next day.
- Moderation. Eat all kinds of foods, but moderate the amounts to help control your calorie intake. You do not need to weigh or measure everything you eat. Watching how much you eat helps you get enough variety without overdoing it on any one specific food or food group. Be especially moderate with foods that are high in fat or added sugars.

READING CHECK

Describe the concept of balance as it relates to food choices.

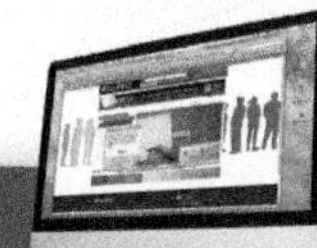

connect ONLINE PROCEDURES

PROCEDURE 9-1

Identifying Nutrients and Food

For health, energy, and growth you need to eat a variety of foods. These foods supply essential nutrients, which are substances that nourish your body.

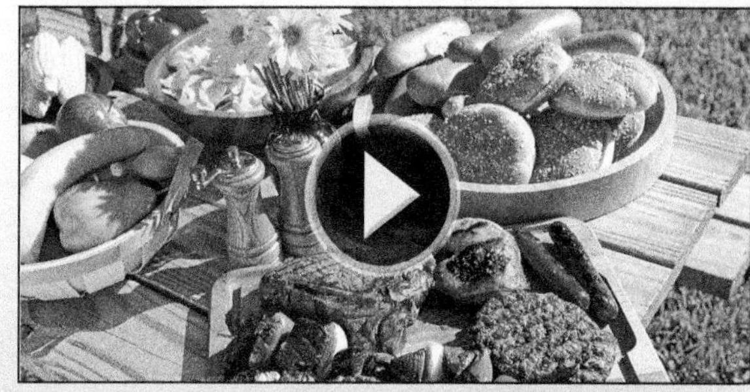

PROCEDURE 9-2

Calculating Your Energy Needs

Calculating your energy needs or the number of calories you should have in a 24-hour period is important to help you maintain your weight and health. BMR determines the number of calories that an individual needs for basic body functions, considering age, height and weight.

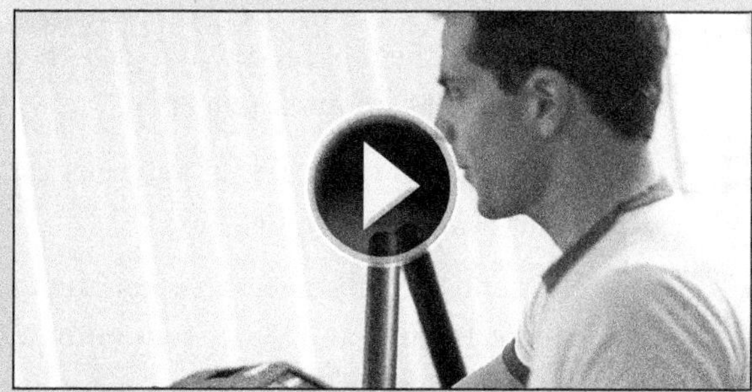

PROCEDURE 9-3

Create a Sample Meal Plan

A meal plan is a menu that you plan in advance. It includes everything you plan to eat or drink. It can be used to help ensure that you are getting nutrients in the right amounts. You can create a meal plan based upon the *Dietary Guidelines* and the *USDA Food Guide.*

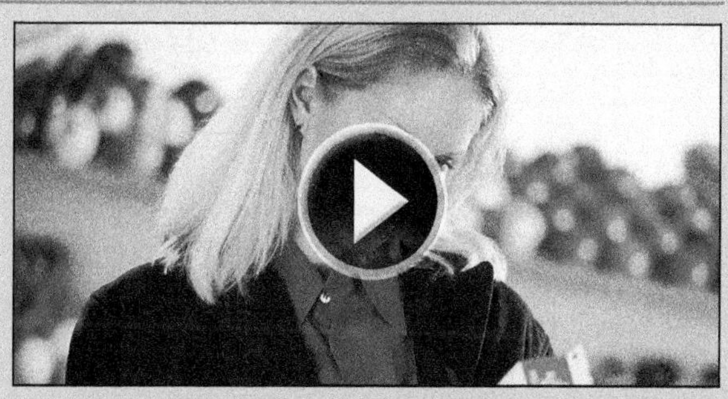

Photos: (t)Purestock/Getty Images, (c)CORBIS, (b)JUPITERIMAGES/ Comstock Images/Alamy

SECTION 9.2 Maintaining Good Nutrition Review

AFTER YOU READ

1. **Select** several nutrient-dense foods.
2. **Evaluate** whether or not you need a dietary supplement. List your reasons.
3. **Identify** the people who have the highest and lowest calorie needs.
4. **Examine** three consequences of poor nutrition.
5. **Explain** how excess amounts of some nutrients can be harmful.
6. **Identify** the three basic principles of healthful eating.

Technology ONLINE EXPLORATIONS

MyPlate

Go the U.S. Department of Agriculture's website for MyPlate. Do the following:

- Review and write down the Tip of the Day.
- Create a plate of food following the guidelines. Write down each food and how much would be on the plate.
- Review the guidelines and determine a weakness you have regarding nutrition and write it down.

CHAPTER 9 Review

Chapter Summary

SECTION 9.1

- Good nutrition is important to sustain life, promote health, and prevent disease. **(pg. 267)**
- For overall health, energy, and growth, you need to eat a variety of foods in moderate yet adequate amounts. **(pg. 267)**
- The six major categories of nutrients are carbohydrates, fats, proteins, vitamins, minerals, and water. **(pg. 267)**
- Nutrients are substances that nourish the body. Their key functions are to provide energy, to build and repair your body, and to keep your body processes running smoothly. **(pg. 267)**
- Even though everyone needs generally the same nutrients for good health, the amounts of nutrients vary depending on the individual. Your energy or calorie needs depend on several factors, including your age, height, weight, level of activity, and gender. **(pg. 276)**

SECTION 9.2

- The *Dietary Guidelines for Americans* and the *USDA Food Guide* are tools to help you design a healthful eating plan that is right for you. **(pg. 277)**
- The major food groups include fruits; vegetables; grains; meat, poultry, fish, dry beans, peas, eggs, nuts, and seeds; and milk, yogurt, and cheese. The largest number of daily servings should come from the fruits, vegetables, and grains groups. **(pg. 278)**
- Getting too few nutrients over a period of time may lead to a nutrient deficiency, which may cause poor health or a lack of energy. Getting too many nutrients can increase your chances of developing health problems. **(pg. 281)**

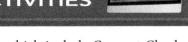

Mc Graw Hill connect™ ONLINE ACTIVITIES

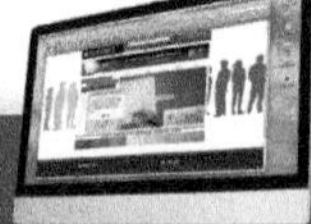

Complete our HST online activities for Chapter 9, which include Concept Check review questions, Reference Flash Cards, and Online Procedures assessment sheets.

- **Concept Check** review questions
- **Reference Flash Cards** medical terminology practice
- **Online Procedures** assessment sheets

9 Assessment

Critical Thinking/Problem Solving

1. You learn that one of your friends who is on the swimming team is taking dietary supplements to help improve his performance. When you question him, you find out that he is taking a multivitamin mineral supplement along with supplements providing extra amounts of vitamin B6 and vitamin C. He is also drinking "protein shakes" made with milk, raw eggs, and protein powder two times a day. What advice can you give him?

2. For breakfast each day, your friend usually eats doughnuts and drinks a bottle of soda. One day after school he complains of feeling tired and weak. What could be his problem?

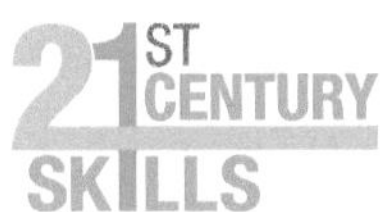

3. **Visualization** Practice using measuring cups and a scale to measure recommended servings of various foods. Compare these servings to your usual helpings. Think of ways to visualize several recommended servings by comparing them to common household items. For example, three ounces of meat is about the size of a deck of cards.

4. **Problem Solving** Obtain nutritional labels from a variety of foods. Review the labels and determine the nutrients available in each. Identify how often the foods should be eaten and how much should be eaten on a regular basis.

5. **Leadership and Responsibility** Write down everything you ate at your last full meal. Be specific by including the amount and the ingredients. Trade your list with a partner. Determine how many servings of each food group your partner consumed. Refer to **Table 9.6** and figure out how many servings of each group your partner will need during the next 24 hours.

6. **Information literacy** Search the Internet for programs designed to analyze your day's food choices. Some programs are low-cost or free. Before you analyze your diet, keep a record of everything you eat and drink for several days. This should detail the specific type of food you eat (low-fat or fat-free milk, fried or boiled egg) and the amounts. Remember to include extras and snacks, such as ketchup on your hamburger or carrot sticks before dinner.

   When you have entered the required information, the computer program will calculate how much of each nutrient your food choices supplied. It may even compare your total daily nutrients to how much you need based on your age and gender.

CHAPTER 10 Vital Signs

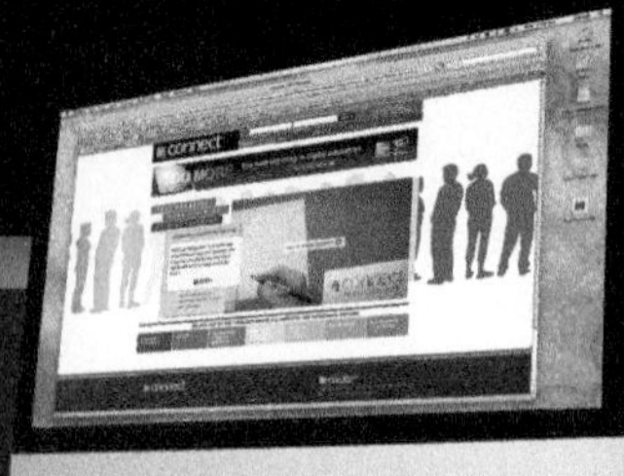

McGraw Hill connect™

It's Online!

- Online Procedures
- STEM Connection
- Medical Science
- Medical Terms
- Medical Math
- Ethics in Action
- Virtual Lab

Essential Question:

How would you expect your vital signs to differ from those of people in other age groups?

Vital signs are indicators of events that happen within the body but might otherwise go undetected. At the doctor's office, or in an emergency situation, collecting a patient's vital signs is often the first act of a health-care practitioner. In this chapter, you will learn to gather the materials necessary to take a patient's vital signs and the procedures that should be followed. Then you will practice taking vital signs of people from different age groups.

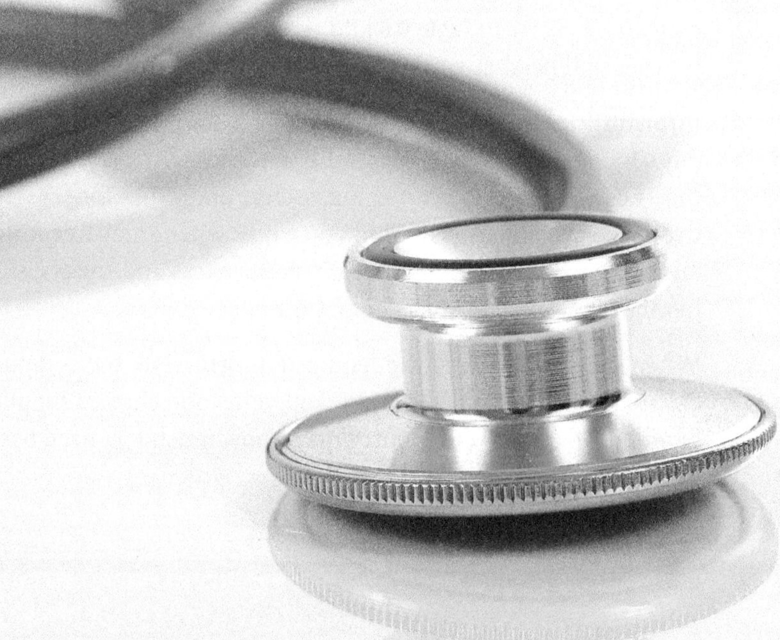

Photo: Nathan Blane/iStock Exclusive/Getty Images

READING GUIDE

OBJECTIVES

After completing this chapter, you will be able to:

- **Discuss** the five vital signs taken by healthcare practitioners and the purpose of each.
- **Define** terms and abbreviations related to gathering vital signs.
- **Distinguish** normal and abnormal values and characteristics of temperature, pulse, respiration, and blood pressure for infants, children, and adults.
- **Analyze** the different methods of measuring temperature and when each method should or should not be used.
- **Assess** sites for taking pulse and blood pressure.
- **List** the effects of high and low blood pressure on the body.

BEFORE YOU READ

Connect Have you ever had your vital signs taken? If so, what did it feel like?

Main Idea

Vital signs are the most important measurements obtained on a client.

Note-Taking Activity

Draw this table. Write key terms and phrases under **Cues**. Write main ideas under **Note Taking**. Summarize the section under **Summary**.

Cues	Note Taking
◦	◦
◦	◦
Summary	

Graphic Organizer

Before you read the chapter, draw a diagram like the one at the right. As you read, write the vital signs covered in this chapter into the diagram.

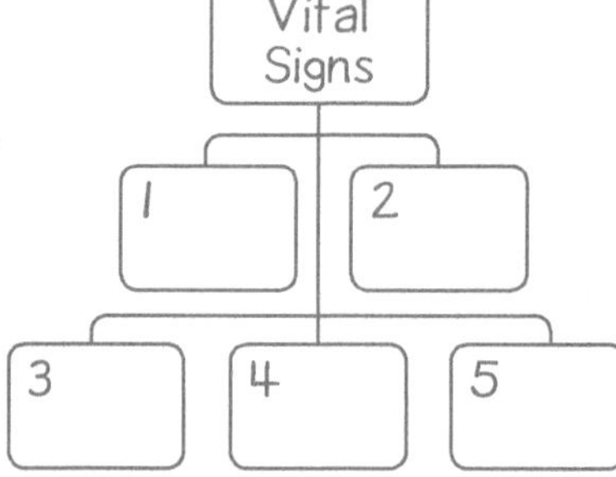

connect
Downloadable graphic organizers can be accessed online.

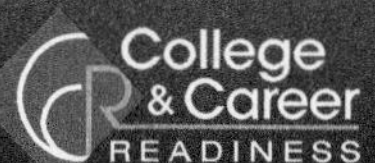

STANDARDS

HEALTH SCIENCE

NCHSE 9.13 Discuss complementary (alternative) health practices as they relate to wellness and disease.

NCHSE 10.11 Apply procedures for measuring and recording vital signs including the normal ranges.

SCIENCE

NSES A Students should develop abilities necessary to do scientific inquiry, understanding about scientific inquiry.

NCHSE *National Consortium for Health Science Education*

NSES *National Science Education Standards*

COMMON CORE STATE STANDARDS

MATHEMATICS

Statistics and Probability

Interpreting Categorical and Quantitative Data S-ID Summarize, represent, and interpret data on a single count or measurement variable.

ENGLISH LANGUAGE ARTS

Writing

Research to Build and Present Knowledge W-8 Gather relevant information from multiple authoritative print and digital sources, assess the credibility and accuracy of each source, and integrate information into the text selectively to maintain the flow of ideas, avoiding plagiarism.

Speaking and Listening

Comprehension and Collaboration SL-2 Integrate multiple sources of information presented in diverse media and formats, including visually, quantitatively, orally.

SECTION
10.1 Vital Signs

Vocabulary

Content Vocabulary

You will learn these content vocabulary terms in this section.

- temperature
- assessment
- vital signs
- oral
- axillary
- tympanic
- temporal
- rectal
- febrile
- pulse
- palpate
- auscultate
- radial
- brachial
- antecubital space
- apical
- stethoscope
- intercostal space
- rhythm
- respiration
- blood pressure (BP)
- systolic blood pressure (SBP)
- diastolic blood pressure (DBP)
- popliteal
- dorsalis pedis
- posterior tibial
- sphygmomanometer
- meniscus

Academic Vocabulary

You will see this word in your reading and on your tests. Find its meaning in the Glossary in the back of the book.

- range

Commonly Measured Vital Signs

What do changes in vital signs suggest?

Temperature, pulse, respiration, blood pressure, and pain **assessment** are the most common **vital signs,** or indicators of events occurring within the body. They are the most important measurements obtained on a patient. They give information about changes within the body and in the environment. Changes in a patient's vital signs may indicate a disease or disorder. Drastic changes can lead to death. These signs are considered vital to life, which is why we use the term vital signs.

Temperature

What is a normal adult temperature?

When someone is ill, body temperature is one of the first vital signs taken. Temperature may be taken from several sites (see **Figure 10.1**):

- **Oral**: within the mouth or under the tongue
- **Axillary**: in the armpit, also known as the axilla
- **Tympanic**: in the ear canal
- **Temporal**: on the side of the forehead near the temple
- **Rectal**: through the anus, in the rectum

Temperature is sometimes taken through monitors that are attached inside or onto the body.

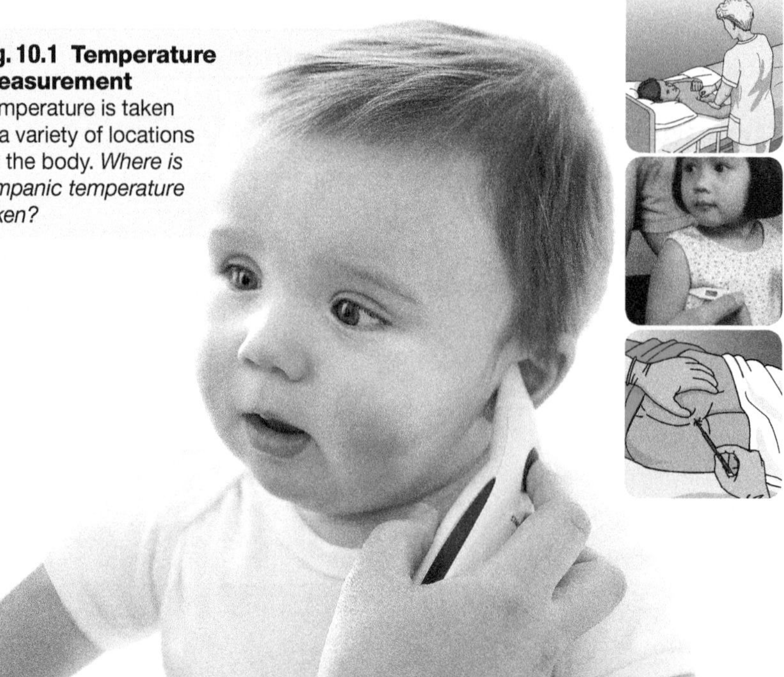

Fig. 10.1 Temperature Measurement Temperature is taken in a variety of locations on the body. *Where is tympanic temperature taken?*

Photos: (l)Science Photo Library RF/Getty Images, (r)Aaron Haupt Photography

Temperature Ranges

A normal adult temperature is 98.6°F or 37°C. When you take a temperature, however, you will find that most people are within a range of 96.8°F to 100.4°F or 36.0°C to 38.0°C. This variation is the result of changes within the body or exposure to the environment, such as:

- Time of day: temperatures are usually lower in the morning and higher in the evening
- Allergic reaction
- Illness
- Stress
- Exposure to heat or cold: temperature is higher when a person is outside in the sun and lower when a person is exposed to cold air

When a temperature is above 100.4°F or 38.0°C, you will document, or write in the patient's chart, that the patient is **febrile.** A person who is febrile is feverish, with a body temperature above normal. If a temperature is within a normal range, the person is afebrile.

Communication & Collaboration

Effective Listening

Healthcare providers need to provide emotional support for patients. One of the first steps to take is to become an effective listener.

Types of Thermometers

Electronic/Digital Thermometers The most common type of thermometer is the electronic/digital thermometers. They come in a variety of types. An electronic thermometer, such as a tympanic thermometer, measures temperature through a probe at the end of the device. Disposable covers are placed over thermometer probes for each patient, to prevent contamination. Smaller electronic/digital thermometers are also available. There are digital thermometers that are disposable. Another type of electronic thermometer used commonly with children is a temporal thermometer (see **Figure 10.2**). Except for patients' homes or other locations outside of a medical facility, glass thermometers are basically a thing of the past. These thermometers used to contain mercury in the bulb but because of the hazards posed by mercury, they are now filled with a non-mercury substance. The substance rises into the glass tube until its level matches the temperature.

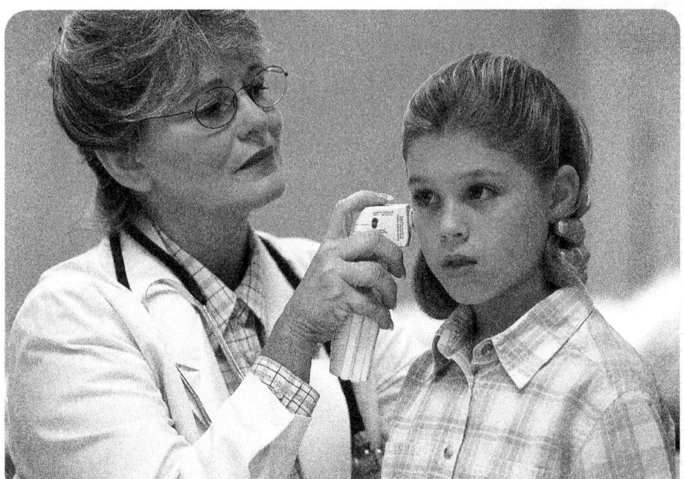

Fig. 10.2 Temporal Electronic Thermometer A temporal scanner is one type of electronic *thermometer. What term refers to a patient whose temperature is above 100.4°F?*

Disposable sheaths or thin plastic covers are placed over glass thermometers for each individual patient, to prevent contamination and avoid having to clean the thermometer after every use.

Disposable single-use thermometers are used more frequently in homes. These thin plastic strips change color according to the temperature of the skin (see **Figure 10.3**).

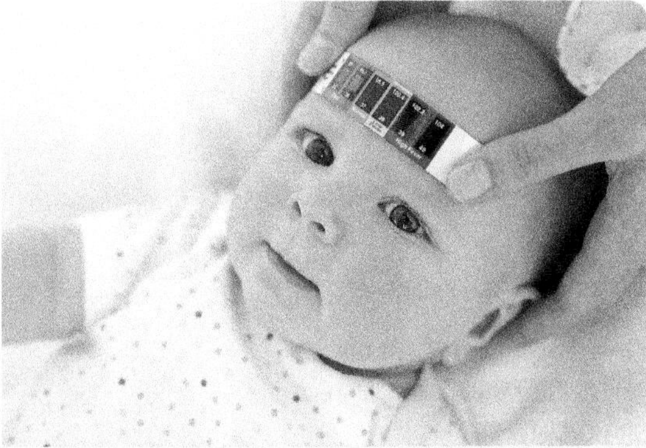

Fig. 10.3 Disposable Thermometer A disposable thermometer strip changes color to indicate the person's temperature. *What does a red reading on a disposable thermometer indicate?*

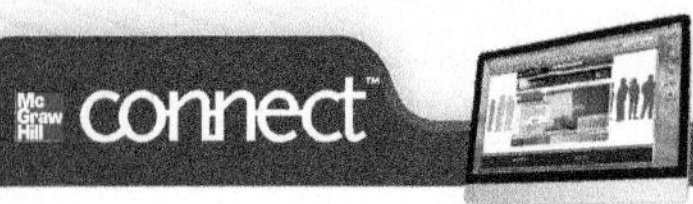

STEM CONNECTION

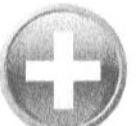

Medical Math

Convert Between Celsius and Fahrenheit
Fahrenheit is a temperature scale based upon 32 degrees as the freezing point and 212 degrees as the boiling point. Celsius, or centigrade, is a temperature scale based upon 0 degrees as the freezing point and 100 degrees as the boiling point (see **Figure 10.4**).

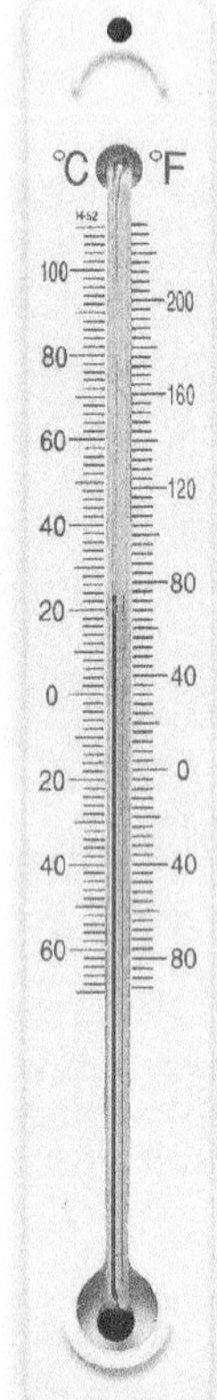

Fig. 10.4 °F Compared to °C Fahrenheit and Centigrade (Celsius) temperature scales. *What are the freezing/boiling points in the Fahrenheit and Celsius temperature scales?*

connect Go online to complete the medical math activity.

Thermometer Handles You will see variations in the color of thermometer handles. A blue handle indicates that the thermometer should be used for oral and axillary temperatures. A red handle indicates that it should be used for rectal temperatures. The colors help in maintaining infection control. There is no difference in their measuring capabilities.

READING CHECK

Recall five common locations where temperature is taken.

Pulse

Have you ever taken your own pulse?

A **pulse** (P) is a wave of blood flow created by the contraction of the heart. Usually, you will check a pulse by using your first two fingers to **palpate,** which means to feel. Sometimes, you will listen for sounds, or **auscultate,** using a stethoscope or an electronic vital signs machine. Pulses are felt or heard where arteries come close to the surface of the skin. These sites are usually named according to the bones or other structures near where they are located.

Pulse Sites

Pulse sites are shown in **Figure 10.5** on page 292 and **Table 10.3** on page 293. The most common pulses assessed are the radial, brachial, and apical.

- The **radial** pulse is best palpated on the inside of the wrist, near the thumb. Use your first and second fingers to feel the pulsation. Do not use your thumb. This is because the thumb can have a rather strong pulse of its own, and you may mistake your pulse rate for the patient's rate.
- In adults, the **brachial** pulse is found in the **antecubital space** of the arm. This is the space on the inside of the bend of the elbow. The brachial pulse site is most often used in very young children, before the brachial muscle is developed. In children, it is in the middle of the inside of the upper arm.
- The **apical** pulse is auscultated with a stethoscope placed on the chest wall. A **stethoscope** is an instrument used to hear body sounds. The apical pulse is found at the apex of the heart, which is located to the left side of the sternum and under the fifth to sixth **intercostal space,** or space between two ribs. In infants and young children, it is closer to the midline of the left chest. This pulse is often taken when assessing infants and young children. For adults, the apical pulse must be taken before certain drugs are administered that may slow the heart rate, such as digitalis.

Characteristics of the Pulse

When you evaluate the pulse, you must always determine the pulse rate. You may also need to evaluate the **rhythm** and volume, and check for bilateral presence.

Pulse Rate Pulse rate is calculated in beats per minute (BPM). The pulse is counted for 15, 20, 30, or 60 seconds. Here is one way to find the pulse rate per minute. Suppose that you counted a rate of 20 beats in 15 seconds. Fifteen seconds is one-fourth of a minute. Or, to put it another way, 15 seconds multiplied by 4 equals 1 minute. So, if you count a rate of 20 beats in 15 seconds, multiply 20 by 4 to get the rate for a minute. In this case, the pulse rate for 20 beats in 15 seconds is 80 beats per minute.

The normal ranges for pulse rate vary according to age and gender. As the cardiovascular system matures, the pulse rate decreases. Women tend to have faster pulse rates than men of the same age. A patient's level of fitness also affects the heart rate. If someone is physically fit, the pulse rate is usually on the low side. Illness and disease can cause variations. **Table 10.1** lists the expected pulse rate ranges of patients by age.

Tachycardia is a pulse rate that is faster than normal. Possible causes of tachycardia are:

- Physical or mental stress such as infection, pain, exercise, and the emotional stress of a crying infant.
- Lack of oxygen or low blood pressure.

Bradycardia is a pulse rate slower than normal. Bradycardia may be seen in patients who are:

- Physically fit athletes
- Taking medication for the heart
- Experiencing a severe lack of oxygen or blood pressure

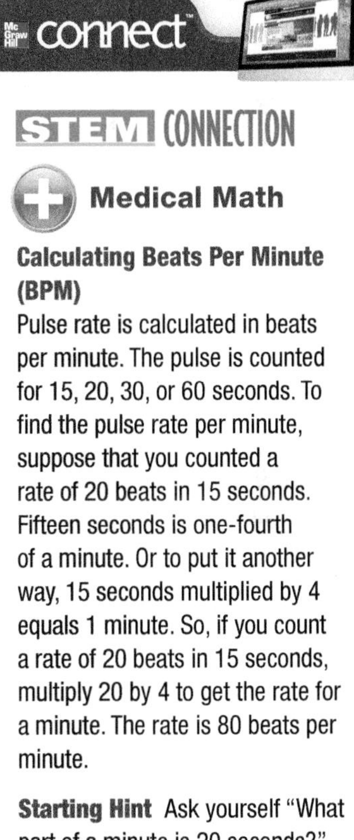

Calculating Beats Per Minute (BPM)

Pulse rate is calculated in beats per minute. The pulse is counted for 15, 20, 30, or 60 seconds. To find the pulse rate per minute, suppose that you counted a rate of 20 beats in 15 seconds. Fifteen seconds is one-fourth of a minute. Or to put it another way, 15 seconds multiplied by 4 equals 1 minute. So, if you count a rate of 20 beats in 15 seconds, multiply 20 by 4 to get the rate for a minute. The rate is 80 beats per minute.

Starting Hint Ask yourself "What part of a minute is 20 seconds?"

Table 10.1 Expected Pulse Rates by Age Group*

Newborn	120 to 160 BPM
1 month to 1 year	80 to 140 BPM
1 to 6 years	80 to 120 BPM
6 years to adolescence	75 to 110 BPM
Adulthood	72 to 80 BPM
Late adulthood	60 to 80 BPM

**Pulse rates vary among individuals. If you obtain a value outside the normal range, re-check your results and check the patient's chart for previous recorded pulse rates.*

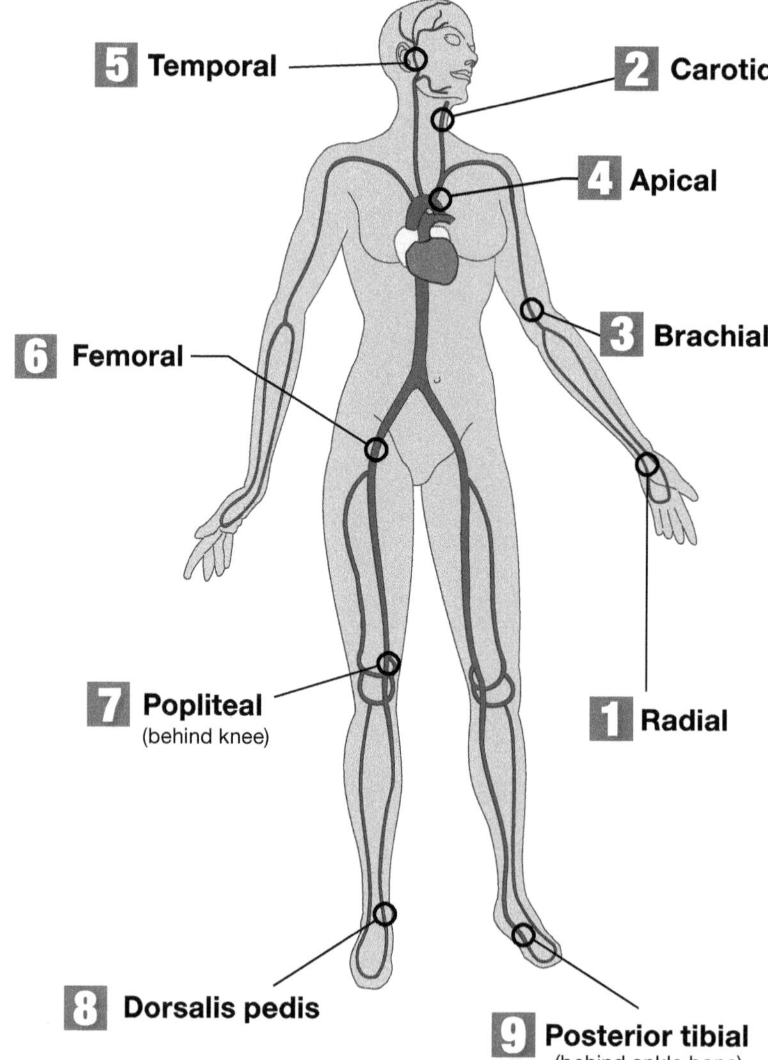

Fig. 10.5 Pulse Sites Pulse can be checked at various locations on the body. *Are pulse rates the same at all body locations?*

Rhythm

Regular

Irregular

Fig. 10.6 Pulse Rhythm Note the rhythm for both pulse and respiration. *How long must the heartbeat of a patient with an irregular heart rhythm be counted to determine an average rate?*

Pulse Rhythm Pulse rhythm is the pattern or regularity of the pulse beat. The pulse should be regular or have evenly paced beats, as shown in **Figure 10.6.** Note in the figure that the regular rate is constant and the irregular rate is variable and inconsistent.

A patient whose heartbeats are irregular may have a dysrhythmia. If a patient of any age has irregular heart rhythm, the heartbeat must be counted for a full minute in order to determine an average rate. When documenting pulse rhythm, you should record the pulse as regular or irregular. An irregular heart rate may be a normal condition that occurs in infants and usually lasts until young adulthood. Certain heart conditions, medications, and lack of oxygen may also cause it.

Pulse Volume The volume of the pulse is also referred to as the strength of the pulse. **Table 10.2** lists the possible measurements of the pulse as it presses against the arterial wall and against your fingertips when you palpate the area. The volume of the pulse can be described using a scale of 0 to 3.

Table 10.2 Scale Used to Describe Pulse Volume

0	Absent, unable to detect
1	Thready or weak, difficult to palpate, and easily stopped by light pressure from fingertips
2	Strong or normal, easily found and stopped by strong pressure from fingertips
3	Bounding or full, difficult to stop with fingertips

Table 10.3 Pulse Sites

PULSE	LOCATION	WHY THIS SITE IS USED
1 Radial	Alongside the radial bone; the area on the thumb side of the patient's wrist is usually assessed.	Common site used to check the pulse manually
2 Carotid	Alongside the trachea and up toward the ear beside the sternocleidomastoid muscle. Placing one finger on the middle of the trachea and then moving the finger down into the groove next to the trachea avoids the large muscle.	Taken on a patient who does not have a noticeable heart-beat. Often used during CPR and when the pulse is weak or blood pressure is low.
3 Brachial	Along the humerus of the upper arm. It is found on the inner aspect of the biceps muscle of infants and young children, in whom this muscle is undeveloped. With older children and adults, it is more easily found in the antecubital space or at the inside of the bend of the elbow	Easily found on infants and children and used often in assessing pulse rate with other vital signs. Site most commonly assessed when obtaining a blood pressure.
4 Apical	At the apex of the heart, which is located on the left side of the chest.	Auscultated with a stetho-scope. Checked in infants and very young children and in adults before certain drugs are administered.
5 Temporal	Next to the front edge of the ears.	Pressure to this area could slow bleeding from the scalp. The temporal artery is also a site used for temperature measurement.
6 Femoral	In the groin or crease between the thigh and lower abdomen.	Most commonly used during invasive surgical procedures; pressure may also be applied here to slow bleeding in a leg.
7 Popliteal	Just behind the knee, toward the midline of the body.	Used to check blood pressure in the leg.
8 Dorsalis pedis	On the dorsal, or top, side of the foot.	Used to check for circulation and nerve function in the feet
9 Posterior tibial	Just behind the medial malleolus (ankle bone), toward the midline of the body.	Used to check for circulation and nerve function in the feet

A pulse that is thready or weak may indicate decreased circulation due to an obstruction of the artery, weak contraction of the heart, or low blood pressure. The strength of the pulse might be rated at 0 or +1. A bounding pulse may indicate high blood pressure or strong contractions of the heart. When pulse rate is recorded according to this scale, it is usually written as +1, +2, and so on.

Bilateral Presence Bilateral means both sides of an object. When you check pulses, they should be found in the same area on both sides of the body and have the same rate, rhythm, and volume on both sides. For example you may check the pulse in both feet of a patient who had surgery in one leg. You would compare the two to determine whether the patient is having any circulation problems in the leg that has been operated on.

READING CHECK

Identify the three most common pulse sites.

Respiration

What counts as one respiration?

Respiration (R) is the act of breathing. It consists of the exchange of oxygen and carbon dioxide between the air and our lungs. Respiration includes breathing in, or inhalation, and then breathing out, or exhalation. One single respiration consists of one inhalation and one exhalation. Therefore, when you count respirations, count one inhalation and one exhalation as one respiration, or a complete breath.

Respiratory Rate

The most common way to assess the respiratory rate (RR) is to observe or feel a patient's chest movement upward and outward for a complete minute. Chest movement in breathing is commonly observed in adults and older children. Younger children, such as those under the age of seven, will use either abdominal movement alone or a combination of chest and abdominal movement.

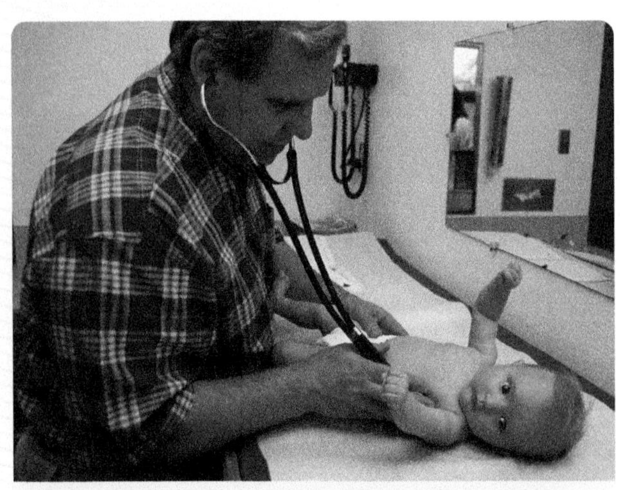

Fig. 10.7 Respirations This pediatrician is listening to an infant's respiration using a stethoscope. *Why would a stethoscope be used to count the respirations of an infant?*

Auscultation with a stethoscope is another way to assess the respiratory rate. This is commonly used with infants, whose rate may be difficult to observe (see **Figure 10.7**). It may also be used with adults, who may alter their breathing when they are aware that you are counting their respiratory rate. One method is to place a warmed stethoscope on the chest wall and tell the patient that you are going to listen to his or her heart.

Characteristics of Respiration

When you assess respiration, you will observe three characteristics: the rate, rhythm, and quality.

Rate of Respiration Respiration rate refers to the number of breaths per minute. A normal adult rate ranges from about 12 to 20 breaths per minute. Respiratory rates decrease as a person increases in size and age. A seven-year-old likely has a faster respiratory rate than an adult. A 100-pound adult would have a faster rate than a 200-pound adult.

An increase above the normal respiratory rate is called hyperventilation. The prefix *hyper-* means above or over. Ventilation refers to the movement of air in and out of the lungs. Possible causes of hyperventilation are:

- Physical or mental stress, such as infection, exercise, or anxiety
- Increase in body temperature
- Lack of oxygen or low blood pressure

A decrease below the normal respiratory rate is called hypoventilation. *Hypo-* means below or under. Possible causes of hypoventilation are:

- Pain medications
- Alcohol
- Decrease in body temperature
- Very low blood pressure
- Severe lack of oxygen

Rhythm of Respiration Respiration rhythm should be regular. Each breath should take the same length of time and be the same amount of time apart; there should be no variation in time and volume from one breath to the next. One type of abnormal respiration is Cheyne-Stokes. This is characterized by shallow breaths that increase to deeper breaths and then decrease to more shallow breaths. Then there is usually a period of apnea, or no breathing, which can last from 5 to 40 seconds.

Quality of Respiration Quality of respiration is seen in volume and effort. Volume is the amount of air taken into the lungs and exhaled from the lungs. It is documented as shallow or deep breathing. Effort is the amount of work the patient uses in order to breathe. If muscle use is observed in the neck, chest, and abdomen during breathing (that is, by muscles not normally essential to the breathing process), this is a sign of labored or difficult breathing, known as dyspnea.

READING CHECK

Identify what it is called if someone is having difficulty breathing, breathing faster than normal, or breathing slower than normal.

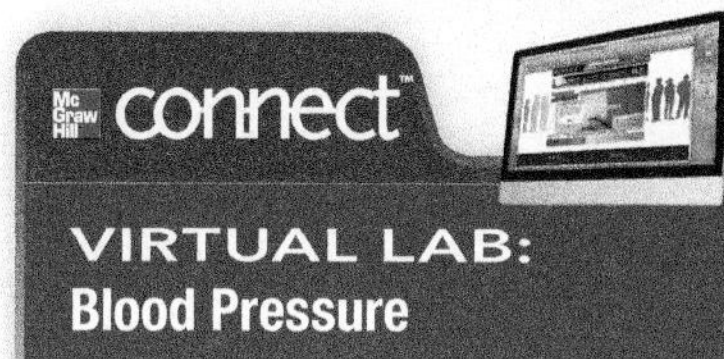

VIRTUAL LAB: Blood Pressure

Question:
How would you expect the vital signs of middle-aged patients to differ from those of teenage patients?

Blood Pressure
Understanding how the heart works is important when taking a patient's vital signs. If you understand the basic workings of the heart, you will better understand what is happening with the blood pressure and pulse readings in patients, especially if they are complaining of symptoms that might be incompatible with healthy heart function.

Go to connect to complete the Virtual Lab on *Blood Pressure.*

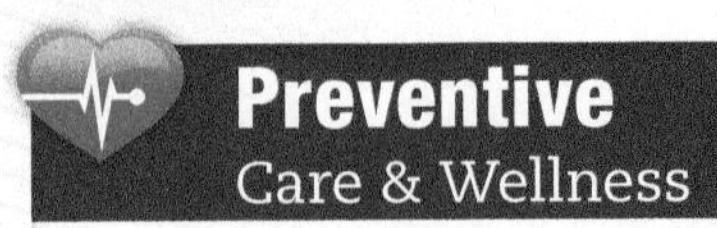

Treating High Blood Pressure

High blood pressure (hypertension) is a silent killer. It can lead to a heart attack or a stroke even when there are no other symptoms. Have your blood pressure checked. If you are found to have hypertension, you will usually have it for life. Medication, losing weight, exercising, and reducing salt intake are methods for treating hypertension. If you are given medication, it must be taken as directed and never discontinued just because you are feeling no symptoms. Always ask your doctor before stopping any medications.

Blood Pressure

Have you ever had your blood pressure taken?

Blood pressure (BP) refers to the amount of pressure exerted on the arterial walls as blood pulsates through them. Two pressures are measured:

- **Systolic blood pressure (SBP)** refers to the pressure exerted on the arteries during the contraction phase of the heartbeat. This number is the higher of the two numbers. The reason for this is that the pressure should be higher in the blood vessels when the heart is contracting.
- **Diastolic blood pressure (DBP)** is the resting pressure on the arteries as the heart relaxes between beats.

Blood pressure is written as a fraction, with the systolic blood pressure in the numerator and the diastolic blood pressure in the denominator. For example, a systolic blood pressure of 120 and diastolic blood pressure of 80 are written as 120/80.

When blood pressure goes above the normal range, it is classified as prehypertension or hypertension. Prehypertension and hypertension frequently do not have symptoms. However, they can lead to other very serious conditions such as a heart attack or a stroke. (See **Table 10.4**). Therefore, it is important to check blood pressure even when thre are no symptoms.

Table 10.4 Expected Blood Pressure Values*

	SYSTOLIC (TOP NUMBER)	DIASTOLIC (BOTTOM NUMBER)
Normal	Less than 120 mm Hg	Less than 80 mm Hg
Prehypertension	121 to 139 mm Hg	80 to 89 mm Hg
Hypertension Stage 1	140 to 159 mm Hg	90 to 99 mm Hg
Hypertension Stage 2	Over 160 mm Hg	Over 100 mm Hg

**As defined by the American Heart Association.*

When blood pressure drops below normal levels (a condition called hypotension), the body attempts to adjust to raise the pressure. Therefore, we see the signs of shock, or a lack of blood flow to the body's tissues. If the blood pressure is 60/34 (very low), the patient may have the following shock symptoms:

- Change in the level of consciousness (awareness)
- Increase in heart rate and respiration rate
- Weak, thready pulses
- Pale, sweaty skin

Sites for Blood Pressure Assessment

Blood pressure can be obtained from any artery. A pulse site is used in the assessment. The safest and most convenient sites for measuring BP are:

- Brachial, on the upper arm, is the most common site for taking vital signs in adults and older children.
- Radial, on the lower arm, is a possible site for infants or patients who have very large upper arms.
- **Popliteal,** on the thigh as an alternative to the arms, is to be used in cases of trauma, disease, medical treatments to arms, or recent mastectomy (breast removal).
- **Dorsalis pedis** and **posterior tibial,** on the lower leg, is a common site for infants when using an automatic blood pressure cuff, because an infant's leg is more accessible and can be held still.

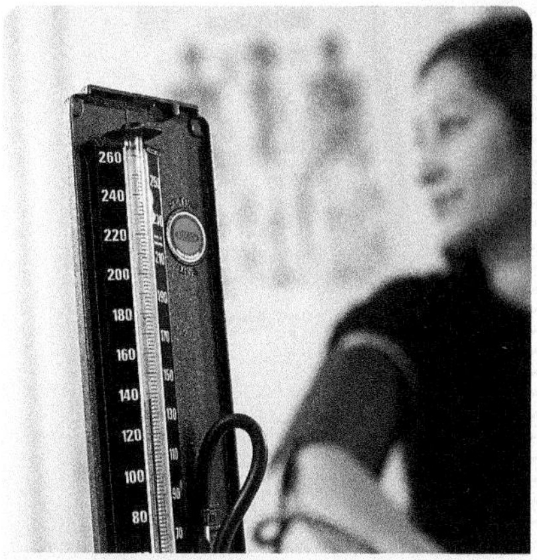

Fig. 10.8 Meniscus When using a columnar gauge, you read the pressure at the meniscus. *Why is it important to read a meniscus at eye level?*

Equipment for Measuring Blood Pressure

A **sphygmomanometer** is the instrument used to measure blood pressure. *Sphygmo* means pulse; *mano* means pressure; and *meter* means measuring device. The sphygmomanometer is commonly referred to as the BP cuff. To take a blood pressure, the BP cuff is placed around an extremity (arm or leg), just above the pulse site. A stethoscope is placed on the pulse site to listen to the sounds or a sphygmomanometer is used to electronically measure the pulse sounds. In either case the cuff is inflated, then the air is released as the healthcare worker listens or the electronic device senses when the pulse begins and ends. These numbers make up the blood pressure value.

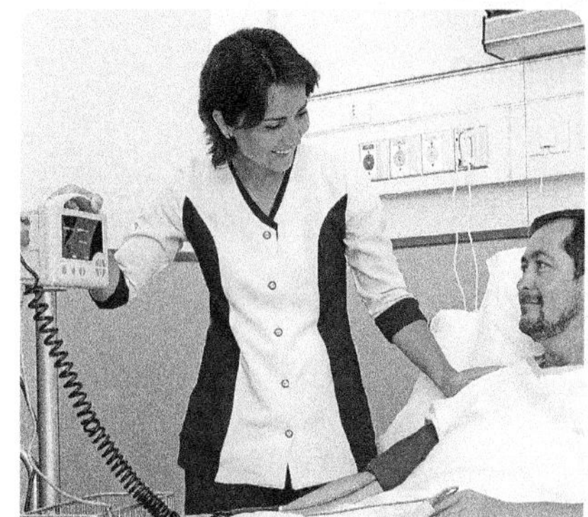

Fig. 10.9 Electronic Blood Pressure Measurement Blood pressure, pulse, and oxygen level are all measured with a sphygmomanometer. *What is another name for this device?*

The Types of Sphygmomanometers There are three basic types of sphygmomanometers.

- Columnar: This is a calibrated glass cylinder that contains a liquid. Since the liquid is within a glass tube, the bottom of the **meniscus** (see **Figure 10.8**) or upper surface of the liquid, forms the indicated point of reference as pressure increases and decreases. Always read the meniscus at eye level for a more accurate measurement.
- Electronic: This has a digital display and may also measure the pulse rate and oxygen level. It does not require the use of a stethoscope (see **Figure 10.9**).
- Aneroid: This is a calibrated dial with a needle that points to numbers on the face of the dial. As the pressure increases, the needle moves around the dial to a higher number and then back down as the pressure decreases (see **Figure 10.10**).

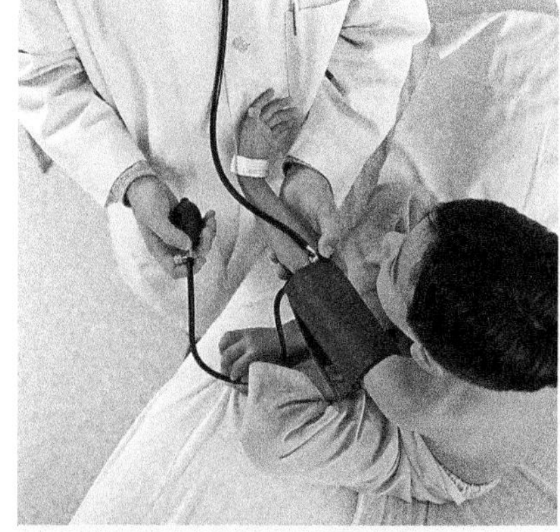

Fig. 10.10 Aneroid Gauge Each line on the aneroid blood pressure gauges indicates 2 mm Hg. *At which pulse site is this medical professional assessing the patient's blood pressure?*

READING CHECK

Classify a blood pressure of 136/78.

Photos: (t)Andrew Brookes, National Physical Laboratory/Photo Researchers, Inc., (c)REB Images/Blend Images/Getty Images, (b)Keith Brofsky/Photodisc/Getty Images

Pain

What is your definition of pain?

Pain is the fifth vital sign. It is frequently checked with the other four vital signs to help determine the condition of a patient. When pain occurs, the patient needs to report the possible cause, location, duration, and the pain quality or rating. The patient may be asked to rate his or her pain on a pain scale. This is a number between 1 and 10 (see **Figure 10.11**).

READING CHECK

Rate from 1 to 10 the pain of a patient who, using the pain scale, points to the face above the word dreadful.

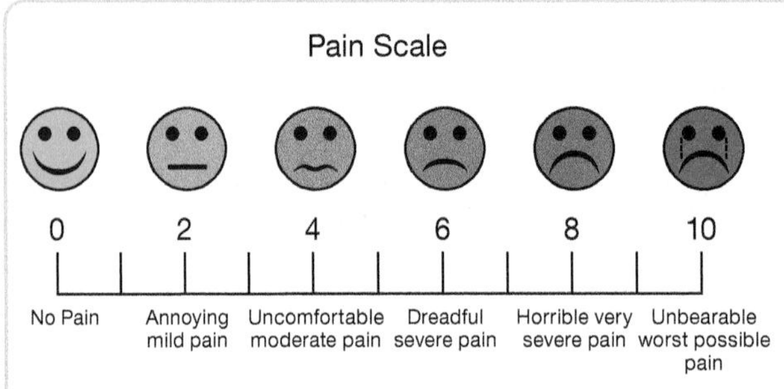

Figure 10.11 Pain Scale A pain scale figure such as this helps the patient to rate his or her pain. *What is the pain scale number for moderate pain?*

SECTION 10.1 Vital Signs Review

AFTER YOU READ

1. **Explain** the difference between palpation and auscultation.
2. **Identify** what the abbreviation BPM represents.
3. **Assess** how a pulse that is strong and easily found should be documented, using the scale in **Table 10.2** on page 292.
4. **Describe** the three characteristics you observe when you assess respiration.
5. **Differentiate** between systolic blood pressure and diastolic blood pressure.
6. **Assess** what a pulse of 102, which is high for an adult, would indicate about a six-year-old child.
7. **Identify** which number in a blood pressure of 140/80 is the measure of pressure caused by heart contraction.
8. **Identify** the unit of measure in which blood pressure is expressed.
9. **Name** the instrument used to listen to blood pressure.
10. **Identify** the fifth vital sign.

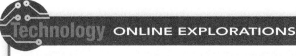

Technology ONLINE EXPLORATIONS

Radial Pulse

Find your radial pulse on both arms. Assess the rate, rhythm, and volume. Practice documenting this assessment. For example:

Radial pulses regular @72 bpm, + 1

SECTION
10.2 Checking Vital Signs

Checking, Documenting, and Recording Vital Signs

What are the vital signs?

Accuracy is of key importance when you measure and record vital signs. When checking vital signs, use this order if possible:

1. Respiration
2. Pulse
3. Temperature
4. Blood pressure
5. Pain

In general, you should perform the vital signs that cause the least discomfort first. For example, a rectal temperature should be done after taking blood pressure, since the procedure to take a rectal temperature is uncomfortable and may increase the blood pressure. If you check the blood pressure before the pulse and respiration rates and a child starts to cry, the pulse and respiration rates may go up as a result. Take the respiration and pulse rates first and at the same time, so the patient remains unaware that you are counting respirations.

When you look for the section of the medical record in which to document vital signs, check for the abbreviations VS (vital signs) or T P R BP (temperature, pulse, respiration rate, blood pressure). Respiration may be abbreviated as RR, for respiratory rate. When documenting vital signs, be sure to use the T P R BP sequence if you are recording only the numbers. For example, use 100.6-72-16-144/88 for the temperature, pulse, respiration rate, and blood pressure, in that order.

In addition to properly recording vital signs in the chart, you should report information about vital signs to your supervisor if requested or if either or both of these results occur:

- The vital sign result falls outside the normal range for the patient.
- The vital sign result is much different from a previous result recorded for the patient.

Measuring and Recording Temperature

When measuring and recording temperature, be sure to use the correct method: oral, axillary, tympanic, temporal, or rectal. Record the temperature location when you record the results. Always check the manufacturer's instructions for the equipment you are using.

Oral Temperatures Oral temperature is one of the most accurate forms of measurements, since it is taken in an area close to blood vessels under the tongue. The thermometer should be placed under

Vocabulary

Content Vocabulary

You will learn this content vocabulary term in this section.

- **alveolar**

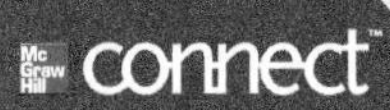
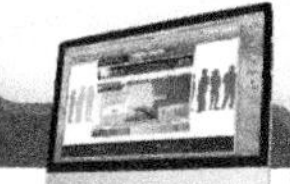

Ethics in Action

Introduction to Confidentiality
Imagine that you have just started working at a hospital with a strict patient confidentiality policy. You overhear a couple of co-workers discussing a patient in the elevator.

Complete the Ethics in Action discussion and research activity on your Healthcare Science Technology connect student page.

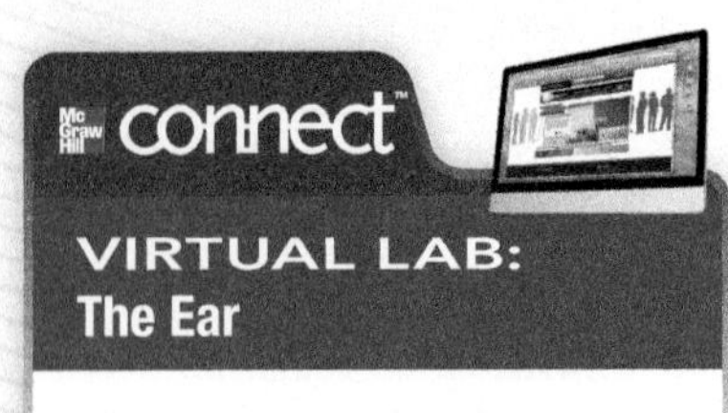

VIRTUAL LAB:
The Ear

The sensation of hearing is the result of a complex process in which sound waves are converted into nerve impulses, which the brain interprets as sound. This animation demonstrates how the human ear processes sound.

Go to connect to complete the Virtual Lab on hearing and the ear.

Teaching Tip
"Normal" vital signs can vary among individuals. Stress to your students the need to know the baseline normal readings for individual patients.

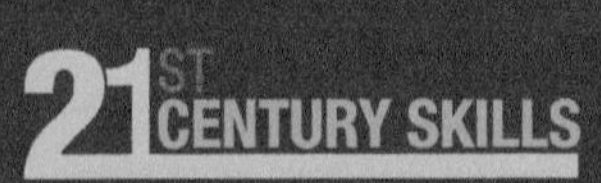

Oral Communication

When measuring vital signs, explain the procedure according to the patient's level of understanding. Do not use technical terms for a child. Even if the patient cannot respond, you should still explain what you are doing. The patient may be able to hear you. If the patient asks you the results of the measurements, be sure you are allowed to tell him or her before you do so. You must find out your role or talk to your supervisor after being asked for results. If you are not allowed to give the patient the results, say, politely, "It is best that you ask [name the physician or other licensed practitioner]."

Follow-up
With a partner, practice explaining to a six-year-old child that you are going to take his or her vital signs.

the tongue in either pocket just off-center in the lower jaw. The patient should hold the thermometer with lips closed. Wait at least 15 minutes after a patient has been eating, drinking, or smoking before taking an oral temperature, or you may obtain an inaccurate result. If necessary, take the temperature using another method.

Other reasons not to take an oral temperature include:

- The patient, such as a young child, is unable to hold the thermometer in his or her mouth.
- The patient might bite the thermometer accidentally if the patient has a history of seizures, is an uncooperative child or adult, is shivering, is a mouth breather, or has suffered trauma to the head.

Tympanic Temperatures A tympanic temperature is the temperature close to the tympanic artery behind the eardrum. Tympanic thermometers are useful with uncooperative patients and with patients who have been eating, drinking, or smoking. Make sure the outer opening of the ear is sealed completely when the probe is in place. Point the thermometer toward the face, to ensure that it is aiming at the eardrum. You may need to tug on the ear to position the thermometer properly.

Reasons not to take a tympanic temperature include:

- Obstruction in the ear canal, such as earwax
- Small ear canals, as in infants and children
- Infection, such as otitis media, or injury of the ear

Rectal Temperatures Rectal temperatures are usually 1°F higher than oral temperatures and are considered the most accurate measurement of body temperature. Gloves are always worn when taking a rectal temperature. The patient is usually placed on his or her left side. This is the preferred position because the rectum is angled in this direction, promoting comfort and preventing accidental puncture of the rectal wall. An infant may be placed on the back with the legs held upward or placed on the belly. The thermometer should be inserted slowly and gently until it can no longer be seen or until you feel resistance, at approximately one inch for adults and ½ inch for infants and small children. When performing a rectal temperature measurement on an infant, have a parent or another healthcare provider assist you. Always hold the thermometer in place while taking temperature here.

Reasons not to take a rectal temperature are:

- A history of cardiac disease. Stimulating the area of the rectum can have an effect on the vagus nerve and cause the heart rate to drop.
- Injury or surgery to the anal or rectal area.
- Recent treatment with chemotherapy, radiation, or medications such as steroids. These treatments can cause tissues to become fragile and more easily damaged.

Axillary Temperatures Have the patient sit or lie down. Place the tip of the thermometer in the middle of the axilla (armpit), with the shaft facing forward. The patient's upper arm should be pressed against his or her side, and the lower arm should be crossed over the stomach to hold the thermometer. The American Academy of Pediatrics advises that the actual body temperature will be 1°F higher than the axillary temperature. Record that the temperature was taken by the axillary method so the licensed practitioner will know to add the degree.

Temporal Temperatures A temporal thermometer measures the infrared heat of the temporal artery and the temperature of the skin at the site where the temperature is taken. These readings are merged together and displayed on the screen. The temporal scanner is a non-invasive and quick procedure for taking temperatures. You stroke the thermometer across the forehead, crossing over the temporal artery. Complete Procedure 10-1 online to practice this skill.

Measuring and Recording Pulse and Respiration

Pulse Count the pulse for one full minute if you are not certain of your accuracy and/or if the pulse is irregular. Do not use your thumb. Adjust the pressure based on the location and strength of the pulse. If you are having difficulty, close your eyes and concentrate on locating the pulse. Complete Procedure 10-2 online to practice this skill.

Respiration Make sure the patient is unaware that you are counting the respiratory rate. Keep your hand on the pulse site or count the respirations while the patient is not looking. Remember that certain factors can increase the respiratory rate. If your patient has just returned from a walk, you will notice an increase. Wait until the patient has been seated for five minutes, if your results are out of the normal range. The pulse and respiration are usually taken together.

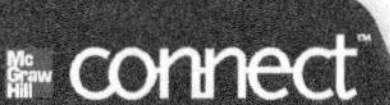
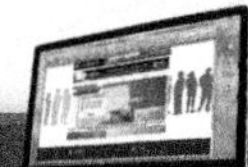

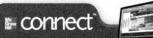

STEM CONNECTION

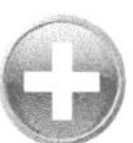

Medical Science

Graphing Vital Signs

Graphs are useful tools because they can provide a great deal of information at a glance. For example, a graph that displays a patient's temperature over a period of several hours will show at a glance if a fever is subsiding. On a simple temperature graph, the vertical line, or axis, represents the patient's temperature, and the horizontal axis represents time.

Go to connect to complete a vital signs graphing exercise.

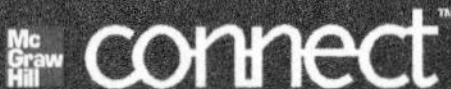
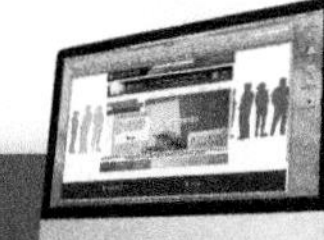

ONLINE PROCEDURES

PROCEDURE 10-1

Measuring and Recording Temperature

Oral temperature is one of the most accurate forms of measurement. Place the thermometer under the tongue just off center in the lower jaw. The patient should hold the thermometer with lips closed. Wait at least 15 minutes after the patient has been eating, drinking, or smoking before taking an oral temperature or you may obtain an inaccurate result.

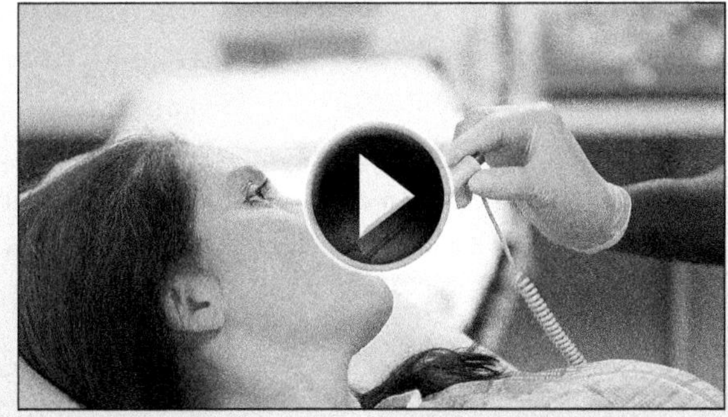

PROCEDURE 10-2

Measuring and Recording Pulse and Respiration

Respirations: Make sure the patient is unaware you are counting respirations. Keep your hand on the pulse site or count the respirations while the patient is not looking. Remember that certain factors can increase respiratory rate.

Pulse: Count the pulse for one full minute if you are not certain of your accuracy and/or if the pulse is irregular. Do not hesitate to count the pulse twice to check your results.

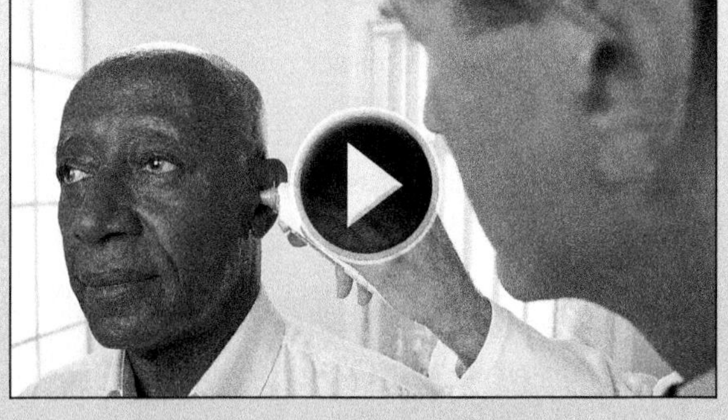

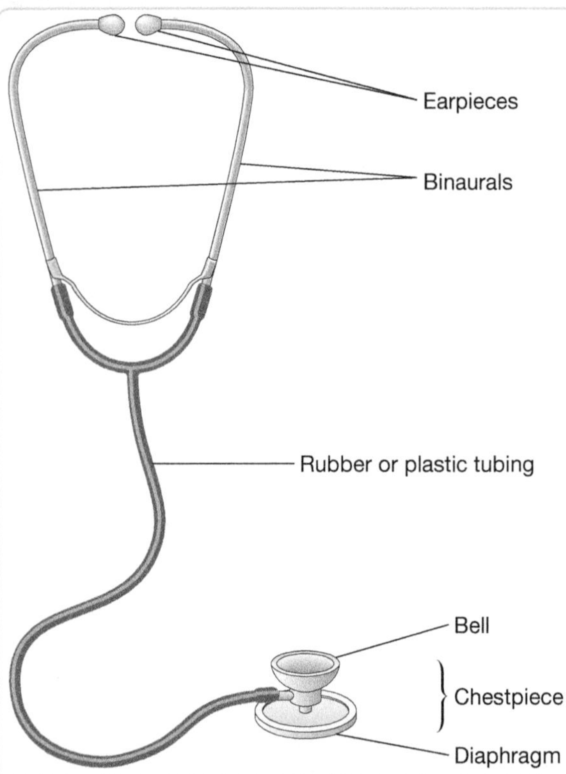

Fig. 10.12 Parts of a Stethoscope The stethoscope amplifies body sounds such as the apical pulse. *Where is the best place to find the apical pulse?*

Apical Pulse The apical pulse is taken in infants, small children and patients with certain cardiovascular diseases. To take an apical pulse, be familiar with the stethoscope and its parts (see **Figure 10.12**). The apical pulse is found just below the breast.

Blood Pressure

To measure blood pressure you must learn to coordinate listening to the sounds and watching the sphygmomanometer while holding the stethoscope and releasing the valve of the bulb. During the procedure, make sure the environment and the patient are quiet.

Use these tips when you listen to blood pressure.

1. The earpieces of the stethoscope should be turned toward your face. The sound will travel better if the earpieces are facing the eardrum.
2. Some stethoscopes have a bell and a diaphragm positioned opposite each other. You can switch between the two by turning the stethoscope.
3. When listening to the sounds, hold the end piece of the stethoscope firmly, just above the connection point to the tubing. Do not put your fingers on the diaphragm or bell.
4. Be sure that the diaphragm is directly over the artery. Before you place the diaphragm, palpate the artery and then place the center of the diaphragm directly over it.

Many blood pressure machines are electronic. These machines are often on a rolling pole and should be plugged into an outlet when not in use. They can be switched to an internal battery so that the machine can be taken into a patient's room. Most machines have functions that allow blood pressure and pulse to be taken at a set frequency—for example, every 15 minutes. Sometimes the machine also measures the blood oxygen level with a device that is attached to the finger. In some cases, a temperature probe is attached.

When manually taking blood pressure, make sure you are using the proper-sized cuff. The bladder inside the cuff should wrap around 80% to 100% of the arm. Place the center of the bladder over the pulse site. Check that you are hearing sound clearly through the stethoscope diaphragm, then place the stethoscope directly over the pulse site. If you are uncertain, remove the cuff, wait one to two minutes, and try again. Complete Procedure 10-4 online to practice this skill.

READING CHECK

Recall whether to take a patient's blood pressure before taking his or her temperature rectally, or in the reverse order.

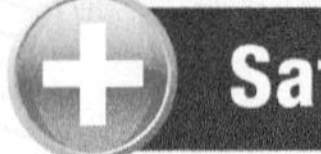

Safety

Special Safety Precautions

- If a woman has had a mastectomy (breast removal), do not take blood pressure in the arm on the side of the mastectomy.
- If a patient has an intravenous infusion (IV) or an injury, do not take blood pressure in the arm or leg where it is located.
- If a patient has a bleeding disorder, do not use an automatic blood pressure machine; there may be excess pressure exerted when the machine cuff inflates.
- When taking two or more blood pressure readings in a row on a patient, take them one to two minutes apart; remove the cuff between inflations.

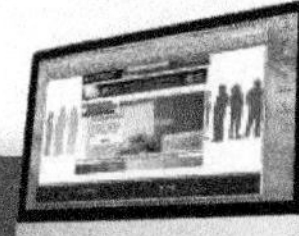

connect ONLINE PROCEDURES

PROCEDURE 10-3

Measuring and Recording Apical Pulse

Tell the patient you are going to listen to the heartbeat through the chest. Before placing the stethoscope against bare skin, rub it on the palm of your hand briskly to warm it up. Complete Procedure 10-3 online to practice this skill.

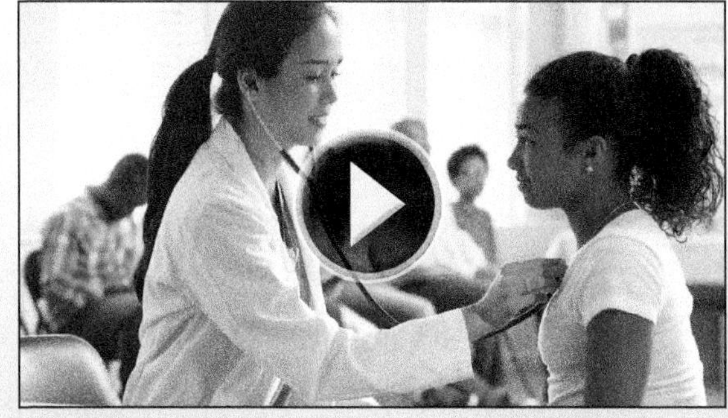

PROCEDURE 10-4

Measuring and Recording Blood Pressure

When you measure and record blood pressure, follow the step-by-step guide in this procedure.

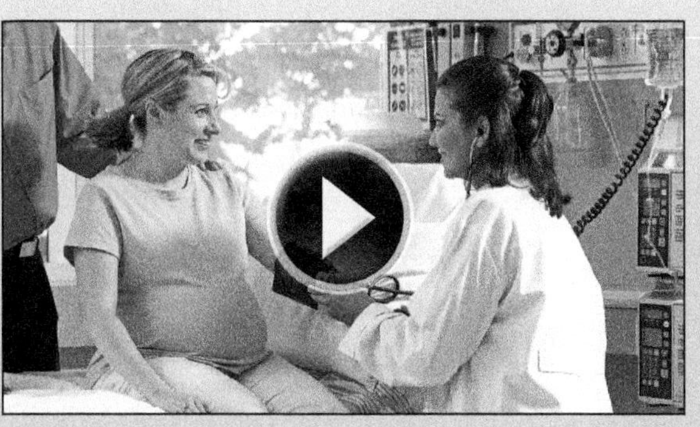

SECTION 10.2 Checking Vital Signs Review

AFTER YOU READ

1. **Define** what T P R BP stands for.
2. **Identify** the location that provides the most accurate result for an oral temperature.
3. **Identify** how long to wait to take the temperature of a patient who just had hot coffee.
4. **Describe** how you can maintain infection control when taking a temperature.
5. **Explain** one reason not to take a tympanic temperature.
6. **Calculate** the heart rate if you have counted 25 beats in 15 seconds.
7. **Indicate** how long you must count the pulse rate if a pulse is irregular.
8. **Explain** when apical pulse is usually taken.

Technology ONLINE EXPLORATIONS

Heart Attack Signs

Visit the National Heart, Lung, and Blood Institute (NHLBI) website and view the *Act in Time to Heart Attack Signs* video (www.nhlbi.nih.gov/health/prof/heart/mi/aitvideo.htm). This video discusses facts related to heart attacks and offers a plan to follow when someone has a heart attack. You may be the one who helps save a life in your family!

CHAPTER
10 Review

Chapter Summary

SECTION 10.1

- Vital signs include measurements of temperature, pulse, respiration, blood pressure, and pain. **(pg. 288)**
- Sites commonly used in assessing body temperature are oral, axillary, tympanic, temporal, and rectal. **(pg. 288)**
- Several pulse sites may be found on the body. The most commonly assessed are the radial for adults and the brachial for children. Characteristics to assess for the pulse are rate, rhythm, volume, and the presence of the pulses on both sides of the body. Pulse is recorded in beats per minute. **(pg. 291)**
- Vital signs change as a person matures. In addition to assessing the value of vital signs, it is important to assess other characteristics such as the rhythm of the pulse. **(pg. 294)**
- Respiration may be observed, or auscultated, with a stethoscope, and is best assessed when the patient is not aware of the observation. Rhythm and quality (effort) are also assessed when respiratory rates are observed. **(pg. 294)**
- Blood pressure is expressed as a fraction, with systolic blood pressure as the numerator (the top number of the fraction) and diastolic blood pressure as the denominator (the bottom number of the fraction). **(pg. 296)**
- Blood pressure may be assessed using the brachial pulse in adults and the dorsalis pedis pulse in young children. The first sound heard while auscultating a blood pressure is the systolic blood pressure, and the last sound heard is the diastolic blood pressure. **(pg. 297)**

SECTION 10.2

- Vital signs are abbreviated as T, P, R or RR, and BP to represent temperature, pulse, respiration rate, and blood pressure. **(pg. 299)**
- When documenting vital signs, use the appropriate terminology and abbreviations. Record measurements in the correct location of the chart and report any abnormal findings to an appropriate supervisor. **(pg. 299)**
- Select the location to take a patient's temperature based upon the patient's age and condition. **(pg. 299)**
- You can be more efficient with the assessment of pulse and respiration by performing the assessments one after the other. This also ensures that the patient is not aware of the respiratory assessment. **(pg. 301)**
- A stethoscope is used to check the apical pulse and with a manual blood pressure measurement. **(pg. 302)**
- Assessment of blood pressure requires coordinating the tasks of listening to the sounds, watching the dial or mercury level, and holding the stethoscope and releasing the valve of the bulb of the sphygmomanometer. **(pg. 302)**

CHAPTER 10 Assessment

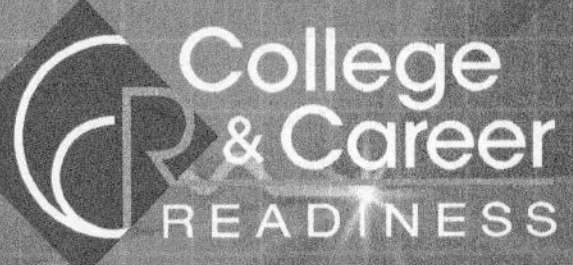

Critical Thinking/Problem Solving

1. You are assisting a nurse who has just received a client from surgery. The client's vital signs must be taken every 15 minutes for the first hour. While taking blood pressure with the automatic blood pressure machine, you see a blood pressure value of 108/110. The client's blood pressure has been averaging around 120/74. What can you do to make sure that this is a correct value?
2. While counting a young child's pulse and respirations, you are having difficulty noting the respiratory rate. What can you do?

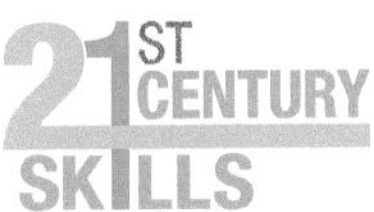

3. **Teamwork** Count your partner's pulse and respiration rate. Have your partner walk or jog in place for three to five minutes. Recount the pulse and respiration rate and note the differences.
4. **Problem Solving** Check your own apical pulse. Have your partner check your radial pulse. Compare the two numbers. Are they the same? If not, check again.
5. **Information Literacy** Visit the National Heart, Lung, and Blood Institute (NHLBI) website and view the *Act in Time to Heart Attack Signs.* This video discusses facts related to heart attacks and a plan to follow when someone has a heart attack. You may be the one who helps save a life in your family.

McGraw Hill connect™ ONLINE ACTIVITIES

Complete our HST online activities for Chapter 10, which include Concept Check review questions, Reference Flash Cards, and Online Procedures assessment sheets.

- **Concept Check** review questions
- **Reference Flash Cards** medical terminology practice
- **Online Procedures** assessment sheets

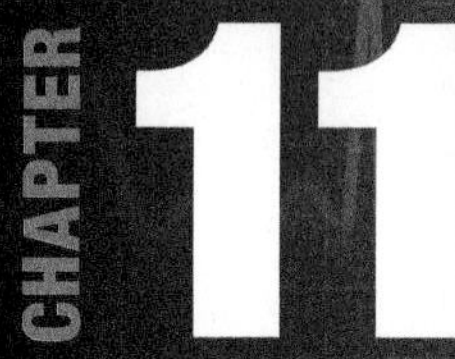

CHAPTER 11 Pharmacology and Medical Mathematics

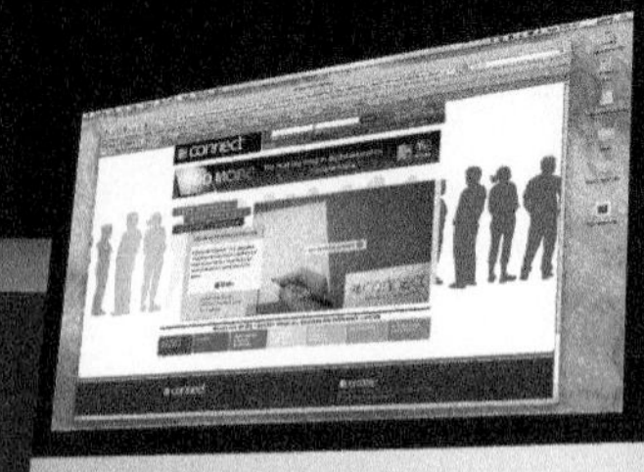

McGraw Hill connect™

It's Online!

- Online Procedures
- STEM Connection
- Medical Science
- Medical Terms
- Medical Math
- Ethics in Action
- Virtual Lab

Essential Question:

How do I safely choose and administer drugs?

This chapter will introduce you to pharmaceutical science. You will learn about medical mathematics and systems of measurement as well as how to calculate a basic medication dosage. Prescription medications and drugs are usually obtained at a pharmacy. Pharmacology is the study of drugs, and covers many specialties. Each adds to our knowledge of how drugs work and how to administer them safely and effectively.

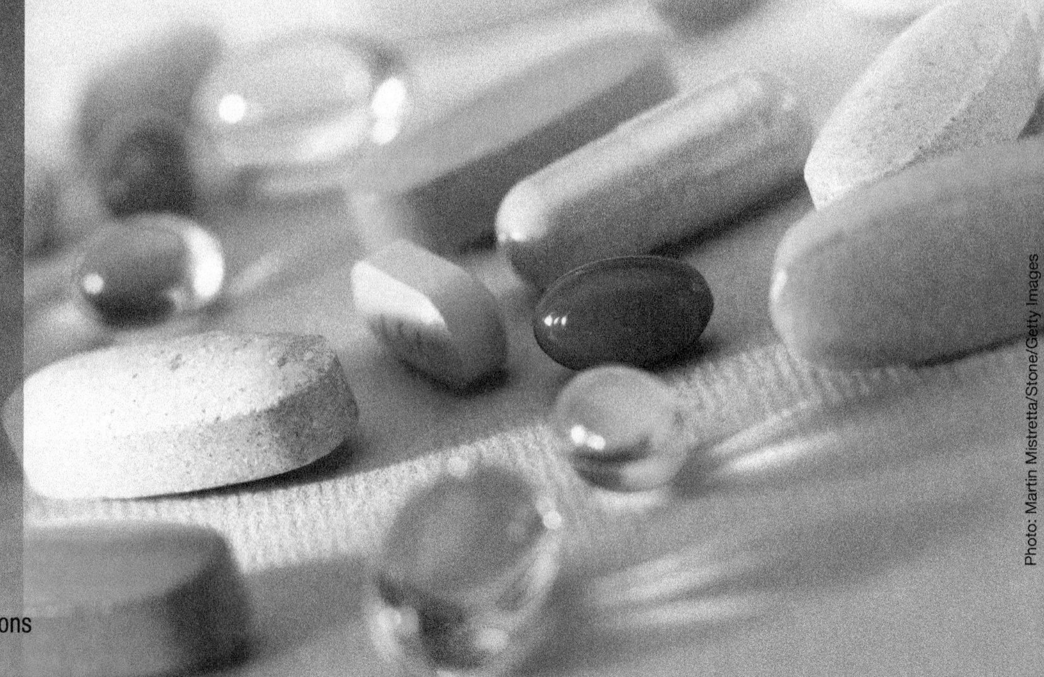

Photo: Martin Mistretta/Stone/Getty Images

READING GUIDE

OBJECTIVES

After completing this chapter, you will be able to:

- **Describe** where drugs come from.
- **Interpret** the mechanism of action of drugs.
- **Categorize** drugs into therapeutic classes.
- **Compare** the advantages and disadvantages of different routes of drug administration.
- **Compare** the four major processes of pharmacokinetics.
- **Compare** units within and among the metric, household, and avoirdupois systems.
- **Calculate** basic medication dosages.

BEFORE YOU READ

Connect How do drugs work?

Main Idea

Healthcare professionals need to know about the types of drugs and how they work in order to best care for their patients.

Note-Taking Activity

Draw this table. Write key terms and phrases under **Cues**. Write main ideas under **Note Taking**. Summarize the section under **Summary**.

Cues	Note Taking
◦	◦
◦	◦
Summary	

Graphic Organizer

Before you read the chapter, draw a diagram like the one to the right. As you read, write the classes of drugs covered in this chapter into the diagram.

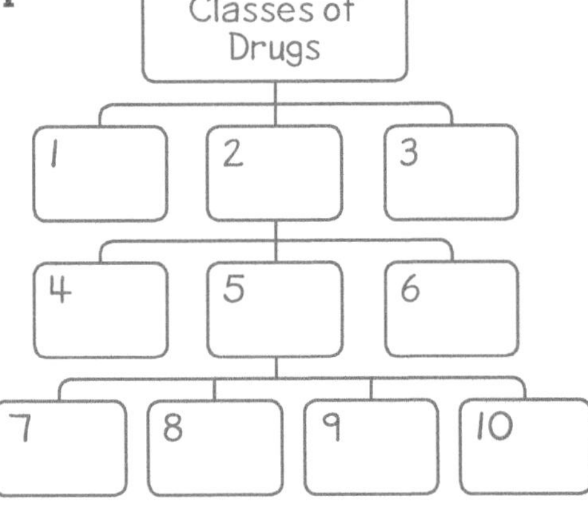

connect
Downloadable graphic organizers can be accessed online.

STANDARDS

HEALTH SCIENCE

NCHSE 1.31 Apply mathematical computations related to healthcare procedures (metric and household, conversions and measurements).

NCHSE 9.11 Apply behaviors that promote health and wellness.

SCIENCE

NSES 1 Develop an understanding of science unifying concepts and processes: systems, order, and organization; evidence, models, and explanation; change, constancy, and measurement; evolution and equilibrium; and form and function.

NCHSE *National Consortium for Health Science Education*

NSES *National Science Education Standards*

COMMON CORE STATE STANDARDS

MATHEMATICS

Number and Quantity

Quantities N-Q 1 Use units as a way to understand problems and to guide the solution of multi-step problems; choose and interpret units consistently in formulas.

ENGLISH LANGUAGE ARTS

Reading

Key Ideas and Details RST-3 Follow precisely a complex multistep procedure when carrying out experiments, taking measurements, or performing technical tasks, attending to special cases or exceptions defined in the text.

Language

Vocabulary Acquisition and Use L-4b Identify and correctly use patterns of word changes that indicate different meanings or parts of speech.

SECTION

11.1 Introduction to Pharmacology

Vocabulary

Content Vocabulary

You will learn these content vocabulary terms in this section.

- **pharmacognosy**
- **mechanism of action (MOA)**
- **pharmacotherapeutics**
- **therapeutic class**
- **binding**
- **lock and key principle**
- **receptor**
- **pharmacology**
- **side effect**

Academic Vocabulary

You will see this word in your reading and on your tests. Find its meaning in the Glossary in the back of this book.

- **channel**

Sources of Drugs

Do you know where drugs come from?

Drugs come from a variety of sources:

- Natural sources such as plants and animals
- Microscopic organisms such as bacteria, fungi, or molds
- Synthetics and bioengineering

Natural Sources

Some drugs are taken from natural sources. **Pharmacognosy** is the study of drugs that are naturally derived from plants or animals.

Modern drug therapy can be traced to the start of recorded history. The oldest known record of herbal medicines is the Ebers Papyrus, produced by the ancient Egyptians. It dates to about 1500 BCE and describes how to prepare different medications such as gargles and ointments from plants believed to have medicinal value.

Many drugs still in use are extracted from plants and animals. Some of these drugs and their uses are listed in **Table 11.1**.

There are problems associated with naturally-occurring drugs. Some are poorly absorbed into the bloodstream or broken down very quickly by the body. Isolating a drug from a plant or animal is often slow and expensive. It may result in a product containing harmful impurities. Also, some naturally-occurring products are extremely scarce.

Even though there can be problems with naturally-occurring drugs, experts in the field of pharmacognosy are still searching for new drugs.

Table 11.1 Common Drugs Obtained from Plants and Animals

SOURCE	DRUG(S)	USE
Poppy	Codeine and morphine	To treat pain
Foxglove	Digitalis	To treat congestive heart failure
Yew	Taxol	To treat cancer
Thyroid gland	Thyroid hormone	As hormone replacement
Stomach	Pepsin	As digestive enzyme

Microscopic Organisms

One of the first drugs that did not come from a plant or animal was penicillin, which is produced by a mold. Sir Alexander Fleming first isolated penicillin in 1928.

Nowadays, most of the drugs used to fight infection are made from microorganisms such as bacteria, fungi, or molds. In fact, all antibiotics are made from these sources. Chemists and molecular biologists make many of these drugs.

Synthetics and Bioengineering

Medicinal chemists have solved many of the problems associated with drugs derived from natural products. Medicinal chemistry modifies natural products by producing them synthetically or by creating new products based on natural products.

Drugs that once had to be injected have now been modified into forms that can be taken orally, inhaled, or applied topically. Synthetic drugs that can be taken once a day have replaced natural forms that had to be taken every four hours.

Aspirin, first patented in 1899, was originally an extract taken from the bark of willow trees. Crude extracts of willow bark had been used to treat pain and fever since early times. However, aspirin sold today is synthetically produced.

Bioengineering applies the most recent methods for developing new sources of medication. With bioengineering, genetically altered bacteria produce drugs that were once available only from animals. The first drug produced by this method was insulin.

Until 1980, diabetics used insulin taken from pigs or cows using a procedure developed by Sir F. G. Banting and Charles Herbert Best. One of the problems with using insulin from these sources was that the insulin was slightly different from human insulin. Some people had severe allergic reactions to animal insulin because their immune systems were reacting to the insulin as if it were foreign. Scientists have since learned how to insert the gene for human insulin into bacteria, turning the bacteria into a microscopic insulin factory. **Figure 11.1** shows how this works.

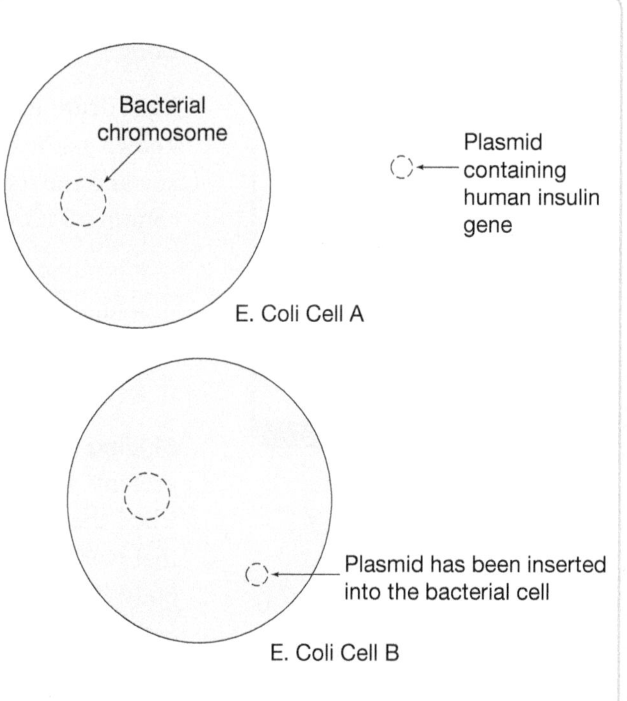

Fig. 11.1 Bioengineering Genetically modified *E. coli* contains the human insulin gene. *What improvements in insulin production have been made possible through bioengineering?*

READING CHECK

Recall three microorganisms that are used to make most of the drugs used to fight infection today.

Pharmacotherapeutics

How do drugs work in your body?

Drugs are chemicals that affect the function of living organisms. They produce their effects by interacting with other chemicals in the body. The term used to describe this is the **mechanism of action (MOA). Pharmacotherapeutics** is the study of the effects of drugs, and

- examines the MOA of drugs.
- describes the effects produced by a drug.
- determines what dose of a drug is needed to produce the desired effect.
- determines what dose of a drug produces toxic effects.

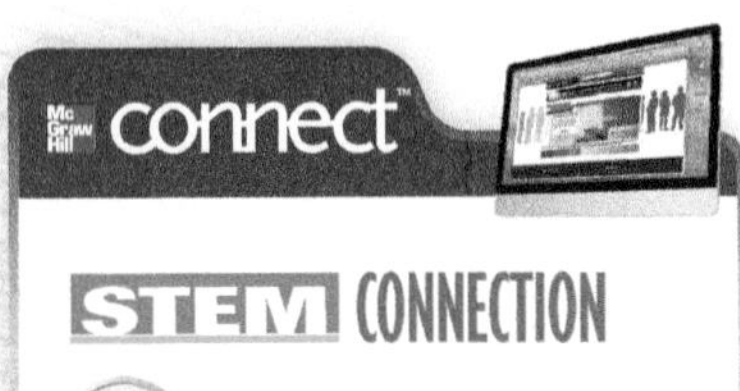

STEM CONNECTION

Medical Science

Chemotherapy
Pharmacotherapeutics uses drugs to restore a process in the body to its state of balance. Chemotherapy uses drugs to kill cells by disrupting an essential process within the cell. There are two main types of chemotherapy, each targeting a different type of cell. They are cancer chemotherapy and antibiotics. Go to connect to learn more about chemotherapy and join a discussion on your group workspace.

Follow-up Give an example of a common condition that is treated by antibiotics. How does the antibiotic kill the infection?

Mechanisms of Action

Drugs that have the same MOA are said to belong to the same **therapeutic class.** That is, they produce their effects in the same way, and have many of the same uses, advantages, and disadvantages. However, each drug within a therapeutic class is a different chemical.

For example, Benadryl® and Claritin® are two drugs used to treat allergies. They belong to the class of antihistamines. All antihistamines work by **binding** to a chemical known as the histamine receptor.

Most drugs use one of four different MOAs. MOAs all rely on what is known as the **lock and key principle** (see **Figure 11.2**). The drug is the key and the lock is the chemical to which the drug binds. The most common MOAs are:

- Binding to and stimulating a receptor in the body
- Binding to and blocking a receptor in the body
- Inhibiting an enzyme
- Decreasing the movement of a chemical across a cell membrane

Binding to and Stimulating a Receptor in the Body Receptors are proteins found in cells. The receptor causes a response within a cell when the receptor is stimulated by a naturally occurring key. Drugs that work according to this MOA imitate the natural key within the body. These drugs are sometimes called agonists or mimetics. Agonists stimulate a receptor. Mimetics mimic a natural key.

Binding to and Blocking a Receptor in the Body Some drugs bind to a receptor without causing a response. This prevents the naturally-occurring key from binding. Drugs that work according to this principle are called antagonists or blockers, because they block the natural key.

Inhibiting an Enzyme Enzymes are proteins in the body that speed up chemical reactions. There are two types of enzymes, anabolic and catabolic. Anabolic enzymes play a constructive role in our body. Catabolic enzymes play a destructive role.

Many drugs work by changing the concentration of these naturally-occurring substances. These drugs increase the concentration of something if they slow its destruction. They decrease the concentration if they slow its production. Drugs that use this MOA are called enzyme inhibitors since they change the effect of an enzyme.

Decreasing the Movement of a Chemical Across a Cell Membrane The cell membrane is the outer covering of the cell. It controls the movement of chemicals into and out of a cell. The membrane does this by using pumps or channels, which are controlled by the cell. Pumps can be turned on or off. Channels can be opened or closed. Pumps and channels have very specific functions. One pump moves sodium, another moves calcium, and so on. These pumps and channels are important to the function of nerve and muscle cells. Some drugs work by inhibiting specific pumps and others block specific channels.

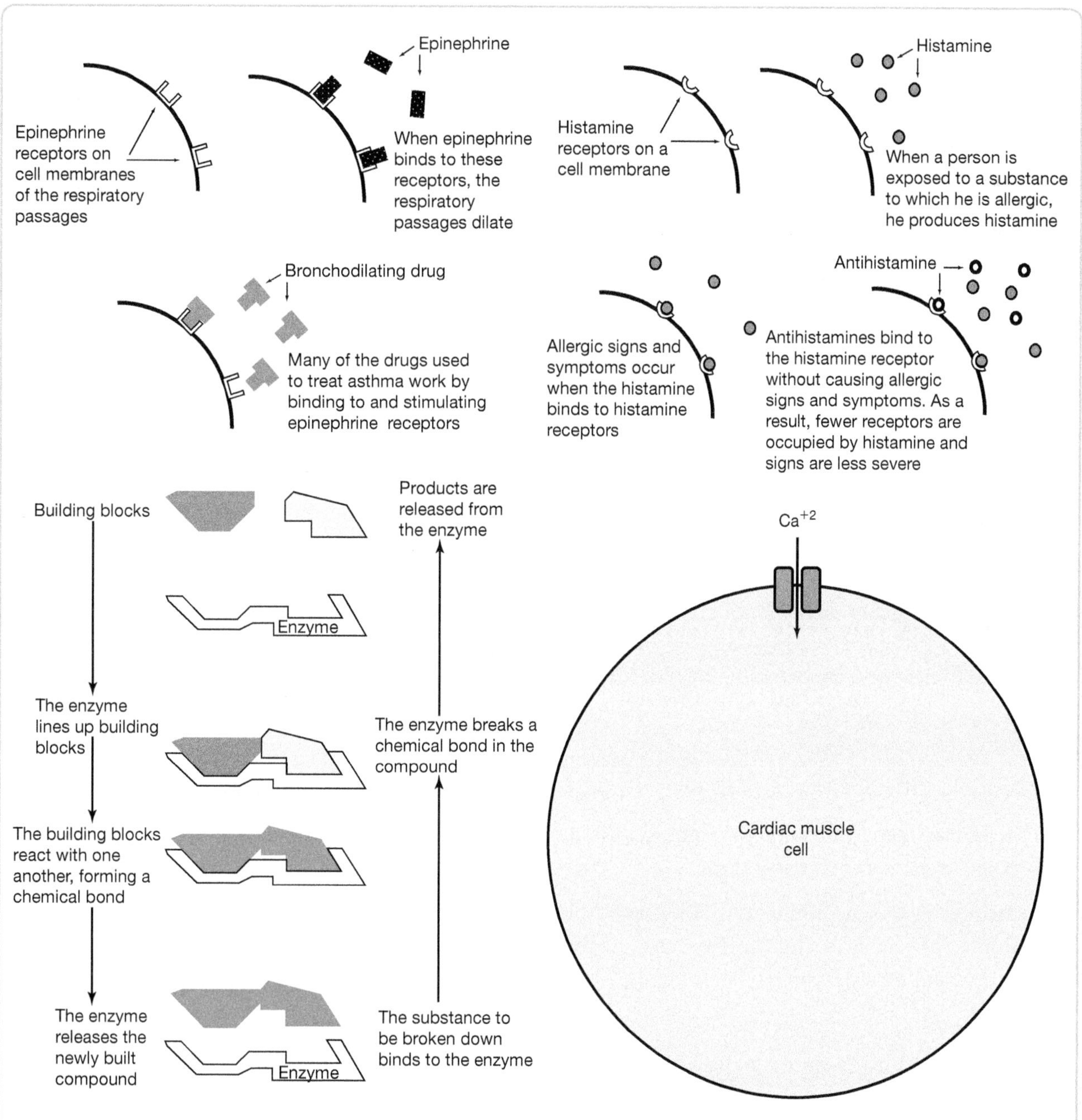

Fig. 11.2. Mechanism of Action The four MOAs. *What is the "lock and key" principle on which the four MOAs rely?*

Side Effects

In spite of all of the advances made in **pharmacology,** many drugs produce undesired effects. Any effect produced by a drug that is not the desired effect is known as a **side effect.** Side effects can be classified into two categories:

- Local side effects
- Systemic side effects

Local Side Effects These side effects occur before a drug is absorbed into the bloodstream. Some drugs, such as aspirin, irritate the lining of the stomach. Inhalers can cause a dry throat or cough. Antibiotics sometimes cause diarrhea when they kill naturally occurring bacteria in our digestive tract. A patch may irritate the skin.

Systemic Side Effects These side effects take place after a drug is absorbed into the bloodstream. Since drugs are not a natural part of our body, occasionally allergic reactions to drugs occur. Most systemic side effects happen because the drug is affecting cells other than the target cells. For example, bronchodilators produce the desired effect by stimulating epinephrine receptors in the respiratory passages. But they also increase the heart rate by stimulating epinephrine receptors in the heart, and they cause insomnia by stimulating epinephrine receptors in the brain.

Side effects will continue to be a problem until science develops a way of delivering drugs only to the desired target within the body.

READING CHECK

Describe the two categories of side effects.

SECTION 11.1 Introduction to Pharmacology Review

AFTER YOU READ

1. **List** four different sources of drugs.
2. **Describe** some advantages that synthetic drugs have over their natural precursors.
3. **Discuss** one drug obtained from a plant or animal. What is it used for? What plant or animal did it come from?
4. **Define** the term "therapeutic class."
5. **Describe** the four MOAs of drugs.
6. **Compare** systemic and local side effects.
7. **Contrast** pharmacotherapeutics and chemotherapy.

Technology ONLINE EXPLORATIONS

Mechanism of Action

Search the Internet for information on the mechanism of action (MOA) of drugs. Find one medication's MOA and create a poster, slide show, or visual presentation for your class.

SECTION

11.2 Classes of Drugs and Routes of Administration

Therapeutic Classes of Drugs

How are drugs grouped together?

This section discusses some common therapeutic classes and routes of administration of drugs.

There are numerous therapeutic classes of drugs. The drugs within the same therapeutic class produce their effect in the same way.

Differences between drugs within a therapeutic class do exist, however. Sometimes clients respond better to one drug than another, even if the drugs are from the same therapeutic class. Although the drugs within a class usually cause the same side effects, the severity or frequency of the side effect may differ. One drug within a class may irritate a client's stomach; another may keep a client awake at night. For example, Benadryl® is more likely to cause drowsiness than Claritin®. A physician considers these differences when deciding which drug from a class is most appropriate for a client.

Some of the common therapeutic classes of drugs include angiotension converting enzyme inhibitors, Beta-1 blockers, Beta-2 agonists, antihistamines, proton pump inhibitors, and statins. For a list of the therapeutic classes and representative drugs, see **Table 11.2** on pages 314 and 315.

Vocabulary

Content Vocabulary

You will learn these content vocabulary terms in this section.

- **vasoconstriction**
- **route of administration**
- **onset of action**
- **parenteral route**
- **gauge**

Academic Vocabulary

You will see these words in your reading and on your tests. Find their meanings in the Glossary in the back of this book.

- **release**
- **trigger**
- **administration**

ACE (Angiotensin-Converting Enzyme) Inhibitors

ACE inhibitors make up a class of drugs that regulate blood pressure by inhibiting the angiotensin-converting enzyme. These drugs are available by prescription only.

Angiotensin is a protein that occurs naturally in the body. It is a powerful vasoconstrictor used by the body to regulate blood pressure. **Vasoconstriction** is a narrowing of blood vessels. When blood vessels become narrow, blood pressure increases.

For that reason, if angiotensin is overactive a client will develop high blood pressure (hypertension). An enzyme called the angiotensin-converting enzyme (ACE) activates angiotensin. If the ACE is inhibited or blocked, the amount of angiotensin produced by the body is reduced. The reduction of angiotensin dilates or widens the blood vessels and lowers blood pressure.

Below you will read brief descriptions of some common therapeutic classes of drugs. **Table 11.2** on pages 314 and 315 shows representative drugs, their indications, and common side effects.

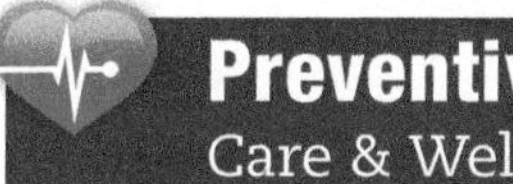

Preventive Care & Wellness

Taking Medications Correctly

Did you know that sometimes taking only part of a medication or taking it the wrong way could do more harm than good? Always follow the instructions or labels on any prescription medication you are given. Do not take old medication and never take someone else's prescription medication. Ask your pharmacist or physician if you have questions or problems.

Table 11.2 Therapeutic Classes and Representative Drugs

THERAPEUTIC CLASS	INDICATIONS	REPRESENTATIVE DRUGS		COMMON SIDE EFFECTS
ACE Inhibitors	Hypertension Congestive Heart Failure	Lisinopril Prinivil® Zetril®	Accupril® Vasotec®	Headache Dizziness
Beta-1 Blockers	Hypertension Rapid heartbeat (tachycardia)	Lopressor® Toprol® Tenormin®		Dizziness Drowsiness
Beta-2 Agonists	Asthma Emphysema	Ventolin® Albuterol Proventil® Brethine®	Serevent® Alupent®	Tremors Increased heart rate Insomnia
Antihistamines	Itching Nasal congestion Seasonal allergies, such as hay fever	Allegra® Benadryl® Claritin® Zyrtec®		Dry mouth Drowsiness
H_2 Antagonists	GERD (gastroesophageal reflux disorder) Gastric ulcers Duodenal ulcers	Tagamet® Pepcid® Zantac®		Diarrhea Headache
Proton pump inhibitors	GERD (gastroesophageal reflux disorder) Gastric ulcers Duodenal ulcers	Prilosec® Prevacid® Aciphex®	Protonix® Nexium®	Diarrhea Headache
Narcotic analgesics	Severe pain	Morphine Codeine Demerol® Hydrocodone	Vicodin® Percodan®	Drowsiness Slow and shallow respirations Constipation
NSAIDs	Mild to moderate pain Inflammation Fever	Aspirin Motrin® Advil® Aleve®	Ibuprofen Naprosyn®	Stomach irritation

Table 11.2 continued

THERAPEUTIC CLASS	INDICATIONS	REPRESENTATIVE DRUGS	COMMON SIDE EFFECTS
Reverse transcriptase inhibitors	HIV infection	AZT Combivir® Sustiva® Retrovir®	Anemia Fever Headache Lack of energy Nausea and vomiting Diarrhea Stomach pain Cough Shortness of breath Sore throat
Statins	High cholesterol	Lipitor® Pravachol® Crestor® Zocor®	Nausea and vomiting Diarrhea Liver damage

Beta-1 Blockers

Epinephrine, which is also called adrenaline, and norepinephrine are chemicals that occur naturally in the body and produce many effects. Normally they are released at a low level. However, they are released at a higher level when a person is startled, frightened, or anxious. One of the effects of epinephrine and norepinephrine is a rapid heartbeat, or tachycardia. They bind to and stimulate beta-1 receptors, which are found in the heart.

Beta-1 blockers are drugs that bind to beta-1 receptors without stimulating them. When they do this, they prevent epinephrine and norepinephrine from binding. This decreases the heart rate. These drugs are available by prescription only. Common side effectives of these drugs are dizziness and drowsiness.

Beta-2 Agonists

Epinephrine causes numerous responses within the body. In the lungs, epinephrine causes the dilation of the bronchioles, or small airways. Epinephrine produces this effect by binding to and stimulating beta-2 receptors on the smooth muscle cells of the bronchioles. Beta-2 receptors are responsible for the function of your smooth muscles. These are the muscles that control body functions but that you do not have control over.

Common side effects of these drugs include tremors, increased heart rate, and insomnia.

Beta-2 agonists are drugs that produce the same effect in the lungs as the naturally occurring epinephrine. They mimic the action of epinephrine by stimulating the beta-2 receptors. They are one of the bronchodilators used to treat the effects of respiratory diseases because they dilate the small airways of the bronchioles. These prescription drugs are available in oral form as tablets or liquids, but are more often prescribed in the form of inhalers.

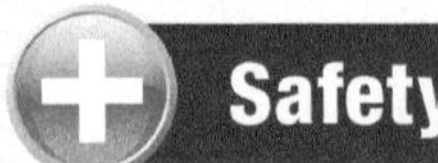

Safety

Check the Label!

Before you give a medication, always read its label. Some medications come in a liquid form, for example, drops for the eyes, which are optic drops, or for the ears, which are otic drops. Because the spelling of "optic" and "otic" is so similar, a mistake in the route of administration could be made. Putting eardrops in an eye could cause severe irritation. Never administer a drug by any route other than what is intended.

Antihistamines

Histamine is a chemical that is released from cells known as mast cells when a person is exposed to an allergen. Allergens are substances that cause allergies. Histamine binds to and stimulates histamine receptors, causing the symptoms associated with an allergy. These include sneezing, runny nose, and watery eyes.

Antihistamines are drugs that bind to histamine receptors but do not stimulate them. The presence of an antihistamine prevents histamine from binding and reduces the symptoms of allergy. Antihistamines are available over the counter or as prescription medication. Common side effects of these medications include dry mouth and drowsiness.

H_2 Antagonists

Histamine is associated with allergies, but also it produces other effects in the body. The presence of food in the stomach triggers the release of histamine, which causes the secretion of hydrochloric acid into the stomach. Histamine produces this effect when it binds to and stimulates H_2 receptors, which are found only in the stomach. Too much histamine can cause an excessive amount of hydrochloric acid in the stomach. This can cause gastrointestinal disorders. H_2 antagonists block these receptors. They do this by binding to the H_2 receptors without stimulating them. This decreases the amount of acid secreted into the stomach following a meal. H_2 antagonists are available by prescription and over the counter.

Proton Pump Inhibitors

Cells in the stomach, called parietal cells, use proton pumps to move hydrogen ions into the cells. The parietal cells use the hydrogen ions when they produce stomach acid. Proton pump inhibitors are drugs that turn off these pumps and thus reduce stomach acid. Proton pump inhibitors are available by prescription and over the counter. Common side effects of these drugs are diarrhea and headache.

Narcotic Analgesics

Endorphins are naturally occurring pain relievers produced by our bodies. They inhibit nerve cells that carry pain impulses to our brain when they bind to and stimulate endorphin receptors in the spine. Narcotic analgesics bind to and stimulate the same receptors. Therefore, they reduce pain. These drugs are the most potent pain medications available and are available by prescription only.

NSAIDs (Nonsteroidal Anti-inflammatory Drugs)

Prostaglandins are chemicals produced in the body that cause the pain and swelling associated with inflammation. One of the enzymes that makes prostaglandins is prostaglandin synthase. Nonsteroidal anti-inflammatory drugs (NSAIDs) inhibit this enzyme, thus reducing the production of prostaglandins and decreasing pain. Prescription and nonprescription NSAIDs are available.

Reverse Transcriptase Inhibitors

The human immunodeficiency virus (HIV) is the virus that causes AIDS. HIV infects the cells of the immune system by injecting a cell with a small piece of its ribonucleic acid (RNA). Inside the cell, RNA is converted into deoxyribonucleic acid (DNA), using an enzyme called reverse transcriptase. The cell produces thousands of new viruses, which infect thousands of other cells. Reverse transcriptase inhibitors decrease the activity of this enzyme, slowing the progress of HIV.

Statins

The leading cause of death in the United States is heart disease, and one of the biggest contributors to heart disease is high cholesterol. The liver produces much of the cholesterol in our body. For some people, diet changes are not sufficient to lower cholesterol levels. One of the enzymes needed by our liver to produce cholesterol is the HMG CoA reductase enzyme. Statins are drugs that inhibit the HMG CoA reductase enzyme, thus reducing the production of cholesterol. They are the most commonly prescribed group of drugs in the United States.

READING CHECK

Explain the function of NSAIDs.

Routes of Administration

How do you take medication?

Routes of administration are the ways used to get a drug into the tissues of the body. The two main routes are:

- Oral, which is by mouth
- Parenteral, which is other than by mouth

Oral Administration

The more common route of administration is oral. A drug administered orally can be a tablet, a capsule, or a liquid. This is more convenient but usually needs 30 to 60 minutes to take effect. Some drugs are placed under the tongue or in the cheek. These will take less time to start working. The time needed before a drug takes effect is known as the **onset of action.**

Parenteral Administration

All other routes of administration are called **parenteral routes** of administration. The onset of action with parenteral administration can be very rapid. For example, drugs administered intravenously can take effect in less than a minute.

Parenteral Routes of Administration There are many parenteral routes of administration (see **Table 11.3**). Some frequently used routes are the metered-dose inhaler, the transdermal patch, injections, and intravenous.

Table 11.3 Parenteral Routes of Administration

ROUTE	DESCRIPTION	APPROXIMATE ONSET OF ACTION	INDICATIONS	EXAMPLES
Buccal	Tablet placed in cheek	Several minutes	When effects of digestion must be avoided	Androgenic drugs
Inhalation	Drug inhaled into the nasal cavity or lungs	Within one minute	For local effects within the respiratory tract	Decongestants, antiasthmatics
Intramuscular (IM)	Drug injected into a muscle	Several minutes	When a drug is absorbed poorly and when high blood levels are desired	Narcotic analgesics, antibiotics
Intravenous (IV)	Drug injected into the blood in a vein	Within one minute	For situations requiring immediate effects or for drugs that are rapidly destroyed in the body	Antiarrhythmics, antibiotics
Rectal	Suppository, cream, or ointment	15 to 30 minutes	For local effect or when client cannot take oral medication	Laxatives, nausea medication
Subcutaneous (subcut)	Drug injected into the fatty layer beneath the skin	Several minutes	When a drug would be inactivated by the gastrointestinal tract	Insulin
Sublingual	Tablet placed under the tongue	Several minutes	When rapid effects are needed	Nitroglycerin
Topical	Creams, ointments, lotions, drops	Within one hour	For local effects on the skin, eye, or ear	Hydrocortisone cream
Transdermal patch	Adhesive patch applied to skin	30 to 60 minutes	When continuous absorption and systemic effects over many hours are needed	Nitroglycerin, estrogen
Vaginal	Suppositories, creams	15 to 30 minutes	For local effects	Antifungal medications for yeast infections

Metered-Dose Inhaler Metered-dose inhalers are used to deliver medications directly to the lungs, through the inhalation route of administration. This route allows for rapid action. Systemic side effects are usually minimal. You will find a discussion of metered-dose inhalers and the procedure for administering the medications they dispense in Chapter 19, Respiratory Care. **Figure 11.3** shows an example of a metered-dose inhaler.

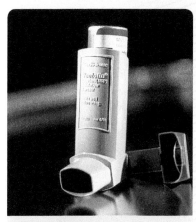

Fig. 11.3 Inhaler This is a metered-dose inhaler. *What is this medication's route of administration?*

Transdermal Patch Patches are designed to deliver a constant amount of drug over an extended period of time, usually 24 hours. When used properly, they are one of the most consistent and convenient dosage forms. An example of a transdermal patch is shown in **Figure 11.4.** For a patch to deliver a drug properly, the following guidelines should be followed:

- Remove the old patch, if any, and discard it.
- Select a site for applying a new patch.
- The site must be hairless.
- The site must be intact, with no cuts, rash, or irritation.
- Apply the patch, making sure that the backing is removed completely and that the patch is in firm contact with the skin.

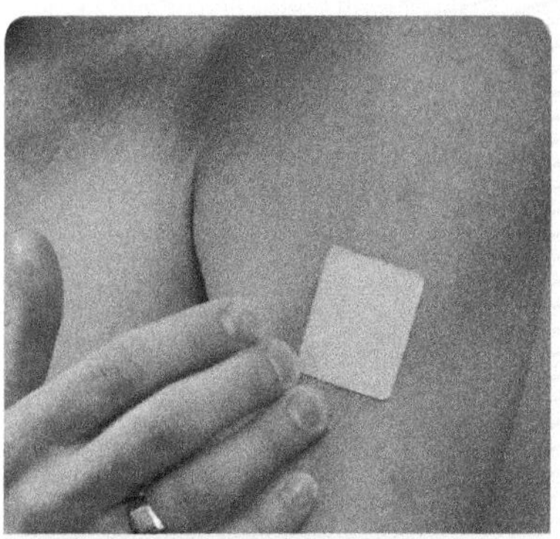

Fig. 11.4 Transdermal Patch A transdermal patch is used to deliver a constant amount of drug. *What are some advantages of using a transdermal patch like this one?*

Injections Injections are given when a rapid effect is needed and when a drug would be destroyed by the digestive system if it were taken orally. An injection is also used when a local effect is desired, such as with a local anesthetic (see **Figure 11.5**). The two most common types of injections are:

- Subcutaneous, an injection into the fatty layer just beneath the skin
- Intramuscular, an injection into a muscle

Subcutaneous, or subcut, injections are given in the upper arm, the thigh, or the abdomen. The needles are normally about ½ inch long and 25 gauge or smaller. **Gauge** is a measurement of the thickness of a needle. No more than 1 mL can be given with a subcut injection.

Intramuscular (IM) injections are normally given into relatively large muscles of the shoulder, buttocks, or outer portions of the thigh. A longer needle must be used, usually 1 to 1½ inches long, 23 gauge or larger. Up to 3 mL of a drug can be given with an IM injection, although injections into the shoulder are limited to 1 mL. Antibiotics and narcotic analgesics are often given by intramuscular injection.

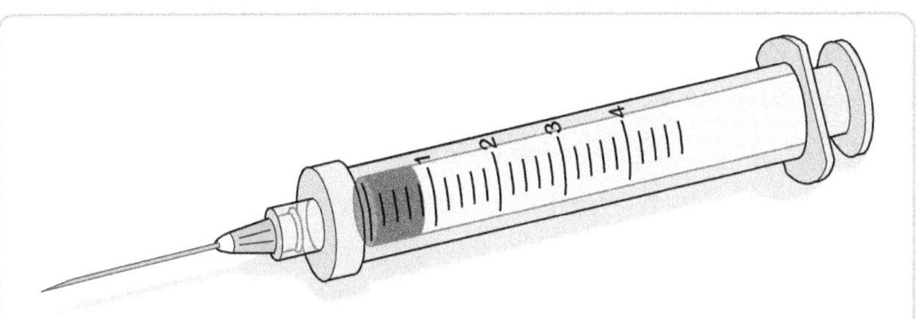

Fig. 11.5 Syringe A shorter needle is used for a subcut injection. *Do you know why?*

Intravenous The intravenous (IV) route is an injection directly into a vein. Medications are delivered by IV when a rapid effect is needed or when the medication would be irritating to subcut or IM tissue. IVs are also used to administer fluids to clients who cannot eat or drink.

READING CHECK

Name four examples of parenteral administration.

Connect ONLINE PROCEDURES

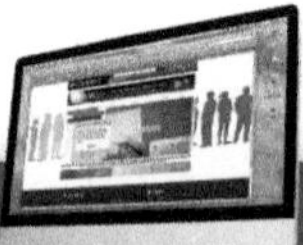

PROCEDURE 11-1

Identifying Medications and their Classifications

Drugs in the same therapeutic class produce their effect on the patient in the same manner. There are numerous therapeutic classes of medications. Each includes various medications. Some are more common than others.

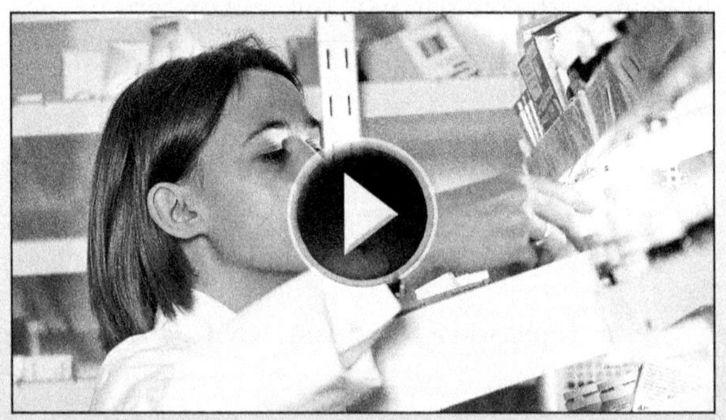

SECTION 11.2 Classes of Drugs and Routes of Administration Review

AFTER YOU READ

1. **Explain** the mechanism of action (MOA) of antihistamines.
2. **Explain** the mechanism of action of aspirin.
3. **Describe** the use of reverse transcriptase inhibitors.
4. **Analyze** how someone can have high cholesterol even on a low-cholesterol diet. What class of medicine would help this client?
5. **Define** the term "parenteral."
6. **Arrange** the following routes of administration in order of onset of action, from fastest to slowest: intramuscular, inhalation, topical, buccal.
7. **Explain** which route of administration is most common. Why?

Technology ONLINE EXPLORATIONS

The Top 50 Medications

Search the Internet to find the 50 most prescribed medications. Create a table similar to **Table 11.2** to share with your class.

Photo: image100/Getty Images

SECTION 11.3

Pharmacokinetics and Dosages

Pharmacokinetics

How do drugs work in the body?

A drug's effects are mainly determined by how much of the drug is in the plasma. Plasma is the liquid part of the blood. The goal of drug treatment is to get the correct plasma concentration. It should be high enough to produce a therapeutic effect but not so high as to cause harm. The range of concentrations (minimum to maximum) that achieves this objective is the **therapeutic range** of a drug. **Figure 11.6** illustrates that range.

Pharmacokinetics is the study of four processes that affect the plasma concentration of drugs. These processes affect which dosage form will be used. They also affect how much drug needs to be administered and how often the drug is given. The four processes, as shown in **Figure 11.7** on page 322, are:

- **A**bsorption
- **D**istribution
- **M**etabolism (transformation)
- **E**limination

You can remember these processes by the first letter of each word: ADME.

Vocabulary

Content Vocabulary

You will learn these content vocabulary terms in this section.

- therapeutic range
- pharmacokinetics
- absorption
- distribution
- metabolism
- elimination
- loading dose
- maintenance dose
- dosage

Academic Vocabulary

You will see this word in your reading and on your tests. Find its meaning in the Glossary in the back of this book.

- chemical

Absorption

Absorption is the process by which a drug enters the blood plasma. For an oral medication to enter the plasma, it must first be dissolved in the fluid in the stomach or intestines. Once dissolved, the drug must pass through the membranes of the gastrointestinal (GI) tract and blood vessels in order to reach the plasma.

Two properties have the greatest impact on how quickly absorption occurs. One is how quickly drugs dissolve. The other is how easily they can move through the cell membranes.

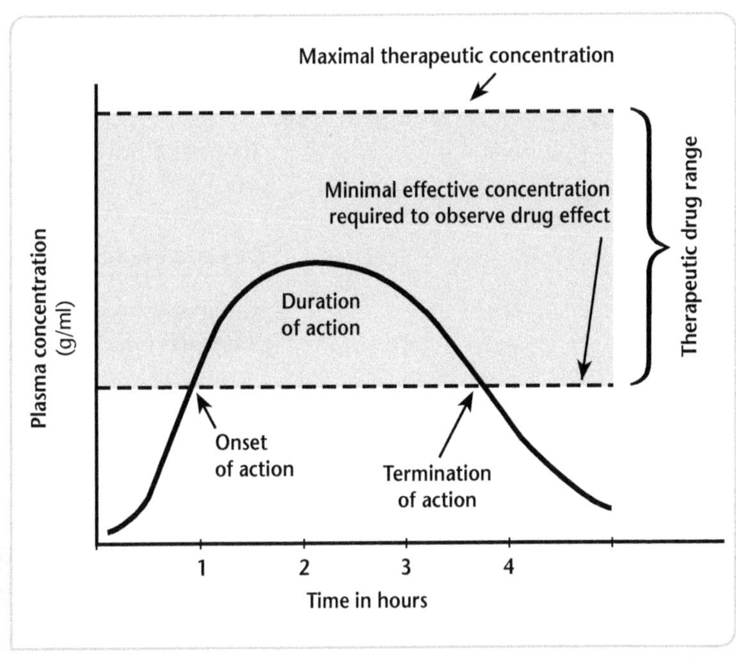

Fig. 11.6 Therapeutic Range Therapeutic range is the range of drug concentration in plasma. *What happens within this range?*

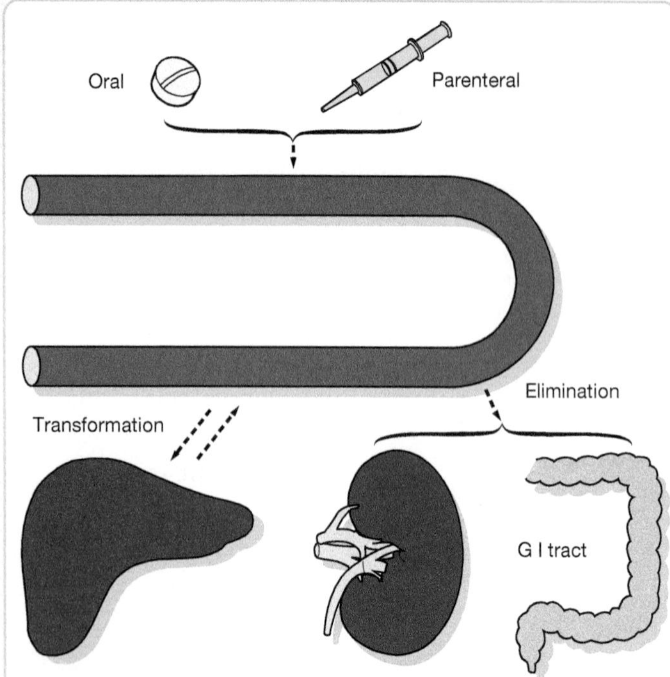

Fig. 11.7 ADME The four processes of pharmacokinetics are absorption, distribution, metabolism (transformation), and elimination. *What are five ways in which drugs are eliminated from the body?*

Distribution

Distribution refers to where the drug goes after entering the plasma. Some of the drug binds to proteins in the plasma. Some of the drug diffuses out of the bloodstream into other tissues. The chemical properties of a drug determine what other tissues a drug will most likely enter. Some drugs concentrate in fatty tissues. Others enter the cerebrospinal fluid. Almost every fluid in the body will contain at least a trace amount of the drug. In most cases, only a small percentage of the drug that is absorbed will reach the site where it will exert its effects.

Metabolism (Transformation)

All the chemical changes in a drug after it has been absorbed into the body take place during **metabolism.**

Metabolism is the chemical change that takes place in a drug after it has been absorbed by the body. The drug **transforms,** or changes, after it has been absorbed.

Most of these chemical changes occur in the liver. Some chemical changes destroy the activity of a drug, but not all do. For example, the liver alters a drug mainly to make the drug more water-soluble, so that it can be more easily removed from the body by the kidneys.

Elimination

Elimination is the process that removes a drug from the body. Most drugs are eliminated primarily in the urine. Smaller amounts of a drug may also be found in feces (stool), sweat, tears, saliva, and breast milk.

READING CHECK

Explain how drugs are eliminated from the body.

Dosages

How do you know how much of a drug to give?

Occasionally a large initial dose of a drug is given, so that the concentration of the drug in the plasma reaches the therapeutic range more quickly. This initial large dose is called a **loading dose.** Smaller doses are then taken at regular intervals to keep the plasma concentration in the therapeutic range. These smaller doses are known as **maintenance doses.**

Effects of Individual Differences on Maintenance Doses

Dosage, or the amount of a drug to be administered, is normally based on the weight of an individual. Body weight is, however, not the only factor that determines the dosage. The amount of a drug and the frequency with which it is administered may be different for two people of the same body weight.

Other factors that influence dosage are the individual's rates of absorption, distribution, metabolism, or elimination of the drug being administered. For example, the rate or amount of absorption of a drug can be affected by the state of the digestive tract, which can be affected by age or disease. Since many drugs tend to concentrate in fatty tissues, one very important factor affecting distribution is the individual's percentage of body fat. In addition to age and weight, malnutrition and dehydration can also affect distribution and, therefore, dosage. Metabolism is most affected by liver disease, and elimination is affected by kidney disease.

Maintenance doses may have to be adjusted for any of the factors described above.

READING CHECK

Recall the factors that affect the amount of a drug to be administered.

SECTION 11.3 Pharmacokinetics and Dosages Review

AFTER YOU READ

1. **Describe** the four processes that contribute to the pharmacokinetic properties of a drug.
2. **Identify** the two properties of a drug that determine how rapidly that drug will be absorbed.
3. **Explain** the difference between a loading dose and a maintenance dose.
4. **List** some factors contributing to individual dosage differences.
5. **Indicate** which organ is responsible for the chemical change, or transformation, of a drug after it has been absorbed by the body.

Technology ONLINE EXPLORATIONS

Dosage Calculation

Search the Internet for a medication that is given in different dosages based upon weight. Try searching for antibiotics, such as amoxicillin or erythromycin. Check for the amount of medication to be given for each kilogram (kg) of weight. Determine how much medication is to be given for a child who weighs 14.5 kg.

SECTION

11.4 Medical Mathematics

Vocabulary

Content Vocabulary

You will learn these content vocabulary terms in this section.

- **metric system**
- **avoirdupois system**

Academic Vocabulary

You will see this word in your reading and on your tests. Find its meaning in the Glossary in the back of this book.

- **volume**

The Metric System

Which metric units have you used to measure items in your science classes?

You will need knowledge of basic medical mathematics in order to enter the field of healthcare. Understanding the systems of measure, mathematical conversions, and basic dosage calculations are also important to practice in the healthcare industry.

The **metric system** is the most widely used system of measurement in pharmacy. The basic units of measure in the metric system are the gram (g), which is used for weight or mass, and the liter (L), which is used to measure volume. The metric system is a decimal system. This means that it is based on multiples of 10.

The dosage of a drug is usually given in milligrams (mg). Liquid medications are often measured in milliliters (mL). When you calculate dosages, you will usually need to know the client's weight in kilograms (kg).

A system of prefixes is used to show how large or small a unit in the metric system is. For example, one unit in the metric system is the meter. The prefix *hecto-* means 100. The prefix *deci-* means a tenth. So a hectometer is 100 meters, and a decimeter is 1/10 (or 0.1) of a meter.

If you must convert from one unit to another within the metric system, you need to know which direction to move the decimal point and how far it needs to be moved.

Table 11.4 lists the metric prefixes from *kilo-* through *milli-*, gives the meaning of each prefix, and shows how the prefixes are combined with the base units for weight and volume.

Table 11.4 Metric Prefixes

	KILO-	HECTO-	DEKA-	NO PREFIX	DECI-	CENTI-	MILLI-
Meaning	×1000	×100	×10		÷10	÷100	÷1000
Abbreviation	k	h	da		d	c	m
Weight	kg	hg	dag	g	dg	cg	mg
Volume	kL	hL	daL	L	dL	cL	mL
	Kate	had	dates	who	didn't	call	much

Converting Between Metric Units of Measure

When you convert from one unit of metric measurement to another, follow these rules.

- Move the decimal to the right if you convert from larger to smaller.
- Move the decimal to the left if you convert from smaller to a larger.

Figure 11.8 will help you determine the direction and the number of places to move the decimal point when you convert between units of metric measurement. For example, milliliter is three places to the right of liter, the basic unit. To convert a quantity from liters (larger) to milliliters (smaller), move the decimal point three places to the right. Similarly, to convert a quantity from grams (smaller) to kilograms (larger), move the decimal point three places to the left.

Now try converting units within the metric system:

Table 11.5 Metric, Household, and Avoirdupois Equivalents

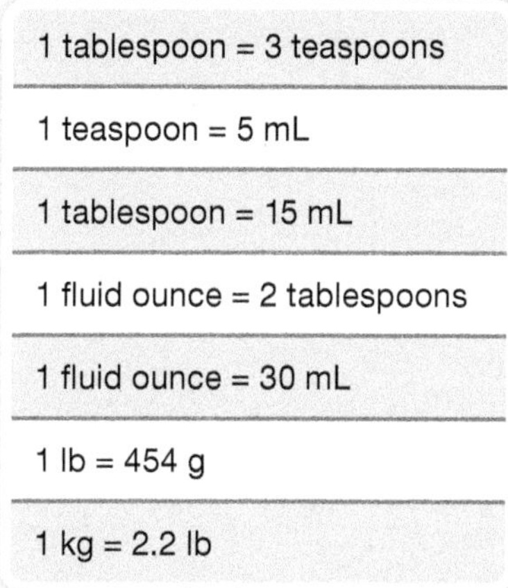

1 tablespoon = 3 teaspoons
1 teaspoon = 5 mL
1 tablespoon = 15 mL
1 fluid ounce = 2 tablespoons
1 fluid ounce = 30 mL
1 lb = 454 g
1 kg = 2.2 lb

Convert 15 g to milligrams (mg)

Follow the rule, by moving the decimal point three steps to the right.

a. First, add a decimal point to the measurement (15 g):
   15. g
b. Since we will need to move the decimal point three places to the right, we will have to add three zeros:
   15.000 g
c. Next move the decimal point three places to the right and change the unit from gram (g) to milligram (mg):
   15,000 mg
d. We have now changed the unit from grams (g) to milligrams (mg):
   15 g = 15,000 mg

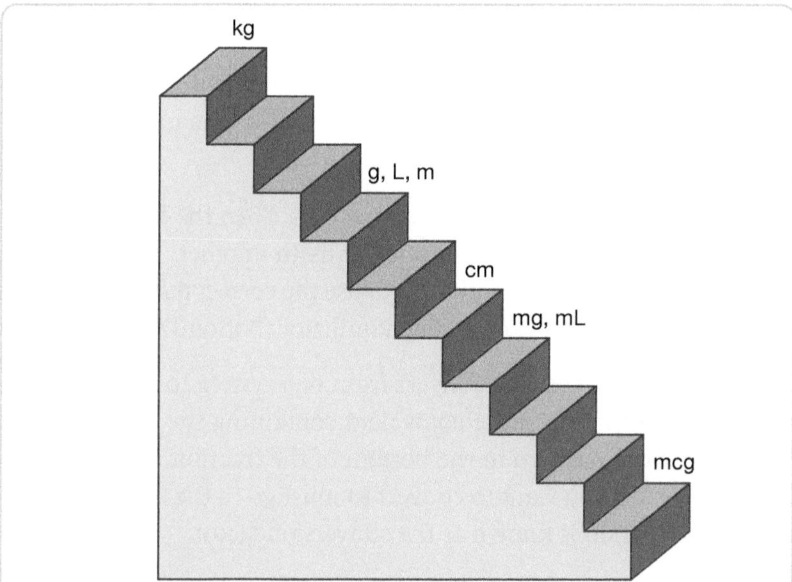

Fig. 11.8 Metric Steps Each step in the diagram represents one decimal place. This helps determine the direction and number of places to move a decimal point during conversion. *What is the unit of measure two steps up from the unit meter?*

Convert 120 grams to kilograms.

We will need to move the decimal point three places to the left to change from grams to kilograms (kg).

a. Move the decimal three places to the left. To do this, add a zero to the right of the decimal point. Also, add a zero to the left of the decimal point. Change the unit. (Note a zero is used to the left of a decimal point when a number is not in this position.)
0.120

b. We have now changed the unit from grams (g) to (kg):
120 g = 0.12 kg

READING CHECK

Describe the relationship to any metric base unit when the prefixes *kilo-*, *centi-*, and *milli-* are added to the unit.

Other Systems of Measure

Do you know the two most common systems in addition to the metric system?

Systems other than the metric system are the household system, the avoirdupois system, and the apothecary system.

The household system of measurement includes measurements used in the kitchen. Examples are the teaspoon and tablespoon.

The **avoirdupois system** measures by units such as the fluid ounce and pound.

The apothecary system is seldom used today. This ancient system is based on the minim (for measuring volume) and grain (for measuring weight).

Converting Between Systems of Measure

You will often find it necessary to convert from one unit of measure to another.

An equivalent can be rewritten as a fraction. Then the fraction can be used to convert from one system of units to another. The key when rewriting equivalents as fractions is to use the correct part of the equivalent in the numerator (top) and denominator (bottom) of the fraction.

Follow this rule when you convert from one system to another using equivalents: The part of the equivalent containing the unit you want to convert ***from*** must go in the bottom of the fraction. The part containing the unit you want to convert ***to*** must go in the top of the fraction. This fraction is known as the conversion factor.

Which conversion factor would you use to convert from kilograms to pounds?

a. Find the equivalent for pounds and kilograms.
1 kilogram (kg) = 2.2 pounds (lb)

b. Rewrite the equivalent as a fraction, putting the unit you are converting from on the bottom and the unit you are converting to on the top. This is the conversion factor to use to convert kilograms to pounds.

$$\frac{2.2 \text{ lb}}{1 \text{ kg}}$$

Which conversion factor would you use to convert from milliliters to fluid ounces?

a. Find the equivalent for milliliters and fluid ounces.
   1 fluid ounce = 30 milliliters (mL)

b. Rewrite the equivalent as a fraction, putting the unit you are converting from on the bottom and the unit you are converting to on the top.

$$\frac{1 \text{ fluid ounce}}{30 \text{ mL}}$$

Using Conversion Factors To convert units, review the following:

Convert 110 pounds to kilograms.

a. Find the equivalent containing pounds and kilograms.
   1 kilogram (kg) = 2.2 pounds (lb)

b. Rewrite the equivalent as a fraction, putting the unit you are converting from on the bottom and the unit you are converting to on the top.

$$\frac{1 \text{ kg}}{2.2 \text{ lb}}$$

c. Set up the problem with the known amount in the numerator. Cancel like units from the numerator and denominator.

$$\frac{110 \cancel{\text{lb}} \times 1 \text{ kg}}{2.2 \cancel{\text{lb}}}$$

d. To arrive at your answer:
   (110 x 1) ÷ 2.2 = 50 kg. 110 lbs is equal to 50 kg.

Convert 12.5 mL to teaspoons.

a. Find the equivalent containing milliliters and teaspoons.
   1 teaspoon = 5 mL

b. Rewrite the equivalent as a fraction, putting the unit you are converting from on the bottom and the unit you are converting to on the top.

$$\frac{1 \text{ teaspoon}}{5 \text{ mL}}$$

   Set up the problem with the known amount in the numerator.

c. Cancel like units in the numerator and denominator.

$$\frac{12.5 \cancel{\text{mL}} \times 1 \text{ teaspoon}}{5 \cancel{\text{mL}}}$$

d. To arrive at your answer:
   (12.5 x 1) ÷ 5 = 2.5. 12.5 milliliters is equal to 2.5 teaspoons.

READING CHECK

Recall the conversion factor you should use when converting from ounces to milliliters.

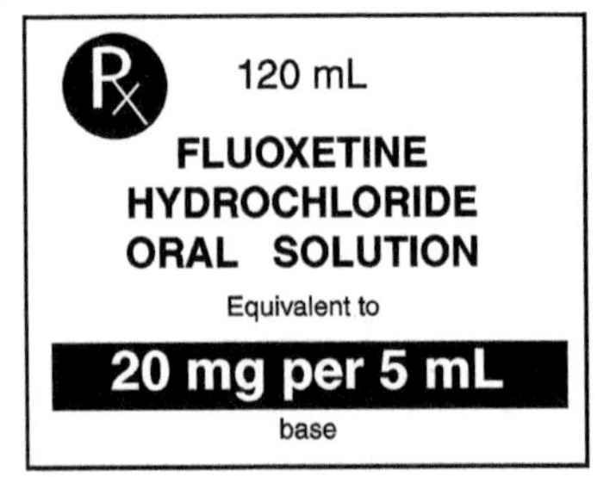

Fig. 11.10 A Fluxotine Hydrochloride Label *How many mg are there in 5 mL of Prozac liquid?*

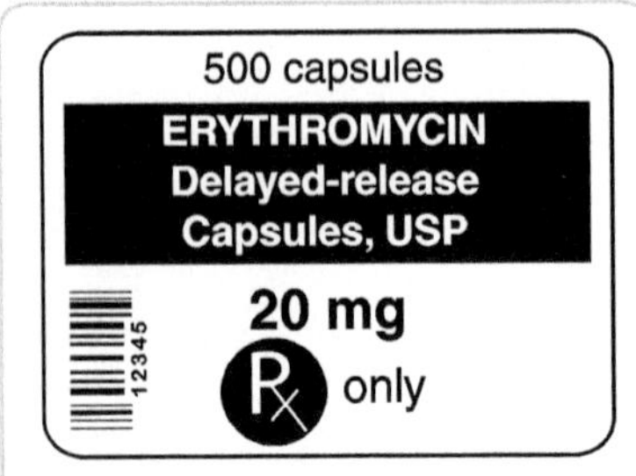

Fig. 11.11 An Erythromycin Label *How many mg are there in each capsule?*

Basic Dosage Calculations

What do you need to know to calculate medication dosages?

Healthcare professionals may be responsible for administering medications, which requires dosage calculations. This should not be taken lightly. Errors can have serious or even fatal consequences.

To administer medication, you must have a physician's order. This is written on the patient's chart or on a prescription form (see **Figure 11.9**). The order should include the following:

- The name of the drug.
- The amount of drug prescribed.
- The frequency with which it should be administered.
- The route of administration.

Be familiar with the order and the label on the drug before calculating any drug dose. Calculate doses using the following proportion:

$$\frac{\text{Known unit (dosage) on hand}}{\text{Known dosage form}} = \frac{\text{Dose ordered}}{\text{Unknown amount to be given}}$$

The parts can be defined as follows:

- **Known unit on hand:** The amount of medication in a particular drug for which the dosage is known. For example, a tablet may contain 10 milligrams (mg) of medicine.
- **Known dosage form:** The form may be 1 tablet or capsule. Another example may be a bottle of cough syrup that indicates that there are 125 mg per 5 mL. The known dosage form is 5 mL.
- **Dose ordered:** The amount of medication ordered.
- **Unknown amount to be given:** This is what you are trying to determine, the amount of medication to be given.

These examples show how to calculate amounts of medication.

Example 1 The order reads "Fluxotine Hydrochloride liquid 40 mg by mouth every day for anxiety." The label reads 20 mg per 5 mL. Calculate the amount of medication to administer (see **Figure 11.10**).

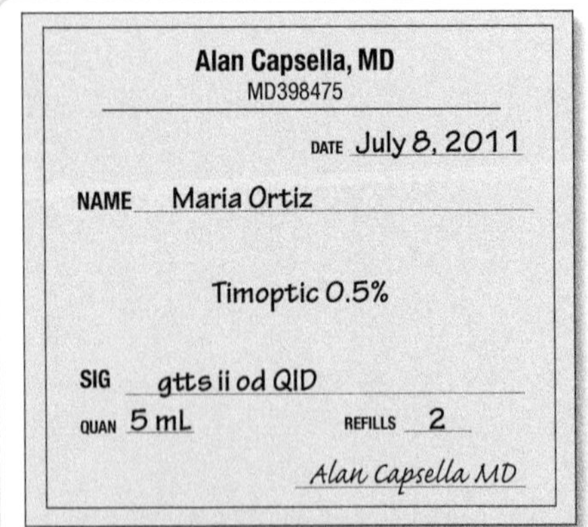

Alan Capsella, MD
MD398475

DATE July 8, 2011

NAME Maria Ortiz

Timoptic 0.5%

SIG gtts ii od QID

QUAN 5 mL REFILLS 2

Alan Capsella MD

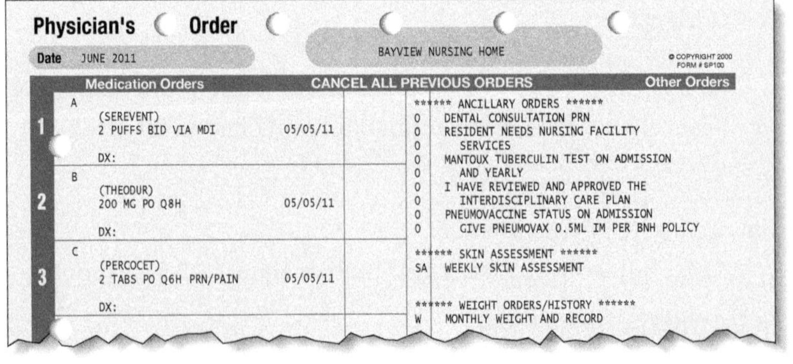

Physician's Order

Date JUNE 2011 BAYVIEW NURSING HOME © COPYRIGHT 2000 FORM # SP100

Medication Orders | CANCEL ALL PREVIOUS ORDERS | Other Orders

1 A (SEREVENT) 2 PUFFS BID VIA MDI 05/05/11 DX:

2 B (THEODUR) 200 MG PO Q8H 05/05/11 DX:

3 C (PERCOCET) 2 TABS PO Q6H PRN/PAIN 05/05/11 DX:

****** ANCILLARY ORDERS ******
O DENTAL CONSULTATION PRN
O RESIDENT NEEDS NURSING FACILITY SERVICES
O MANTOUX TUBERCULIN TEST ON ADMISSION AND YEARLY
O I HAVE REVIEWED AND APPROVED THE INTERDISCIPLINARY CARE PLAN
O PNEUMOVACCINE STATUS ON ADMISSION
O GIVE PNEUMOVAX 0.5ML IM PER BNH POLICY
****** SKIN ASSESSMENT ******
SA WEEKLY SKIN ASSESSMENT
****** WEIGHT ORDERS/HISTORY ******
W MONTHLY WEIGHT AND RECORD

Fig. 11.9 Physician's Orders Physician's orders are necessary to administer medication. *What are the similarities and differences between these two physician's orders?*

- 20 mg/5 mL = 40 mg/? mL
- Known unit on hand = 20 mg
- Known dosage form = 5 mL
- Dose ordered = 40 mg
- Unknown amount to be given = ?
- Cross-multiply: 20×? = 5 × 40
- 20 × ? = 200
- Divide by 20: ? = 10 mL

Example 2 The order reads "Erythromycin® delayed-release capsules 500 mg by mouth every 12 hours." Referring to **Figure 11.11,** calculate the dose as shown below.

- Known unit on hand = 250 mg
- Known dosage form = 1 capsule
- Dose ordered = 500 mg
- Unknown amount to be given = ? capsules
- 250 mg/1 capsule = 500 mg/? capsules
- Cross-multiply: 250 × ? = 1 × 500
- 250 × ? = 500
- Divide by 250: ? = 2 capsules

125mg/5ml
AMOXICILLIN/
CLAVULANATE POTASSIUM
FOR ORAL SUSPENSION
Reconstituted, each 5 mL contains:
AMOXICILLIN, 125 mg
as the trihydrate
CLAVULANIC ACID, 31.25 MG
as clavulanate potassium
75mL (when reconstituted)

Fig. 11.12 An Augmentin® Label. *How many mg are there in 5 mL of this medication?*

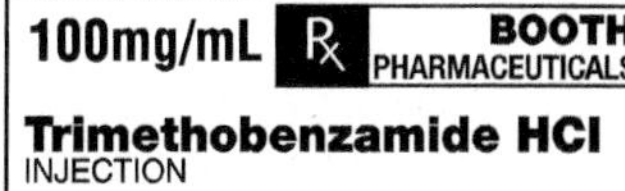

Fig. 11.13 A Tigan® Label. *How many mg are there in 1 mL of this medication?*

READING CHECK

Identify two things you must know before calculating any drug dose.

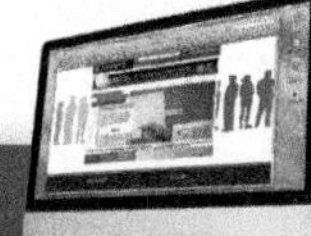

connect ONLINE PROCEDURES

PROCEDURE 11-2

Using the Metric System

The metric system is the most widely used system of measurement in pharmacy. This system was established in 1960 to make units of measurement for the metric system standard throughout the world.

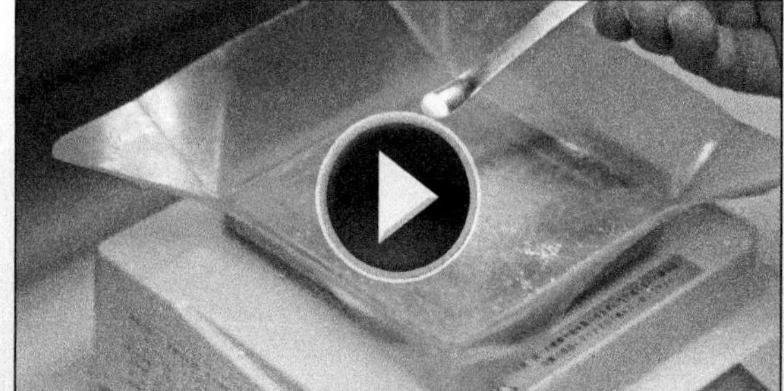

PROCEDURE 11-3

Identifying Metric Abbreviations

The meter, gram, and liter are the basic units of the metric system. The meter and gram are abbreviated with lowercase letters, but liter is abbreviated with an uppercase L. This minimizes the chance of confusing the lowercase letter L (l) with the digit 1.

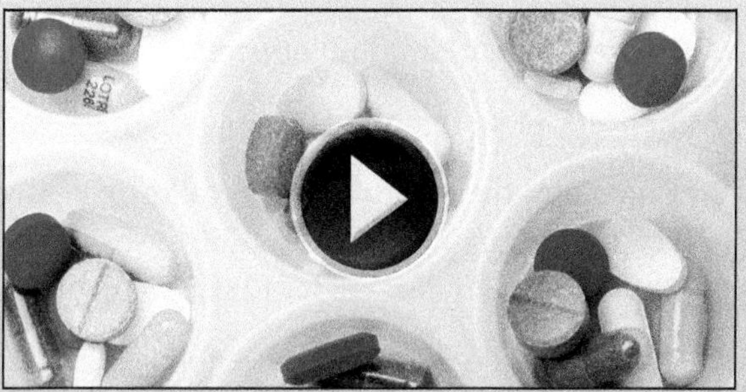

Photos: (t)amana images inc./Alamy, (b)Image Source

Mc Graw Hill connect

ONLINE PROCEDURES

PROCEDURE 11-4

Converting Between Metric Measurements

Length is used to express measurements such as patient height, infant head circumference, and lesion or wound size. Weight and volume measurements are frequently used when you calculate dosages. Most dosages and drug strengths are expressed using the metric system. Converting measurements may be necessary.

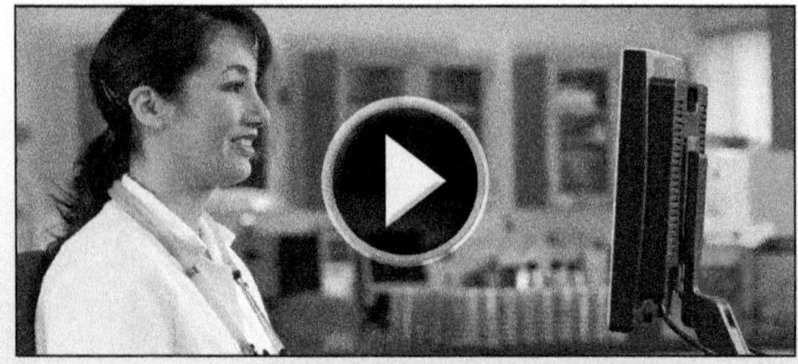

PROCEDURE 11-5

Recognizing Equivalent Measurements

Unlike the metric system, neither the avoirdupois system nor the household system is based on multiples of 10. Sometimes it will be necessary to convert units from one system to another. Keep in mind that equivalent measures are approximations and not exact.

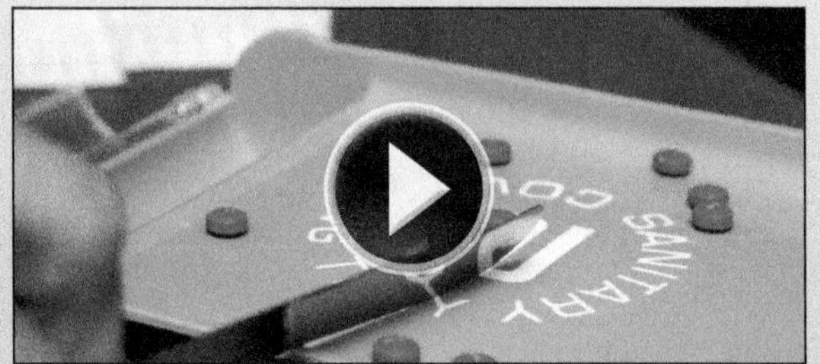

PROCEDURE 11-6

Converting by the Proportion Method

First write a conversion factor with the units needed in the numerator and the units you are converting from in the denominator. Next, write a fraction with the unknown (x) in the numerator and the number you need to convert in the denominator. Third, set the two factors up as a proportion. Cancel units and cross-multiply. Then solve for the unknown.

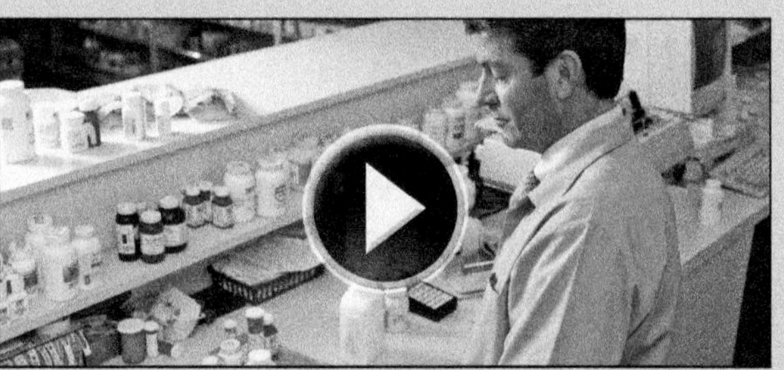

Photos: (t)Huntstock/Getty Images, (c)C. Sherburne/PhotoLink/Getty Images, (b)CORBIS

SECTION 11.4 Medical Mathematics Review

AFTER YOU READ

1. **Express** 1 gram in milligrams.
2. **Express** 123.4 mL in liters.
3. **Express** 120 mL in fluid ounces.
4. **Express** 44 kg in pounds.
5. **Calculate** the dose for the following: (see **Fig. 11.12**): "Augmentin® liquid 250 mg by mouth 3 times a day." Label reads "125 mg/5 mL."
6. **Calculate** the dose for the following: (see **Fig. 11.13**: "Tigan® injection 200 mg intramuscularly 3 times a day." Label reads "100 mg/mL".

Technology ONLINE EXPLORATIONS

Unit Conversions

Search the Internet for a tool to help you convert units of measure. Use it to perform the following conversions:

- 24 decigrams to milligrams
- 212 milliliters to deciliters
- 1412 centimeters to meters
- 14 lbs to ounces
- 30 cm to inches

CHAPTER 11 Review

Chapter Summary

SECTION 11.1

- Naturally occurring drugs are obtained from numerous sources, including plants, animals, and bacteria. Scientists can produce or modify drugs through chemical means or by genetic means. **(pg. 308)**
- The mechanism of action, or MOA, of a drug describes how it produces its desired effect. All MOAs are based on the lock and key principle, in which the drug acts as the key. **(pg. 310)**
- Pharmacotherapeutics is the study of the effects of drugs. **(pg. 310)**
- Any effect produced by a drug that is not the desired effect is known as a side effect. Side effects can be classified as either local or systemic. **(pg. 312)**

SECTION 11.2

- There are numerous therapeutic classes of drugs. Drugs within a therapeutic class share many of the same properties and are generally used to treat the same conditions. **(pg. 314)**
- The various ways in which a drug can be given are known as routes of administration. Each route has advantages and disadvantages. **(pg. 317)**

SECTION 11.3

- Pharmacokinetics is the study of the four processes—absorption, distribution, metabolism (transformation), and elimination—that affect how the dosage of a drug is determined. **(pg. 321)**
- Sometimes a large initial dose, called a loading dose, of a drug is given, so that the concentration of the drug in the patient's plasma reaches the therapeutic range more quickly; afterward, smaller doses, called maintenance doses, are taken at regular intervals to keep the plasma concentration in the therapeutic range. **(pg. 322)**

SECTION 11.4

- The most commonly used system of measurement is the metric system. The dosage of a drug is usually given in milligrams (mg); liquid medications are often measured in milliliters (mL). **(pg. 324)**
- Systems other than the metric system are the household system, the avoirdupois system, and the apothecary system. **(pg. 326)**
- Doses must be calculated with accuracy using the following formula:

$$\frac{\text{Known unit (dosage) on hand}}{\text{Known dosage form}} = \frac{\text{Dose ordered}}{\text{Unknown amount to be given}}$$ **(pg. 328)**

CHAPTER 11 Assessment

Critical Thinking/Problem Solving

1. Your grandmother is taking nitroglycerin for her heart condition. One day while you are visiting, you see her get a large glass of water and swallow her nitroglycerin pill. Did she take her pill correctly? If not, how would you explain the method and importance of taking the pill correctly?
2. A client has been taking the medication Vasotec® for hypertension. He has a pulse of 110 bpm and is complaining that he has a headache. What can be done to help this client?
3. A client has been suffering from sneezing, watery eyes, and nasal congestion during hay fever season. What medications would you advise for this client? What are the possible side effects?

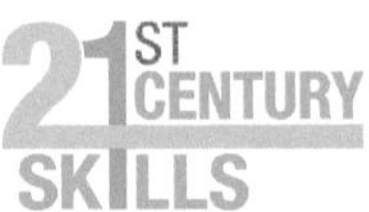

4. **Teamwork** Working in teams of three or four, role-play the four mechanisms of action (MOAs) that are described in Section 1 of this chapter. Assign each of your team members a role and give him or her a label. Perform your MOA drama for the class.
5. **Listening** Obtain syringes and sterile water. Under the direction of your teacher, work in pairs and practice giving SC and IM injections to tomatoes and oranges.
6. **Information Literacy** Using the Internet, find at least one additional medication for each of the classes discussed in Section 11.3 of this chapter. You may try searching for words such as "medication," "drugs," or "therapeutic classes." You may also search for the name of each therapeutic class; for example, narcotic analgesics.

Mc Graw Hill connect™ ONLINE ACTIVITIES

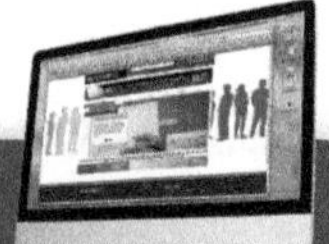

Complete our HST online activities for Chapter 11, which include Concept Check review questions, Reference Flash Cards, and Online Procedures assessment sheets.

- **Concept Check** review questions
- **Reference Flash Cards** medical terminology practice
- **Online Procedures** assessment sheets

CHAPTER

12 Legal and Ethical Responsibilities

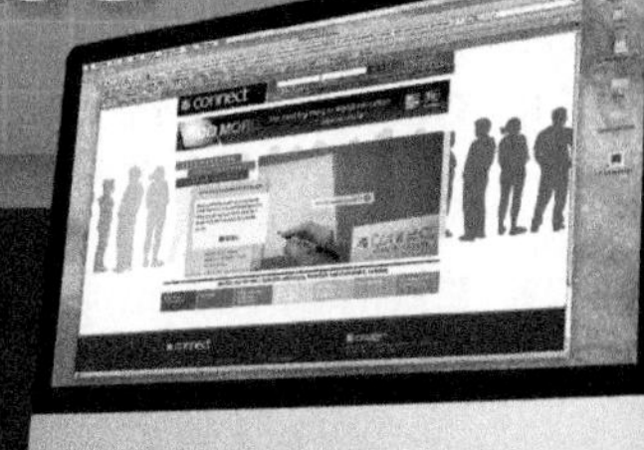

Essential Question:

How will legal and ethical considerations affect how you make decisions as a healthcare professional?

If you intend to become an effective and successful healthcare professional, you must be familiar with certain legal and ethical standards and follow them when performing your duties in the workplace. These standards will be your professional guidelines.

The following sections explain the ways in which written laws and unwritten behavior guidelines affect us all.

Mc Graw Hill connect™

It's Online!

- Online Procedures
- STEM Connection
- Medical Science
- Medical Terms
- Medical Math
- Ethics in Action
- Virtual Lab

Photo: Tetra Images/Terra/CORBIS

READING GUIDE

OBJECTIVES

After completing this chapter, you will be able to:

- **Contrast** laws, morals, and ethics.
- **Explain** the purpose of professional codes of ethics.
- **Define** the term standard of care.
- **Describe** informed consent.
- **Discuss** the importance of confidentiality and HIPAA for healthcare professions.
- **Explain** what an advance directive is.
- **Compare** a living will, a durable power of attorney, and a healthcare proxy.
- **Describe** clients' rights and responsibilities.
- **Name** the qualities of a successful healthcare worker.

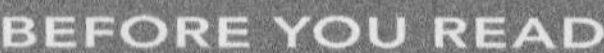

Connect How closely do your own morals and ethics match those of the healthcare field?

Main Idea

Healthcare professionals must understand and act according to the accepted morals, laws, and ethics related to their occupation in all aspects of their work, including working with clients, procedures, or records.

Note-Taking Activity

Draw this table. Write key terms and phrases under **Cues**. Write main ideas under **Note Taking**. Summarize the section under **Summary**.

Cues	Note Taking
○ ○	○ ○
Summary	

Graphic Organizer

Before you read the chapter, draw a diagram like the one to the right As you read, write the legal and ethical responsibilities covered in this chapter into the diagram.

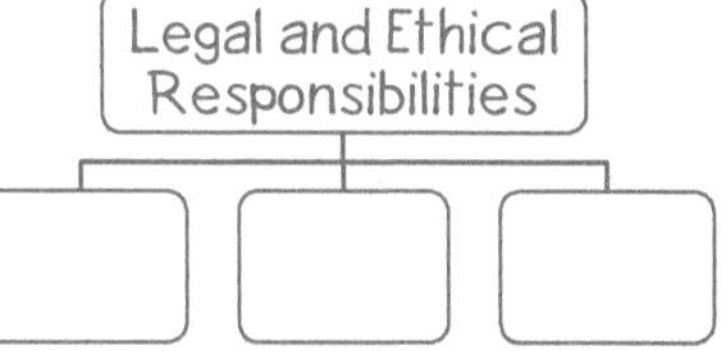

connect
Downloadable graphic organizers can be accessed online.

STANDARDS

HEALTH SCIENCE

NCHSE 5.12 Apply procedures for accurate documentation and record keeping.

NCHSE 6.12 Recognize ethical issues and their implications related to healthcare.

SCIENCE

NSES F Develop understanding of personal and community health; population growth; natural resources; environmental quality; natural and human-induced hazards; science and technology in local, national, and global challenges.

NCHSE *National Consortium for Health Science Education*

NSES *National Science Education Standards*

COMMON CORE STATE STANDARDS

MATHEMATICS

Statistics and Probability

Making Inferences and Justifying Conclusions S-IC Make inferences and justify conclusions from sample surveys, experiments, and observational studies.

ENGLISH LANGUAGE ARTS

Conventions of Standard English

Vocabulary Acquisition and Use

L-6 Acquire and use accurately a range of general academic and domain-specific words and phrases sufficient for reading, writing, speaking, and listening at the college and career readiness level; demonstrate independence in gathering vocabulary knowledge when considering a word or phrase important to comprehension or expression.

SECTION
12.1 Legal and Ethical Standards

Understanding Laws, Morals, and Ethics

What is the difference between law and ethics?

Although we may not often think about the way we behave, in our daily lives we are all affected by standards of behavior. What are the sources of these standards? As this chapter shows, the main sources are:

- Laws made by governing bodies
- Rules of behavior established by the society in which we live
- Personal feelings of right and wrong

Laws

Laws are needed if society is to function smoothly. A **law** is a rule of conduct or action. They are enacted and enforced by a controlling authority, such as the federal, state, or local government. There are penalties for breaking the law. Depending upon the severity of the crime, penalties may include jail time, fines, community service, or probation.

Criminal Laws Criminal laws protect members of society from certain harmful acts of others. A crime is committed when the law is broken. A criminal act may be one of

- commission, if there is a law forbidding a certain act.
- omission, in violation of a law requiring a certain act.

Criminal laws are passed at local, state, and federal levels. They generally carry stricter penalties for offenders than civil statutes do.

Civil Laws Civil laws are concerned with private rights and remedies. Under civil law, a person may sue another person, a business, or the government. Some examples of the causes of civil disputes are:

- Contract violation
- Slander or libel
- Trespassing
- Product liability
- Automobile accidents
- Family matters, such as divorce, child support, and child custody

Court judgments in civil cases often require that money be paid to the injured party.

READING CHECK

Compare the penalties in a criminal case with court judgments in a civil case.

Vocabulary

Content Vocabulary

You will learn these content vocabulary terms in this section.

- **law**
- **tort**
- **negligence**
- **medical malpractice**
- **morals**
- **licensure**
- **registration**
- **certification**
- **reciprocity**
- **standard of care**
- **scope of practice**
- **liable**
- **law of agency**
- **informed consent**
- **confidentiality**
- **privileged communication**

Academic Vocabulary

You will see these words in your reading and on your tests. Find their meanings in the Glossary in the back of the book.

- **civil**
- **license**

Civil law includes a general category of law known as torts. A **tort** is broadly defined as a civil wrong committed against a person or property, excluding breach of contract. A tort may have caused physical injury, resulted in damage to someone's property, or deprived someone of his or her personal liberty and freedom.

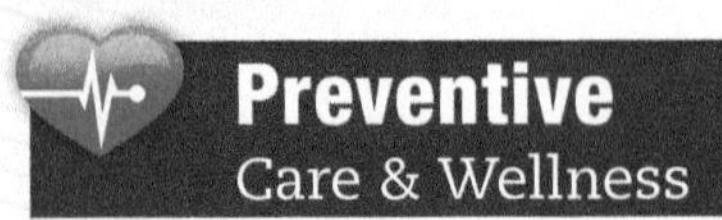

Organ Donation

Although we do not like to think about our own death, there is one way to help others even after death. This is by donating your organs.

If an organ is healthy, it can be given to someone in need of an organ transplant. Another form of donation is for medical research. Medical donations can help find cures for hereditary diseases and discover safe and effective drugs and therapies to treat disease and illness.

Planning to donate in advance helps to ease the burden on families and offers direction during a very difficult time. In many states you can simply check a box on your driver's license application.

Torts may be intentional (willful) or unintentional (accidental). Intentional torts may also be crimes. Therefore, they may be prosecuted in both civil and criminal courts.

Unintentional torts are acts that are not intended to cause harm. However, they are committed "unreasonably," or without regard for the consequences. Therefore in legal terms, an unintentional tort is caused by **negligence.**

In healthcare, negligence is often called **medical malpractice.** Negligence is the most common unintentional tort that occurs in the healthcare delivery system. Negligence is charged when a healthcare practitioner fails to exercise ordinary or expected care and a client is injured or sustains damages of some sort as a result. The practitioner who is charged with negligence may have performed an act that a reasonable person, in similar circumstances, would probably not have performed. In other cases, the practitioner may have failed to perform an act that a reasonable person would have performed. The phrases "didn't intend to do it" or "should have known better" best describe a negligent act.

In a lawsuit involving medical malpractice, the plaintiff (the person bringing the lawsuit) must prove that the defendant (the person facing the charges):

- Owed a *duty* to the plaintiff, which in the context of healthcare means that a healthcare practitioner/client relationship had existed. This means that the client was being treated in a medical setting.
- Was *derelict*, or did not live up to the obligation of caring for the client (or plaintiff).
- Committed a breach of duty that directly *damaged* the client (or plaintiff).

According to the legal principles of negligence, the "three Ds" of negligence listed above—duty, derelict, damage—must be present for a lawsuit to have merit. For example, a healthcare practitioner is not necessarily liable (legally responsible) for a poor outcome when delivering healthcare. Many clients do not recover, but this does not mean that they were the victims of malpractice. A healthcare practitioner is liable only if it can be established that they were negligent in the delivery of professional services and caused injury to a client through that negligence.

The people most likely to be charged with negligence, or medical malpractice, are physicians, but other healthcare practitioners may also be subject to such charges.

Medical practice acts are state statutes that govern medical practice. The medical practice acts in all fifty states are similar to one another. The acts

- cover requirements and methods for licensing healthcare providers.
- establish medical licensing boards.
- list the grounds for revoking licenses.

Medical practice acts protect the public from dishonest or unqualified people who might try to sell worthless healing devices, practice medicine without the proper license, or otherwise defraud the public.

Morals and Ethics

Morals and ethics also affect your work in a healthcare profession.

Morals are formed from your personal values and reflect your concept of right and wrong. You develop moral values through the influence of family, culture, and society. Acting morally toward others involves treating them the way you would like to be treated.

Ethics are standards of behavior developed as a result of your moral values. Ethics are not the same as laws. In some circumstances, however, ethics may govern behavior more strictly than laws do. For example, it is not against the law for you, as a healthcare professional, to accept a tip from a client, but your sense of ethics may prevent you from accepting that tip. In other words, an unethical act is not necessarily illegal. (Keep in mind, that an illegal act is always unethical.)

Your personal moral values are always at work as you make decisions in your daily life. Your values will help you deal compassionately and fairly with others in your job as a healthcare worker.

For further guidance, most healthcare organizations have established codes of ethics to help their professional members with difficult decisions. For example, the American Nurses' Association (ANA) has a Code for Nurses. In addition, formalized codes of ethics have been issued by the American Society of Radiologic Technologists (ASRT), the American Association of Medical Assistants (AAMA), and many other organizations that represent specialized healthcare professions.

The first known code of ethics was developed around 400 B.C.E. by Hippocrates, a Greek physician known as the father of Western medicine. It was called the Hippocratic Oath. **Figure 12.1** is a translation of the oath from its original Greek. The oath is a pledge that physicians have traditionally recited, in part, during medical school graduations. For most of us, the wording of this ancient oath is difficult to understand. The *Code of Medical Ethics: Current Opinions with Annotations,* issued by the American Medical Association (AMA), provides a detailed code of ethics for all modern physicians. See Table 12.1 for a comparison of law, ethics, and moral values.

I swear by Apollo the physician and Asklepios, and Health, and All-Heal, and all the gods and goddesses, that, according to my ability and judgment.

I will keep this Oath and this stipulation — to reckon him who taught me this Art equally dear to me as my parents, to share my substance with him, and relieve his necessities if required; to look upon his offspring in the same footing as my own brothers, and to teach them this Art, if they shall wish to learn it, without fee or stipulation; and that by precept, lecture, and every other mode of instruction, I will impart a knowledge of the Art to my own sons, and those of my teachers, and to disciples bound by a stipulation and oath according to the law of medicine, but to none others.

I will follow that system of regimen which, according to my ability and judgment, I consider for the benefit of my patients, and abstain from whatever is deleterious and mischievous, I will give no deadly medicine to any one if asked, nor suggest any such counsel; and in like manner I will not give to a woman a pessary to produce abortion. With purity and holiness I will pass my life and practice my Art.

I will not cut persons labouring under the stone, but will leave this to be done by men who are practitioners of this work. Into whatever houses I enter, I will go into them for the benefit of the sick, and will abstain from every voluntary act of mischief and corruption; and, further, from the seduction of females or males, of freemen and slaves. Whatever, in connection with my professional practice, or not in connection with it, I see or hear, in the life of men, which ought not to be spoken of abroad, I will not divulge, as reckoning that all such should be kept secret. While I continue to keep this Oath unviolated, may it be granted to me to enjoy life and the practice of the Art, respected by all men, in all times! But should I trespass and violate this Oath, may the reverse be my lot!

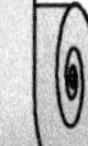

Fig. 12.1 The Hippocratic Oath
Who recites this oath?

Table 12.1 Law, Ethics, and Moral Values

	LAW	ETHICS	MORAL VALUES
Definition	Set of governing rules	Standards of behavior that reflect moral values	Concept of right and wrong formed through influence of family, culture, and society
Main purpose	To protect the public	To raise standard of competence	To serve as a guide for personal conduct
Purpose	To promote smooth functioning of society	To build values and ideals	To serve as a basis for forming personal code of ethics
Penalties or consequences	Upon conviction in civil or criminal court: fines, imprisonment, loss of professional license, or other penalty determined by courts	Suspension or eviction from professional society membership, as decided by peers	Difficulty in getting along with others

Noncompliance

There are penalties for noncompliance with legal responsibilities and ethical standards. Penalties for breaking the law are usually stricter than those for unethical behavior. Noncompliant healthcare workers may face fines or prison sentences and can lose their licenses to practice.

Members of professional organizations such as the AMA or AAMA who are accused of unethical conduct may face a peer council review and censure or expulsion from the group. Professional organizations, however, cannot revoke a member's license to practice. Only the state can revoke a license to practice.

READING CHECK

Explain how liability could be established in a medical malpractice case.

Licensure, Registration, and Certification

Do you know the differences among licensure, registration, and certification?

Depending on the state and job classification, members of a healthcare team may be licensed, registered, or certified to perform specific duties. Each state's medical practice acts define the requirements for each job classification or profession.

Licensure

Licensure is required for certain professions within a state. All states require that physicians, nurses, and many other healthcare workers have licenses to practice in that state. Persons who do not meet state standards for a license may not legally practice.

Registration

Registration means that a person's name has been listed in an official registry or record as having satisfied the standards for a certain healthcare occupation. For some, all you need to do is add your name to the list in the registry. In this case, unregistered workers are not barred from working if they are otherwise qualified. Therefore, registration is not required in order to practice.

A second way to become registered as a worker in a healthcare occupation is to fulfill certain educational requirements and/or pay a registration fee. When there are specific requirements for registration, unregistered individuals may not work at the job, even if they have qualifying education and experience. In this case, registration is required.

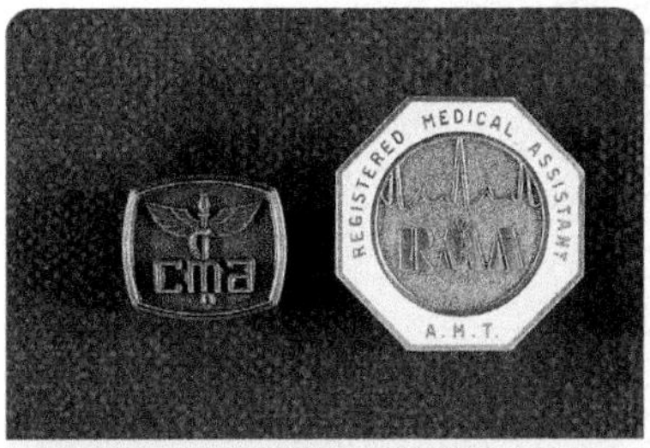

Certification

Certification is usually voluntary and national in scope. Certification by a professional organization is most often achieved by taking an examination. Passing the examination shows that an applicant has attained a certain level of knowledge and skill. Since the process is voluntary, lack of certification does not prevent an employee from practicing the profession if he or she is otherwise qualified. **Figure 12.2** illustrates both certification and registration pins.

Fig. 12.2 Certification Medical assistants certified by the Certifying Board of the American Association of Medical Assistants wear the pin on the left. Medical assistants who are registered (RMA) by the American Medical Technologies organization wear the pin on the right.

For those healthcare professions that require a state license, such as physician, registered nurse, or licensed practical or vocational nurse, **reciprocity** may be granted. This means that a state licensing authority will accept a person's valid license from another state without requiring reexamination.

READING CHECK

Identify how the requirements for licensure, registration, or certification are established.

Standard of Care and Scope of Practice

How do the standard of care and scope of practice relate?

According to the legal doctrine of standard of care, healthcare workers should perform only those duties that fall within the scope of their license or job description. **Standard of care** is the level of performance expected of a healthcare professional in carrying out his or her duties. It is based upon the individual's **scope of practice.** The scope of practice is based upon job description, level of training, and qualifications. In **Figure 12.3,** a technician carries out a test that is within her scope of practice.

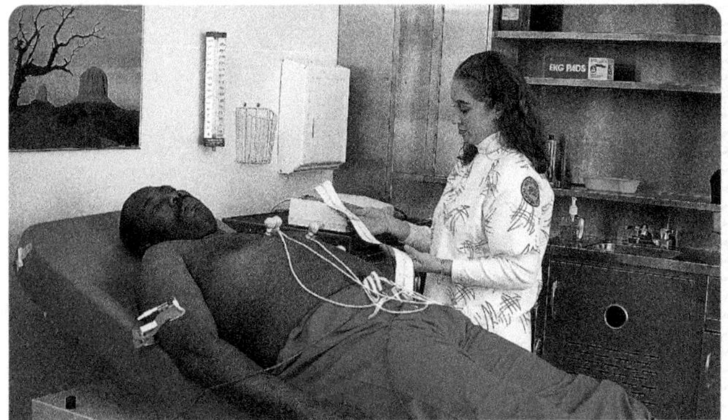

Fig. 12.3 Scope of Practice This electrocardiograph technician is operating an electrocardiograph machine. *Why is this duty within her scope of practice?*

The standard of care expected of a healthcare professional also depends upon the professional's job classification. For example, physicians are held to a higher standard of care than nurses. Registered nurses are held to a higher standard of care than licensed practical/vocational nurses. Medical assistants are held to a higher standard of care than nursing assistants, and so on. Individuals who are specially trained to perform specific tasks, such as physicians, nurses, or medical assistants, are held to a standard of care that is consistent with their training.

Standard of care is an important legal concept. If a healthcare worker performs a procedure that is not within the scope of his or her practice and causes injury to a client, the healthcare worker may be found **liable,** or legally responsible, if a lawsuit is filed.

For example, suppose that on a busy day in a medical office, a certified medical assistant (CMA) is asked to start an IV on a client. According to her state's laws, starting an IV is not within the CMA's scope of practice, but she believes that she is capable and since the office is short-handed, she complies.

Over the next two weeks, the client develops an infection at the site where IV was started and must be hospitalized. The infection finally heals, but the client's arm is permanently scarred. Because of the infection and scarring, the client then decides to sue the physician who is the medical assistant's employer. The medical assistant is liable for her actions and, in the event of a lawsuit, could be held to the standard of care of a registered nurse, who, by the scope of his or her practice, is qualified to start an IV.

Standard of care and scope of practice legally define what members of a healthcare profession can and cannot do. The concepts help to define each professional's role on the healthcare team. If you are a healthcare practitioner, working within your scope of practice fulfills two important job requirements. It ensures that you

- do not injure clients or put them at risk by performing procedures that are beyond your ability, and
- will not be held to a standard of care that is beyond your training, experience, and job description if a legal situation arises.

The Law of Agency

The **law of agency** is closely linked to the concept of standard of care. According to this legal doctrine, an employer is legally liable for acts performed by employees. In the example above, under the law of agency, the physicians affiliated with the medical office that hired the medical assistant could also be held liable in the case of a lawsuit.

READING CHECK

Evaluate what could happen if a healthcare worker performs a procedure that is not within his or her scope of practice.

Informed Consent

Do you know who can give informed consent for a medical procedure?

For many procedures and tests, such as surgery or some kinds of blood tests, clients must sign a consent form. The form gives consent for the procedure or test to be performed.

Healthcare professionals in charge of documenting treatment should include in a client's medical record the signed consent form and a statement saying that the client was properly informed before signing the consent form. This is known as **informed consent. Figure 12.4** shows a sample consent form.

It is not enough to hand a client a brochure or information sheet about his or her condition. This does not meet the requirements for informed consent. To make an informed decision regarding treatment, the client needs to be told:

- The proposed methods of treatment
- Why the treatment is necessary
- The risks involved in the proposed treatment
- All available alternative types of treatment
- The risks of any alternative methods of treatment
- The risks involved if treatment is refused

Adults who are considered to be of sound mind are usually able to give informed consent. Some people cannot legally be expected to give informed consent. These groups include, for example:

Minors Minors are individuals who are under the age of majority. In most states, this is under the age of 18. In other states, it is under the age of 21. Exceptions can include minors who live away from home and support themselves. Other exceptions are those who have been judged by the court to be mature minors. They may be considered emancipated. They have the right to seek birth control or care during pregnancy, treatment for reportable communicable diseases, or treatment for drug- or alcohol-related problems without first obtaining parental consent.

AUTHORIZATION FOR
DISCLOSURE OF THE RESULTS OF THE
HIV ANTIBODY BLOOD TEST

A. AUTHORIZATION

I hereby authorize Hamilton County Public Hospital to furnish to

____

(Name of person or entity who is to receive results)

the results of my blood test for antibodies to HIV.

B. USES

The Receiver may use the information for the following purpose(s):

____

____

C. RESTRICTIONS

This authorization is being given with the understanding that the Receiver will be informed in writing by the Hospital that state law protects the confidentiality of this information and prohibits any further disclosure of the information without my specific, written consent, or as otherwise permitted by law. The Receiver will be informed that a general authorization for the release of medical or other information is not sufficient for this purpose.

D. DURATION

This authorization shall become effective immediately and shall remain in effect indefinitely or until ____________________, whichever is shorter.
(Date)

__________________ Date

__________________ Patient's signature

__________________ Print name of patient

Fig. 12.4 Informed Consent A sample consent form.
Who cannot sign a consent form?

Mentally Incompetent Individuals Persons judged by the court to be insane, senile, mentally disabled, or under the influence of drugs or alcohol cannot give informed consent. In these cases, a competent person may be designated by a court to act for the individual.

Speakers of a Foreign Language When a client does not speak or understand English, an interpreter may be necessary in order to inform the client and obtain consent for treatment.

READING CHECK

Recall where the client's consent form should be placed after it has been signed.

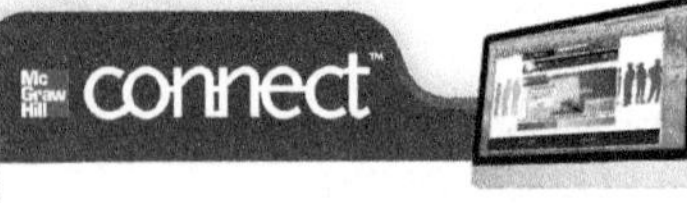

Ethics in Action

Technology and Confidentiality Great contributions have been made by technology in the area of creating, maintaining, and transporting clients' medical information. You should be aware, however, of some of the disadvantages of using this technology, especially where confidentiality is concerned.

Go to connect for guidelines related to confidentiality and information technology, then answer the questions.

Confidentiality

Do you know when you should and should not share client information?

Clients have a legal and ethical right to have all personal medical information kept private. By law, this information comes under the heading of "privileged communication." It is both unethical and illegal for a healthcare worker to not observe **confidentiality.**

The term **privileged communication** refers to information that is held private within a protected relationship, such as that between a physician and client. Laws that govern this vary from state to state. In most states, clients may sue healthcare workers who violate client confidentiality and cause damage to the client. In many states, physicians and other healthcare workers who breach confidentiality can lose their licenses.

Keeping client medical information confidential means:

- Not informing any unauthorized person about the information contained in a client's medical records
- Not showing written information to an unauthorized third party
- Taking proper precautions when communicating such information over a computer, telephone, or fax machine

In some instances, information may be given to a third party, such as an insurance company representative. In this case, the written consent of the client or his or her legal representative must be obtained in advance. **Figure 12.5** shows a sample release form.

Here are some guidelines to follow if you have access to client information:

- Do not decide whether information is confidential on the basis of whether you approve of, or agree with, the views or morals of the client.
- Do not reveal financial information about a client. This information is also confidential.

I authorize: Name of person or institution ______________________ (Provider of information)

Street address ______________________

City, State, Zip Code ______________________

To release medical information to:

Name of person or institution: ______________________ (Recipient of information)

Street address ______________________

City, State, Zip Code ______________________

Attention: ______________________

Nature of information to be disclosed:

- ☐ Clinical notes pertaining to evaluation and treatment
- ☐ Other, please specify ______________________

Purpose of disclosure:

- ☐ Continuing medical care
- ☐ Second opinion
- ☐ Other, please specify ______________________

This authorization will automatically expire one year from the date of signature, unless specified otherwise ______________________

This consent may be revoked at any time by sending written notice to the above-named provider of information. Any release of information made prior to the revocation of this compliant authorization is not a breach of confidentiality. Disclosed information may be reviewed by contacting the provider of information.

Patient's name ______________________

Signature of patient or legal guardian ______________________ Date ______________________

Complete address ______________________

Relationship, if not the patient ______________________ Patient's date of birth ______________________

SPECIFIC CONSENT FOR RELEASE OF INFORMATION
PROTECTED BY STATE OR FEDERAL LAW

Iowa law (and in some cases federal law) provides special confidentiality protection to information relating to substance abuse, mental health, and HIV-related testing. In order for information to be released on this subject matter, this specific authorization and the above authorization must be signed:

I authorize release of information relating to:

☐ Substance abuse (alcohol/drug abuse)
Signature of patient or legal guardian

______________________ Date ______________________

☐ Mental health (includes psychological testing and mental health counseling)
Signature of patient or legal guardian

______________________ Date ______________________

☐ HIV-related information (AIDS-related testing)
Signature of patient or legal guardian

______________________ Date ______________________

Date information is sent ______________________ Sent by (name) ______________________

To the recipient of this information: This information has been disclosed to you from records protected by federal confidentiality rules. The federal rules prohibit you from making further disclosure without additional consent.

Fig. 12.5 Consent to Release Information A sample release form. *When might a client sign this form?*

- When talking on the telephone, do not use the client's name or otherwise disclose confidential information if others in the room might overhear.
- Use caution in giving the results of medical tests to clients over the telephone. Avoid having others overhear the information. When leaving a message on an answering machine or with voice mail, ask the client to return a call regarding a recent visit or appointment on a specific date. Do not mention the nature of the call.
- Do not leave medical charts or insurance reports where clients or others can see them.
- Do not release information if the client has not given written permission to release it.
- Do not talk about clients in public places, such as the cafeteria or elevator.

Confidentiality for client medical records may be waived under the following circumstances:

- When a third party requests a medical examination, such as a pre-employment examination, and that party pays the client's bill.
- When a client sues a physician or other healthcare practitioner for malpractice.
- When the client signs a waiver allowing the release of information.

READING CHECK

Identify some consequences for violating client confidentiality.

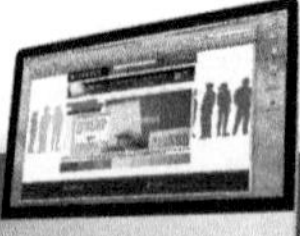

connect ONLINE PROCEDURES

PROCEDURE 12-1

Recognizing Informed Consent

Informed consent involves the patient's legal and ethical rights to receive all information relative to their condition. A decision regarding treatment should be based upon that knowledge. Informed consent also proves that a patient was not forced into treatment. Some people cannot legally be expected to give informed consent.

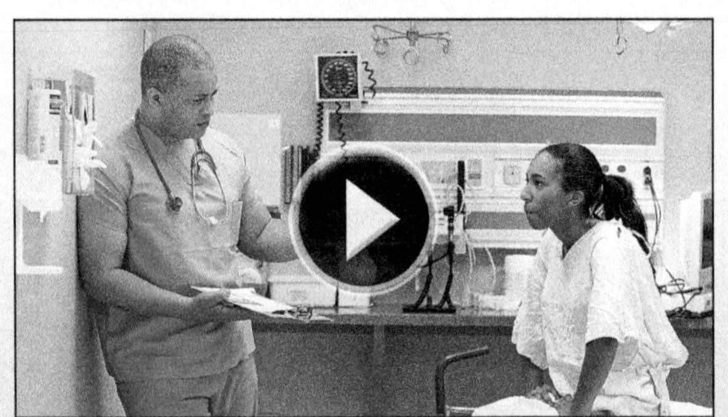

SECTION 12.1 Legal and Ethical Standards Review

AFTER YOU READ

1. **Explain** the difference between law and ethics.
2. **Define** the following terms: licensure, registration, and certification.
3. **Explain** why standard of care and scope of practice are important legal concepts for healthcare professionals.
4. **Assess** why is it important that you, as a healthcare worker, protect the confidentiality of client medical information.
5. **List** some of the information you must share with a client to ensure that the client is giving informed consent.

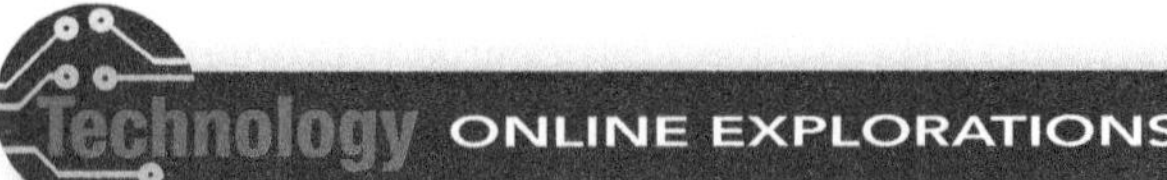

Technology ONLINE EXPLORATIONS

Medical Malpractice

Search the Internet for a medical malpractice case. Review the case, determining what happened and the outcome of the case. Try to find cases against individuals in the healthcare profession you are considering, if possible in the same state where you intend to practice.

SECTION

12.2 Medical Records and Policies

Medical Records

Have you ever seen your own medical record?

A medical record is the data recorded when a client seeks treatment. Informed consent and privileged communication are critical factors when medical records are prepared, stored, and released. All healthcare facilities are required to keep accurate medical records.

These records also provide:

- A format for tracking and documenting a client's health data
- Documentation of a client's lifelong healthcare
- A basis for managing a client's healthcare
- Background information in the event of a lawsuit
- Clinical data for education, research, statistical tracking, and assessing the quality of healthcare

A client's medical record is very important. Information should be correctly and carefully recorded. Records may be kept on paper, microfilm, or digital storage devices.

Clients own the information in their medical records. However, the records themselves are the property of the facility where they were created. For example, a physician in private practice owns the records. Records in a clinic are property of the clinic. Hospital records are the property of the admitting hospital. State laws differ, but usually clients may obtain copies of their medical records if they sign a release form.

Correcting a Medical Record

If you make an error in a printed medical record, it should be corrected in a certain way. If the records were ever used in a lawsuit, it should not look as though they were falsified. Follow these guidelines when correcting errors in a client's medical record:

- Draw a line through the error, making sure that it is still legible. Do not completely cover up or erase the incorrect information.
- Write or type in the correct information above or below the original line or in the margin. If necessary, attach another sheet of paper with the correction on it. Note in the record "See attached document A" to indicate where the corrected information can be found.
- Make a note near the correction explaining why it was made. You might write "error, wrong date" or "error, interrupted by a phone call." Do not make changes in the record without noting the reason.

Vocabulary

Content Vocabulary

You will learn these content vocabulary terms in this section.

- **protected health information (PHI)**
- **individual identifiable health information (IIHI)**
- **advance directive**
- **living will**
- **durable power of attorney**
- **healthcare proxy**

Academic Vocabulary

You will see these words in your reading and on your tests. Find their meanings in the Glossary in the back of the book.

- **data**
- **error**
- **use**

- Enter the date and time and initial the correction.
- If possible, ask another staff member or the physician to witness and initial the correction to the record when you make it.

READING CHECK

Analyze how you would go about making a needed correction to a medical record.

Health Insurance Portability and Accountability Act

Have you ever heard of HIPAA? If so, in what circumstances?

All healthcare facilities had to be compliant with the Health Insurance Portability and Accountability Act (HIPAA) by 2003. This law states that all patients have rights regarding their health information, which is known as **protected health information (PHI)**. A patient's PHI is stored in the patient's record chart. Federal law protects the individual's rights to know how her or his PHI is used and disclosed.

The use of PHI is the employment, application, utilization, sharing, examination, or analysis of **individual identifiable health information (IIHI)**. For example, when a medical assistant enters a patient's health insurance number for payment information, the patient's PHI is used.

The term "disclosure" means the release or transfer in any way of patient IIHI beyond the confines of the healthcare practice to which the information was given. For example, when a medical assistant gives patient information to another medical office to which the patient is being referred, PHI is being disclosed.

Clients have the following rights under HIPAA law:

1. **The right to notice of privacy practices.** Because it is unlikely that patients will read federal laws, the law states it is the healthcare facility's responsibility to give each patient a copy of the laws that protect them concerning their PHI. Patients must receive a written notice of privacy practices on their first visit to a healthcare provider. They should sign a form stating they have received this information. This signed and dated form must be carefully filed in the patients' medical record, and updated regularly.
2. **The right to limit or request restriction on their PHI and its use and disclosure.** This means that patients can limit how a facility uses their medical information, and how much of that information is shared. For example, a patient with a history of sexually transmitted disease may not wish to have that information released to the orthopedic physician who is setting his broken arm. In general, only the minimal amount of patient information should be released to meet the current needs of the patient. This is a general rule called the "Need to Know."

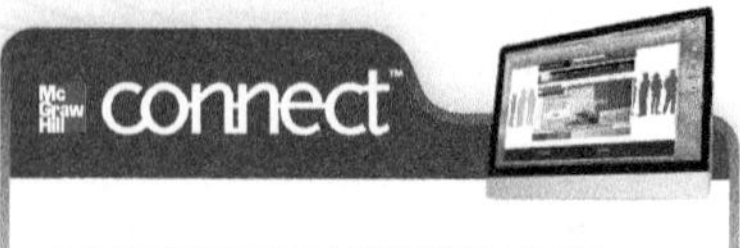

STEM CONNECTION

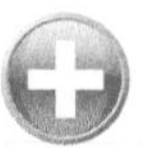

Medical Math

Converting from 12-Hour to 24-Hour Time
Many facilities use the 24-hour clock, known as "military time" or "international time." Knowing this time may be required as part of your duties for charting client information.

12-hour time is written with the hour first, followed by a colon, and then the minutes. It also includes the letters A.M. and P.M. 24-hour time is always four digits and does not include the colon. The first two digits are the hour, and the second two digits are the minutes. For example, nine thirty-nine a.m. would be written as follows.:

12-hour time: 9:39 A.M.
24-hour time: 0939

Go to connect to complete the related activity.

3. **The right to confidential communications.** This means that patients can request to receive PHI otherwise than during a medical appointment. For example, your patients may request that you call them at a variety of different numbers, including home, work, or cell phone number. The patient does not have to explain the request. The law says you must make a reasonable effort to communicate with the patient in a confidential manner as the patient requests.

4. **The right to inspect and obtain a copy of their PHI.** This means that patients have a right to request and receive a copy of their own medical records. It is important to always follow the protocols established in your office for medical record copying. It is considered an acceptable practice to act on a request within 30 days of the request, and to charge a reasonable fee to cover the expense for copying supplies and labor.

5. **The right to request an amendment to their PHI.** Healthcare providers have the right to require that a request to amend a record be made in writing. However, the request may be denied if the healthcare provider receiving the request is not the original recorder of the PHI, or if the PHI is believed to be accurate and complete. All requests for amendment and response must be carefully documented and filed in the patient's medical record.

6. **The right to know if their PHI has been disclosed and why.** Providers are required to keep a written record of every disclosure made of a patient's PHI. You must also keep a written record of any request by the patient for this information and the response of the healthcare provider. This information is usually filed in the patient's medical record. When making a disclosure of information, always record the date of the disclosure, the name and address of the person receiving the PHI, a brief summary of the information released, and the purpose of the disclosure.

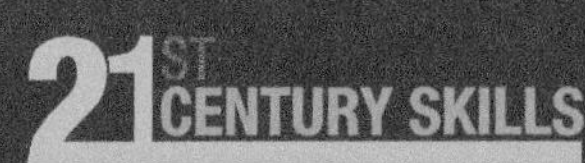

Communication

Have you ever had a teacher tell you how important it is to write clear, correctly-spelled papers for his or her class? Now think about a client's record. As a legal document, it may be read by many people and may even be read in court. Misspelled words, improper grammar, or incomplete information could end up being an embarrassment to you or your place of employment. More important, these errors could be detrimental to a legal case.

Follow-up

What is wrong with the following entry on a client's medical record? "Client complans of headake & dizziness and taking med, but pain ain't gone."

READING CHECK

Identify what is included in a patient's PHI.

Advance Directives

Do you know anyone who has completed an advance directive?

An important document to include in your clients' medical records is their advance directive. An **advance directive** is a legal document that makes known a person's wishes about life-support measures and other medical procedures. An advance directive will come into force when a client is unable to speak for him- or herself. Clients in all states have the legal right to execute advance directives. Examples of advance directives are:

- A living will
- A durable power of attorney
- A healthcare proxy

Living Will

A **living will** provides instructions directly to physicians, hospitals, and other healthcare providers involved in a client's medical treatment. **Figure 12.6** shows a sample living will. A living will may describe situations when treatment should be discontinued, such as a coma, brain death, or terminal conditions. It may also detail which treatments or medications to suspend. When a client's medical condition reaches a certain stage, for example, he or she may not wish to be treated with kidney dialysis, placed on a respirator, or given drugs for pain. In addition, the living will may list other measures that should not be used, such as emergency surgery in certain circumstances and cardiopulmonary resuscitation (CPR). When hospital clients specify they are not to be revived if their heart stops, Do Not Resuscitate (DNR) orders may be issued, in accordance with their wishes.

Durable Power of Attorney

The **durable power of attorney** is not specifically a medical document, but it may serve that purpose. It gives one person, called the designee, the authority to make a variety of legal decisions on behalf of another person, called the grantor. It takes effect when the grantor cannot make decisions, because of a coma, mental incompetence, or some other reason.

The document may limit the rights and responsibilities of the designee. It may also give specific instructions regarding the grantor's medical preferences and other wishes. Standard power of attorney forms are available from many sources, including online. The format and contents of these forms are established by state law.

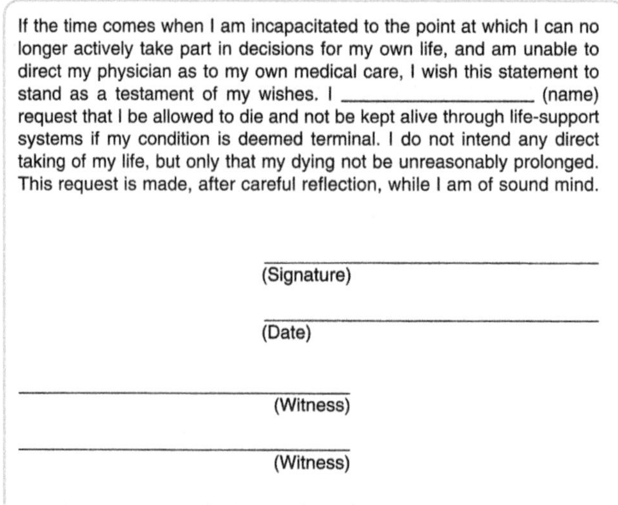

If the time comes when I am incapacitated to the point at which I can no longer actively take part in decisions for my own life, and am unable to direct my physician as to my own medical care, I wish this statement to stand as a testament of my wishes. I ____________________ (name) request that I be allowed to die and not be kept alive through life-support systems if my condition is deemed terminal. I do not intend any direct taking of my life, but only that my dying not be unreasonably prolonged. This request is made, after careful reflection, while I am of sound mind.

____
(Signature)

____
(Date)

____
(Witness)

____
(Witness)

Fig. 12.6 Living Will A sample living will. *What is the purpose of a living will?*

Healthcare Proxy

A **healthcare proxy,** or healthcare power of attorney, is also called an end-of-life document. Like the durable power of attorney, a healthcare proxy is state-specific. With a healthcare proxy, clients specify their wishes and designate an agent to make medical decisions for them if they lose the ability to reason or communicate. Like the living will, this document outlines care and treatment that the client wishes to permit or exclude. It also outlines the specific responsibilities and authority of the proxy (chosen representative).

Organ Donor Directive

Clients may want to donate organs for transplantation or medical research. Some states allow drivers to fill out an organ donation form when they apply for a driver's license. Some people carry an organ donor card. **Figure 12.7** illustrates a sample donor card.

READING CHECK

List three examples of advance directives.

UNIFORM DONOR CARD

Of ____________________
Print or type name of donor

in the hope that I may help others, I hereby make this anatomical gift, if medically acceptable, to take effect upon my death. The words and marks below indicate my desires.

I give: (a) ☐ any needed organs or parts
(b) ☐ only the following organs or parts

____
Specify the organ(s) or part(s)

for the purposes of transplantation, therapy, medical research or education:
(c) ☐ my body for anatomical study if needed.

Limitations or special wishes, if any: ____________________

Front of card

Signed by the donor and the following two witnesses in the presence of each other:

Signature of Donor ____________________
Date of Birth of Donor ____________________
Date Signed ____________________
City and State ____________________
Witness ____________________
Witness ____________________

THIS IS A LEGAL DOCUMENT UNDER THE UNIFORM ANATOMICAL GIFT ACT OR SIMILAR LAWS.

Back of card

Fig. 12.7 Organ Donation A donor card. *How can donating your organs help others?*

Client Autonomy

Do clients have the right to know if anyone involved in their care is a student or resident?

Clients have important rights and key responsibilities that provide them with autonomy. Autonomy is the freedom to govern one's own moral and legal affairs.

The American Hospital Association (AHA), a national organization that represents hospitals and their patients, has developed a *Patient Care Partnership* document. This plain-language brochure informs patients about what they should expect during a hospital stay with regard to their rights and responsibilities (see **Figure 12.8** on page 349).

Clients' Rights

When clients enter a facility to receive medical care, they have rights. Healthcare providers understand client rights as required by their state. Typically, a patients' bill of rights states the client has a right to

- receive considerate and respectful care.
- receive complete and current information concerning diagnosis, treatment, and prognosis.

- know the identity of physicians, nurses, and others involved in his or her care, and know when those involved are students or trainees.
- know the immediate and long-term costs of treatment choices.
- receive information necessary to give informed consent prior to the start of any procedure or treatment.
- draw up an advance directive concerning treatment or be able to choose a representative to make decisions regarding care.
- refuse treatment to the extent permitted by law.
- receive every consideration of his or her privacy.
- be assured of confidentiality.
- obtain reasonable responses to requests for services.
- obtain information about his or her healthcare, review his or her record, and have any information explained or interpreted.
- know when treatment is experimental and be able to consent or decline to participate.
- expect reasonable continuity of care.
- ask about and be informed of the existence of any business relationships between the hospital and others that may influence the client's treatment and care.
- know which hospital policies and practices relate to client care, treatment, and responsibilities.
- be informed of available resources for resolving disputes, grievances, and conflicts.
- examine the bill, have it explained, and be informed of available payment methods.

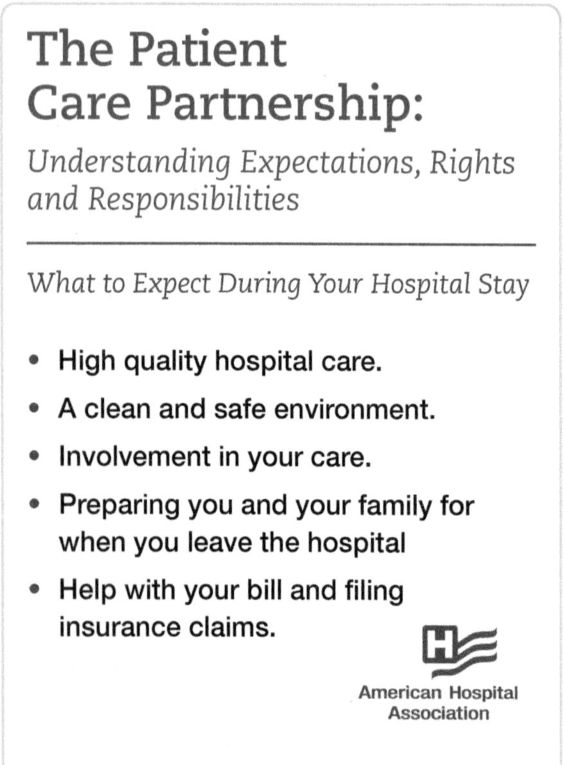

The Patient Care Partnership:

Understanding Expectations, Rights and Responsibilities

What to Expect During Your Hospital Stay

- High quality hospital care.
- A clean and safe environment.
- Involvement in your care.
- Preparing you and your family for when you leave the hospital
- Help with your bill and filing insurance claims.

American Hospital Association

Fig. 12.8 Client Autonomy The Patient Care Partnership document from the American Hospital Association. *What is the purpose of this document?*

Clients' Responsibilities

Healthcare workers should also know that clients have certain responsibilities when they seek medical care. Clients are responsible for

- providing information about past illnesses, hospitalizations, medications, and other matters related to their health status. If an incorrect diagnosis is made because a client fails to give the physician the proper information, the physician is not liable.
- participating in decision making by asking for additional information about their health status or treatment when they do not fully understand information and instructions.
- providing healthcare agencies with a copy of their written advance directive, if they have any.
- informing physicians and other caregivers if they anticipate problems in following a prescribed treatment.

- following the physician's orders for treatment. If a client willfully or negligently fails to follow the physician's instructions, that client has little legal recourse. Remember, though, that the client has the right to refuse treatment to the extent permitted by law.
- providing healthcare agencies with necessary information for insurance claims, and working with the healthcare facility to make arrangements to pay fees when necessary.

READING CHECK

Name two client responsibilities that can absolve a physician of liability if they are not performed.

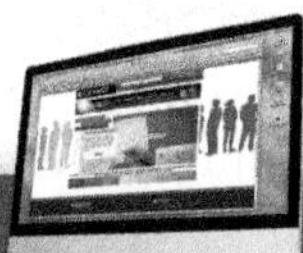

connect ONLINE PROCEDURES

PROCEDURE 12-2

Recording Information on a Medical Record

As a healthcare worker, you may be asked to record information on a client's medical record or to update existing records. For legal protection, as well as for continuity of care, a complete, accurate, and timely record of client medical care must be kept. Entries in the medical record must be objective and concise. Do not add personal judgments, observations, attempts at humor, or abbreviations not accepted by the healthcare facility where you are employed.

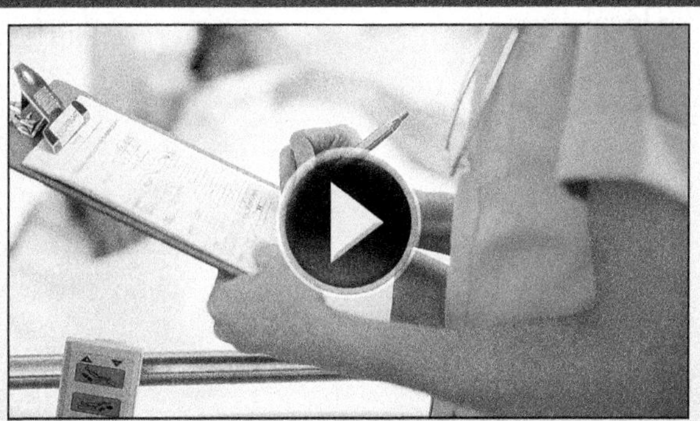

Go to connect to complete Procedure 12-2.

SECTION 12.2 Medical Records and Policies Review

AFTER YOU READ

1. **Name** five purposes served by clients' medical records.
2. **Recall** who owns a client's medical record.
3. **Explain** how errors made in recording information in a medical record can be corrected.
4. **Explain** the purpose of HIPAA.
5. **Define** "advance directive" and name three examples.
6. **Discuss** client rights and responsibilities.

Technology ONLINE EXPLORATIONS

HIPAA

Search the Internet for more information about HIPAA. Based on your research, create a list of guidelines that the healthcare professional must follow in order to be compliant with HIPAA.

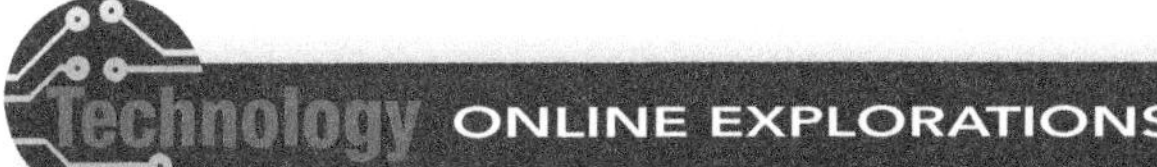

Photo: Getty Images/OJO Images

SECTION
12.3 Qualities for Success

Vocabulary

Content Vocabulary

You will learn this content vocabulary term in this section.

- **The three Cs**

Academic Vocabulary

You will see this word in your reading and on your tests. Find its meaning in the Glossary in the back of the book.

- **legal**

Qualities for Success

Which of your personal qualities do you feel make you well-suited for a healthcare career?

Before you can practice legal and ethical responsibilities, you must first practice qualities for success. These qualities say a lot about your legal, ethical, and moral character. They demonstrate your ability to be successful in the healthcare field. The first responsibility of the healthcare profession is always to provide competent, courteous healthcare to clients. People who are most likely to achieve this goal have certain characteristics, called **the three Cs,** which are:

- Courtesy
- Compassion
- Common sense

The three Cs are vital to the professional and personal success of healthcare workers. Other qualities that are helpful to those who choose to work in the healthcare field are:

- A relaxed attitude when meeting new people
- A willingness to learn new skills and techniques
- An aptitude for working with the hands
- Empathy for others
- Good communication and listening skills
- Patience in dealing with others
- The ability to work as a member of a healthcare team
- Proficiency in English, science, and mathematics
- Tact
- The ability to keep information confidential
- The ability to leave personal concerns at home
- Trustworthiness
- A sense of responsibility

As a healthcare professional, you will interact with a wide variety of people, including clients, employers, coworkers, insurance representatives, and medical equipment and product salespeople. To deal comfortably and competently with clients and others, you will need to practice the three Cs and develop the other qualities listed above.

As part of your qualities for success, you must follow the rules and regulations at your place of employment. This includes specific requirements regarding your appearance. Healthcare facilities may require you to wear a uniform or a lab coat. Depending upon where you are employed, you may be required to avoid nail polish, jewelry (including body piercings), or heavy perfumes and powders. Not wearing nail polish helps prevent the spread of nosocomial infections. In addition, you may be asked to wear a name pin. Name pins worn by all will enhance security. These policies are written and enforced for your protection and the protection of your clients.

Responsibilities to Employers

As an employee in a healthcare facility (or in any other job), you should deal morally, ethically, and legally with your employer. For instance, when you apply for a position as a healthcare worker, you should provide accurate, honest information about your qualifications for the job. This information should include a detailed account of your education, past work experience, and any specialized training you have received that is relevant to the position. More information about obtaining a job is presented in Chapter 13, Communication and Employability Skills.

Once hired, you are obligated to report for work on time each day, properly dressed and groomed, and ready and willing to accept your day's assignments.

Healthcare professionals should stay current in their field, by:

- Attending seminars and continuing education courses
- Subscribing to professional journals
- Obtaining in-house training

They need to do this to fulfill license renewal requirements.

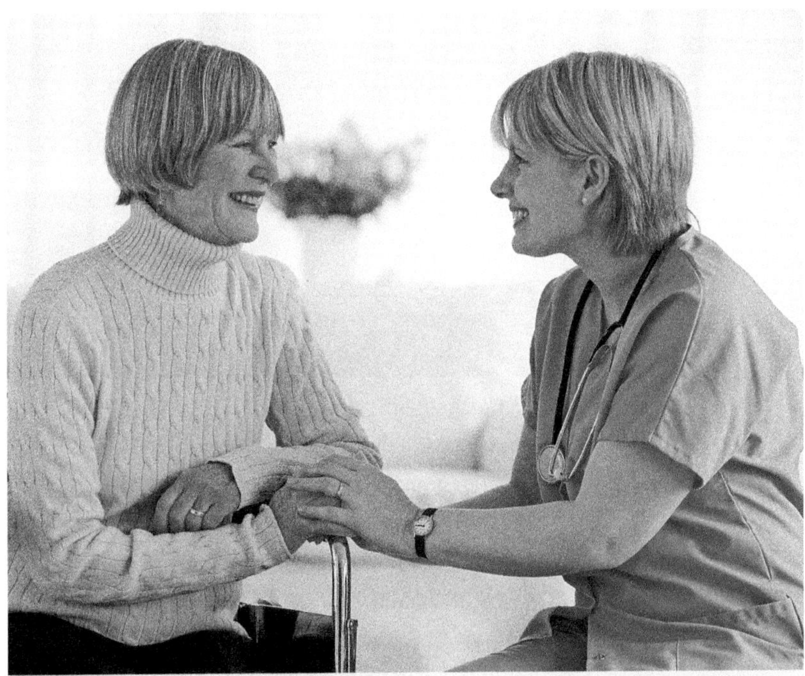

Fig. 12.9 Listening Effective care giving includes listening to the client. *How can you improve your listening skills?*

Photo: Tetra Images/CORBIS

21ST CENTURY SKILLS

Listening

As a healthcare worker, you may often find that the most valuable service you can perform is listening to clients. **Figure 12.9** puts this into context. Instead of ignoring clients as you concentrate on your assigned tasks, be available, within reasonable limits, to listen if they seem eager to talk.

21st CENTURY SKILLS

Working as a Team Member

When you accept a position as a healthcare worker, you automatically become a member of a team. The members of the team may change from day to day, depending upon the medical situation. The team's goal is always the same—to provide quality healthcare for clients that will

- help clients get well and/or stay well.
- contribute to diagnosing diseases or conditions.
- make clients more comfortable or otherwise improve the quality of their lives.

To achieve these goals, you must demonstrate the ability to work with others, help set goals, and help plan strategies to meet these goals.

The Healthcare Team

Workers in healthcare facilities are members of a healthcare team. The team members must be capable of working cooperatively with others so that clients will receive the best possible care.

Chapter 13 discusses how to be a good team member. The healthcare team includes, but is not limited to:

- Physicians
- Registered nurses
- Licensed practical nurses
- Licensed vocational nurses
- Dietitians
- Physical therapists
- Occupational therapists
- Respiratory therapists
- Electrocardiography technicians
- X-ray technicians
- Medical transcriptionists
- Nursing assistants

READING CHECK

Explain why good listening skills are important in healthcare.

SECTION 12.3 Qualities for Success Review

AFTER YOU READ

1. **Examine** your own personal qualities for success.
2. **Name** some responsibilities that a healthcare worker owes to his or her employer.
3. **Relate** qualities for success to your legal, ethical, and moral responsibilities as a healthcare professional.
4. **Describe** some of the ways you can be a good team member.
5. **Illustrate** some of the ways you can remain current in your chosen healthcare field.

ONLINE EXPLORATIONS

Active Listening

Being an effective listener is essential to the healthcare professional. Use the Internet to learn more about this skill. Search for "active listening," "effective listening," "improving my listening skills," and other similar phrases. Find an online exercise, game, or other resource with which to practice active listening with your classmates, family, or friends.

CHAPTER
12 Review

Chapter Summary

SECTION 12.1

- Laws are a set of governing rules. Criminal laws protect members of society from certain harmful acts of others. Civil laws are concerned with private rights and remedies. **(pg. 335)**
- Ethics are standards of behavior that reflect moral values. Morals are our concept of right and wrong, and are formed through the influence of family, culture, and society. **(pg. 336)**
- Negligence—known in the healthcare field as medical malpractice—is the tort most likely to affect healthcare practitioners. **(pg. 336)**
- Standard of care and scope of practice are legal concepts dictating that healthcare practitioners may perform only those duties prescribed by their education, training, and job description. **(pg. 339)**
- Informed consent means that healthcare clients have a legal and ethical right to receive all information relative to their condition before they consent to medical treatment. **(pg. 341)**
- Clients have a legal and ethical right to have all personal medical information kept private and confidential. **(pg. 342)**

SECTION 12.2

- For legal reasons and for continuity of care, information must be correctly recorded in clients' medical records. **(pg. 345)**
- Clients have the right to prepare advance directives, which include a living will, a durable power of attorney, and a healthcare proxy. **(pg. 347)**
- Clients have important rights when they enter a healthcare facility such as a hospital. Such rights are listed in a document provided by the American Hospital Association. **(pg. 349)**
- Clients also have responsibilities, such as providing accurate and complete information about their medical history to healthcare workers and participating in decision making regarding their care. **(pg. 350)**

SECTION 12.3

- To provide competent care to clients, a healthcare practitioner should work on the three Cs—courtesy, compassion, and common sense. **(pg. 352)**
- Healthcare professionals stay current in their field by attending seminars and continuing education courses, subscribing to professional journals, and through in-house training. **(pg. 353)**

CHAPTER 12 Assessment

Critical Thinking/Problem Solving

What would you say or do in each of the following situations?

1. You are a medical assistant. An attorney telephones your office and demands to know whether or not a certain client is being treated by one of the physicians who employs you.
2. You are a registered nurse. Your neighbor asks you to tell her the diagnosis for a man who is a mutual acquaintance, because she fears that she was exposed to his disease and wonders if it is contagious.
3. A client of the medical office where you work asks that his records be sent to another physician.

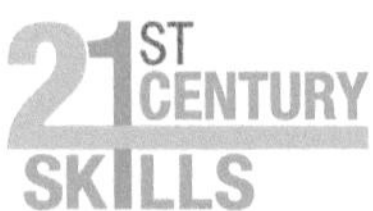

4. **Teamwork** Working in pairs, select a career that you would like to pursue. Determine what your workplace appearance for that career should be and decide why. Present your career appearance to the class.
5. **Listening** With a partner, describe in detail a very embarrassing or exciting moment in your life. Have your partner retell the story. Did he or she really hear what you said?
6. **Information Literacy** Go online to find a case currently in the news concerning medical negligence or malpractice. Write a paragraph summarizing the case. Include your opinion or projection of the outcome.

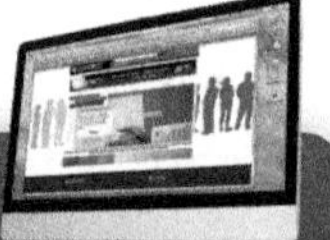

connect ONLINE ACTIVITIES

Complete our HST online activities for Chapter 12, which include Concept Check review questions, Reference Flash Cards, and Online Procedures assessment sheets.

- **Concept Check** review questions
- **Reference Flash Cards** medical terminology practice
- **Online Procedures** assessment sheets

CHAPTER

13 Communication and Employability Skills

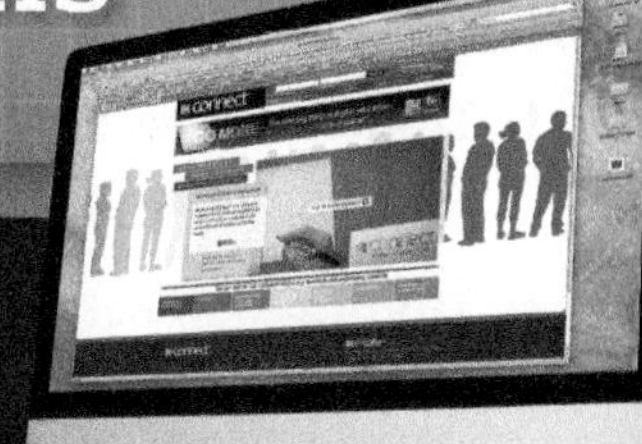

Essential Question:

What characteristics do employers look for in an effective healthcare worker?

Why do we work? The importance of making enough money to meet our needs cannot be overlooked, but there are many other reasons to have a job. Jobs provide money to meet basic needs and enjoy recreation, benefits like insurance and retirement programs, part of our sense of identity, personal fulfillment, social contact, and structure for our time.

Getting a job requires time and effort. You must display the traits discussed in Section 13.2 and use these traits to help you keep the job and be successful in it.

McGraw Hill connect™

It's Online!

- Online Procedures
- STEM Connection
- Medical Science
- Medical Terms
- Medical Math
- Ethics in Action
- Virtual Lab

READING GUIDE

OBJECTIVES

After completing this chapter, you will be able to:

- **Demonstrate** the elements of communication.
- **Distinguish** between subjective and objective information.
- **Identify** barriers to communication.
- **List** the elements of professionalism.
- **Apply** critical thinking and problem-solving skills.
- **Discuss** strategies for time and stress management.
- **Compare** the characteristics of a good team member and a good team leader.
- **Explain** the importance of respecting diversity.
- **Analyze** the strategies for finding a job.
- **Prepare** a résumé and cover letter.
- **Demonstrate** how to approach a job interview.
- **Describe** the procedure for leaving a job.

BEFORE YOU READ

Connect What are some things you should do to prepare for your healthcare career job search?

Main Idea

A successful career in healthcare involves more than knowledge of body systems and procedures. The way in which you present yourself to a prospective employer and clients is vital to a successful job search and healthcare career.

Note-Taking Activity

Draw this table. Write key terms and phrases under **Cues**. Write main ideas under **Note Taking**. Summarize the section under **Summary**.

Cues	Note Taking
○	○
○	○
Summary	

Graphic Organizer

Before you read the chapter, draw a diagram like the one to the right. As you read, write the topics covered in this chapter into the diagram.

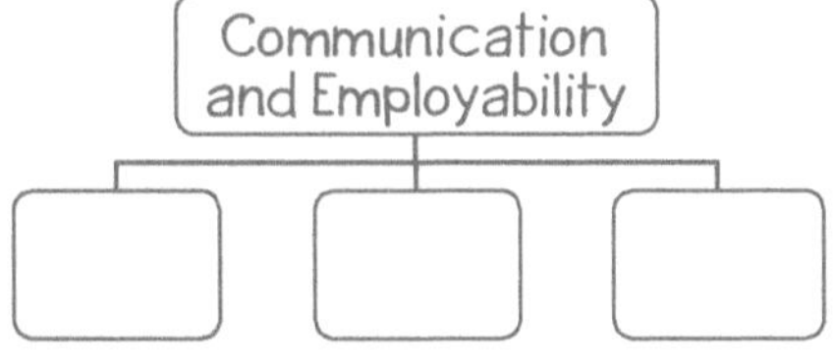

connect

Downloadable graphic organizers can be accessed online.

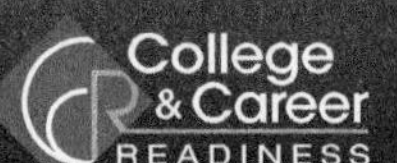

STANDARDS

HEALTH SCIENCE

NCHSE 2.12 Recognize barriers to communication.

NCHSE 2.15 Apply speaking and active listening skills.

SCIENCE

NSES A Develop abilities necessary to do scientific inquiry, understandings about scientific inquiry.

NCHSE *National Consortium for Health Science Education*

NSES *National Science Education Standards*

COMMON CORE STATE STANDARDS

MATHEMATICS

Number and Quantity

Quantities N-Q Reason quantitatively and use units to solve problems.

ENGLISH LANGUAGE ARTS

Writing

Production and Distribution of Writing W-4 Produce clear and coherent writing in which the development, organization, and style are appropriate to task, purpose, and audience.

Production and Distribution of Writing W-5 Develop and strengthen writing as needed by planning, revising, editing, rewriting, or trying a new approach, focusing on addressing what is most significant for a specific purpose and audience.

Speaking and Listening

Presentation of Knowledge and Ideas SL-6 Adapt speech to a variety of contexts and communicative tasks, demonstrating command of formal English when indicated or appropriate.

SECTION

13.1 Communication

The Communication Process

Are you a good communicator?

Employment in healthcare requires knowledge of the process of communication. Communication is vital in the field of healthcare. since miscommunication in healthcare can lead to serious physical and legal consequences. Healthcare professionals must be good communicators to be successful. Communication is the process by which we assign and convey meaning in an attempt to create a shared understanding.

Communication comes in many forms, including oral, written, and nonverbal (including electronic). It usually is made up of five components: the sender or source, the message, the receiver, feedback, and noise.

The sender is the information source. The receiver decodes the message. Feedback is the verbal or nonverbal response to the sender. The receiver uses feedback to indicate his or her understanding of the message. Anything that distorts the message or feedback is noise (see **Figure 13.1**). Consider the **verbal communication** below. Fernando, who works in a physical therapy office, is speaking with Mrs. Riveria, a patient who is being treated for a back injury.

Fernando: The physical therapist says you're making progress and you can do some simple exercises at home. I'd like to go over them and give you a sheet that illustrates the exercises. How does that sound?

Mrs. Riveria: I'm a little nervous about doing exercises. I still have some pain when I bend over.

Fernando: I understand. It's important, though, to start using those muscles again. Why don't you show me where it hurts? Then we can go over proper body mechanics, such as bending down to pick something up and getting in and out of chairs, the car, and bed. Then we'll just start with one or two of the exercises and save the rest for next time, when you're feeling more ready.

Mrs. Riveria: Yes, I only feel up to doing a little bit today.

Fernando (the source) gives a verbal message (about back exercises) to the client (the receiver). The patient gives feedback by drawing attention to her pain and uneasiness about certain movements. The giving

Vocabulary

Content Vocabulary

You will learn these content vocabulary terms in this section.

- **verbal communication**
- **nonverbal communication**
- **feedback**
- **aphasia**
- **objective comment**
- **subjective comment**

Academic Vocabulary

You will see these words in your reading and on your tests. Find their meanings in the Glossary in the back of the book.

- **component**
- **distort**

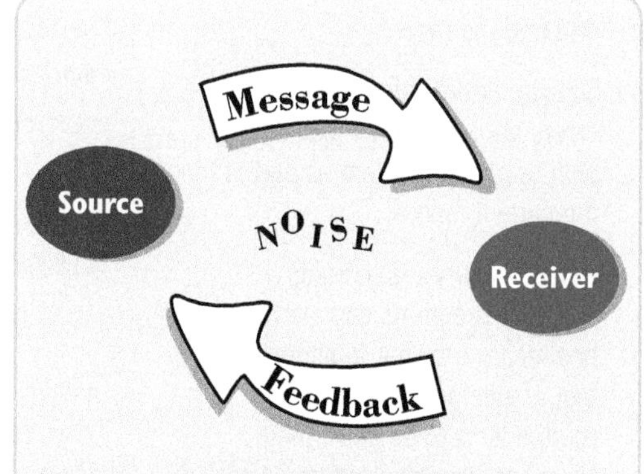

Fig. 13.1 The Communication Process Noise distorts the message or feedback. *What are some examples of "noise" in the communication process?*

and receiving of information continues until the communication is finished. If Mrs. Riveria had been hard of hearing or very uncomfortable, or could not receive the message for some other reason, this exchange would have been noise, not communication.

Nonverbal Communication

In **nonverbal communication,** signals provide information. Nonverbal communication is often thought to be the more honest and universal of the two forms of communication. Nonverbal communication usually supports verbal communication. When verbal and nonverbal communication do not match, confusion and misunderstanding result.

Feedback

Feedback is very valuable. It tells the sender whether or not the receiver got the message that the sender intended. Feedback may change the course of communication. Feedback can be verbal or nonverbal. Feedback for written communication usually is not immediate. It is critical, therefore, that written communication be as clear as possible.

Communication Problems

Anything that interferes with communication can lead to a lack of understanding or misinterpretation of the message. This is considered the "noise" in the communication process. Communication problems occur often in the healthcare field. Clients are often physically ill and emotionally upset when a healthcare worker is attempting to communicate with them. Clients may have difficulty concentrating or paying attention.

In addition to general communication problems, healthcare has its own specialized language, as discussed in Chapter 5, Medical Terminology. Clients often do not understand medical terms. They may have sensory impairments such as poor hearing, poor vision, confusion, and speaking problems. For example, people who have had a stroke sometimes suffer from **aphasia.** Aphasia is an impairment of the ability to communicate through speech, writing, or signs. Clients might be confused because they suffer from Alzheimer's disease, or their medications may affect their mental processes. If English is not the client's first language, this might add to the communication problems.

Regardless of the situation, it is your responsibility to make sure that the client understands the information being given and that you understand what the client wants to convey. You may need to use special techniques to communicate with some clients (see **Table 13.1**).

Good Communication

Good listening skills are an important part of communication. Always try to face the client. Lean forward and make eye contact. Watch closely for any discrepancy between verbal and nonverbal messages.

21ST CENTURY SKILLS

Electronic Health Records

The federal government is encouraging all healthcare entities to switch to **electronic health records (EHRs)** by 2014. Electronic health records (EHRs) are essentially a computer-based or digital recording of patient information. They are also called computer records, electronic medical records (EMRs), electronic charts, and computer health records. EHRs provide several important advantages over paper records.

- **Access** Electronic records can be accessed by healthcare providers at various locations, including the medical records department, the laboratory, and even the pharmacy.
- **Availability** Information is immediately available, so healthcare providers do not have to wait for the paper document to be written and sent. The data are entered and then immediately viewed at any electronic record location.
- **Security** Electronic records provide security through special passwords for each individual entering the records.
- **Safety** Patient identification errors are reduced by including a picture of each patient as part of the patient record.
- **Extra features** Electronic software programs can alert the healthcare provider to abnormal test results or to the need for routine tests to be performed. More sophisticated programs can document health trends, provide voice recognition, and convert notes to complete sentences.

Figure 13.2 shows effective verbal and nonverbal communication. Try to provide visual feedback by nodding and using other body language. Give verbal feedback by saying "yes" or "I don't understand." To be sure that you correctly received the client's message, summarize in your own words the message as you heard it. Ask whether that is what he or she meant.

You have already learned that clients have the right to informed consent. To be informed, they must be given information that they can understand. Many healthcare facilities employ medical interpreters who explain procedures and information in each client's own language.

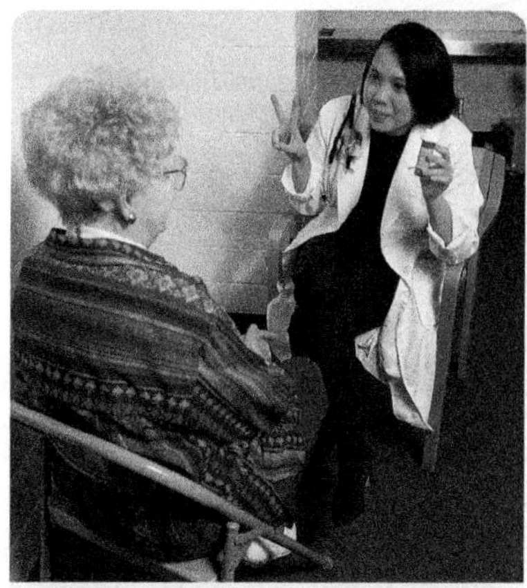

Fig. 13.2 Verbal and Nonverbal Communication Whenever possible, use both verbal and nonverbal communication. *How do good listening skills contribute to good communication?*

READING CHECK

Explain why communication is vital in the field of healthcare.

Table 13.1 Overcoming Communication Problems

PROBLEM	SOLUTION
Client does not hear well.	Be sure the client knows you are approaching. Face the client and speak clearly.
	Be sure the client's hearing aid is adjusted properly. Speak louder, but don't shout.
	Increase your nonverbal communication. "Show" the client what she or he needs to know. Use feedback to be sure that communication has taken place correctly.
Client does not see well.	Speak clearly. Remember that the client cannot see your nonverbal communication.
	Announce yourself when entering the room, and make it clear when you are leaving the room. Explain any unusual noises.
	Do not shout. The client may not see well, but may be able to hear just fine.
	Use plenty of feedback to be sure that communication has taken place correctly.
Client is confused.	Be sure to announce yourself when you enter the room, and make it clear when you are leaving the room.
	Remain calm. Be patient. The client may need extra time to think or respond.
	Keep your messages short and simple. Use whatever form of communication works best for the client.
	Use plenty of feedback to be sure that communication has taken place correctly.
Client has aphasia or a similar problem.	Face the client and speak slowly and clearly. Be patient. The client needs extra time.
	Use both verbal and nonverbal communication.
	Use closed questions whenever possible, so that the client does not need to express complex thoughts. Closed questions are those that may be answered with "yes" or "no," "now" or "later," or a similar brief response.
	Be aware that client may use incorrect words that might change his or her meaning.
	Use plenty of feedback to be sure that communication has taken place correctly.

Photo: Cliff Moore

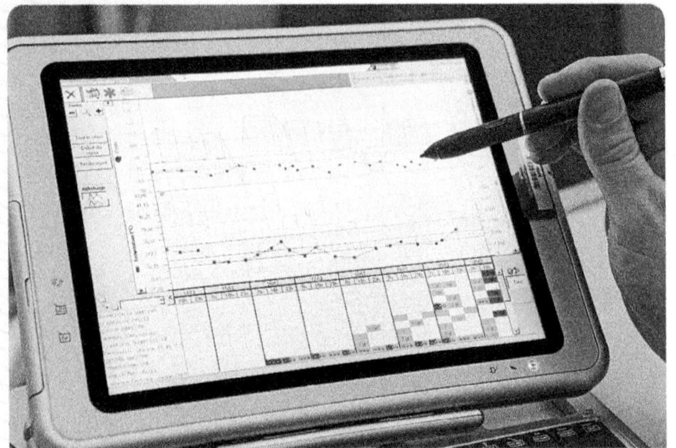

Fig. 13.3 Electronic Health Record Electronic health records have become very common and provide many advantages over a written healthcare record. *What are the advantages of such a system over paper records?*

Written (Electronic) Communication

What client information can be stored electronically?

Nearly everything that happens in healthcare is recorded in some way. A client's health record is an ongoing document of his or her healthcare. A health record may be either written or electronic. Electronic health records have become very common and provide many advantages over a written healthcare record (see **Figure 13.3**). These advantages include the following:

- Records of the client's care and billing are more complete and better coordinated.
- Fewer medical records are lost, because all materials are in electronic format and will be backed up electronically.
- Charts are easier to read and understand. Charts may even be highlighted in color, to improve understanding.
- Charts are easier to access after hours.
- Access to the record may be granted to more than one person at a time.
- Patient education materials are easier to access.

See **Procedure 13-1** to learn more about using electronic health records.

Whether the chart is written or electronic, you should follow these rules:

- Never chart anything until you actually do it.
- Be objective and precise when you chart. **Objective comments** are based upon facts, not opinions. **Subjective comments** are opinions or perceptions. For example, do not chart "the patient was angry." You should write instead, "The patient said, 'Get out of my room right now.'" The first example is subjective; it is an opinion. The second indicates objectively what happened.
- Use only abbreviations approved by your employer.
- List events in chronological order.

For paper charts, you should follow these additional guidelines:

- Use the ink color recommended by your place of employment.
- Always initial or sign what you record.
- Never leave a space between what you have charted and your initials or signature.
- Do not black out an error, use correction fluid to correct it, or erase it. Score through the error with a single line, making sure that it is still legible. Correct written errors according to workplace policy.

READING CHECK

Recall which special guidelines apply to paper charts.

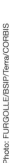

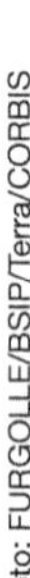

Telephone Etiquette

Do all healthcare professionals answer the phone?

Regardless of where you are employed, you will probably have work-related telephone conversations. Use the following guidelines when receiving a telephone message.

- Answer promptly.
- Identify the facility or organization, and state your name.
- Speak clearly and use a friendly, professional tone.
- Take a clear, concise message if the call is for someone else.
- Return calls as soon as practical.

READING CHECK

Identify what to state when answering the telephone.

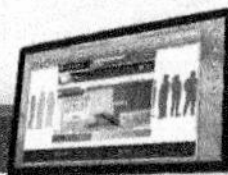

connect

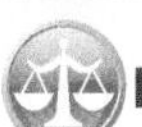

Ethics in Action

Confidentiality The need for absolute confidentiality when communicating client information cannot be stressed too strongly. Confidentiality is so important that healthcare employers have policies calling for the dismissal of anyone who violates this principle.

Go to connect to complete the Ethics in Action discussion and research activity.

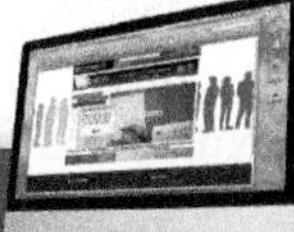

connect ONLINE PROCEDURES

PROCEDURE 13-1

Using Electronic Health Records

Nearly everything that happens in healthcare is recorded in some way. Electronic health records are very common and provide a lot of advantages. Electronic health records will eventually be the only method of maintaining health records because of these advantages.

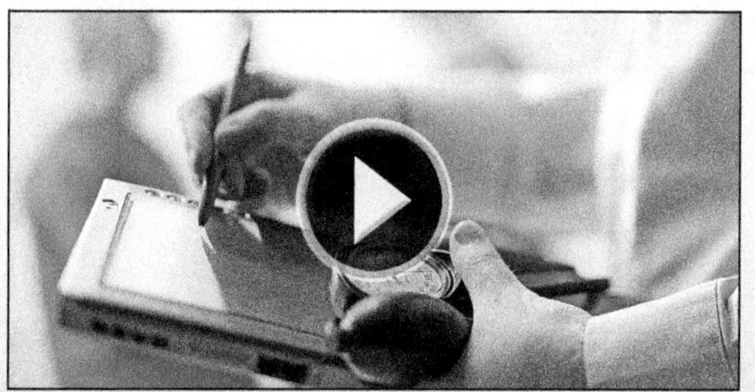

SECTION 13.1 Communication Review

AFTER YOU READ

1. **Identify** the five basic elements of communication.
2. **Describe** four communication problems you might encounter with clients and list three possible solutions to each problem.
3. **Assess** the advantages of electronic health records.
4. **List** at least four rules of charting.
5. **Demonstrate** the procedure for receiving a telephone message.

Technology ONLINE EXPLORATIONS

Communication

Search online for information about any of the communication-related topics listed below. Write a one-page summary of the information that you find, including some type of visual element such as a photo, drawing, map, or diagram, to present to your class.

- The communication process
- Interpersonal communication
- Barriers to communication
- Charting techniques
- Telephone etiquette

Photo: Comstock/Getty Images

SECTION

13.2 Employment Skills and Personal Traits

Vocabulary

Content Vocabulary

You will learn these content vocabulary terms in this section.

- **consensus**
- **passive personality**
- **aggressive personality**
- **assertive personality**
- **diversity**
- **stereotype**
- **sexual harassment**

Academic Vocabulary

You will see this word in your reading and on your tests. Find its meaning in the Glossary in the back of the book.

- **specific**

Basic Skills

Do you have the skills needed to be employed in the healthcare profession?

In addition to excellent communication skills, to enter the healthcare industry you must have a specific set of skills and personal traits. This section discusses basic skills for a healthcare professional and desirable personal traits for a member of a healthcare team. Having these skills will provide you with a strong foundation for finding and keeping employment and advancing on the job.

- **Basic skills:** Reading, writing, speaking, listening, and knowing arithmetic and mathematical concepts
- **Thinking skills:** Reasoning, making decisions, solving problems, thinking creatively, and knowing how to learn
- **Personal qualities:** Responsibility, flexibility, honesty, reliability, and a commitment to quality and excellence
- **Interpersonal skills:** Negotiating, exercising leadership, participating in teams, serving clients, teaching others new skills, and working with diversity
- **Information skills:** Obtaining and evaluating data, interpreting and communicating information, and using computers
- **Systems:** Understanding systems, monitoring and correcting system performance, and improving and designing systems
- **Resources:** Identifying, organizing, planning and allocating money, time, energy, materials, and personnel
- **Technology utilization skills:** Selecting technology, applying technology to a task, and troubleshooting technology

READING CHECK

List the basic skills that employers expect employees to have as a foundation.

Math, Science, and Technology

Do you enjoy learning and working with math, science, or technology?

Employment in the healthcare field requires some knowledge of math, science, and technology. Here are some of the skills you will need.

Basic Math Skills

Employment in the healthcare field requires math knowledge that includes the abilities to

- use the metric system, a system based on counting by 10s that is the standard system in health technology.
- add, subtract, multiply, and divide.
- work with percentages and decimals.

Basic Science Skills

The amount of scientific knowledge you will need varies greatly depending upon the area of healthcare you pursue. In some cases, you will need an in-depth knowledge of all the areas listed below. In other cases, you may need only a minimal understanding. Most healthcare professionals need at least a basic knowledge of anatomy and physiology, biology, microbiology, chemistry, and physics.

Technology

Today, all healthcare workers must be able to use computers and be familiar with software applications.

Keyboarding Keyboarding is required for almost every healthcare occupation. The two most important keyboarding skills are speed and accuracy. The best way to enhance these skills is by practicing at every opportunity. In addition, basic knowledge of common software programs, e-mail, and the Internet is always valuable and often essential.

E-mail Many healthcare facilities use e-mail to communicate with clients. Using e-mail in a business setting is a little different from sending e-mail or an IM to a friend. Here are some tips.

- Address the person by his or her last name. For example, write "Dear Ms. Garcia," not "Hi, Mary."
- Remember that e-mail is not secure. Do not reveal private or confidential information in an unencrypted e-mail.
- Use good spelling and grammar.
- Be courteous and state your message clearly.

Electronic records Many healthcare organizations use specialized programs for maintaining records, tracking costs, billing, and other functions. Information is often transferred by computer from one part of the organization to another or from one facility to another. This speeds up communication, reduces paperwork, and is more efficient than traditional methods of information processing. Healthcare professionals typically receive on-the-job training in the use of the specific programs used at a healthcare facility.

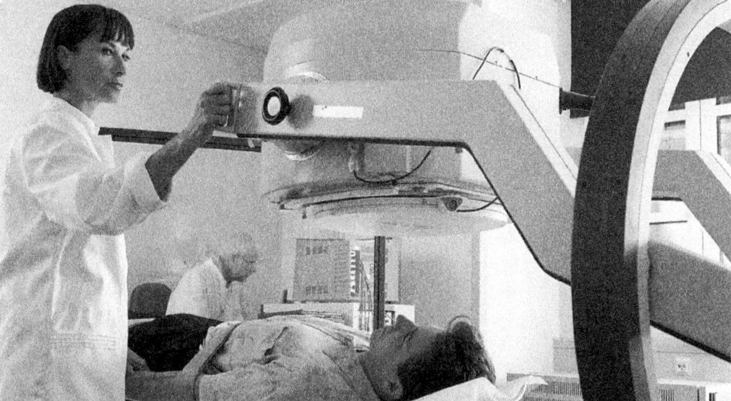

Fig. 13.4 Technology Skills Technology is used in all aspects of healthcare. *What basic technology skills will you need to work in healthcare?*

Photo: Comstock Images/Jupiter Images/Getty Images

This includes electronic health records. However, it is much easier to learn new programs if you already have a solid background in basic computer operations.Most of the high-tech machines used in healthcare rely on computers. Imaging machines such as MRIs, CAT scans, and ultrasound (shown in **Figure 13.4**) are based on computers. Many laboratory tests are performed with computers. When you choose an occupation in healthcare, you will receive training in using the technology in that field.

READING CHECK

Analyze why healthcare workers need to be computer literate.

Professionalism

What professional behaviors do you display?

Certain qualities distinguish workers who behave professionally from those who just "get by." Professionalism includes the following:

- Dependability: being timely, accurate, and conscientious.
- Responsibility: being prepared to be held accountable for your actions.
- Integrity: being honest, truthful, and reliable.
- Self-motivation: performing work without constant supervision.
- Discretion: using good judgment in what you say or do, especially regarding confidentiality.
- Patience: being tolerant of challenging people and situations.
- Competence: being able to perform the job effectively.
- Contributions to the profession: maintaining membership and active participation in professional organizations.

READING CHECK

Identify the professional qualities that are most likely to lead to a successful career in healthcare.

Critical Thinking and Problem Solving

How do you solve problems?

Critical-thinking and problem-solving skills often make the difference between an average worker and an excellent employee. Critical thinking involves the ability to:

- analyze situations.
- determine which aspects of a situation are most important.
- reach conclusions that go beyond the obvious.

Critical Thinking

What variables must be considered when solving a problem using critical thinking?

Critical thinking includes factual problem identification and creative decision-making skills. It is the ability to see the whole picture and to reach reasonable conclusions based on the most important facts. See **Figure 13.5** for more information on this essential skill.

Problem solving can be broken down into a step-by-step approach.

- Identify the problem and define it clearly.
- Identify the circumstances that affect the problem.
- Clarify the objectives to be achieved.
- List as many potential solutions and strategies as possible.
- Analyze the potential solutions and strategies.
- Implement the strategy that appears to be the best solution.
- Evaluate the results and repeat the steps as needed.

READING CHECK

Describe how creativity contributes to critical thinking.

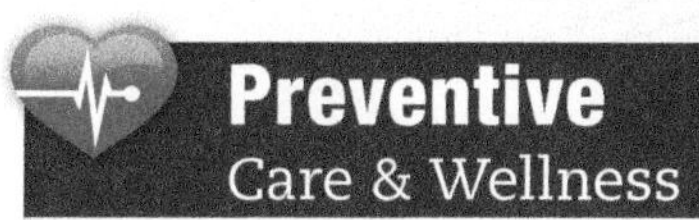

Stress

Excessive stress can contribute to ill health or even cause certain diseases. Some stressful events cannot be prevented, so prepare yourself whenever you can. Once stress has occurred, try these simple stress busters:

- Take a brisk walk, run, or jog.
- Go to a movie.
- Bake a cake.
- Call a friend.
- Listen to your favorite music.
- Close your eyes and take some deep breaths.

Time Management

Do you ever run out of time?

The healthcare work environment is exceptionally busy and challenging. Job satisfaction may be increased by knowledge and use of time management strategies.

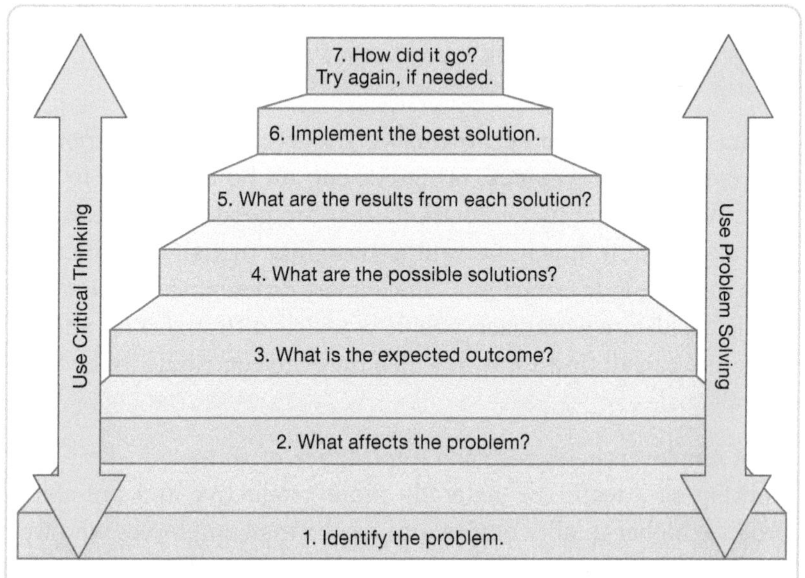

Fig. 13.5 Steps to Problem Solving A healthcare professional needs to be a good problem solver. *What are the consequences of not thinking critically?*

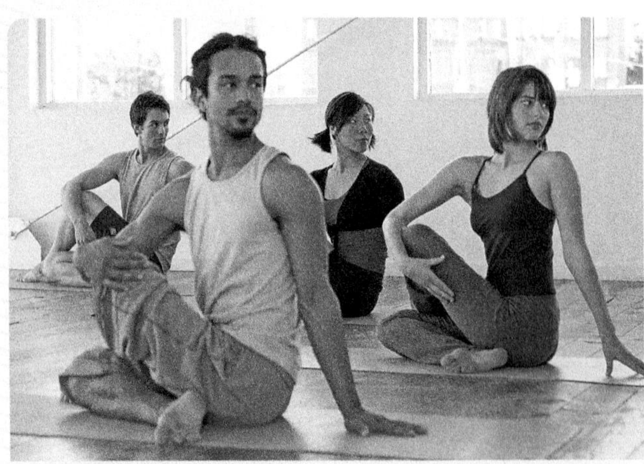

Fig. 13.6 Stress Relief Exercise relieves stress. *What kinds of stress-reducing activities do you enjoy?*

Here are some time management tips.

- Make a list of the tasks you need to do.
- If tasks need to be done at a specific time, put them in chronological order.
- Prioritize tasks according to their importance.
- Group tasks in terms of location or similarity of activity.
- Allow extra time for the unexpected.
- Start on the highest-priority task to avoid playing catch-up later.

Properly managing your time will also help reduce stress. It is difficult to eliminate stress entirely in this fast-paced world, but stress management is essential to your physical and mental well being. Here are some strategies for stress management (see **Figure 13.6**).

- Balance work with enjoyable non-work activities.
- Schedule "play" time as a routine part of your activities, not as an "add-on."
- Schedule time for regular exercise.
- Take time for specific relaxation activities such as meditation.
- Do not try to solve all your problems at once.
- Eat nutritious meals and avoid junk food.
- Avoid using alcohol or other drugs in an attempt to relax.

READING CHECK

Recall which personal habits are important to stress management.

Teamwork

What type of personality do you have?

Groups just work together. Teams work together with a common goal and come to a **consensus,** or agreement, on how they are to function. Team players make decisions that are good for the team, and operate as a unit. It is important to recognize that all team members have something to contribute. Since many different skills are needed in the healthcare workplace, people of widely differing skills and personalities can all find a way in which they can contribute to the team's overall goals.

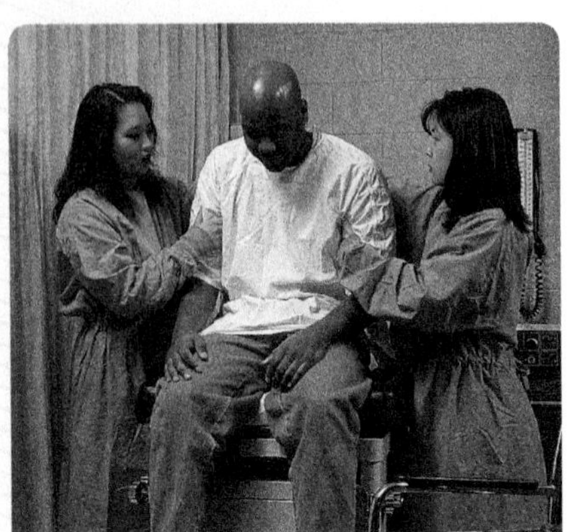

Fig. 13.7 Teamwork Most employers recognize the importance of teamwork. *Why is it important to work together?*

Most employers recognize the importance of teamwork. Employees working as a team are generally more productive and are able to produce higher-quality output and results than employees who work independently. Job satisfaction also tends to be higher when employees work together as part of a team. See **Figure 13.7** for an illustration of teamwork.

Groups of people who have similar jobs often work very closely together to provide services to clients. Small teams are clustered with other teams to create the entire healthcare team. In teamwork, individuals come together to reach goals that are shared by all. There is a division of labor that results in the efficient handling of tasks that need to be completed. Remember that clients and their families should always be part of the team.

How can you be a good team player?

- Learn what your personal responsibilities are and be dependable in carrying them out.
- Participate in the decision-making process to the fullest extent possible.
- Once decisions are made, support those decisions even if you do not fully agree.
- If you are asked to do something that violates your personal ethics, tell your team members that you cannot participate.
- When possible, take the initiative to do things that need to be done even if they are not your direct responsibility.
- Help other people grow by teaching them things that they do not know.
- Without violating confidentiality, share information that will help others improve at their jobs.
- Practice good communication skills, especially active listening.
- Change is the only constant. Be willing to accept change.
- Be assertive, not aggressive or passive. (These personality traits are discussed below.)
- Be willing to accept input from others.
- Be honest.

Personality Traits

Three common personality traits affect how we relate to others in groups:

- People with a **passive personality** tend to put the needs of others ahead of their own needs, even when doing so is harmful to themselves.
- People with an **aggressive personality** tend to put their own needs ahead of the needs of others and to push others out of the way in order to get what they want.
- People with an **assertive personality** stand up for their own rights, but recognize and respect the rights and needs of others. In a work environment, team members who are assertive help facilitate a more cohesive and successful effort. In addition, assertive people feel better about themselves (see **Figure 13.8**).

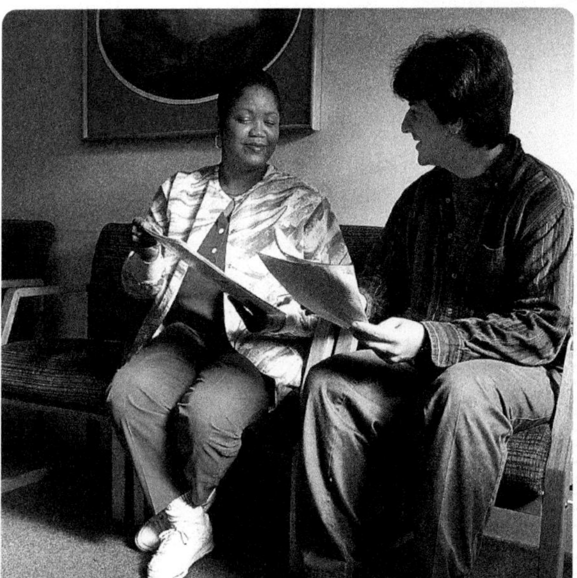

Fig. 13.8 Asserting Your Rights Assertive people know and understand their rights. *How can you find out about your rights as a client?*

Photo: Kathy Sloane

In order to work as a member of a team, you should recognize the ways in which you relate to the world. You should also recognize that different people relate to the world in different ways. Differences in perceptions and attitudes have a major impact on how we approach our lives and our work. It is useful to examine your basic personal tendencies and preferences, to help understand how you will function as a team member. One way to do this is to determine your personality type, using one of many available tools. The Myers-Briggs Type Indicator and the Keirsey Temperament Sorter, both based on the work of psychologist Carl Jung, are two of the better-known tools for profiling personality types.

READING CHECK

List the advantages of having an assertive personality.

Leadership

What does it take to be a leader?

Sometimes terms such as "manager," "director," or "supervisor" are used as synonyms for "leader." But these terms do not have the same meaning. A leader is someone who is able to influence others to work toward a common goal. Many people are leaders, even though their names do not appear on an organization chart. On the other hand, some people who hold positions of authority may not be especially good leaders.

One basic requirement for being a good leader is to be a good follower. Although that may sound contradictory, qualities such as a willingness to be supervised and a willingness to follow directions are important aspects of leadership. Although there is no magic formula for defining leadership, some traits of effective leaders are

- A desire to achieve personal and organizational goals
- Confidence based on a true understanding of a situation
- An ability to work with others and influence them to accomplish goals
- An ability to communicate appropriately
- An ability to accommodate change
- Integrity
- Willingness to accept responsibility
- Recognition that goals are achieved through the efforts of the team

Team Building

Good leaders help their teams become effective. An effective team accomplishes tasks well and makes the best use of each member's abilities.

A leader cannot build a team on his or her own. Everyone needs to participate. The leader's responsibility is to create a climate that encourages and values good teamwork. Leaders need to

- make sure team members know their jobs and carry out their responsibilities (see **Figure 13.9**).
- encourage each member to contribute.
- foster good communication and mutual trust.
- help their team members set worthwhile and attainable goals.

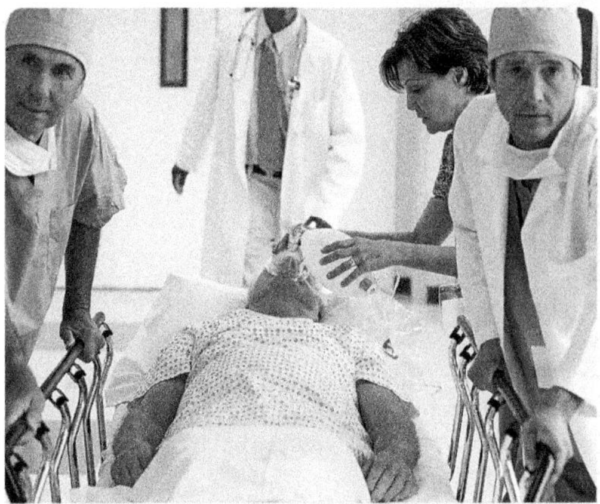

Fig. 13.9 Teamwork in Action Team members working as a unit. *Why is it important to accept responsibility on the job?*

Goal Setting

Leaders help their team members set personal and team goals. Having goals helps people understand what is expected of them. It provides a way to measure progress and identify areas for improvement.

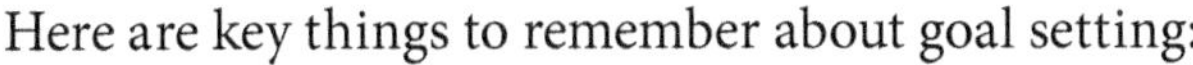

Here are key things to remember about goal setting:

- Goals should be challenging but not impossible to attain.
- Individuals should have input into setting their personal and team goals.
- Goals need to be measurable.
- Once goals have been set, a plan must be developed to turn those goals into actions. An action plan outlines what will be done, who will do it, in what order, and when.
- Leaders need to meet with individuals and teams to evaluate progress. Were goals met? What was done well? What needs improvement? The evaluation provides the basis for setting new goals.

READING CHECK

Explain how goals help professionals succeed.

Understanding and Respecting Diversity

How are you diverse from others?

Have you heard the expression "It takes all kinds"? Part of teamwork is understanding people who are different from you and respecting their right to be different. After all, from their point of view, you are the one who is different! **Diversity** can mean differences in age, gender, race, ethnicity, physical ability, sexual orientation, religious beliefs, values, goals, or personality. To understand diversity, you should have open communication with people who are different from you. How can you understand if you do not learn? Being respectful does not mean that you have to agree with the lifestyles and beliefs of others. It means that you accept the idea that others have every right to be different from you. **Figure 13.10** on page 372 shows an example of accepting diversity.

Photo: Fuse/Getty Images

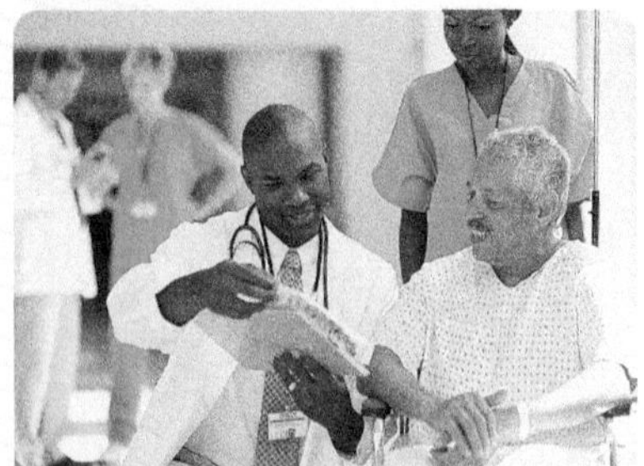

Fig. 13.10 Diversity Healthcare professionals may encounter clients of various ages. *How can you respect diversity?*

The list below gives some ideas that may help you understand and respect diversity.

- Increase your awareness of diversity. Communication will help you learn about individual similarities and differences.
- Increase your awareness of your own feelings. Everyone has biases. People tend to **stereotype** others, and this can lead to discrimination. Examine your own biases. Are they realistic?
- Look at individuals. As you learn about people as individuals, any group stereotypes you may have often begin to break down.
- Value differences. A major part of the team concept is that all participants can contribute. People who are different from you have unique contributions to make.
- In healthcare, it is especially important that you provide quality services in a respectful manner to people who are different.

Sexual Harassment

A final word about respecting others concerns sexual harassment. **Sexual harassment** is an unwanted communication or act of a sexual nature. It is damaging to individuals and to the organization, and can have serious professional and legal consequences. Most organizations have written policies covering sexual harassment and procedures for reporting and dealing with it. Make it clear that you will have no part in sexual harassment, and that you know these policies and procedures.

READING CHECK

Suggest how stereotypes can be countered.

SECTION 13.2 Employment Skills and Personal Traits Review

AFTER YOU READ

1. **Describe** the basic skills required for all workers.
2. **Describe** some uses of technology a healthcare professional should know.
3. **Explain** six attributes of a professional.
4. **List** the seven steps needed to solve a problem.
5. **Identify** time management strategies.
6. **Write** a short essay on the value of teamwork.
7. **Select** three characteristics of an effective leader.
8. **Choose** four attitudes or strategies that can help you understand and respect people who are different from you.

Technology ONLINE EXPLORATIONS

Team Leadership

Working with classmates, search the Internet for information about leadership skills. Prepare a skit for the class that demonstrates team building and goal setting.

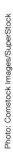

Photo: Comstock Images/SuperStock

SECTION

13.3 Getting and Keeping a Job

Determining Your Skills

Do you know what career you would like to enter when you graduate?

It is important to evaluate your interests and aptitudes, to help you decide what kinds of jobs would be satisfying to you. Many tools are available to help you evaluate what your interests are. Try some of them. No assessment tool can fully define your interests and capabilities, but you may be able to develop a general idea.

Your attitude, or how you view yourself and your relationships with others, is also important. In fact, your attitude may have a bigger effect on your success than any other factor. If you have a positive attitude toward life, your behavior on the job will probably be positive as well. Coworkers and clients will be affected by your attitude. Also, your satisfaction with your work will depend on your attitude toward the job. The benefits of a positive attitude cannot be overstated.

Vocabulary

Content Vocabulary

You will learn these content vocabulary terms in this section.

- **networking**
- **discrimination**
- **résumé**
- **cover letter**
- **portfolio**

Academic Vocabulary

You will see these words in your reading and on your tests. Find their meanings in the Glossary in the back of the book.

- **attitude**
- **participate**

Job-Seeking Strategies

How do people find jobs?

When you hear about a job that interests you, it is important to evaluate and interpret the information. Consider the following:

- Where is the job? If the job is not located in your community, are you willing and able to move?
- What education, training, or previous work experience is required? Do you have those qualifications? If not, do you have other qualifications that could make you a good candidate for the job?
- Is it a full-time or part-time job? What are the hours?
- What are the salary and benefits? How do these compare with similar jobs at other places?
- Research the company that is hiring. How can you determine if the information you found on that company is reliable?

There are many ways to find out about job listings. Each approach has advantages and disadvantages. Employment agencies provide assistance for a fee. The employer often pays the fee, but sometimes the applicant has to pay it. Classified advertisements in newspapers are a good source of job listings. Job fairs are conducted on college campuses and elsewhere. They provide a way for job seekers to have direct contact with representatives from many different organizations.

The Internet

A tremendous amount of job information is available on the Internet. Classified advertising from major newspapers is generally accessible for no charge. Companies, facilities, and organizations also post employment opportunities on their websites. Be careful, though—not all online information is accurate and reliable.

Personal Contact

The very best help you will ever have in your job search is personal contact. It is extremely useful to have someone of influence working to help you get a job. Letters of recommendation are the simplest form of this type of contact. Cultivate relationships with respected people and, when the time is right, ask if you can use them as references. These people might be teachers or respected people in the community or the healthcare field.

Networking

Networking is the regular communication you have with your personal and professional contacts. It can be a very efficient way of finding a job. Get acquainted with people whose job interests are similar to yours. Such contacts are valuable when you look for a job. Let's say that one of your classmates is working for a hospital and you apply for a job at that facility. Having that person "put in a good word" for you can make all the difference. Of course, you still need to be qualified for the job and to present yourself well.

One way to expand your network of contacts is by joining student organizations such as SkillsUSA and the Health Occupations Student Association (HOSA). You can increase your contacts through the activities of organizations such as these, especially when you attend their regional, state, or national meetings.

Hiring Practices

Many laws, regulations, and initiatives affect the way hiring is done. You may have heard of some of them already. Examples are the Equal Opportunity Employment Act, affirmative action, and the Americans with Disabilities Act.

In many announcements of open positions, you will see a statement about the hiring practices of the organization. An example of such a statement is "Hiring is done without regard to race, color, religion, national origin, sex, age, or disability." In other words, the organization is stating that it will not practice **discrimination** based on those criteria when it hires people.

READING CHECK

Summarize some of the benefits of networking.

The Job Application

Why is it important to keep your résumé up to date?

Most organizations require you to submit a job application as the first step in applying for a position. The application form is obtained at the facility or online. It is an official document and it represents you; therefore, it must be accurate. False or misleading information may be considered fraudulent and could lead to dismissal.

The majority of applications contain the same information. The information is generally the same as the contents of your résumé. Do not write "See résumé" on the form. Prepare your résumé first, and use it as a guide for completing the application.

When preparing your application, include the same terminology that is found in the job posting. The computer parameters will include these key words for selecting applications. Applications are also completed online. Remember that most electronic versions do not offer a spell check utility! Whether completing the form electronically or by pen, ensure that words are spelled correctly and the overall appearance is neat. Read and follow instructions carefully. Submit the application as directed. **Procedure 13-2** guides you through the application process.

READING CHECK

Explain how to use a résumé to complete a job application.

Résumés

Why do you need a résumé?

You should develop a résumé when you are preparing to apply for a job. A **résumé** is a brief representation of your credentials. It summarizes your education, experience, and other background. The résumé allows the prospective employer to learn about your qualifications in the shortest time possible. The résumé should be accompanied by a cover letter.

The purpose of the résumé and letter is to convince the employer that you have the necessary qualifications for the job and that you should be interviewed. There are many different styles of résumés. Word processing programs often have résumé guides that can help you develop a format. But, however you set up your résumé, you should follow some general rules:

- Use some type of outline format.
- Leave plenty of "white space" to give the résumé an uncluttered look.

- Provide your name, address, phone number(s), and e-mail address at the top of the page.
- List information in chronological order beginning with the most recent. If there are any gaps in the chronology, be prepared to explain them in an interview.
- List your education.
- List your work experience, including volunteer experience if it is related to the job for which you are applying.
- When appropriate for the job, list activities, honors, and membership in organizations.
- Be sure that there are no errors in the document. Have someone else look it over: two heads are better than one.

While there are varying opinions as to the format and details that should be included in résumés, most entry-level résumés should be limited to one page. Remember, the people reading your résumé are usually very busy. It is generally in your favor to keep your résumé concise, and to use a clean, straightforward design and layout. **Figure 13.11** shows a sample résumé.

READING CHECK

List three types of information that must be included on a résumé.

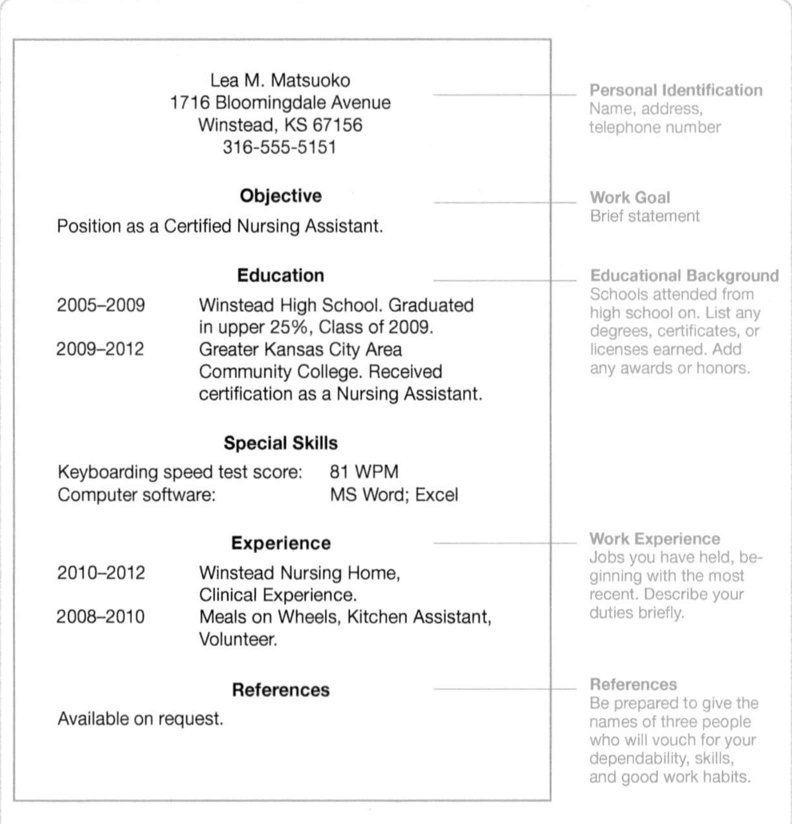

Lea M. Matsuoko
1716 Bloomingdale Avenue
Winstead, KS 67156
316-555-5151

Objective

Position as a Certified Nursing Assistant.

Education

2005–2009 Winstead High School. Graduated in upper 25%, Class of 2009.
2009–2012 Greater Kansas City Area Community College. Received certification as a Nursing Assistant.

Special Skills

Keyboarding speed test score: 81 WPM
Computer software: MS Word; Excel

Experience

2010–2012 Winstead Nursing Home, Clinical Experience.
2008–2010 Meals on Wheels, Kitchen Assistant, Volunteer.

References

Available on request.

Fig. 13.11 The Résumé Résumés present employment information in a standardized format. *What essential information is found in this résumé?*

Cover Letters

Is it important to write a cover letter when applying for a job?

A **cover letter** allows you to briefly introduce yourself to a prospective employer. **Figure 13.12** shows a sample cover letter. Follow these guidelines when writing one.

- Address the letter to a specific person, if possible.
- Make sure that the letter is error-free and in correct business letter format.
- In the opening of the letter, state that you are applying for a job, what job you are interested in, and how you heard about it.
- Briefly explain why you believe that you are qualified for the job.
- End the letter with a statement indicating your willingness to be interviewed and to provide additional information, including references.

Remember that the goal of the cover letter is to get the employer to read your résumé.

READING CHECK

Identify what makes a cover letter successful.

Portfolios

Have you begun to compile your personal portfolio?

An important item to have available when applying for employment is your personal portfolio. A **portfolio** is a collection of materials that exhibits your efforts, progress, and achievements in one or more areas.

July 2, 2011
Dr. Sonia Murphy
North Clinic Health Care
2331 Terrace Street
Chicago, Illinois 69691

Dear Dr. Murphy:

Mr. David Leeland, Director of Internship at Bakers College, gave me a copy of your advertisement for a nursing assistant. I am interested in being considered for the position.

Your medical office has an excellent reputation, especially regarding health care for women. I have taken several courses in women's health and volunteer at the hospital in a women's health support group. I believe I can make a significant contribution to your office.

My work experiences have provided valuable hands-on opportunities. In addition to excellent office skills, including computer programming, I have clinical experience and people skills. I speak Spanish and have used it often in my volunteer work.

I have paid for most of my college education. My grades are excellent and I have been on the Dean's list in my medical and health classes. I have also completed advanced computer and advanced office procedures classes.

I will call you on Tuesday, July 22, to make sure you received this letter and to find out when you might be able to arrange an interview.

Sincerely,

Lea M. Matsuoko

Lea M. Matsuoko
1716 Bloomingdale Avenue
Winstead, KS 67156
Home phone: 316-555-5151
e-mail: leam@aol.com

Fig. 13.12 The Cover Letter A cover letter allows you to briefly introduce yourself to a prospective employer. *What information is found in this cover letter?*

In addition to your résumé, the following are some examples of items that should be in your portfolio.

- Cover sheet to identify yourself
- Table of contents
- Letter of introduction
- Academic and practical skills list
- Letters of recommendation
- Special interests and awards received in or out of school, including volunteer work and club membership

Building and maintaining a portfolio will help with future employment and education.

READING CHECK

List three components of an employment portfolio.

The Interview

What should you take away from an interview as a job candidate?

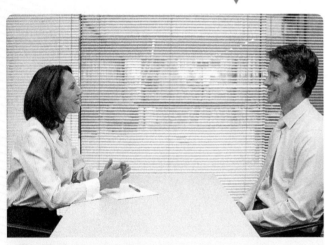

Fig. 13.13 The Job Interview Interviews can be stressful. *What are the important things to remember about a job interview?*

If the prospective employer believes your credentials are strong enough, you will be asked to interview. The interview might be with one person, or a committee may interview you. The impression you make will influence your chance of getting the job. Many factors affect hiring decisions, so do not pressure yourself to be perfect. **Figure 13.13** gives you an idea of a typical interview.

Do not forget that the interview is a two-way street. You should be confident that you are a strong candidate for the position. The interview is an opportunity to impress the employer with your qualifications and professional demeanor. It is also a time for you to learn more about the employer and the specifics of the job. You cannot make a well-informed decision about whether or not you want the position until after the interview.

Most interviews are friendly, but do not be surprised if you are given a problem to solve using critical thinking. Sometimes employers want to know how you conduct yourself under pressure. Practicing prior to the interview is helpful. Although you cannot predict the exact questions that might be asked, you can develop answers to questions that probably will be asked in some form. Here are some examples:

- "Tell me how your background has prepared you for this position."
- "Do you prefer working alone or as a member of a team?"
- "What is it about the position or our company that attracts you?"

- "How does this position fit into your long-term plans?"
- "Give me examples of how you have used the skills required by this position in the past."

You should also be ready to ask some questions of your own. Prior to the interview, research the organization and the position. Visit the organization's website, to learn about the organization's goals. Emphasize your knowledge of the organization during the interview.

Do not assume that you need to practice good social skills only during the interview. During your visit to a facility, treat everyone you encounter with respect and courtesy. Athough they may not participate in the interview, they might influence the people who are hiring.

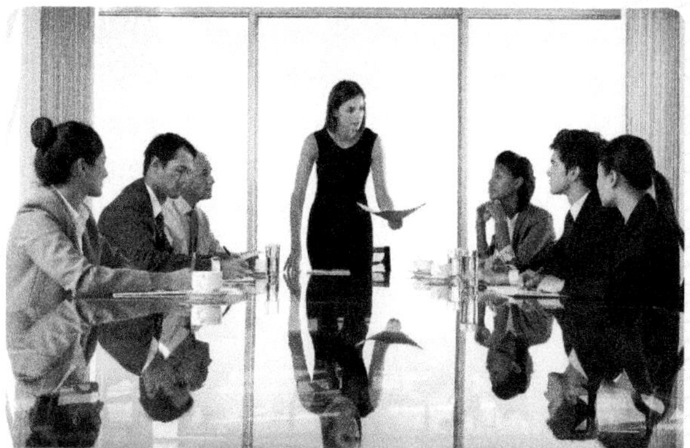
Fig. 13.14 Dress for Success Appropriate attire is important. *How can you find out what is the proper attire at a particular job site?*

It is essential to dress appropriately for the interview. Your attire should be as formal as, or a little more formal than, the attire you will wear on the job. Refer to **Figure 13.14** for an example of appropriate attire. In some settings, workers wear "scrubs," which are durable garments designed to withstand repeated washing. However, even if that is the case, you should wear office attire to the interview.

You may visit the organization in advance to see how people dress. However, neat and clean clothing is mandatory for the interview. Be sure that you are clean and you have combed your hair and brushed your teeth prior to the interview. The way you dress, posture, and body or breath odor will convey a message. Make the message a positive one.

READING CHECK

Name the types of questions you should prepare for an interview.

Adapting to Change

How do you deal with change?

In today's world, most people will change jobs and even careers numerous times during their working lives. Changes in technology, the economy, and society bring about changes in the job market. Old jobs disappear or transform. Entirely new jobs are created.

How can you stay employed when the job market keeps changing? The key is to adapt. Prepare yourself for new challenges and opportunities.

- Continuously improve your skills and learn new skills.
- Keep up with technology.
- Stay networked. Even if you have a good job, you may be looking for work tomorrow.

Performance Evaluations

Have you ever had your performance evaluated by an employer?

Most employees receive periodic performance evaluations. In many workplaces, this is done after your first 90 days and then once each year after that. Try to approach reviews without being defensive. Take pride in the things you do well, and show that you are willing to learn and improve.

If an employer has a complaint about your performance, he or she is required to let you know about that complaint according to the rules of due process. Most places of employment have established policies that require employees be given verbal and written notices before they can be "let go."

READING CHECK

Summarize the ideal mindset for approaching a performance review.

Leaving a Job

Why would you leave a job?

Most people have several jobs in their lifetime. You will probably leave a job for other opportunities. There are proper ways to do this (see **Figure 13.15**).

Some guidelines for leaving a job are listed below.

- Give the employer enough notice to replace you. Two weeks is considered minimum notice.
- Provide your employer with a letter stating that you are leaving and what the last day of your employment will be.
- If you are dissatisfied with the job, the resignation letter is not the place to express your dissatisfaction. Most employers conduct exit interviews that give the employee an opportunity to express any disappointments that he or she has had. It is unwise to express hostility, either in the resignation letter or in the exit interview.

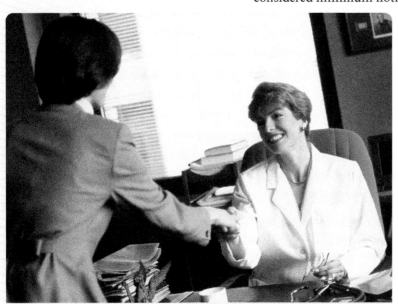

Fig. 13.15 Leaving a Job Leave on good terms. *What should you do to be sure that you could be rehired?*

Photo: Ariel Skelley/CORBIS

- Thank the employer for the opportunities you were given.
- Submit the letter to your supervisor before you tell your coworkers that you will be leaving.
- Offer to help a new person transition to your job.
- It is often easier to find a job if you have one. Therefore, it is best to get the new job before giving notice of your resignation.

READING CHECK

Analyze why it is a good idea to be helpful to your employer during the resignation process.

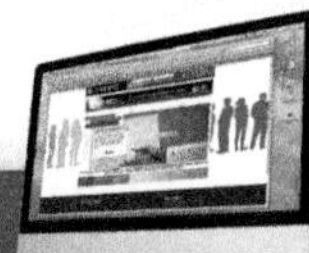

connect™ ONLINE PROCEDURES

PROCEDURE 13-2

Completing a Job Application

Most organizations require you to submit a job application as the first step in the application process. The form can be obtained at the facility or online. It is an official document and it must be accurate. False or misleading information may be considered fraudulent and could lead to dismissal.

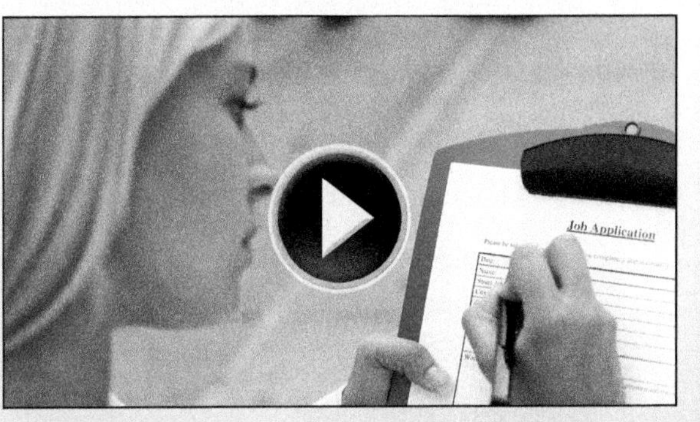

SECTION 13.3 Getting and Keeping A Job Review

AFTER YOU READ

1. **Name** five benefits other than money that a job provides.
2. **List** at least three strategies for finding a job.
3. **List** four facts that should be included on a résumé.
4. **Write** a paragraph explaining how and why you would research a company before an interview.
5. **Describe** five steps you should take when you leave a job.

Technology ONLINE EXPLORATIONS

Employment Legislation

Search the Internet for the Equal Opportunity Employment Act, affirmative action, and the Americans with Disabilities Act. You will find the most accurate information on government (.gov) websites. Write a brief paragraph describing why you think these acts or initiatives are necessary and how they might affect you when you apply for a job.

Photo: Winston Davidian/Photodisc/Getty Images

CHAPTER 13 Review

Chapter Summary

SECTION 13.1

- The elements of communication usually consist of sender, receiver, feedback, and message. Avoid miscommunication by following basic guidelines. **(pg. 359)**
- Barriers to communication prevent a message from being received. **(pg. 360)**
- Objective comments are factual and are based on concrete examples. Subjective comments tend to be an opinion or idea. **(pg. 362)**

SECTION 13.2

- Qualities such as dependability, integrity, self-motivation, patience, and competence are the marks of a true professional. **(pg. 366)**
- Your ability to use critical thinking skills will influence your job success. **(pg. 366)**
- Managing your time can improve your effectiveness as a healthcare employee. **(pg. 367)**
- People working as a team are usually more successful than people working independently at meeting organizational goals. **(pg. 368)**
- To be a successful member of a team, you need to respect human differences. **(pg. 371)**

SECTION 13.3

- There are several ways to find a job, but personal contacts are especially important. **(pg. 374)**
- Usually the first information a prospective employer has about you comes from your application form, résumé, or cover letter. **(pg. 375)**
- When interviewing, be professional in your manner and the way you dress to present yourself in the most positive way. **(pg. 378)**
- When leaving a job, give adequate notice in writing, and make sure that you leave the job in a spirit of goodwill. **(pg. 380)**

Mc Graw Hill connect™ **ONLINE ACTIVITIES**

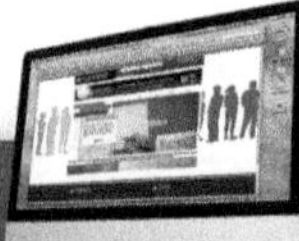

Complete our HST online activities for Chapter 13, which include Concept Check review questions, Reference Flash Cards, and Online Procedures.

- **Concept Check** review questions
- **Reference Flash Cards** medical terminology practice
- **Online Procedures** assessment sheets

CHAPTER
13 Assessment

Critical Thinking/Problem Solving

1. As a nursing assistant, you have the following duties this evening. It is now 4 P.M.
   - Feed four debilitated clients at 5 P.M.
   - Take vital signs on eight clients at 8 P.M.
   - Do range-of-motion exercises with four clients between 6 and 8 P.M.
   - Provide evening care to ten clients at the clients' bedtimes, which vary.
   - Give bed baths to three clients.

   Just as you begin, one of the clients falls and appears to be injured. What should you do? How will you organize your time to complete the above tasks?

2. You are the only registered nurse on duty at a nursing home. It is 4 P.M. Two nursing assistants are working. One RN is on call, but she told you she has evening plans.

   Your duties are to do the following:
   - Administer medications to twelve clients at 5 P.M., eight clients at 8 P.M., and three clients at 10 P.M.
   - Administer an intravenous medication to a client starting at 6 P.M. This takes an hour and must be checked every 10 minutes by a registered nurse.
   - Change the dressings on a client's open wound every three hours.
   - Complete several reports that were due last week.

   You learn that a client is being transferred to your facility and will be there in an hour. Determine your priorities. How will you organize your time?

3. Consider the scenario presented in Question 2. Which of the stress management tips in this chapter might be useful in this situation? Which would not? Explain.

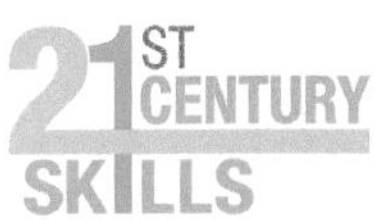

4. **Teamwork** Choose a place of employment where you would like to work. With a partner, role-play a job interview at that facility. Use the interviewer questions in this chapter and compose at least two more questions related to that job. Determine where you and your partner could improve your interview skills. Write a summary.

5. **Communication** Prepare an e-mail to Ms. Mary Scott to let her know that her appointment has been changed from 2 P.M. this Tuesday to 3 P.M. next Tuesday.

6. **Information Literacy** Using the Internet, research jobs in healthcare. Prepare a résumé and cover letter for a job opening that interests you.

UNIT 2

Careers in Therapeutic Services

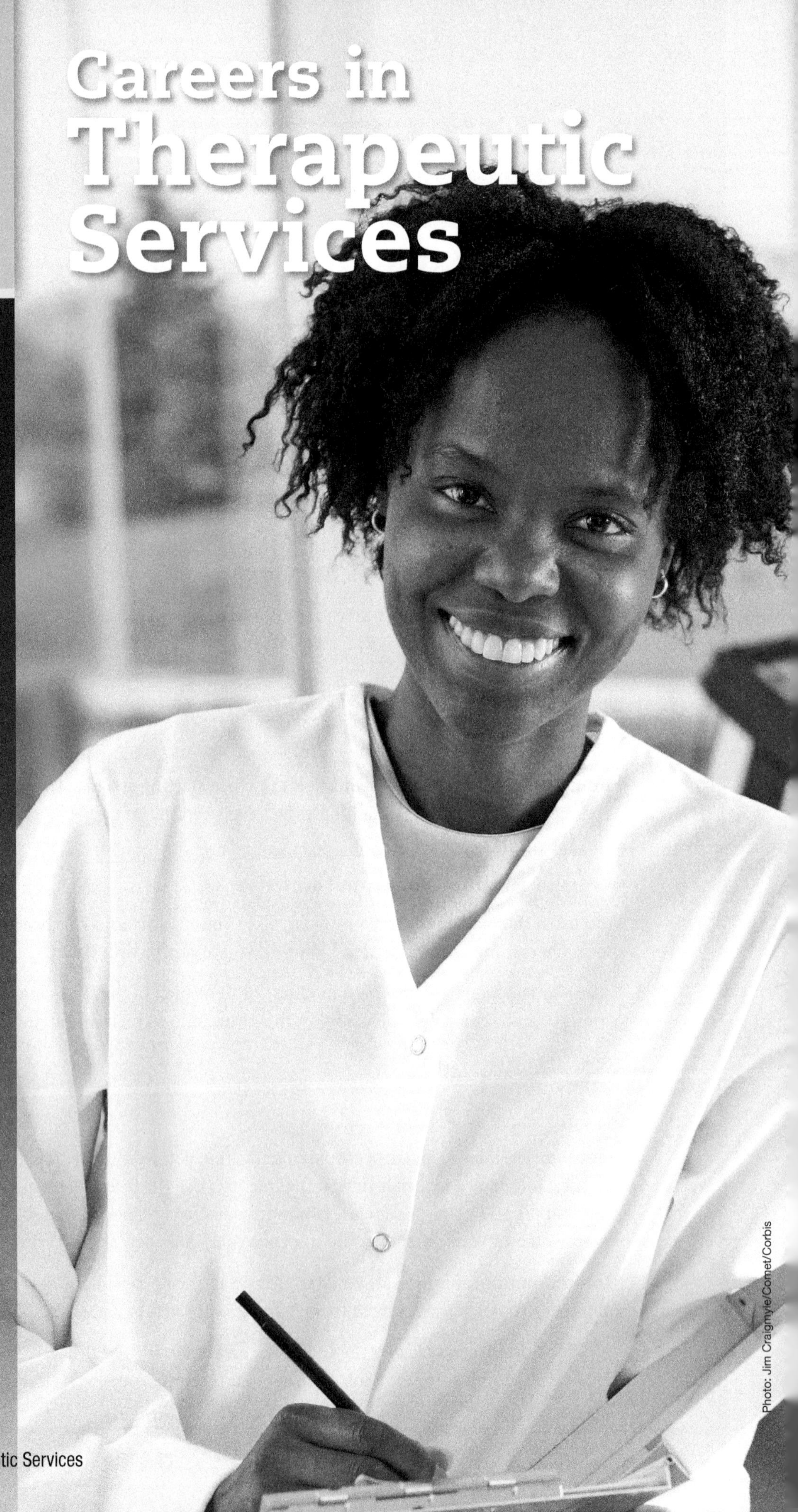

Photo: Jim Craigmyle/Comet/Corbis

CHAPTER **14** Emergency Medical Services

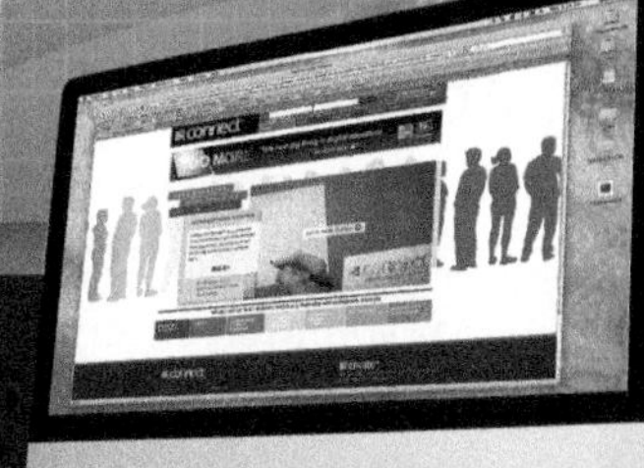

Essential Question:

How do the educational requirements and job responsibilities for emergency medical responders, emergency medical technicians, and paramedics differ?

Every day, all across the United States, sick and injured people call for help. The men and women of emergency medical services (EMS) answer those calls. They respond to all kinds of incidents, from falls to gunshot wounds to emergency childbirth. Each incident requires a prompt and competent response from an emergency medical services provider who gives care at the scene of the incident and during transport to a medical facility.

McGraw Hill connect™

It's Online!

- **Online Procedures**
- **STEM Connection**
- **Medical Science**
- **Medical Terms**
- **Medical Math**
- **Ethics in Action**
- **Virtual Lab**

Photo: ER Productions/Spirit/CORBIS

READING GUIDE

OBJECTIVES

After completing this chapter, you will be able to:

- **Compare** the roles of an emergency medical responder, emergency medical technician, advanced emergency medical technician, and paramedic.
- **Practice** safety rules when using oxygen for therapy.
- **Identify** the purpose of a nasal cannula and nonrebreather mask.
- **Define** the role of the automated external defibrillator in cardiac arrest.
- **Recall** the safety requirements for operating an AED.
- **Identify** situations requiring the use of an AED.
- **Demonstrate** one emergency medical services procedure.

BEFORE YOU READ

Connect Have you ever seen an emergency medical professional in action? How quickly was he or she able to decide on the appropriate procedure?

Main Idea

The calls to which an emergency medical service provider responds require prompt medical care. The four main professions in this area are emergency medical responder, emergency medical technician, advanced emergency medical technician, and paramedic.

Note-Taking Activity

Draw this table. Write key terms and phrases under **Cues**. Write main ideas under **Note Taking**. Summarize the section under **Summary**.

Cues	Note Taking
o o	o o
Summary	

Graphic Organizer

Before you read the chapter, draw a diagram like the one to the right. As you read, write the main occupations covered in this chapter into the diagram.

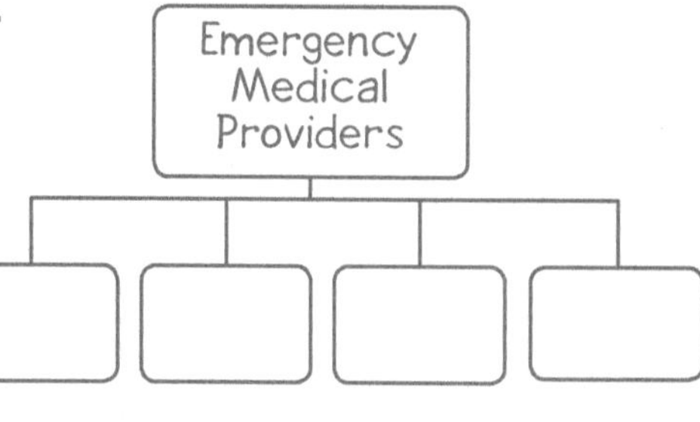

connect

Downloadable graphic organizers can be accessed online.

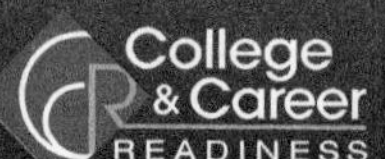

STANDARDS

HEALTH SCIENCE

NCHSE 1.21 Describe common diseases and disorders of each body system (prevention, pathology, diagnosis, and treatment).

NCHSE 2.22 Use medical abbreviations to communicate information.

SCIENCE

NSES A Develop abilities necessary to do scientific inquiry, understandings about scientific inquiry.

NCHSE *National Consortium for Health Science Education*

NSES *National Science Education Standards*

COMMON CORE STATE STANDARDS

MATHEMATICS

Geometry

Modeling With Geometry G-MG 2 Apply concepts of density based on area and volume in modeling situations (e.g., persons per square mile, BTUs per cubic foot).

ENGLISH LANGUAGE ARTS

Writing

Text Types and Purposes W-3 Write narratives to develop real or imagined experiences or events using effective technique, well-chosen details, and well-structured event sequences.

Speaking and Listening

Presentation of Knowledge and Ideas SL-5 Make strategic use of digital media (e.g., textual, graphical, audio, visual, and interactive elements) in presentations to enhance understanding of findings, reasoning, and evidence and to add interest.

SECTION

14.1 Careers in Emergency Medical Services

Emergency Medical Careers

What do you think is the most challenging aspect of an emergency medical services career?

The number of jobs in emergency medical services (EMS) has risen due to increased call volume from the aging population. **Table 14.1** on page 388 gives more information about these occupations.

The four most common careers in emergency medical services are

- Emergency Medical Responder (EMR)
- Emergency Medical Technician (EMT)
- Advanced Emergency Medical Technician (AEMT)
- Paramedic

Vocabulary

Content Vocabulary

You will learn these content vocabulary terms in this section.

- **cervical collars**
- **basic life support (BLS) skills**

Academic Vocabulary

You will see this word in your reading and on your tests. Find its meaning in the Glossary in the back of the book.

- **assess**

Emergency Medical Responder

Which organizations employ emergency medical responders?

EMRs are the first professionals to arrive at the scene of an incident. They gain access to patients, assess their illness or injury, and provide emergency care. EMRs may be firefighters, law enforcement officers, or private citizens who have passed an approved EMR program.

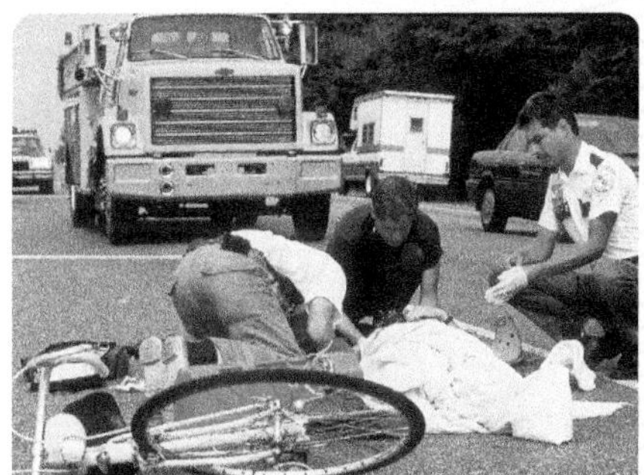

Fig. 14.1 Emergency Medical Responder Emergency medical responders are often those who arrive first at the scene of an accident. *What are the responsibilities of the Emergency Medical Responder (EMR)?*

Responsibilities of the Emergency Medical Responder

Upon arrival the EMR will evaluate the scene for safety and

- determine the total number of patients.
- identify the cause of the injury or the nature of the illness.
- request additional help if necessary.

The EMR's primary duties, as shown in **Figure 14.1**, are to

- gain access to the patient, using simple tools when necessary.
- determine what is wrong and provide emergency medical care.
- move patient only when necessary, without causing further injury.
- transfer the patient and whatever patient information they have to more highly trained personnel when they arrive at the scene.

READING CHECK

Recall when an EMR should move a patient.

Photo: Kenneth Murry/Photo Researchers

Table 14.1 Overview of Careers in Emergency Medical Services

OCCUPATION	EDUCATION REQUIREMENT	CERTIFICATION OR LICENSING AGENCY	JOB OUTLOOK
Emergency Medical Responder (EMR)	A minimum of 48 hours in an approved training program.	Certification through each state's department of health or certification through the National Registry of EMTs.	EMRs are usually employees of industry, or police or fire departments; outlook is based upon location.
Emergency Medical Technician (EMT)	A minimum of 150 hours in an approved training program, including at least ten hours of internship with ten patient assessments.	Certification through each state's department of health or certification through the National Registry of EMTs.	EMT jobs are expected to grow about as fast as average for all occupations through 2018.
Advanced Emergency Medical Technician (AEMT)	Additional approved training with a minimum of 150 to 250 hours total instruction including classroom, practical, clinical, and field internship.	Certification through each state's department of health or in some states certification through the National Registry of EMTs.	AEMT jobs are expected to grow about as fast as average for all occupations through 2018.
Paramedic	Additional approved paramedic training equal to 1000 hours or more including classroom, practical, clinical, and field internship. Completion of program may lead to a two-year associate degree or higher.	State certification. Some states require the National Registry EMTs certification exam, Paramedic.	Paramedic jobs are expected to grow about as fast as average for all occupations through 2018.

Emergency Medical Technicians

What physical abilities are required of emergency medical technicians?

A 911 operator dispatches Emergency Medical Technicians (EMTs) to an incident. They often work with fire and police personnel. EMTs work in many environments and in all types of weather. They may be called upon at any hour. Once at the scene, the EMT

- assesses the situation to determine if it is safe.
- takes appropriate precautions including infection control.
- interviews and examines the patient.
- seeks medical advice, if needed, from doctors or nurses by radio or telephone.
- provides appropriate out-of-hospital care according to established local procedures and guidelines.
- transports the patient to a medical facility.

EMTs use a variety of equipment. Backboards and **cervical collars** are used to immobilize neck, back, or spinal injuries. Automated external defibrillators (AEDs) help restore the normal heart rhythm of a cardiac arrest patient.

Advanced EMTs (AEMT) and paramedics start intravenous lines (IVs) and administer various medications. They also secure the patient's airway with advanced airway equipment. After providing emergency care and loading the patient into the ambulance, one EMT drives while the other EMT continues to administer medical care in the back of the ambulance.

Some EMTs are volunteers, while others have full-time or part-time positions with local city or county governments. Other employers of EMTs include private or independent ambulance companies, hospitals, emergency helicopter programs, industries, or correctional facilities.

The EMT's work environment is both physically strenuous and mentally stressful. It often involves life-and-death situations with injured and sick patients. Despite this, many EMTs find the profession exhilarating and challenging and value the opportunities they are given to help others.

Some characteristics of successful EMTs include emotional stability, exceptional manual dexterity, agility, physical coordination, and the ability to lift and move heavy loads. They must also have good eyesight.

Many EMTs advance to become supervisors, operational managers, administrative directors, dispatchers, instructors, registered nurses, or physician assistants. Others move into sales and marketing of EMS and fire equipment. A number of EMTs eventually leave the profession to return to school to become physicians, respiratory therapists, nurses, or other kinds of allied health professionals.

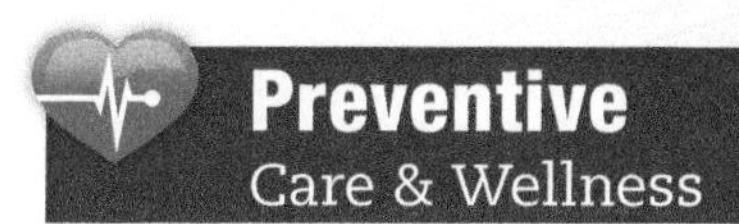

Allergic Reactions

Allergic reactions can range from a runny nose to an anaphylactic reaction, which is a life-threatening reaction that interferes with breathing. Substances in the environment such as dust or pollen usually cause simple reactions such as a headache, sneezing, and a runny nose. These symptoms are usually treated with antihistamines. An EpiPen, which injects epinephrine, is used to prevent a severe anaphylactic reaction in an individual who is severely allergic. Those severe reactions can result from many events, such as eating the wrong food or suffering a bee sting. Those individuals should have an EpiPen with them at all times.

Responsibilities of the EMT

In most regions in the United States, the EMT is the minimum level of certification for ambulance personnel. Certification as an EMT requires completion of the EMT National Standard training program sponsored by the U.S. Department of Transportation (DOT) or equivalent. Equivalent programs must be approved by a state emergency medical services program or other authorized agency.

Individuals with EMT credentials provide **basic life support (BLS) skills.** These are skills essential to maintain life. BLS skills include the use of oral and nasal airways, application of a cervical spine immobilization collar, use of the AED, assisting a patient with administration of his or her own medications—such as nitroglycerine, an EpiPen, or a metered-dose inhaler—and immobilization of injuries to the arms or legs.

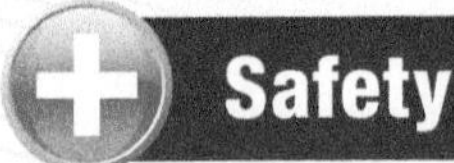

Safety

Preparing for a Disaster

A disaster is a sudden event that causes great damage, loss, or destruction. Individuals in the healthcare profession must be prepared for such events, which can be due to weather, a natural event such as an earthquake or hurricane, terrorism, or accidents. In addition to firefighters and police, emergency medical personnel and other healthcare personnel play a vital role in responding to a disaster situation. City, county, state, and federal agencies assist as necessary to coordinate the response to the event. Frequently, communities conduct disaster drills to test their ability to respond to an emergency. Disaster drills are essential to the safety and welfare of the community. As a healthcare professional, you will be asked to participate in these drills.

In general, the job responsibilities of the EMT include:

- Ensuring his or her own personal safety as well as the safety of the crew, patient, and bystanders.
- Examining and interviewing the patient to determine what emergency care is appropriate.
- Providing patient care based on interview and examination findings.
- Lifting, moving, and transporting the patient to a medical facility.
- Transferring care of the patient to the medical staff at the receiving medical facility.
- Speaking on behalf of the patient by reporting concerns and findings to the receiving medical staff.

Advanced Emergency Medical Technicians

How do the skills of an AEMT differ from those of an EMT?

In addition to the qualifications of the EMT, the Advanced EMT (AEMT) has the emergency skills to evaluate and manage trauma accidents, cardiac, respiratory, and other medical emergency situations.

Responsibilities of the AEMT

An AEMT performs the same basic skills as the EMT. However, the AEMT has had additional training and possesses additional skills. The Advanced EMT can

- administer certain medications beyond those permitted at the EMT level.
- start an IV (intravenous) line.
- give a medication using a mechanical IV Pump.
- set up and maintain a Manual/Automated Transport Ventilator.

READING CHECK

List the additional skills that an AEMT may have that an EMT may not have.

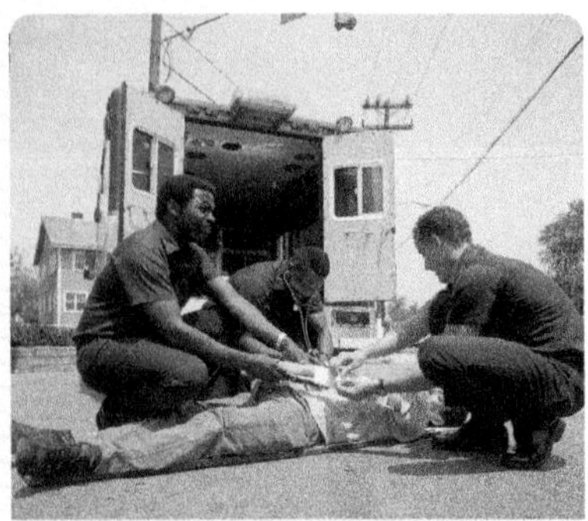

Fig. 14.2 Paramedics Paramedics assist accident victims. *How are the responsibilities of the paramedic different from those of the EMR?*

Photo: Tim Courlas

The Paramedic

How does a person become certified as a paramedic?

The level of Paramedic represents the highest level of training among EMS professionals. **Figure 14.2** shows some of the paramedic's duties. Paramedic training follows or exceeds the U.S. DOT National Standard Paramedic curriculum. Training programs can last two years or longer. They are normally given in a college setting, and many paramedic students earn an associate degree or higher. Preparation includes extensive course work: skills practice labs, hospital clinical rotations, and fieldwork. Such preparation prepares the paramedic student to take the National Registry of Paramedic Examination to become certified as a Paramedic. Because of the intensive preparation, almost all paramedic positions are paid. In addition to the skills performed by the Advanced EMT, paramedics may administer medications by the oral, intravenous, subcutaneous, intramuscular, and intraosseous routes of administration, perform advanced airway techniques, and use monitors and other complex medical equipment.

Additional Paramedic Skills

The roles and responsibilities of the paramedic (and the AEMT) include not only patient care but also various responsibilities prior to, throughout, and following an emergency response. Among the essential responsibilities are the following:

- A thorough understanding of the local EMS system's policies and procedures
- Ability to use local communication systems, including radios and communication protocols
- Strong leadership skills, including self-confidence, inner strength, decision-making skills, and willingness to accept responsibility
- Ability to size up the scene and the safety of self, crew members, patient, and bystanders
- Expertise to examine and interview the patient
- Assignment of priorities of care, development of an action plan, and performance of emergency care

READING CHECK

Recall why the job of paramedic is rarely a volunteer position.

SECTION 14.1 Careers in Emergency Medical Services Review

AFTER YOU READ

1. **Explain** what an EMR does.
2. **Recall** where EMRs are employed.
3. **Analyze** the differences between the roles and responsibilities of an EMT and those of a paramedic.
4. **Identify** the educational requirements needed to become a paramedic.
5. **List** five skills that every emergency medical professional should know.

Technology ONLINE EXPLORATIONS

Emergency Response

Research the Internet for information related to emergency services response to chemical or biological terrorism events. Review EMS personnel training requirements, preparations to respond, identification of and response to an incident, and other essential information. Prepare a written report, poster, or slide presentation of your findings to present to the class.

SECTION
14.2 Emergency Medical Services Procedures

Vocabulary

Content Vocabulary

You will learn these content vocabulary terms in this section.

- **mechanism of injury**
- **nature of illness**
- **sign**
- **oropharyngeal airway**
- **nasopharyngeal airway**
- **gag reflex**
- **nonrebreather mask**
- **nasal cannula**
- **defibrillator**
- **placenta**
- **umbilical cord**
- **amniotic sac**
- **labor**
- **crowning**

Academic Vocabulary

You will see these words in your reading and on your tests. Find their meanings in the Glossary in the back of the book.

- **resources**
- **objectives**
- **document**
- **integrated**

Patient Assessment Process

Why is it so important to assess the scene when providing emergency services?

The assessment process performed by EMRs and EMS providers consists of seven main steps. The steps in order are:

1. Scene Size-Up
2. Primary Assessment
3. History Taking
4. Secondary Assessment
5. Reassessment
6. Communication
7. Documentation

Scene Size-Up

The primary focus of this portion of the assessment is safety. It includes the following evaluations.

- Ensure safety of the scene.
- Take standard precautions.
- Determine the mechanism of injury or nature of illness.
- Identify the number of patients.
- Consider the need for specialized resources or assistance.

Evaluation of the scene begins before contact is made with an injured or sick patient. EMRs and EMTs are expected to provide assistance to others in need. However, they must ensure their own safety before and during emergency care. Examples of scene hazards include wrecked motor vehicles that may be leaking flammable liquids, downed power lines, hazardous materials, and angry or combative people.

Always survey each scene for potential hazards. If you observe hazards that you cannot handle, call for assistance, perhaps from firefighters or police. Assuring your personal safety and the safety of team members, the patient, and bystanders is of paramount importance.

After assessing scene safety, EMTs take standard precautions as determined by the nature of the incident. These precautions include wearing latex or non-latex gloves or other personal protective equipment (PPE), such as eye protection, face shields, and protective gowns.

EMRs and EMTs also make a note of the **mechanism of injury** for a trauma patient, and the **nature of illness** for a medical patient. These observations provide clues to the types of injuries or problems the patient may be experiencing. The mechanism of injury is defined as the force that caused the injury. For example, was the patient shot by a gun? Did the patient fall? Did a car strike the patient? Where is the site of the injury? Signs at the scene provide clues that suggest specific injuries to the patient. For example, a cracked windshield implies that the patient was not wearing a seat belt and struck the windshield. Injuries may include damage to the head, skull, or neck.

The nature of illness such as chest pain, shortness of breath, or abdominal pain assists the provider in determining the specific problem. For example, a patient with chest pain is assumed to be having a heart attack.

The remainder of the scene evaluation includes specifying the number of patients involved and the need for additional resources and assistance.

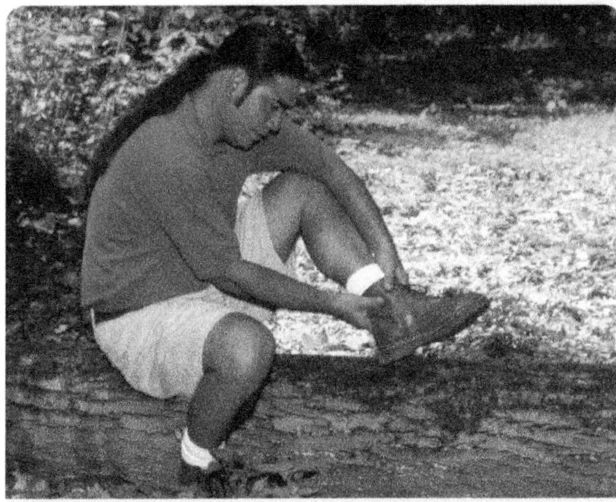

Fig. 14.3 Hiker Study the behavior of this hiker as he takes a break from hiking. *What is your general impression of this patient?*

Following a survey of the scene and execution of safety measures, the EMR or EMT makes contact with the sick or injured patient.

Primary Assessment

The next action performed is a primary assessment of the patient to detect and correct any life-threatening problems involving the airway, breathing, and circulation. This is essential to the patient's survival. There are seven components of the primary assessment.

1. Form a general impression.
2. Determine the level of responsiveness.
3. Assess the airway and identify and treat life-threatening problems associated with it.
4. Assess breathing and identify and treat life-threatening problems associated with it.
5. Assess circulation, including the presence of a pulse, major bleeding, skin color, temperature and moisture, and identify and treat any life-threatening problems.
6. Perform a rapid body scan.
7. Make a decision regarding the urgency of the patient's condition.

General Impression and Level of Responsiveness EMRs and EMTs form a general impression of the patient's surroundings and condition. This includes the patient's level of responsiveness, level of distress, facial expressions, age, ability to talk, and skin color. If the mechanism of injury suggests an injury to the spine, apply manual immobilization of the neck to protect the spine and prevent further movement. If the patient is unresponsive, tap the patient's shoulder and ask, "Are you OK?" See **Figures 14.3** and **14.4** to form an impression of two patients.

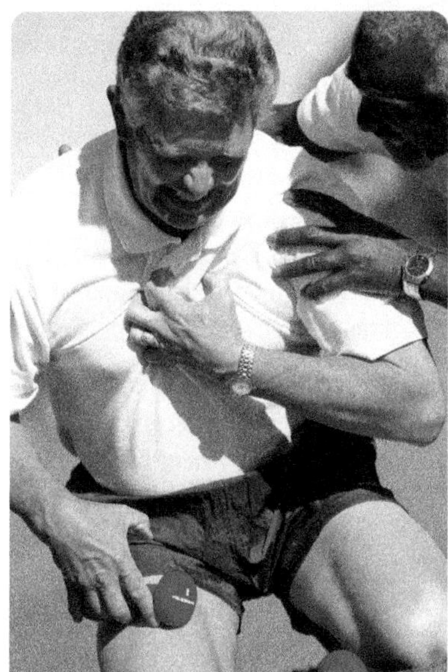

Fig. 14.4 Exercising Study the behavior of this man as he shows discomfort while exercising. *What is your general impression of this patient?*

Assess the Airway Check to see if the patient's airway is open. If the patient is awake, alert, and talking, the airway is open, the patient is breathing, and there is a pulse. If the patient is unresponsive, it will be necessary to open the airway using the head tilt/chin lift maneuver or the jaw thrust, depending on whether there is a suspected neck injury.

21ST CENTURY SKILLS

Communicating with Injured Patients and Family

Learning to communicate with a patient or family in crisis is difficult and often requires years of experience. These guidelines may be helpful for EMRs and EMTs.

- **Obtain the patient's first and last name.** Address patients by their last names unless the patient gives permission to use the first name. For example, say "How do you feel, Mr. Diaz?" or "Can you bend your leg, Ms. Kurlansky?" Never call patients by any slang terms or use addresses such as "honey," "sweetie," or "pal."
- **Be considerate and respectful.** Take care of the patient as you would like to be cared for.
- **Be aware of your body language and position.** If safety considerations permit, position yourself at or below the eye level of the patient. This stance is less intimidating. Do not stand with your arms crossed because this sends a message to the patient that you are uninterested.
- **Use eye contact.** Make frequent eye contact with your patient. This lets him or her know that you are interested in and attentive to his or her needs.
- **Be honest.** Attempt to answer the patient's questions honestly without scaring him or her. Let the patient and family know that you are doing everything possible to help. As you perform a procedure, let the patient and family know what you are doing. If you are going to cause pain, let them know, but tell them that you will be as gentle as possible.
- **Listen.** Be attentive to what the patient and family members have to say. Do not interrupt unless it is necessary.

Assess Breathing Ask yourself if the patient is breathing. Is the patient breathing adequately? If there is no breathing, then rescue breaths are required. If there is inadequate breathing, the patient could require oxygen therapy or breathing assistance using a bag-valve-mask.

Assess Circulation Does the patient have a pulse? Do you see any serious external bleeding? Correct any significant bleeding using direct pressure and dressings. Observe the color, temperature, and moisture of the patient's skin. Normal skin is pink, warm, and dry. Abnormal skin colors are pale, ashen, red, or cyanotic (bluish). Abnormal skin temperatures are cold, cool, or hot. The skin should not be clammy or moist. Changes in skin color, temperature, and moisture may suggest sudden or ongoing illness or injuries.

For an unresponsive patient, promptly determine the level of responsiveness. If there is no response, determine the presence of breathing. If the patient's breathing is absent or gasping, check for a pulse. If the pulse is absent immediately start chest compressions. (For details on providing CPR, see Chapter 4, Emergency Preparedness).

Perform a Rapid Scan of the Body The rapid body scan follows the assessment of the patient's airway, breathing, and circulation status after life-threatening problems have been identified and treated.

Begin your rapid scan by starting at the head and performing the following steps. Perform this assessment rapidly, taking only about 90 seconds.

1. **Head.** Begin by looking at and feeling the patient's head for deformities, bruises, open wounds, tenderness, depressions, and swelling. Check the ears and nose for blood as well as clear fluid. Check the mouth for bleeding, loose teeth, or other foreign bodies.
2. **Eyes.** Gently open the eyes and compare the pupils. They should be the same size.
3. **Neck.** Look and feel for deformities, bruises, depressions, open wounds, tenderness, and swelling. Check for a medical alert pendant.
4. **Chest.** Look and feel for deformities, bruises, open wounds, tenderness, depressions, and swelling.
5. **Abdomen.** Look and feel for deformities, bruises, open wounds, tenderness, depressions, and swelling.
6. **Pelvis.** Look and feel for deformities, bruises, open wounds, tenderness, depressions, and swelling. Gently press downward on the pelvis to check for pain. Gently grasp the upper thighs and press inward to check for pain.
7. **Arms.** Look and feel for deformities, bruises, open wounds, depressions, tenderness, and swelling. If injury does not prevent your doing so, check for movement and sensation. Have conscious patients wiggle their fingers, or touch a finger and have them identify which finger was touched.

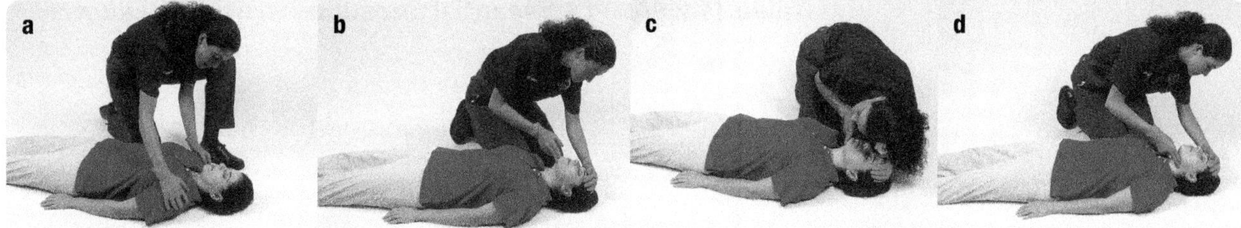

Fig. 14.5 Primary Assessment This responder is demonstrating four of the parts of a primary assessment. That assessment includes: 1. Form a general impression. 2. Determine level of responsiveness. Tap and ask. (a, above) 3. Assess the airway and open if needed. (b, above) 4. Assess breathing. (c, above) 5. Assess circulation (d, above) including presence of pulse, major bleeding, skin color, temperature, and moisture. 6. Perform a rapid body scan. 7. Determine urgency of the patient's condition. *When should you perform a primary assessment?*

8. **Legs.** Look and feel for deformities, bruises, open wounds, depressions, tenderness, and swelling. If the injury does not prevent your doing so, check for movement and sensation. Have conscious patients wiggle their toes. Touch a toe and have them identify the toe. If the patient can wiggle his or her toes, as well as identify a toe touched, it can be assumed that the nerve pathways to that extremity are intact and no damage has occurred at this time.
9. **Back.** Slide your hand under the patient's back as far as it will go without moving the patient. Look and feel for bleeding, deformities, bruises, open wounds, depressions, tenderness, or swelling.

Assess Priority Determine the priority and urgency of the patient's condition and seek immediate and appropriate transport to a medical facility (see **Figure 14.5**).

History Taking: Present History and SAMPLE History

Find out the patient's chief complaint. What is his or her reason for seeking emergency assistance? If time and the patient's condition permit, you should then obtain additional information about the patient's present and past medical problems and conditions. This information should include both objective and subjective information. Objective information is factual information that may be gained by a sign. A **sign** is something that you see, hear, feel, or smell, such as a bruise, pale skin, a deformity, or gurgling sounds. Subjective information is information provided by the subject, which may include symptoms that you are not able to observe. Examples of symptoms that may not be observable include dizziness, chest pain, headache, nausea, or fatigue.

The acronym SAMPLE is an easy way to remember the essential questions to ask the patient about his or her current problem and any past medical problems or conditions. If the patient is not able to provide this information quickly, ask these questions of any friends, coworkers, or family members who may be present (see **Table 14.2** on page 396).

Table 14.2 **SAMPLE** Essential questions to ask the client.

S	Signs and Symptoms "What is your complaint?" "What seems to be bothering you today?" "What is wrong?"
A	Allergies "Are you allergic to any medications? What are they?"
M	Medications "What prescription and over-the-counter medications are you taking?"
P	Pertinent Past Medical History "Have you ever had this problem before? What was the diagnosis?" "What other medical problems do you have?"
L	Last Oral Intake "When did you last eat or drink anything? What was it?"
E	Event Preceding "What were you doing when this happened?" "How did it happen?"

Secondary Assessment

Vital signs are indicators of events occurring within the body. They include pulse, respiration, blood pressure, skin color, temperature, and condition, and the pupils' size and reaction to light. A complete set of vital signs is taken and recorded for each client.

If time permits, an EMT or paramedic will perform a detailed full body scan or, in some situations, a focused assessment of the client in the ambulance on the way to the hospital. These scans are used to identify further injury or illness and include a careful and systematic looking at, feeling, and listening to the client.

Reassessment

No assessment is ever complete. While taking care of and providing emergency care to the sick or injured client, there is always a need to reevaluate the primary assessment, chief complaint, vital signs, and emergency treatments. It is important to note continuously any changes that occur while the client is in your care.

Communication

EMRs and EMTs must converse with the client and his or her family. They must also communicate with dispatchers, deliver a radio or cell phone report to the hospital, and give a verbal transfer or hand-off report to the hospital staff. Communication skills, especially interpersonal skills, are vital to these professions.

Documentation

The last component of an EMS or EMR call is to document what he or she did. This requires a written report that describes the physical findings of the client examination, procedures performed, medications given, vital signs, and the name, age, and address of the client.

READING CHECK

Identify the primary focus of the scene size-up.

Airway Management

What is an airway adjunct and how is it used?

EMS training places great emphasis on airway assessment and management. The primary assessment directs EMRs and EMTs to find, aggressively treat, and manage all life-threatening problems involving airway, breathing, and circulation.

Our airway is the passageway by which air enters and exits the body. Its structures include the nose, mouth, pharynx, larynx, trachea, bronchi, and lungs. Trauma or disease in these structures limits our ability to move air into or out of our airway. One of the greatest threats to our airway is the tongue. In an unconscious client, the tongue can fall back into the mouth, blocking the airway. Thus, maneuvers such as the head tilt/chin lift or the jaw thrust are used to open the airway of an unconscious client. These maneuvers are described in Chapter 4, Emergency Preparedness. EMRs and EMTs determine which airway maneuver is most appropriate. The head tilt/chin lift is the preferred method for situations not involving trauma. The jaw thrust maneuver is used to open the airway of clients suspected of having a neck or back injury. This opens the airway without moving the head or neck.

Airway Adjuncts

A device called an airway adjunct assists in maintaining an open airway. EMRs and EMTs use two common adjuncts: the **oropharyngeal airway** adjunct and the **nasopharyngeal airway** adjunct. The oropharyngeal airway adjunct is inserted into the mouth of an unconscious client. It prevents the tongue from falling back onto the pharynx. The nasopharyngeal airway adjunct is inserted into one nostril, rests in the pharynx, and prevents the tongue from becoming an airway obstruction.

Before inserting an airway adjunct, you must carry out all basic life support assessments and procedures, including opening the airway and assessing for breathing and signs of circulation.

Oropharyngeal Airway Adjunct (OPA) The oropharyngeal airway adjunct (OPA) is a curved plastic device with a flange at the mouth opening. Several sizes are shown in **Figure 14.6.** The flange rests on the client's teeth, to prevent the OPA from slipping into the mouth.

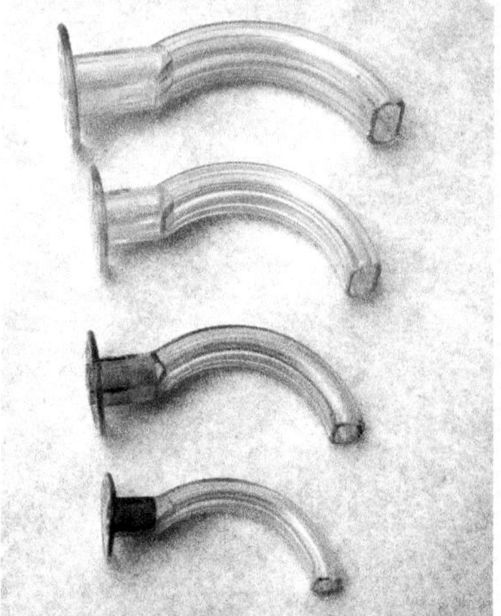

Fig. 14.6 OPAs Shown are four sizes of oropharyngeal airway adjuncts. *With which clients are these airways adjuncts most effective?*

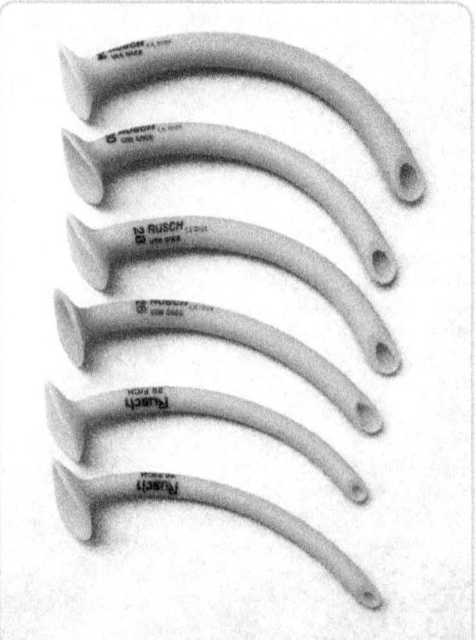

Fig. 14.7 NPAs A variety of sizes of nasopharyngeal airway adjuncts are shown. *With which clients are these airways most effective? Why?*

This airway adjunct is most effective on unresponsive patients with no gag reflex. The **gag reflex** causes retching and vomiting when something is placed far back in the mouth. In states of unresponsiveness, this reflex usually disappears. If an OPA is inserted into the mouth of a patient with a gag reflex, the patient may retch and vomit. If this happens, remove the OPA immediately. See **Procedure 14-1** to learn more about using an OPA.

An oropharyngeal airway adjunct should be correctly sized for the patient. A correctly sized OPA will extend from the corner of the patient's mouth to the tip of his or her earlobe.

Nasopharyngeal Airway Adjunct (NPA) NPAs are least likely to cause a gag reflex in most patients. Because they are not likely to make the patient gag, they are the airway adjuncts of choice in cases of seizure, stroke, and injuries of the mouth, when the patient's teeth are tightly clenched, and when a responsive patient is having difficulty maintaining his or her airway. However, never use an NPA where there is a suspected head injury accompanied by clear fluid (cerebrospinal fluid) draining from the nose. Nasopharyngeal airway adjuncts are made of soft latex and come in a variety of sizes, shown in **Figure 14.7.** See **Procedure 14-2** to learn more about using an NPA.

READING CHECK

Name the condition in which a patient is least likely to have a gag reflex.

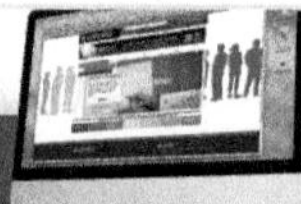

connect ONLINE PROCEDURES

PROCEDURE 14-1

Inserting an Oropharyngeal Airway Adjunct

The oropharyngeal airway adjunct (OPA) is a curved plastic device with a flange at the mouth opening. An oropharyngeal airway adjunct should be correctly sized for the patient. A correctly sized OPA will extend from the corner of the patient's mouth to the tip of his or her earlobe.

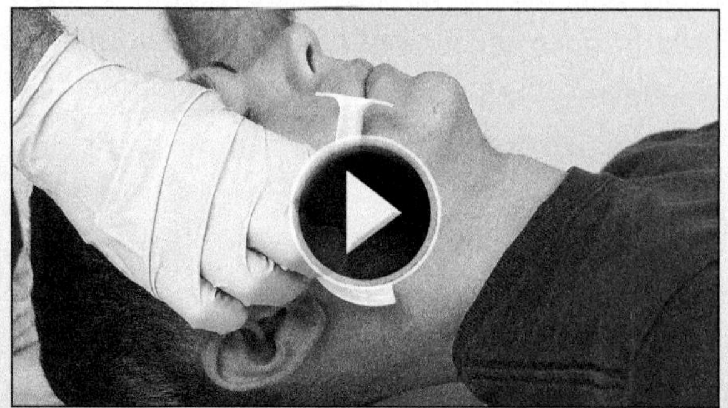

PROCEDURE 14-2

Inserting a Nasopharyngeal Airway Adjunct

Nasopharyngeal airway adjuncts (NPA) are made of soft latex and come in a variety of sizes. NPAs are least likely to cause a gag reflex in most patients. Do not use an NPA for a suspected head injury accompanied by clear fluid (cerebrospinal fluid) draining from the nose.

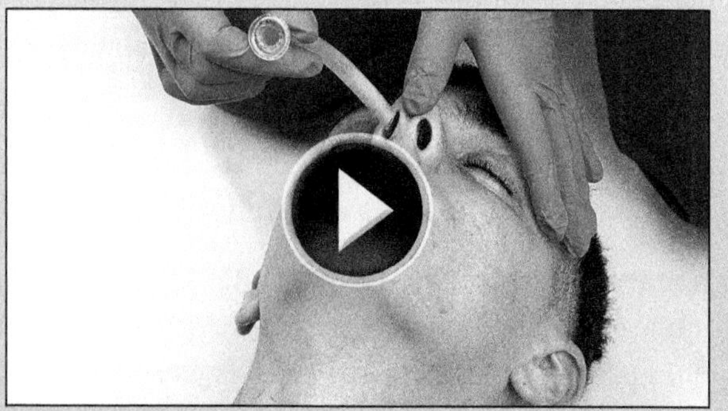

Oxygen Therapy

Which conditions require oxygen therapy?

Oxygen administration is the single most important treatment provided by both EMRs and EMTs. The way in which oxygen is administered by respiratory therapists is discussed in Chapter 19, Respiratory Care. Our atmosphere normally provides 21 percent oxygen. Certain illnesses and injuries, however, place tremendous stress on our body, which may require supplemental oxygen at the scene of the injury or illness. Conditions that require supplemental oxygen include:

- **Respiratory or cardiac arrest** CPR performed correctly is at best 35 percent effective. To improve the odds, provide supplemental oxygen.
- **Heart attack** A heart attack places tremendous stress on the heart's ability to pump blood. The circulated blood needs additional oxygen to support the body's functions.
- **Shock** Shock of any type reduces the flow of oxygen to our cells. Lack of oxygen increases the likelihood of tissue death. Supplemental oxygen reduces the risk of shock.
- **Severe blood loss** Major bleeding results in a loss of the red blood cells that carry oxygen to the tissues. Supplemental oxygen helps the remaining blood cells carry more oxygen.
- **Various lung disease or disorders** Any condition that affects the lungs' ability to exchange oxygen ultimately inhibits our ability to breathe. Supplemental oxygen helps ensure that the body tissues are receiving adequate oxygen.
- **Stroke** A stroke stresses the body and may deprive cell tissues of needed oxygen. Supplemental oxygen helps ensure that tissues are receiving the oxygen they need.
- **Drug overdose** Certain drugs suppress our ability to breathe and consequently reduce the amount of oxygen reaching the cells. Supplemental oxygen ensures that deprived cells will receive the needed oxygen.
- **Severe bone injuries** Injuries may produce shock, requiring the patient to have supplemental oxygen.

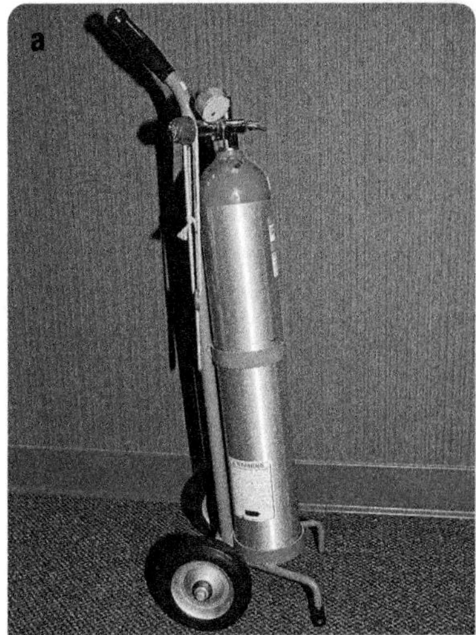

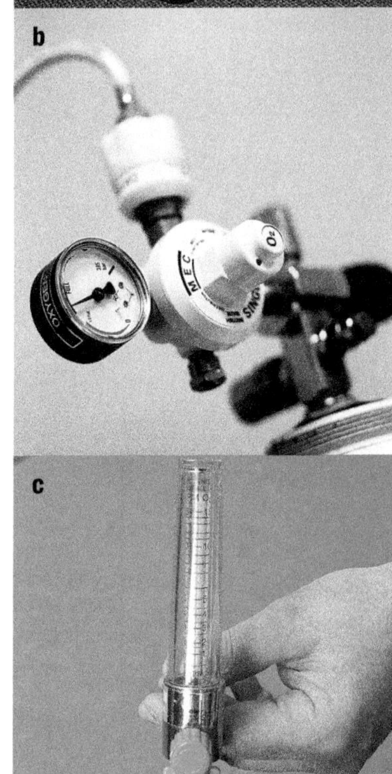

Fig. 14.8 Oxygen Equipment (a) oxygen cylinder (b) oxygen regulator (c) oxygen flow meter. *What are some conditions that may require supplemental oxygen?*

Photos: (t)Wallace Weeks/Alamy, (c)MARK SYKES/Science Photo Library/Alamy, (b)McGraw-Hill Companies, Inc./Scott Thompson, photographer

Oxygen Therapy Equipment

Oxygen delivery requires the following equipment (see **Figure 14.8**):

Oxygen Cylinders EMRs and EMTs use oxygen that is stored in portable oxygen cylinders. The cylinder is a seamless steel or lightweight alloy container filled with oxygen under pressure, equal to approximately 2000 pounds per square inch (psi) of pressure when full. Common portable cylinders include the D cylinder, which contains 350 liters of oxygen, and the E cylinder, which contains 625 liters of oxygen. For identification purposes, oxygen cylinders are usually green and white, although some may be unpainted steel or aluminum.

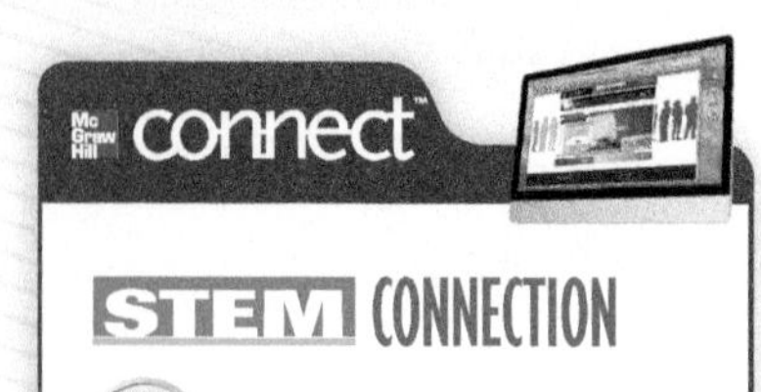

STEM CONNECTION

Medical Science

PSI (Pounds Per Square Inch)
Air pressure is the pressure exerted by air molecules striking a surface. The measurement of pounds per square inch (psi) is one type of air pressure scale.

Go to connect to learn how to measure psi in healthcare equipment.

Oxygen cylinders have a safe residual pressure of 200 psi. Safe residual pressure is the lowest pressure at which a cylinder can safely deliver oxygen to a patient. Most EMRs and EMS agencies replace or recharge the tanks when they reach around 500 psi. This precaution provides an additional margin of safety. See **Procedure 14-3** to learn more about preparing an oxygen cylinder.

Safety must always be a prime concern when working with oxygen and oxygen cylinders. The following list of cautions is an absolute necessity to ensure a safe environment.

- Be sure there is a metal-bound elastometric sealing washer (gasket), which assures an airtight seal between the collar of the regulator and valve stem. Nylon or plastic crush gaskets are no longer recommended. If used, crush gaskets can only be used once and then must be replaced.
- Never allow smoking in areas where oxygen is being administered. Oxygen increases the combustibility of other materials.
- Never allow oxygen cylinders, regulators, or delivery devices to be exposed to oil, grease, or other petroleum products. This can cause a fire or, worse, an explosion.
- Never drop an oxygen cylinder or allow it to fall.
- Never leave an oxygen cylinder upright without securing it.
- Never use adhesive tape of any type on an oxygen tank. The adhesive can react with the oxygen and cause a fire.
- Always handle an oxygen cylinder with extreme care. The cylinder is under extreme pressure, and if it is punctured or if the valve becomes broken, there is sufficient projectile force to make the cylinder capable of penetrating a concrete wall.

Oxygen Regulator The oxygen regulator is an essential link between the oxygen cylinder and delivery device. Without a regulator, the oxygen coming from the cylinder is under too great a pressure for the patient to use safely. An oxygen regulator for sizes D and E portable cylinders has a yoke and pin-indexed safety system that works only with an oxygen tank. It reduces the flow out of the tank to a safe pressure of 40 to 70 psi. Before connecting a regulator, open the valve on the oxygen for slightly less than a second to clear any dirt or dust.

Oxygen Flow Meter The flow meter is generally integrated into the regulator. It controls the oxygen flow from the tank, measured in liters per minute. Two regulator types are used for portable D and E cylinders, the Bourdon Gauge flow meter and the constant flow selector valve. Both allow oxygen flow rates of 15 to 25 liters per minute.

Oxygen Delivery Device Oxygen is administered to patients by two methods, directly through a bag-valve mask, or using either a **nonrebreather mask** or a **nasal cannula.** A nonrebreather mask delivers high concentrations of oxygen, up to 80 to 90 percent at a flow rate of 12 to 15 liters per minute, to a breathing patient. These devices are best suited for patients who exhibit signs of inadequate breathing and are short of breath, complain of chest pains, or are suffering from severe injuries and altered mental states.

For patients who cannot tolerate a face mask, the nasal cannula is used. A nasal cannula delivers an oxygen concentration of 24 to 44 percent at a flow rate of 1 to 6 liters per minute. See **Procedure 14-4** to learn more about providing oxygen.

READING CHECK

Summarize the chief safety concerns when working with oxygen.

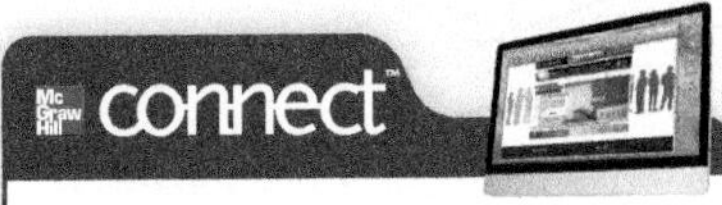

STEM CONNECTION

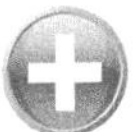

Medical Science

Oxygen's Role in Supporting Life

Oxygen therapy, or supplemental oxygen, is the most widely used therapy for people both in and out of the hospital.

Go to connect to learn more about oxygen's life-supporting role and its use in medical environments.

The Automated External Defibrillator (AED)

How do AEDs save lives?

A key function of the EMR or EMT is the primary assessment of each patient to find and treat any life-threatening conditions. He or she checks for spontaneous breathing and signs of circulation. If a patient lacks these signs, the EMR or EMT provides CPR and early defibrillation. This, along with early advanced prehospital care, improves the chance of survival for patients who face sudden cardiac arrest.

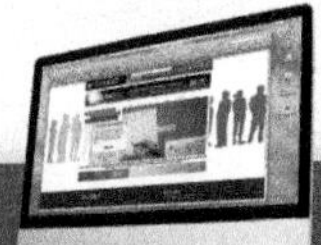

connect ONLINE PROCEDURES

PROCEDURE 14-3

Preparing an Oxygen Cylinder

An oxygen cylinder is a seamless steel or lightweight alloy container filled with oxygen under pressure. This pressure is approximately 2000 pounds per square inch (psi) when full. To administer oxygen you must be able to prepare the oxygen cylinder.

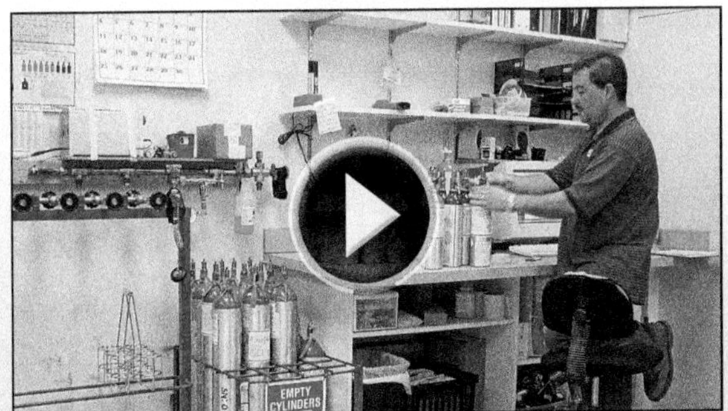

PROCEDURE 14-4

Providing Oxygen

Oxygen is administered to patients by two methods. First, oxygen is directly connected to a bag-valve mask device to assist patients who are not breathing or who have inadequate breathing. Second, oxygen is administered to patients who are breathing but need supplemental oxygen to improve their condition. Supplemental oxygen is given to these patients using either a nonrebreather mask or a nasal cannula.

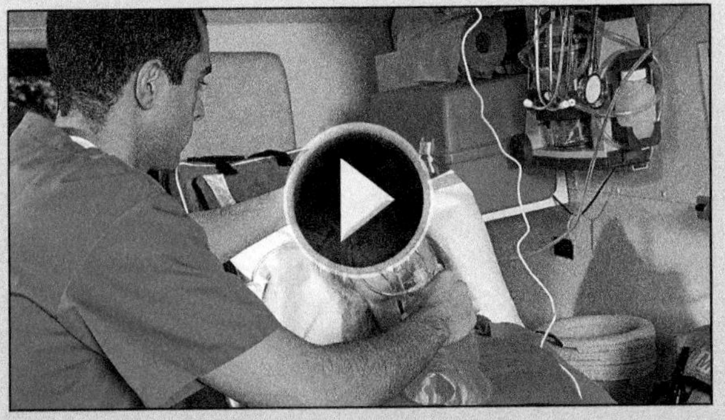

Photos: (t)Wallace Weeks/Alamy, (b)IS854/Image Source/Alamy

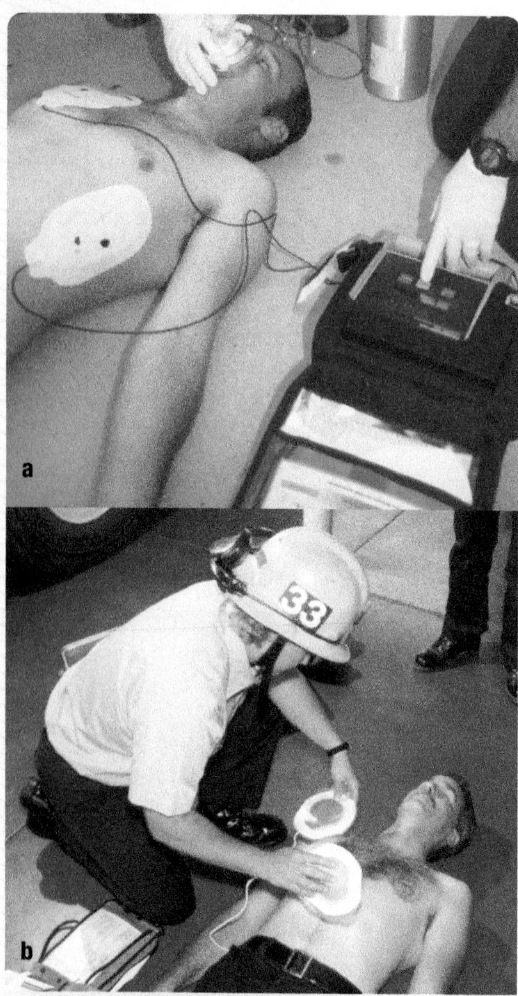

Fig. 14.9 Automated External Defibrillator (AED) (a) AED device connected to a patient. (b) AED chest pads. *How are AED pads attached to the chest?*

Ventricular fibrillation (V-fib or VF) is an abnormal heart rhythm. It is the most common cause of cardiac arrest. During VF, the heart rhythm becomes chaotic and the heart does not pump blood efficiently. The treatment for VF is defibrillation using a device called a **defibrillator.** It works by delivering an electrical shock to the heart to interrupt the chaotic rhythm. This allows the heart's natural rhythm to resume. Defibrillators are effective only if used within minutes of the patient's collapse from sudden cardiac arrest. The American Heart Association recommends that a patient in sudden cardiac arrest receives the first shock within five minutes after collapse. Survival rates of up to 49 percent have been reported following immediate use of a defibrillator.

There are two main types of defibrillators. The manual defibrillator requires the operator to view the patient's heart rhythm on a heart monitor, interpret the rhythm, decide if it is a shockable rhythm, apply electrode gel to the paddles, charge the defibrillator's paddles, and deliver the shock. This type of defibrillator requires extensive training in recognition of heart rhythms and proper use of the defibrillator.

Both EMRs and EMTs are trained in the use of the automated external defibrillator (AED). This is a computerized defibrillator programmed to recognize VF and another lethal rhythm, ventricular tachycardia (V-tach or VT), when the heart is beating abnormally fast. The AED is extremely reliable, easy to operate, and may be used by other individuals such as security guards, airline crews, and others after only a few hours of AED training. **Figure 14.9(a)** shows an example of an AED.

The AED may be used immediately after a witnessed cardiac arrest. However, it is recommended that at least two minutes of CPR be performed prior to using the AED after an unwitnessed cardiac arrest.

How Does the AED Work?

The AED is a computerized defibrillator that

- analyzes the heart rhythm.
- recognizes a rhythm that requires shock, such as VF or VT.
- advises the EMR or EMT, through voice prompts or flashing or lighted buttons, that the rhythm should be shocked.
- automatically charges to the appropriate shock energy level.

The AED comes in two types: the semiautomatic and the fully automatic. Fully automatic AEDs are rarely used. When properly attached to a patient's heart, a fully automatic AED can analyze the patient's heart rhythm, determine whether it is shockable, charge itself, and deliver the shock, all without the operator's intervention. The semiautomatic defibrillator requires the operator to push a button when the AED is fully charged.

To use the AED, the EMR or EMT must attach adhesive electrode pads to the patient's chest in a specific arrangement determined by the manufacturer. There are illustrations on the electrode's packing that show where to attach pads. After the pads are attached, as shown in **Figure 14.9b,** the AED will analyze the rhythm of the patient's heart and determine whether a shock is required. If a shock is required, the AED automatically charges to a preset energy level.

If the AED is semiautomatic, the EMR or EMT then presses the SHOCK button, and an electrical charge is delivered to the patient's heart by way of the AED's electrode wires attached to the chest.

After the shock, the EMR or EMT must resume CPR and follow the instructions given by the AED. The AED will advise the operator to stop every few minutes, so that it can reanalyze the heart rhythm.

When to Use an AED

Use an AED only in cases of sudden cardiac arrest. Before attaching an AED, determine whether the following signs are present:

- No response to voice or touch stimulation. Patient does not respond after you have tapped him or her on the shoulder and called out.
- No spontaneous breathing or abnormal breathing, meaning that the patient is gasping for breath.
- No pulse.

Special Considerations for AED Use

There are situations that may require you to change the way you use an AED. You will need to modify procedures if

- the patient is wet, lying on a wet surface, or in water. If the patient is lying in water, move him or her to a dry area before attaching the AED. Wipe the patient's chest dry before placing the electrodes.
- the AED is an older model. Older AEDs are intended for use on the adult patient but may, in extreme circumstances, be used on a child from one year of age to puberty. Newer AED's, however, are configured for both adults and children and will probably include pads for both.
- the patient is a child. Even on a newer-model AED, it may be necessary to use different cables, insert a key, or turn a switch to activate the child AED feature. Adult pads may be used on a child, but never use a child's pads on the adult patient. Some AED pads require the EMR or EMT to place a pad on the child's chest and one on the back. Be sure to follow the pictures on the AED pads.
- the patient has a pacemaker or an internal defibrillator with a battery pack. This will be visible as a lump under the skin about two inches long in the upper part of the chest or abdomen, usually on the left side. If you see this lump, avoid placing the pads directly on top of the device, if this is possible while still maintaining proper pad placement.

- the client is lying on a metal surface, such as on a bleacher seat, metal bench, or stretcher. Do not allow the electrodes to touch the metal surface.
- the client is wearing medication patches, such as a nitroglycerin patch. Immediately remove any patch on the chest and wipe the area clean before applying the AED pads.

General Principles for AED Use

Follow these general principles when using the AED:

- One EMR or EMT will operate the AED; the other will perform CPR.
- Defibrillation always comes first. Never delay applying an AED if the client has no spontaneous breathing or lacks signs of circulation.
- Know your AED.
- Do not touch the client when the AED is analyzing the client's rhythm.
- Be sure to say "Clear" and be sure everyone is clear of the client before delivering each shock.
- Periodically check your AED's battery. An AED defibrillator will not work if the battery power is low.

Operational Steps for AED Use

Figure 14.10 illustrates the sequence of steps for operating an AED. These steps are listed here.

1. Turn on the AED. To turn on an AED, you will need to press the power switch, lift the monitor cover, or lift the screen to the "up" position.
2. Attach pads to the client's chest and attach leads to the AED.
3. Remain clear of the client and allow the AED to analyze the client's heart rhythm. In other words, do not touch the client when the AED is analyzing the heart rhythm.
4. Remain clear of the client and deliver a shock if indicated. Under no circumstances should you or anyone else touch the client when a shock is being delivered.

The steps described above are the general steps for attaching and using any type of AED. **Procedure 14-5** explains, in general terms, how to operate a semiautomatic defibrillator. Your local operational protocols and procedures will determine the sequence of steps for you to follow when using your specific model of AED. Always refer to the manufacturer's manual and your local EMS guidelines for the defibrillator you will use.

READING CHECK

Recall how soon after cardiac arrest an AED should be employed.

STEPS IN USING AN AUTOMATED EXTERNAL DEFIBRILLATOR

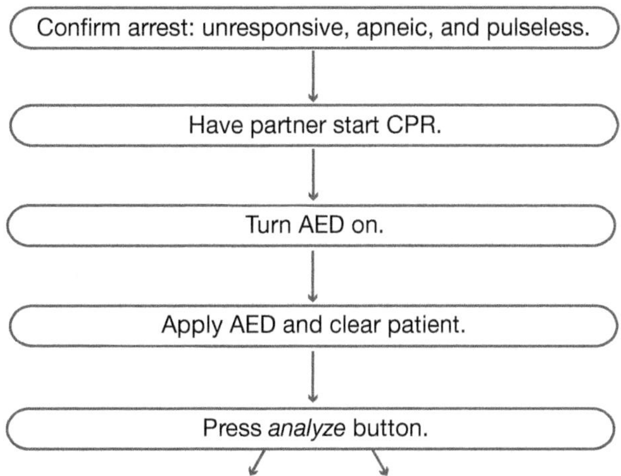

Confirm arrest: unresponsive, apneic, and pulseless.
Have partner start CPR.
Turn AED on.
Apply AED and clear patient.
Press *analyze* button.

Shock indicated (SI)

- Deliver 3 shocks in succession as long as AED gives *SI* message.
- Check pulse.
- If no pulse, CPR × 1 minute.
- Press *analyze* button.
- If *SI*, deliver 3 more shocks in succession as long as AED gives *SI* message.
- After 6 shocks, prepare to transport client. Follow local protocols for additional shocks.

No shock indicated (NSI)

- Check pulse. If none, CPR × 1 minute.
- Press *analyze* button.
- No shock indicated *(NSI).*
- Check pulse. If none, CPR × 1 minute.
- Press *analyze* button.
- No shock indicated *(NSI).*

Check pulse. If none, do CPR and transport.

Notes:

When a *no shock indicated (NSI)* message appears, check for a pulse. If the client regains a pulse, check breathing. Ventilate with high-concentration oxygen, or give oxygen by nonrebreather mask as needed.

If you initially shock the client and then receive an *NSI* message before giving six shocks, follow the steps for *no shock indicated* shown above in the right-hand column.

If you initially receive an *NSI* message and then on a subsequent analysis receive a *shock indicated (SI)* message, follow the steps for *shock indicated* in the above left-hand column.

Occasionally you may need to shift back and forth between the two columns. If this happens, follow the steps until one of the indications for transport (described below) occurs.

Transport as soon as one of the following occurs:
- You have administered six shocks.
- You have received three consecutive *NSI* messages (separated by one minute of CPR).
- The client regains a pulse.

If you shock the client out of cardiac arrest and he or she arrests again, start the sequence of shocks from the beginning.

Fig. 14.10 Sequence of Steps Shown are the steps for using an AED. *While the EMT operates the AED, what should another EMT or EMR on the scene be doing?*

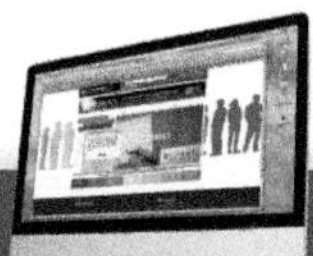

connect ONLINE PROCEDURES

PROCEDURE 14-5

Operating the Semiautomatic Defibrillator

A defibrillator works by delivering an electrical shock to the heart. Defibrillators are effective only if used within minutes of the client's collapse from sudden cardiac arrest. Automated External Defibrillators (AEDs) are found in many public locations. If AEDs are used, survival rates from sudden cardiac arrest improve.

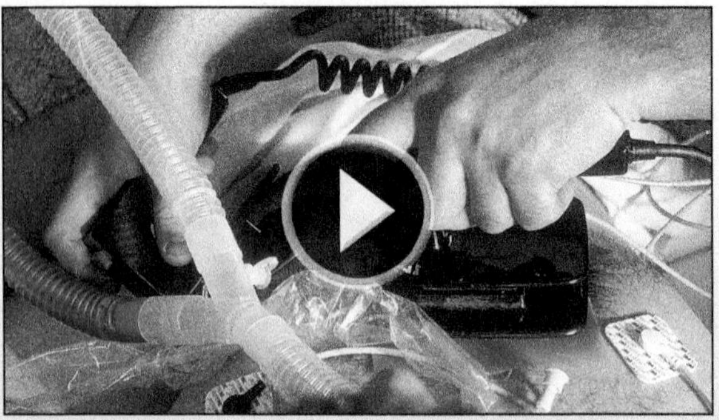

Spinal Immobilization Skills

What are the signs of a spinal injury?

Injury to the head and neck can occur in many ways. The head of an unrestrained occupant in a motor vehicle may strike the windshield. The head of a diver may strike the bottom of a pool. These forces can inflict injury to the underlying bony structures of the head, neck, and spinal cord. Injury may also occur when a patient falls from a significant height and lands in a standing position. Injuries to the spinal column may impair breathing and lead to paralysis and death. The most common causes of spinal injury are

- automobile or motorcycle collisions.
- shallow water diving accidents.
- falls.
- in children, falls from heights two to three times the child's height; falls from a tricycle or bicycle; being struck by a motor vehicle.

Common signs and symptoms of spinal injury include the following:

- Paralysis to the arms and/or legs
- Weakness, tingling or numbness, loss of feeling in the arms or legs
- Pain or tenderness along the back of the neck or spine
- Pain with or without movement
- Loss of bowel or bladder control
- Difficult or labored breathing with little or no movement of the chest

EMRs and EMTs are trained to assess for signs of these injuries. When they are found or suspected, specific procedures are followed to prevent further injury. Manual stabilization of the head, neck, or spine is the first procedure performed when an injury to the spinal column is suspected based upon the signs and symptoms listed above. See **Procedure 14-6** to learn more about stabilization of the head and neck.

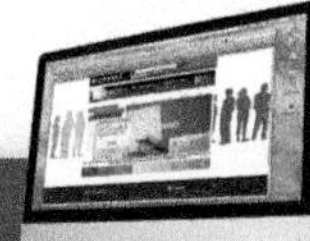

Connect ONLINE PROCEDURES

PROCEDURE 14-6

Manual Stabilization of the Head and Neck

The object of this procedure is to maintain the patient's head and neck motionless in a neutral, inline position. In this position, the head is facing forward, not turned to either side, nor tilted forward or backward. Applying manual stabilization prevents further movement of the head and neck and is used for possible head or neck injury.

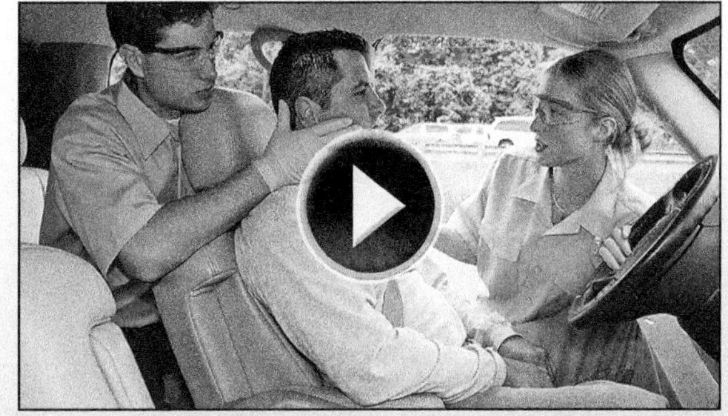

Emergency Childbirth

How long can labor last?

Before the early 1900s, most babies were born at home. Then mothers began having their babies in hospitals or birthing centers. Sometimes childbirth still occurs outside a medical facility. For this reason, EMRs and EMTs must know procedures for both normal and abnormal deliveries. However, unless delivery is expected to take place within a few minutes, the mother should be transported to a hospital.

Anatomy and Physiology

It takes nine months for a baby to develop and be born. This is called the gestation period. These nine months are divided into three trimesters. Review the information about these trimesters in Chapter 8, Human Growth and Development. Also review the information about the female reproductive system in Chapter 6, Human Structure and Function. This information is important to know when going through the procedures for emergency childbirth, as shown in **Procedure 14-7**.

Attached to the wall of the uterus is a special organ called the **placenta** (see **Figure 14.11**). The placenta acts as an exchange area between mother and fetus. It allows oxygen and nutrients to cross from the mother's circulation to nourish the fetus. Likewise, carbon dioxide and other wastes cross over from the fetus's circulation to the mother's circulation, to be eliminated by the mother. Since the placenta is required only during pregnancy, it is expelled after the birth of the infant.

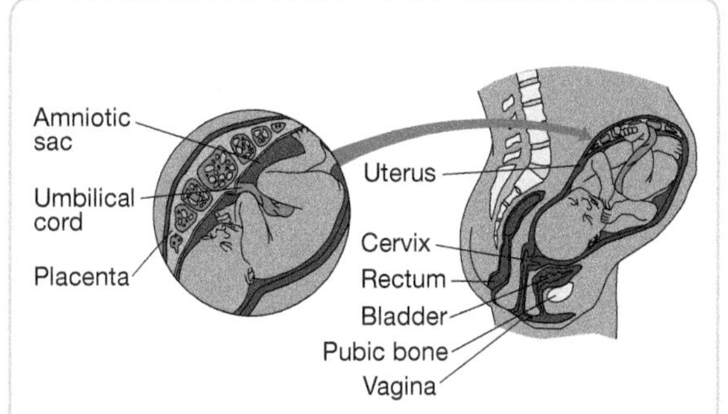

Fig. 14.11 Placenta Attached to the wall of the uterus is a special organ called the placenta. *What is the role of the placenta in the process of pregnancy?*

The fetus receives nourishment and expels waste through blood vessels found in its **umbilical cord,** a cordlike structure that links the fetus's navel and the placenta.

a

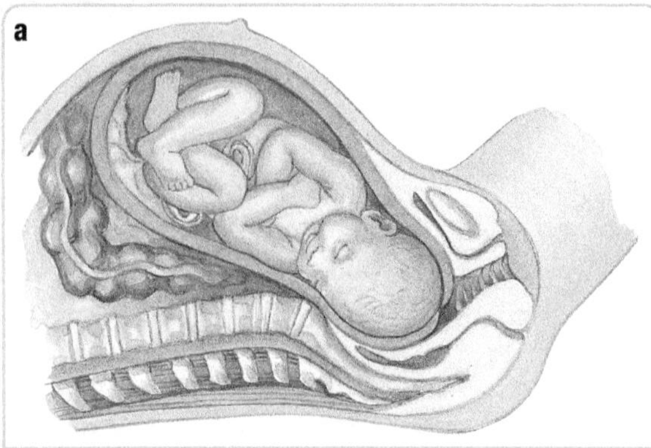

b

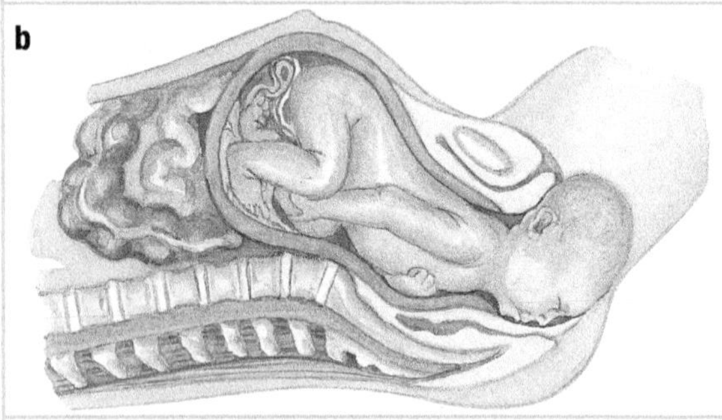

c

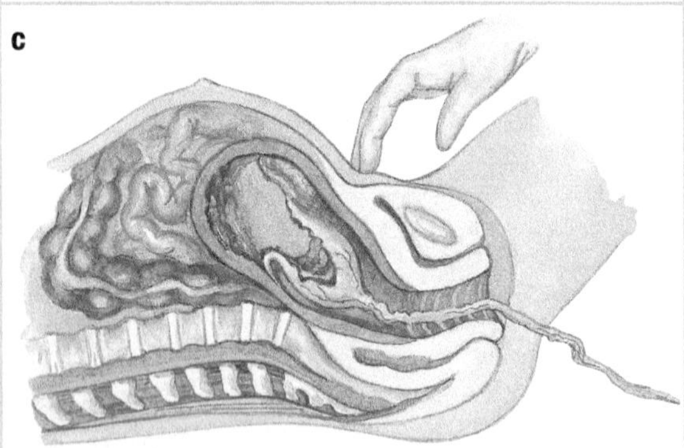

Fig. 14.12 Stages of Childbirth (a) First stage: beginning of contractions until full cervical dilation. (b) Second stage: baby enters birth canal and is born. (c) Third stage: placenta is delivered. *What is the definition of labor?*

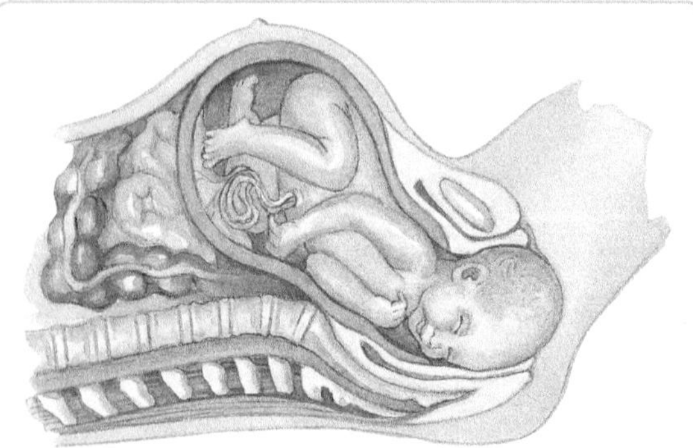

Fig. 14.13 Crowning Delivery is imminent when crowning is observed. *What is crowning?*

During its period of development inside the uterus, the fetus is enclosed and protected by a thin, membranous sac known as the **amniotic sac.** This sac contains approximately one to two liters of amniotic fluid. The amniotic sac allows the fetus to freely float during development and acts as a cushion to protect it from outside blows and shocks. Just before the birth of the baby, the amniotic sac breaks, releasing the fluid through the vagina.

During the ninth month of pregnancy, both the fetus and the mother's uterus and other organs prepare themselves for delivery. The fetus, which has been developing in an upright position, gradually turns completely over until the head is pointing downward. It is now ready to be born. Similarly, the uterus prepares for the day it will contract and push the baby out through the vaginal canal and into the world. This process is known as **labor.** There are three stages of labor. Understanding these three stages will help you to determine the urgency of a patient's impending delivery. **Figure 14.12** shows these stages.

- **First Stage.** The first stage of labor begins with regular contractions of the uterus and the thinning and gradual dilation of the cervix and ends with full dilation of the cervix. Cycles of contractions, along with labor pains, start far apart and become shorter as delivery becomes imminent. These contractions range from being 30 minutes apart to being three minutes apart or less. As contractions occur, the cervix thins and dilates further, to allow passage of the infant through the neck of the uterus. A woman may be in labor for 24 hours or more, or for less than four hours. The length of labor is usually longer for first-time mothers. The first stage of labor ends with full dilation of the cervix. In addition to these events, there may be a watery or bloody discharge of mucus and a rupture of the amniotic sac if it did not break at the onset of labor. Both events are normal.
- **Second Stage.** The second stage is the period that extends from when the baby enters the birth canal until the time it is born. During this stage, contractions become intense and frequent. The mother will express a need to push and move her bowels, as the baby's head puts pressure on her rectum. The moment of delivery is nearing. Delivery is imminent when **crowning** is observed. Crowning, as shown in **Figure 14.13,** occurs when the baby's head first bulges from the vaginal opening. The second stage ends when the baby is born.

- **Third Stage.** The third stage of labor starts after the delivery of the infant and lasts until the delivery of the placenta and umbilical cord have been completed. Contractions will continue a little longer as the uterus prepares to deliver the placenta. This period can last ten to twenty minutes and concludes with the delivery of the placenta.

READING CHECK

Explain the function of the amniotic sac.

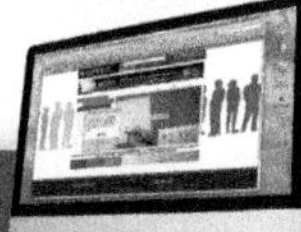

connect ONLINE PROCEDURES

PROCEDURE 14-7

Emergency Childbirth During a Normal Delivery

Sometimes childbirth occurs outside a medical facility. For this reason healthcare professionals must know procedures for both normal and abnormal deliveries. However, unless delivery is expected to take place within a few minutes, the mother should be taken to a hospital.

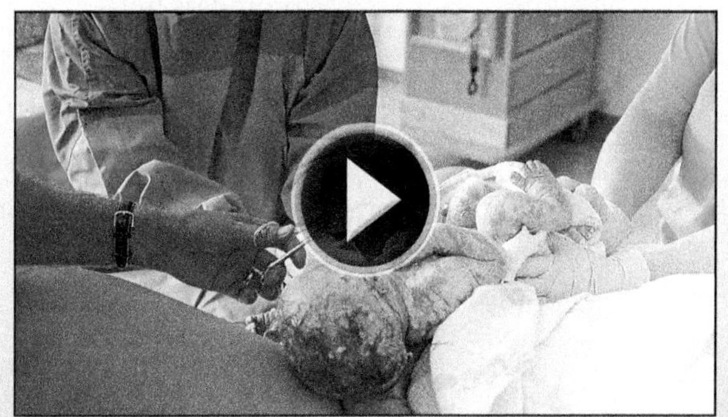

SECTION 14.2 Emergency Medical Services Procedures Review

AFTER YOU READ

1. **Explain** the importance of considering the mechanism of injury when evaluating a trauma client.
2. **List** the steps of the rapid body scan.
3. **Name** three situations in which oxygen therapy would be appropriate.
4. **List** the steps to follow in applying an AED.
5. **Define** the three stages of labor.
6. **Identify** the anatomic structures of a mother's body that are associated with pregnancy.

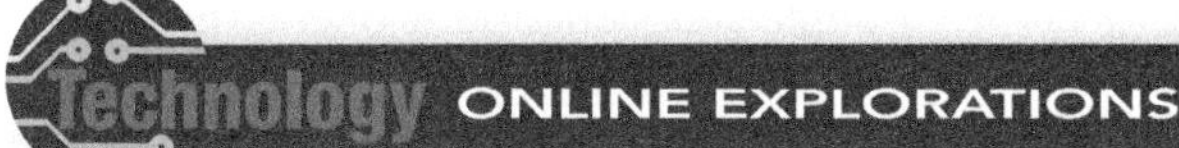

EMS Careers

Choose a career in EMS, then make a list of the steps necessary to enter the career you have chosen. Search the websites of the American Red Cross, American Heart Association, National Highway Traffic Safety Administration, or the National Safety Council to obtain your information.

Photo: Darren Mower/Vetta/Getty Images

CHAPTER

14 Review

Chapter Summary

SECTION 14.1

- EMRs, EMTs, AEMTs, and paramedics are healthcare providers trained to assist and provide emergency care to those who become sick or injured outside of a hospital or medical care setting. **(pg. 387)**
- Emergency service providers must safely gain access, determine what is wrong, provide emergency care, lift and move the patient, and transport the patient to an appropriate medical facility. **(pg. 387)**
- Emergency service provider skills are varied and include learning to size up a scene, assessing a patient for life-threatening conditions as well as for other less dangerous conditions, taking vital signs and medical history, and communicating findings both orally and in writing to other healthcare providers. **(pg. 388)**
- An AEMT performs the same basic skills as the EMT. However, the AEMT has had additional training and possesses additional skills. **(pg. 390)**
- The level of Paramedic represents the highest level of training among EMS professionals. **(pg. 390)**

SECTION 14.2

- EMS providers perform a seven-step assessment before providing emergency services. **(pg. 392)**
- Essential procedures carried out by EMRs, EMTs, and paramedics include maintaining the airway with airway adjuncts, administering supplemental oxygen, and using an AED. **(pg. 397)**
- Some additional skills of emergency service providers include spinal immobilization and procedures for emergency childbirth. **(pg. 406)**

Mc Graw Hill connect™ **ONLINE ACTIVITIES**

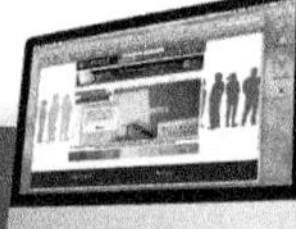

Complete our HST online activities for Chapter 14, which include Concept Check review questions, Reference Flash Cards, and Online Procedures assessment sheets.

- **Concept Check** review questions
- **Reference Flash Cards** medical terminology practice
- **Online Procedures** assessment sheets

CHAPTER

14 Assessment

Critical Thinking/Problem Solving

1. You are called to help a patient who has just passed out in a cafeteria. As you approach the patient, what should you consider? Why would it be important for you to assess this patient thoroughly? What would you include in this assessment, and why?

2. You are preparing to assist a patient who has experienced cardiac arrest by using an AED. As you bare the patient's chest in preparation to attach the AED's electrodes, you notice that the patient's chest is extremely hairy in the areas where the electrode pads are to be placed. You are not sure if the pads will make proper contact with the skin. What should you do?

3. You are responding to a patient who is lying on the floor of a home. The patient does not respond after you have tapped her on the shoulder and called out, but she is gasping for breath and has a weak pulse. Should you use an AED in this situation?

4. You are called out for "boy fallen." As you approach the scene, you find a 12-year-old boy lying at the base of a tree. The boy tells you he fell from one of the branches about halfway up the tree. He says he landed on both feet and then fell forward, catching himself with his hands.

   a. The boy tells you that his hands, feet, neck, and legs hurt a lot. Which bones or joints may have been injured?

   b. Why would it be important to assess this patient thoroughly?

   c. What would you include in this assessment?

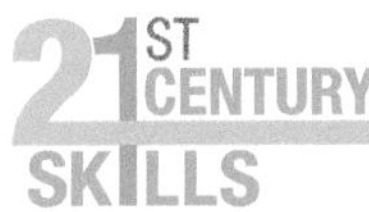

5. **Problem Solving** With a student acting as a patient, practice the steps for operating an AED. Use paper for electrodes and a small box as your AED; **NEVER practice with a real AED.**

6. **Teamwork** With a partner, practice the initial assessment and focused exam. Practice obtaining a history and taking vital signs.

7. **Information Literacy** Go online and search for the requirements in your state to become a first responder. Locate a program or programs in your area for training EMRs, EMTs, AEMTs, and/or paramedics. Learn the requirements for obtaining certification in each of these careers as part of your exploration of the healthcare field.

CHAPTER 15 Nursing

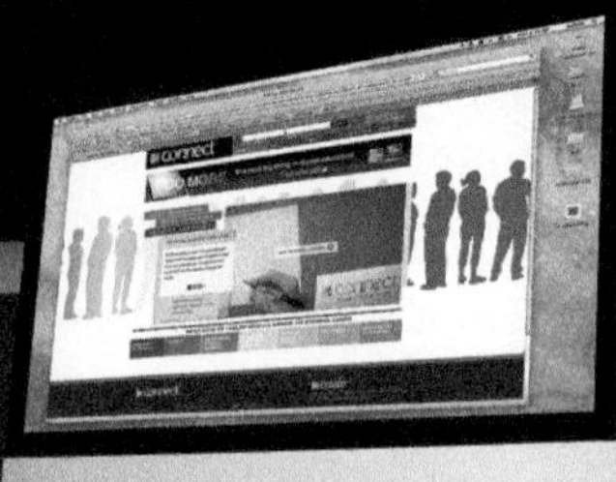

McGraw Hill connect™

It's Online!

- Online Procedures
- STEM Connection
- Medical Science
- Medical Terms
- Medical Math
- Ethics in Action
- Virtual Lab

Essential Question:

What are the educational requirements for a nursing career?

The nursing profession offers many career options. Job opportunities for those who have nursing skills are expected to grow faster than average in the future. One of the reasons for this explosive growth is the large number of people who are retired or near retirement age and will often need more healthcare as they age. Also, many current nursing professionals are reaching retirement age. They will be replaced by younger workers. In many of the entry level nursing personnel areas, there is a high rate of turnover. This creates a need for newly trained individuals.

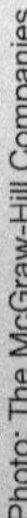

Photo: The McGraw-Hill Companies Inc.

READING GUIDE

OBJECTIVES

After completing this chapter, you will be able to:

- **Explain** the roles and responsibilities of unlicensed personnel who perform nursing duties, including certified/certificated nursing assistants, home health aides, dialysis technicians, patient care technicians, and surgical technicians.
- **Differentiate** between the roles and responsibilities of licensed nurses, including licensed practical nurses and licensed vocational nurses, registered nurses, and advanced practice nurses.
- **Demonstrate** 34 nursing procedures.

BEFORE YOU READ

Connect Have you ever received medical care from a member of the nursing profession? How would you describe that experience?

Main Idea

With the growing need to provide patient care in the most cost-effective manner possible, the role of nurses is continually being re-examined. As a result, many basic nursing tasks are now being performed by people who are trained in those tasks but do not have the complete training of a licensed nurse.

Note-Taking Activity

Draw this table. Write key terms and phrases under **Cues**. Write main ideas under **Note Taking**. Summarize the section under **Summary**.

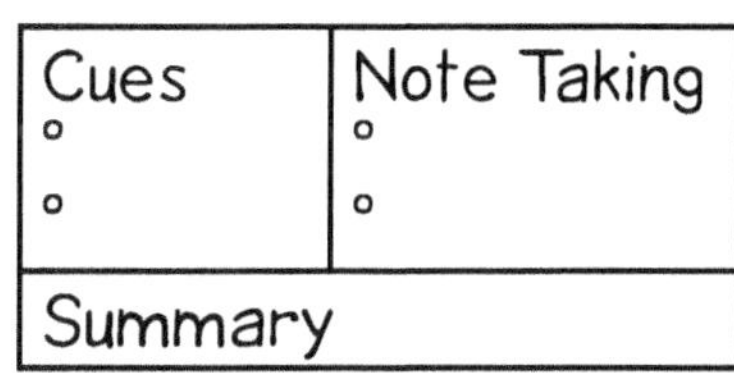

Graphic Organizer

Before you read the chapter, draw a diagram like the one to the right. As you read, write the careers covered in this chapter into the diagram.

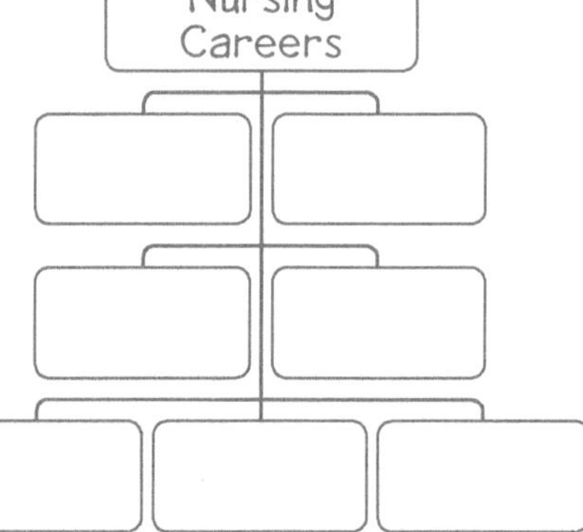

connect

Downloadable graphic organizers can be accessed online.

STANDARDS

HEALTH SCIENCE

NCHSE 1.13 Analyze basic structure and function of the human body.

NCHSE 1.22 Recognize emerging diseases and disorders.

SCIENCE

NSES A Develop abilities necessary to do scientific inquiry, understandings about scientific inquiry.

NCHSE *National Consortium for Health Science Education*

NSES *National Science Education Standards*

COMMON CORE STATE STANDARDS

MATHEMATICS

Number and Quantity

Quantities Reason quantitatively and use units to solve problems.

ENGLISH LANGUAGE ARTS

Reading

Integration of Knowledge and Ideas R-7 Integrate and evaluate multiple sources of information presented in diverse formats and media (e.g., quantitative data, video, multimedia) in order to address a question or solve a problem.

Speaking and Listening

Presentation of Knowledge and Ideas SL-6 Adapt speech to a variety of contexts and communicative tasks, demonstrating command of formal English when indicated or appropriate.

SECTION 15.1 Careers in Nursing

Vocabulary

Content Vocabulary

You will learn these content vocabulary terms in this section.

- **certified nursing assistant**
- **certificated nursing assistant**
- **Omnibus Budget Reconciliation Act (OBRA)**
- **ambulate**
- **long-term care facility**
- **patient care technician (PCT)**
- **licensed practical nurse (LPN)**
- **licensed vocational nurse (LVN)**
- **advocate**

Academic Vocabulary

You will see these words in your reading and on your tests. Find their meanings in the Glossary in the back of the book.

- **research**
- **minimal**
- **period**
- **monitoring**
- **options**

Nursing Careers

What kind of nursing career might be the best match with your personality and talents?

The nursing profession can be divided into two main areas: unlicensed nursing personnel and licensed personnel.

The unlicensed nursing personnel discussed in this chapter are:

- Certified or certificated nursing assistant
- Home health aide
- Dialysis technician
- Surgical technician
- Patient care technician

The licensed nursing personnel discussed in this chapter are:

- Licensed practical nurse or licensed vocational nurse
- Registered nurse
- Advanced practice nurse

Table 15.1 gives information about these occupations. The paragraphs that follow discuss them in greater detail.

Unlicensed Nursing Personnel

When would it be appropriate to use unlicensed nursing personnel?

The increasing need to provide care in the most cost-effective manner is causing the role of nurses to be re-examined.

Many basic nursing tasks can be safely performed by people who have specific training to do those tasks. This type of training does not take the amount of time or expense that it takes to become a licensed nurse. Those who are trained to do some of the basic nursing tasks but who are not licensed are called unlicensed nursing personnel.

Licensed nurses supervise unlicensed nursing personnel and delegate tasks to them. This reduces costs. **Figure 15.1** on page 416 shows an example of a person working as unlicensed nursing personnel.

The biggest issues here are deciding what to delegate and how much supervision is needed. The National Council

Table 15.1 Overview of Nursing Occupations

OCCUPATION	EDUCATION REQUIREMENT	CERTIFICATION OR LICENSING AGENCY	JOB OUTLOOK
Certified or certificated nursing assistant	Federal law requires at least 75 hours of training and passing of a competency evaluation that includes knowledge and skill tests.	The department of health in each state is responsible. In many states the department contracts this responsibility to another agency.	Expected to grow faster than average because of aging of the United States population and a high turnover rate.
Home health aide	On-the-job training is accepted in some states. Other states require formal training. If agencies receive reimbursement from Medicare, federal law suggests at least 75 hours of training.	The National Association for Home Care offers national certification.	One of the fastest-growing occupations because of turnover rate and the large population of aging individuals.
Dialysis technician	16 to 18 weeks of training.	The Nephrology Nursing Certification Commission offers certification for clinical hemodialysis technicians after a training program, six months of experience, and passing an exam. The National Nephrology Certification Organization offers certification in clinical nephrology technology after 12 months' experience and passing its examination. The Board of Nephrology Examiners for Nursing and Technology offers certification after 12 months' experience and passing its examination.	Faster than average growth because the number of patients on dialysis is increasing and dialysis technicians are replacing registered nurses in treatment centers.
Surgical technician	9 to 24 months' training and education in a program accredited by the Commission on Accreditation of Allied Health Education Programs.	Liaison Council on Certification for the Surgical Technologist.	Faster than average growth because of increases in surgical procedures and the large number of aging individuals.
Licensed practical nurse/licensed vocational nurse (LPN/LVN)	Approximately one year of education. All states require the LPN/LVN to pass a licensing examination.	License varies from state to state. Licenses may be issued by a state board of nursing or the department of labor's licensing and regulation agency.	Average growth.
Registered nurse (RN)	Two to five years of education. All states require the RN to graduate from a nursing program and pass a licensing examination.	License varies from state to state. Licenses may be issued by a state board of nursing or the department of labor's licensing and regulation agency.	Faster than average growth because of the variety of positions available, the addition of new positions, and an aging population of nurses presently employed.
Advanced practice nurse	Registered nurse degree plus one to two years of graduate-level education.	Many professional associations provide certificates. Each state differs in licensure.	Increasing growth due to increase in independent practice in rural areas and lower cost than that related to a physician.

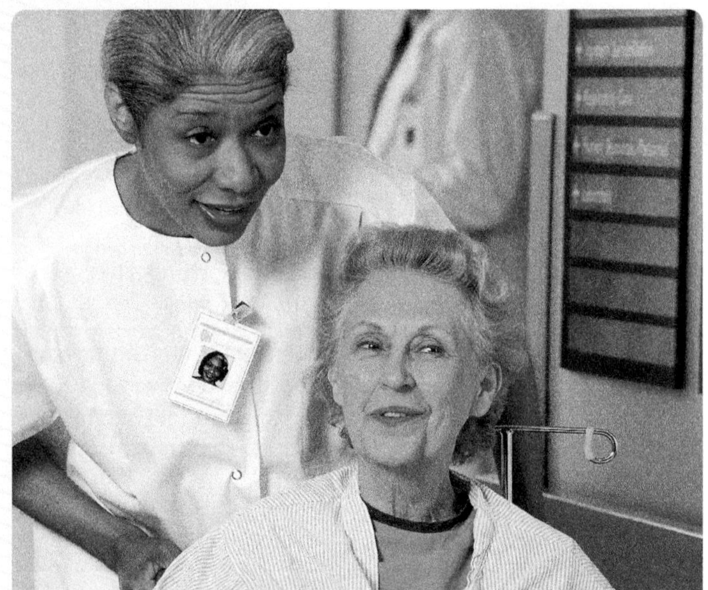

Fig. 15.1 Unlicensed Nursing Personnel Unlicensed personnel provide care to patients in long term, acute and residential care facilities. *How do unlicensed personnel help control healthcare costs?*

of State Boards of Nursing has conducted research on the tasks that are safe to delegate to unlicensed personnel. Some healthcare facility administrators believe fairly complex tasks can be delegated to unlicensed staff, but more research is needed. Often healthcare providers find themselves caught between their employer's wishes and their own ideas about how care should be provided.

The Certified or Certificated Nursing Assistant

State law, not the federal government, regulates nursing certification. Since state laws vary, unlicensed personnel have different titles from state to state. The titles **certified nursing assistant** or **certificated nursing assistant** are often used. Unlicensed individuals rely on the training and practices of the person who delegates tasks to them.

Minimum requirements for nursing assistant training were written into federal law in the 1986 **Omnibus Budget Reconciliation Act (OBRA).** This act specifies that training include at least 75 hours of education for individuals who work in a long-term care facility (nursing home). It also specifies the evaluation or testing that must be performed after the training has been completed. Each state department of health establishes training and testing standards and sets up a state registry. The health department may perform this duty internally, or it may contract the responsibility to another entity.

A high school diploma is often not required to train to become a certified or certificated nursing assistant. Usually, the training is minimal, but minimum standards must be met. Assistants who complete their training and successfully pass the federally required test are placed on a state registry. This allows the individual to practice in that state only. If a nursing assistant moves to another state, he or she may be required to take another test or complete more training.

The Nursing Assistant's Job Responsibilities Certified or certificated nursing assistants take care of people in a variety of facilities, including hospitals, nursing homes, and residential care facilities. They perform basic care tasks that are delegated to them by licensed nurses, and they work directly under the supervision of licensed nurses.

Nursing assistants are often the primary care givers. They frequently have more personal contact with patients than any other care provider. Many times, they develop close long-term relationships with patients. The care they provide makes a tremendous difference in the quality of life for elderly, ill, or disabled people. Patient safety, both physical and psychological, is of the highest concern for nursing assistants.

Utmost care must be taken to ensure patient confidentiality. This is important in order to protect people from the harm that can be done if personal information is inappropriately revealed. Also, accurate communication, both written and verbal, is very important.

Certified or certificated nursing assistants work mainly in three types of facilities including acute care, long-term care, or residential care.

Job Responsibilities in Acute Care Certified or certificated nursing assistants may work in acute care facilities such as hospitals. Acute care patients usually have an immediate problem, such as a broken bone or infection, and their stay is normally short. Relationships with these patients differ from the ones developed in long-term or residential care. The most important responsibilities of a certified or certificated nursing assistant are to protect patient safety and report any significant changes. Some of the tasks delegated to nursing assistants include:

- Answering call signals from patients' rooms
- Setting up rooms for new admissions
- Keeping patient rooms neat, especially to ensure safety
- Delivering messages, supplies, and equipment
- Serving and assisting with meals
- Assisting with daily personal care
- Assisting with toileting
- Making beds
- Assisting with bathing and/or showering
- Providing oral care
- Assisting with skin care
- Helping with shaving
- Taking and reporting vital signs
- Reporting any changes in the patient's condition
- Helping patients transfer (from bed to chair, for example) and/or **ambulate** (walk)

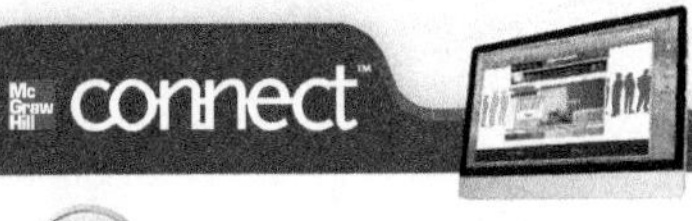

Ethics in Action

Scenarios to Consider You are having lunch in the cafeteria when a coworker enters and sits down beside you. He asks about your assigned patients for the shift. You know that patient confidentiality is a legal right. Someone in the cafeteria might overhear confidential information if you discuss it with your coworker in that setting. Also, it is never acceptable to talk about patients with anyone who is not directly involved with their care.

Go to connect to read more about this and other similar ethical challenges, and complete the related activity.

Job Responsibilities in Long-Term Care As the population ages, more and more people will need to enter a long-term care facility, or nursing home. A **long-term care facility** is a healthcare facility for patients who do not require acute care but are unable to live alone (see **Figure 15.2**). It is very important that the certified or certificated nursing assistant contribute to a respectful, caring, and dignified environment.

Patients may spend years in the same facility. The facility becomes their home. At times, this is difficult, for the patients may be disagreeable and the duties may be unpleasant. Nursing assistants in these facilities perform the same duties as an acute care nursing assistant.

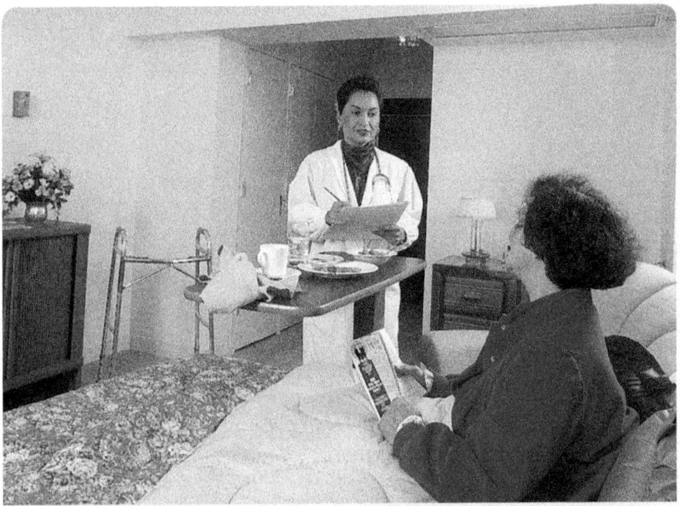

Fig. 15.2. A Long-Term Healthcare Facility A healthcare worker interacts with a resident of a long-term care facility. *Do you know any other names for long-term care?*

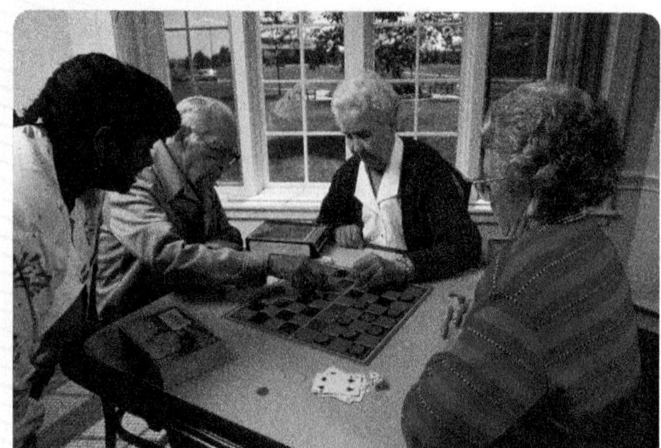

Fig. 15.3 Residential Care Facilities
Residential care facilities are homes for individuals who are able to handle many of their own basic needs. *What is the difference between residential and long-term care?*

Additional duties in long-term care may include:

- Emptying bedpans
- Cleaning incontinent patients
- Reporting significant changes, including changes in mental status or self-care capabilities

Job Responsibilities in Residential Care Residential care facilities are homes for individuals who cannot take care of themselves in their own home but are able to handle many of their own basic needs. Therefore, they do not require the level of care provided in a long-term facility. For the most part, residential care facilities resemble a home situation. Clients generally have a bedroom that may be private or shared, a communal dining area, a communal area for visiting or watching TV, and planned recreation and exercise. Residential care facilities may be small, with as few as five or six clients, or they may be large facilities with as many as 100 clients or more. Some are very homelike and comfortable. Others resemble luxury hotels and are located in elegant settings. **Figure 15.3** shows a typical residential care facility.

Individuals may live for months or years in residential care, and long-term relationships may develop between the nursing assistants, clients, and their families. The work can be very satisfying and rewarding. In addition to the responsibilities described for acute and long-term care facilities, the nursing assistant in a residential care facility may be responsible for:

- Assisting with medications
- Assisting with taking clients shopping or on other outings
- Providing assistance with transportation to medical appointments

The Home Health Aide

Home health aides work with clients in their homes. The clients may be elderly, disabled, or ill, but they are able to live safely in their own homes instead of in a care facility. A home healthcare client may live alone or with family. However, such clients require more care than family or friends are able to provide. **Figure 15.4** shows a client who is receiving home healthcare.

Home health aides may do a lot of driving during the course of the day. Some home health aides work for a long time in a home in which a member of the family has a chronic condition. Some home healthcare clients have an acute illness but may need help for just a short period while they recover.

A home health aide might go to the same home every day or might visit several homes during one day. Aide assignments can even change daily. Some clients' homes are neat and comfortable, whereas others may be untidy or depressing. Some clients are pleasant and very appreciative of the help the home health aide provides. Other clients

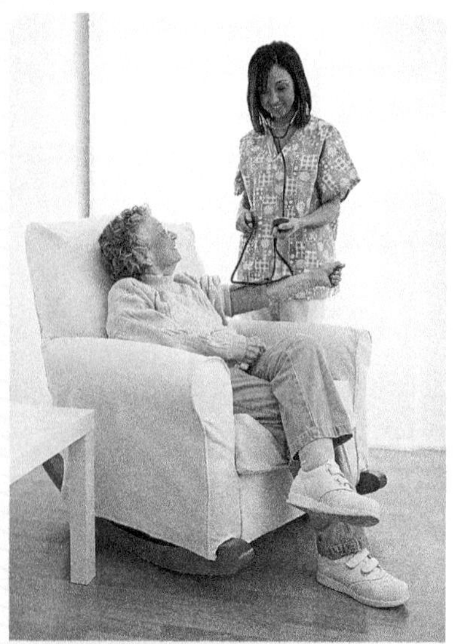

Fig. 15.4 Home Healthcare
Home health aides work with clients in their homes. *How might care in a client's home differ from care in a healthcare facility?*

may be angry, confused, and hard to care for. Working in the client's home environment may have dangers. The supervising nurse should assess each home for dangerous situations before the home health aide begins his or her visits.

The home health aide usually works on an independent basis. He or she works alone, with visits from a supervisor at set intervals. The supervisor is usually a home health nurse, who writes detailed plans of care for the aides to follow. The supervisor also works with the home health aides to make sure that they are comfortable in providing a given level of care.

The Home Health Aide's Job Responsibilities Home health aides provide basic health-related care in the client's home. These tasks may include:

- Performing all tasks outlined for a certified or certificated nursing assistant
- Assisting with medications
- Assisting with personal care such as cooking meals; helping with eating, bathing, and dressing; light housekeeping; laundry; and changing bed linens
- Assisting with shopping and taking clients to medical appointments
- Helping the client to remain safe in his or her home

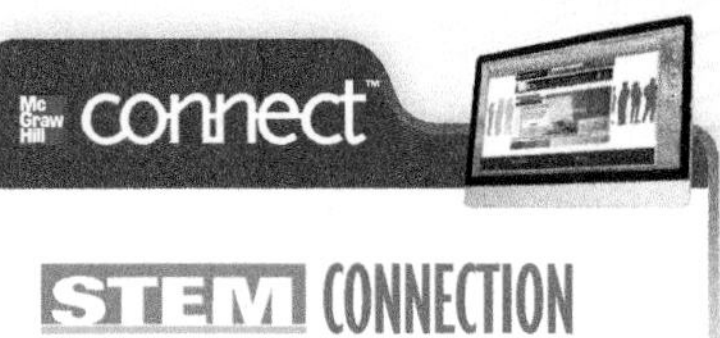

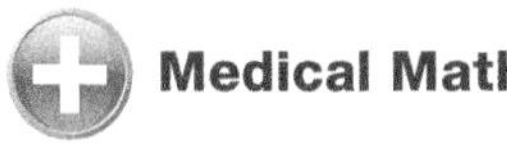

Medical Math

Metric and Avoirdupois Measurements

To perform accurate intake and output measurements, you must be able to convert measurements from avoirdupois to metric. The ounce (oz), teaspoon (tsp), and tablespoon (T) are avoirdupois measurements for fluids. Milliliters (mL) and the cubic centimeter (cc) are metric measurements for fluids. Milliliters and cubic centimeters are exactly the same amount.

Go to connect to complete the Metric and Apothecary Measurements activity and worksheet.

The Dialysis Technician

Dialysis technicians are also known as hemodialysis or renal dialysis technicians. These technicians operate kidney dialysis machines. The machines filter the blood of patients whose kidneys are not working correctly. This process is done to filter out waste products and extra fluids from the patient's blood. Dialysis technicians may work directly with the patients who are receiving treatments, or they may work with the equipment only, performing maintenance and repairs on it.

The Dialysis Technician's Job Responsibilities Dialysis technicians work in outpatient dialysis clinics and acute care settings in which dialysis is performed. They must know all about the dialysis equipment and the scientific basis for dialysis. Dialysis technicians work in clean, comfortable environments with seriously ill patients. Since the work requires contact with blood and blood products, the risk of exposure to infectious disease is high. Strict observance of sterilization procedures and standard precautions can decrease the risk of disease transmission.

Responsibilities may vary according to the state laws and facility policy. It is imperative that dialysis technicians know these laws and policies. The work of the technician may include any or all of the following:

- Preparing the equipment
- Obtaining and recording patients' weight and vital signs before the procedure

- Administering local anesthetics and medications before, during, or after the procedure
- Beginning the procedure
- **Monitoring** the patient and machine during the procedure
- Observing the patient during the procedure for signs or symptoms of an adverse reaction
- Administering emergency care if there is an adverse reaction to any medication or to the procedure. Emergency care may include performance of basic cardiopulmonary resuscitation
- Cleaning the equipment after the procedure
- Training patients to perform their dialysis treatments at home

The Surgical Technician

Surgical technicians are also known as operating room technicians. They assist during surgical procedures, with supervision from surgeons, registered nurses, and others. Surgical technicians work in clean, well-lit places. This type of work requires standing and walking for long periods. It also requires wearing special clothing. Often, surgical technicians work a 40-hour week, Monday through Friday. However, the job may also require surgical technicians to be on call for nights, weekends, and holidays.

To work as a surgical technician, one must be able to handle instruments safely and quickly. There is a chance of exposure to communicable diseases during surgical procedures. Also surgical technicians may be exposed to unpleasant sights, odors, or materials. It is not a profession for anyone who does not like the sight of blood.

The Surgical Technician's Job Responsibilities Most surgical technicians work in the operating or delivery room of acute care facilities. However, there are job positions in outpatient surgery centers, working for physicians and dentists. Also, some specialty physicians may hire a surgical technician to work exclusively with them on specific teams, such as transplant teams.

The surgical technician may help set up an operating room before surgery. He or she may assist during operations by handing instruments and other supplies to the surgeon or surgical team and/or their assistants. Other duties of the surgical technician may include:

- Performing sterilization procedures to maintain the environment required for safe surgery
- Maintaining knowledge of what surgical tools are required during surgery
- Knowing the order in which surgical tools are required during surgery
- Setting up and testing non-sterile equipment
- Preparing patients' surgical sites by shaving, cleaning, and disinfecting
- Taking patients' vital signs

- Checking medical charts to provide information to the surgeon or surgical team
- Transporting patients to a recovery room
- Cleaning and restocking surgical suites after procedures

The Patient Care Technician

The **patient care technician (PCT)**, or patient care assistant, is responsible for providing assistance to doctors, nurses, and other support staff while also interacting directly with the patient. The patient care technician is a critical member of the healthcare team.

Patient care technicians focus on recording vital health information, collecting samples, and assisting patients. The education and job responsibilities vary between states and healthcare facilities.

If you are interested in becoming a patient care technician, you must first complete a one or two-year PCT certificate program, which is offered through community colleges or vocational schools. In addition, most programs require students to obtain at least 40 hours of clinical experience prior to the program's completion. The employment rate and job prospects for patient care technicians have increased and are expected to continue growing.

The Patient Care Technician's Job Responsibilities Job responsibilities for a PCT will vary based upon the state and place of employment. Here is a list of some common patient care technician responsibilities.

- Providing basic nursing care duties
- Taking and recording health information such as weight, height, and vital signs
- Performing electrocardiograms (ECGs)
- Inserting and removing urinary catheters
- Obtaining blood specimens

READING CHECK

Explain why nursing is such a growing field.

Licensed Nursing Personnel

In what situations are licensed nurses required?

Licensed nursing personnel take courses after high school and must pass a test upon completion. These individuals are licensed by a state agency. They are held accountable for their practice through standards, which are set by the state agency. Licensed nurses belong to professional groups, which also set practice standards. The training and job duties of licensed nurses are similar throughout the field of nursing. As licensed nurses gain more training, they usually take on more duties and receive more pay.

21ST CENTURY SKILLS

Communicating Respect and Empathy

Kind, empathetic communication can help reduce fear in people who are undergoing great change in their lives. Patients who are being admitted or transferred may be sick, scared, in pain, or just uncomfortable. Patients who are being discharged may be apprehensive about returning home. Healthcare providers cannot change the situation, but they can listen. Often the simple act of quietly holding a hand and attentively listening allows a patient to know that someone cares. Open-ended questions such as "How are you feeling?" may encourage patients to talk to you and help them work through their feelings of grief and loss.

Follow-up: What would your response be to a fearful patient?

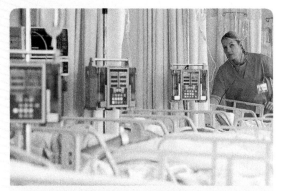

Fig. 15.5 LPN/LVN Licensed Practical Nurses and Licensed Vocational Nurses can work in acute care hospitals such as this one. *How is an LPN/LVN supervised?*

The Licensed Practical or Vocational Nurse

Licensed practical nurses (LPNs) are also known as **licensed vocational nurses (LVNs).** They perform nursing care for patients under the supervision of a physician or registered nurse. Most LPNs and LVNs receive training in vocational or technical schools. Programs have both a classroom or online component and a clinical component. In the classroom or online, practical nurses study basic nursing concepts and healthcare subjects. In the clinical component, they practice under the supervision of an instructor who is a registered nurse. All states require practical nurses to pass a licensing examination. **Figure 15.5** shows one place of employment for an LPN/LVN.

The LPN/LVN's Job Responsibilities The licensed status of practical or vocational nurses means that they are responsible for assessing patients' conditions and providing the necessary care. Most LPN/LVNs provide basic bedside care and are responsible for the safety of the patient. They practice independently but under the supervision of a physician or registered nurse. In some states LPN/LVNs may receive training that allows them to be supervisors in long-term care facilities.

Some of the duties of the LPN/LVN are:

- Taking vital signs
- Treating bedsores (decubitus ulcers)
- Administering injections
- Giving enemas
- Administering medications
- Applying dressings
- Applying ice packs and hot water bottles
- Inserting and caring for urinary catheters
- Assessing patients for effects of medication and treatments
- Assisting with meals
- Recording intake and output of food and liquids
- Helping with all personal needs of patients
- Helping with emotional needs of patients
- Assisting with the delivery of infants
- Caring for and feeding infants
- Supervising nursing assistants
- Helping evaluate patient needs and developing care plans
- Making appointments and keeping records in physicians' offices
- Teaching patients how to care for themselves

The Registered Nurse

Registered nurses (RNs) work with patients to promote health. They also may work as educators to help prevent diseases and to help patients cope with an existing illness.

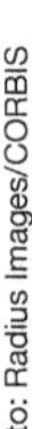

All states require registered nurses to graduate from an approved nursing program. **Table 15.2** gives a brief description of the education needed to qualify as a registered nurse. All registered nurses must pass a national licensing examination, and they must also be licensed in the state in which they are working. Each state has its own licensing requirements. The trend, however, is for states to grant reciprocity. This means that if a nurse is licensed in one state, other states will recognize his or her license so that the nurse can practice in another state without having to go through the licensing process again.

Table 15.2 Nursing Education and Training

LEVEL OF EDUCATION	LENGTH OF PROGRAM	LOCATION OF EDUCATION
Diploma	2 to 3 years	Hospitals
Associate degree (AD)	2 years	Community college or private proprietary school
Bachelor of Science in Nursing degree (BSN)	4 to 5 years	College or university

Registered nurses work independently or in a team setting. Their license allows them to provide nursing care without supervision. However, they must communicate and work with other members of the healthcare team such as physicians, therapists, medical social workers, aides, and dietitians.

The Registered Nurse's Job Responsibilities The responsibilities of a registered nurse range from basic patient care to administrative positions. But above all other responsibilities, the registered nurse is a patient advocate. As an **advocate,** he or she tries to ensure that the patient's needs are being met. **Figure 15.6** shows an RN acting as a patient advocate.

All registered nurse careers have similar duties. However, specific work areas have slightly different focuses, some of which are listed below.

Hospital nurses

- provide all levels of care given by LPN/LVNs.
- provide bedside nursing care.
- start intravenous (IV) infusions.
- carry out medical regimens as ordered by physicians.
- supervise LPN/LVNs and unlicensed assisting personnel.

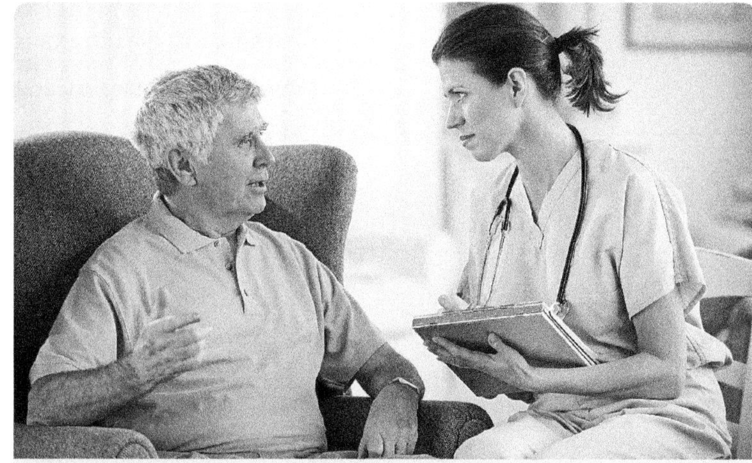

Fig. 15.6 The RN as a Patient Advocate The responsibilities of a registered nurse range from basic patient care to administrative duties. *What does it mean to be a patient advocate?*

Photo: Ietra Images/Getty Images

Safety

Avoiding Back Injury

One of the major hazards faced by nursing personnel is back injury caused by positioning, lifting, and moving patients. Back injury is the number one cause of workers' compensation claims for both licensed and unlicensed healthcare personnel. Healthcare providers can avoid many accidental injuries by being aware of and using proper body mechanics and following procedures properly.

Office nurses

- provide care for patients in an outpatient setting.
- prepare patients for examinations.
- assist physicians with examinations.
- administer injections and intravenous solutions.
- perform wound care.
- assist with minor surgeries.
- maintain documentation.
- perform routine specimen collection and lab work.

Nursing home nurses

- manage the nursing care for patients.
- fill management positions.
- participate in staff education.
- handle administrative and supervisory duties.
- assess patients' medical conditions.

Home health nurses

- provide periodic care to clients in their homes.
- assess the home environment for safety.
- teach clients how to care for themselves and teach their family members how to care for the clients.
- supervise the home health aide, who may be an LPN/LVN.

Public health nurses

- work with selected populations to improve the health of the community at large.
- educate community members in health maintenance, disease prevention, nutrition, and child care.
- provide health screenings.

Occupational or industrial nurses

- provide workplace care to employees and customers.
- assess and educate on health hazards found in the workplace.
- assist with health examinations.

Head nurses or supervisory nurses

- manage the department.
- plan work schedules and assign duties.
- plan and monitor the budget.
- supervise all personnel.
- maintain all required records.

The Advanced Practice Nurse

Registered nurses who successfully complete additional training requirements may obtain an advanced practice certificate or degree.

Advanced practice nurses work under the supervision of a physician to provide basic medical care. They are able to diagnose and treat common ailments. Nurse practitioners and other advanced practice nurses are allowed to prescribe medications with the approval of a physician.

These are some common specialties of advanced practice nurses.

- Clinical nurse specialists specialize in a specific nursing area such as gerontology (care of older patients) or neonatology (care of newborn infants).
- Certified registered nurse anesthetists have additional training in the use of anesthesia. They work in surgical suites under the supervision of an anesthesiologist.
- Certified nurse-midwives assist with the delivery of infants. They have training and expertise in the delivery process.

The Advanced Practice Nurse's Job Responsibilities Advanced practice nurses perform many duties and have many options, depending on their specialty. Nurse practitioners often work in areas where there is little access to traditional healthcare. They may work in a physician's office alongside the physician. Clinical nurse specialists may work in a hospital setting or in an outpatient area with specific categories of patients. Certified registered nurse anesthetists work in a surgical area. Certified nurse-midwives work in acute care settings, clinics, or homes.

The main responsibility of the advanced practice nurse is to protect the safety and health of the patients.

21ST CENTURY SKILLS

Nursing Care Needed

From 2004 to 2008, over 400,000 nurses were licensed to practice. However, during that same time, the total number of practicing nurses only grew by about 150,000. Nurses are retiring faster than new nurses are being licensed.

Advanced practice nurses are needed for the training of new nurses, but many nurses are not choosing to further their education to advanced practice.

The aging baby boomer population and healthcare reform are increasing the demands for nursing personnel at all levels. All of these factors continue to make opportunities in the field of nursing excellent!

READING CHECK

Explain who provides licensing for licensed practical nurses, registered nurses, and advance practice nurses.

SECTION 15.1 Careers in Nursing Review

AFTER YOU READ

1. **Examine** the difference between licensed and unlicensed nursing personnel.
2. **Identify** the main responsibilities of the certified or certificated nursing assistant.
3. **List** the locations where a certified or certificated nursing assistant might work.
4. **Explain** how the work of a home health aide differs from that of a nursing assistant.
5. **Compare** an advanced practice nurse with a licensed practical or vocational nurse.
6. **Describe** the main responsibility of the registered nurse regarding patients.
7. **Describe** the training required to become an advanced practice nurse.

Technology ONLINE EXPLORATIONS

Nursing School Research

Go online to compare three different schools that provide nursing education. Determine what is needed to enter the program, the length and type of the program, and what type of degree or certificate will be provided. Create a report about your findings, and then determine which school you would prefer to attend and why.

SECTION
15.2 Basic Nursing Procedures

Vocabulary

Content Vocabulary

You will learn these content vocabulary terms in this section.

- **decubitus ulcer**
- **open beds**
- **closed beds**
- **occupied bed**
- **intake and output**
- **fluid balance**
- **perineum**
- **incontinent**
- **phlebitis**
- **thrombophlebitis**
- **indwelling urinary catheter**

Academic Vocabulary

You will see this word in your reading and on your tests. Find its meaning in the Glossary in the back of the book.

- **assigned**

Hand Hygiene

How does proper hand hygiene benefit healthcare workers?

One of the greatest threats to nursing personnel and patients is the transmission of disease and infection. The most effective measure healthcare workers can take to prevent transmission of infection or disease is proper hand hygiene. The Centers for Disease Control and Prevention recommends a specific hand-washing procedure or the use of alcohol-based hand rubs. Healthcare workers should perform hand hygiene every time they finish working with one patient, before moving on to the next. They should perform hand hygiene after using the restroom, after breaks, if they touch any contaminated item, and before they perform any kind of care. **Figure 15.7** shows a healthcare worker practicing hand washing.

READING CHECK

Identify when healthcare workers should perform hand hygiene.

Making an Open or Closed Bed

How does proper bed-making technique benefit the healthcare professional?

Making a bed seems simple. Why is it so important to patients? First, patients are more susceptible to injury than healthy individuals. A fold in a sheet can cause a life-threatening open sore. This open sore is known as a **decubitus ulcer** or bedsore. Even if a patient does not develop a bedsore, lying in a soiled or untidy bed is unpleasant. Also, because healthcare employees make many beds, they must conserve energy and reduce stress on their backs. Therefore, it is important to know how to make beds properly.

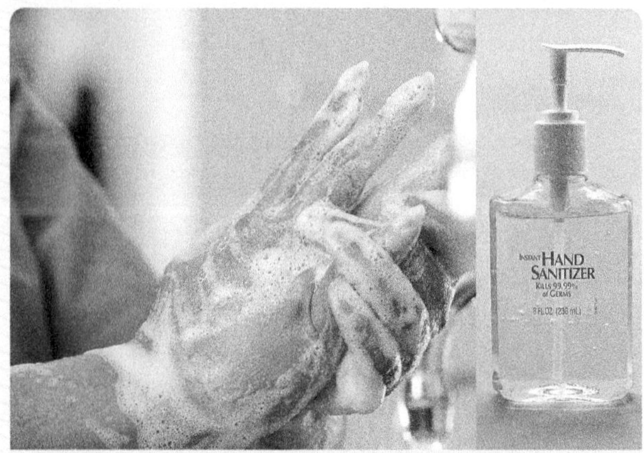

Fig. 15.7 Hand Hygiene Shown is one step of proper handwashing technique. *How does hand hygiene help to ensure your patient's safety?*

Open beds are beds that are used by a patient but are unoccupied when they are made. The top sheets and blanket are turned back for when the patient needs to get into the bed.

Photos: (l)CORBIS, (r)Richard Hutchings

Closed beds are those that are in readiness for the next patient. The top sheets and blankets are not turned down. A closed bed remains "closed" until a new patient is assigned to it. It is important to follow a facility's policy on cleaning or sterilizing a mattress between patients, especially if the previous patient had any type of infection or open wound.

The procedure for making a closed or open bed is the same. The difference is how the mattress is cleaned and how the top linens are set (see **Figure 15.8**). Each facility has specific procedures about which linens are used to make beds.

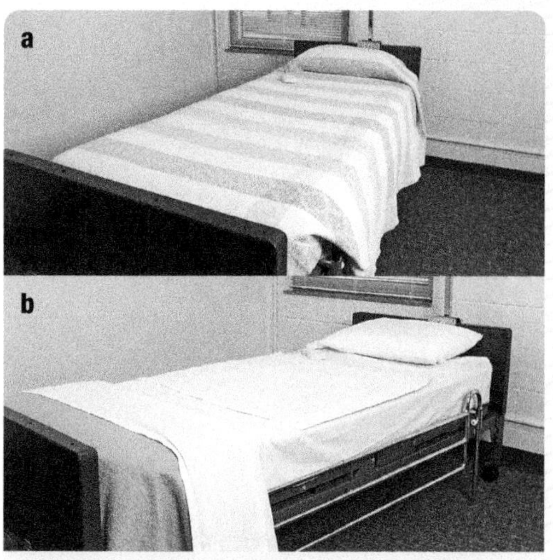

Fig. 15.8 Making a Bed (a) A closed bed is made in readiness for the next patient. (b) An open bed is being used by a patient but is currently unoccupied. *What is the purpose of an open bed?*

READING CHECK

Identify the main difference between open and closed beds.

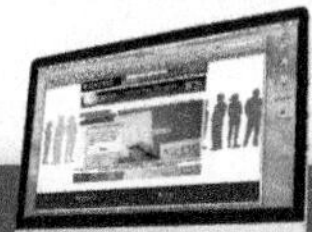

connect ONLINE PROCEDURES

PROCEDURE 15-1

Admitting a Patient

Patients may be apprehensive about being admitted to a facility. They may be feeling sadness and grief because of losing their independence and being away from home. It is important to make them feel as comfortable and welcome as you can. You can do this with a positive, friendly attitude and kindness. Your empathy and attitude can make all the difference in the world to the person who is being admitted.

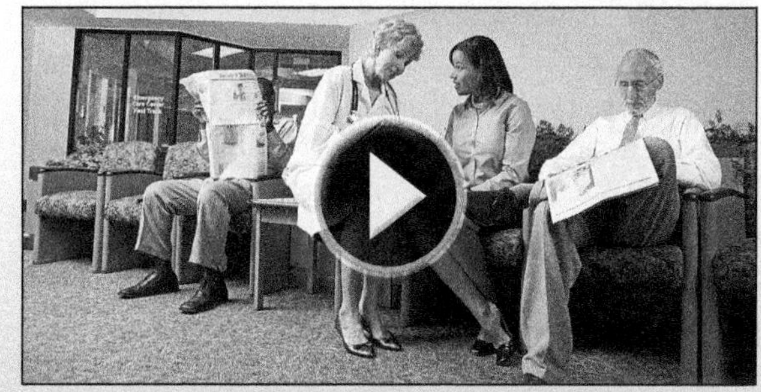

PROCEDURE 15-2

Transferring a Patient

When moving a patient from one room to another, one unit to another, or into a different facility, explain as many times as needed why the change is being made. The change may be due to a request from a family member, patient, healthcare worker, or it may be due to a change in health. It is important that the patient knows that the move is a positive one.

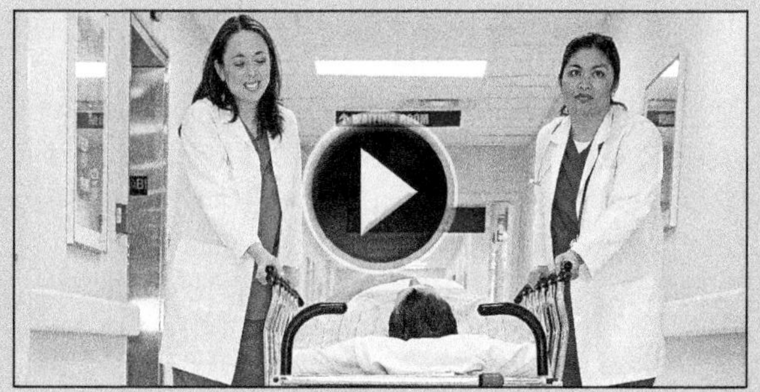

PROCEDURE 15-3

Discharging a Patient

Whether a patient is better and able to go home, or the patient is discharged from one facility in order to transfer to another facility, the physician should write the discharge order, and the supervising nurse should be responsible for the process.

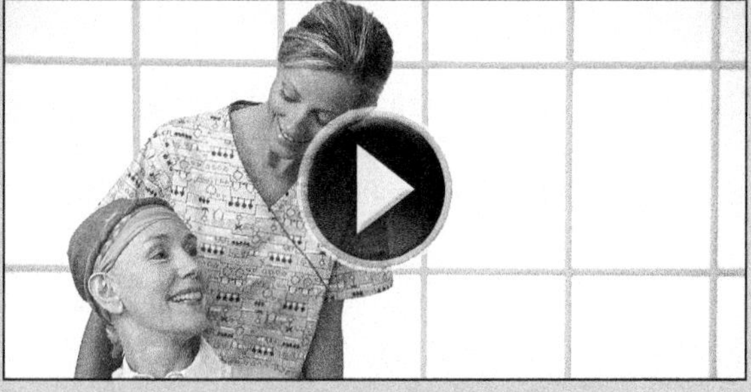

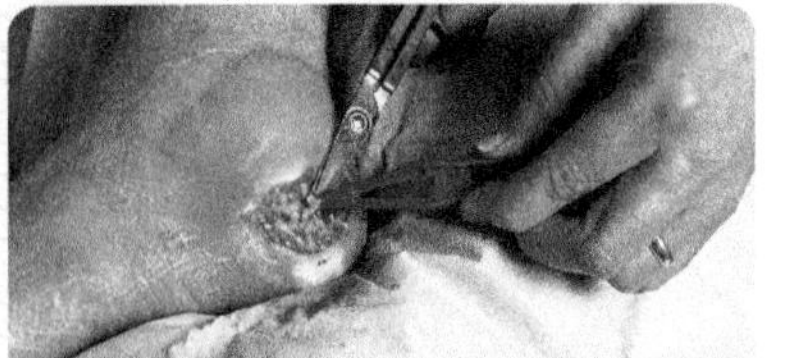

Fig. 15.9 Bedsores Shown is a bedsore or decubitus ulcer. *What can be done to prevent bedsores such as this?*

Preventing Bedsores

Decubitus ulcers, or bedsores, are lesions that come from continual pressure on flesh over bony prominences or friction from bed linens, poor circulation, emaciation, obesity, or failure to keep bed linens dry and free of wrinkles. Encouraging a patient to turn, or turning an immobile patient, is important to prevent bedsores. Massaging areas prone to skin breakdown is also helpful (see **Figure 15.9**).

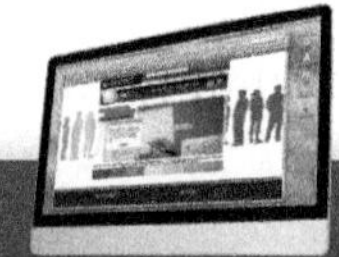

connect ONLINE PROCEDURES

PROCEDURE 15-4

Making an Open or Closed Bed

Open beds are beds that are being used by a patient but are unoccupied when they are being made. The top sheets and blanket are turned back in readiness for the patient. Closed beds are made in readiness for the next patient. These beds are made after a patient is discharged or moved.

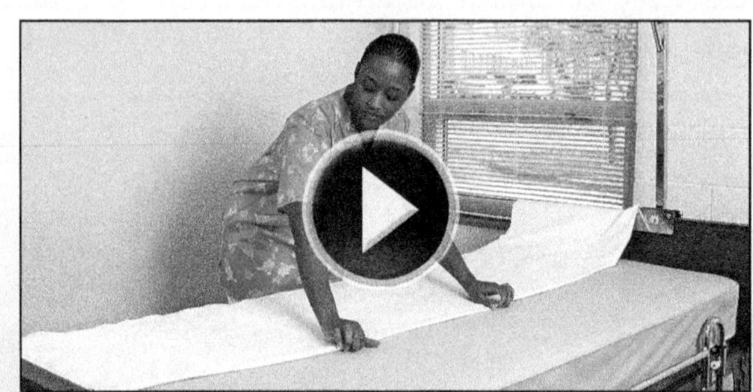

PROCEDURE 15-5

Changing an Occupied Bed

Sometimes patients cannot get out of the bed for one reason or another. In this case fresh linens must be placed on the bed while the patient is in the bed. This is called an occupied bed.

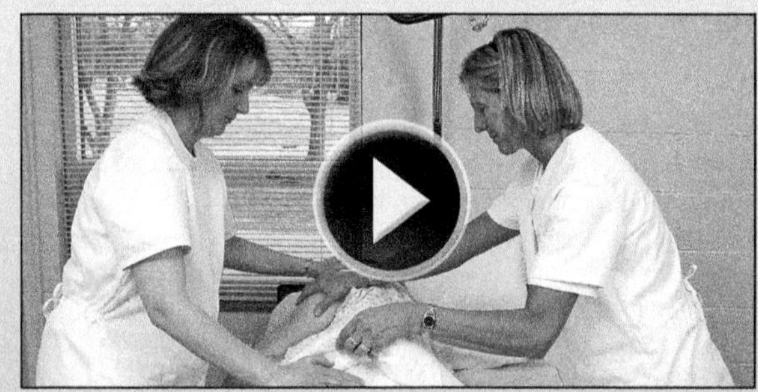

PROCEDURE 15-6

Measuring Oral Fluid Intake

Accuracy counts when you measure **intake and output** to assess **fluid balance.** Cups and glasses used in healthcare facilities hold a specific amount of fluid. Certain foods such as broth and gelatin are measured as fluid intake. When patients are unable to excrete excess fluid, they may have too much fluid and develop edema, or swelling.

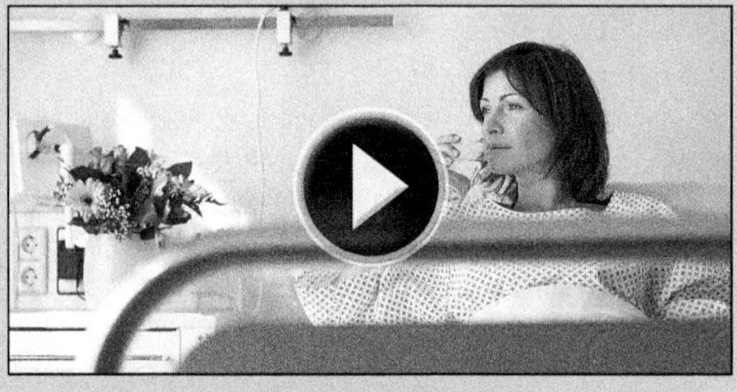

PROCEDURE 15-7

Measuring Urinary Fluid Output

Urinary output must also be measured with accuracy. Standard precautions, including the use of gloves, are necessary when handling urine or other fluid output.

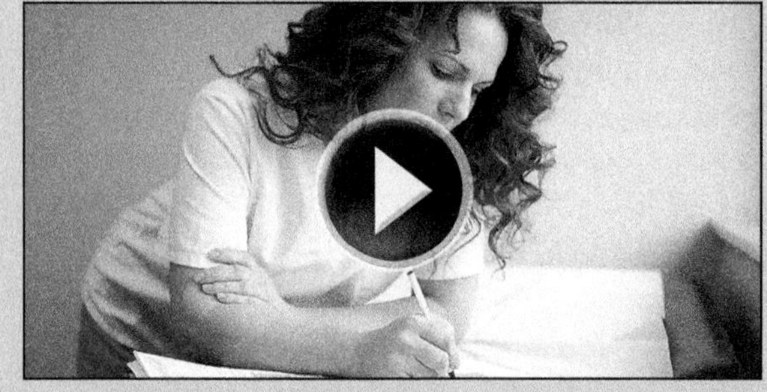

Transporting Patients

Sometimes patients need to be moved to other parts of a facility for diagnostic or therapeutic procedures. It may also be necessary to transfer patients from one healthcare facility to another. These patients may be on ventilators, require monitoring equipment, or may be receiving intravenous drugs. Do not transport patients who are using additional equipment if you have not been trained and authorized to do so.

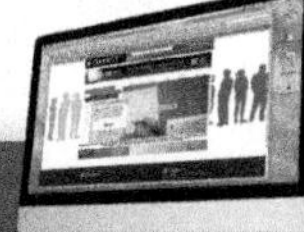

Mc Graw Hill connect™ ONLINE PROCEDURES

PROCEDURE 15-8

Positioning Patients

When positioning patients, always remember to use good body mechanics to prevent injury to yourself and the patient. In addition, ask for help if you have to move a patient who is heavy or is unable to assist.

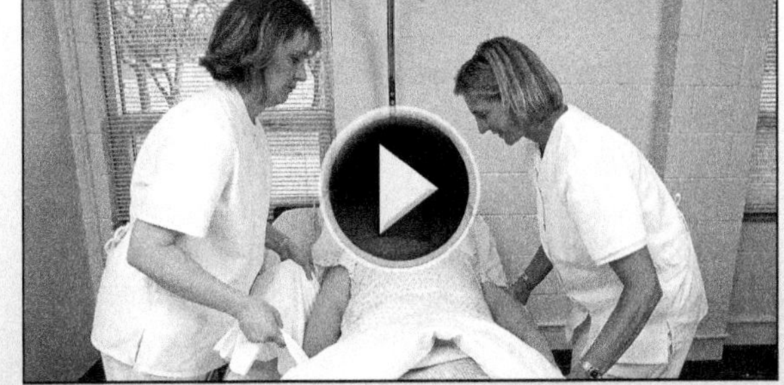

PROCEDURE 15-9

Moving a Patient up in Bed with the Patient's Assistance

Patients who are in bed tend to gravitate toward the bottom of the bed. This puts them out of proper alignment, and they become very uncomfortable. At times, it is necessary to move them up in the bed. Use good body mechanics and get assistance when needed.

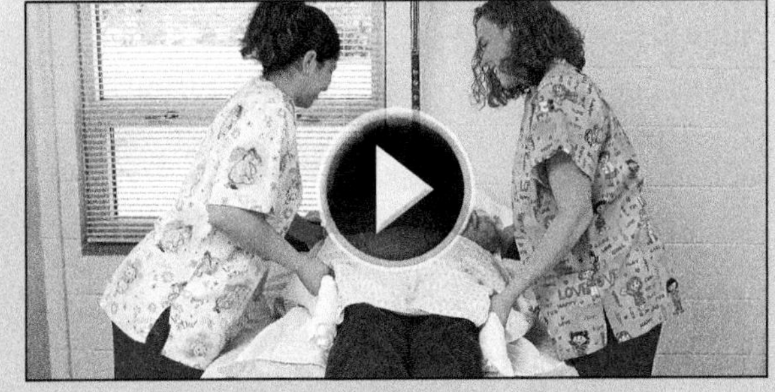

PROCEDURE 15-10

Moving a Patient up in Bed Using a Turn or Lift Sheet

Using a turn sheet when you are moving a patient up in bed makes the task easier and helps prevent back injury. A turn or lift sheet is positioned under the patient, from the shoulders to the upper thighs. It may be a flat sheet folded or a special smaller sheet.

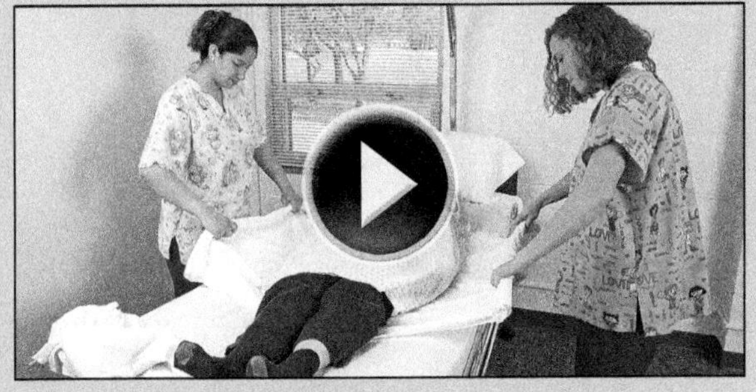

PROCEDURE 15-11

Transferring a Patient Using a Mechanical Lift

Mechanical lifts supply assistance in transfers. Safety is the utmost concern. You should be familiar with the brand of lift you are going to use. Read the directions on the machine or in the policy manual, or see the manufacturer's directions before you start.

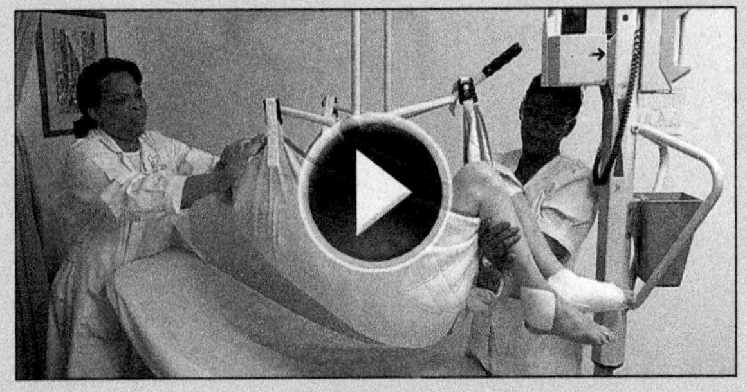

Photos: (t to b)McGraw-Hill Companies, Inc./Scott Thompson, photographer, McGraw-Hill Companies, Inc./Scott Thompson, photographer, McGraw-Hill Companies, Inc./Scott Thompson, photographer, Lou Bopp/Lou Bopp Photography

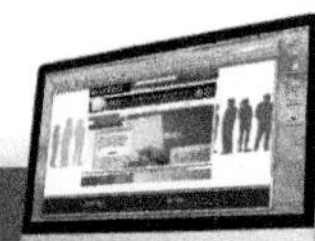

connect ONLINE PROCEDURES

PROCEDURE 15-12

Transferring a Patient into a Wheelchair

Assisting a patient into a wheelchair requires the use of good body mechanics. Be certain you know where the brakes of the wheelchair are before you start the procedure.

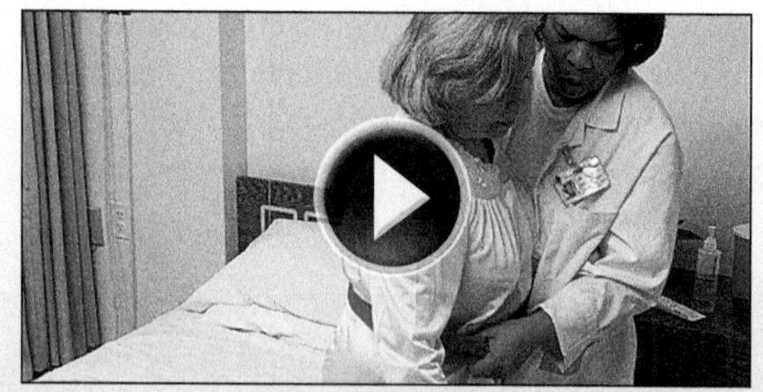

PROCEDURE 15-13

Transferring a Conscious Patient from a Bed to a Stretcher

When a patient is conscious (awake), he or she may be able to assist during the transfer between a bed and a stretcher. Make sure the patient remains safe throughout the procedure. In addition, you should protect yourself from injury by having someone assist you with the procedure.

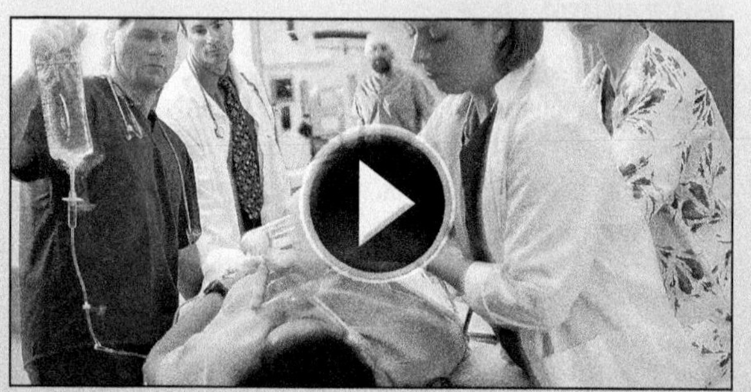

PROCEDURE 15-14

Transferring an Unconscious Patient from a Bed to a Stretcher

When transferring a patient who is unconscious (not awake) or one who cannot assist, you will need at least three healthcare personnel. The effort to move the patient must be well coordinated to ensure safety of both the patient and the healthcare personnel.

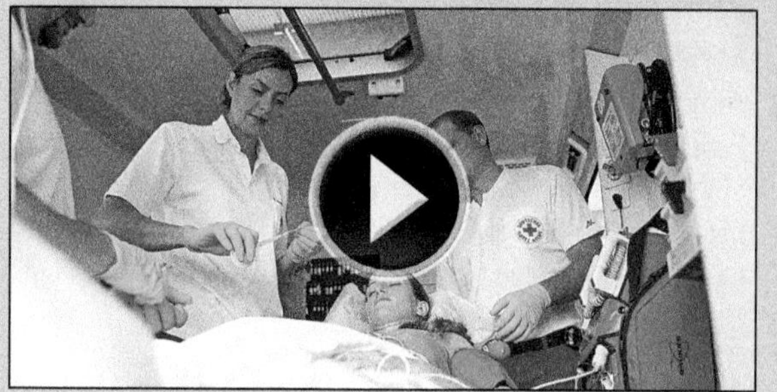

PROCEDURE 15-15

Assisting with a Bath or Shower

When assisting a patient to bath or shower provide for safety. Test the water temperature. Make sure that the patient can reach the emergency signal light if you are going to leave the room. Follow the safety policy at your facility.

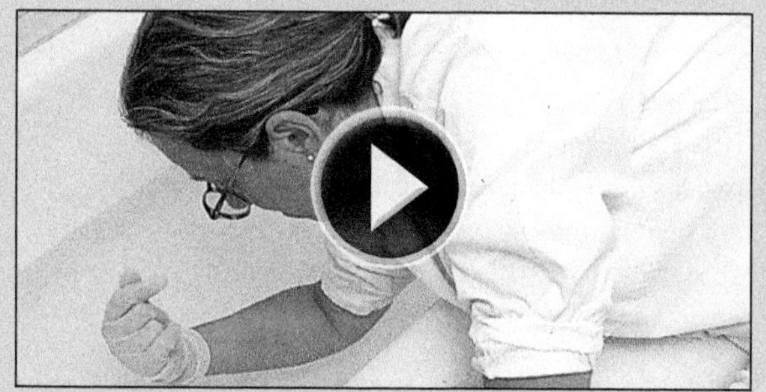

PROCEDURE 15-16

Performing a Partial Bed Bath

If a patient cannot get out of bed, you may need to assist with a partial bed bath. Your job is to provide all the needed equipment and clean the areas that the patient is unable to reach.

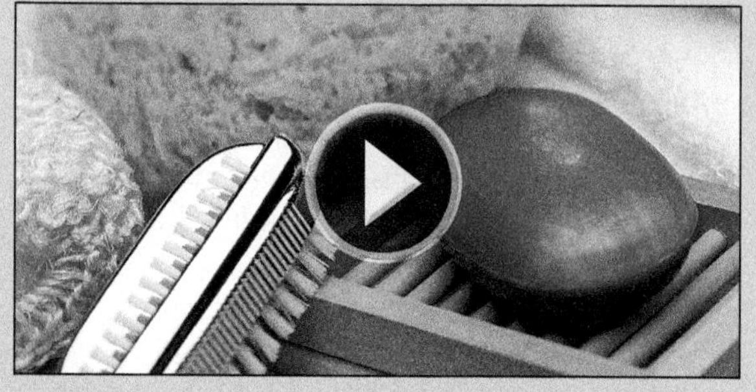

Photos: (t to b)Lou Bopp/Lou Bopp Photography, Photodisc/Getty Images, Jochen Sand/Digital Vision/Getty Images, Lou Bopp/Lou Bopp Photography, Kevin Jordan/Getty Images

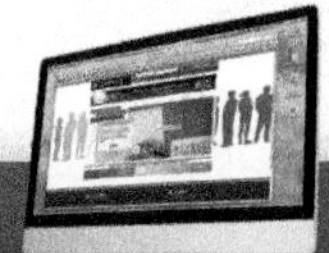

connect ONLINE PROCEDURES

PROCEDURE 15-17

Performing a Complete Bed Bath

A complete bed bath is performed on patients who cannot get out of bed or assist with the bathing process. Provide for safety and comfort by ensuring that the water temperature is correct, changing the water frequently, wearing gloves, and keeping the side rail up on the opposite side of the bed.

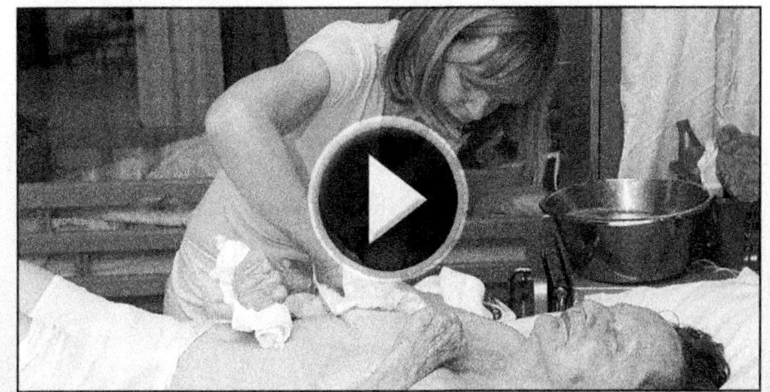

PROCEDURE 15-18

Providing Denture Care

If a patient has dentures (false teeth) you may need to assist with cleaning them and help the patient rinse his or her mouth. Be extra careful when handling dentures to prevent dropping them.

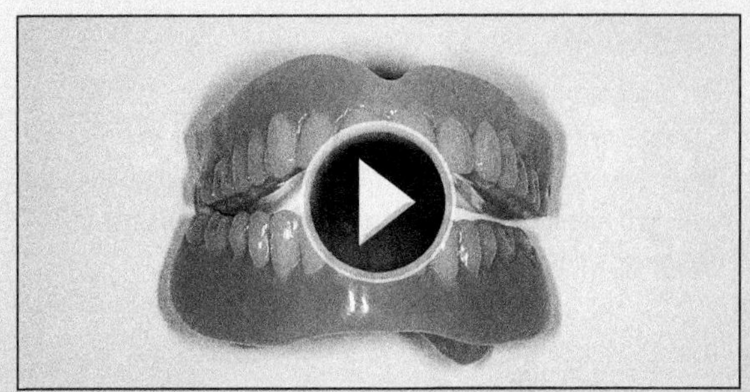

PROCEDURE 15-19

Assisting with Oral Care

Daily oral care helps to improve overall health. So oral care for patients must always be completed. When you assist a patient with oral care, encourage the patient to be as independent as possible.

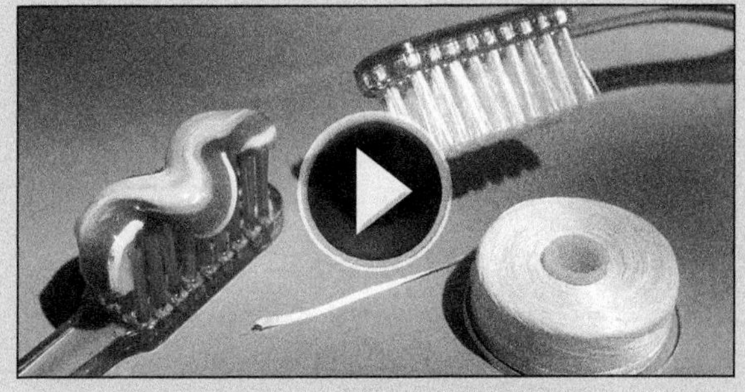

PROCEDURE 15-20

Performing Oral Care on a Helpless Patient

Patients who are unable to perform any care may need total assistance with oral care. Use standard precautions and wear gloves during this procedure.

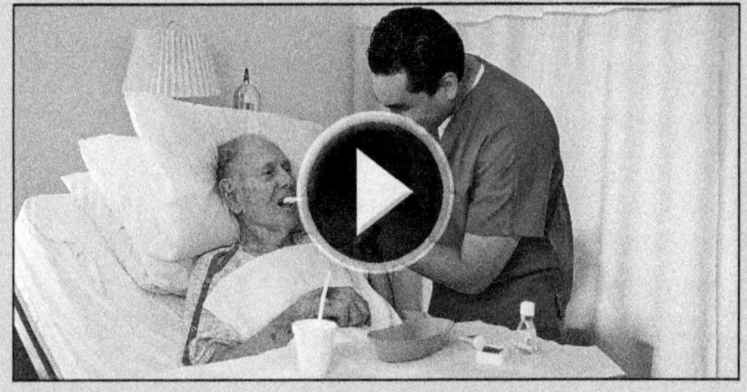

PROCEDURE 15-21

Nail Care

Clean, neat nails add to a patient's sense of self-esteem and may prevent injury from scratching. Before providing nail care always make sure it is in your scope of practice. Some patients can only have their nails cared for by a licensed practitioner.

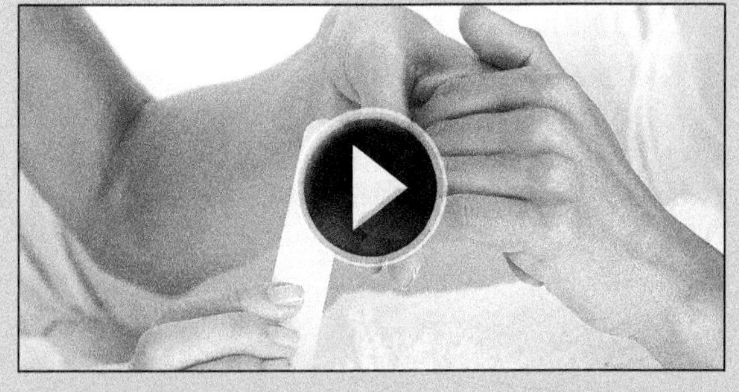

Photos: (t to b)Horacio Sormani/Photo Researchers, Inc., Image Source/Getty Images, Ingram Publishing, McGraw-Hill Companies, Inc./Tim Fuller, photographer, PhotoAlto/Alix Minde/Getty Images

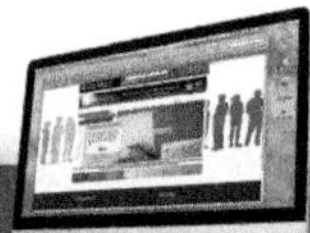

PROCEDURE 15-22

Shampooing a Bed-Bound Patient's Hair

Some patients may be unable to perform hair care for themselves. After being bed bound for several days, a patient will appreciate having his or her hair washed, dried, and even styled. If your patient can respond, allow him or her to decide how the hair should look.

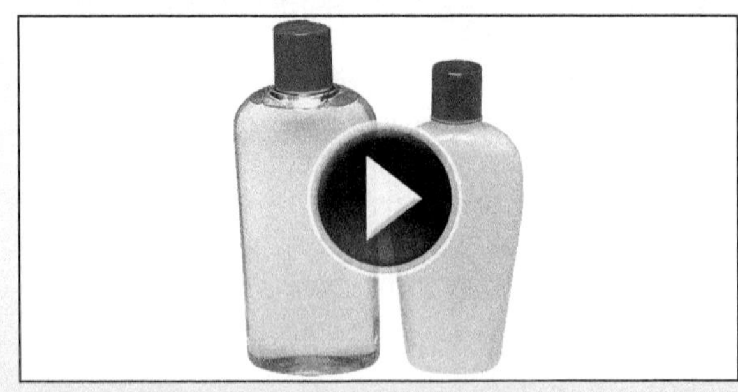

PROCEDURE 15-23

Brushing or Combing a Patient's Hair

Having one's hair combed and neat promotes self-esteem. Be sure to ask patients if they want their hair combed before visiting hours or for special occasions. Allow patients to decide how they want their hair to look.

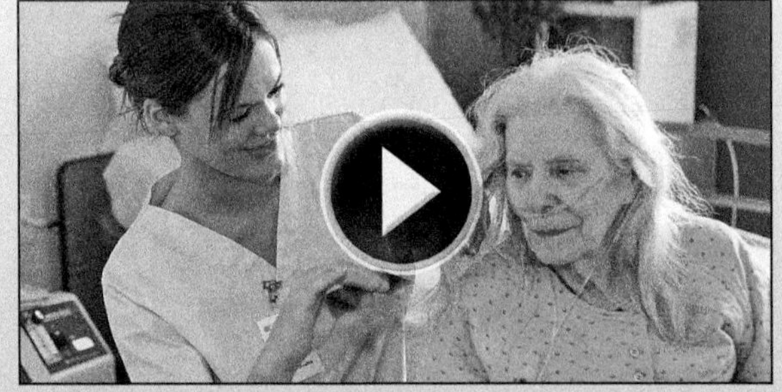

PROCEDURE 15-24

Assisting a Patient with Shaving

Most males and some females like to shave as part of their daily grooming routine. You should always find out from the patient how he or she likes to shave. There may be personal or religious reasons for shaving choices. Always make sure the patient has been assessed and that you may shave him or her safely. In addition, allow the patient to perform as much of the shaving as possible.

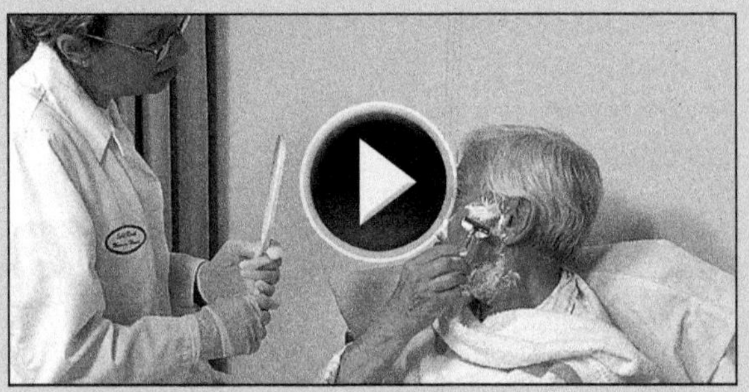

PROCEDURE 15-25

Providing Female Perineal Care

The **perineum** is the area of the body around the genitals and rectum. These areas are moist and not exposed to air, so pathogens can grow easily. Some clients may be **incontinent**, and this increases the risk of infection. The perineum should be cleaned once daily as part of the daily bath, or more often if necessary.

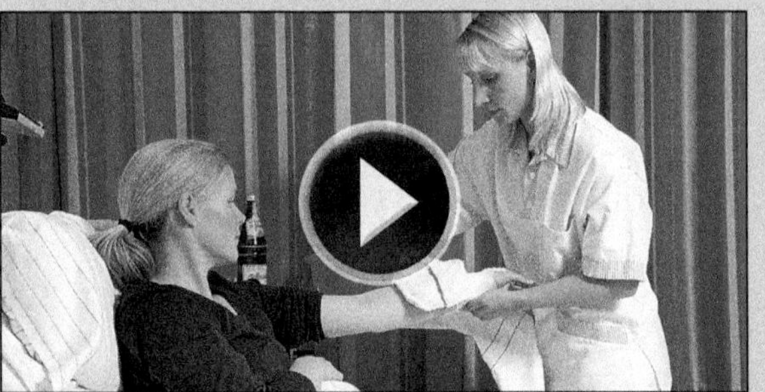

PROCEDURE 15-26

Providing Male Perineal Care

The perineum is the area of the body around the genitals and rectum. For the male patient, this includes the penis, the foreskin if the patient is not circumcised, the scrotum, and the anal area.

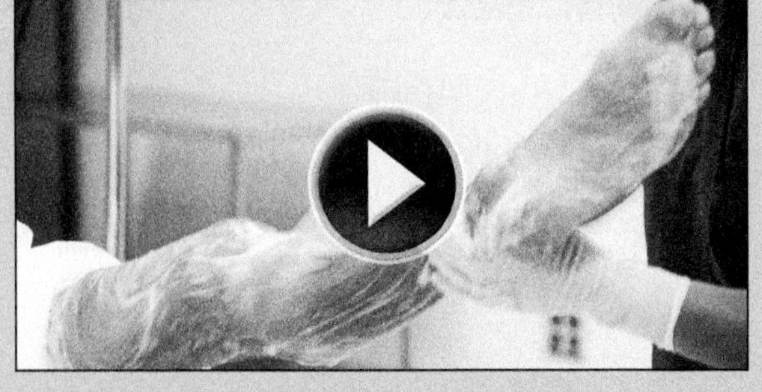

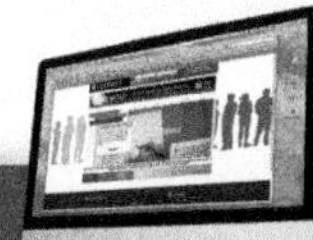

connect ONLINE PROCEDURES

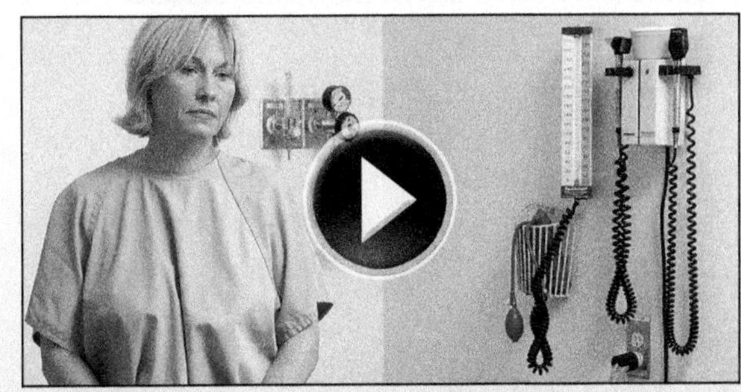

PROCEDURE 15-27

Changing a Patient's Gown

Gowns are used instead of clothes in some facilities. They should be changed daily and any time they become soiled.

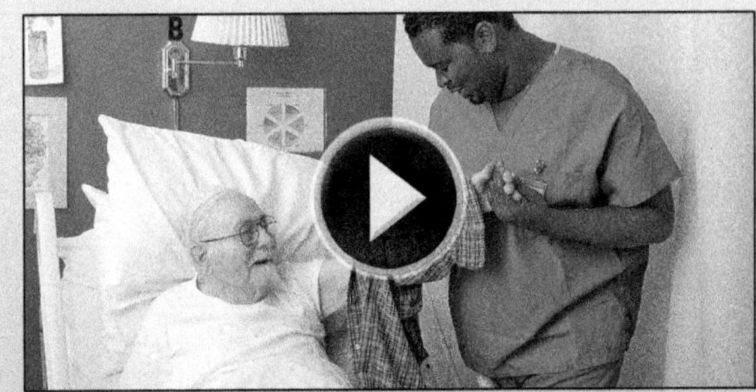

PROCEDURE 15-28

Undressing and Dressing a Patient Who Has Limited Use of Limbs

Patients may have limited movement of their arms for many reasons. For example, they may have an intravenous infusion (IV) or have had a stroke. These patients need extra assistance when changing their clothes or gown.

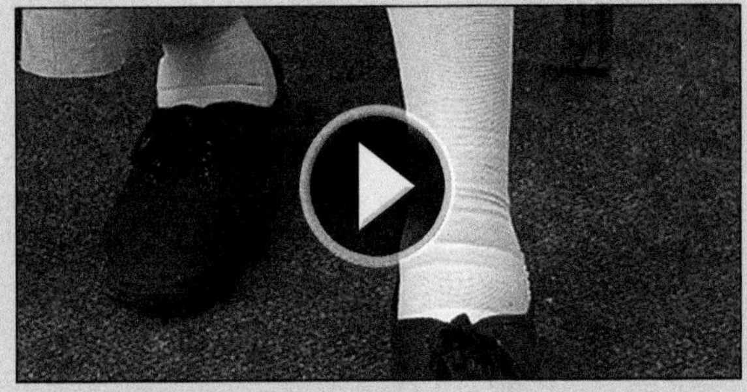

PROCEDURE 15-29

Applying Elastic Stockings

Elastic stockings are used on patients to improve the circulation in the legs and to help with conditions such as **phlebitis** (an inflammation of the veins) and **thrombophlebitis** (a blood clot in the vein). They are used only when ordered by a physician. Putting them on is a bit different from putting on socks because of how tight the elastic stockings are.

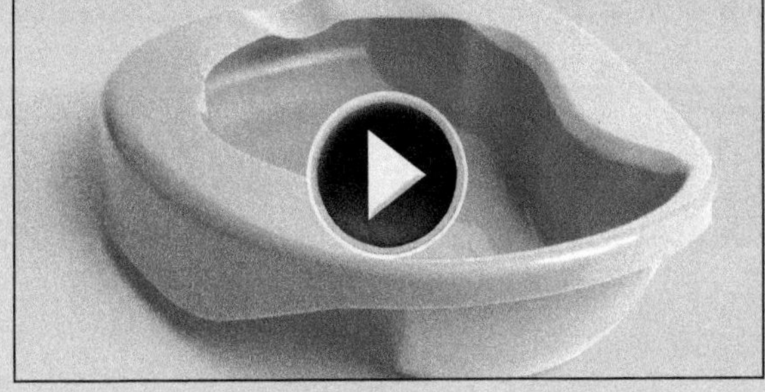

PROCEDURE 15-30

Providing and Removing a Bedpan

Bedpans are used for patients who cannot get out of bed. Providing comfort and assistance will make the task easier for the patient. You will need to assist them on and off the bedpan and with any other special needs.

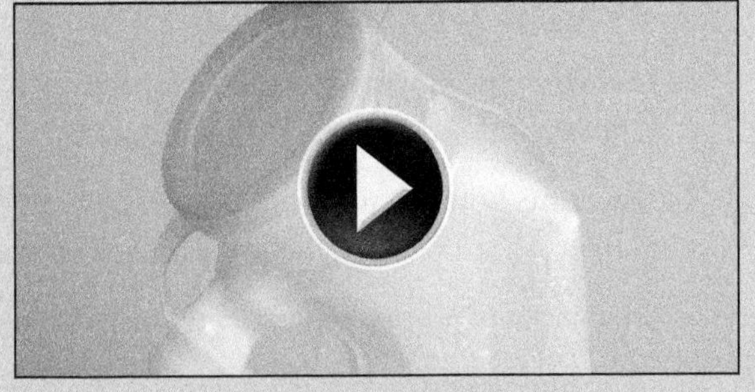

PROCEDURE 15-31

Providing and Removing a Urinal

When providing and removing the urinal, you must provide for privacy and assist as needed. In addition, always follow standard precautions to prevent infection.

Photos: (t to b)UpperCut Images/Getty Images, McGraw-Hill Companies, Inc./Kevin May, photographer, Lou Bopp/Lou Bopp Photography, Spencer Grant/PhotoEdit, Spencer Grant/PhotoEdit

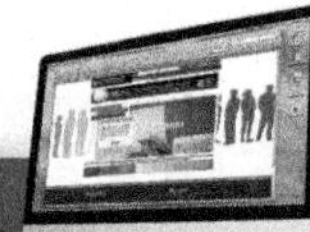

Mc Graw Hill connect™ ONLINE PROCEDURES

PROCEDURE 15-32

Providing Indwelling Catheter Care

When a catheter is inserted into the urethra to drain urine there is a great chance of infection for the patient. Use standard precautions and provide at least daily cleaning and care for an **indwelling urinary catheter.**

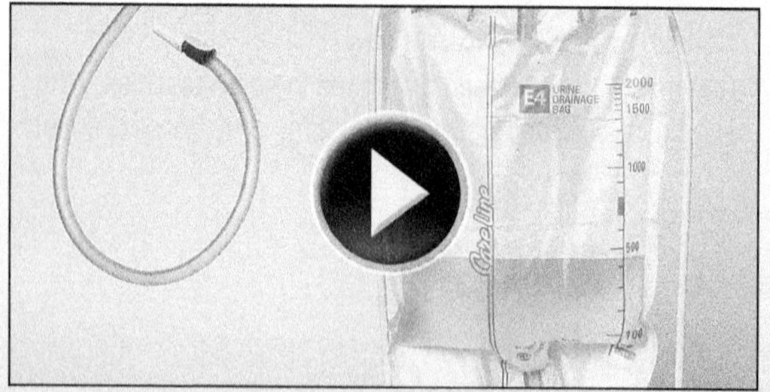

PROCEDURE 15-33

Emptying a Catheter Drainage Bag

When an indwelling catheter is in place it must be able to drain properly. If the tubing is kinked or blocked, complications can occur. Use gloves and perform hand hygiene when caring for a catheter.

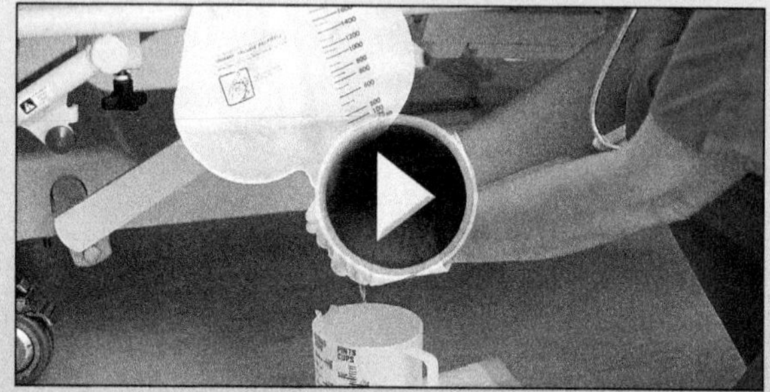

PROCEDURE 15-34

Assisting with a Bedside Commode

Bedside commodes are used for patients who are unable to travel to the restroom. The patient may need assistance when transferring to the bedside commode. Use good body mechanics.

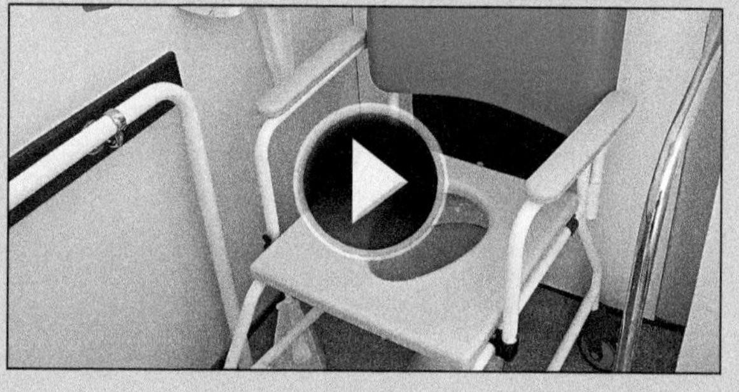

Photos: (t)Dorling Kindersley/Getty Images, (c)Beau Lark/CORBIS, (b)Chris Howes/Wild Places Photography/Alamy

SECTION 15.2 Basic Nursing Procedures Review

AFTER YOU READ

1. **Explain** how the nursing assistant's attitude affects a patient's healthcare.
2. **Identify** the most important procedure that reduces the risk of disease transmission.
3. **Describe** how to protect yourself and your patients when you lift, move, or transfer them.
4. **Discuss** why proper bed making is important.
5. **Describe** what to do before you empty urine from a catheter, bedpan, urinal, etc.

Technology ONLINE EXPLORATIONS

Job Research

Go online to research local job possibilities in the field of nursing. Determine where you would most like to be employed, then contact the facility to find out which skills you will need.

CHAPTER
15 Review

Chapter Summary

SECTION 15.1

- Nursing assistants, home health aides, dialysis technicians, surgical technicians, and patient care technicians are all unlicensed nursing personnel. The educational requirements and places of employment for these workers vary. Nursing assistants work in acute care, long-term care, or residential care facilities. Home health aides work in the home. **(pg. 414)**
- Certain basic procedures are performed by unlicensed personnel. Licensed personnel must delegate these procedures. **(pg. 414)**
- The licensed practical or vocational nurse (LPN/LVN) is trained for about one year. These nurses perform nursing care under the supervision of a physician or a registered nurse (RN). **(pg. 415)**
- The training and education needed to become a registered nurse can take from two to five years. All nurses must pass an examination to obtain a license in the state in which they wish to practice. **(pg. 415)**
- The care that RNs provide includes all the nursing functions. In addition, a primary responsibility of an RN is to be a patient advocate. **(pg. 423)**
- Advanced practice nurse training includes education as an RN plus specialized knowledge in the area of practice. **(pg. 424)**

SECTION 15.2

- The most effective measure that healthcare workers can take to prevent transmission of infection or disease is to perform proper hand hygiene. **(pg. 426)**
- Do not transport patients who are using additional equipment if you have not been trained and authorized to do so. **(pg. 429)**

Mc Graw Hill connect™ **ONLINE ACTIVITIES**

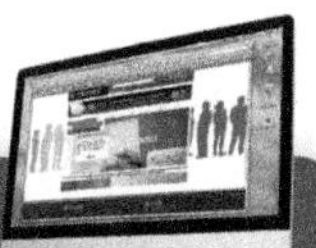

Complete our HST online activities for Chapter 15, which include Concept Check review questions, Reference Flash Cards, and Online Procedures assessment sheets.

- **Concept Check** review questions
- **Reference Flash Cards** medical terminology practice
- **Online Procedures** assessment sheets

CHAPTER

15 Assessment

Critical Thinking/Problem Solving

1. You work in a long-term care facility as a certified nursing assistant. A patient is angry with her roommate, who is sometimes confused and touches the patient's possessions. The angry patient says, "If she goes through my drawers one more time, I'm going to slap her!" What should you do?
2. You work in an acute care facility. One of your patients is dying, and he tells you that he is afraid to be alone. His family is not available, and your other patients need your attention. What could you do to help this patient?
3. Practice dressing a patient with a weakness on one side of the body by placing a gown or large shirt over your partner's clothing. Now, practice undressing a patient by removing the gown or shirt from your partner. Do not assist each other. Was it uncomfortable not to dress or undress yourself? Imagine what it would be like if the weakness were a permanent condition.
4. Obtain the necessary equipment to perform nail care on a partner. See Procedure 15-21 on p. 431. How did it feel to care for another person's nails? Did you enjoy it? Why or why not?

21ST CENTURY SKILLS

5. **Teamwork** Working with a partner, go online to compare two different nursing careers. Create a chart showing the job responsibilities, education, licensing requirements, and places of employment. Determine which career you might want to enter and explain the reasons for your choice, including the job outlook.
6. **Teamwork** With a partner, practice verbal and nonverbal communication required to perform the procedures in this chapter. Practice how you would introduce yourself and explain each of the procedures. Describe what you would do if the patient were unable to respond.
7. **Information Literacy** Go online to research a chronic disease or illness that is common among patients in nursing homes or residential care facilities. Sample key words are diabetes, Alzheimer's, chronic obstructive pulmonary disease (COPD), senile dementia, osteoporosis, and congestive heart failure (CHF). Write a report describing the disease and its symptoms. Discuss how you would feel if you had the condition or disease.

CHAPTER 16 The Clinical Office

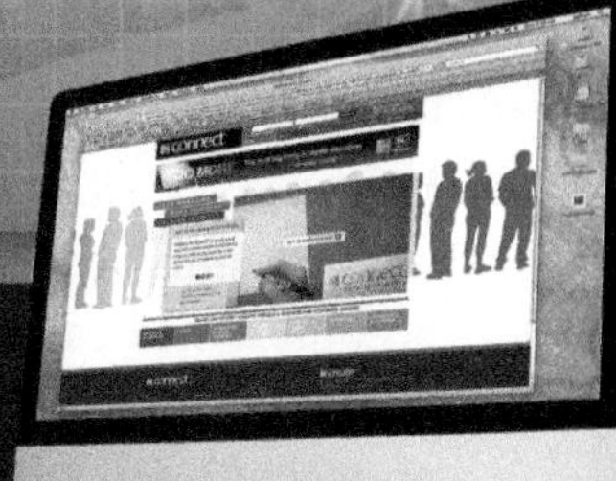

Essential Question:

For what kinds of care might you expect to see a medical assistant, physician assistant, and physician?

Working in a clinical office requires excellent interpersonal skills, a caring attitude, and a willingness to continue learning about new equipment and procedures. Career opportunities in a clinical office include work as a medical assistant, as a physician assistant, and as a physician.

McGraw Hill connect™

It's Online!

- Online Procedures
- STEM Connection
- Medical Science
- Medical Terms
- Medical Math
- Ethics in Action
- Virtual Lab

Photo: Ross M Horowitz/The Image Bank/Getty Images

READING GUIDE

OBJECTIVES

After completing this chapter, you will be able to:

- **Indicate** the educational requirements needed to become a medical assistant, physician assistant, and physician.
- **Compare** the job responsibilities of the medical assistant, physician assistant, and physician.

- **Describe** the licensure, certification, and credentialing of the clinical office professional.
- **Identify** various medical specialties.
- **Differentiate** between administrative duties and clinical duties in the office.
- **Relate** basic anatomy to the common skills needed in the clinical office.
- **Explain** five clinical office procedures.

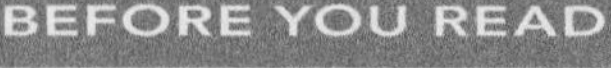

BEFORE YOU READ

Connect What have your experiences in a clinical office been? What roles did the clinical office personnel play in those experiences?

Main Idea

With the growing need to provide patient care in the most efficient and cost-effective manner possible, various medical office tasks are now divided among people with specific qualifications so that the physician will be able to see the maximum number of patients in a working day.

Note-Taking Activity

Draw this table. Write key terms and phrases under **Cues**. Write main ideas under **Note Taking**. Summarize the section under **Summary**.

Cues	Note Taking
o	o
o	o
Summary	

Graphic Organizer

Before you read the chapter, draw a diagram like the one to the right. As you read, write the clinical office careers covered by this chapter into the diagram.

Clinical Office Personnel

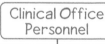

connect Downloadable graphic organizers can be accessed online.

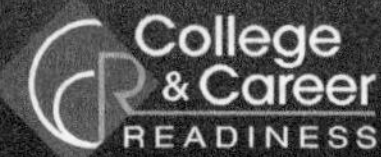

College & Career READINESS

STANDARDS

HEALTH SCIENCE

NCHSE 1.13 Analyze basic structure and function of the human body.

NCHSE 1.22 Recognize emerging diseases and disorders.

SCIENCE

NSES 1 Develop an understanding of science unifying concepts and processes: systems, order, and organization; evidence models, and explanation; change constancy, and measurement; evolution and equilibrium; and form and function.

NCHSE *National Consortium for Health Science Education*

NSES *National Science Education Standards*

COMMON CORE STATE STANDARDS

MATHEMATICS

Number and Quantity

Quantities N-Q 3 Choose a level of accuracy appropriate to limitations on measurement when reporting quantities.

ENGLISH LANGUAGE ARTS

Reading

Integration of Knowledge and Ideas R-7 Integrate and evaluate multiple sources of information presented in diverse formats and media (e.g., quantitative data, video, multimedia) in order to address a question or solve a problem.

Speaking and Listening

Presentation of Knowledge and Ideas SL-6 Adapt speech to a variety of contexts and communicative tasks, demonstrating command of formal English when indicated or appropriate.

SECTION 16.1 Careers in the Clinical Office

The Clinical Office

What does the term "clinical" mean to you?

Healthcare changes rapidly, and skills become outdated quickly. However, if you enjoy a fast-paced environment, working in a clinical office can be very rewarding as a healthcare career. **Figure 16.1** shows a typical clinical office. Three occupations are common to the clinical office:

- The clinical medical assistant
- The physician assistant
- The physician

Table 16.1 on page 440 gives information about these occupations. A detailed discussion of the three occupations follows.

Vocabulary

Content Vocabulary

You will learn these content vocabulary terms in this section.

- **chief complaint**
- **dermatology**
- **gastroenterology**

Academic Vocabulary

You will see these words in your reading and on your tests. Find their meanings in the Glossary in the back of the book.

- **accommodate**
- **similar**

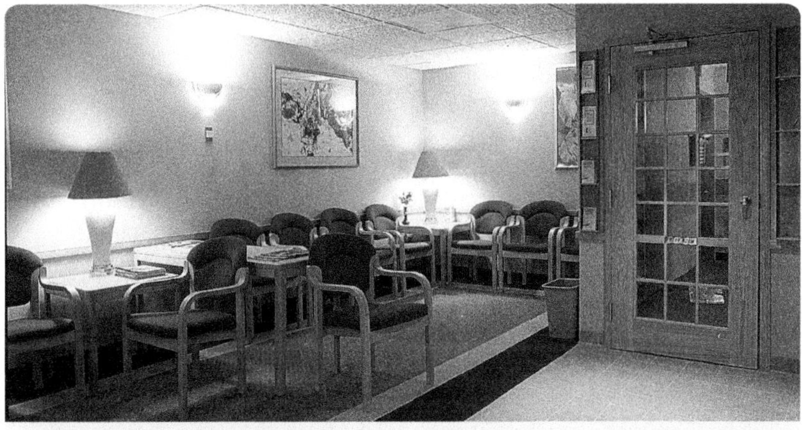

Fig. 16.1 Reception Area The patient reception area in the clinical office must be comfortable and safe. *Why should patients feel comfortable as they wait in this office?*

The Medical Assistant

What clinical skills does a medical assistant perform?

The well-trained medical assistant (MA) is an asset to a medical facility. Medical assistants typically work under the direction of a physician or other licensed healthcare professionals. MAs do not diagnose diseases or prescribe medications. However, their skill in routine clerical and clinical duties is invaluable. They help maintain an efficient and organized office. Taking blood pressure and other vital signs on patients (see **Figure 16.2**) is an important clinical skill of the medical assistant.

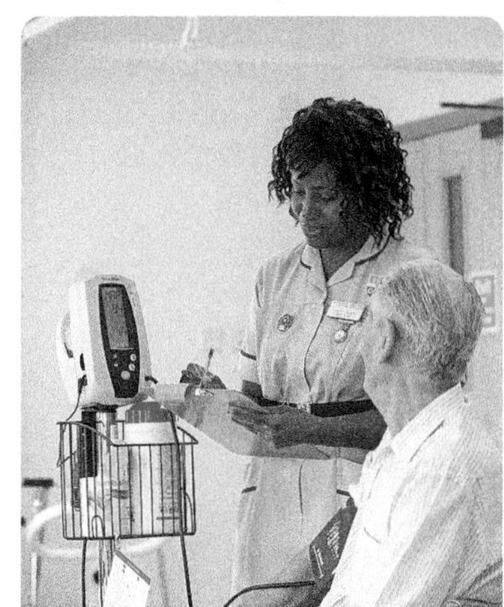

Fig. 16.2 Medical Equipment The clinical medical assistant may use an electronic blood pressure device like this one to measure the blood pressure and pulse. *What are these measurements called?*

Table 16.1 Overview of Occupations in a Clinical Office

OCCUPATION	EDUCATIONAL REQUIREMENTS	CERTIFYING OR LICENSING AGENCY	JOB OUTLOOK
Medical assistant	Short term (one year or less) training programs at vocational-technical or private schools and two-year associate degree programs are available.	Students completing formal programs accredited by the Commission on Accreditation of Allied Health Education Programs (CAAHEP) or the Accrediting Bureau of Health Education Schools (ABHES) may become certified or registered. Registered Medical Assistants (RMAs) are credentialed by the American Medical Technologists (AMT) organization. Certified Medical Assistants (CMAs) are credentialed by the American Association of Medical Assistants (AAMA).	One of the fastest-growing occupations in the United States over the 2008 to 2018 decade.
Physician assistant	Four-year bachelor's degree or master's degree programs are most common. Education requirements, training, and scope of practice vary from state to state.	Physician assistants must pass the Physician Assistants National Certifying Examination administered by the National Commission on Certification of Physician Assistants (NCCPA) and offered to students graduating from accredited programs.	Faster than average growth especially in rural and inner-city areas.
Physician	A bachelor's degree, the completion of four years of medical school, and the completion of a three- to eight-year residency or internship after medical school are the minimum educational requirements for a medical doctor (M.D.) or doctor of osteopathy (D.O.).	Physicians receive a license after graduating from an accredited school and passing an examination. Individual states administer the examination, which is prepared by the state board of medical examiners.	Faster than average growth due to growth in the aging population. Opportunities in rural and low-income areas are very good.

Medical assisting is one of the fastest-growing careers. Medical assistants may work in a small office or in a large clinic. Some MAs work for healthcare specialists such as optometrists and podiatrists.

State laws may define the duties of an MA. An MA's education is typically short-term private or vocational-technical school training, or a two-year degree. Employers recognize the importance of formal training and/or certification and prefer to hire MAs who have these qualifications.

Formal MA programs include a clinical experience known as an externship or practicum. During this time students gain on-the-job administrative and clinical experience in an office, using skills they learned in the classroom. **Figure 16.3** shows an MA putting information into an electronic health record. Students who complete programs accredited by CAAHEP (Commission on Accreditation of Allied Health Education Programs) or ABHES (Accrediting Bureau of Health Education Schools) are eligible to take the national certification examination administered by the American Association of Medical Assistants (AAMA) or the American Medical Technologist (AMT) organization. The MA may then add the CMA (certified medical assistant) or RMA (registered medical assistant) credential after his or her name. Although the credential is not always required for employment as an MA, it demonstrates to the physician that the MA has met certain standards of competence.

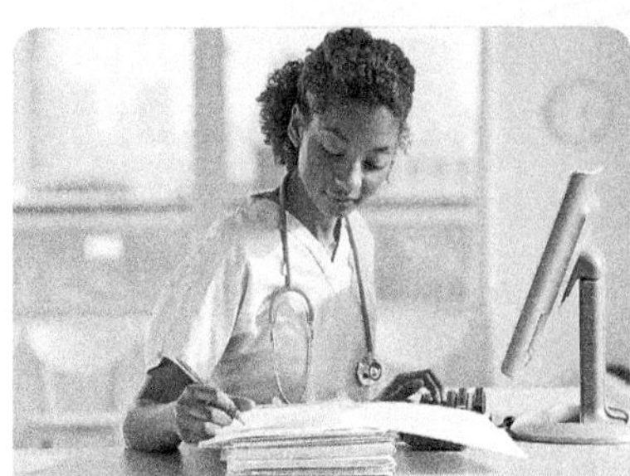

Fig. 16.3 Medical Assistant A medical assistant is putting information into an electronic health record. *Would this be considered an administrative skill or a clinical skill?*

Job Responsibilities of the Medical Assistant

Medical assistants are multi-skilled professionals trained to perform a variety of tasks competently and efficiently. Other healthcare team members, such as nurses, may be at ease when performing clinical tasks but uncomfortable doing administrative tasks such as billing and insurance claims. The medical receptionist or insurance specialist may feel comfortable performing administrative duties but not comfortable performing clinical tasks. However, MAs are trained to work in both the administrative and clinical areas. This flexibility makes the MA a valuable employee.

The MA must have excellent communication skills, both written and verbal, and must interact with many types of people during the average workday. For example, the MA may have to calm an angry patient who does not understand an insurance or billing problem, provide reassurance to an anxious patient, or explain a physician's orders to a hearing- or visually-impaired patient. The MA may order medications from a pharmacist, as directed by a physician, may speak with an insurance company representative regarding a claim, or may listen to a visiting pharmaceutical sales representative describe the latest drug therapies. **Figure 16.4** shows an MA performing an important clinical duty.

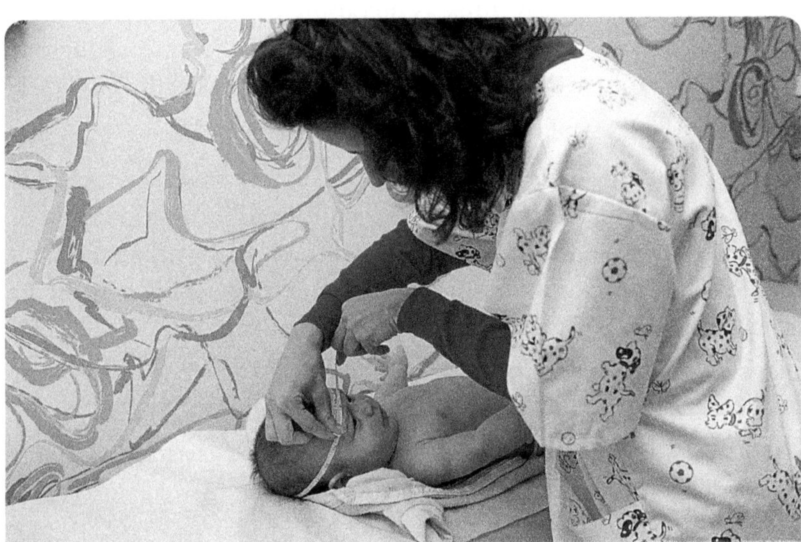

Fig. 16.4 Measurements This MA is measuring the circumference of a baby's head. *What specialty office does she work in?*

21ST CENTURY SKILLS

Verbal and Nonverbal Communication

The written and verbal communication needed by the PA or MA are extremely important, but listening and nonverbal communication skills are equally important. To be an effective communicator, you need to become an active listener. Active listening skills include the following techniques: assuming a position equal to that of the speaker; establishing eye contact; making brief, encouraging comments such as "umm-hmm," "Please go on," or "I see"; nodding; making reflective comments; restating the speaker's statement; and summarizing the speaker's statement. Gaining insight into your own behavior and learning to use nonverbal communication skills will help you to interact effectively in both social and professional situations.

Follow-up:
How will enhancing your knowldge of nonverbal communication, including facial expressions, body expression, and spatial proximity, improve your skills as an MA?

Some of the administrative skills required of the MA are the following:

- Operating and maintaining office equipment
- Scheduling patients for appointments
- Maintaining financial and medical records
- Ordering supplies
- Completing general office correspondence for the physician
- Processing insurance claims and patient billing

Some of the clinical skills required of the MA are the following:

- Obtaining patients' medical records
- Documenting the patient's reason for coming into the office, or the **chief complaint**
- Taking and recording vital signs and other pertinent data
- Administering medications
- Obtaining blood or other specimens for testing either in the office or in a laboratory
- Processing specimens obtained from the patient for the outside laboratory
- Performing visual and hearing screening tests
- Assisting the physician with minor office procedures
- Removing sutures
- Making sure that the patient receives instructions and schedules follow-up appointments
- Cleaning the examination room after the patient leaves
- Processing simple X-rays according to state laws (This requires additional training and certification in general radiology.)

Much of a routine day for an MA involves interacting with people and educating patients according to the physician's orders. A busy clinical office may see 60 to 90 patients in one day. It is the MA who makes sure the day runs as smoothly as possible. Of course, like any healthcare professional, the MA must be flexible enough to accommodate office emergencies and be ready to assist the physician in an efficient and competent manner during busy days.

In the clinical office, the MA may work 40 hours a week and, depending upon the medical practice, some evenings and Saturday hours too. In addition, the well-trained MA can work on many administrative tasks even when the physician is not in the office. This is likely to increase the efficiency and organization of the medical office.

READING CHECK

Identify some clinical tasks that the medical assistant might perform.

The Physician Assistant

What tasks of a physician can be performed by a physician assistant?

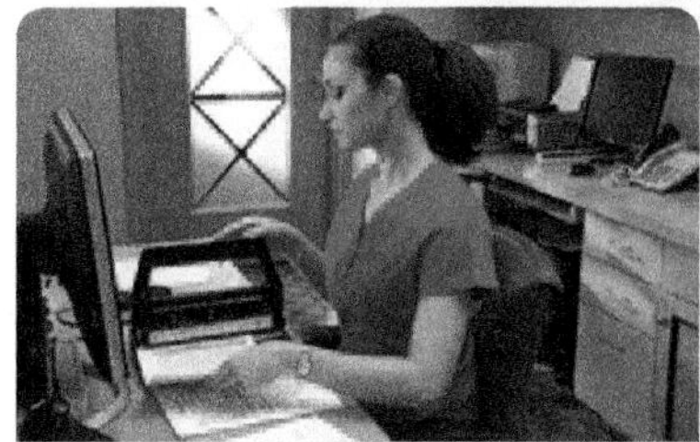

Fig. 16.5 Physician Assistant The physician assistant regularly discusses care and treatment with the patient. *What are the typical education requirements for becoming a PA?*

A physician assistant (PA) works under the direct control of a licensed physician. **Figure 16.5** shows a PA meeting with a patient.

States regulate PA training. All states require students to complete a formal education program. This takes at least four years and includes classroom and clinical training. Admission requirements vary among schools. Most require general education and work experience such as

- college credit.
- an associate or bachelor's degree.
- evidence of knowledge in specific areas.
- documented experience working with patients in a healthcare environment.

High school courses such as biology, chemistry, and math may be required for admission into a PA program. Graduates earn a bachelor's or master's degree.

Physician assistant graduates must pass the Physician Assistants National Certifying Examination, which is administered by the National Commission on Certification of Physician Assistants (NCCPA). Upon passing it, the student may use the credential PA-C (physician assistant-certified) after his or her name and obtain employment as a PA. Physician assistants must maintain their certification by completing additional education and training throughout their career. The PA must take a recertification examination every six years.

Although PAs must work under the supervision of a physician, many work in geographical areas where physicians are in short supply. In this situation, the PA may see the supervising physician only once or twice a week. The supervising physician will be available to the PA by phone or electronically, as needed or as required by state law.

Job Responsibilities of the Physician Assistant

Physician assistants perform functions that a licensed physician performs. Although duties of the PA may be limited by the supervising physician or state law, skills used by the PA include:

- recording patients' medical histories.
- performing physical examinations.
- ordering laboratory and X-ray procedures.
- interpreting the results of laboratory and X-ray tests.
- prescribing appropriate medications and treatments.
- suturing lacerations.
- applying splints or casts to musculoskeletal injuries, as shown in **Figure 16.6.**

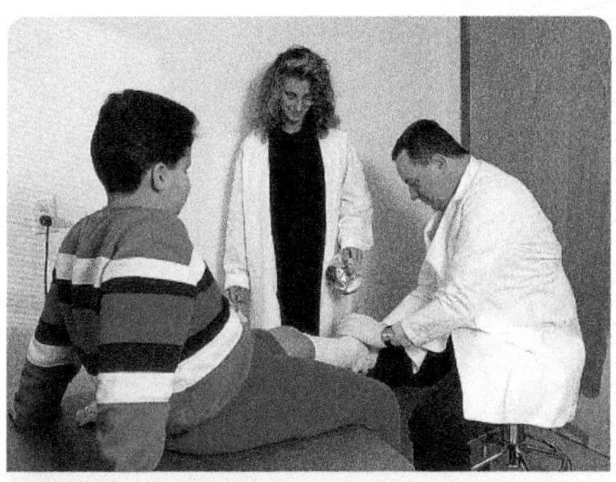

Fig. 16.6 Applying a Cast The PA in this picture is applying a cast and giving instructions to the young patient on how to care for it. *What are other skills often used by the PA?*

READING CHECK

Recall how physician assistant graduates obtain certification.

The Physician

What is a residency?

Physicians are among the highest paid professionals in the healthcare field. The required education and training are also the longest. Most physicians are doctors of medicine (M.D.), but some are doctors of osteopathic medicine (D.O.).

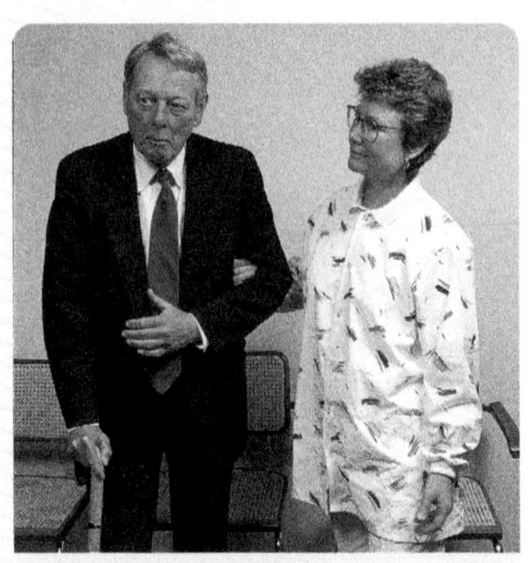

Fig. 16.7 Specialties Some physicians specialize in geriatrics, or the care of the older patient. *Can you name two other physician specialties?*

Family practice physicians meet most of the healthcare needs of patients of all ages. Some doctors, though, prefer to focus on one type of care. They may specialize by patient area or by body system. For example, pediatrics deals with the treatment of children. Geriatrics focuses on older adults. (see **Figure 16.7**). **Dermatology** deals with treatment related to the skin. **Gastroenterology** deals with disorders of the stomach and intestines.

Though all physicians receive similar training, physicians who specialize may be required to have more education and training. A physician may take an examination to become certified in a specialty, or board certified. The physician may use board certification to advertise his or her medical practice.

After four years of college and acceptance into a medical school, the student must complete an additional four years of medical training. The first two years of this training is in the classroom, learning more about the body and how it works (anatomy and physiology), microorganisms (microbiology), diseases (pathology), and drugs (pharmacology). The remaining two years are spent working in a hospital setting under the supervision of an experienced physician. The student learns how to treat patients with various diseases and illnesses. **Figure 16.8** shows a group of students learning how to diagnose and treat patients.

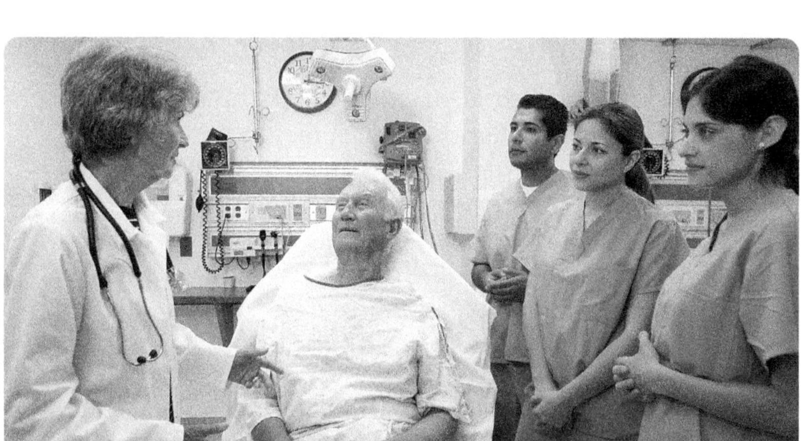

Fig. 16.8 Collaboration These medical students are learning practical information about diagnosing and treating patients. *What communication skills are important when dealing with patients?*

In the United States, all physicians must be licensed to practice medicine. This examination consists of an oral and a written part. Once the physician has passed the examination, he or she is licensed and may use the title M.D. or D.O.

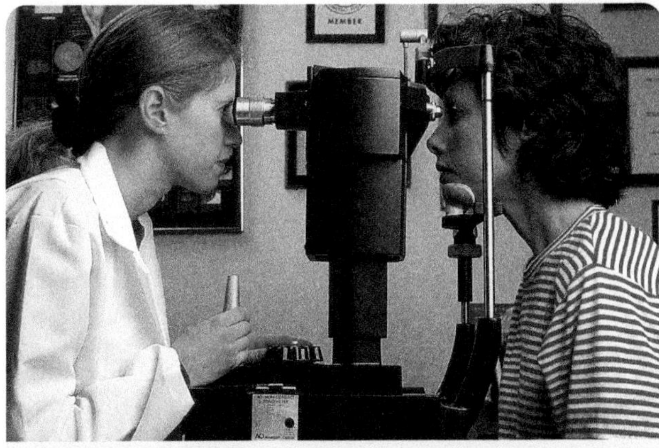

Fig. 16.9 Ophthalmology The patient shown here is having a test done to measure the pressure on the inside of the eye, using a tonometer. *What board certification might this physician have?*

A new physician must continue learning by entering a residency or internship. This is on-the-job training during which the skill of diagnosing and treating ill and injured patients is further developed. During the residency or internship, physicians are "rotated" through several areas of the hospital, including obstetrics and gynecology, the emergency room, pediatrics, orthopedics, and surgery. Many physicians seek additional training and certification to increase their skill in a particular area after completing the residency or internship. There are 24 specialty boards. The physician in **Figure 16.9** is specialized in ophthalmology.

The 24 specialty boards are:

- Allergy and immunology
- Anesthesiology
- Colon and rectal surgery
- Dermatology
- Emergency medicine
- Family practice
- Internal medicine
- Medical genetics
- Neurological surgery
- Nuclear medicine
- Obstetrics and gynecology
- Ophthalmology
- Orthopedic surgery
- Otolaryngology
- Pathology
- Pediatrics
- Physical medicine and rehabilitation
- Plastic surgery
- Preventative medicine
- Psychiatry and neurology
- Radiology
- Surgery
- Thoracic surgery
- Urology

Job Responsibilities of the Physician

Years of dedication are required of the student who wants to become a physician, but there are also many rewards. A physician may expect a long career that involves challenges and a sense of accomplishment.

Besides having the dedication and motivation to spend many years in formal education and training, physicians must also keep abreast of the ever-changing healthcare environment. The physician must be able to communicate clearly and efficiently with a variety of people, including:

- Patients
- Nurses
- Medical assistants
- Physician assistants
- Pharmacists
- Laboratory personnel
- Medical supply salespeople
- Other healthcare team members

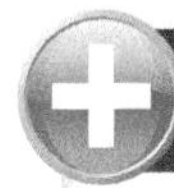

Safety

Patient Safety – Patients with Disabilities

A patient with a physical disability may or may not need additional assistance. Make sure the patient with a disability has assistance consistent with his or her abilities. On the other hand, do not assume that a patient with a disability needs or wants assistance.

Photo: Terry Wild Studio

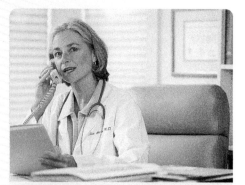

Fig. 16.10 Communication This physician is communicating with a pharmacy about a patient's medication order. *What communication skills must the physician have?*

Communication with these individuals may be verbal or written. The physician must be quick to adapt from using medical language, which is understood mainly by healthcare personnel, to explaining complicated instructions or laboratory results to an anxious patient or family member. In **Figure 16.10**, a physician is discussing a patient's medication with a pharmacist.

There is no "typical" day for the physician, but some responsibilities that may be similar regardless of the physician's specialty are:

- Obtaining a patient's medical history
- Performing a physical examination
- Listening to heart and lung sounds for abnormalities
- Performing minor in-office medical procedures
- Prescribing medications to prevent or treat a variety of medical conditions
- Ordering laboratory or radiology tests to assist in diagnosing various diseases
- Consulting with other physicians or healthcare team members
- Interpreting laboratory results
- Educating patients
- Making purchasing decisions: medical equipment, computers, and other items

In addition, physicians must be able to perform competently and quickly under stress. Even the most routine day can quickly become chaotic if there is an emergency.

READING CHECK

List several fields of specialization for physicians.

SECTION 16.1 Careers in the Clinical Office Review

AFTER YOU READ

1. **Describe** the two credentials an MA can obtain.
2. **Compare** the roles and responsibilities of an MA, a PA, and a physician.
3. **Contrast** the various administrative and clinical tasks performed in a clinical office.
4. **Identify** which of the three medical personnel discussed in this chapter can diagnose illness and prescribe medication. Explain your answer.
5. **Describe** the steps physicians must take to become trained and licensed.

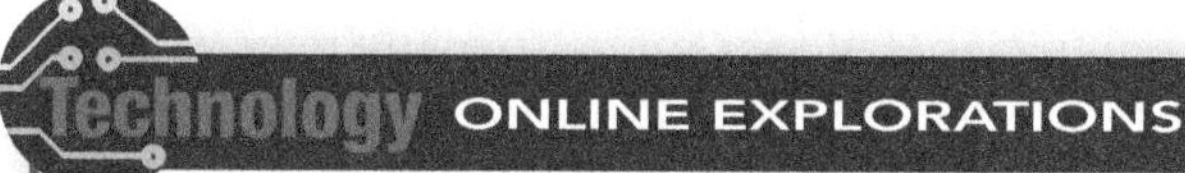

M.D. or D.O.?

Go online to find a college or university that has a medical school program for the medical doctor (M.D.) and a college or university that has a program for the doctor of osteopathy (D.O.). Compare the programs in terms of length and course requirements. Write a short summary of your findings, comparing the schools and the classes required of the M.D. and the D.O.

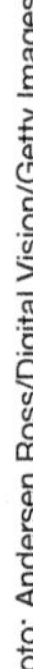

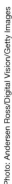

SECTION 16.2 Clinical Office Procedures

The Gynecological Exam

Why are regular gynecological exams important?

The gynecological examination is necessary for females who are over 18 or are sexually active. The Pap smear, which detects cancer of the cervix, is frequently part of this examination. "Pap" is short for Papanicolaou, the name of the physician who developed the test. Results are reported as: negative or normal; ASCUS (atypical squamous cells of undetermined significance, or cells that just look odd); CIN I, which is mild dysplasia; CIN II, which is moderate dysplasia; and CIN III, which is severe dysplasia or a cancerous condition. Regular gynecological exams are very important. Early detection and treatment of sexually transmitted diseases, abnormal Pap tests, and uterine, ovary, or breast lumps greatly improve the health and wellness of all females.

Vocabulary

Content Vocabulary

You will learn these content vocabulary terms in this section.

- **scalpels**
- **sutures**
- **Mayo stand**
- **vial**
- **diluent**
- **ampule**
- **intramuscular (IM)**
- **intradermal (ID)**
- **subcutaneous (subcut)**
- **dorsogluteal**
- **vastus lateralis**
- **deltoid**

Academic Vocabulary

You will see this word in your reading and on your tests. Find its meaning in the Glossary in the back of the book.

- **method**

Assisting with Office Surgery

How does a clinical assistant help the patient during a minor surgical procedure?

Many physicians perform minor surgical procedures in the office. The clinical office staff is responsible for setting up the treatment area and the surgical tray. The surgical tray holds the instruments, such as **scalpels,** scissors, curettes, and grasping instruments, that will be used in the procedure (see **Figure 16.11**).

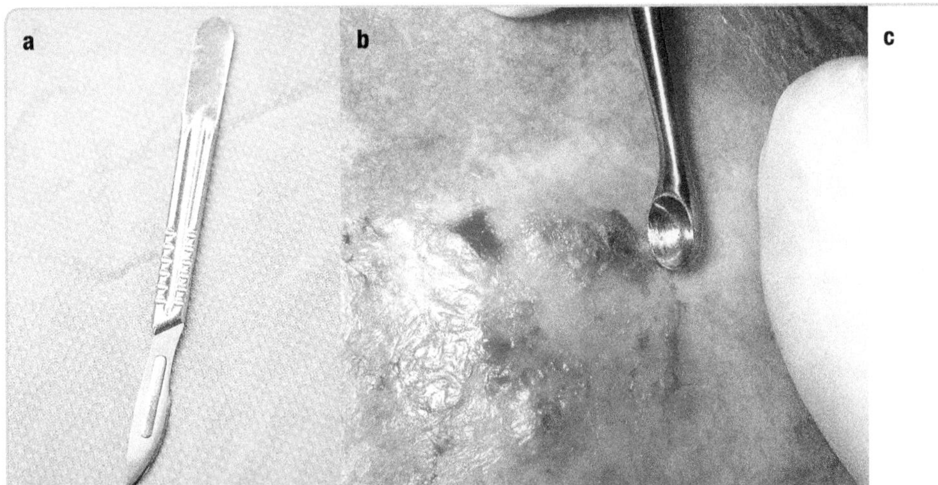

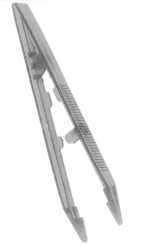

Fig. 16.11 Surgical instruments It may be the responsibility of the MA to set up the sterile tray with all sterile items before the minor office procedure. Items on a sterile tray include (a) scalpels, (b) curettes, and (c) instruments for grasping. *What are the assistant's other responsibilities related to these procedures?*

Photos: (l to r)Dynamic Graphics/Jupiter Images, The McGraw-Hill Companies, Inc./Ken Karp photographer, Medical-on-Line/Alamy

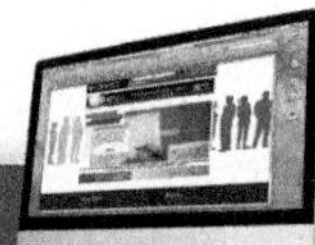

connect ONLINE PROCEDURES

PROCEDURE 16-1

Positioning Patients for a Physical Examination

Patients are placed in various positions depending upon the type of examination or treatment they will be receiving. Provide for comfort and safety and assist the patient as needed.

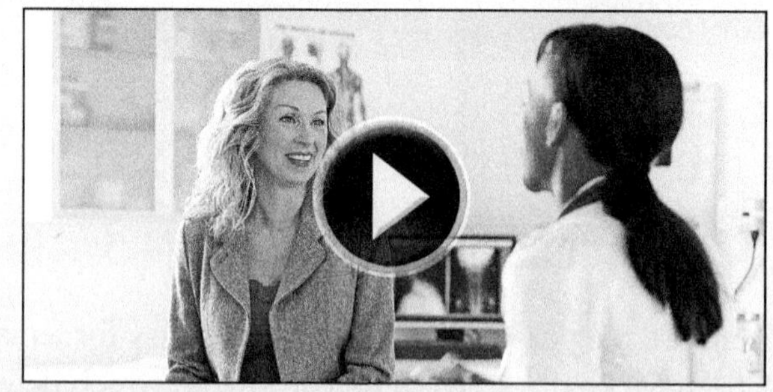

PROCEDURE 16-2

Assisting with Gynecological Examinations

A gynecological (GYN) exam should be done yearly on women. The examination is done to check for any abnormalities to the female organs including abnormal growths. It also includes a Pap smear, which checks for cervical cancer.

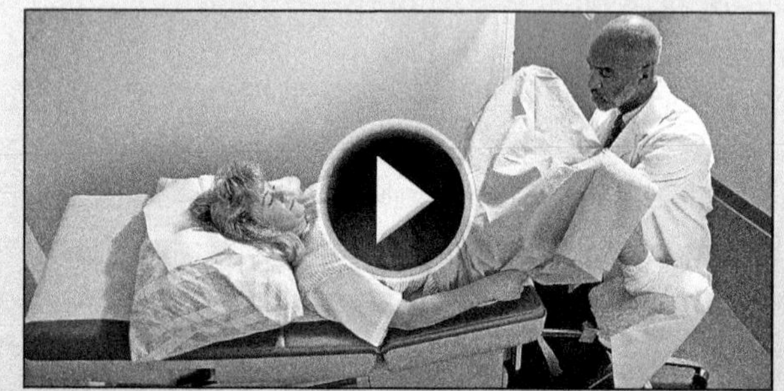

PROCEDURE 16-3

Obtaining a Throat Culture

When a patient complains of upper respiratory symptoms, such as a sore throat, the physician often orders a throat culture to determine whether pathogens are in the pharynx. The culture must be processed and tested after it is obtained.

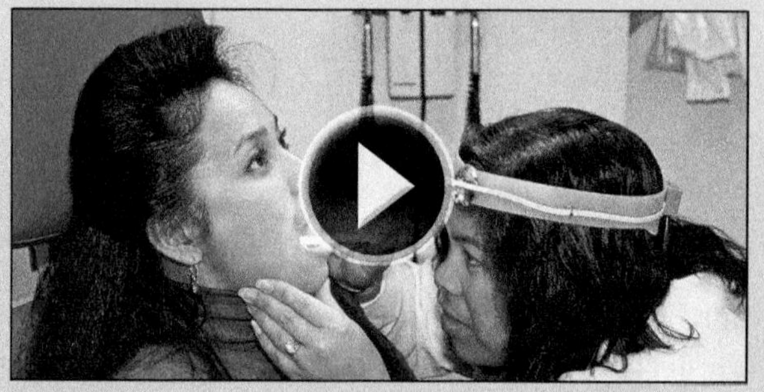

PROCEDURE 16-4

Collecting a Clean-Catch Urine Specimen

A clean-catch urine specimen is done to reduce the number of contaminants in the specimen. The patient will need to be instructed on the proper procedure to ensure accurate results.

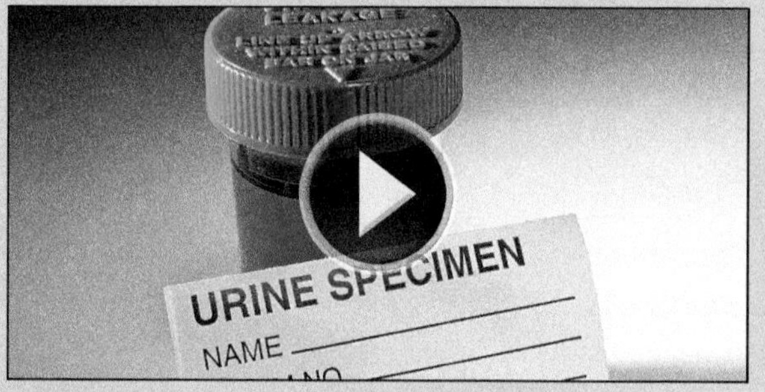

PROCEDURE 16-5

Applying Bandages

Bandages are used to hold dressings in place or to provide support to an injured area of the body. Often, bandage material is packaged in rolls in individual sterile packages. If a wound is to be covered, a sterile dressing must be used.

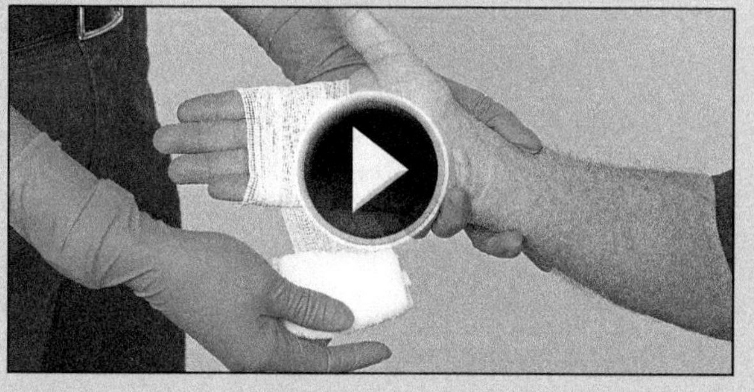

Photos: (t to b)Thomas Barwick/Getty Images, Photodisc/Getty Images, Royalty-Free/CORBIS, Spike Mafford/Getty Images, The McGraw-Hill Companies, Inc./Rick Brady, photographer

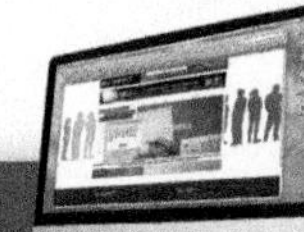

connect ONLINE PROCEDURES

PROCEDURE 16-6

Measuring Blood Glucose

Glucometers are easy to use and give rapid results, usually within 1 to 3 minutes. All machines have specific instructions and timings that need to be followed for accurate results. Although a variety of machines are available, all glucometers are battery operated and use a small sample of whole blood from a capillary finger stick.

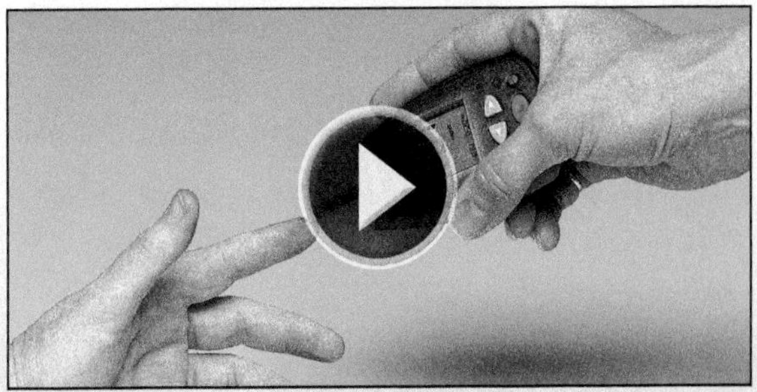

PROCEDURE 16-7

Removing Sutures

The physician determines when **sutures** should be removed. However, it may be the responsibility of the office staff to remove them. Any wound that is open or draining purulent material (pus) should be reported to the physician before the sutures are removed. In most cases the physician will observe the sutures before you remove them.

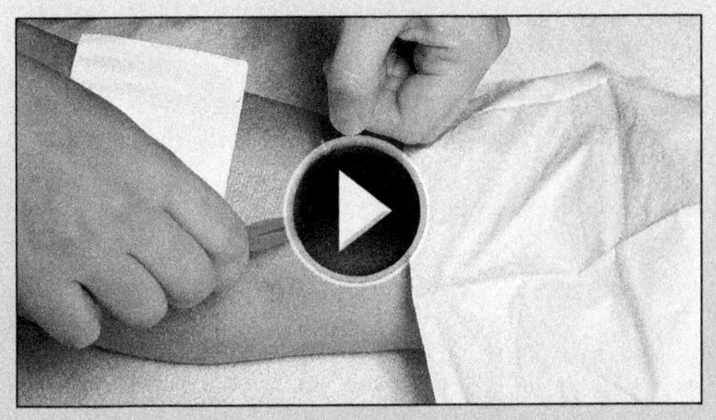

The physician is responsible for explaining the procedure to the patient. The assistant prepares the patient and makes sure the consent form has been signed. During the procedure, the assistant reassures the patient and assists the physician. After the procedure, the patient is given instructions for wound care.

Remember the following points during an in-office surgical procedure. If a sterilized pack is used, it is opened, and its inside wrapper becomes the sterile field. Otherwise, spread a sterile drape over the **Mayo stand** and place sterile supplies on the drape (see **Figure 16.12**). Items that cannot be placed on the sterile field are placed on a side table or countertop. Drop Sterile items onto the field without touching them or use transfer forceps to place them on the sterile field.

If a specimen is obtained, hold the specimen container so the physician can place the tissue in it without touching the outside rim with the tissue (see **Figure 16.13**). Sharps should be placed in a puncture resistant container with the biohazard symbol (see **Figure 16.14** on page 450).

READING CHECK

Summarize the process of preparing a sterile field.

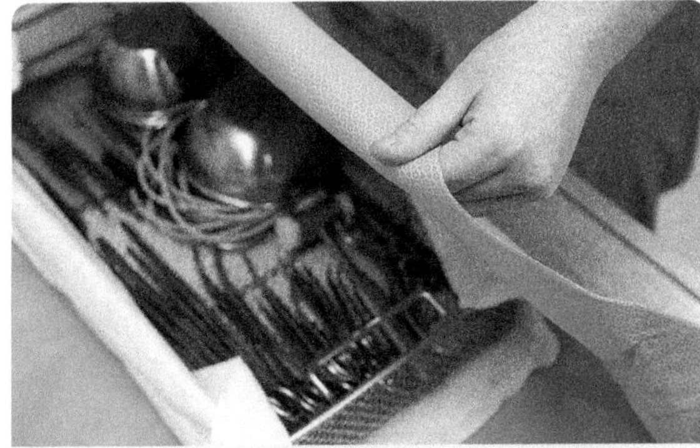

Fig. 16.12 Sterile items The inside wrapper of the sterilized pack becomes the sterile field once it is opened. *What should you use if you need to place a sterile item on a sterile field?*

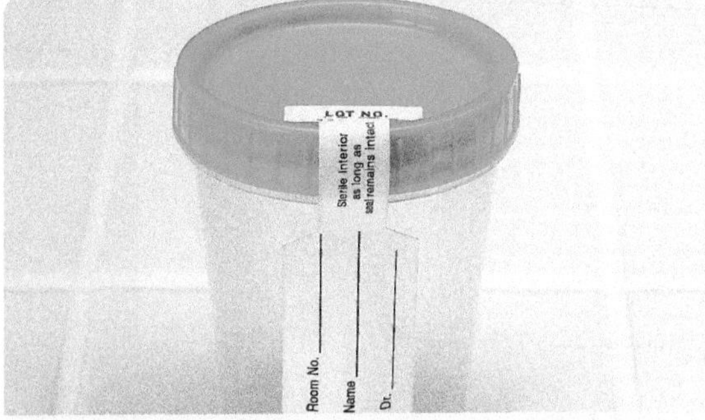

Fig. 16.13 Specimen container The container is held so that the physician can place the tissue in it without touching the outside rim with the tissue. *Why is it important not to touch the rim?*

Photos: (t to b)McGraw-Hill Companies, Inc./Kevin May, photographer, Image Source/Getty Images, Oberhaeuser/Caro/Alamy, Steven Puetzer/Iconica/Getty Images

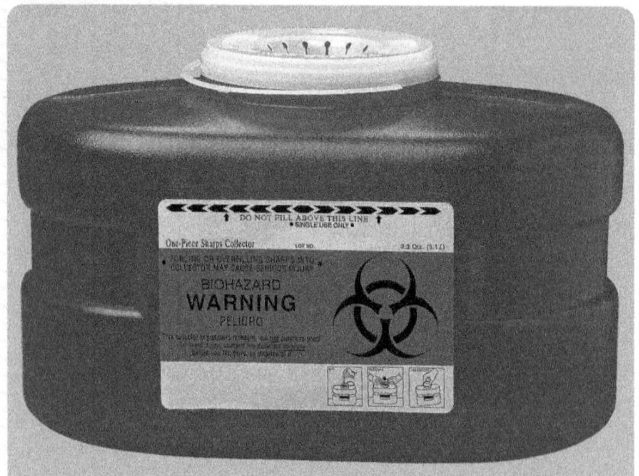

Fig. 16.14 Sharps Container All biohazard sharps containers should be puncture resistant. *Why is this an important feature?*

Injections

How is the correct needle chosen for a specific injection?

Medication for injection is administered in liquid form, measured in milliliters. The healthcare professional responsible for administering medications must accurately calculate the dosage ordered (see Chapter 18, Pharmacy). This calculation is based on how the medication is supplied or reconstituted into liquid form. Always check the route of administration by referring to a drug reference book. The healthcare professional should also review the medication before administration. A reliable source, such as a drug reference book or trusted website, should be used to verify drug names, dosages, side effects, and contraindications before any medication is administered. The Physicians' Desk Reference is available online or in book form (see **Figure 16.15**).

Employees in clinical offices are often required to administer medications. These should be kept in an area inaccessible to unauthorized persons and should be checked regularly for outdated drugs. Stored medication must be categorized, either alphabetically or according to the drug classification.

The two types of containers most frequently used to store medications are vials and ampules. A **vial** is a small glass bottle with a rubber stopper. Vials may contain powdered medication that must be mixed with a **diluent** (liquid) before use. An **ampule** is a small glass container with a narrow neck.

Injections of medications into a muscle are called **intramuscular (IM)** injections. **Intradermal (ID)** injections are made into the superficial layer (dermis) of the skin. **Subcutaneous (subcut)** injections are made into the soft tissue beneath the skin (see **Figure 16.16**).

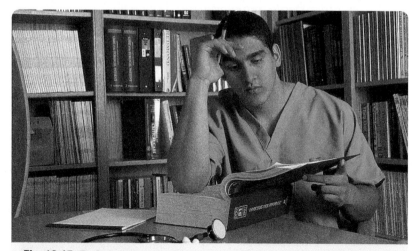

Fig. 16.15 Reference It is important to verify drug names, dosages, side effects, and contraindications before administering any medication to a patient. *What reference book is this medical office employee most likely referring to before administering a medication?*

Some intramuscular injections must be given in large muscles such as the **dorsogluteal** or **vastus lateralis,** and others may be given in the **deltoid** muscle. The amount of medication to be administered also determines the injection site. No more than one milliliter of medication should be injected into the deltoid muscle, but the dorsogluteal and vastus lateralis muscles can hold up to three milliliters. Subcutaneous and intradermal injections should be less than 1 milliliter.

The method of injection determines the length and gauge of the needle used. The gauge is a measurement of thickness. Subcutaneous injections are given with needles about $\frac{1}{2}$ inch long and 25 gauge or smaller.

Always put a new, sterile needle on the syringe before giving the injection. A sharp needle causes the patient less pain. Rub the site for injection with vigor. Friction cleanses, and surface pressure and local irritation reduce the patient's discomfort when the needle is inserted.

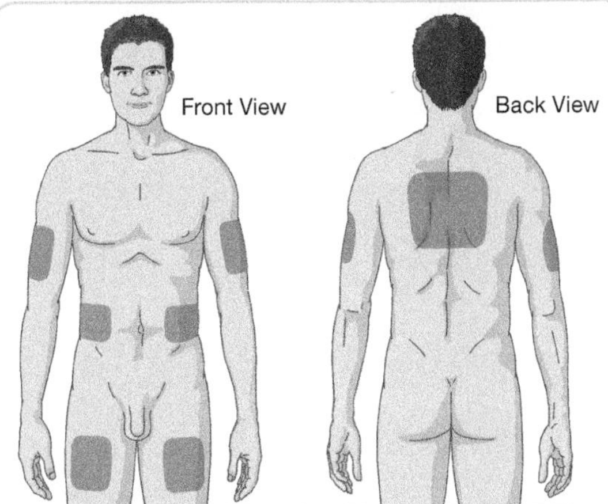

Fig. 16.16 Injections Three common sites for administering intramuscular injections are: the gluteus medius, the deltoid, and the vastus lateralis. Note that bony landmarks must be palpated to locate the muscle. The shaded areas shown in this figure, on the anterior of this body, are suitable for subcutaneous injections. Medication injected into the dermal layer of the skin correctly will produce a reddish raised wheal. *How much medication can be injected into the vastus lateralis or dorsogluteal muscles?*

READING CHECK

Explain how to prepare a site for an injection.

SECTION 16.2 Clinical Office Procedures Review

AFTER YOU READ

1. **Explain** the role of the employee in a clinical office with regard to safety when positioning a patient for an examination.
2. **List** the positions in which it would be appropriate to place a patient for an examination of the abdomen.
3. **Identify** the supplies necessary for a gynecological examination.
4. **Describe** what you would do in this procedure: While you are obtaining a throat culture, the patient gags and the swab touches the uvula.
5. **Analyze** why it is important to start and stop the flow of urine before obtaining the urine for the clean-catch urine specimen.
6. **List** the signs indicating that a bandage has been applied to an extremity too tightly.
7. **Describe** what a glucometer is and why it must be calibrated.
8. **Identify** one instrument used to cut or dissect.
9. **Name** some common sites for IM, and subcut injections.

Technology ONLINE EXPLORATIONS

Blood Testing

Do you know anyone who has to draw blood to test blood sugar? Go online to research other ways to monitor blood sugar. Identify at least one method that does not use blood. In a short report, give the name of the equipment and the manufacturer, the equipment's status (whether it has government approval), and a picture with a brief description.

CHAPTER

16 Review

Chapter Summary

SECTION 16.1

- The medical assistant (MA) works under the supervision of a physician and may be responsible for administrative and/or clinical duties in the physician's office. The MA may receive training on the job or may attend a formal program. The MA who graduates from an accredited program is eligible to take the national certification examination. **(pg. 439)**
- The physician assistant (PA) works under the supervision of a physician. Most PAs earn a bachelor's or master's degree. **(pg. 443)**
- The certified PA performs many of the clinical procedures that a physician would normally perform. The physician may or may not be present when the PA performs these procedures. **(pg. 443)**
- Physicians can be trained as M.D.s or D.O.s. Both types of physicians are qualified to practice medicine, including diagnosing diseases, prescribing medications, and performing surgery. **(pg. 444)**
- All physicians must be licensed to practice medicine in the United States. The education and training for a physician take about eight years plus several years of practical experience known as an internship and/or residency. **(pg. 444)**

SECTION 16.2

- Proper positioning and draping are essential and depend upon the examination to be performed. **(pg. 448)**
- Patient privacy must be maintained throughout the gynecological examination. **(pg. 448)**
- A throat specimen may reveal the presence of streptococcal bacteria. This test can be performed by using a rapid detection test, inoculating a culture plate, or sending the specimen to an outside lab for testing. **(pg. 448)**
- The patient should be instructed in the proper procedure for collecting a clean-catch urine specimen. **(pg. 448)**
- Minor surgery is performed in the physician's office or clinic. Many materials are used that must be kept sterile until use. **(pg. 449)**
- Medications and dosages must be checked carefully before administering any type of injection including IM, or subcut. **(pg. 450)**

CHAPTER

16 Assessment

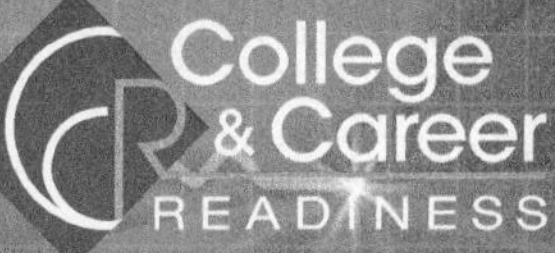

Critical Thinking/Problem Solving

1. You are preparing to assist with an examination. The patient complains of pain while you are positioning him in Sims' position. What will you do?
2. You are getting ready to teach a patient how to obtain a clean catch-urine specimen when she states "I know how to do it, just give me the cup." What should you do?
3. What symptoms might a patient with a urinary tract or a kidney infection exhibit?
4. What area of medicine would you like to learn more about? Select an area and discuss the particular skills you would need to be able to work in that field of medicine.

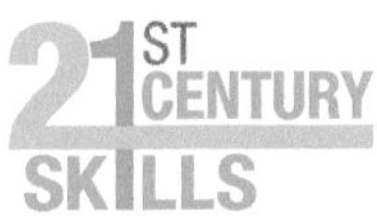

5. **Problem Solving** Review the seven examination positions described in Procedure 16-1. Place yourself or a partner in each of these positions. On paper, list the type of examination or procedure that might be performed for each position.
6. **Information Literacy** Obtain medical history forms and practice taking a medical history from a partner. Follow the communication techniques in this chapter.
7. **Problem Solving** Use a stethoscope to listen to a partner's breathing and heartbeat.
8. **Organization** Identify various instruments used during an examination.
9. **Teamwork** With a partner, obtain cotton-tipped applicators and culture plates and practice streaking a culture. If equipment is not available, use paper and pencil.
10. **Information Literacy** Research the professional organizations for the medical assistant (American Association of Medical Assistants) and the physician assistant (American Academy of Physician Assistants). Find the code of ethics for each. In teams, create posters comparing these professions. Include the code of ethics.

McGraw Hill connect™ ONLINE ACTIVITIES

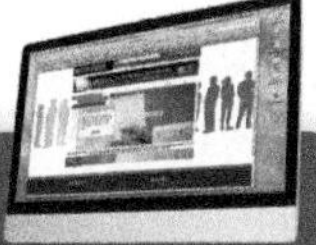

Complete our HST online activities for Chapter 16, which include Concept Check review questions, Reference Flash Cards, and Online Procedures assessment sheets.

- **Concept Check** review questions
- **Reference Flash Cards** medical terminology practice
- **Online Procedures** assessment sheets

CHAPTER 17 Mental Health

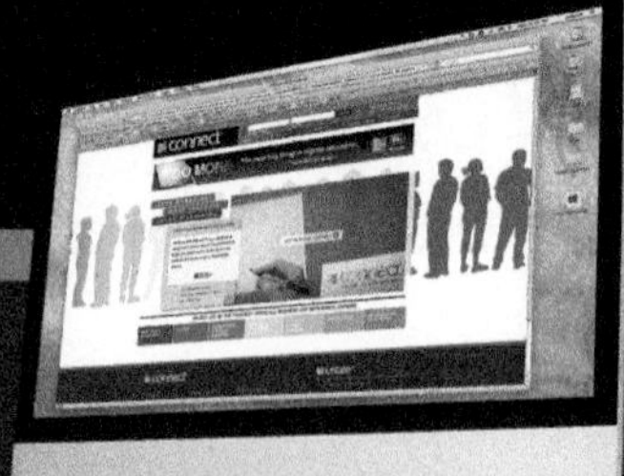

McGraw Hill connect™

It's Online!

- Online Procedures
- STEM Connection
- Medical Science
- Medical Terms
- Medical Math
- Ethics in Action
- Virtual Lab

Essential Question:

How has the approach to treating mental illnesses changed in recent years?

Mental disorders are often hard to diagnose, and in the past those disorders were sometimes mistaken for social problems. The field of mental healthcare today includes many different occupations. Changing attitudes have created a wide range of opportunities for careers in the mental health field.

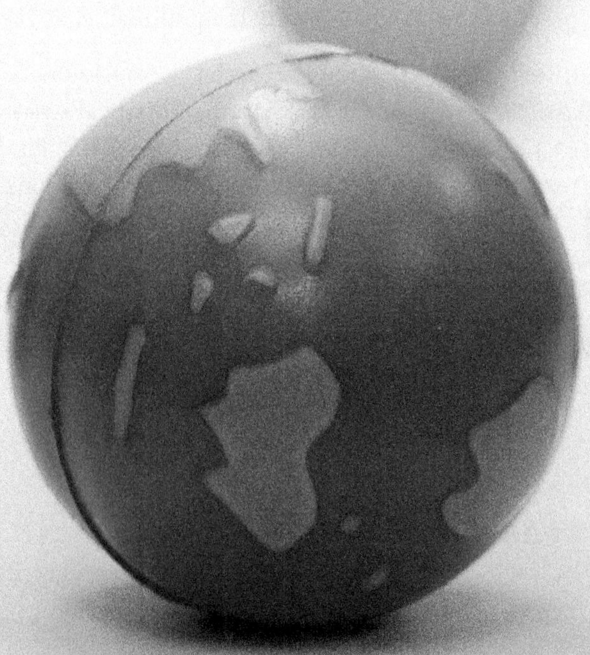

Photo: The McGraw-Hill Companies Inc.

READING GUIDE

OBJECTIVES

After completing this chapter, you will be able to:

- **Identify** the roles and responsibilities of personnel in mental healthcare, including mental health aides and mental health technicians.
- **Compare** the roles and responsibilities of licensed mental healthcare professionals, including psychologists, psychiatrists, social workers, and counselors.
- **Discuss** safety and legal issues related to the use of restraints.
- **Explain** the use and purpose of reality orientation.
- **Describe** the tasks performed during postmortem care.

BEFORE YOU READ

Connect What do you already know about the duties of healthcare professionals in various mental healthcare fields?

Main Idea

Even more than in other healthcare fields, communication skills and a genuine desire to understand the emotions of the patient are vital to professionals in the mental healthcare field.

Note-Taking Activity

Draw this table. Write key terms and phrases under **Cues**. Write main ideas under **Note Taking**. Summarize the section under **Summary**.

Cues	Note Taking
o	o
o	o
Summary	

Graphic Organizer

Before you read the chapter, draw a diagram like the one below. As you read, write the main careers covered by the chapter into the diagram.

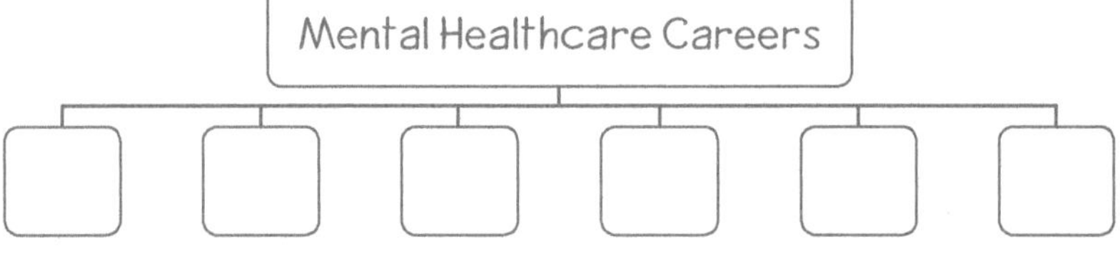

connect
Downloadable graphic organizers can be accessed online.

STANDARDS

HEALTH SCIENCE

NCHSE 2.15 Apply speaking and active listening skills.

NCHSE 4.31 Discuss levels of education, credentialing requirements, and employment trends in healthcare.

SCIENCE

NSES F Develop understanding of personal and community health; population growth; natural resources; environmental quality; natural and human-induced hazards; science and technology in local, national, and global challenges.

NCHSE *National Consortium for Health Science Education*

NSES *National Science Education Standards*

COMMON CORE STATE STANDARDS

MATHEMATICS

Statistics and Probability

Making Inferences and Justifying Conclusions S-IC 6 Evaluate reports based on data.

ENGLISH LANGUAGE ARTS

Writing

Production and Distribution of Writing W-6 Use technology, including the Internet, to produce, publish, and update individual or shared writing products, taking advantage of technology's capacity to link to other information and to display information flexibly and dynamically.

Speaking and Listening

Presentation of Knowledge and Ideas SL-6 Adapt speech to a variety of contexts and tasks, demonstrating command of formal English when indicated or appropriate.

SECTION

17.1 Careers in Mental Healthcare

Vocabulary

Content Vocabulary

You will learn these content vocabulary terms in this section.

- **therapeutic communication**
- **developmentally disabled**
- **cerebral palsy**
- **autism**
- **geropsychology**
- **neuropsychology**

Academic Vocabulary

You will see these words in your reading and on your tests. Find their meanings in the Glossary in the back of this book.

- **significant**
- **technique**
- **intervene**

Opportunities in Mental Health

Which of the careers in the mental health field is most interesting to you?

Mental healthcare is provided in the most efficient and cost-effective manner possible. Unlicensed mental health aides and technicians perform many non-medical duties. But many patients need assessment and treatment plans that require oversight from licensed personnel with specific training. **Table 17.1** gives information about these occupations. A detailed discussion of the occupations follows.

The mental healthcare occupations discussed in this chapter are:

- Mental health aide
- Mental health technician
- Social worker
- Counselor
- Psychologist
- Psychiatrist

The Mental Health Aide

Have you ever spoken to a counselor or other mental healthcare professional?

Mental health aides may work directly or indirectly with patients. When they work directly with patients, they might provide transportation or emotional support. They may monitor patients' daily activities. They may telephone or visit patients' homes or they may assist with activities of daily living (ADLs). The mental health aide doing this type of work may be employed in a variety of settings, such as an office, clinic, hospital, group home, shelter home, day workshop, or a patient's home (see **Figure 17.1**).

A mental health aide who works indirectly with patients may review Medicaid applications for eligibility. They also may arrange transportation or assist with healthcare visits. Mental health aides may work as social service assistants or case manager aides.

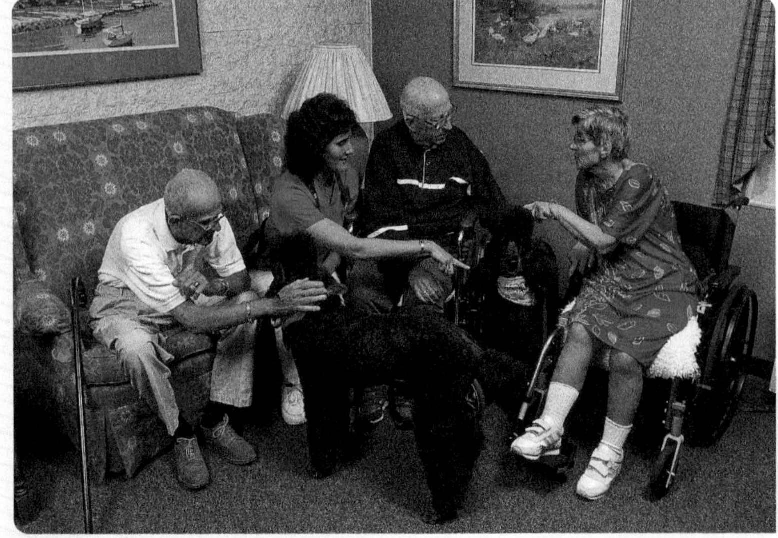

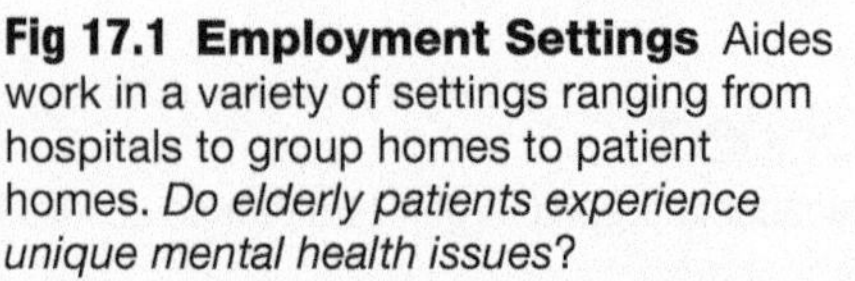

Fig 17.1 Employment Settings Aides work in a variety of settings ranging from hospitals to group homes to patient homes. *Do elderly patients experience unique mental health issues?*

Photo: Lou Bopp/Lou Bopp Photography

Table 17.1 Overview of Mental Healthcare Occupations

OCCUPATION	EDUCATIONAL REQUIREMENTS	CERTIFICATION OR LICENSING AGENCY	JOB OUTLOOK
Mental health aide (psychiatric aide)	Usually requires training beyond high school in a certificate program.	No certification or licensing may be required or offered.	Growth in this area is expected to be below average.
Mental health technician (psychiatric technician)	On-the-job training or formal one- to two-year training programs are offered. In many states, an associate degree in social or behavioral science is required.	License and certification requirements vary from state to state. Some states do not require a license. Certain states require graduation from an accredited educational program consisting of at least 1,530 hours of classroom training, clinical experience, and a test.	Growth in this area is expected to be below average.
Social worker	Minimum requirement of a bachelor's degree for entry into the field. Many positions require a master's degree.	All states and the District of Columbia require licensing for social workers. The National Association of Social Workers offers certification, as does the Academy of Certified Social Workers.	Growth is faster than average because the population is aging.
Counselor	Some states require master's degrees; others may require a bachelor's degree with additional coursework. The amount of education required depends on the state and area of counseling specialty.	The National Board for Certified Counselors offers general practice credentials. The Commission on Rehabilitation Counselor Certification certifies rehabilitation counselors. The National Board for Certified Counselors, Inc. certifies mental health counselors.	Growth is faster than average for vocational and educational counselors. Job growth for rehabilitation and mental health counselors is expected to remain strong. Job openings are increasing in rural areas.
Psychologist	Postgraduate work leading to a doctoral degree is usually required. Psychologists who have a Ph.D. usually work in clinical positions. An average of five to seven years of graduate school is required for a doctoral degree. Educational specialists with an Ed.S. degree are qualified to work as school psychologists.	Each state establishes individual licensing requirements. In general, requirements vary according to the type of position.	Jobs for psychologists are expected to grow about as fast as average. It is predicted that those with doctoral degrees who specialize in counseling or mental health will have increased opportunities.
Psychiatrist	Undergraduate degree in premedicine, plus four years of medical school and an additional three to eight years of internship and residency are required. Psychiatrists have either an M.D. or D.O. with specialization in mental healthcare.	All states and U.S. territories require psychiatrists to be licensed. All psychiatrists must graduate from an accredited medical school and pass an examination.	Jobs for psychiatrists are expected to grow faster than average with the rising awareness of the importance of mental health and the increase in the aging population. Opportunities will be very good in rural and low-income areas.

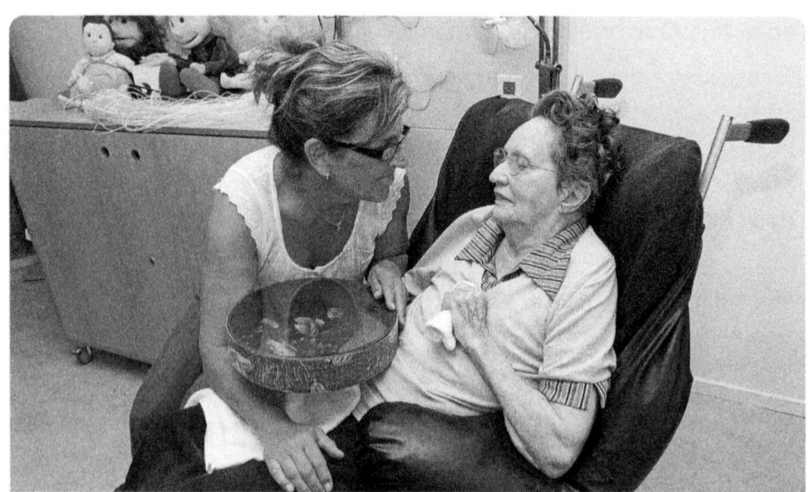

Fig. 17.2 Mental Health Aide A mental health aide works with a patient. *How can mental health aides assist with patients' emotional needs?*

They may also work as social worker assistants or community support assistants (see **Figure 17.2**).

In general, you do not need a two- or four-year college degree to work as a mental health aide. However, some employers require a certificate or training beyond high school. In some cases, mental health aides must first qualify as nursing assistants.

The Job of the Mental Health Aide

Most mental health aides work 40 hours per week. Those working in a clinical position may work evenings, nights, or weekends.

The work can be very satisfying. It can also be tremendously draining as working with mental illnesses can be difficult. Patients may be withdrawn, uncommunicative, unpredictable, depressed, or violent. A mental health aide must have great patience and greatly enjoy helping people.

Aides must also have strong communication skills. Communication is one of the most important tools used in mental healthcare. These providers must be able to communicate with their patients and with other members of the healthcare team. **Figure 17.3** illustrates therapeutic communication, which is discussed further on the next page.

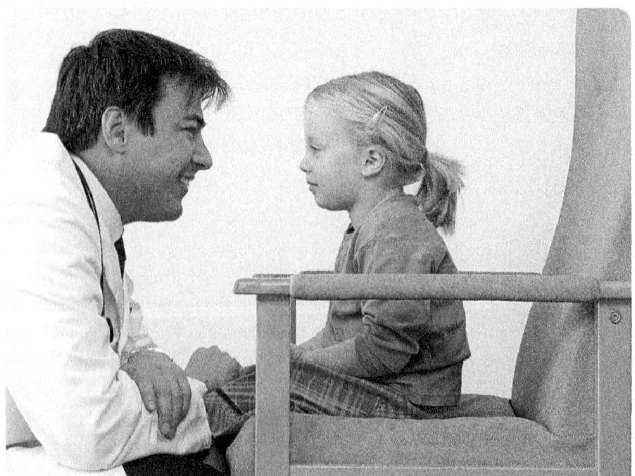

Fig. 17.3 Therapeutic Communication Therapeutic communication is the ability to communicate with patients in terms that they can understand. *How might this professional communicate with this child differently than with an adult patient?*

Mental healthcare professionals must be responsible and adhere strictly to proper behavior. This is because the mental healthcare provider is often a role model for patients. The behavior of the healthcare provider may be incorporated into the patient's behavior.

Mental health aides who work in the clinical field may work with patients to provide assistance with the everyday activities of daily living. They may work in acute care facilities, shelter homes, group homes, long-term care facilities, or patients' homes.

The best job opportunities are expected to be in residential care facilities and private social service agencies.

Mental health aides assist with emotional and/or physical needs. Often the aide is the person who spends the most time with a mentally ill patient and frequently develops a close relationship with the patient. This can be especially therapeutic for the mentally ill patient.

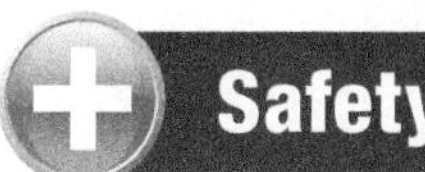

Healthcare Costs and Patient Safety

Rising healthcare costs and the need to contain and reduce those costs create patient safety dilemmas. Through the use of mental health aides and technicians, quality care can be provided to patients in a cost-effective manner. However, the protection of patients and healthcare professionals must remain a top priority. A trained and licensed individual educated in specific mental healthcare methods must assess each patient and determine if it is safe for a mental health aide or technician to provide care. Even after that determination has been made, specially trained and licensed personnel must continually direct and supervise the care.

The Job Responsibilities of the Mental Health Aide

The most important responsibilities of the mental health aide are to protect patient safety and report any significant changes to the supervisor. Mental health aides may do tasks similar to those delegated to nursing assistants. In addition, mental health aides may be asked to:

- Assess patients' needs
- Assist patients with finances
- Maintain case records
- Report progress to supervisors
- Provide emotional support
- Resolve conflicts with other people
- Help patients with medical forms
- Organize and lead group activities
- Assist patients who are in need of counseling
- Assist patients in finding community resources
- Talk with family members
- Help patients to become involved in their own care

Therapeutic Communication Techniques

Mental healthcare professionals must practice **therapeutic communication,** that is, communicate with patients in terms that they can understand. At the same time, it is important to feel at ease and comfortable with what is said. Therapeutic communication techniques help to improve communication with patients and involve the following communication skills.

- **Be silent.** Silence allows the patient time to think without pressure.
- **Accept.** Acceptance lets the patient know you are really listening. It shows that you have heard the patient and are following their thought pattern. Some indicators of acceptance include nodding; saying "Yes," "I understand," and other such phrases; and the use of body language.
- **Give Recognition.** Show patients that you are aware of them by stating their name in a greeting and by noticing positive changes. You are recognizing the patient as a person or individual.
- **Offer Self.** Make yourself available to the needs of the patient.
- **Give a Broad Opening.** Let the patient take the initiative in starting a topic. Ask open-ended questions, such as "Is there something you'd like to talk about? or "Where would you like to begin?"
- **Offer General Leads.** Give the patient encouragement to continue by making comments such as "Go on" or "And then?"

Preventive
Care & Wellness

Stress Management

There are two kinds of stress. Good stress is associated with the hormone epinephrine and can sharpen attention. Bad stress is linked to the hormone cortisol and is associated with negative emotions, including feeling frazzled or overwhelmed. Manage stress by converting bad stress to good stress. Here are some suggestions.

1. Ask questions. You will feel in better control.
2. Do not spend time worrying about things you cannot control.
3. Always have a "Plan B," or another method of handling a difficult situation.
4. Maintain a positive attitude. Optimism is a source of good stress.
5. Keep things in perspective.
6. Prepare for difficult situations. This summons good stress.
7. Learn how to relax. Become aware of your muscles, posture, and breathing.
8. Make regular time for yourself.

- **Make Observations.** Make your perceptions known to the patient. Say things like, "You appear tense today" or "Are you uncomfortable when you…?" By calling patients' attention to what is happening to them, you encourage them to notice it for themselves, so that they can describe it to you.
- **Encourage Communication.** Ask patients to verbalize what they perceive. Make statements such as "Tell me when you feel anxious" or "What is happening?" Patients should feel free to describe their perceptions to you, and you must try to see things as they do.
- **Mirror.** Restate what the patient has said, to demonstrate that you understand.
- **Reflect.** Encourage patients to think through and answer their own questions. A reflecting dialogue may go like this: Patient—"Do you think I should tell the doctor?" Healthcare professional—"Do you think that you should?" Reflecting questions or statements back to patients helps them feel that their opinions are of value.
- **Focus.** Focusing encourages the patient to stay on the topic.
- **Explore.** Encourage patients to express themselves in more depth. Try to get as much detail as possible about a patient complaint, but avoid probing and prying if the patient does not wish to discuss it.
- **Clarify.** Ask patients to explain themselves more clearly if they provide information that is vague or not meaningful.
- **Summarize.** This involves organizing and summing up the important points of a discussion and gives the patient an awareness of the progress being made toward greater understanding.

READING CHECK

Name some ways in which mental health aides work directly with patients.

The Mental Health Technician

How much experience do you have with developmentally disabled people?

Mental health technicians may also work with the **developmentally disabled.** People who are developmentally disabled have a condition caused by a congenital anomaly, trauma, deprivation, or disease. The condition is characterized by various problems, including an interrupted sequence and rate of normal growth, development, and maturation. These patients may have mental retardation or may be afflicted with **cerebral palsy, autism,** or behavioral disorders. Cerebral palsy is a condition that is characterized by various problems such as mental retardation, epilepsy, and motor impairment. Autism is a self-centered mental state that can involve inaccessibility, aloneness, rage reactions, and language disturbances. People suffering from autism may have birth defects or brain injuries. It generally affects a person's ability to socialize, communicate, and understand appropriate behavior.

The Job of the Mental Health Technician

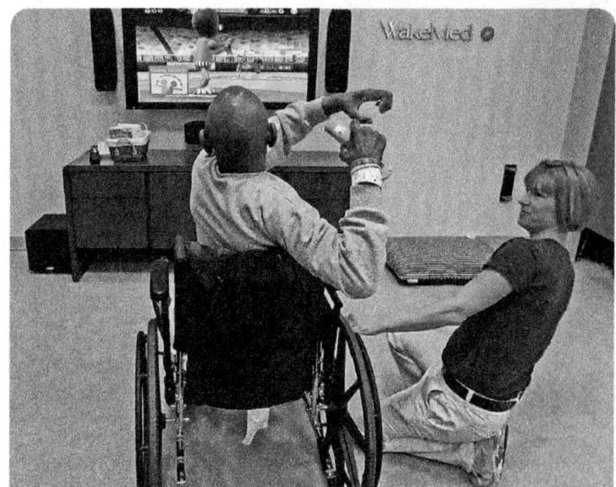

Fig. 17.4 Mental Health Technician Mental health aides and technicians may participate in social and recreational activities with patients. *What is the value of the healthcare worker's participation in activities?*

Mental health technicians may work in the same areas as aides, or they may specialize in crisis intervention, substance abuse, or children's problems. Mental health technicians may work in crisis centers, substance abuse facilities, hospitals, social service centers, schools, or community mental health programs. Technicians observe and record patient behavior and present their findings to counselors, nurses, or other healthcare professionals.

In addition to helping patients dress, bathe, groom, and eat, mental health technicians socialize with patients. They also lead patients in educational and recreational activities (see **Figure 17.4**). Technicians may play games with patients, watch television with them, or participate in group activities, such as sports or field trips. They observe and report physical or behavioral signs that might be important to the professional staff. They accompany patients to and from examinations and treatments. Because they have such close contact with patients, mental health technicians can have a great deal of influence on their outlook and treatment.

Job Responsibilities of a Mental Health Technician

Responsibilities for mental health technicians vary according to the work setting and level of training. They may perform any of the following tasks depending upon their expertise and place of employment.

- Interview patients and their families and record information.
- Help develop and implement patient treatment plans.
- Observe patients and report any meaningful changes or developments to the professional staff.
- Lead individual and group counseling sessions, and therapy activities.
- Teach skills that help patients resolve problems that affect their day-to-day life.
- Check and record patients' vital signs.
- Assist supervisors in giving prescribed medication.
- Provide nursing care.

READING CHECK

Describe three responsibilities of a mental health technician.

Photo: Sara D. Davis/Stringer/Getty Images

The Social Worker

What people do social workers help?

Social workers help patients solve personal and family problems. They often work with patients who have social problems or who have a

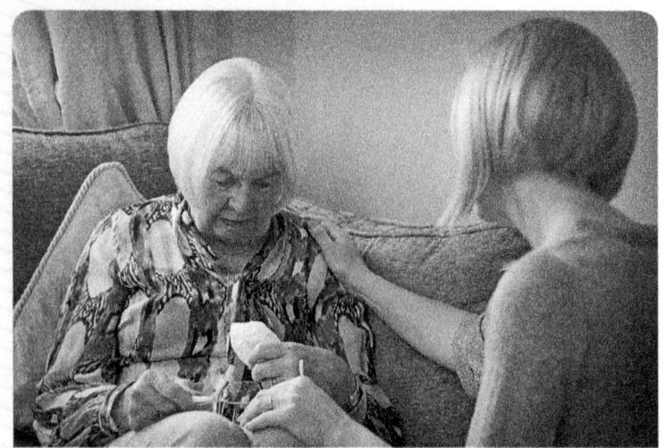

Fig. 17.5 Social Work Some social workers may work in long-term care to support patients who are grieving over the loss of their independence. *What are two other job responsibilities of a social worker?*

life-threatening disease. Such patients may have poor housing and/or be unemployed. They may not have any job skills and may be in financial distress (see **Figure 17.5**). Social workers also help patients living in inappropriate conditions. These conditions may involve abusive situations, which include spousal abuse or child abuse.

The Job of the Social Worker

Social workers help patients find resources for their mental and physical care, and may provide clinical counseling. They may work with community organizations to find patients good living accommodations. They may make referrals to other healthcare professionals, who provide patient support services. In those cases, the social worker follows up with patients to make sure those professionals are providing what is needed.

Social workers often provide case management for patients. They help patients direct their own healthcare and mental health treatments.

Social workers perform their duties in many different places. They may work for a state, city, or private group. If they work independently, they usually have an office. However, they may go to patients' homes, community settings, mental health centers, clinics, schools, correctional facilities, long-term care facilities, and acute care facilities.

Many positions for social workers are in hospitals, long-term care facilities, and community mental health agencies. They also help patients transition from living in a facility to living in the community.

Many times, social workers operate in emotionally charged situations. As such, they must be emotionally mature and able to view situations objectively. They must be able to work independently and behave responsibly. They must be able to work with patients without judging them.

The Job Responsibilities of the Social Worker

Social workers perform a great many tasks and duties, including activities to help patients with daily living. Social workers may delegate certain tasks to other healthcare providers. They work with the aged, and help deal with problems, such as poverty, crime, juvenile delinquency, mental illness, and social crisis. They may make a referral to a home health agency in order to obtain assistance with therapy, nursing care, or activities of daily living (ADL). They may also

- perform direct counseling.
- assist patients in finding effective solutions and community resources.
- refer patients to specialists.
- assist patients with eligibility requirements for community services.
- provide emotional support during a crisis.
- evaluate individuals in the criminal justice system and perform pre-sentencing assessments.
- arrange adoptions and foster homes.

- investigate reports of abuse and neglect.
- help patients cope with chronic, acute, or terminal illness.
- assess and diagnose student problems.
- work in employee assistance programs.
- develop social education programs.

READING CHECK

Describe three social worker responsibilities.

The Mental Health Counselor

Do you know your school counselor's educational background?

Counselors work in many settings (see **Figure 17.6**). They may be in schools or colleges, rehabilitation programs, or industrial or vocational settings. Or they may work as mental health counselors. In general, they help patients with personal, educational, or mental health problems.

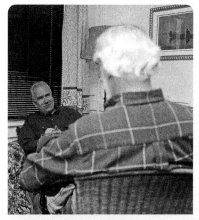

Fig. 17.6 Counselor A mental health counselor deals with patient problems daily. *Is counseling still necessary for older adults?*

Nearly two-thirds of counselors have master's degrees but, these degrees may be in many different areas. They may be in student affairs, elementary or secondary schooling, or career counseling. They may be in gerontology or in marriage, family, or community counseling. Substance abuse, rehabilitation, mental health, and psychology are other possible areas in which a counselor may be qualified to work.

Most states have requirements for credentialing, licensing, certification, or registration. It is important for counselors to know the regulations of the states in which they want to practice.

The Job of the Mental Health Counselor

People who plan to become counselors should first choose an area in which they wish to work. They may then direct their careers through the college courses they take. Counselor careers include the following.

- School and college counselors work with students to assess their abilities and develop plans for their education. Counselors help with career information, job search skills, or college information.
- Employment counselors assist patients with career decisions.
- Rehabilitation counselors help patients with social and/or vocational disabilities. They assess the strengths and limitations of patients. They also help patients develop and follow a rehabilitation plan.
- Mental health counselors may work with patients who are trying to deal with addictions, substance abuse, thoughts of suicide, stress, or a lack of self-esteem. Problems may be associated with aging, physical and mental diseases, or personal relationships. The mental health counselor works with other members of the mental health treatment team, including psychiatrists, psychologists, social workers, psychiatric nurses, and other counselors.

21st CENTURY SKILLS

Dealing with Anger

One job responsibility of a counselor or other mental healthcare professional is to help patients handle conflict without turning to violence. Violence usually occurs because of anger, which is a normal—and usually healthy—emotion. But when anger gets out of control and becomes destructive, it can lead to problems on the job, in personal relationships, and in the overall quality of life.

A mental healthcare employee must be able to control their anger and handle conflicts with patients and coworkers. Conflicts occur frequently in life, but must be dealt with correctly. Effective conflict resolution is a method of handling difficulties in a manner that is non-violent and constructive. Some tips for dealing with conflict include:

- Be understanding. Look at the situation from all points of view. People want to feel safe, understood, and respected. Put yourself in their shoes before you react.
- Think "win-win" and be prepared to compromise. Believe that there is a solution that will satisfy both parties. Use statements such as "I'd like to see if we can make this work for all of us" or "How can everyone come out of this on the positive side?"
- Make suggestions or proposals rather than demands. Brainstorm creative possibilities.
- If a compromise cannot be achieved, give the situation some time. Walk away or put some distance between the parties. Take the time to let everyone calm down. During that time, creative solutions may occur to you.
- In some situations, it may be best to "agree to disagree" and then move on to another topic.

The Job Responsibilities of the Mental Health Counselor

In general, the duties the mental health counselor may perform are:

- Assess abilities and personality characteristics
- Develop plans to help patients achieve goals
- Interview patients
- Meet with patients in counseling sessions
- Perform diagnostic tests
- Assist patients with common social and behavioral personal problems
- Offer drug and alcohol prevention programs
- Assist patients in anger management, helping them handle conflict without resorting to verbal or physical violence
- Identify abuse situations and intervene in them as appropriate
- Help patients overcome the effects of disabilities
- Assist patients who are addicted to various substances
- Work in suicide prevention programs
- Assist patients with stress management
- Help patients deal with problems of self-esteem

READING CHECK

List three job responsibilities of the counselor.

The Psychologist

Does your school have a psychologist on staff?

Psychologists are social scientists. They study human behavior and the mind. They work in many areas. A psychologist can be a research psychologist or a clinical psychologist. Most psychologists practice in clinical areas. They may also be consultants.

The Job of the Psychologist

Psychologists may specialize in a clinical area of practice. They may work in counseling centers, clinics, or acute care facilities. Their responsibilities are varied. They may help mentally and/or emotionally disturbed patients design plans to deal with the activities of daily living. They may help patients who are ill adjust to life changes. They also may help people to work through a personal crisis. **Figure 17.7** shows a counseling session.

Clinical psychologists may specialize in studying the mind and behavior of elderly patients in a specialty called **geropsychology.** A specialty dealing with patients who have neurological disorders is called **neuropsychology.** They may also choose counseling psychology, school psychology, experimental psychology, and a variety of other specialties.

The type of work psychologists do determines their work environment. Many psychologists have their own offices and set their own hours. Some psychologists work during the evening because that is when patients are available for appointments. Psychologists who work in an acute care setting may work evenings too, as well as weekends and holidays. Psychologists who are members of college and university faculties teach and may spend time in research activities. Some psychologists even testify as expert witnesses in court cases.

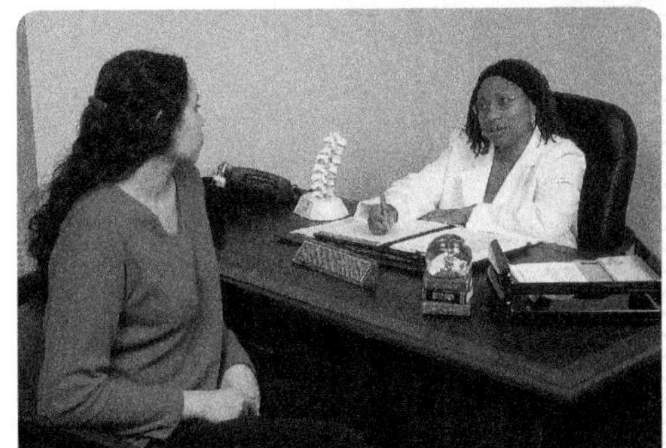

Fig. 17.7 Psychologists Psychologists may specialize in a number of different fields. *What types of patients do psychologists see?*

The Job Responsibilities of the Psychologist

It is impossible to list all the varied duties and responsibilities of a psychologist. However, there are certain key roles that are performed by most psychologists. Some job responsibilities are listed below.

- Perform diagnostic tests
- Provide individual, family, or group psychotherapy
- Assist patients with behavior modification
- Work with healthcare professionals on plans of care
- Teach and research
- Develop health promotion programs
- Work with patients who have had strokes or head injuries
- Work with elderly patients
- Assist people who are in crisis
- Assess students' behavioral problems
- Assist teachers and parents in dealing with children's issues
- Work with patients who have substance abuse problems
- Work with students with disabilities, or who are gifted and talented
- Assess a patient's interactions with others
- Study group behavior

READING CHECK

Name two possible psychologist job responsibilities.

The Psychiatrist

What is the difference between a psychiatrist and a psychologist?

Psychiatrists are physicians. They are either medical doctors (M.D.s) or doctors of osteopathic medicine (D.O.s), who have specialized in mental healthcare.

The Job of the Psychiatrist

In many cases, a psychiatrist heads up the mental health team. He or she is in charge of patient assessment and diagnosis. The psychiatrist

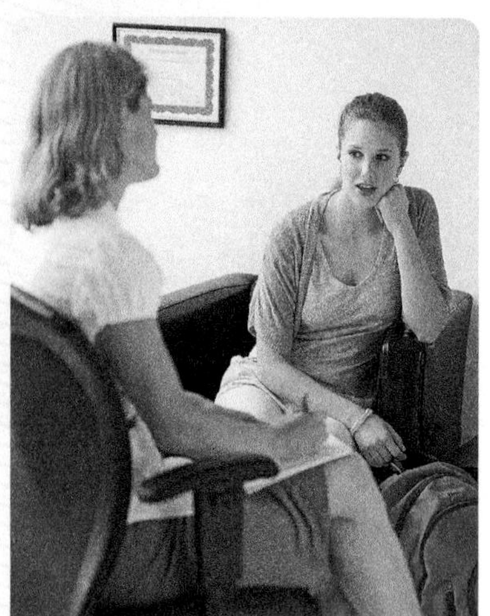

Fig. 17.8 **Psychiatrist** The psychiatrist is often the head of a mental health team. *What are the psychiatrist's major responsibilities as head of the mental healthcare team?*

also oversees the patient's plan of care. The rest of the mental healthcare team reports findings to the psychiatrist, who is responsible for making changes in treatment (see **Figure 17.8**).

Psychiatrists, like most physicians, work long hours. Many psychiatrists work in private practice, either with partners or alone. It can take between 11 and 16 years to complete the training to become a psychiatrist.

All states require physicians and psychiatrists to be licensed. Psychiatrists must graduate from an accredited medical school, pass a licensing examination, and complete a residency. However, each state has established individual licensing requirements.

The Job Responsibilities of the Psychiatrist

Individuals who want to practice as psychiatrists must be self-starters, have a strong desire to help people, and be able to deal with the pressure and workload of the required schooling. There may be many specific duties. A few are listed below.

- Diagnose and treat mental illnesses
- Prescribe medications
- Examine and administer treatments
- Perform diagnostic tests and interpret results
- Healthcare counseling
- Assist with personal crises
- Help develop plans for the activities of daily living
- Provide emergency mental and physical healthcare

SECTION 17.1 Careers in Mental Healthcare Review

AFTER YOU READ

1. **Describe** the main responsibilities of the mental health aide.
2. **Identify** some important personal characteristics needed by a mental healthcare professional.
3. **Compare** the duties of a mental health aide and a mental health technician.
4. **Discuss** how the duties of all mental healthcare professionals may overlap.
5. **Identify** the most important duty of all mental healthcare professionals.
6. **Explain** the main difference between a psychiatrist and a psychologist.
7. **Demonstrate** three therapeutic communication techniques.

Technology ONLINE EXPLORATIONS

Mental Healthcare Groups

Research the Internet or another source for mental healthcare consumer groups. Are any groups active in your area? Write a short paper on why you think a group like this might be needed. Include in your report an account of the activities of the group.

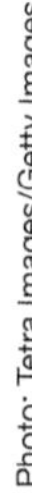

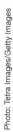

SECTION

17.2 Mental Health Procedures

Physical Restraints

When can physical restraints be used?

Restraints are anything that impedes a patient's movements. They may be physical or chemical. Restraints may not be used unless specific conditions are met. Patients have the right to be free from restraints and abuse, and the right to participate in activities. Restraints may violate either or both of these rights.

Restraints must be used sparingly and only under a physician's orders. They should be used only as needed to protect the patient or others from harm. When possible, try calming a patient. Restraints may be used to help prevent patients from falling out of bed, falling while walking, scratching at wounds, or pulling out IVs.

Bedside rails are considered restraints. Quarter side rails that only block half of one side of the bed may be used. In many facilities, keeping side rails up for those with mental problems is considered a standard of care. When using side rails, never leave a side rail down when you are not directly at the bedside and facing the bed.

Before any type of restraint is used, all other methods of ensuring patient safety must be assessed. Attempts to calm the patient should be made (see **Figure 17.9**).

See **Procedure 17-1** to learn more about using restraints. The restraints may be risky for some patients. Their use may also have legal implications for the healthcare professional. Here are some safety rules to follow.

- Make sure you use the right size and type of restraint. If you have not been trained in applying restraints, ask a supervisor for directions.
- Make sure the patient is in a comfortable position after the restraint is applied. Check to see that the patient can move the body part that is restrained. Check that circulation below the restraint is good, and the patient can breathe easily. Notify a supervisor of any issues.
- Make sure that the patient's needs are taken care of while restrained. The restraint must be loosened or taken off at least every two hours.
- Never tie restraints to a bed's side rail. Use quick-release ties so the restraint can be removed quickly. Make sure scissors are available in case the restraint needs to be cut. Keep scissors in a safe place.

Vocabulary

Content Vocabulary

You will learn these content vocabulary terms in this section.

- **extremity**
- **reality orientation**
- **Do Not Resuscitate (DNR)**
- **postmortem care**

Academic Vocabulary

You will see this word in your reading and on your tests. Find its meaning in the Glossary in the back of this book.

- **inevitable**

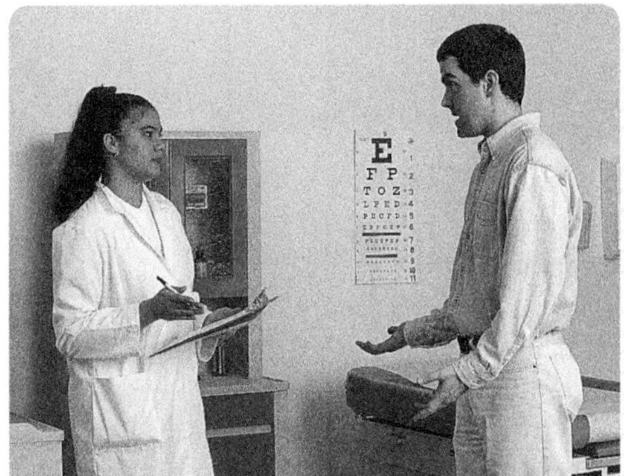

Fig. 17.9 Calming Patients Patients often become frustrated or agitated. *How would you deal with an agitated patient?*

Photo: David Kelly Crow

- Never leave a patient unattended when restraints are removed.
- Document all information concerning restraints completely.

READING CHECK

Explain why all other methods of ensuring patient safety should be assessed and eliminated before any type of restraint is used.

Depression

Have you ever felt depressed?

Feeling depressed and being in a mental state of depression are not the same. Individuals who have depression often see the world in bleak and hopeless terms. They can withdraw from social contact and may be unable to work or function in a family setting. Depression can result from a physical ailment or be a reaction to a medication.

Feeling depressed can be, but is not always, a sign of the mental state of depression. Usually, people who feel depressed are still able to function. In contrast, a mental state of depression is long-lasting, and in serious cases results in an inability to function. Suicidal thoughts and suicide attempts may occur. Depression is a common mental disorder that is usually curable with therapy and medication.

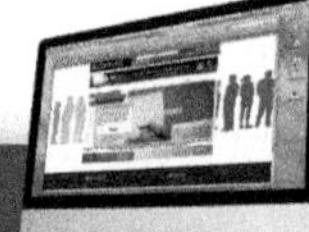

connect ONLINE PROCEDURES

PROCEDURE 17-1

Applying a Physical Restraint

Physical restraints must be used sparingly and only when a physician orders them. If used, restraints should be applied only as needed to protect the patient or others from harm. Restraints may be used to help prevent patients from falling out of bed, falling while walking, scratching at wounds, pulling out IVs, or harming themselves or others.

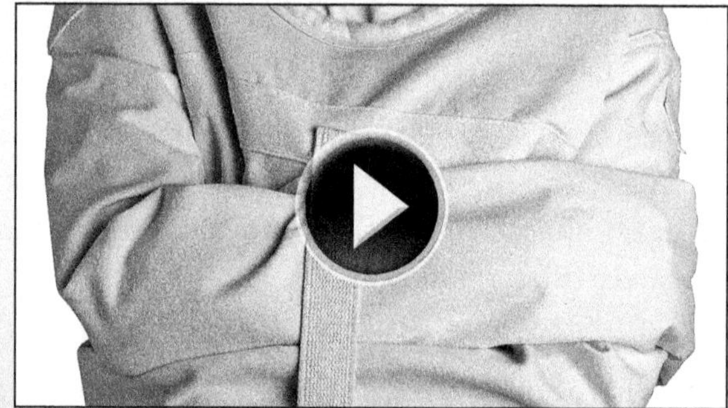

PROCEDURE 17-2

Administering Chemical Restraints

Unless a patient presents a clear and present danger that cannot be treated through other means, chemical restraints should not be used. There are strict rules on who may and may not administer chemical restraints, which are medications. If you are adequately trained and your state and facility permit you to administer medications, practice caution.

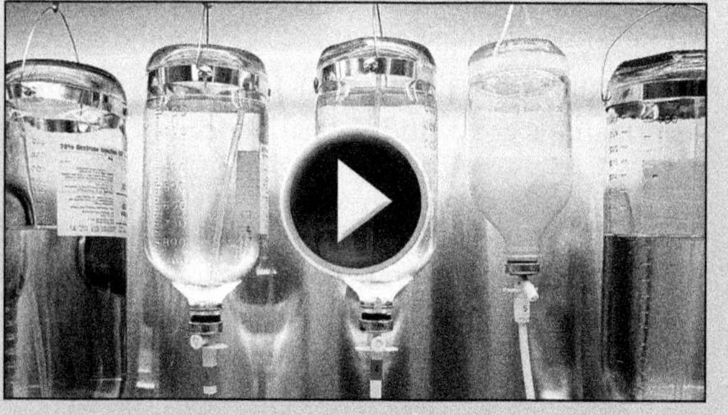

Photos: (t)Brand X Pictures/Getty Images, (b)PhotoLink/Photodisc/Getty Images

Chemical Restraints

Do you know when chemical restraints may be used?

Healthcare professionals must make sure that patients' rights to freedom of movement are respected. Unless a patient presents a clear and present danger that cannot be treated through other means, chemical restraints should not be used. There are strict rules on who may and may not administer chemical restraints, which are medications.

Administering medication is serious business. See **Procedure 17-2** to learn how to use this skill. If you are adequately trained and your state and facility permits you to administer medications, practice caution. Remember these points:

- A physician or authorized prescriber must prescribe the medication. That physician or another licensed practitioner is responsible for explaining the medication and its effects to you and the patient.
- Any time a medication is given, patient rights for medication administration must be followed.
- Positive identification with two patient identifiers is mandatory. Check an identification bracelet or have the patient show you some type of identification. If you are not 100 percent certain that you have correctly identified the patient, do not give the medication.
- If you are giving a medication, make sure that it is taken. Do not leave it at the bedside or assume that the patient has swallowed it. Observe the patient until you are certain that the medicine is taken.

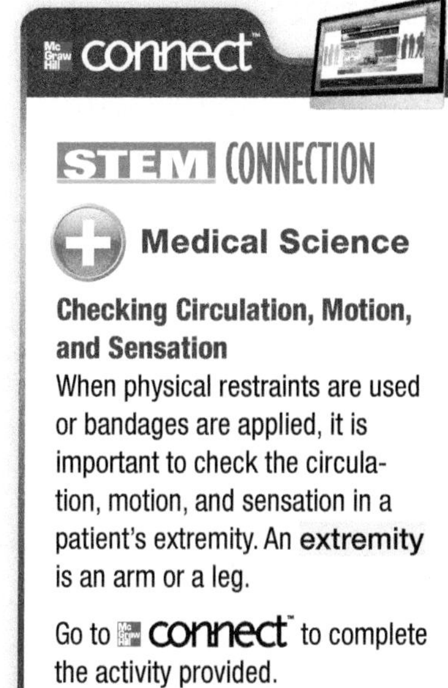

connect
STEM CONNECTION
Medical Science
Checking Circulation, Motion, and Sensation
When physical restraints are used or bandages are applied, it is important to check the circulation, motion, and sensation in a patient's extremity. An extremity is an arm or a leg.
Go to connect to complete the activity provided.

READING CHECK

Describe the only situation in which chemical restraints should be used.

Reality Orientation

How can a medical professional help a confused patient?

People with mental health disorders sometimes become confused. They may react inappropriately to activities going on around them. They may be unable to focus on what they are doing. They may become lost and wander. They may not be able to follow directions.

However, diseases such as Alzheimer's and depression may have the same results. Older people may become confused for many reasons such as illness, new surroundings, and dehydration.

You can use a variety of methods to help confused patients. One technique is called **reality orientation,** which is helping the patient

21ST CENTURY SKILLS

Effective Listening

Healthcare professionals need to provide emotional support for patients. One of the first steps to take is to become an effective listener.

Effective listening requires active listening. To listen actively takes time and effort. We are all busy, and often what we are thinking about interferes with our active listening.

become aware of his or her surroundings, the date and time, and other information about his or her present situation (see **Procedure 17-3**).

If the healthcare professional remains calm and reassuring, the patient is less likely to feel threatened. Loud noises, the use of force, and scolding may increase a patient's anxiety and confusion. Always approach the patient from the front so as not to startle them. Speak slowly and clearly. Make sure that the patient understands what you are saying.

Sometimes patients will respond to a gentle touch. Try holding the patient's hand, patting or rubbing their back, or even singing softly. However, be alert to patients who might become violent. Do not touch them if it seems to increase their distress. Always encourage patients to express their feelings. Try to distract those who become disruptive.

READING CHECK

Recall three reasons why older people might become confused.

Postmortem Care

Do you know the five stages of grief and loss?

An inevitable part of healthcare is that sometimes patients will die. Providing care for patients who are dying can be very difficult.

connect ONLINE PROCEDURES

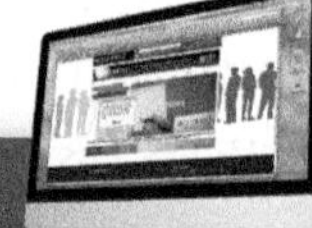

PROCEDURE 17-3

Providing Reality Orientation

Elderly patients or those who have mental health disorders sometimes become confused. They may react inappropriately to activities going on around them. They may be unable to focus on what they are doing. They may become lost and wander. They may not be able to follow directions. In these cases reality orientation may be useful.

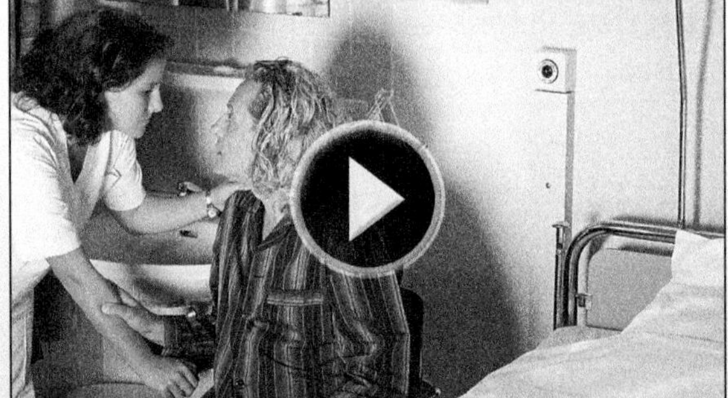

PROCEDURE 17-4

Providing Postmortem Care

Postmortem care is provided to patients after they die to help maintain their dignity and appearance. You should not provide postmortem care until you are instructed to do so. If the family members wish to view the body, it is important that the body be neat and clean.

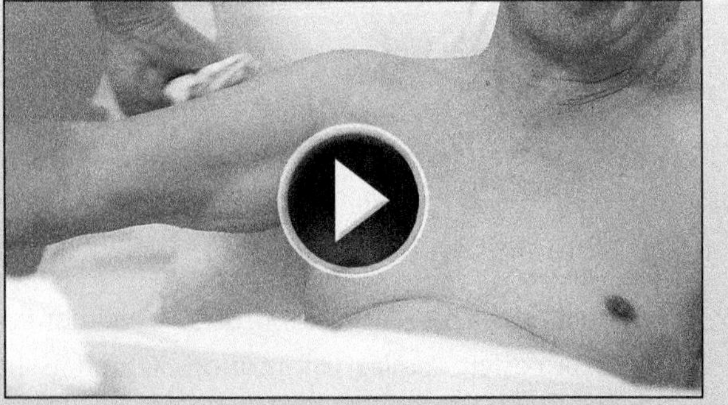

Photos: (t)Color Day Production/Riser/Getty Images, (b)Dex Image/Alamy

Dr. Elisabeth Kübler-Ross studied the emotions of dying patients. She identified the stages people go through prior to death. These five stages of grief and loss are denial, anger, bargaining, depression, and acceptance. Review these when you prepare to care for dying patients. See the 21st Century Skills box at right for a description of each stage.

Understanding these stages will help healthcare professionals to support their patients. Care providers may also feel grief when they care for dying patients and may experience the stages themselves.

Healthcare professionals must deal with their own thoughts about death. Never avoid a dying patient. Often the most helpful thing you can do is to sit and listen, hold a patient's hand, or just be there.

It is important to ensure that a dying patient's wishes are respected. All patients have the right to a **Do Not Resuscitate (DNR)** order, or a No Code order. This means that no extraordinary measures will be taken to prevent a patient's death. The patient can request several different levels of care during this time. Know what each patient's request is. If you are unsure, check with your licensed supervisor.

When a patient dies, a physician or supervising nurse must certify the death. The doctor or the nurse is also responsible for notifying the patient's family. When a patient dies, there is no pulse, respiration, or blood pressure. The eyes will be fixed and dilated.

Postmortem care is provided after a patient dies to help maintain dignity. Do not provide postmortem care until you are instructed to do so. If family members wish to view the body, it is important that it be neat and clean. See **Procedure 17.4** for more about postmortem care.

21ST CENTURY SKILLS

Communication

Understanding the Stages of Grief, Death, and Loss are invaluable to healthcare professionals as they deal with dying patients and their loved ones.

Denial Periods of disbelief; generally temporary

Anger Sudden realization of what is really happening; causes anger, temper tantrums, and fits of rage.

Bargaining Making deals with God, physicians, clergy, and family members; hoping for just a little more time or to survive until a scheduled event.

Depression Withdrawal, lethargy and sobbing

Acceptance Being at peace; Able to make arrangements for funeral or burial requests.

READING CHECK

Explain what a DNR order means.

SECTION 17.2 Mental Health Procedures Review

AFTER YOU READ

1. **Discuss** how restraints may violate a patient's rights.
2. **Discuss** how it might feel to be restrained against your will.
3. **Explain** how a mental healthcare professional can help patients with reality orientation.
4. **Analyze** why it would be important to report a patient's confusion to a supervisor if that patient is not normally confused.
5. **Identify** the five stages of grief and loss.

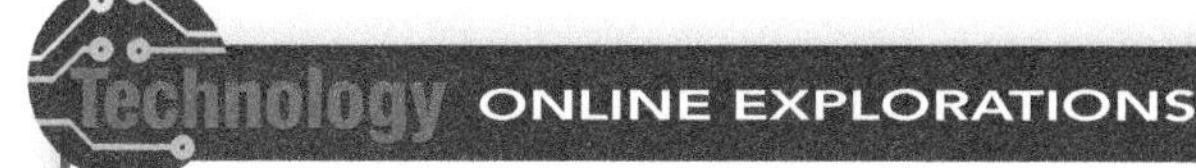

Grief and Loss

Search online for more information about the stages of grieving. Review each stage carefully. Have you ever lost someone in your life? Relate each stage of grieving to your own personal experience in coming to terms with loss.

CHAPTER 17 Review

Chapter Summary

SECTION 17.1

- Mental health aides may work directly with patients, or they may arrange care for them. The most important responsibilities of the mental health aide are to protect patient safety and report significant changes to a supervisor. **(pg. 456)**
- Mental health technicians usually have more formal education, training, and responsibilities than mental health aides. Technicians observe and record patient behavior and present their findings to counselors, nurses, and other professionals. **(pg. 460)**
- Social workers help patients solve personal and family problems. They can choose from many different areas in which to work. Social workers may work directly or indirectly with clients. **(pg. 461)**
- Counselors work with patients to help solve personal and family problems. Counselors can specialize in many different areas. Their duties depend upon the area in which they practice. Most counselor positions require a master's degree in a related field. **(pg. 463)**
- Psychologists are social scientists who study human behavior and the mind. They may work directly with patients, providing them mental healthcare. They may work indirectly with patients by doing research or teaching. In general, a doctorate is required to qualify as a psychologist. **(pg. 464)**
- Psychiatrists are physicians who specialize in mental healthcare. The education required is extensive. All states require that psychiatrists be licensed. The psychiatrist frequently heads up the mental healthcare team. **(pg. 465)**

SECTION 17.2

- Restraints impede a patient's movements. Concern for patients' rights prohibits the use of restraints unless very specific conditions are met. Many safety and legal issues must be considered when restraints are used. Unless a patient presents a clear and present danger that cannot be handled through other means, restraints should not be used. **(pg. 467)**
- People who are confused react inappropriately to stimuli in the environment. Reality orientation is one technique used to help patients who are confused. **(pg. 469)**
- Caregivers must be emotionally able to deal with death. They must respect patients' wishes regarding care as their death approaches. Postmortem care is preparing the body for the family to view and for transportation to the morgue. **(pg. 471)**
- Patient dignity and rights must be maintained in all healthcare settings. It is important for the mental healthcare professional to know what patients' rights are and to protect those rights. **(pg. 471)**

CHAPTER 17 Assessment

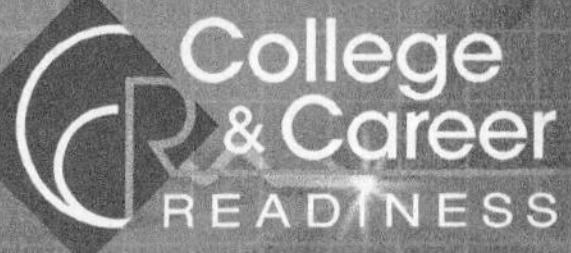

Critical Thinking/Problem Solving

1. The patient you are working with, a child, tells you that his caretaker hit him last night and he is afraid to go home. You know the caretaker and you do not believe that she is capable of such an action. What should you do?

2. A new employee who is working as a mental health technician says, "Let's put a restraint on our patient. He has really been a lot of trouble lately, and he may fall out of bed." What should you say or do?

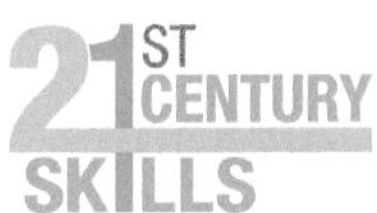

3. **Listening** Practice effective and reflective listening. Question a partner about an event that caused him or her to feel excited, happy, or depressed. After the partner has described those feelings, reflect back to him or her, in your own words, what you believe you heard. Give your partner time to think about what you just said. Did you really understand what he or she was describing? Were you communicating and listening effectively?

4. **Teamwork** With two partners, practice providing emotional support for a dying patient and his or her family. Take turns role-playing the caregiver, patient, and family member.

5. **Teamwork** Obtain a restraint and apply it to a partner. Remove the restraint. Next, have your partner apply the restraint to you and then remove it. Imagine that you are a patient and write a short paragraph about how it feels to be in a restraint. Describe some of the dangers that might be present when you are in the restraint.

6. **Information Literacy** Search online for a specific mental health disease or disorder. Develop a multimedia presentation or brochure that could be used to teach the general public about the condition.

McGraw Hill connect™ ONLINE ACTIVITIES

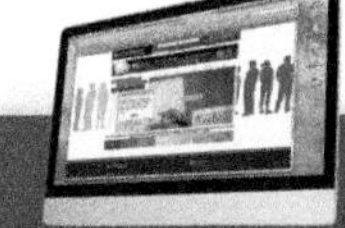

Complete our HST online activities for Chapter 17, which include Concept Check review questions, Reference Flash Cards, and Online Procedures assessment sheets.

- **Concept Check** review questions
- **Reference Flash Cards** medical terminology practice
- **Online Procedures** assessment sheets

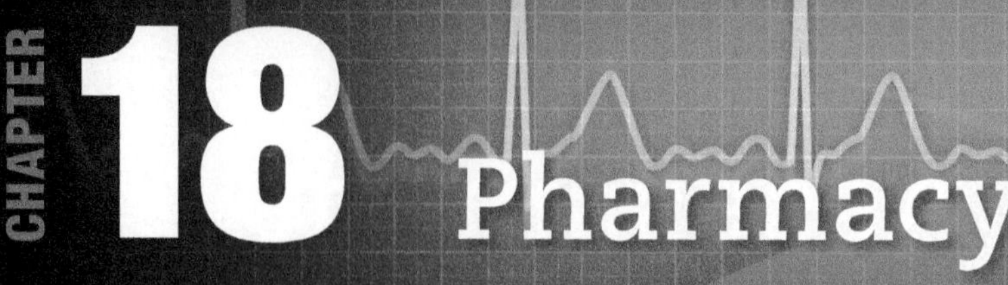

CHAPTER 18 Pharmacy

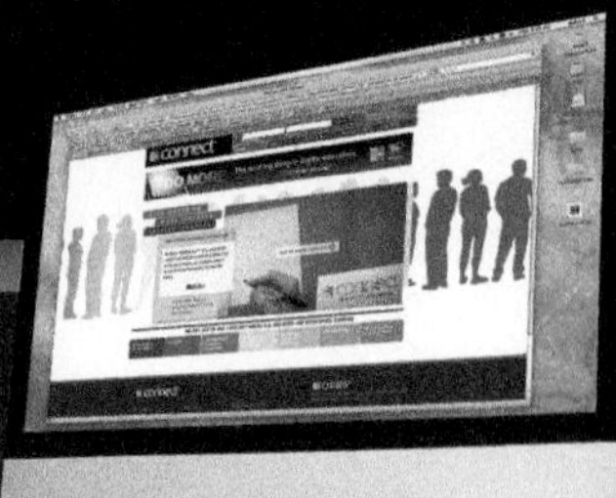

McGraw Hill connect™

It's Online!

- Online Procedures
- STEM Connection
- Medical Science
- Medical Terms
- Medical Math
- Ethics in Action
- Virtual Lab

Essential Question:

Have you ever had a prescription filled at a pharmacy?

Pharmacists, pharmacy aides, and pharmacy technicians play a vital role in providing medications prescribed by physicians. Pharmacy workers measure and fill prescriptions; advise patients on usage, drug interactions, and possible side effects; and provide information about over-the-counter drugs. In this chapter, you will learn about the activities and responsibilities of pharmacy employees.

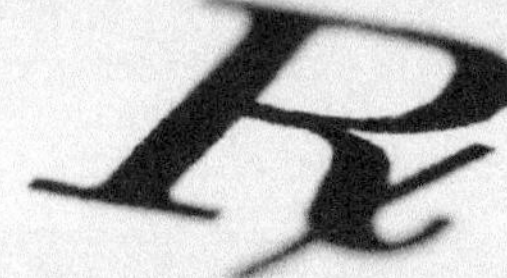

Photo: Tom Grill/Photographer's Choice RF/Getty Images

READING GUIDE

OBJECTIVES

After completing this chapter, you will be able to:

- **Compare** the roles and responsibilities of the pharmacy aide to those of the pharmacy technician.
- **Describe** the education and responsibilities of the pharmacist.
- **Identify** the pharmacy specialty areas.
- **Describe** the additional career opportunities available in the field of pharmacy.
- **Demonstrate** two pharmacy procedures to your classmates.

BEFORE YOU READ

Connect Have you ever talked with a member of a pharmacy staff before making a purchase?

Main Idea

Pharmacy aides, pharmacy technicians, and pharmacists all play essential roles in providing both medication and advice about medication to patients.

Note-Taking Activity

Draw this table. Write key terms and phrases under **Cues**. Write main ideas under **Note Taking**. Summarize the section under **Summary**.

Cues	Note Taking
o	o
o	o
Summary	

Graphic Organizer

Before you read the chapter, draw a diagram like the one to the right. As you read, write the pharmacy careers and procedures covered by the chapter into the diagram.

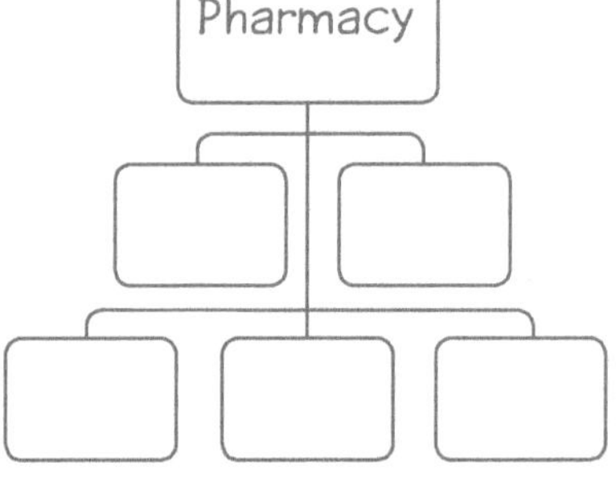

connect

Downloadable graphic organizers can be accessed online.

STANDARDS

HEALTH SCIENCE

NCHSE 1.31 Apply mathematical computations related to healthcare procedures (metric and household, conversions and measurements).

NCHSE 11.11 Identify records and files common to the healthcare setting.

NCHSE 11.21 Communicate using technology (fax, e-mail, and Internet) to access and distribute data and other information.

SCIENCE

NSES F Develop understanding of personal and community health.

NCHSE *National Consortium for Health Science Education*

NSES *National Science Education Standards*

COMMON CORE STATE STANDARDS

MATHEMATICS

Number and Quantity

N-Q Quantities Reason quantitatively and use units to solve problems.

ENGLISH LANGUAGE ARTS

Speaking and Listening

Comprehension and Collaboration SL-2 Integrate multiple sources of information presented in diverse media or formats (e.g., visually, quantitatively, orally) evaluating the credibility and accuracy of each source.

Writing

Research to Build and Present Knowledge W-9 Draw evidence from literary or informational texts to support analysis, reflection, and research.

SECTION 18.1 Careers in Pharmacy

Vocabulary

Content Vocabulary

You will learn these content vocabulary terms in this section.

- **pharmacy aide**
- **pharmacy technician**
- **pharmacist**
- **franchise**

Academic Vocabulary

You will see these words in your reading and on your tests. Find their meanings in the Glossary in the back of this book.

- **diverse**
- **diminish**

The Pharmacy Aide

What makes the pharmacy aide position a good entry-level job?

Pharmacy is a diverse field, involving professionals in many different areas who have a wide variety of educational backgrounds. The most familiar and visible members of the pharmaceutical industry are the individuals who fill or assist in filling prescriptions and who educate the client on how to use medications safely and correctly. These are **pharmacy aides, pharmacy technicians,** and **pharmacists,** the professionals licensed to prepare and dispense drugs.

Pharmacy aides help licensed pharmacists with clerical duties. Aides often are clerks or cashiers. Their chief duties are to answer telephones, and handle billing and payments. They also stock shelves. They may work closely with pharmacy technicians, who usually perform more complex tasks than aides. In some states, however, their duties overlap.

Most pharmacy aides have at least a high school diploma and receive informal on-the-job training. Formal pharmacy aide training is also sometimes offered in technical high schools. Previous experience as a cashier may be an advantage to those seeking jobs as pharmacy aides.

Table 18.1 Overview of Pharmacy Careers

OCCUPATION	EDUCATIONAL REQUIREMENTS	CERTIFICATION OR LICENSING AGENCY	JOB OUTLOOK
Pharmacy Aide	Technical or on-the-job training	None	Average growth due to the increased pharmacy needs of a larger and aging population and to the increasing use of medication
Pharmacy Technician	Technical or college training of six months to two years, ending with either a certificate or associate degree	Pharmacy Technician Certification Board	Much faster than average due to the needed expansion of retail pharmacies and other employment settings as a result of population growth and aging
Pharmacist	A minimum of six years at an accredited school of pharmacy, to earn a master's degree or doctorate. Must serve an internship under a licensed pharmacist	Examination required, regulated by each state	Average growth due to the increased pharmacy needs of a larger and aging population and to the increasing use of medication

Job Responsibilities of the Pharmacy Aide

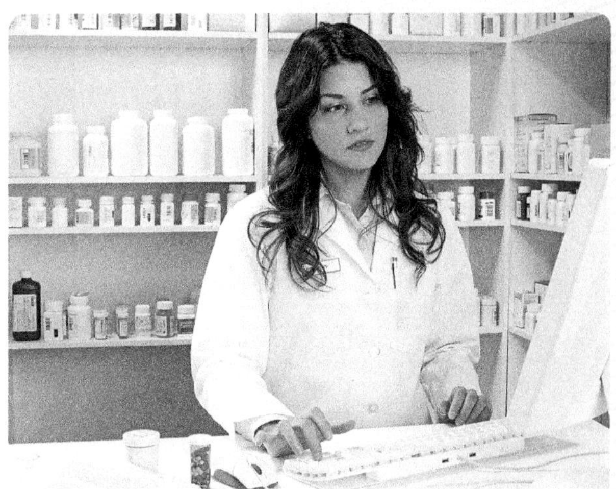

Fig. 18.1 Pharmacy Aide Skills A pharmacy aide at work. *Why would a pharmacy aide need to know how to use a computer?*

To be a successful pharmacy aide, you must have the following qualities and background:

- Strong customer service and communication skills
- Experience using a computer (see **Figure 18.1**)
- Organizational skills, dedication, a friendly manner, and a sense of responsibility
- Willingness and ability to follow directions
- No prior record of drug or substance abuse
- Ability to work in a team with technicians and pharmacists
- Ability to perform repetitious work accurately
- Good basic mathematical skills and good manual dexterity
- Neat appearance, and the ability to deal pleasantly and tactfully with customers

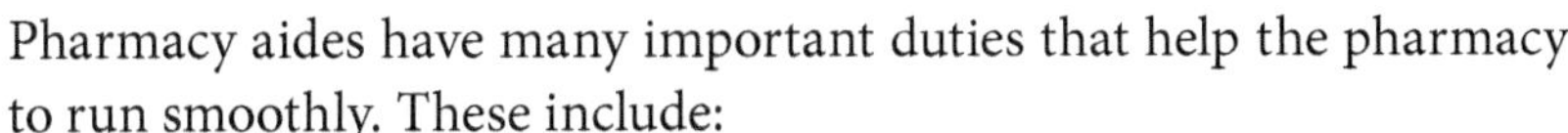

Pharmacy aides have many important duties that help the pharmacy to run smoothly. These include:

- Establishing and maintaining client profiles
- Preparing insurance claim forms
- Stocking and taking inventory of prescription and over-the-counter medications
- Maintaining inventory and informing the supervisor of stock needs
- Cleaning pharmacy equipment
- Helping with the maintenance of equipment and supplies
- Managing the cash register

READING CHECK

List several of the retail-oriented tasks of a pharmacy aide.

The Pharmacy Technician

How does a pharmacy technician assist the pharmacist?

Pharmacy technicians work in a hospital or a retail pharmacy, under the direction of a pharmacist. Their main role is to help the pharmacist.

Pharmacy technicians prepare and fill prescriptions. They may issue medicine and also label and store supplies. Like other professionals in this field, they must be able to communicate well with people from diverse backgrounds. They must also be able to assist with the administrative and clerical tasks required to keep the pharmacy operating smoothly.

Photo: upiterimages/Comstock Images/Getty Images

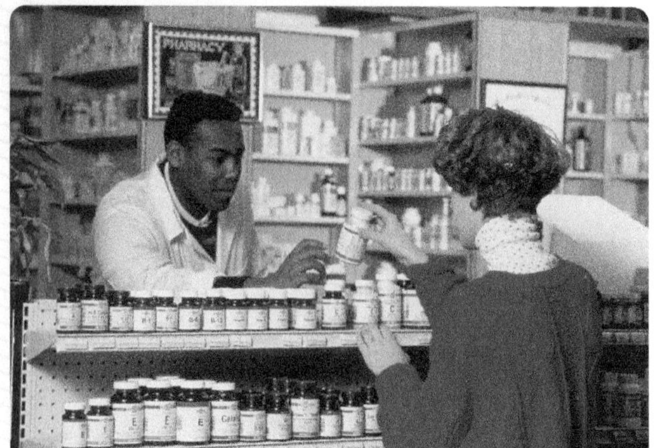

Fig. 18.2 Pharmacy Jobs Many pharmacies employ a pharmacist and a pharmacy technician or pharmacy aide. *What are three duties performed by the technician?*

Job Responsibilities of the Pharmacy Technician

As a pharmacy technician, you will need to know the basics such as reading, filling, and dispensing prescriptions. When preparing medication, you will

- receive prescriptions or requests for prescription refills when there is no change to the prescription (see **Figure 18.2**).
- verify the accuracy and completeness of the prescription information.
- retrieve, count, pour, weigh, measure, and sometimes mix the medication.
- prepare the prescription labels.
- select the type of container.
- affix the prescription and auxiliary labels to the container.

A pharmacy technician also has many other duties, including:

- Answering the phone and performing other clerical duties
- Referring any questions regarding prescriptions, drug information, or health matters to a pharmacist
- Completing claim forms, and billing insurance companies to ensure that payment is received for medications
- Preparing intravenous medications and chemotherapy
- Establishing and maintaining client profiles
- Taking inventory of both prescription and non-prescription medications
- Ordering new supplies of medications as needed
- Maintaining the pharmacy equipment

READING CHECK

Summarize the tasks that a pharmacy technician performs when filling prescriptions.

The Pharmacist

How does a pharmacist help customers?

Registered pharmacists must earn a doctor of pharmacy degree (PharmD) from an accredited college of pharmacy. The PharmD program will take six to seven years. The first two years are considered prepharmacy, which is similar to premed. The student then applies to enter the pharmacy program. Admission is limited and highly competitive. The final stage of the student's education is clinical training when the student works as a pharmacy intern. Intern positions place the student in a number of different settings. These settings usually include both a community (retail) pharmacy and a hospital pharmacy.

Safety

Checking the Prescription

As a pharmacy aide or technician, you must always have the pharmacist do a final check on any medication that you have assisted in preparing. Do not provide the medication to the client or the hospital floor without the pharmacist's final check and approval.

After earning a degree, graduates take the state pharmacy board examination to become licensed as a pharmacist. Most pharmacists work in either a hospital or a community pharmacy.

Job Responsibilities of the Pharmacist

The most important responsibility of the pharmacist is to provide clients the correct medication in the correct amount. In addition, the pharmacist has many other responsibilities, some of which are listed here.

- Advise physicians and other health practitioners on the selection, dosages, interactions, and side effects of medications
- Counsel clients and answer questions about prescription drugs, including questions on possible adverse reactions or interactions
- Provide information about non-prescription drugs and make recommendations after asking a series of health questions, such as whether the customer is taking any other medications
- Complete third-party insurance forms and other paperwork
- Hire and supervise personnel and oversee the general operation of the pharmacy
- Prepare sterile solutions
- Purchase medical supplies
- Provide specialized services to help clients with smoking cessation and conditions such as diabetes, asthma, and high blood pressure
- Assess, plan, and monitor drug programs or regimens
- Evaluate drug use patterns and outcomes for clients in hospitals or managed care organizations
- Teach pharmacy students serving as interns in preparation for graduation and licensure
- Delegate prescription-filling and administrative tasks, and supervise their completion

READING CHECK

Recall some responsibilities of a pharmacist that involve the pharmacy's other personnel.

Preventive Care & Wellness

Drug Interactions

Drugs can sometimes interfere with each other, creating serious medical problems. Drug interactions will vary according to the dosage, age, sex, and overall health of the client. Follow these general rules:

- Ask a physician or pharmacist before consuming alcohol while taking any drug.
- Avoid cigarettes when taking certain drugs. Cigarettes can **diminish** the effectiveness of medication or create added hazards with certain medications.
- Avoid caffeine and alcohol, which can affect the action of some drugs.
- Consult a doctor before using medications during pregnancy.
- Consult a doctor before taking any medications—including vitamins, nutritional supplements, over-the-counter medications, and herbal remedies—before combining them or taking them along with medication.

Work Locations

Are pharmacists business owners?

Pharmacy employees may choose to work in many settings. Two of the most common are community (retail) pharmacies and hospital pharmacies.

Community or Retail Pharmacies

Community or retail pharmacies may be independently owned, part of a chain, or a franchise (see **Figure 18.3**).

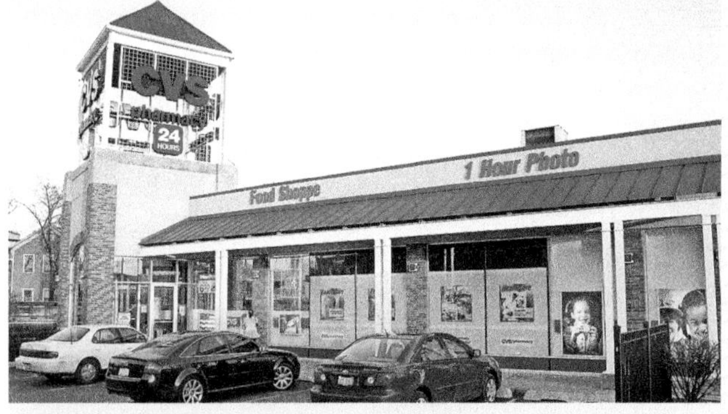

Fig. 18.3 Types of Pharmacies This is a CVS pharmacy. *What type of pharmacy is this?*

Independently owned pharmacies are not affiliated with any regional or national company. Often, they are owned by the pharmacist. A chain is a group of businesses of the same kind that are under the same ownership, or management. Many are part of a drug store chain. Grocery store and discount store chains may also have pharmacies.

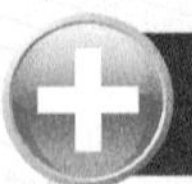

Safety

Hazardous Drugs

In a pharmacy, you may be exposed to hazardous drugs and/or materials. These require special handling to avoid personal injury or property damage. The hazardous drugs or materials may be corrosive or cytotoxic. Corrosive materials are substances that can damage body tissues. Cytotoxic materials are substances that are poisonous to cells. For example, anti-neoplastic drugs are cytotoxic. These medications are used to treat cancer and are most commonly found in hospital pharmacies. Adverse health effects from both acute and chronic exposures have been shown to occur in healthcare personnel. You should know the standard operating procedures, work practices, and protective equipment used to minimize the risk of exposure to hazardous drugs or materials, and receive appropriate training from your place of employment.

A **franchise** is an agreement that allows an individual or a group to use a company's name and sell its goods or services. It combines the qualities of an independent business and a large retail chain. The pharmacists who own franchises hire and supervise personnel, and oversee the business operations.

Hospital Pharmacies

A hospital pharmacy offers 24-hour service. Typically, a pharmacist is on duty at all times. As in a retail pharmacy, a hospital setting requires the pharmacist to prepare medications for clients and to counsel them on medications when they are about to be discharged from the hospital. Unlike a retail pharmacy, the hospital pharmacy prepares IV (intravenous) medications, stocks the nursing stations, and may deliver medications to clients' rooms.

One of the most important duties of a hospital pharmacist is to stay well informed through education and networking. Pharmacists are expected to be able to provide information to physicians, and to advise them on appropriate and affordable medication therapy.

READING CHECK

Recall some job responsibilities that are unique to the hospital pharmacist.

Additional Pharmacy Career Opportunities

Why might a pharmacy technician want to become a pharmaceutical representative?

Pharmaceutical companies have research and development positions for those with health science backgrounds. Researchers help develop new medications. They also refine or improve existing ones. Company representatives are the link between drug companies and healthcare workers. They inform healthcare workers about new medications. Each of these roles is vital to the proper delivery of drug therapy.

Pharmaceutical Researchers

Pharmaceutical researchers usually have a graduate degree (either a master's degree or a Ph.D.) in a biological or chemical science. A person with a bachelor's degree must complete two or three additional years of college to earn a master's degree. It takes three or four additional years of college to earn a Ph.D. A researcher works as a part of a team in developing new medications, and each member of the team will have his or her own area of expertise. The ultimate goal of the pharmaceutical researcher is the development or refinement of drug therapies that will address unmet medical needs (see **Figure 18.4**).

Pharmaceutical Representatives

Pharmaceutical representatives usually have an associate's or bachelor's degree in a health field, and some training in business as well. Some pharmacy technicians and other healthcare professionals decide to change jobs to become representatives.

Before they can begin working for a pharmaceutical company, they will receive intensive training and education on the company's products. They distribute this information to healthcare workers by traveling to pharmacies, clinics, and hospitals to meet with doctors, nurses, and pharmacists.

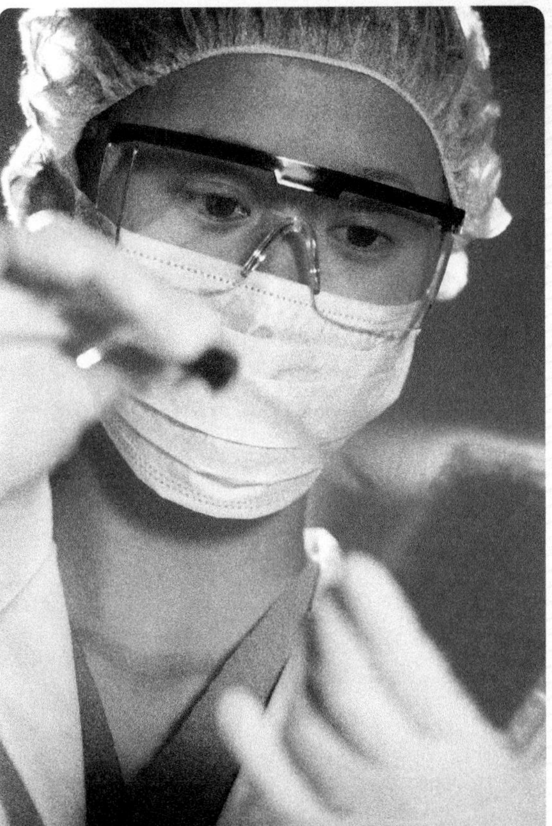

Fig. 18.4 Pharmaceutical Research A pharmaceutical researcher in a laboratory. *What is the main goal of a pharmaceutical researcher?*

Photo: Comstock Images/PictureQuest

READING CHECK

Identify the professional goal of the pharmaceutical researcher.

SECTION 18.1 Careers in Pharmacy Review

AFTER YOU READ

1. **Explain** the difference between a pharmacy aide and a pharmacy technician.
2. **Indicate** what would you say to client who asked you (the pharmacy aide) how much of a medication he or she should take.
3. **Indicate** how long it takes to complete a degree to become a pharmacist.
4. **Compare and contrast** hospital pharmacies and retail pharmacies.
5. **Identify** the degree needed to become a pharmaceutical researcher.
6. **Analyze** the role of a pharmaceutical representative.

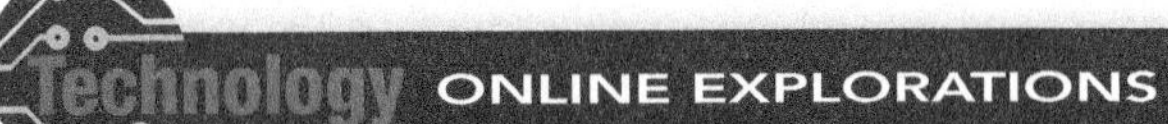

State Requirements

Determine the requirements for pharmacy aides and technicians in your state. Go online to locate a school for pharmacy technicians. Then find out whether you qualify to apply and how long the course of study takes to complete.

SECTION 18.2 Pharmacy Procedures

Vocabulary

Content Vocabulary

You will learn these content vocabulary terms in this section.

- **United States Pharmacopeia (USP)**
- **National Formulary (NF)**
- **over-the-counter (OTC) medication**
- **prescription medication**

Regulations and Procedures

What information can be found on drug labels?

Ordering, handling, and dispensing medications are the primary responsibilities of those who work in pharmacies. Following proper procedures is essential.

Federal Regulations

Since 1906, when the landmark Pure Food and Drug Act was passed, numerous laws have been enacted to regulate the composition, uses, names, labeling, and testing of drugs. Federal agencies, including the Food and Drug Administration (FDA) and the Drug Enforcement Administration (DEA) have been established to ensure that these laws are followed, and to investigate violations of these laws. **Table 18.2** summarizes the most important drug-regulation laws.

Table 18.2 Federal Law and Regulating Agencies

LEGISLATIVE ACT	ENFORCEMENT AGENCY
Pure Food and Drug Act of 1906 required drugs to meet official standards.	Bureau of Chemistry; later, Food and Drug Administration (FDA)
Food, Drug, and Cosmetic Act (FDCA) of 1938 replaced the 1906 act and includes additional regulations.	FDA
Comprehensive Drug Abuse Prevention and Control Act (CDAPCA) of 1970 requires the industry to maintain physical security and strict records for certain drugs.	Drug Enforcement Administration (DEA)
The Controlled Substances Act, Title II of the CDAPA, regulates manufacture and sale of narcotics and controlled drugs.	DEA
Drug Regulation and Reform Act of 1978 permits shorter investigation time for new drugs.	FDA
Orphan Drug Act of 1983 speeds up drug availability for clients with rare diseases.	FDA
Drug Price Competition and Patent Term Restoration Act of 1984 permits generic companies to produce generic equivalents without costly clinical trials.	FDA
Omnibus Budget Reconciliation Act of 1987 protects patient rights in long-term care facilities.	The Centers for Medicare and Medicaid Services (CMS)
Omnibus Budget Reconciliation Act of 1990 requires pharmacists to perform drug reviews and offer counseling on all medications to all patients.	CMS
Health Insurance Portability and Accountability Act (HIPAA) of 1996 protects a patient's protected health information (PHI).	Office for Civil Rights (OCR)

Drug Labels

In order to select the appropriate medication for a prescription, it is necessary to understand the information that appears on the drug label. Understanding this information is also very important for non-prescription medications. The following items are examples of information found on the drug label (see **Figure 18.5**).

- **Drug Name.** This usually includes the trade name (brand name) and the generic name. The brand name is registered with a specific company and is spelled with a capital letter. The generic name is the drug's official medical name found in the **United States Pharmacopeia (USP)** or **National Formulary (NF).** Both of these are national listings of medications. For example, Tylenol® is the brand name and acetaminophen is the generic name of a medication commonly used for pain and fever.
- **Form of the drug.** Manufacturers offer the same drugs in different forms. For example, penicillin may be dispensed as tablets, capsules, or a liquid.
- **Total number or volume in the container.** This is the total number of tablets or capsules, or the amount of liquid in the container.
- **Route of administration.** This is the way medication is to be taken. For example, it can be taken by mouth, as ear drops, as eye drops, or by other methods such as an injection, or topical (for creams and ointments).
- **Warnings.** These may include such statements as "May be habit forming," "High potency," "Not safe for pregnant women," "Avoid sunlight when taking this medication," "Do not operate heavy machinery when taking this medication," or "Take with food."
- **Storage information.** Some drugs may need to be stored in the refrigerator or away from light.
- **Manufacturing information.** This includes the name of the manufacturer and the expiration date of the medication.

NDC 0591-0385-01 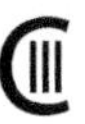

100 Tablets

Hydrocodone Bitartrate and Acetaminophen Tablets USP

7.5 mg-500 mg

℞ only

Booth

Fig. 18.5 Drug Label Drug labels provide pharmacists and consumers with important information. *Which items of information on this drug label can you identify?*

Packaging

Oral medications are sometimes packaged in unit-dose containers (see **Figure 18.6**). Although the box or other container is labeled, each dose of the medication is contained in a small foil or plastic package. They are most frequently dispensed by a hospital pharmacy, when the pharmacist is restocking the nursing care station medication cart.

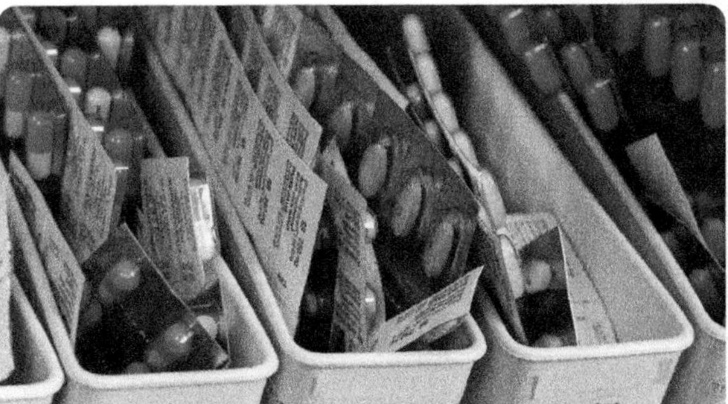

Fig. 18.6 Unit-Dose Packaging Unit dose packages separate each dose in plastic or foil. *Where are these containers most frequently dispensed?*

Non-prescription medications and prescription medications often are packaged in multiple-dose containers, which contain a number of doses of the medication (see **Figure 18.7**).

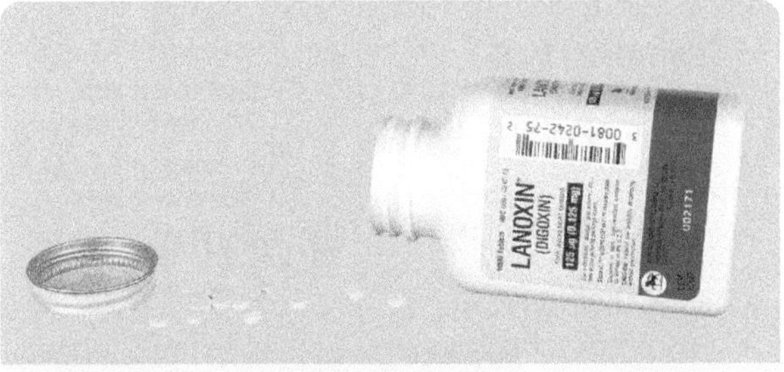

Fig. 18.7 Multiple-Dose Bottles Large bottles of multiple-dose medications are used to prepare prescriptions. *Do you know how to get medication out of this bottle without touching the pills?*

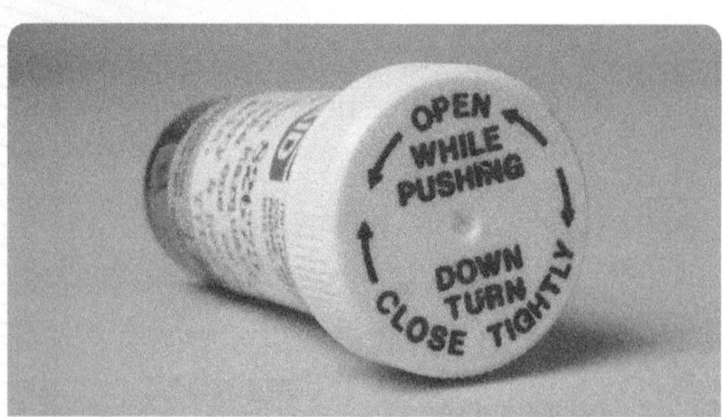

Fig. 18.8 Packaging A child-resistant container. *Why are child-resistant containers used?*

Child-Resistant Containers

Child-resistant containers are designed to be difficult for a child to open (see **Figure 18.8**). The Poison Prevention Act of 1970 requires, with some exceptions, that prescription drugs be packaged in child-resistant containers. However, if a physician orders or a client requests a non-child-resistant container, this is allowed. Clients who receive medication in a non-child-resistant container usually have to sign to acknowledge that they have requested such a container.

Over-the-Counter (OTC) Medications

Over-the-counter (OTC) or "non-prescription" medications are any medications that can be dispensed without a prescription. Caution should always be used when taking OTC medications, especially when not directed to do so by a physician. OTC medications can have side effects and also may interfere with other medication taken. Also, an OTC medication can be the same drug as a prescription medication, but in a lower dose (see **Figure 18.9**). For example, the drug Motrin (generic name ibuprofen) comes in an over-the-counter strength of 200 milligrams (mg). The prescription strength for this medication is 800 milligrams (mg).

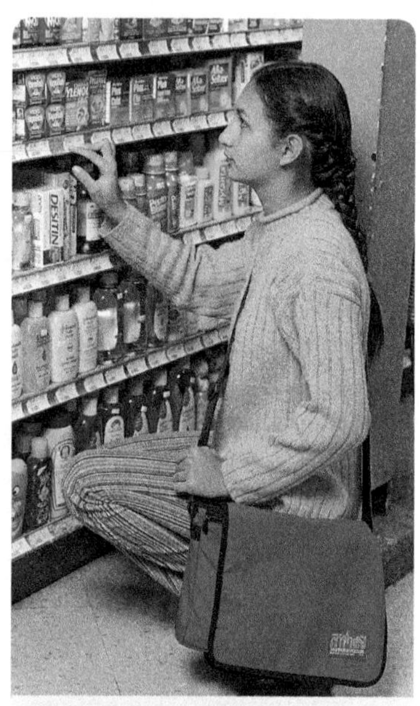

Fig. 18.9 Over-the-Counter Medications OTC medications can be dispensed without a prescription. *Why should you use caution when taking these medications?*

Ellen Trent, MD
14 Southwood Blvd.
Georgetown, Co 12345
989-555-1234

Name of the patient

Prescribed Date July 2, 2012

Name Arthur Simons DOB 4/29/49

Address

Rx: Doxycycline 100 mg — Drug and dose

QUANTITY: #20 — Quantity to dispense

SIG: cap I po BID pc — Instructions to appear on label

Refills 0 — Number of refills permitted

MD123456 — Prescriber ID — Prescriber number

E Trent MD — Signature — Physician name

Fig. 18.10 A Prescription for Medication *Why is a prescription necessary for certain medications?*

Prescription Medications

Prescription medications are sometimes also called legal drugs. **Figure 18.10** shows what a prescription might look like. These drugs can only be dispensed with a prescription and the label must state "Caution: Federal Law Prohibits Dispensing Without Prescription." Prescription drugs with the potential for abuse are classified under the Comprehensive Drug Abuse Prevention and Control Act of 1970.

Controlled Substances The Comprehensive Drug Abuse Prevention and Control Act (CDAPCA) of 1970 was created to combat and control drug abuse. The drugs and drug products that come under the jurisdiction of the CDAPCA are divided into five schedules, or categories, as

Photos: (t)Doug Martin, (b)McGraw-Hill Companies Inc./Ken Karp, photographer shown in **Table 18.3.** Controlled substances are placed on these schedules based upon their potential for abuse.

READING CHECK

Describe some common containers and packages used for medications.

Table 18.3 Controlled Substances Schedule Medications

Schedule I Substances:	No accepted medical use in the United States and a high abuse potential.	Examples: dihydromorphine heroin LSD
Schedule II Substances:	High abuse potential, with severe psychic or physical dependence liability. Schedule II controlled substances consist of certain narcotic, stimulant, and depressant drugs.	Examples: codeine hydromorphone (Dilaudid®) meperidine (Demerol®) methylphenidate (Ritalin®) oxycodone (Percodan®)
Schedule III Substances:	Abuse potential is less than that of substances in Schedules I and II. Includes compounds containing limited quantities of certain narcotic and non-narcotic drugs.	Examples: amobarbital compounds Fioricet® paregoric pentobarbital compounds secobarbital compounds Tylenol® with codeine
Schedule IV Substances:	Abuse potential is less than those substances listed in Schedule III.	Examples: alprazolam (Xanax®) chlordiazepoxide (Librium) detropropoxyphene (Darvon®) diazepam (Valium) flurazepam (Dalmane) lorazepam (Ativan®) meprobamate (Equanil, Miltown) midazolam (Versed®) phenobarbital
Schedule V Substance:	Less abuse potential than those substances listed in Schedule IV. Consist primarily of preparations containing limited quantities of certain narcotic and stimulant drugs, generally for antitussive (cough suppressant), antidiarrheal, and analgesic (pain relieving) purposes.	Examples: buprenorphine Lomotil® propylhexedrine

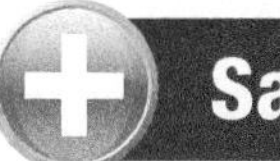

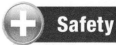

Safety

Customer Comments, Questions, and Complaints

Always take seriously a client who comments, questions, or complains about medication in any way. For example, if a client states that the pill looks "different," that he or she is having abnormal symptoms, or wants to know what to use to treat a cold, you should take the statement or question seriously. Always explore comments, questions, and/or complaints further and refer them to the pharmacist. It is never your responsibility to answer any questions. It is, however, your responsibility to notify the pharmacist that a comment, question, or complaint has been expressed.

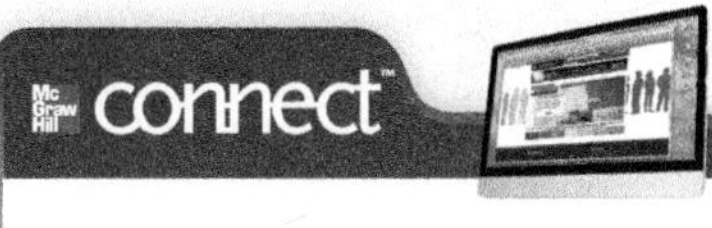

STEM CONNECTION

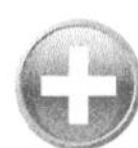

Medical Math

Estimating the Wait Time for Clients

When a client is going to wait to pick up a prescription, he or she usually wants to know roughly how long it will take. You will need certain information before you can give the client an estimate.

connect Go online to learn how to estimate the time it will take to fill a prescription.

connect ONLINE PROCEDURES

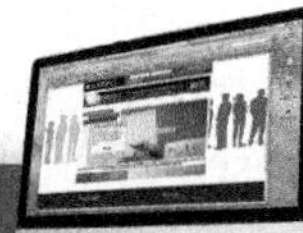

PROCEDURE 18-1

Reviewing Prescriptions and Medication Orders

For retail or community pharmacies, physician orders are given as prescriptions. Physician orders in a hospital are usually written on a medication order sheet. Both forms are written to include the drug, dose, route, frequency, and additional instructions.

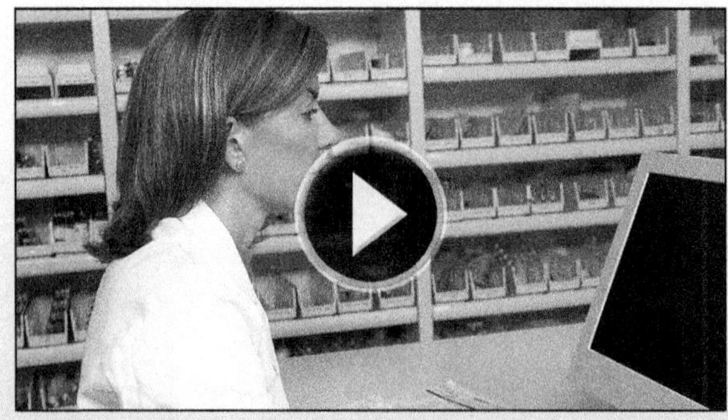

PROCEDURE 18-2

Creating a Patient Profile and Handling a Prescription

When working in a retail or independent pharmacy, you may be responsible for creating the patient profile and handling the prescription. The regulations governing your responsibilities vary based upon the size of the pharmacy, level of training, and your place of employment. Use this procedure as a guideline, and follow the facility's policies and procedures.

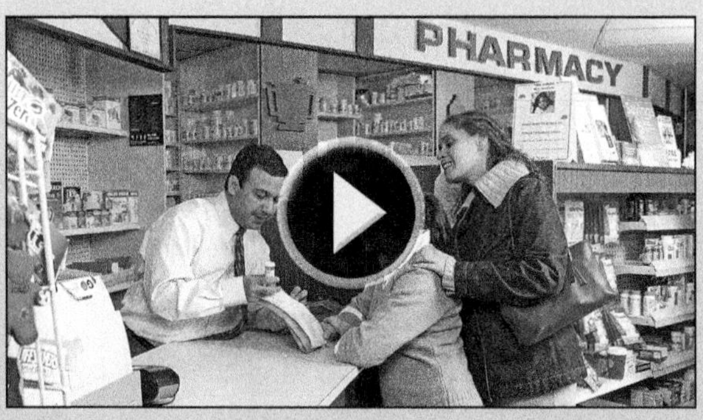

SECTION 18.2 Pharmacy Procedures Review

AFTER YOU READ

1. **Explain** why federal laws were passed regarding medications.
2. **Identify** the law and the agency that regulate the manufacture and sale of narcotics.
3. **Contrast** the generic name and the trade name of a drug.
4. **Describe** where unit dose medication packages are most commonly used.
5. **Explain** what a client who does not want a child-resistant container would have to do.
6. **Identify** two reasons for caution with OTC medications.
7. **Distinguish** between an OTC medication and a prescription medication.
8. **Indicate** some of the warnings that can be found on a prescribed medication label.
9. **Identify** at least three trade names and their corresponding generic names from the five controlled substance schedules.
10. **Name** the parts of a prescription.
11. **Analyze** what must you be able to do prior to receiving and handling a prescription.

Technology ONLINE EXPLORATIONS

Common Prescriptions

Go to the website www.rxlist.com. Look for the list of the top 200 prescription medications. Create a prescription for five of these medications. Be certain to include all the information required on a prescription.

Photos: (t)image100/Alamy, (b)McGraw-Hill Companies Inc./ Ken Karp, photographer

CHAPTER
18 Review

Chapter Summary

SECTION 18.1

- The pharmacy aide and the pharmacy technician may perform some of the same duties, depending on the state where they are working. However, pharmacy technicians usually perform more complex tasks. **(pg. 476)**
- The most important responsibilities for a pharmacist are to provide the correct medication for each client and to offer teaching and counseling regarding medications. **(pg. 479)**
- Two main pharmacy specialty areas are community, or retail, pharmacies and hospital pharmacies. **(pg. 479)**
- A pharmaceutical researcher may have a science degree, usually a Ph.D., and develops or improves medications, **(pg. 480)**
- A pharmaceutical representative may travel to various locations to promote and sell drugs manufactured by a specific pharmaceutical company. **(pg. 481)**

SECTION 18.2

- The drugs and drug products that come under the jurisdiction of the CDAPCA are divided into five categories or schedules. **(pg. 484)**
- When you review a prescription or physician order, all of the elements on that order must be legible and accurate. The client must be asked for identifying information. The pharmacist should be notified if any information about the medication is not legible. **(pg. 486)**
- You must know the following to create a client profile: identifying information, insurance and/or billing information, medical history, medication/prescription history, prescription preference, and refusal of information signature (if applicable). **(pg. 486)**

Mc Graw Hill connect™ ONLINE ACTIVITIES

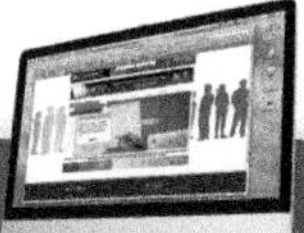

Complete our HST online activities for Chapter 18, which include Concept Check review questions, Reference Flash Cards, and Online Procedures assessment sheets.

- **Concept Check** review questions
- **Reference Flash Cards** medical terminology practice
- **Online Procedures** assessment sheets

CHAPTER 18 Assessment

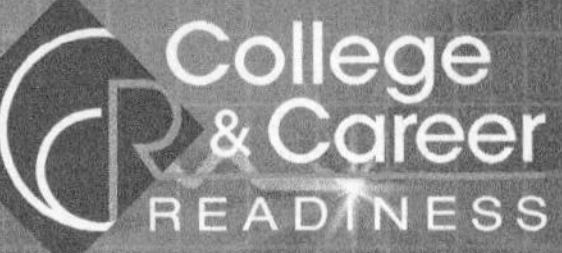

Critical Thinking/Problem Solving

1. You are a pharmacy technician. A client calls to say that she is "feeling funny" after taking one dose of a prescribed medication that she has never taken before. What should you do?
2. You are a pharmacy technician. A client asks you how much Tylenol she should take for a headache. What should you say?
3. You are a pharmacy technician and need to be alert for forged prescriptions. What might you look for when receiving a prescription to verify that it has not been forged?
4. Read the following physician orders. See Table 5.1 in Appendix B to review medical abbreviations
   a. Take Lipitor 80 mg po q am
   b. Promethazine 2 mL IM q4h prn for nausea

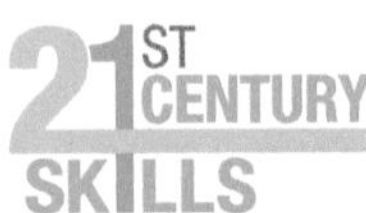

5. **Teamwork** Obtain a blank copy of a client profile. With a partner, role-play a pharmacy technician and a pharmacy client. Complete the client profile and then reverse roles.
6. **Information Literacy** Obtain copies of the *United States Pharmacopeia* (USP) and the *National Formulary* (NF). With a partner or in groups, look up common medications as assigned by your teacher. Prepare an oral presentation to discuss the medication or medications you researched.
7. **Information Literacy** Obtain a completed prescription and/or physician order. Identify each of the elements on the prescription or physician order as listed in **Procedure 18-1**.
8. **Information Literacy** Physician prescriptions can be now filled using the Internet. Go online to identify at least three websites on which you can have a prescription filled. Choose one such site and write a step-by-step summary of how the process works on that site. Explain how security is maintained so that the prescription is filled correctly and the medication goes to the correct client. Give your opinion as to how simple or complicated it is to fill a prescription on that site. Your report should also give your ideas on how the Internet could affect employment in the field of pharmacy.

CHAPTER 19 Respiratory Care

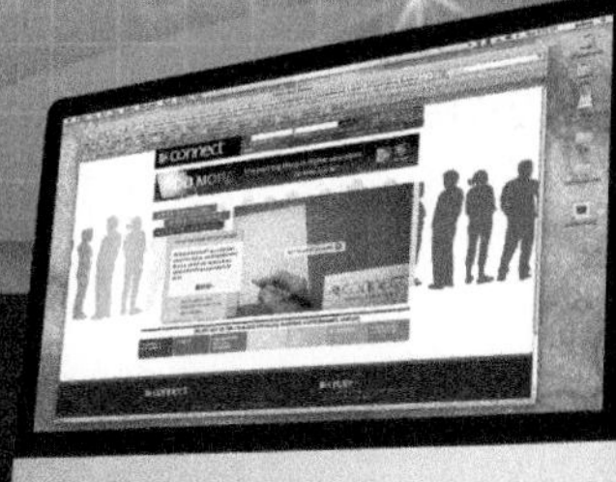

Essential Question:

How can breathing difficulties affect your entire body?

The basic goal of respiratory therapists is to help patients breathe more easily through the prevention and treatment of lung disease. They work in various settings, including hospitals, skilled nursing facilities, and patients' homes. Oxygen therapy, medicated aerosols, and hyperinflation therapy are three treatments for respiratory conditions that are discussed in this chapter.

McGraw Hill connect™

It's Online!

- **Online Procedures**
- **STEM Connection**
- **Medical Science**
- **Medical Terms**
- **Medical Math**
- **Ethics in Action**
- **Virtual Lab**

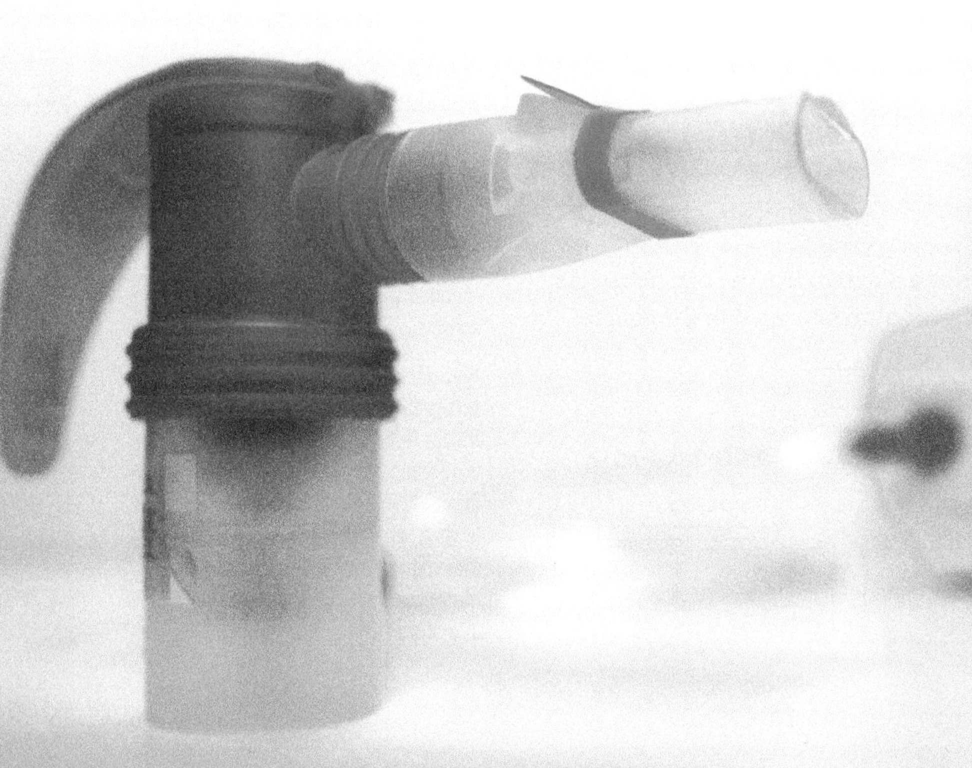

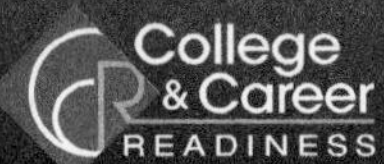

READING GUIDE

OBJECTIVES

After completing this chapter, you will be able to:

- **Recall** the respiratory system and its function.
- **Discuss** the services provided by respiratory care professionals.
- **Compare** diagnostic and therapeutic procedures performed by a respiratory therapist.
- **Describe** the therapeutic effects and hazards of oxygen therapy.
- **Arrange** to provide oxygen.
- **Compare** the advantages and disadvantages of aerosolized medications.
- **Evaluate** the outcomes of medicated aerosol therapy.
- **Explain** reasons for performing hyperinflation therapy.

BEFORE YOU READ

Connect Have you ever had a serious breathing problem? How did this affect your ability to function?

Main Idea

Respiratory therapists help people breathe more easily by providing respiratory care and helping to prevent lung disease.

Note-Taking Activity

Draw this table. Write key terms and phrases under **Cues**. Write main ideas under **Note Taking**. Summarize the section under **Summary**.

Cues	Note Taking
o o	o o
Summary	

Graphic Organizer

Before you read the chapter, draw a diagram like the one below. As you read, write the careers and procedures covered in the chapter into the diagram.

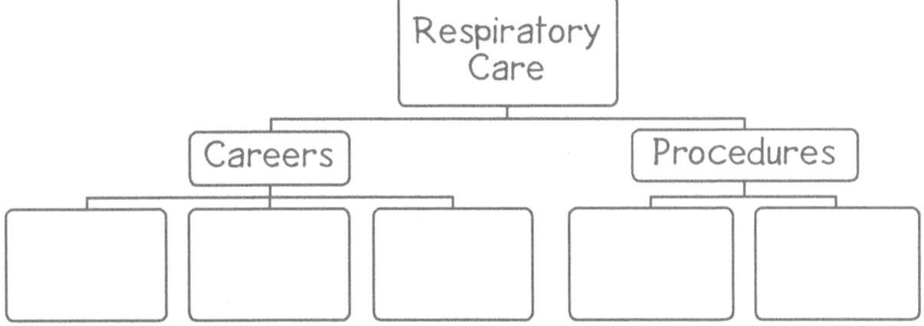

connect
Downloadable graphic organizers can be accessed online.

STANDARDS

HEALTH SCIENCE

NCHSE 1.22 Recognize emerging diseases and disorders.

NCHSE 9.11 Apply behaviors that promote health and wellness.

SCIENCE

NSES E Develop abilities of technological design, understandings about science and technology.

NCHSE *National Consortium for Health Science Education*

NSES *National Science Education Standards*

COMMON CORE STATE STANDARDS

MATHEMATICS

Number and Quantity

Quantities N-Q 3 Choose a level of accuracy appropriate to limitations on measurement when reporting quantities.

ENGLISH LANGUAGE ARTS

Speaking and Listening

Comprehension and Collaboration SL-2 Integrate multiple sources of information presented in diverse media or formats (e.g., visually, quantitatively, orally) evaluating the credibility and accuracy of each source.

Reading

Integration of Knowledge and Ideas R-7 Translate quantitative or technical information expressed in words in a text into visual form (e.g., a table or chart) and translate information expressed visually or mathematically (e.g., in an equation) into words.

SECTION
19.1 Careers in Respiratory Care

The Respiratory Therapist

How can healthcare professionals help patients breathe more easily?

There must be an exchange of **oxygen** and **carbon dioxide** in the lungs to support life. The role of the respiratory system is to provide oxygen to the body tissues and remove the waste gas, carbon dioxide. People who have respiratory diseases often have the scary experience of not being able to get enough oxygen.

Respiratory therapists help patients breathe more easily through prevention and treatment of lung disease, working in various settings such as hospitals, skilled nursing facilities, and patients' homes. The common credentials (see **Table 19.1**) for a respiratory therapist are:

- Certified respiratory therapist (CRT)
- Registered respiratory therapist (RRT)
- Pulmonary function technologist

Many respiratory therapists belong to the **American Association for Respiratory Care,** a professional society for respiratory therapists, managers of respiratory and cardiopulmonary services, and educators who provide respiratory care training.

Vocabulary

Content Vocabulary

You will learn these content vocabulary terms in this section.

- **oxygen**
- **carbon dioxide**
- **American Association for Respiratory Care**
- **sleep apnea**

Academic Vocabulary

You will see this word in your reading and on your tests. Find its meaning in the Glossary in the back of this book.

- **priority**

Table 19.1 Overview of Respiratory Occupations

OCCUPATION	EDUCATIONAL REQUIREMENTS	CERTIFICATION OR LICENSING	JOB OUTLOOK
Certified Respiratory Therapist (CRT)	Two- or four-year degree. Program must be approved by the Committee on Accreditation for Respiratory Care (CoARC).	National Board of Respiratory Care (NBRC) certification upon passing of entry-level CRT examination.	Faster than average growth due to rising age of population; technological advances in the treatment of heart attacks, cancer, and accident victims; and environmental problems.
Registered Respiratory Therapist (RRT)	Two-year associate degree or four-year degree. Program must be approved by CoARC.	National Board of Respiratory Care (NBRC) certification upon receipt of CRT credential and passing of one additional examination.	Faster than average growth, for the reasons given above.
Pulmonary Function Technologist	Two- or four-year degree plus additional training and experience.	Receipt of CRT or RRT credential plus passing additional examination.	Faster than average growth, for the reasons given above.

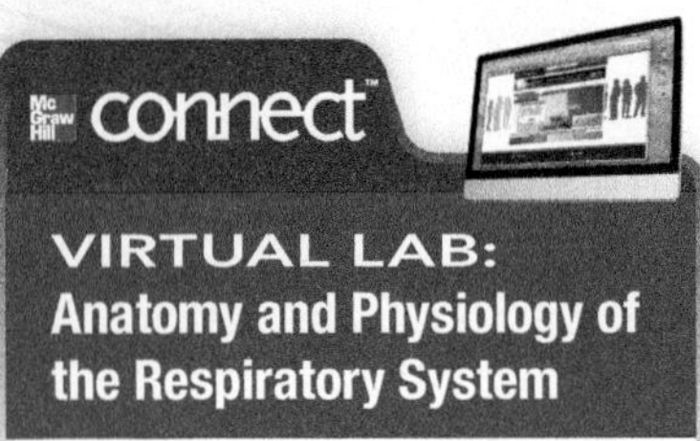

VIRTUAL LAB: Anatomy and Physiology of the Respiratory System

The respiratory system consists of:

- The upper air passages, which includes the nose, mouth, and trachea (windpipe)
- The lungs
- The bloodstream
- Muscles used to inhale and exhale

connect Go online to learn how the respiratory system brings oxygen into the body and expels carbon dioxide from the body.

The Certified Respiratory Therapist and the Registered Respiratory Therapist

There are two main levels of respiratory care. A certified respiratory therapist (CRT) is the entry-level position. The other level is a registered respiratory therapist (RRT). To obtain either of these, you must graduate from a two- or four-year Committee on Accreditation for Respiratory Care (CoARC) approved program and pass the National Board for Respiratory Care (NBRC). Respiratory care practitioner applies to both levels and is also used by many states for licensure.

With additional training, you may

- perform specialized sleep studies that diagnose the cause of **sleep apnea** (a halt in breathing during sleep).
- perform metabolic assessment studies.
- perform cardiac functioning tests, such as electrocardiography, Holter monitoring, hemodynamics, and cardiac stress testing.
- specialize in working with infants and children as a perinatal, neonatal, or pediatric care specialist.

All respiratory therapists must have cardiopulmonary resuscitation (CPR) certification, and many get advanced cardiac life support (ACLS) certification.

The Pulmonary Function Technologist

A respiratory therapist can choose to become a pulmonary function technologist. This requires passing a test that proves you can perform a pulmonary function test (PFT). PFTs are assessment tools that help a therapist detect the presence of lung disease or measure the effect of a known disease on lung function. The test helps measure the effects of occupational and environmental exposure, and evaluate disability or impairment. In addition, it helps the therapist determine the effects of therapy and assess the risk for surgery.

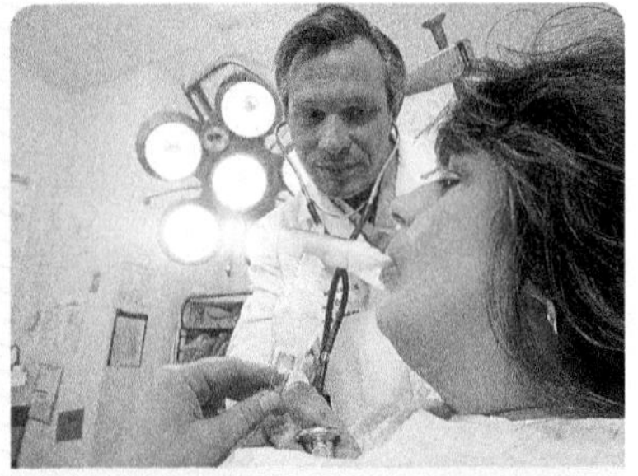

Fig. 19.1 Respiratory Therapy Respiratory technologists assess the need for therapeutic respiratory procedures. *How can a respiratory therapist help patients with lifestyle changes?*

Job Responsibilities of the Respiratory Technologist

The basic responsibilities of all respiratory technologists personnel are to assess the need for therapeutic respiratory procedures (see **Figure 19.1**), determine the potential benefits of the therapy, and monitor the outcome of the therapy to determine whether the treatment objectives were met.

Respiratory therapists help educate patients and their families in living with respiratory problems. They also work in the community.

They conduct smoking cessation clinics, asthma awareness camps, and lung disease management programs.

READING CHECK

Explain the purpose of the pulmonary function test.

Respiratory Diagnosis and Therapy

What life-support activity is performed by respiratory therapists?

Many respiratory therapy procedures involve assessing the condition of the lungs, helping the lungs oxygenate the blood and tissues, and evaluating the lungs' ability to rid the body of carbon dioxide. Respiratory diagnostic and therapeutic procedures help the ventilatory, or breathing, process work as well as possible.

Respiratory Diagnostic Procedures

Diagnostic procedures are used to help assess the level of lung function and determine whether specific types of illness or conditions are present. The most frequently used diagnostic tests performed by respiratory therapists are listed in **Table 19.2.**

Table 19.2 Respiratory Diagnostics

TEST	PURPOSE
Arterial blood gas analysis	To assess levels of oxygen, carbon dioxide, and other elements in the bloodstream.
Pulmonary function testing	To determine impaired functioning and diagnose disease by measuring lung volumes and flow rates.
Pulse oximetry	To measure the level of oxygen-carrying capabilities in the blood.
Auscultation	To listen with a stethoscope for normal and abnormal lung sounds.
Capnography	To measure the amount of exhaled carbon dioxide to assess the level of ventilation.

Respiratory Therapeutic Procedures

Respiratory therapists prevent and treat lung disease by using a number of therapies. **Table 19.3** on page 494 lists the main therapeutic procedures and gives a basic description of them.

Mechanical Ventilation During mechanical ventilation, a patient is attached to a machine that helps them breathe (see **Figure 19.2** on page 494). Mechanical ventilation is used for two main reasons:

- When other respiratory procedures fail to keep the lungs from moving enough oxygen into the bloodstream and from removing enough carbon dioxide from the lungs
- When a patient goes into respiratory arrest, which means that the patient has stopped breathing

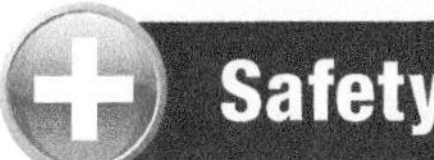

Safety

Secondhand Smoke

If you do not smoke but are regularly exposed to secondhand smoke, you may experience

- increased risk of lung cancer over those not exposed to smoke.
- an increased frequency of respiratory infections, such as bronchitis and pneumonia.
- an increased risk of asthma.
- acute, sudden, and occasionally severe reactions, including eye, nose, throat, and lower respiratory tract symptoms.

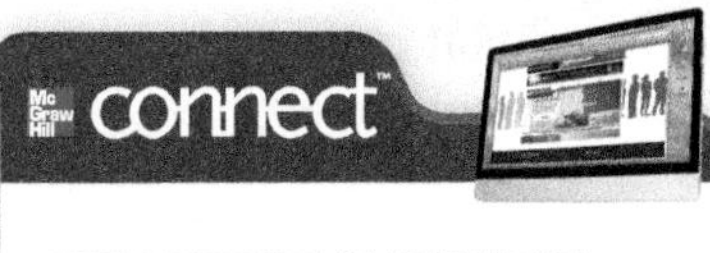

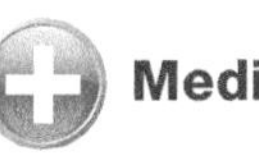

STEM CONNECTION

Medical Science

How the Airways Work
For respiration to work well, the airways must be kept open. Airways consist of the nasal passages, oral cavity (mouth), pharynx (throat), larynx (voice box), trachea (windpipe), bronchi (the main airways in the lungs), and alveoli (the gas exchange units).

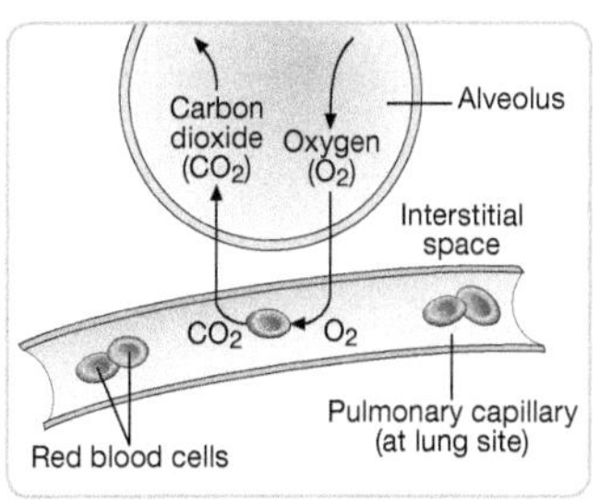

connect Go online to learn how the respiratory therapist works to keep the airway lining of patients functioning properly.

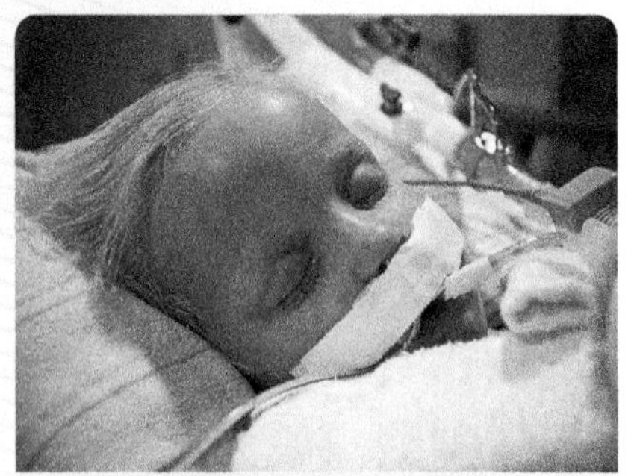

Fig. 19.2 Ventilators Ventilators are attached to the patient's mouth, nose, or throat to assist breathing or take over when a patient is in respiratory arrest. *In what other situations may a ventilator be used?*

The respiratory therapist manages life-support ventilators that take over the work of the lungs until they can recover. Once this advanced life support treatment has begun, it must be carefully monitored. Patient response, comfort, and psychological support must be a priority.

The decision to begin or withdraw advanced life support is not an easy one. Patients who have a living will or advanced directives can decide what they want to have done in this situation. In addition, some patients request a Do Not Resuscitate (DNR) order (see Chapter 17, Mental Health) that must be honored by healthcare practitioners.

READING CHECK

List tests used to evaluate the performance of the lungs.

Table 19.3 Respiratory Therapies

THERAPY	DESCRIPTION
Oxygen therapy	Provides supplemental oxygen to lungs.
Aerosol therapy	Provides medication and/or additional humidity to airways.
Hyperinflation (lung expansion) therapy	Prevents and treats lung collapse.
Chest physical therapy	Aids in lung hygiene; may include postural drainage, percussion, breathing retraining, and coughing.
Suctioning	Applies negative pressure directly to the airways to remove secretions.
Mechanical ventilation	Controls or supports the patient's breathing by providing advanced life support.

SECTION 19.1 Careers in Respiratory Care Review

AFTER YOU READ

1. **Assess** the primary role of a respiratory therapist.
2. **Describe** two levels of a respiratory therapist and the state educational requirements for each level.
3. **Identify** the additional certifications available after becoming a respiratory therapist.
4. **Discuss** some reasons why the need for respiratory therapists will increase in the future.
5. **List** three places where you can seek employment after graduating from a respiratory therapy program.

Technology ONLINE EXPLORATIONS

Respiratory Therapist

Go online to determine the following:

1. How long would it take you to become a respiratory therapist in your state?
2. Where is the closest school for respiratory therapy?
3. What is the name of the school?
4. What are the admission requirements for entering that school?
5. What credential or credentials would you have when you graduated?

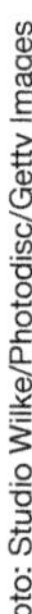

SECTION **19.2** Respiratory Care Procedures

Oxygen Therapy

Is oxygen a drug?

Certain lung diseases or conditions can hinder a person's ability to take in oxygen or transfer it into the bloodstream. Common diseases, such as chronic bronchitis, can lower the level of oxygen in the blood. When this happens, the patient often needs supplemental oxygen. In this context, oxygen is considered to be a drug. Therefore, a doctor's order is needed before it can be given to a patient. The order specifies the amount of oxygen to be given. Respiratory therapists and EMS personnel can administer oxygen. The procedure for providing oxygen is found on page 401 of Chapter 14, Emergency Medical Services.

Reasons for Oxygen Therapy

How will you know if a patient needs more oxygen? There are three main reasons for oxygen therapy.

Low Levels of Oxygen in the Blood (Hypoxemia) The amount of oxygen in the blood can be determined by analyzing a blood sample from an artery. The amount of oxygen in the blood of a normal adult is between 80 to 100 mm Hg.

Another way to find out how much oxygen is in the blood is to use a device called a **pulse oximeter** (see **Figure 19.3**), which uses infrared technology to measure how saturated the red blood cells are with oxygen. The normal adult saturation should be at least 95 percent. A patient with a lower blood saturation value may require additional oxygen. The oxygen saturation measurement is abbreviated SpO_2.

Work Demands of Breathing Oxygen therapy is used to decrease the work of breathing. Having to work hard for each breath puts a great strain on the body. A patient who is short of breath is consuming a lot of oxygen by working the respiratory muscles hard just to survive.

In most cases, the rate and depth of breathing must increase in order to bring in more oxygen. This means that a patient lacking in oxygen must breathe more rapidly and deeply than normal. Common signs that the respiratory muscles are being overworked include:

- An increase in the rate and depth of breathing
- The use of accessory muscles, in this case muscles other than the diaphragm, such as the intercostal muscles, to breathe
- Cyanosis, or a bluish skin color, which indicates low levels of oxygen or hemoglobin

Vocabulary

Content Vocabulary

You will learn these content vocabulary terms in this section.

- **pulse oximeter**
- **chronic obstructive pulmonary disease (COPD)**
- **simple mask**
- **oxygen toxicity**
- **atelectasis**
- **bronchodilate**
- **lung expansion therapy**

Academic Vocabulary

You will see this word in your reading and on your tests. Find its meaning in the Glossary in the back of this book.

- **device**

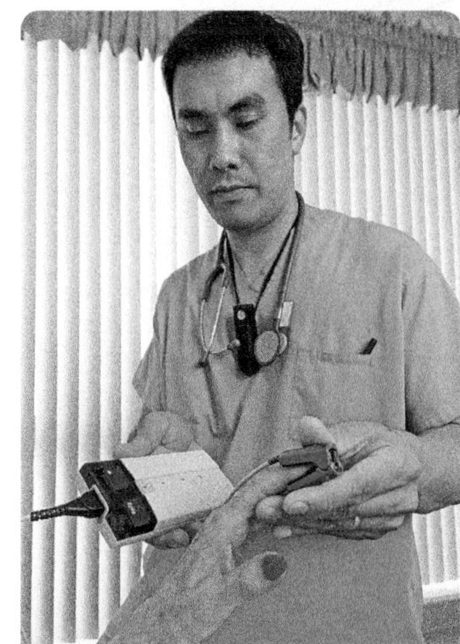

Fig. 19.3 Pulse Oximeter Normal pulse oximetry readings are 95 to 99 percent. A level below 95 percent may indicate a need for treatment. *How does the pulse oximeter work?*

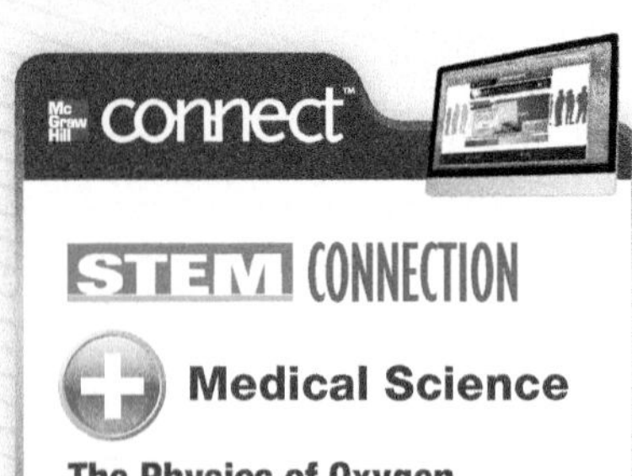

STEM CONNECTION

Medical Science

The Physics of Oxygen
To find out how much oxygen is in the red blood cells, a blood sample is drawn from a patient. The purpose of the test is to measure arterial blood gas. This means that the blood sample is analyzed to find out how much pressure is being exerted by the oxygen dissolved in the blood.

connect Go online to learn about the pressure oxygen exerts in the bloodstream.

Stress of the Heart Another purpose for oxygen therapy is to relieve the work of the heart, to prevent it from being further stressed. The heart pumps the blood containing oxygen to the tissues of the body. When oxygen levels in the blood are decreased, the heart tries to correct this situation by increasing its pumping force and rate. But an increase in the heart's pumping force and rate means that the heart needs more oxygen because it is working harder. In other words, low oxygen levels in the blood cause a "vicious circle." Patients who have cardiac conditions often need oxygen therapy because their hearts have an increased workload and are under stress.

Oxygen Delivery Devices

Various devices are available to provide supplemental oxygen. Increasing the percentage of oxygen we breathe increases the amount of oxygen that gets into the lungs and bloodstream. Recall that the atmosphere around us is 21 percent oxygen. For people who are not getting enough oxygen, it is possible to increase the amount of oxygen from about 24 percent to as much as 100 percent, depending on the device used.

After you determine that a patient needs oxygen therapy, the next step is to decide what device to use to provide the needed amount. Low-flow oxygen delivery systems are most commonly used. This device provides some of the oxygen the patient needs. The rest comes from breathing the air. Two common devices used to deliver oxygen are the nasal cannula and the simple mask.

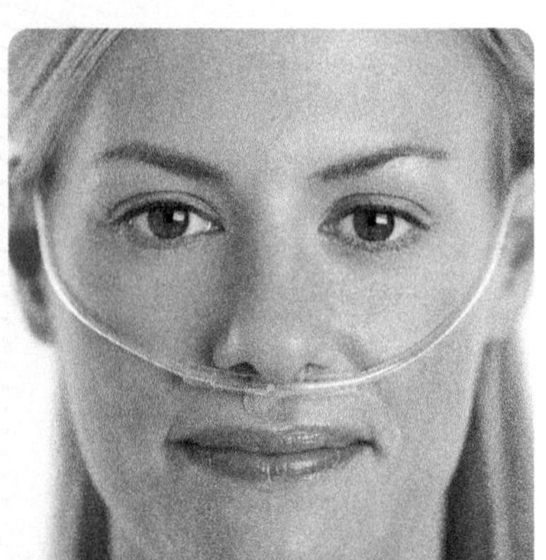

Fig. 19.4 Nasal Cannula The nasal cannula oxygen delivery device is used in the hospital and at home. *What is one advantage of this device?*

Nasal Cannula The nasal cannula (see **Figure 19.4**) is a commonly used device to provide low-flow oxygen therapy. It carries supplemental oxygen through small-diameter flexible plastic tubing. The tubing has two short extensions that are inserted into the nostrils. The nasal cannula is lightweight, easy to use, and well tolerated by most patients. The main advantage is that a patient can eat and speak comfortably when it is in use. This device can deliver from one to six liters per minute of supplemental oxygen. **Table 19.4** lists the approximate oxygen percentages per liter flow.

Table 19.4 Approximate Oxygen Percentages per Liter Flow

LITER FLOW	OXYGEN %	LITER FLOW	OXYGEN %
1	24	4	36
2	28	5	40
3	32	6	44

The nasal cannula is often used for long-term oxygen therapy for patients with **chronic obstructive pulmonary disease (COPD)** because they usually have long-term or chronic hypoxemia, or lack of oxygen in the blood. COPD is a disease of the airways such as emphysema. In these cases, an oxygen tank may be attached to a walker with a tube leading from the tank to the nasal cannula.

Simple Mask A **simple mask** (see **Figure 19.5**) is designed to fit over a patient's nose and mouth and provides a reservoir of oxygen. With this device, the amount of oxygen delivered varies for a number of reasons. The most common reason is the difficulty in getting a tight seal between the mask and the face.

The simple mask is often used for emergencies and short-term therapies. It can deliver between 35 and 50 percent of oxygen, depending upon the patient's ventilation rate and depth.

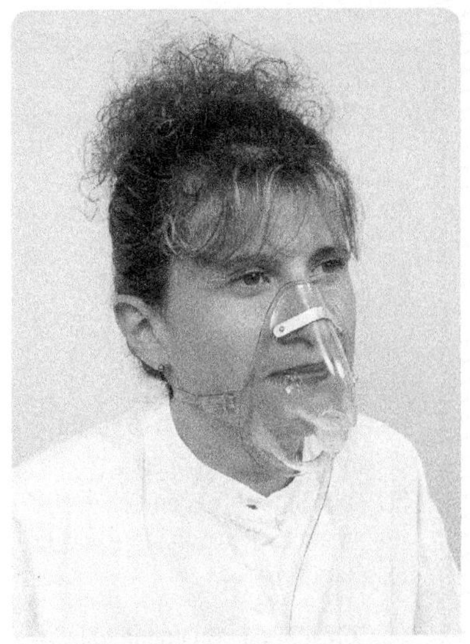

Fig. 19.5 Simple Mask A simple mask gives slightly higher oxygen percentages than the nasal cannula. *Why do oxygen percentages vary with this device?*

Monitoring Oxygen Therapy

One of the most important jobs of the respiratory therapist is to determine if oxygen therapy is working. If oxygen therapy is effective, the following improvements should take place:

- The patient should think more clearly and become less restless and agitated, because more oxygen is reaching the brain.
- Shortness of breath will decrease. The patient will breathe more easily. The patient's color may improve. This will be noticeable in the skin, lips, nail beds, and mucous membranes.
- Vital signs should come closer to normal. When a patient is suffering from hypoxemia, the heart increases its rate to try to send more oxygen to the tissues. The lungs also increase their rate and depth of breathing in an attempt to make up for low levels of oxygen. When oxygen therapy is correctly applied, the heart rate and respiratory rate should move toward their normal levels.
- The oxygen value obtained from a test of arterial blood gas (PaO_2) will rise to an acceptable level for that particular patient. A normal value is 80 to 100 mm Hg for most patients.
- An improvement in the pulse oximetry values, which measures the amount of hemoglobin saturated with oxygen (SpO_2).

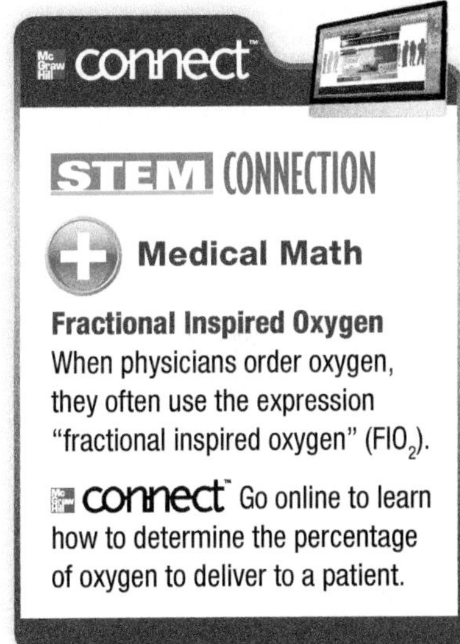

STEM CONNECTION

Medical Math

Fractional Inspired Oxygen
When physicians order oxygen, they often use the expression "fractional inspired oxygen" (FIO_2).

connect Go online to learn how to determine the percentage of oxygen to deliver to a patient.

Hazards of Oxygen Therapy

As you know, oxygen is considered a drug. If oxygen is not correctly delivered, harmful effects may occur. Some of the hazards of oxygen therapy are listed here.

- **Oxygen toxicity** is a serious, life-threatening condition that may occur if too much oxygen is delivered for too long a period of time. If a normal person breathes 100 percent oxygen for longer than 12 to 24 hours, they will show early signs of oxygen toxicity. Some of these symptoms are sore throat, difficulty with breathing, a cough, and chest discomfort. Lung tissue is eventually damaged.
- Retinopathy of prematurity (ROP) is caused by high oxygen levels in infants. ROP is a disorder of the retina, the innermost layer of the eye, and it may lead to blindness. Oxygen is often administered to premature infants to help them breathe because their lungs are not fully developed. However, when too much oxygen is delivered, serious or permanent eye damage may occur. Maintaining oxygen levels no higher than 80 mm Hg can prevent this damage.

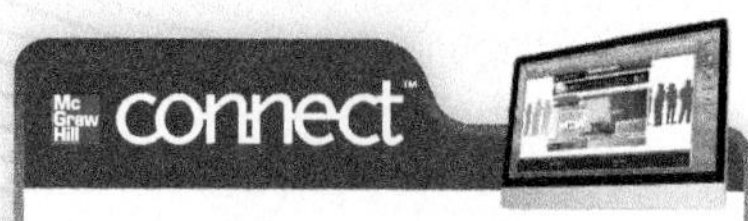

STEM CONNECTION

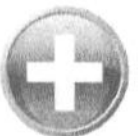

Medical Math

Calculating Oxygen Delivery
Here is a rule of thumb for determining how much oxygen is delivered through a nasal cannula. For each liter of oxygen delivered, the amount of oxygen increases by about four percent.

connect Go online to learn how to calculate the percentage of oxygen delivered through a nasal cannula.

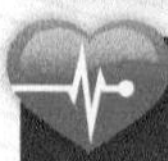

Preventive Care & Wellness

Smoking

Smoking causes many lung diseases such as emphysema, chronic bronchitis, and lung cancer. As a respiratory therapist, you should be actively involved in smoking education and cessation programs. Here are some ways to help you or someone you know stop smoking.

- Write down the reason or reasons you want to quit.
- Know that it will take effort to quit smoking.
- Realize that half of all adult smokers have quit, and you can, too!
- Get help if you need it.
- Stay away from places or things that are most likely to make you want to smoke.
- Plan ways to handle stress: chew gum, take deep breaths, exercise.
- If you blow it, do not beat yourself up. Just start again.
- When you succeed, reward yourself with a favorite activity.
- Stay hydrated by drinking water and fruit juice. Avoid caffeine.

- **Atelectasis,** or lung collapse, can occur when high concentrations of oxygen reduce the amount of nitrogen in the lungs. Nitrogen is a gas that keeps the lungs open.

READING CHECK

Recall the three main reasons for providing oxygen therapy.

Medicated Aerosol Therapy

Why might antibiotics be delivered as an aerosol?

Sometimes a patient needs medication delivered directly into the lungs. Several devices can do this in the form of an aerosol or mist that can be inhaled directly into the lungs. **Figure 19.6** shows a nebulizer device for infants. Medicated aerosols open up the airways. They are called bronchodilators. To **bronchodilate** is to open up the airways.

Bronchodilators are used when the airways become constricted, as in an asthma attack. The main advantage of a medicated aerosol is that the medication is delivered directly and quickly to where it is needed. Also, side effects are minimal. A side effect is any effect caused by a drug other than its intended effect. They often happen because a drug travels through the bloodstream. Since aerosols do not travel throughout the body but are inhaled into the lungs, it is less likely that they will cause unwanted effects such as nausea, vomiting, or diarrhea.

The Advantages of Aerosolized Medications

Some advantages of using an aerosolized medication are:

- Smaller doses of a drug can be used because it is inhaled directly into the lungs. If the drug were taken orally, it would have to first travel through the stomach and intestines. Then, it would make its way into the bloodstream, where it might be diluted. Finally, it would act on the lungs.
- Inhaled aerosols can act very quickly. The lungs have a large surface area with a rich blood supply that permits the fast absorption of the drug.
- Side effects are reduced.
- It is convenient, easy, and painless.
- It can be used at home, thus reducing hospital admissions.

The Disadvantages of Aerosolized Medications

Aerosolized medications do have disadvantages, such as the following:

- It is difficult to administer the correct dosage each time, because many factors influence how much of the drug actually reaches the airway.

- It is sometimes difficult to teach patients how to use the aerosol device correctly.
- Healthcare providers may not know how to properly use or instruct the patient on the proper technique for using the aerosol device.

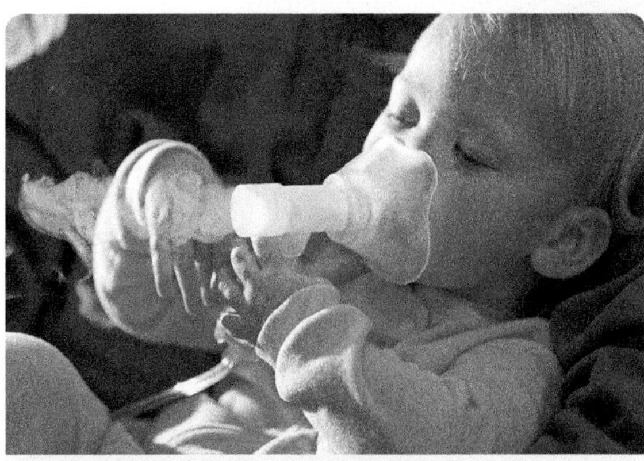

Fig. 19.6 Nebulizer for Infants The infant pacifier nebulizer is used to deliver medication. The liquid is suspended into particles in the chamber. *Why might an infant need a nebulizer?*

Types of Drugs Given by Aerosol

A number of drugs can be delivered by aerosolized medications. Here are some examples that are also discussed in more detail below.

- Nasal decongestants
- Bronchodilators
- Antiasthmatics
- Corticosteroids
- Mucolytics
- Antimicrobials

Nasal Decongestants Nasal decongestants are available in squeeze bottles, which can be bought over the counter. These decongestants contain vasoconstrictors, which are drugs that decrease the flow of blood to the vessels of the nose. Decreasing the flow of blood makes the vessels shrink. Once this happens, the nasal passages open up and air can flow more easily.

Bronchodilators Bronchodilators are drugs that increase the diameter of the airways of the lungs. When the airways of the lungs become narrow, breathing becomes difficult. Patients whose airways have become narrow may have excessive secretions or bronchospasms. The use of bronchodilators makes breathing easier.

Antiasthmatics Asthma attacks are often caused by allergic reactions. Antiasthmatic drugs reduce the allergic response. They can be used to prevent attacks or decrease the number of attacks in patients who suffer from allergic asthma.

Corticosteroids Corticosteroids are drugs that may be inhaled. They are used for anti-inflammatory maintenance therapy, often for moderate to severe persistent asthma. They help when airways become swollen and can help prevent or reduce what is called late-phase asthma. This can be severe and may occur hours after an initial asthma attack.

Mucolytics Mucolytics are drugs used to break down secretions within the lungs. When secretions are broken down, it is easier for them to be expectorated, or coughed out. Mucolytics are used to treat excessive, thick secretions that can often occur in patients who have lung disease.

Antimicrobials Aerosolized antibiotics, which are antimicrobials, are used to treat a number of bacterial and fungal pulmonary infections. In recent years, aerosolized antibiotics have also been used to treat viral infections.

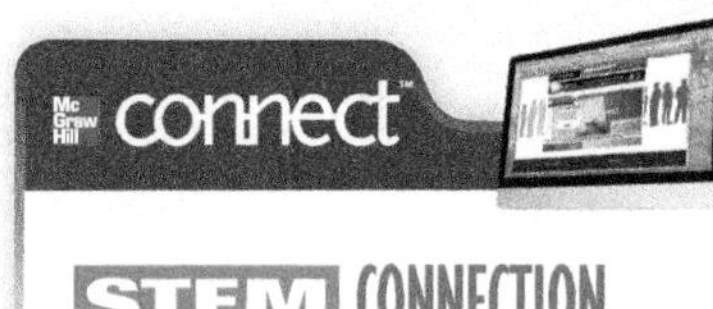

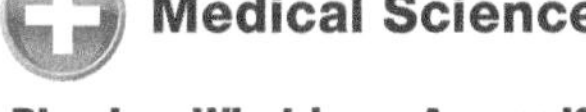

Medical Science

Physics: What Is an Aerosol?
An aerosol is a suspension of a liquid or a solid in a gas. Aerosols exist around us in everyday life. Pollen, mist, dust, smoke, fog, smog, and even a sneeze are aerosols. In a hospital setting, medicated or therapeutic aerosols are administered by the use of nebulizers. A nebulizer is a device that disperses liquid into small particles and suspends the particles in a gas to be breathed into the lungs.

connect Go online to learn about the importance of the size of aerosol particles that are to be deposited in the lungs.

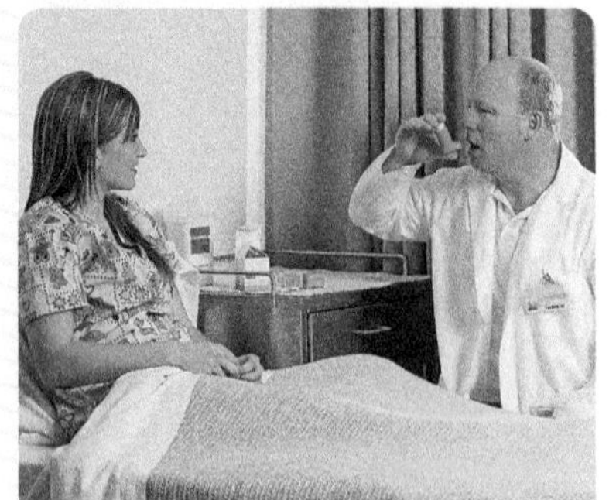

Fig. 19.7 Metered Dose Inhaler The most commonly used aerosol medication delivery device is the metered dose inhaler (MDI). *What is a metered dose?*

Aerosol Drug Delivery System

It is very important to teach patients the proper technique for using an aerosol device because the aim is to maximize the amount of medication that actually gets into the lungs.

Several types of aerosol devices are available, but the metered dose inhaler (MDI) is used most frequently.

The Metered Dose Inhaler A metered dose inhaler (MDI) is a small portable pressurized device that delivers medication to the lungs. A metered dose is a measured amount of medication. An MDI consists of a canister that contains a pressurized gas propellant and medication. When the canister is turned upside down and depressed, a metered dose is delivered through the mouthpiece in the form of an aerosol, which must then be breathed in (see **Figure 19.7**).

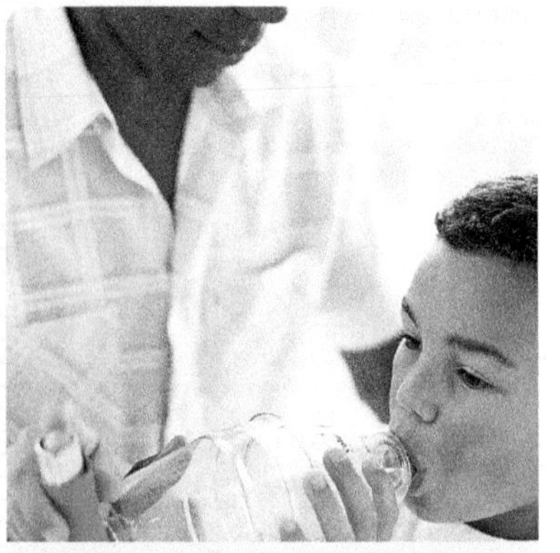

Fig. 19.8 MDI Spacers Several types of spacers or chambers can be added to MDIs to make them easier to use and more effective. *What are two ways in which these accessories make an MDI more effective?*

Several add-on devices can make an MDI more effective and easier to use. Spacers, holding chamber, and extension device are names for equipment often used with the MDI to administer drugs (see **Figure 19.8**). The advantages of using these accessories are:

- The aerosol is directed into the patient's mouth. Without the accessory, the MDI must be held away from the mouth. Therefore, the add-on device prevents the aerosol from inadvertently being sprayed into the patient's eyes or face.
- The spacer add-on helps make the particle size of the aerosol consistent. This means that more particles are able to get deep into the lungs.
- An accessory device can make it easier to use an MDI properly. When the patient first tries to use an MDI, it is hard to avoid having the aerosol particles become deposited in the mouth rather than breathed in. With the add-on device, the aerosol is created in the chamber. This gives the patient more time to inhale the particles into the lungs, rather then allowing them to be deposited in the mouth.

Mc Graw Hill connect™ ONLINE PROCEDURES

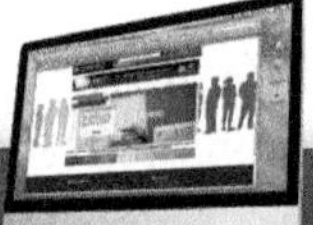

PROCEDURE 19-1

Delivering a Metered Dose Inhaler Treatment

Sometimes a patient needs medication delivered directly into the lungs. A metered dose inhaler (MDI) is one type of device that delivers medication in the form of an aerosol or mist that can be inhaled directly into the lungs. Medicated aerosols open up the airways.

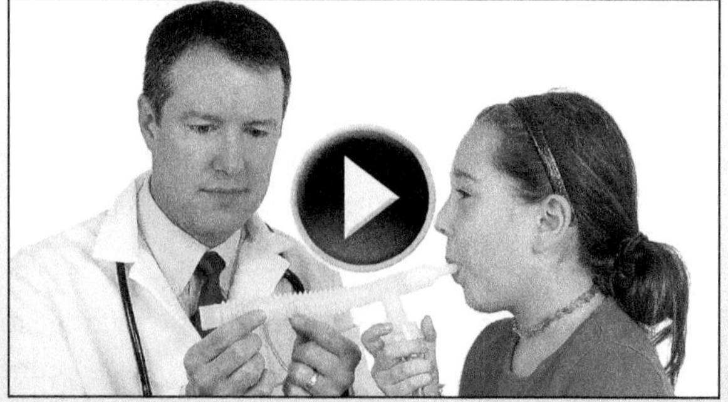

Evaluating Aerosol Therapy

An important job of the respiratory therapist is to determine if an aerosol treatment is producing the desired results. To do this, you must assess the patient and establish a baseline before treatment. A baseline is a list of observations you make at the start, so that you will have a basis for comparison after treatment. Your baseline and post-treatment assessment should include the following:

- Listen to the breath sounds before treatment, and note any improvement after treatment. For example, did abnormal breath sounds such as wheezes diminish after the treatment? This would indicate that the airways opened as the result of treatment.
- Administer a pulmonary function test before and after treatment. This will help you determine whether the rate and volume of air going in and out of the lungs increased after treatment. If there has been an increase, this indicates that ventilation has improved.
- Ask the patient if he or she feels better after the treatment. Check the patient's appearance. Does he or she seem to have less shortness of breath? Is he or she able to speak more easily? Has his or her color improved? Did he or she cough up any secretions after the treatment?

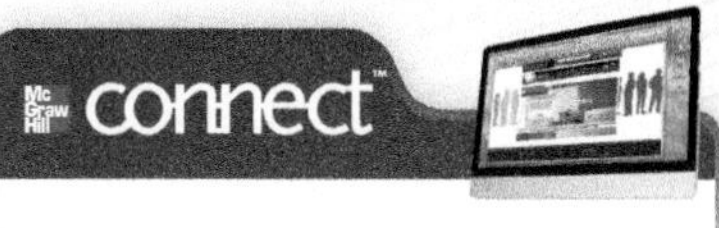

STEM CONNECTION

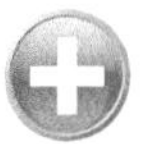

Medical Science

Oxygen in the Bloodstream
A condition called hypoxemia exists when there are low levels of oxygen in the blood. Oxygen, a gas, is dissolved in blood, which is a liquid. The oxygen is carried in the bloodstream. It becomes attached to the hemoglobin molecule of the red blood cell.

connect Go online to learn more about how oxygen is supplied to body tissues and organs.

READING CHECK

Summarize how you would determine the effectiveness of aerosol therapy.

Hyperinflation Therapy

Which patients are at greatest risk of lung collapse?

Hyperinflation therapy involves treatments designed to prevent or treat lung collapse. This therapy is also called **lung expansion therapy.** Atelectasis, partial or full lung collapse, is usually the result of a blockage of the airways. This can be caused by tumors or large amounts of mucus in the airways that prevent ventilation to an area of the lung.

Lung collapse can develop when a patient consistently breathes small amounts of air and does not fully expand his lungs. It usually occurs when such a patient is sedated or is in pain. Preventing or treating lung collapse requires deep breathing or secretion removal to keep the airways open at all times.

Indications for Hyperinflation Therapy

Anything that impairs a patient's ability to take deep breaths and cough makes the patient a candidate for hyperinflation therapy.

Some examples for hyperinflation therapy are patients who

- have had surgery of the chest wall or the upper abdominal region.

- are heavily sedated.
- have neuromuscular disease.
- have spinal cord injuries.
- are bedridden.
- have a history of chronic lung disease that causes excessive mucus production, such as chronic bronchitis or cystic fibrosis.

Incentive Spirometry

The most common hyperinflation therapy is incentive spirometry (IS). Incentive spirometry is performed using devices that give the patient a visual clue by showing the patient the numbers signifying volume. The patient can see when the desired volume or flow has been reached. Coach the patient to take slow deep breaths followed by a five- to ten-second holding of the breath. This breathing pattern is called sustained maximal inspiration (SMI). **Figure 19.9** shows an incentive spirometry device.

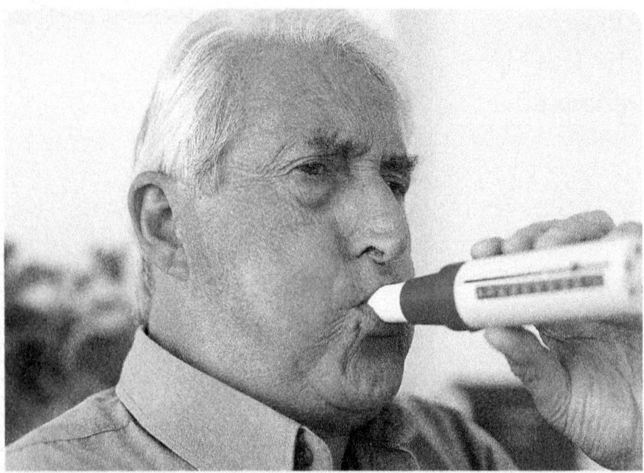

Fig. 19.9 Incentive Spirometer The incentive spirometer device gives the patient a visual target goal or volume to reach. *What visual target does the patient see?*

Indications for Incentive Spirometry The main reason to use incentive spirometry is to prevent or treat existing atelectasis. Patients who may be prone to atelectasis include those who

- have had upper abdominal surgery.
- have had thoracic (chest) surgery.
- have chronic obstructive pulmonary disease (COPD) and are undergoing or have undergone surgery.
- have been bedridden for extended periods of time.
- are heavy smokers and are undergoing or have undergone surgery.

Incentive spirometry can also be used as a preventive measure for patients who may be at risk for the development of atelectasis.

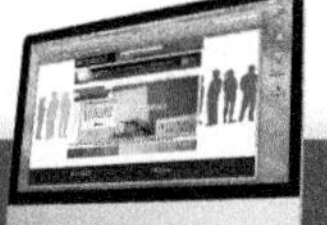

Mc Graw Hill connect™ ONLINE PROCEDURES

PROCEDURE 19-2

Administering Incentive Spirometry (IS)

The most common hyperinflation therapy is incentive spirometry (IS). Incentive spirometry is performed using devices that give the patient a visual clue by showing the patient the numbers signifying volume. The patient can see that the desired volume or flow has been reached.

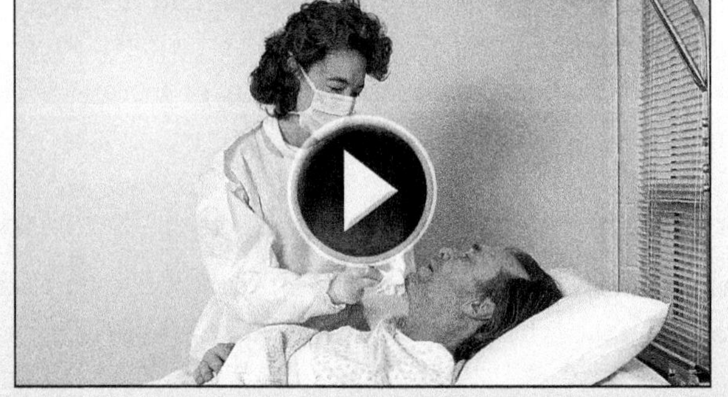

Indications for preventive use include:

- The presence of conditions that predispose the patient to atelectasis, such as upper abdominal surgery, thoracic surgery, or surgery in patients who suffer from chronic obstructive pulmonary disease (COPD)
- The presence of a restrictive lung disorder associated with quadriplegia or a dysfunctional diaphragm

Contraindications for Incentive Spirometry Patients who should not be treated with incentive spirometry are those who

- cannot be instructed or supervised on the proper use of the device.
- are unconscious patients or unable to cooperate.
- are not able to deep breathe effectively (achieving a vital capacity of less than 10 cc/Kg or who achieve less than $\frac{1}{3}$ of their predicted inspiratory capacity).

READING CHECK

Analyze the primary reason for using incentive spirometry.

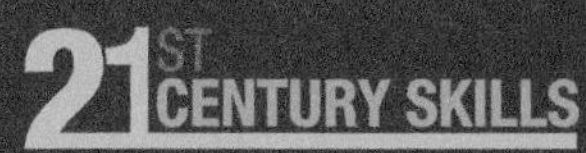

Teamwork and Scope of Practice

Healthcare providers must understand and follow their scope of practice, which legally defines what people in a particular profession may and may not do. It helps define your role on a healthcare team and makes teamwork possible among various healthcare professions. In most states, the scope of practice for respiratory therapy is defined by the medical board. The board may certify healthcare workers and issue licenses to practice within the state.

SECTION 19.2 Respiratory Care Procedures Review

AFTER YOU READ

1. **Review** the common signs indicating that a patient is having difficulty breathing and may require oxygen therapy.
2. **Illustrate** how to monitor the effectiveness of oxygen therapy.
3. **Compare** the advantages and disadvantages of aerosol therapy.
4. **Name** three types of medications that can be aerosolized and inhaled into the lungs.
5. **Explain** why atelectasis (lung collapse) happens.
6. **Evaluate** what type of therapy would be required for the following patients:
   a. A patient with chronic obstructive pulmonary disease.
   b. A patient who is having an asthma attack.
   c. A patient who has lung disease and has just had surgery.

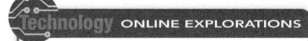

Technology ONLINE EXPLORATIONS

Patient Brochure

Go online to research a diagnostic test or therapeutic procedure that a respiratory therapist may perform. Develop a one-page patient brochure or teaching sheet about that test or procedure.

CHAPTER

19 Review

Chapter Summary

SECTION 19.1

- The role of the respiratory system is to provide oxygen to the body tissues and remove the waste gas, carbon dioxide. **(pg. 491)**
- Upon graduation from a two- or four-year educational program, you may take examinations for two different levels of credentials. Passing the entry-level examination given by the NBRC qualifies you as a certified respiratory therapist (CRT). You may also take an additional test to become an advanced practitioner or registered respiratory therapist (RRT). **(pg. 492)**
- Additional training and certification opportunities include pulmonary function testing and perinatal-neonatal specialized credentials. In addition, many therapists are cross-trained in areas such as sleep studies, cardiac stress testing, administering ECGs, and hemodynamic monitoring. **(pg. 492)**

SECTION 19.2

- Oxygen therapy may be used in situations when the lungs are not delivering adequate oxygen into the bloodstream. Various oxygen delivery devices may be used. The patient must be monitored to determine how well the oxygen therapy is working and to prevent any harmful side effects from occurring. **(pg. 495)**
- Medicated aerosols can be delivered directly into the lungs. The major group of drugs used as medicated aerosols are bronchodilators, which open up the airways and make it easier for the patient to breathe. The most common type of aerosol device is the metered dose inhaler (MDI). **(pg. 498)**
- Hyperinflation therapy is a way to fully expand the lungs and prevent or treat lung collapse. The medical term for lung collapse is atelectasis. Incentive spirometry (IS) is the most common type of hyperinflation therapy. **(pg. 501)**

McGraw Hill connect™ ONLINE ACTIVITIES

Complete our HST online activities for Chapter 19, which include Concept Check review questions, Reference Flash Cards, and Online Procedures assessment sheets.

- **Concept Check** review questions
- **Reference Flash Cards** medical terminology practice
- **Online Procedures** assessment sheets

CHAPTER 19 Assessment

Critical Thinking/Problem Solving

1. Your patient is receiving oxygen through a simple mask and still appears to be short of breath. What might be the problem? What can be done to fix it?
2. What role does the diaphragm play in respiration? What would happen if your patient's diaphragm were paralyzed?
3. Search online for information about two common acute respiratory diseases that can occur in children or adults—respiratory syncytial virus (RSV) and acute respiratory distress syndrome (ARDS). Choose one, and find out its cause, prevention, and treatment. Develop an educational brochure or presentation to teach the public about these respiratory problems.
4. Obtain a drug reference book or go online to find one trade name and the generic and chemical names of the types of drugs given by aerosol that are listed on page 499. Refer to Chapter 18, Pharmacy, to review the definitions of the terms trade name and generic name.

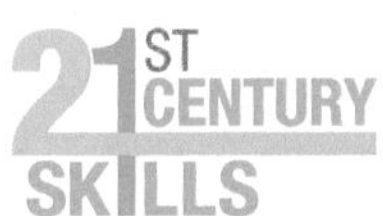

5. **Problem Solving** Using a placebo inhaler, demonstrate the proper technique for administering a metered dose inhaler (MDI). With a partner, explain and perform the MDI on each other.
6. **Teamwork** In pairs, try this activity to get an idea of what it is like to have restricted breathing. Breathe only through a soda straw placed in the mouth and not through the nose. Do a few ordinary activities such as walking and going up and down a staircase to see how it feels. Report the sensations to your partner.
7. **Teamwork** The respiratory therapist must be able to listen to the lungs and identify normal and abnormal breath sounds. Using a stethoscope, listen to your partner's lungs. Move the stethoscope around and listen carefully. You should be able to hear three types of normal breath sounds.
8. **Information Literacy** Go online to find more information about normal and abnormal breathing sounds. Find an Internet site that provides the actual sounds so that you can determine the three types of normal breathing sounds.
9. **Information Literacy** As a respiratory therapist, you should have an excellent understanding of the risk factors of lung disease and its prevention. Use the website of the American Lung Association to learn more about lung disease and its prevention.

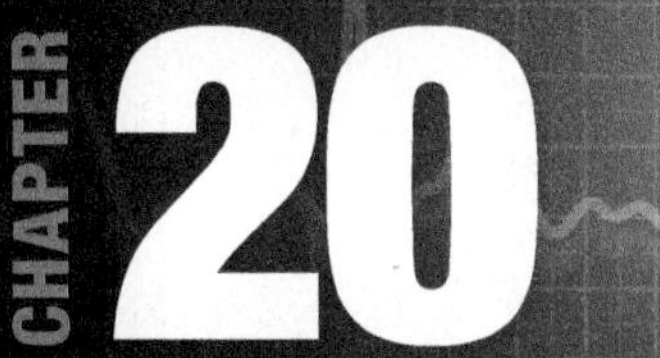

CHAPTER 20 Rehabilitation

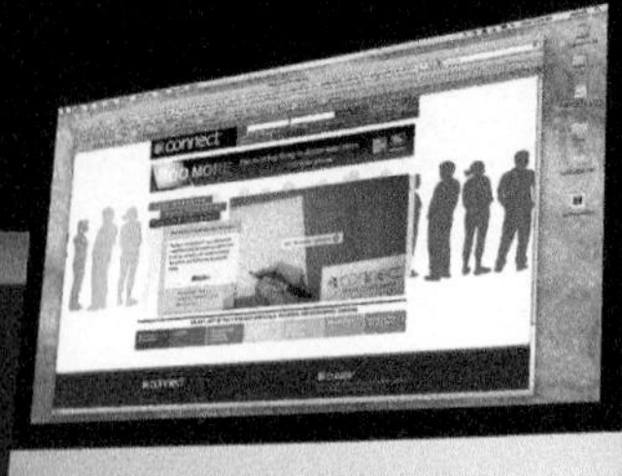

connect

It's Online!

- Online Procedures
- STEM Connection
- Medical Science
- Medical Terms
- Medical Math
- Ethics in Action
- Virtual Lab

Essential Question:

How can working with a physical therapist benefit someone who was injured in an accident?

Healthcare professionals in rehabilitation work with patients and their families after disabling injuries or chronic illnesses. They become involved soon after the injury or illness has occurred, and continue their efforts after the patient goes home. In addition to introducing the career choices available in this field, this chapter will provide some background on types of rehabilitation and specific rehabilitation procedures.

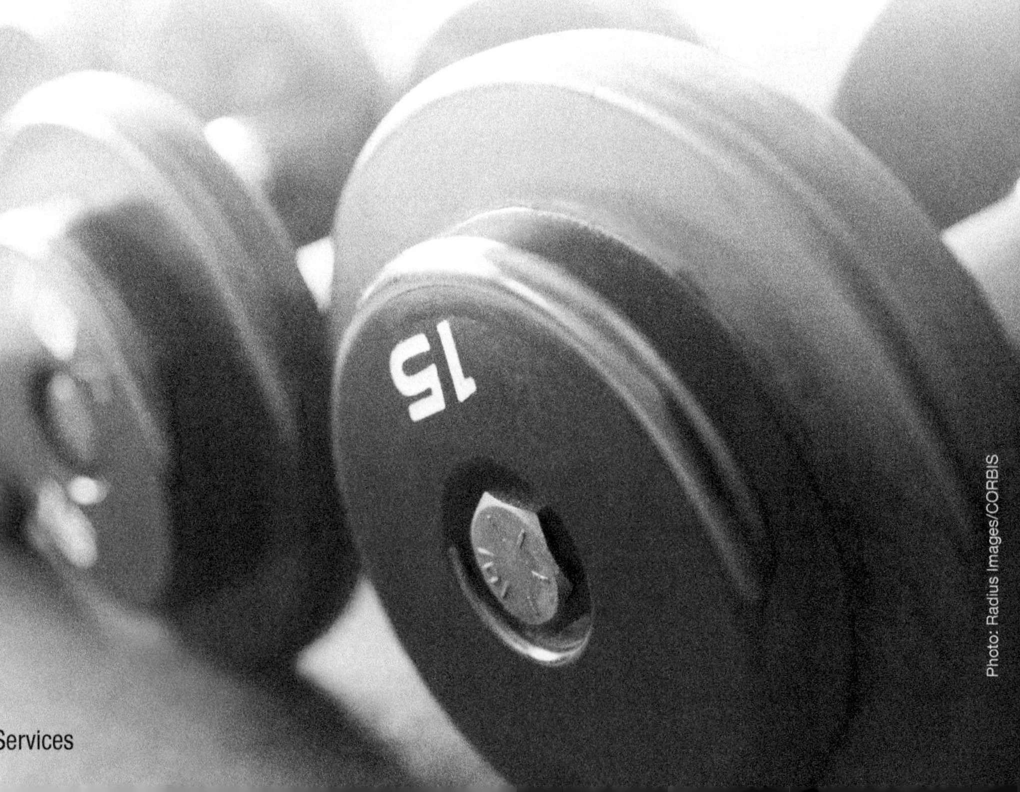

Photo: Radius Images/CORBIS

READING GUIDE

OBJECTIVES

After completing this chapter, you will be able to:

- **Explain** the goal of rehabilitation.
- **Examine** the roles and responsibilities of individuals working in the field of rehabilitation.
- **Compare** careers in occupational therapy and recreational therapy.
- **Describe** the roles and responsibilities of a speech-language pathologist and an audiologist.
- **Illustrate** the use and practice of communicating with sign language.
- **Demonstrate** eight rehabilitation procedures successfully.

BEFORE YOU READ

Connect What are some careers that help people overcome physical injuries, disabilities, and communication problems?

Main Idea

Rehabilitation workers help people recover from accidents, overcome disabilities, and improve their ability to communicate. They help individuals with physical or mental disabilities lead active, productive lives.

Note-Taking Activity

Draw this table. Write key terms and phrases under **Cues**. Write main ideas under **Note Taking**. Summarize the section under **Summary**.

Cues	Note Taking
◦ ◦	◦ ◦
Summary	

Graphic Organizer

Before you read the chapter, draw a diagram like the one below. As you read, write the rehabilitation careers and procedures covered in the chapter into the diagram.

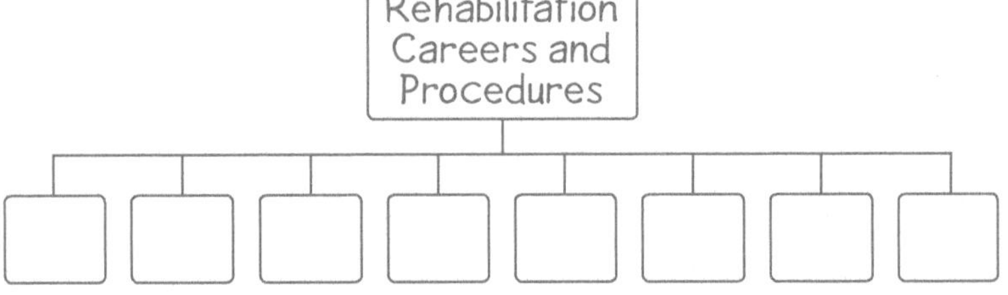

connect
Downloadable graphic organizers can be accessed online.

STANDARDS

HEALTH SCIENCE

NCHSE 1.13 Analyze the basic structure and function of the human body.

NCHSE 2.12 Recognize barriers to communication.

SCIENCE

NSES F Develop understanding of personal and community health; population growth; natural resources; environmental quality; natural and human-induced hazards; science and technology in local, national, and global challenges.

NCHSE *National Consortium for Health Science Education*

NSES *National Science Education Standards*

COMMON CORE STATE STANDARDS

MATHEMATICS

Number and Quantity

Quantities N-Q 1 Use units as a way to understand problems and to guide the solution of multi-step problems; choose and interpret units consistently in formulas; choose and interpret the scale and the origin in graphs and data displays.

ENGLISH LANGUAGE ARTS

Language

Conventions of Standard English

L-1a Apply the understanding that usage is a matter of convention, can change over time, and is sometimes contested.

Language

Vocabulary Acquisition and Use

L-5 Demonstrate understanding of figurative language, word relationships, and nuances in word meanings.

SECTION

20.1 Careers in Rehabilitation

Vocabulary

Content Vocabulary

You will learn these content vocabulary terms in this section.

- **mobility**
- **electrotherapy**
- **tinnitus**
- **cleft palate**
- **audiometer**
- **cochlear implant**

Academic Vocabulary

You will see this word in your reading and on your tests. Find its meaning in the Glossary in the back of this book.

- **restore**

Physical Therapy Careers

How do physical therapists help their patients have a better quality of life?

Healthcare professionals who have careers in rehabilitation help people who have been disabled by sickness, an injury, or a birth defect. Their goal is to help such people develop or recover as many of the abilities for the activities of daily living (ADL) as possible. Activities of daily living are the patient's routine daily activities, such as dressing and bathing.

Physical therapists are experts in examining and treating problems that affect patients' abilities to move well and function (see **Figure 20.1**). An important part of anyone's health is to be able to maintain an upright posture. People also need to move their arms and legs freely in order to perform many tasks and activities. Oxygen is the "fuel" of muscles and movement, but cardiac and pulmonary problems may change the body's ability to use oxygen. People can learn to live with medical conditions if they are able to continue a somewhat normal routine.

Physical Therapy Aide

Physical therapy aides, under the supervision of a physical therapist or physical therapy assistant, help make therapy sessions productive. They usually are responsible for keeping the treatment arca clean and organized and preparing for each patient's therapy.

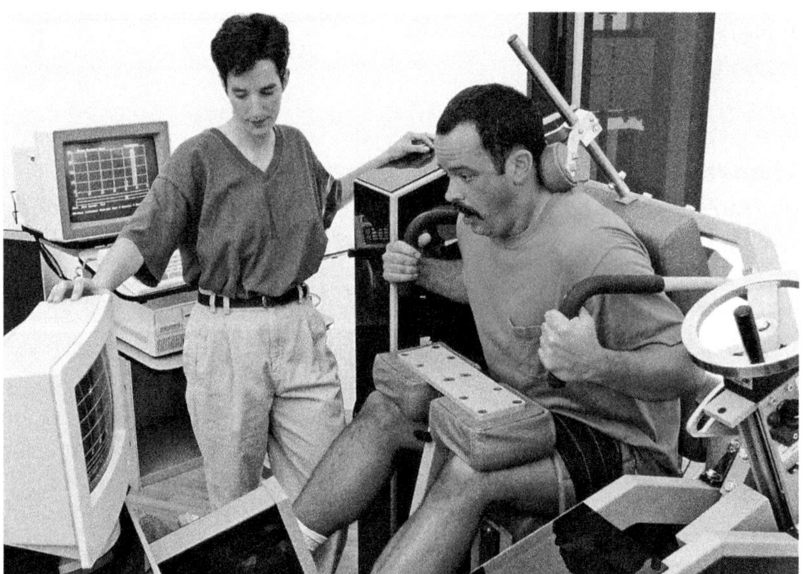

Fig. 20.1 Physical Therapy A physical therapist working with a patient. *How long does it take to become a physical therapist?*

Photo: Keith Brofsky/Photodisc/Getty Images

Table 20.1 Overview of Rehabilitation Careers

OCCUPATION	EDUCATIONAL REQUIREMENTS	CERTIFICATION OR LICENSING AGENCY	JOB OUTLOOK
Physical therapy aide	High school diploma	No licensing or certification is required.	Keen competition because of the large pool of qualified individuals
Physical therapy assistant (PTA)	Completion of a two-year associate degree program in an accredited junior, community, or technical college	Licensing or certification is not required in all states. Complete information may be obtained from state licensing boards.	Faster than average because of aging population and the increased need of physical therapists for assistants
Physical therapist (PT)	Degree from an accredited physical therapist education program. Such programs are offered in many colleges and universities.	A national licensure examination must be passed.	Faster than average because of aging population and increased insurance payments to physical therapists
Occupational therapy aide	On-the-job training in most facilities	No certification or licensure is required.	Keen competition because of the large pool of qualified individuals
Occupational therapy assistant (OTA)	An associate degree or certificate program from an accredited community or technical college	Must pass a national certification examination.	Faster than average because of growth in the number of individuals with disabilities
Occupational therapist (OT)	A degree from an accredited educational program	Must pass a national certification examination.	Faster than average because of growth in the number of individuals with disabilities
Recreational therapist	Bachelor's degree preferred; associate degrees accepted in a few states	The National Council for Therapeutic Recreation Certification (NCTRC) provides certification after the applicant passes a written test and completes an internship.	Slower than average because of change of emphasis from inpatient to outpatient care; better prospects for individuals with a bachelor's degree
Speech-language pathologist	Master's degree from a college or university that offers accredited communication programs	Certification by the American Speech-Language-Hearing Association is required after passing a national examination.	Faster than average because of hearing loss in the aging population
Audiologist	Master's degree with clinical experience. A doctorate in audiology (Au.D.) requires four years of postgraduate work.	Certification by the American Speech-Language-Hearing Association when applicants with a master's degree pass a national examination. This is now being phased out and replaced by a required Au.D. degree.	Much faster than average because of hearing loss in the aging population

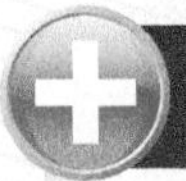

Safety

Crutches

Certain safety guidelines must be followed when a patient is using crutches.

1. Before giving crutches to the patient, make sure that the crutches have been fitted properly. The patient is measured and fitted for crutches by a therapist or other licensed personnel.
2. Check the crutches for cracks, bends, worn tips, and loose bolts. Replace the crutches with another pair if you find any problems.
3. **CAUTION:** Make sure that the patient is wearing flat shoes with nonskid soles.
4. Warn the patient that nerve damage can occur if weight is supported constantly on the arm rests.
5. Explain that the patient must use shoulder and arm strength to swing up to and through the crutches, stopping slightly in front of the crutches.
6. Check to make sure that the patient is not moving too far forward at one time.
7. Warn the patient that the length of steps should be limited. If the patient attempts to move the crutches too far forward, he or she can easily lose his or her balance and fall.

When patients need assistance moving to or from a treatment area, aides transport them in a wheelchair or give them a shoulder to lean on. Because they are not licensed, aides do not perform the clinical tasks of a physical therapy assistant. Physical therapy aides may also perform clerical tasks, such as ordering supplies, answering the phone, and filling out insurance forms.

Physical Therapy Assistant

A physical therapy assistant performs components of physical therapy procedures. Physical therapy assistants provide services that improve **mobility,** relieve pain, and prevent or limit permanent physical disabilities.

Two-year associate degree programs for physical therapy assistants are offered in junior, community, and technical colleges. Programs are divided into academic study and clinical experience. Before students begin their clinical field experience, many programs require that they complete a semester of anatomy and physiology and have certifications in CPR and first aid. Both educators and prospective employers view the clinical experience as essential in ensuring that students understand the responsibilities of a physical therapy assistant.

Physical Therapist

Physical therapist (PT) programs start with basic science courses—including biology, chemistry, and physics—and then introduce specialized courses, such as biomechanics, microanatomy, human growth and development, manifestations of disease, examination techniques, and therapeutic procedures. Many programs require experience as a volunteer in a physical therapy department of a hospital or clinic.

Physical therapists examine patients' medical histories and measure their strength, range of motion, balance and coordination, muscle performance, respiration, and motor function. They evaluate a patient's ability to be independent and to reenter the community or workplace after injury or illness. Physical therapists develop treatment plans that include a treatment strategy, its purpose, and an anticipated outcome.

Physical therapists are key members of the medical teams that evaluate and treat injured or disabled patients. They treat a wide variety of patients, including orthopedic, pediatric, and geriatric patients. The types of treatment physical therapists use include therapeutic exercise, massage, and the application of heat, cold, **electrotherapy,** and ultrasound. Physical therapists also plan, administer, and evaluate rehabilitation services and provide consultative, preventive, educational, and research services.

Career opportunities for physical therapists are varied. Physical therapists practice in school settings, private medical practices, sports rehabilitation centers, nursing homes, home health agencies, and industry, as well as more traditional acute care settings such as hospitals and rehabilitation centers. Opportunities are available in administration, research, teaching, and serving as an officer in the armed forces.

READING CHECK

Name the types of treatment performed by physical therapists.

Occupational Therapy Careers

Where are occupational therapy aides usually trained?

During World War I (1914–1918), recovering wounded soldiers often remained in the hospital for a long time. It was found that patients who were given handwork to do and tools to do it with recovered faster than those who did not. This led to the first schools of occupational therapy. The National Society for the Promotion of Occupational Therapy was formed in 1925. It is now the American Occupational Therapy Association.

The occupational therapy team first assesses a patient's physical or mental problems. They then help the patient regain, develop, or master skills. The first focus for a patient with a physical disability is to perform daily activities such as dressing, grooming, bathing, and eating. The goal for all patients is to function on their own, and live a useful and satisfying life.

Occupational Therapy Aide

Occupational therapy aides receive most of their training on the job rather than in a classroom. They prepare materials and assemble equipment used during treatment. Often they are responsible for telephone duties, restocking and ordering supplies, and filling out insurance forms and other paperwork. Aides are not licensed. By law, they are not allowed to perform as wide a range of tasks as are occupational therapy assistants.

Occupational Therapy Assistant

An occupational therapy assistant (OTA) typically works under the direction of an occupational therapist. OTAs receive an associate's degree or a certificate from an accredited community college or technical school.

The certified occupational therapy assistant helps patients with rehabilitative activities outlined in a treatment plan. This plan is developed in collaboration with the occupational therapist. Activities may range from teaching the proper method of moving from a bed into a wheelchair to the best way to stretch and loosen the muscles of the hand. Assistants monitor patients' rehabilitative activities, provide encouragement, and record the patient's progress for the therapist. They often document treatment for billing to the patient's health insurer.

21ST CENTURY SKILLS

Rehabilitation Recordkeeping

In the rehabilitation field, the process of recording a patient's activities and progress is essential. Accurate records are necessary for evaluating patients, billing, and reporting to physicians. These records help pinpoint problems and justify the cost of treatment when applications for reimbursement are submitted to insurance carriers. With electronic health records, in many cases the physician or other healthcare professional can view an electronic record of the patient's progress.

Follow-up

List any information that you think would be included in the record for a patient who was in a motorcycle accident and required physical therapy for two broken legs.

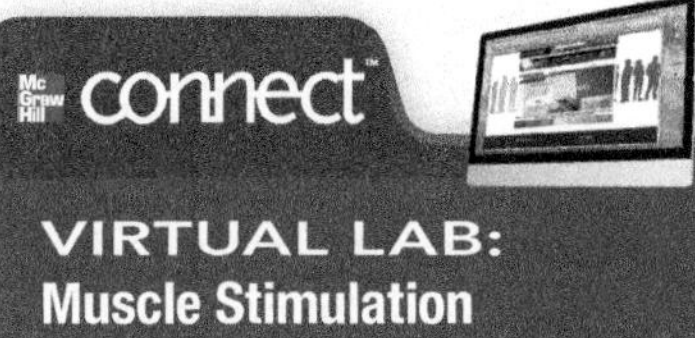

VIRTUAL LAB: Muscle Stimulation

In some states and healthcare facilities, only physical therapists, registered nurses, or other licensed personnel may perform range-of-motion exercises on the head and neck. Before you perform these exercises on any patient, check to be sure that you are legally authorized to do so.

Go to connect online to view the Virtual Lab and complete the assignment.

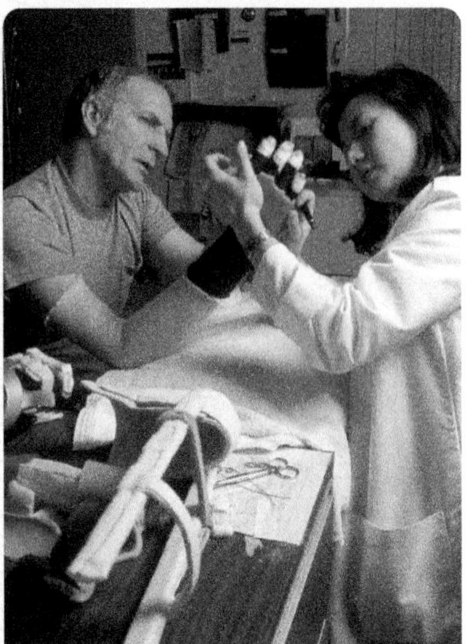

Fig. 20.2 Occupational Therapy An occupational therapist with a patient. *What types of patients may benefit from occupational therapy?*

Occupational Therapist

Occupational therapists (OTs) help patients develop, recover, maintain, or improve their ability to perform tasks in their daily living and working environments. They help patients improve basic motor functions and reasoning abilities. They also help patients compensate for permanent loss of function. The goal of an OT is to help patients live independent, productive, and satisfying lives. **Figure 20.2** shows an occupational therapist working with a patient.

Occupational therapists assist patients in performing all types of activities, from using a computer to meeting daily needs such as dressing, cooking, and eating. Physical exercises may be used to increase strength and dexterity. Paper-and-pencil exercises may be used to improve visual acuity. A patient who has short-term memory loss, for instance, might be encouraged to make lists to aid recall.

Patients who have permanent functional disabilities, such as spinal cord injuries, cerebral palsy, or muscular dystrophy, require adaptive equipment such as wheelchairs and splints. Therapists develop computer-aided adaptive equipment and teach patients how to use it. This enables patients to communicate better and to control other aspects of their environment.

Occupational therapists may work exclusively with patients in a particular age group or with patients who have particular disabilities. For example, in schools they evaluate children's abilities, recommend and provide therapy, modify classroom equipment, and in general, help children participate as fully as possible in school programs and activities. Occupational therapy is also beneficial to the elderly population. Therapists help senior citizens lead more active and independent lives through a variety of methods, including the use of adaptive equipment.

Occupational therapists in mental health settings treat individuals who are mentally ill, mentally challenged, or emotionally disturbed. They may also work with individuals who are dealing with alcoholism, drug abuse, depression, eating disorders, or stress-related disorders. Occupational therapists help with time management skills, budgeting, shopping, homemaking, use of public transportation, etc.

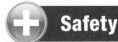

Safety

Caring for a Hearing Aid

Remember these important points:

- Do not drop a hearing aid. It is a fragile instrument.
- Do not expose the hearing aid to heat or moisture. Remove it before a bath or shower.
- Do not get lotions, sprays, or shampoos on the hearing aid. They can clog the mechanism.
- Do not let a patient wear a hearing aid when sleeping.

READING CHECK

List some areas of specialization as an occupational therapist.

Recreational Therapy

How can recreation help people with disabilities?

Recreational therapy came into being in the late 1940s and early 1950s, based on the premise that the use of recreation as a therapy tool has

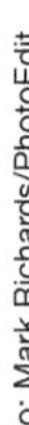

great merit. Recreational therapy involves recreation as treatment for ill or disabled patients. It helps ease the effects of illness or disability and restore the patient's function.

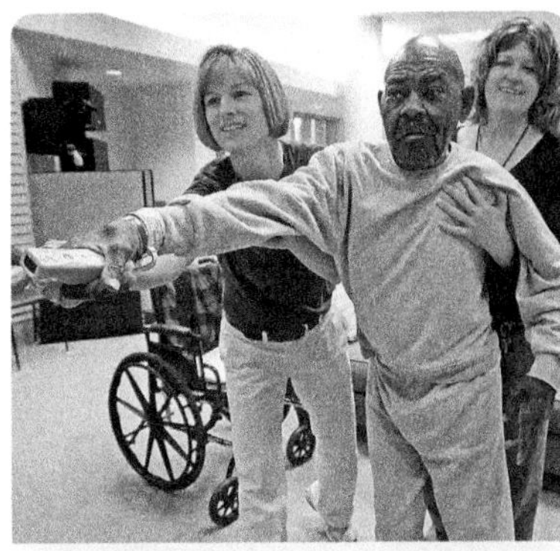

Fig. 20.3 Recreational Therapy Recreational treatment using a Wii video-game system. *What advantages does this type of therapy have over a game of cards?*

Recreational Therapy Careers

Recreational therapists provide recreation treatment activities to help with physical and mental problems. They also help support the emotional well-being of patients. Treatment may include the use of arts and crafts, music, drama, animals, sports, and games (see **Figure 20.3**). Recreational therapists should not be confused with recreation and fitness workers, who organize recreational activities primarily for enjoyment.

The goal of this type of therapy is to help patients reduce depression, stress, and anxiety. Recreational therapists help individuals recover basic motor functioning and reasoning abilities, build confidence, and socialize effectively. Such therapy fosters greater independence and helps reduce or eliminate the effects of illness or disability. In addition, recreational therapists help integrate people with disabilities into the community by assisting them in the use of community resources and recreational activities.

In long-term recreational care facilities, recreational therapists use leisure activities, especially structured group programs, to improve and maintain the residents' general health and well-being. **Figure 20.4** shows a recreational therapist working with patients.

Most employers prefer to hire candidates who are certified therapeutic recreation (CTR) specialists and have a bachelor's degree. An associate degree in recreational therapy; training in art, drama, or music therapy; or qualifying work experience may be sufficient for activity director positions in nursing homes or for similar job opportunities.

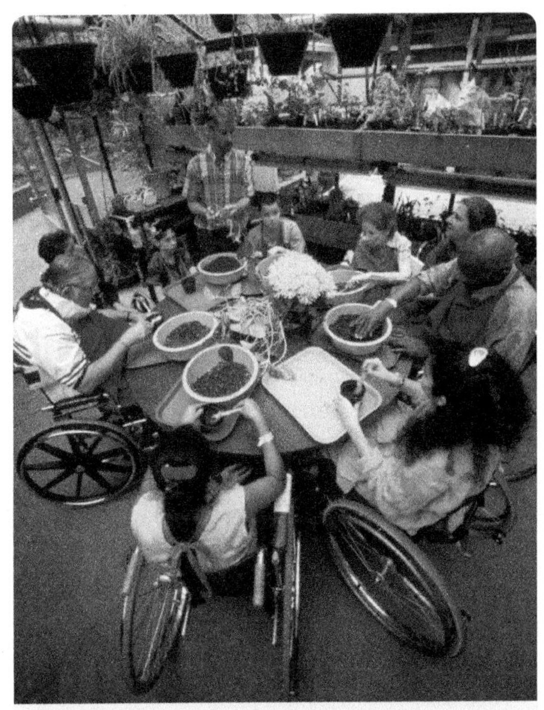

Fig. 20.4 Group Program Group recreational therapy. *What are the benefits of recreation?*

READING CHECK

Explain when the field of recreational therapy first emerged.

Speech, Language, and Hearing Careers

What physical conditions can impede verbal communication?

Language is vital to learning and working. There are many ways to express language, including speaking, using sign language, and writing. Speech-language pathologists assess, treat, and prevent communication and swallowing disorders.

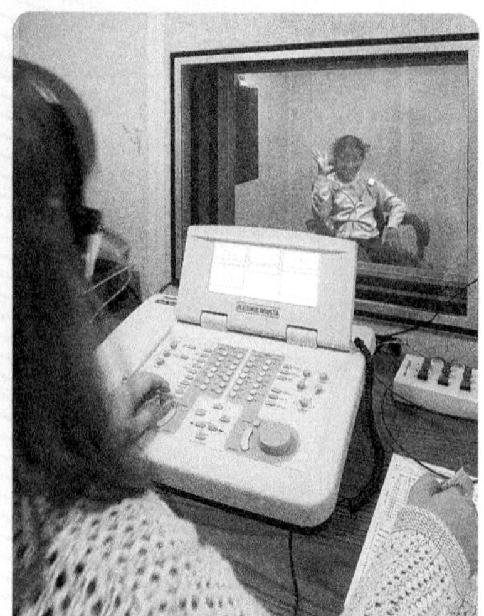

Fig. 20.5 Hearing Testing An audiologist with a patient. *What types of problems do audiologists treat?*

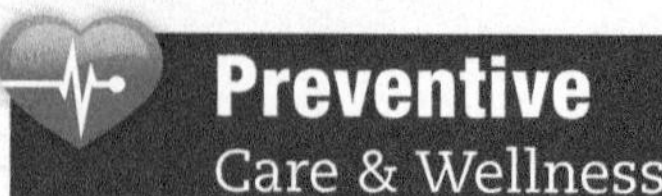

Preventive Care & Wellness

Protecting Your Hearing

The ear is composed of numerous delicate structures designed to carry sound waves to the brain. The hair cells in the inner ear are particularly important because they stimulate the auditory nerve, which transmits impulses to the brain. The brain then translates auditory impulses into the sounds we hear. Repeated exposure to too much noise can result in gradual hearing loss. Over time, excessive noise exposure can even result in permanent hearing loss. Think about that every time you turn up the volume of music, especially when you are wearing ear buds. If you must be exposed to loud noises, always use ear protection.

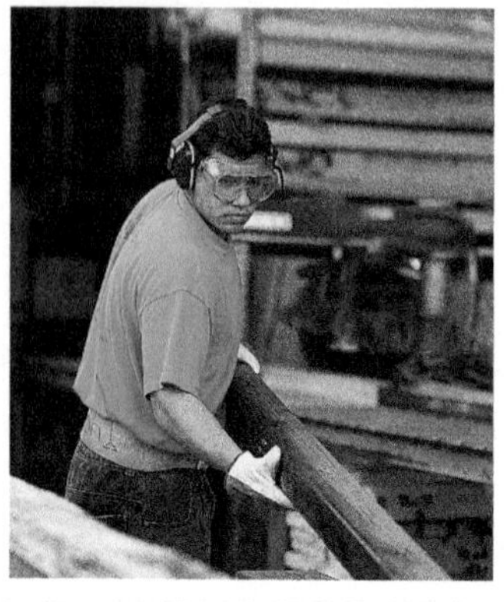

Audiologists assess and treat hearing- and balance-related problems. They select and fit devices to treat hearing loss. They also conduct research on problems such as **tinnitus** (ringing in the ear), hearing loss, and impaired balance. **Figure 20.5** shows an audiologist with a patient.

A certified speech-language pathologist or certified audiologist usually must obtain a master's degree. In a few states, noncertified audiologists and speech-language pathologists who have a bachelor's degree are also permitted to practice.

Speech-Language Pathologist

Speech-language pathologists work with patients who have a variety of speech and language difficulties. Some patients, for example,

- cannot make speech sounds or cannot make them clearly.
- have problems with speech rhythm and fluency, such as stuttering.
- have voice quality problems, such as inappropriate pitch.
- have difficulty understanding and producing language.
- wish to improve communication impairments, such as attention, memory, and problem-solving disorders.
- have oral motor problems with eating and swallowing.

These problems can result from many conditions including hearing loss, brain injury or deterioration, cerebral palsy (a condition involving impaired muscular abilities or paralysis), stroke, **cleft palate** (a condition in which the two plates that form the roof of the mouth are not completely connected), cognitive disabilities, and emotional problems. The causes of these problems may be congenital, developmental, or acquired. Speech-language pathologists use written and oral tests as well as special instruments to diagnose the nature and extent of impairment. They record and analyze speech, language, and swallowing irregularities. They then develop an individualized plan of care.

For patients who have little or no speech capability, speech-language pathologists may teach them alternative communication methods, including automated devices and sign language. They teach these patients how to make sounds, improve their voices, or increase their skills to communicate more effectively. Speech-language pathologists help patients develop, or recover, reliable communication skills, so that they can perform their educational, vocational, and social roles.

Speech-language pathologists must keep records on the initial evaluation, progress, and discharge of patients. They counsel patients and their families concerning communication disorders, and teach them how to cope with the stress and misunderstandings that often accompany those disorders. They work with family members to change behavior patterns that hinder communication and treatment.

Audiologist

Audiologists work with people who have hearing, balance, and related problems. They work in a variety of settings, often as a member of an interdisciplinary team that plans and implements treatment for children and adults of all ages.

Audiologists use a device called the **audiometer** (see **Figure 20.6**). Audiologists measure the loudness at which a patient begins to hear sounds, the patient's ability to distinguish between sounds, and the extent of the patient's hearing loss. They interpret these results to make a diagnosis and determine a course of treatment.

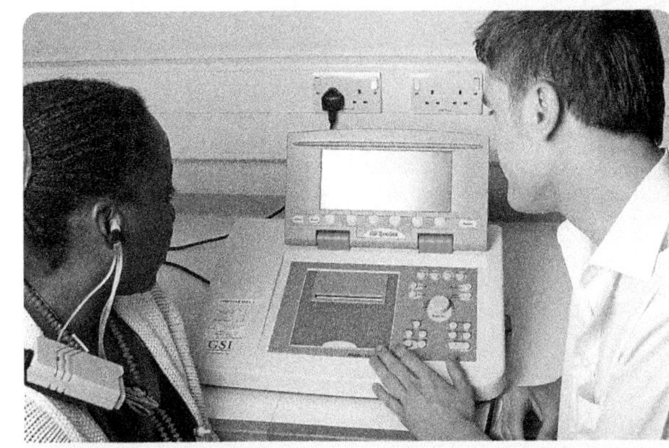

Fig. 20.6 Audiometer Audiometers are used to measure hearing. *What are some causes of hearing disorders?*

Hearing disorders can result from a variety of causes, such as trauma at birth, viral infections, genetic disorders, exposure to loud noise, and aging. Treatment may include examining and cleaning the ear canal, fitting and dispensing hearing aids or other assistive devices, and audiologic rehabilitation. The term "audiologic rehabilitation" refers to auditory training or instruction in speech or lip reading.

Audiologists may fit and dispense hearing aids. They fit and tune **cochlear implants** (devices that partially restore the ablity to hear) and help patients adjust to listening with implant amplification systems. They also measure noise levels in workplaces and conduct hearing-protection programs. Audiologists may work in hearing clinics or may independently develop and implement treatment programs.

READING CHECK

Summarize possible components of a speech-language pathologist's treatment plan.

SECTION 20.1 Careers in Rehabilitation Review

AFTER YOU READ

1. **Identify** the healthcare professionals who might be included on a rehabilitation team.
2. **Describe** how the goals of rehabilitation are accomplished.
3. **Name** the career that requires a period of volunteering before an applicant can be admitted to a professional educational program.
4. **Indicate** the name of the other workers with whom recreational therapists are sometimes confused.
5. **Select** three problems that could make it necessary for a patient to require speech therapy.
6. **Identify** the kinds of problems that patients of audiologists have.

Technology ONLINE EXPLORATIONS

Career Investigation

Select the career in rehabilitation that interests you the most. Research that career online and create a complete job description for it. Then visit a facility that has one or more employees in the rehabilitation field you have chosen. Interview a professional in the field and compare his or her duties with the job description you created. What was the same? What was different?

SECTION

20.2 Rehabilitation Procedures

Vocabulary

Content Vocabulary

You will learn these content vocabulary terms in this section.

- range-of-motion (ROM) exercise
- contracture
- transfer (gait) belt
- crutches
- cane
- walker
- otoscope
- audiogram
- decibel (dB)
- American Sign Language (ASL)

Academic Vocabulary

You will see this word in your reading and on your tests. Find its meaning in the Glossary in the back of this book.

- range

Range-of-Motion Exercises

What are contractures?

Each joint in our body has a range of motion (ROM). Sometimes patients have an illness or disability that requires long periods of immobility or bed rest. During this time it is vital that all their joints be moved through their full range of motion. **Range-of-motion (ROM) exercises** help to maintain muscle tone and joint flexibility. They also prevent **contractures,** the permanent shortening of muscles due to lack of use. Healthcare professionals such as therapy and nursing personnel may be asked to help patients perform the exercises. In most cases, a physician or therapist details the joints to be moved and the number of times each movement should be performed, as well as the number of times per day each group of exercises should be performed. As described in **Table 20.2,** the movements in the range-of-motion exercises have special names based upon the way the joint moves.

There are three categories of range-of-motion exercises, which vary according to the patient's physical abilities. Those categories are

- **Active range of motion:** The patient is able to move the joint or extremity (limb) without assistance.
- **Active assisted range of motion:** The patient has limited ability to move the joint or limb and needs some assistance.
- **Passive range of motion:** The patient is unable to move the joint or limb, so the healthcare worker moves it for him or her.

READING CHECK

Name the type of patient who requires the most assistance when performing range-of-motion exercises.

Table 20.2 Range-of-Motion Movements

MOVEMENT NAME		ACTION EXAMPLES
Abduction	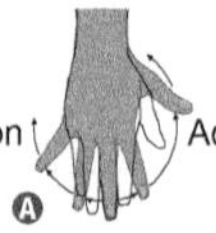	**Action:** Moving away from the body **Example:** Shoulder, hip, ankle, fingers, and toes
Adduction	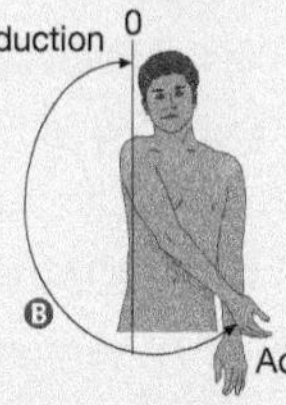	**Action:** Moving toward the body **Example:** Shoulder, hip, ankle, fingers, and toes

Table 20.2 Range-of-Motion Movements (continued)

MOVEMENT NAME	ACTION EXAMPLES
Extension 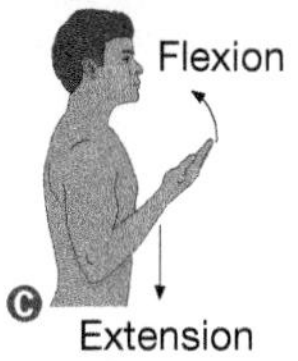	**Action:** Straightening **Example:** Hinge joints: hip, knee, shoulder, elbow, wrist, neck, back, fingers, and toes
Flexion 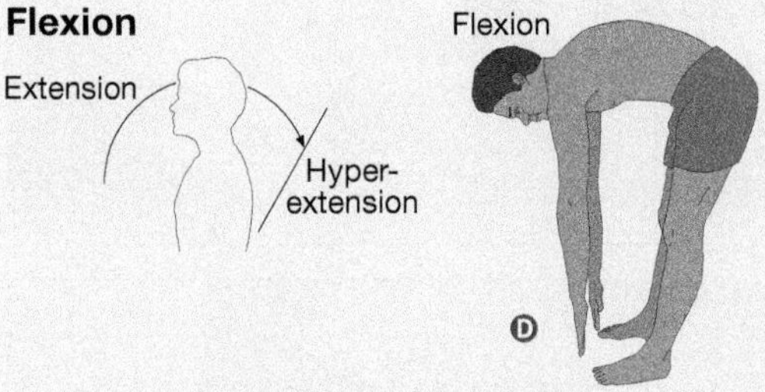	**Action:** Bending **Example:** Hinge joints: knee, elbow, and waist
Hyperextension 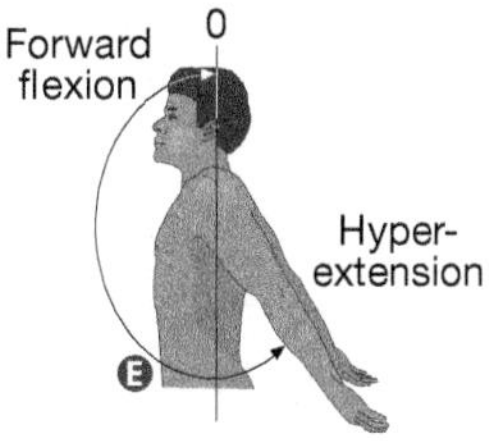	**Action:** Excessive straightening **Example:** Neck and wrist
Inversion and Eversion 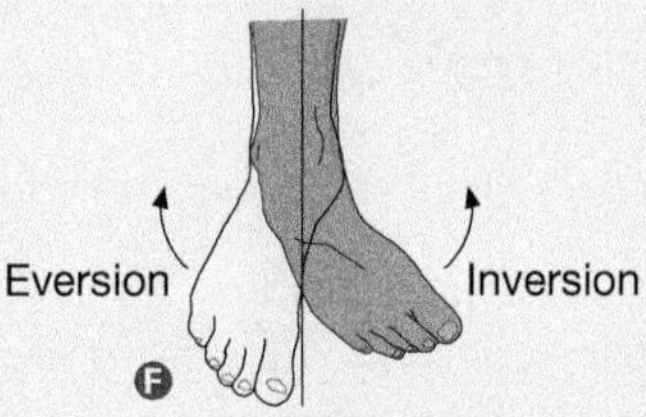	**Action: (Inversion)** Moving toward the inside **Example:** Foot and ankle **Action: (Eversion)** Moving toward the outside **Example:** Foot and ankle
Dorsiflexion 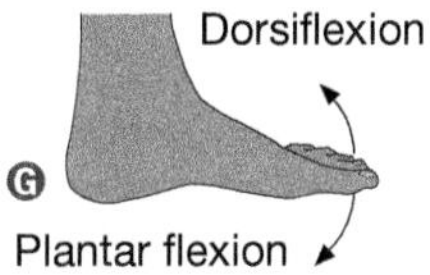	**Action:** Bending backward **Example:** Ankle
Rotation 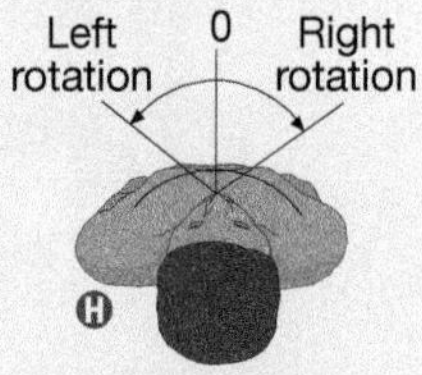	**Action:** Turning on an axis **Example:** Ankle, shoulder, and hip
Internal and External Rotation 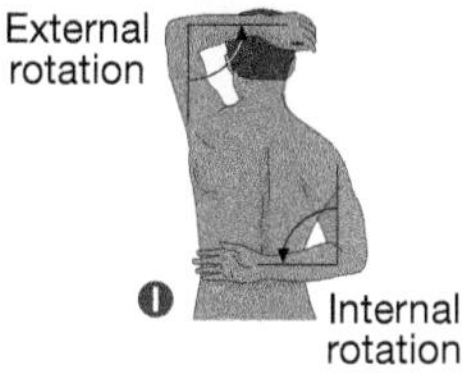	**Action:** (Internal) Turning inward **Example:** Hip and shoulder **Action:** (External) Turning outward **Example:** Hip and shoulder
Pronation and Supination 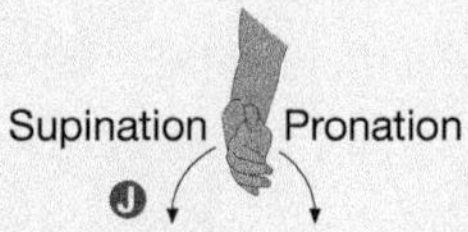	**Action:** (Pronation) Turning downward **Example:** Forearm **Action:** (Supination) Turning upward **Example:** Forearm

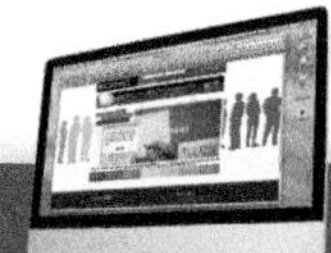

connect ONLINE PROCEDURES

PROCEDURE 20-1

Performing Range-of-Motion Exercises

Range of motion relies on muscle flexibility, which is possible due to the elasticity of the muscles. Elasticity can be defined as the ability of muscles to regain their true size and shape after being stretched or otherwise deformed. When a patient has been confined to bed rest for an extended time ROM becomes even more important.

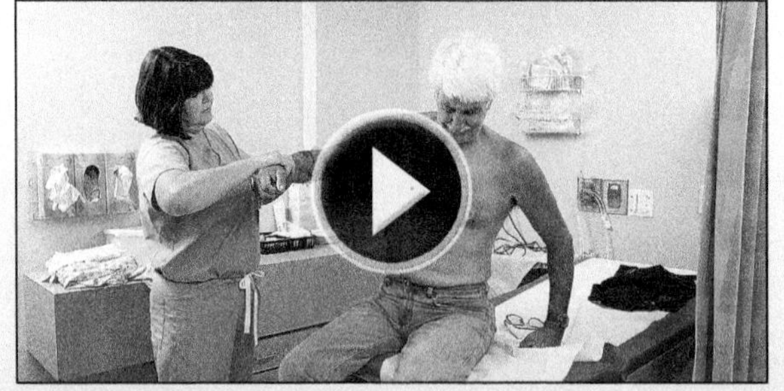

PROCEDURE 20-2

Ambulating a Patient with a Transfer (Gait) Belt

A **transfer, or gait, belt** is a band of fabric or leather that is positioned around a patient's waist during transfers or ambulation. It provides additional support for the patient. The transfer belt gives the patient a sense of security and stabilizes the patient's center of balance.

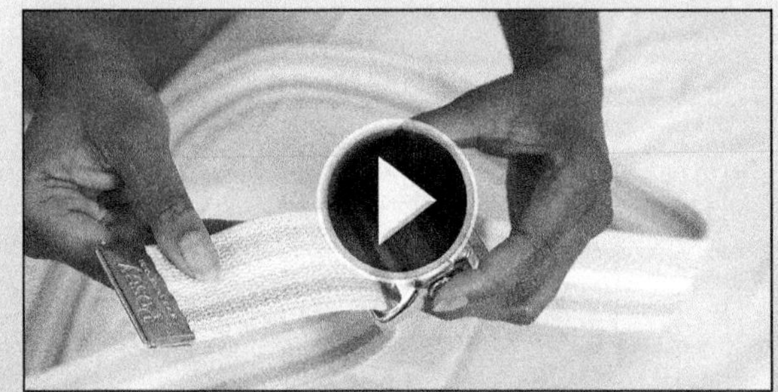

PROCEDURE 20-3

Ambulating a Patient with Crutches

Crutches are a walking aid for patients who are unable to use one leg or who need to gain strength in both legs. Crutches are used to reduce the weight load on one leg and broaden the support base to improve balance and stability. A therapist or other authorized individual fits the crutches to the patient and teaches the appropriate gait.

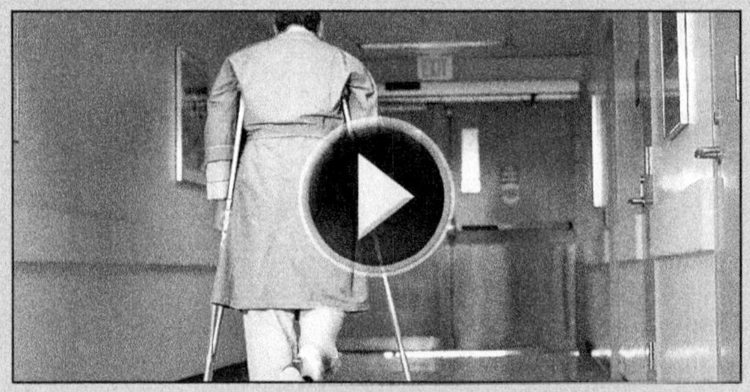

PROCEDURE 20-4

Ambulating a Patient with a Cane

A **cane** is another type of walking aid. Canes help patients who have weakness on one side of the body gain balance and support. Patients who need maximum support should use a three- or four-point cane. Patients who need less support may use a single-point cane.

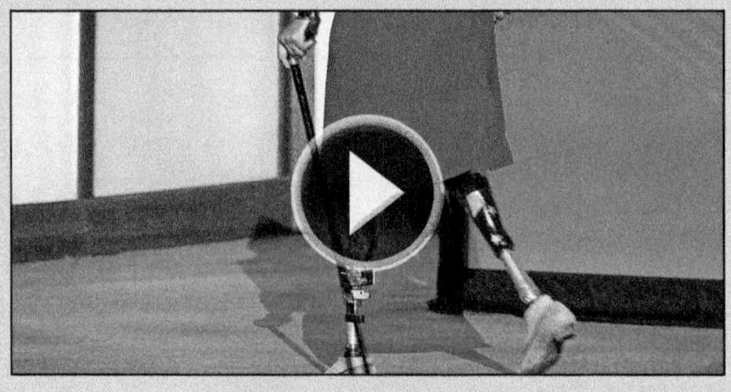

PROCEDURE 20-5

Ambulating a Patient with a Walker

A **walker** is a support device with a frame, handgrips, and four points at the bottom. Walkers provide more support than a cane or crutches can. Walkers are usually made of a lightweight yet sturdy material, such as aluminum.

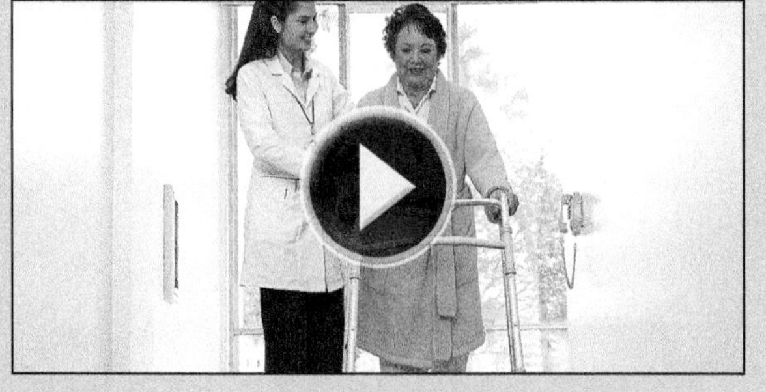

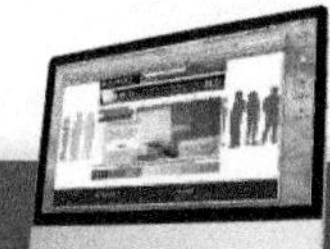

connect ONLINE PROCEDURES

PROCEDURE 20-6

Helping a Patient Who Is Falling

Falls can happen for a number of reasons. Some falls are preventable, and some are not. Even with prevention efforts, sometimes a patient who is standing or walking may begin to fall. Your most important concern should be for the patient's safety.

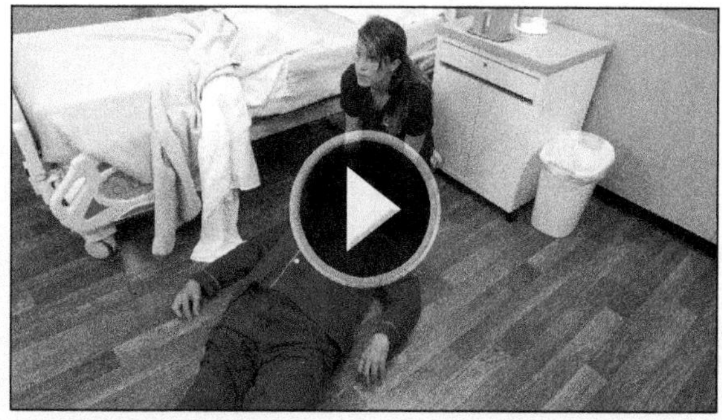

PROCEDURE 20-7

Assisting with an Examination of the Ear

The ear might be examined in a routine physical or when disease processes are suspected. They are usually examined with an instrument called an **otoscope,** a handheld instrument with a tiny light and a cone-shaped plastic tip called an ear speculum.

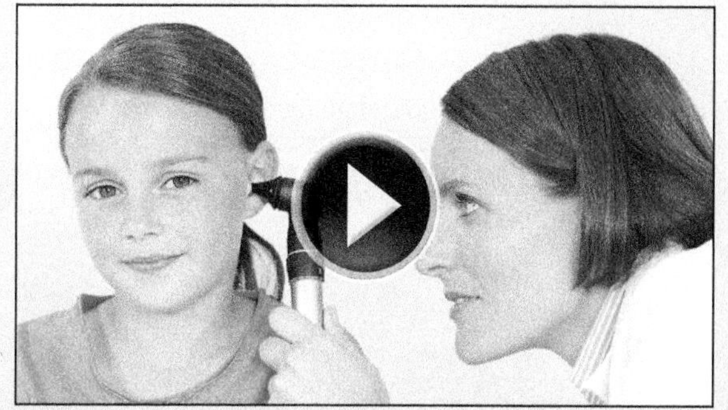

Testing Hearing

How is it possible to measure how well another person can hear?

More than 40 million people in the United States suffer from hearing loss. Hearing loss is therefore one of the most widespread chronic healthcare problems in society. With today's technology, an audiologist can determine whether hearing loss is present, even in newborns. With early detection, a child may be helped to develop language and speech despite the loss of hearing.

After using an **otoscope** (an instrument with a light and a cone-shaped tip called an ear speculum; see **Figure 20.7**) to examine the outer and middle ear (see **Procedure 20-7** to learn more about this process), an audiologist may use several tests to find out which tones, sounds, and words a patient can or cannot hear. These tests are usually given in a soundproof room using electronic equipment. The patient is asked to signal when he or she hears tones through an earphone that delivers sounds to the patient. When the test is completed, the results are printed on a graph called an **audiogram** (see **Figure 20.8** on page 520), a tool used to determine the extent of hearing loss. It shows the point at which the patient begins to hear low pitches or frequencies.

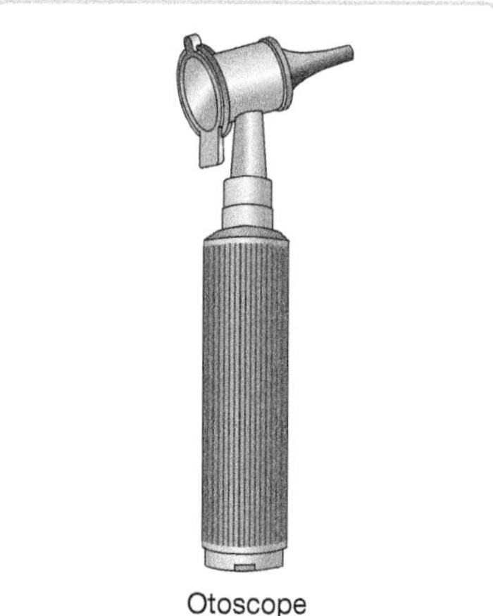

Fig. 20.7 Otoscope An otoscope is an instrument for examining the ear. *What parts of the ear can be examined with an otoscope?*

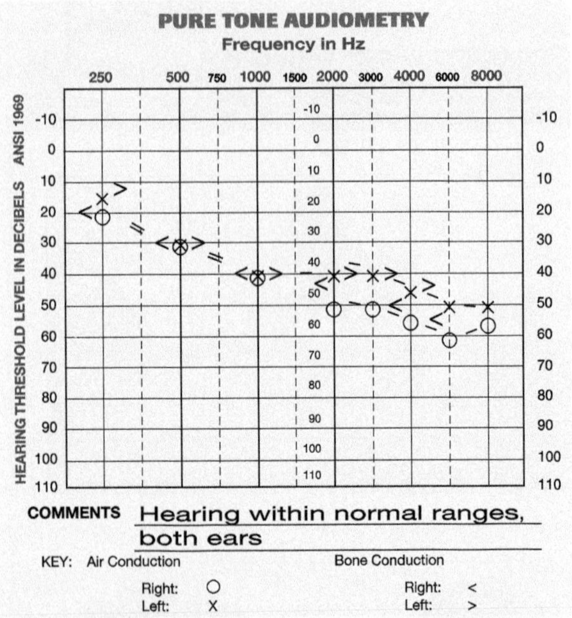

Fig. 20.8 Audiogram Audiogram results indicate the level at which the patient begins to hear sound. *What instrument is used to measure hearing?*

Hearing is not measured in percentages. Instead, it is measured in an arbitrary unit of loudness called the **decibel (dB)**. A normal conversation is measured at approximately 60 dBs. There are three types of hearing loss:

- Conductive hearing loss occurs when the eardrum, bones, and membranes do not properly transmit vibrations to the cochlea. The cochlea, a cone-shaped tube, is a portion of the inner ear and contains the receptor for hearing. Causes include traumatic head injury or birth defects.
- Sensorineural hearing loss is characterized by deterioration of the cochlea. The aging process and excessive exposure to loud noise cause this type of hearing loss. This type of damage is permanent.
- Mixed hearing loss involves a combination of both conductive and sensorineural hearing loss.

READING CHECK

Identify the physical conditions that can cause hearing loss.

Sign Language

How many English words can be signed?

Although **American Sign Language (ASL)** is similar to the spoken language, it is not just a form of English and has its own distinct grammatical structure. ASL is not auditory but visual. It is made up of precise hand shapes and movements.

American Sign Language was developed by American deaf people to communicate with each other. Standardization of the language began

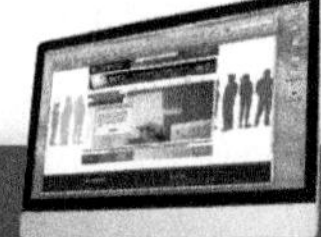

Mc Graw Hill connect™ ONLINE PROCEDURES

PROCEDURE 20-8

Removing and Inserting a Hearing Aid

A hearing aid is a device that can amplify sound waves in order to help a deaf or hard-of-hearing person hear more clearly. It can help most people with hearing loss understand speech better and achieve better communication. More than 1000 different models of hearing aids are available in the United States. Most of these must be removed for the following activities and reinserted later: cleaning, battery changes, bathing, and sleeping. You may have to assist a patient who is unable to remove and insert his or her own hearing aid.

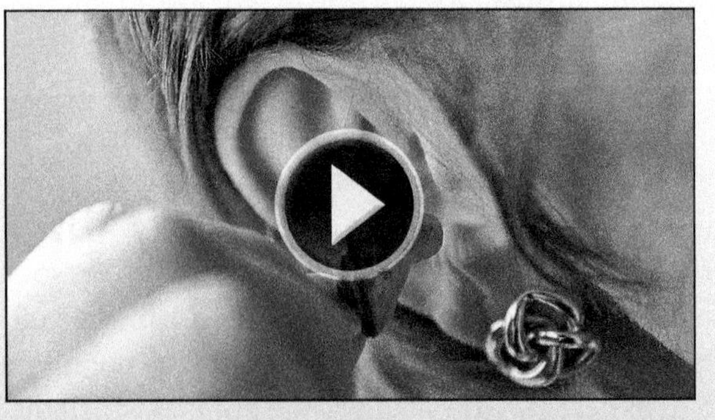

Photo: Jack Star/PhotoLink/PhotoDisc/Getty Images

in 1817, when Thomas H. Gallaudet and Laurent Clerc opened the first school for the deaf in the United States. Students then spread the use of ASL to other parts of the United States and to Canada.

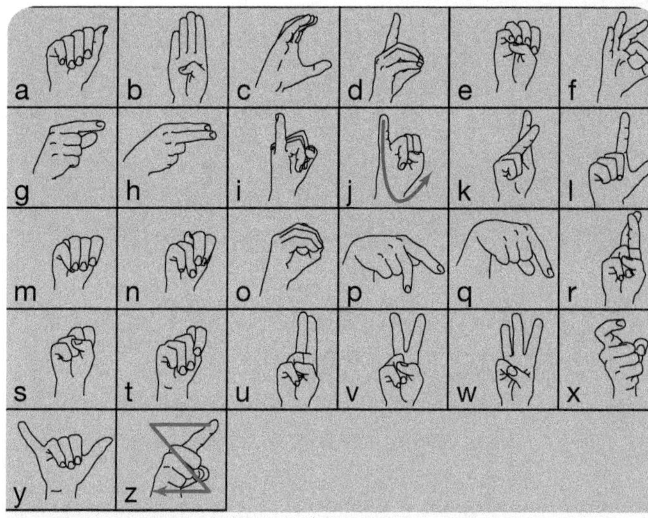

Fig. 20.9 Signs These are the letters of the American Sign Language (ASL) Alphabet. *Can you sign your own name?*

In the late 1800s, deaf people were discouraged from using ASL. Many well-meaning but misguided educators believed that the only way for deaf people to fit into the hearing world was through speech and lip-reading. These educators insisted that deaf children try to learn to speak English. Some even went so far as to tie down a deaf child's hands. Since the 1960s, there has been a tremendous growth in the number of sign language classes taught in the United States. ASL (see **Figure 20.9**) expresses many concepts with single gestures. It is not necessary to reproduce every word in a spoken English-language sentence in gestures. Sign language includes the full English alphabet, numbers, and well over 1200 words or phrases communicated by using the hand gestures only.

READING CHECK

Identify some differences between spoken English and sign language.

SECTION 20.2 Rehabilitation Procedures Review

AFTER YOU READ

1. **Indicate** the muscle condition that may be caused by long periods of immobility.
2. **Select** three types of range-of-motion exercises.
3. **Explain** the purpose of a transfer (gait) belt.
4. **Indicate** the warning that should be given to a patient preparing to walk on crutches.
5. **Analyze** how a cane helps a patient.
6. **Predict** what might happen if a patient slides a walker rather than lifting it forward.
7. **Describe** what must happen before a patient who has fallen can be moved.
8. **Identify** what redness or fluid in the eardrum might indicate.
9. **Name** what the decibel measures.
10. **Explain** how a hearing aid should be cleaned.
11. **Recall** the great achievement of Thomas Gallaudet and Laurent Clerc.

Technology ONLINE EXPLORATIONS

Hearing Loss

Research online for information about causes of hearing loss. Create a list of at least ten common causes. Determine whether you may be at risk for hearing loss. If so, explain why you may be at risk. If you believe you are not at risk, explain why.

CHAPTER 20 Review

Chapter Summary

SECTION 20.1

- The primary goal of rehabilitation is to restore a patient to the highest possible level of functioning for that individual and to maintain the patient at that level. **(pg. 508)**
- Physical therapists examine and treat problems that affect patients' abilities to move well and to function in their daily lives. **(pg. 510)**
- Occupational therapists help patients improve their ability to perform tasks in their daily living and working environments. Recreational therapists improve functioning and independence and provide recreational resources and opportunities in order to improve health and well-being. Both types of healthcare workers help patients to reduce or eliminate the effects of illness or disability. **(pg. 512)**
- Speech-language pathologists assess speech and language development, and treat language and speech disorders. Audiologists assess, treat, and rehabilitate deficits in hearing and balance. **(pg. 514)**

SECTION 20.2

- It is important to understand the positive aspects of exercise and the possible complications of immobility. **(pg. 516)**
- Skill in performing range-of-motion exercises is needed to prevent harm to patients during these exercises. **(pg. 516)**
- Proper techniques must be used to ambulate patients. **(pg. 518)**
- Although the technique for assisting a patient who is falling is important, it is more important to prevent a fall. **(pg. 519)**
- A licensed healthcare giver uses an otoscope to examine the ears. **(pg. 519)**
- An audiogram is a tool used to determine the extent of hearing loss. **(pg. 519)**
- Hearing aids are fragile and expensive, and should be handled carefully. If possible, the patient should insert and remove his or her own hearing aid. **(pg. 520)**
- American Sign Language is visual, with a distinct grammatical structure. **(pg. 520)**

Mc Graw Hill connect™ ONLINE ACTIVITIES

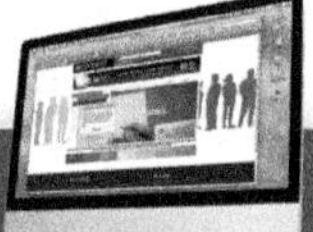

Complete our HST online activities for Chapter 20, which include Concept Check review questions, Reference Flash Cards, and Online Procedures assessment sheets.

- **Concept Check** review questions
- **Reference Flash Cards** medical terminology practice
- **Online Procedures** assessment sheets

CHAPTER

20 Assessment

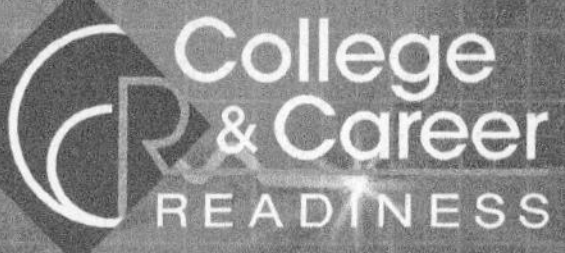

Critical Thinking/Problem Solving

1. What should be done if a patient refuses to perform range-of-motion exercises?
2. If a person has had a spinal cord injury causing paralysis of both legs, what types of therapists might care for him or her?
3. How do the duties of a PT and an OT differ? How are they similar?
4. If a person using crutches complains of pain or numbness in the axilla, arm, or hand, what might be causing the problem?
5. You enter a patient's room and find him sitting on the floor. What should you do?
6. While assisting a female patient into the shower, you notice that she has a hearing aid in place. What should you do?
7. Obtain crutches and practice the five types of gait discussed in **Procedure 20-3**.

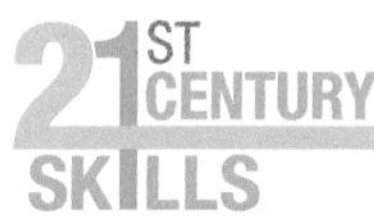

8. **Teamwork** With a partner, take turns pretending to have a disability. Use earplugs to simulate a hearing deficit, or use some type of brace, cast, or crutches. Try to do activities such as using a telephone, combing your hair, or putting on a coat. Write a summary of how you felt, what difficulties you encountered, and how you were treated by others. Include why the field of rehabilitation is or is not important.
9. **Teamwork** Using the movements described in **Table 20.2** on pages 516–517, exercise your own or a partner's joints to the full range of motion. Make a list of the movements performed by each joint. For example: Elbow—flexion and extension.
10. **Information literacy** Review **Figure 20.9** on page 521, which shows the ASL alphabet, or do a search for an online sign language dictionary. Practice signing your name, a word, or a complete sentence. Show a partner what you have practiced.
11. **Information literacy** Choose a rehabilitation career field. Visit the website of its professional association. List the advantages and disadvantages of your chosen field. Consider the entrance and educational requirements, job responsibilities, and rewards and challenges of the job. Review your list and decide if you are interested in entering this field. Here are some associations to investigate:
    - American Physical Therapy Association
    - American Occupational Therapy Association
    - American Therapeutic Recreation Association
    - American Speech-Language-Hearing Association

CHAPTER 21 Sports Medicine

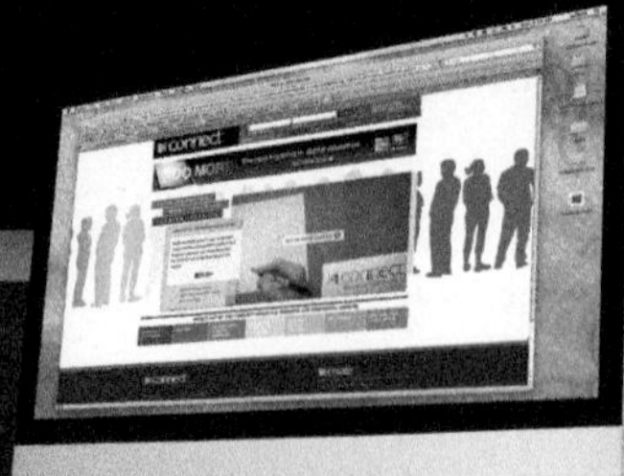

McGraw Hill connect™

It's Online!

- Online Procedures
- STEM Connection
- Medical Science
- Medical Terms
- Medical Math
- Ethics in Action
- Virtual Lab

Essential Question:

What types of athletes are most likely to need the help of sports medicine professionals?

The need for sports medicine personnel will continue to grow as more people recognize the benefits of exercise. The healthcare professionals covered in this chapter—sports medicine technicians, certified personal trainers, certified athletic trainers, certified strength and conditioning specialists, exercise physiologists, and sports physical therapists—have at least one thing in common: They all improve fitness through exercise. People working in sports medicine may have once been athletes or may feel a need to stay close to athletic settings. Whatever the reasons for their career choices, they all work to help clients of all ages and fitness levels achieve their potential.

Photo: Stefan Obermeier/imagebroker/Alamy

READING GUIDE

OBJECTIVES

After completing this chapter, you will be able to:

- **Compare** the job duties of a sports medicine technician, certified personal trainer, certified athletic trainer, certified strength and conditioning specialist, exercise physiologist, and sports physical therapist.
- **Identify** settings where sports medicine professionals work.
- **Compare** the job duties of a personal trainer to those of a strength and conditioning specialist.
- **Recognize** the uses of hot versus cold modalities.
- **Identify** the situations in which hot or cold modalities should and should not be used.
- **Explain** the components of proper physical fitness.
- **Calculate** a target heart rate.
- **Perform** four sports medicine procedures.

BEFORE YOU READ

Connect Have you ever been injured while playing sports? If so, how was your injury treated?

Main Idea

Professionals in sports medicine help both athletes and non-athletes recover from injuries and improve their physical fitness.

Note-Taking Activity

Draw this table. Write key terms and phrases under **Cues**. Write main ideas under **Note Taking**. Summarize the section under **Summary**.

Cues	Note Taking
o o	o o
Summary	

Graphic Organizer

Before you read the chapter, draw a diagram like the one below. As you read, write the names of the sports medicine careers covered in the chapter into the diagram.

Sports Medicine careers

connect

Downloadable graphic organizers can be accessed online.

STANDARDS

HEALTH SCIENCE

NCHSE 1.11 Classify the basic structural and functional organization of the human body (tissue, organ, and system).

NCHSE 1.31 Apply mathematical computations related to healthcare procedures (metric and household, conversions and measurements).

NCHSE 7.22 Apply principles of body mechanics.

SCIENCE

NSES F Develop understanding of personal and community health; population growth; natural resources; environmental quality; natural and human-induced hazards; science and technology in local, national, and global challenges.

NCHSE *National Consortium for Health Science Education*

NSES *National Science Education Standards*

COMMON CORE STATE STANDARDS

MATHEMATICS

Number and Quantity

Quantities N-Q Reason quantitatively and use units to solve problems.

Statistics and Probability

Interpreting Categorical and Quantitative Data S-ID Summarize, represent, and interpret data on a single count or measurement variable.

ENGLISH LANGUAGE ARTS

Speaking and Listening

Comprehension and Collaboration SL-2 Integrate multiple sources of information presented in diverse media or formats (e.g., visually, quantitatively, orally) evaluating the credibility and accuracy of each source.

SECTION 21.1 Careers in Sports Medicine

Vocabulary

Content Vocabulary

You will learn these content vocabulary terms in this section.

- **hydrocollator**
- **body mass index (BMI)**
- **strength**
- **aerobic exercise**
- **anaerobic exercise**
- **modalities**
- **ergonomics**
- **sprains**
- **strains**
- **kinesiology**
- **VO2 max test**
- **proprioception**
- **passive range of motion**

Academic Vocabulary

You will see this word in your reading and on your tests. Find its meaning in the Glossary in the back of the book.

- **implementing**

Sports Medicine Technician

How does the sports medicine technician help maintain training facilities?

As the demand for sports physical therapists grows, so will the need for sports medicine technicians. These technicians aid therapists and trainers with basic tasks, such as applying hot and cold packs or placing a client in a sports whirlpool. Technicians also monitor clients as they perform therapeutic exercises and pay close attention to proper form as well as the correct speed, range of motion, and number of repetitions and sets.

Often, a certified or licensed professional will treat more than one client at a time. They may also need to spend extended time with a specific client. To assist, the technician may watch the other clients. However, the technician is there to supervise, not modify, the exercises.

Many sports medicine technicians are high school and college students interested in a career in physical therapy, athletic training, or a related field. Shadowing a professional or working as a technician gives insight into clinics and what job duties staff members perform.

Many sports medicine programs for physical therapy or athletic training prefer or require a candidate to have logged a certain number of volunteer hours in a clinical or hospital setting before applying to an undergraduate or graduate program. See **Table 21.1** for an overview of sports medicine careers.

The Job of the Sports Medicine Technician

Sports medicine technicians perform many duties at the beginning of the day, including opening the clinic, retrieving client records, filling the whirlpool and setting the temperature, putting linens on treatment tables, and reviewing overnight messages from clients.

During the day, the technician may perform the following tasks:

- Apply hot and cold packs
- Assist clients in and out of the whirlpool
- Monitor clients as they perform exercises
- Change linens after treatments
- Inform therapists of client arrival
- Take phone calls from clients who are making or canceling appointments

Table 21.1 Overview of Sports Medicine Careers

OCCUPATION	EDUCATIONAL REQUIREMENTS	CERTIFICATION OR LICENSING AGENCY	JOB OUTLOOK
Sports Medicine Technician	Technicians are usually at least 14 years old and interested in a sports medicine career field. On-the-job training is usually available.	None	Faster than average growth due to the growing need for assistance by sports medicine professionals.
Certified Personal Trainer	Varies from passing the National Strength and Conditioning Association's certification exam to a four-year undergraduate degree. Certification in cardiopulmonary resuscitation (CPR) is usually required. Must earn continuing education units every two to three years.	The National Strength and Conditioning Association, National Federation of Professional Trainers, Aerobics and Fitness Association of America, American College of Sports Medicine, and American Council on Exercise	Faster than average growth due to the increased understanding of the benefits of exercise.
Certified Athletic Trainer	A four-year undergraduate degree, usually in a sports medicine discipline such as kinesiology or exercise physiology. May be followed by a two-year graduate degree. CPR certification is usually required.	National Athletic Training Association (NATA) Certification Board States may also require certification through their exams and in-state licensure or registration.	Faster than average growth due to the increased awareness of the benefits of exercise and a growth in the number of injuries associated with exercise.
Certified Strength and Conditioning Specialist	A four-year undergraduate degree or the status of senior at an accredited college or university. Certification in CPR is required. Must complete six continuing education units, as defined by NSCA, every three years	National Strength and Conditioning Association (NSCA)	Faster than average growth due to the increased understanding of the benefits of exercise.
Exercise Physiologist	A Master of Science degree to assist in research. A Ph.D is required for independent research positions.	None	Faster than average growth due to increased research and interest in supplements and extremes of environment on the human body.
Sports Physical Therapist	A minimum of three years of undergraduate prerequisites before starting a graduate program. Most programs are at the master's level and some are doctoral programs.	Individual state Boards of Physical Therapy/ Medicine	Faster than average growth due to an aging population, realization of the benefits of exercise, and a growth in the number of injuries associated with exercise.

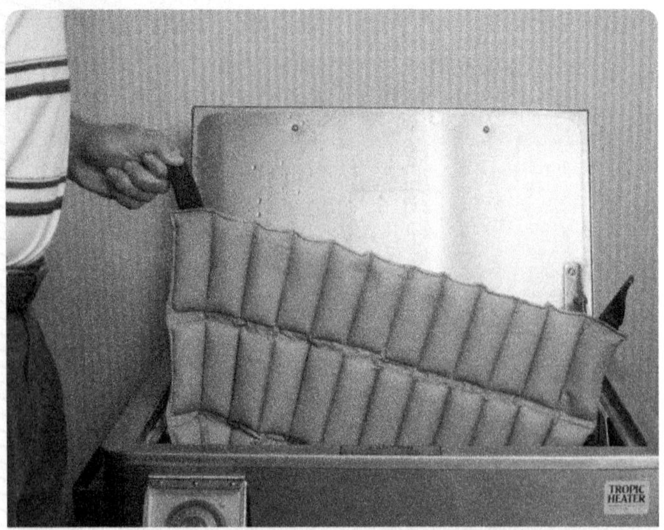

Fig. 21.1 Hydrocollator Shown is a hydrocollator with gel-filled packs. *What is this machine used for?*

- Retrieve equipment needed by the therapists
- Periodically clean the **hydrocollator** (see **Figure 21.1**), which holds and heats gel-filled packs for hot therapy

At the end of the day, the technician may:

- Drain and clean the whirlpool
- Wipe down equipment and treatment tables
- Shut down the computers and file completed paper records
- Discard used linens
- Close the clinic

READING CHECK

Explain how a job as a sports medicine technician can help prepare you for other careers in sports medicine.

Certified Personal Trainer

Why does a personal trainer need to consider the client's self-esteem?

More people are joining health clubs to lose weight, lower their cholesterol and/or blood pressure, and improve their overall level of fitness as well as their appearance. A record number of Americans today are obese. This means that they have a **body mass index (BMI)** of 30 or greater. The BMI is a number that indicates the relationship between weight and height. The higher the BMI, the greater the risk of chronic disease.

This index to measure obesity is classified as follows.

- A BMI of less than 20 is considered underweight.
- A BMI of 20 to 25 is considered normal weight.
- A BMI of 25 to 30 is considered overweight.
- A BMI of 30 to 40 is considered obese.
- A BMI of greater than 40 is considered severely obese.

The certified personal trainer (CPT) sets up and monitors a workout schedule and diet, both of which are designed to meet the specific goals of each client. Some people may want to lose fat but gain muscle mass. Others need to tone existing muscle while not putting on more weight.

Still other clients may want to improve their cardiovascular fitness, which may lead to lower blood pressure and a decrease in heart disease, heart attacks, and strokes. Physically active people are also interested in improving their **strength,** or muscular ability.

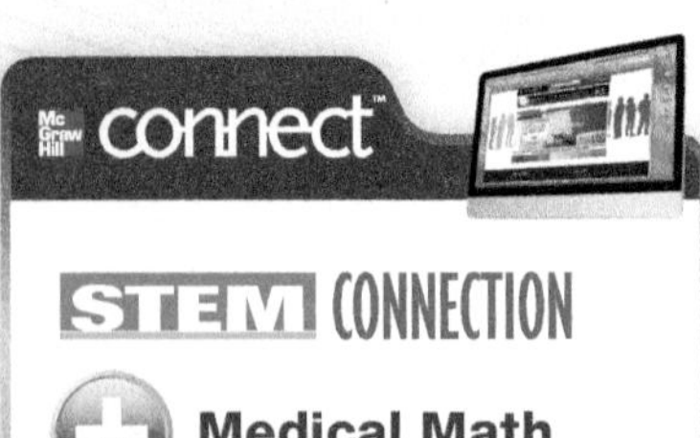

STEM CONNECTION

Medical Math

Target Heart Rate and Body Fat Percentage

As a sports medicine employee or volunteer, you may direct clients during aerobic exercises. When a client requires primarily aerobic exercises, it will be important to establish a target heart rate while exercising. If the client's heart rate is too low, fat burning will not occur and the client will not lose weight. If the heart rate is too high, exercise will not be sustained long enough to cause the body to burn fat. It is also helpful to know how to determine body fat percentage. This is the percentage of a person's total body weight comprised of fat.

connect Go online to learn how to calculate a client's heart rate and body fat percentage.

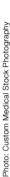

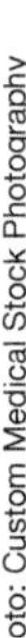

To best serve clients, the CPT must also be knowledgeable about proper eating habits. An exercise regimen will not meet its intended goals if proper nutritional guidelines are not followed.

Because of the one-on-one nature of the job, a CPT should have a healthy lifestyle that can serve as an example to a client. What would you think if your trainer looked more out of shape than you? You would likely have less respect for that trainer's advice.

Empathy and enthusiasm are two other traits a good CPT should have. Some clients may feel self-conscious about their physical appearance or may never have exercised. Proper reassurance and encouragement helps make the transition to a new lifestyle more enjoyable and, therefore, easier (see **Figure 21.2**). It should be the goal of the CPT to eventually make the client independent in his or her workouts and eating habits.

CPTs come from a wide variety of backgrounds and educational levels. Knowledge of exercise is just as important as academic training. If the CPT does not know the proper technique of an exercise, he or she will not be able to assist the client. This could eventually result in an injury or prevent the athlete from meeting his or her goals.

Fig. 21.2 Personal Trainer This client is working out with the help of a certified personal trainer. *Why do you think it is important to show enthusiasm while working with a client?*

The Job of the Personal Trainer

Most personal trainers work at health clubs or other fitness facilities. When clients first meet with a CPT, the trainer will generally take a medical history and physical inventory of measurements including:

- Height
- Weight
- Resting heart rate
- Resting blood pressure
- Body fat percentage
- Circumferential measurements of the arms, thighs, chest, waist, and hips
- Flexibility

These measurements will be used as a baseline to set goals and gauge the client's progress.

Once the CPT and client have finalized short- and long-term goals, a schedule of supervised workouts is developed. Time spent with a client is normally billed by the hour. Workouts may vary in length from 30 minutes to two hours and may occur two to five days a week.

Depending on the goals, exercises may be aerobic, anaerobic, or a combination of the two. **Aerobic exercise** is cardiovascular in nature; it focuses on fat loss or muscle toning. **Anaerobic exercise** focuses on increasing muscle mass. A combination of both provides a balanced fitness approach.

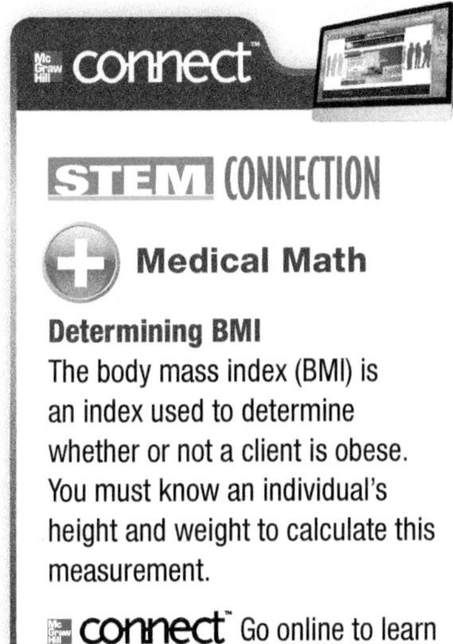

STEM CONNECTION

Medical Math

Determining BMI

The body mass index (BMI) is an index used to determine whether or not a client is obese. You must know an individual's height and weight to calculate this measurement.

connect Go online to learn how to calculate a client's body mass index.

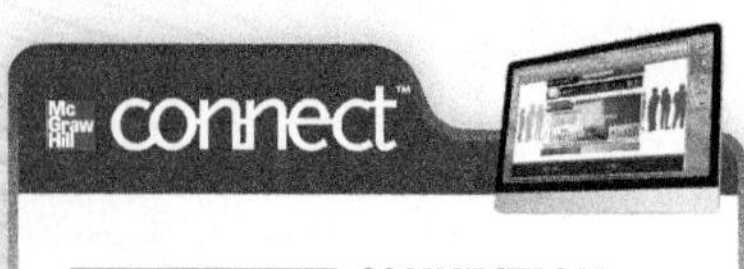

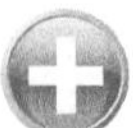

STEM CONNECTION

Medical Science

Aerobic and Anaerobic Exercise

During exercise, two main processes for muscular energy generation occur. For this reason, exercise can be classified as either aerobic or anaerobic.

connect Go online to learn more about the two types of exercise and how they benefit the body.

To assist the client in reaching goals, a personal trainer's job includes deciding the best types of exercises, knowing the proper form and execution of each exercise, and recognizing adverse effects.

In some cases, certified personal trainers also study to become registered dieticians. For more information on the job of the dietician, see Chapter 32, Dietetics.

READING CHECK

Identify the most common goal of a personal trainer's clients.

Certified Athletic Trainer

Why must an athletic trainer be able to think and react quickly?

Certified athletic trainers (ATC) assess, evaluate, and provide treatment for acute sports injuries that occur on the playing field. The evaluation process is a vital part of their duties. ATCs also help injured players learn rehabilitation techniques, which will often take place in a training room or a sports medicine facility.

In addition to exercise, certified athletic trainers use a variety of other **modalities**, or methods of treatment. For example, they may apply cold, heat, or ultrasound to the injured area. Taping, bracing, and padding may be used to protect the injured area. The goal is to enable the athlete to resume his or her sport safely.

Once the student has graduated from an accredited athletic training program, he or she must pass a certification exam consisting of three sections. The first section of the exam is multiple-choice, evaluating the candidate's basic knowledge learned during the program.

The second section is a practical portion based on psychomotor skills, such as manual evaluation and treatment techniques, anatomical landmark palpation, taping procedures, and padding.

The last section is a written simulation consisting of eight scenarios and is used to evaluate the candidate's decision-making skills, particularly in injury management.

The Job of the Certified Athletic Trainer

There are a variety of settings in which athletic trainers work, but the majority of these fall into four main categories:

- Educational facilities such as high schools, colleges, and universities
- Outpatient sports medicine physical therapy clinics
- Professional sports teams
- Industrial/ergonomic settings and corporate wellness centers

Often, the first two categories overlap when the ATC is at a sports medicine facility. These facilities are usually contracted by an educational institution to provide athletic training services. Many ATCs also teach and provide after-school training for an additional financial consideration, much like teachers who coach sports.

Ergonomics relates to the design of work areas to accommodate human physical characteristics. The ultimate objective is to decrease on-the-job injuries. One aspect of ergonomics that an athletic trainer can assist with is teaching proper body mechanics for lifting, sitting, bending, or any other action a worker may perform during the workday.

In any of the settings mentioned, the ATC may perform the following:

- Provide immediate acute care for injuries, including icing, splinting, controlling bleeding, and performing CPR
- Assess injured players to determine whether they are capable of participating in a practice or game without risk of further injury
- Apply braces, tape, or other materials to injured or noninjured players to minimize the risk of sprains, strains, tears, or fractures during practice or competition
- Relay verbal and/or written evaluations of the athlete's condition to the athlete, coach, team physician, and/or the athlete's family
- Conduct athlete rehabilitation and reconditioning
- Educate athletes on the prevention of injuries

An ATC should possess several key skills in order carry out his or her job responsibilities successfully.

- **Good listening skills.** ATCs must know exactly what happened when an athlete is injured. Information may come from the athlete, other players, referees, or anyone else who witnessed the injury.
- **Finely tuned manual skills.** The ATC must perform many hands-on tests to assist in assessing the injured.
- **Excellent communication skills.** The ATC is usually the first person on the scene when an athlete is injured. After making an initial assessment, the ATC then relays the information to the appropriate medical personnel. The ATC must quickly and concisely explain which body part is injured and how severe the injury is.
- **Ability to think and respond quickly and appropriately.** Occasionally, an ATC's decisions will mean the difference between life and death for a severely injured athlete or in the ability of the athlete to continue playing his or her sport in the future. A quick and accurate evaluation of the injury is of critical importance.
- **Organization and management skills.** It is important that all assessments and treatments be documented and that complete and accurate medical files be kept on every athlete.

READING CHECK

Name the four settings in which most athletic trainers work.

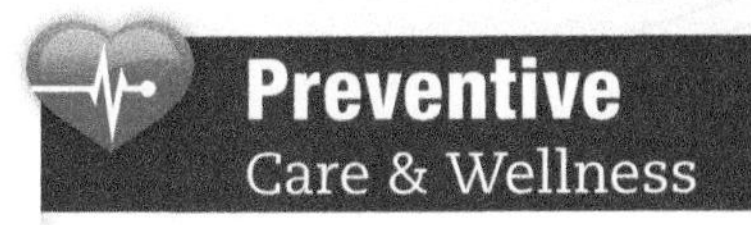

Preventive
Care & Wellness

Why Physical Activity?

Physical activity contributes to health by decreasing the risk for cardiovascular disease and reducing the amount of bone loss associated with aging. Physical activity also helps the body use calories more efficiently, thereby helping in weight loss or weight maintenance. It can increase basal metabolic rate, reduce appetite, and help in the reduction of body fat.

Certified Strength and Conditioning Specialist

How do you assess the performance of an individual athlete?

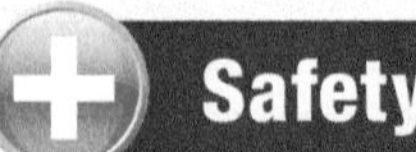

Safety

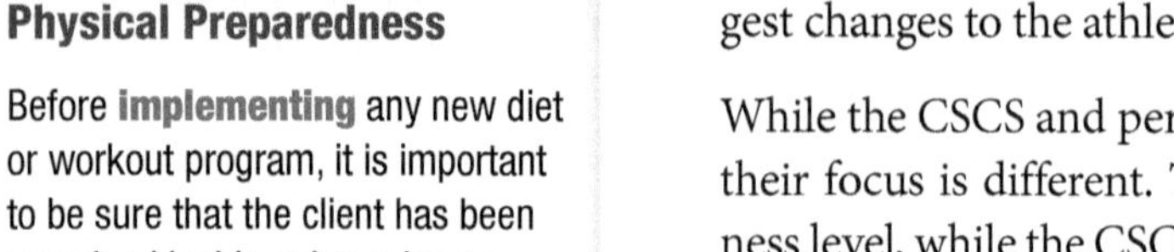

Physical Preparedness

Before **implementing** any new diet or workout program, it is important to be sure that the client has been examined by his or her primary care physician and is cleared for participation in the program.

Athletes who want to improve in their sports often seek the help of a certified strength and conditioning specialist (CSCS). These specialists study the athlete's performance, looking for weak points. They then suggest changes to the athlete's training program.

While the CSCS and personal trainer need the same type of knowledge, their focus is different. The CPT works to enhance a person's total fitness level, while the CSCS focuses on helping an athlete improve specific skills for a given sport. There is some overlap in their methods and both can work in many settings. The National Strength and Conditioning Association (NSCA) certifies both.

Certification may be required. A strong educational background in the exercise science of **kinesiology,** which is the study of body movement, or a related field is highly recommended. The CSCS exam consists of a multiple-choice test in two parts. One part of the exam covers the candidate's scientific knowledge in such areas as body energy systems and muscular anatomy. The other part explores practical applications and proper exercise execution. In order to maintain certification, the CSCS is required to complete six continuing education units every three years.

connect

STEM CONNECTION

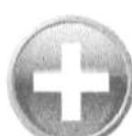

Medical Science

Sprains and Strains

When an individual injures a body part, there are several possible injury types. Two very common types are **sprains** (tears in ligaments) and **strains** (injury to a muscle instead of a ligament).

connect Go online to learn more about what causes sprain and strain injuries.

The Job of the Certified Strength and Conditioning Specialist

Frequently, the CSCS is employed in settings where there are sports teams, either at the high school level or, more frequently, at the college and professional levels. The CSCS helps to improve athletic performance through proper physical conditioning.

When preparing the athlete in the preseason, the postseason, and during the sport's regular season, the CSCS will perform some or all of the following.

- Make a physical assessment of players like the one a personal trainer makes of clients
- Observe the athlete's technique in doing the exercises and make corrections as needed
- Be sure proper eating habits are followed to enhance exercise recovery and maximize performance
- Put the athlete through a series of tests to determine where there is a weakness in performance. Examples of those tests include the vertical jump; 40-yard dash; 12-minute run for distance; and maximum lifting ability for the bench press, squat, pull-up, and other related tests.

High school coaches with CSCS certification provide young athletes with a good introduction to sport and exercise (see **Figure 21.3**). If the CSCS works in a college setting, he or she will be knowledgeable about the conditioning of athletes in a variety of sports. For example, the training for a tennis player will likely differ from that of a swimmer. At the professional level, the CSCS only has to focus on one sport. Quite often, he or she is considered part of the coaching staff. There is a great deal of pressure on the CSCS to be sure the team is appropriately conditioned.

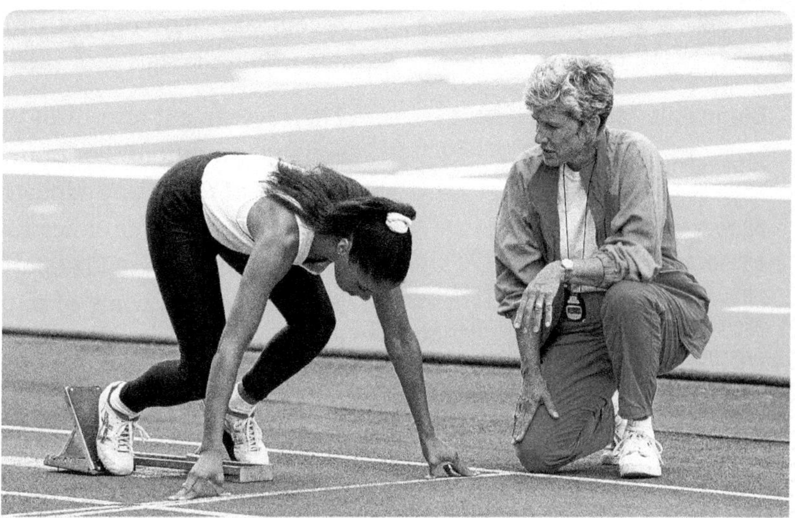

Fig. 21.3 Evaluating the Situation This CSCS is working with a high-school athlete. *What type of tests does the CSCS use to measure an athlete's ability?*

READING CHECK

Summarize how a certified strength and conditioning specialist helps athletes improve their performance.

Exercise Physiologist

Why do corporations and government agencies hire exercise physiologists?

Exercise physiologists research the effects of exercise on the human body. They explore topics such as which proteins make up muscle and how much oxygen an athlete uses.

They may work for a large vitamin and nutritional supplement company, where their research helps produce new products. For example, they may help create a new protein mix to help an athlete recover from workouts. Or they may help design a new carbohydrate drink.

They may also work as teachers, helping students apply their knowledge to research projects.

Hospitals use exercise physiologists for cardiac rehabilitation. Here, clients with cardiac problems may undergo testing from an exercise physiologist supervised by a physician. Exercise physiologists also monitor the exercise programs of clients recovering from a heart attack (see **Figure 21.4**). The client's activity level is regulated and increased according to data collected.

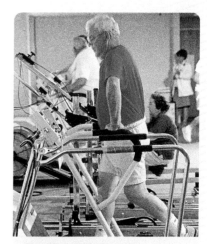

Fig. 21.4 Monitoring Recovery Exercise physiologists monitor clients in facilities such as a cardiac rehabilitation center. *Why is the number of cardiac rehabilitation centers increasing?*

Corporate wellness centers also provide an increasing number of opportunities for exercise physiologists. Businesses recognize that having healthy employees often results in less lost work time due to injury or illness, higher productivity, and decreased insurance costs.

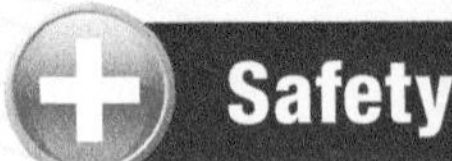

Safety

Diagnostic Testing of Clients

Never perform a VO2 max test on an individual with a history of cardiovascular disease. This test measures cardiovascular fitness and requires a high level of exercise and intensity. Clients with previous cardiovascular disease should instead be tested with an exercise electrocardiograph or stress test.

A company may contract with an exercise physiologist or it may hire one to join the staff.

The government also hires physiologists to test human responses to extreme conditions. For example, the military may need to know how a pilot will react to a sudden change in atmospheric pressure if something happens to his or her aircraft or how an astronaut's bone density changes during extended periods of time in microgravity. As you can see, there are a variety of settings and employment opportunities for exercise physiologists.

The Job of the Exercise Physiologist

Cardiac rehabilitation is a strong employment area for exercise physiologists. As a large segment of the population ages, the incidence of cardiac-related problems is also likely to increase. Stress tests and exercise electrocardiography are used to determine whether there are early indications of heart disease. (This testing will be discussed further in Chapter 26, Medical Testing.) An exercise physiologist may assist with this test and perform the following tasks:

- Explain the procedure and progression of the test
- Attach the electrodes to the client
- Observe the physiological reactions to the test, including heart rate and rhythm
- Stop the test if the client has an adverse reaction

A **VO2 max test** is similar to a stress test. The analysis can be used to gauge cardiovascular fitness by assessing the athlete's efficiency of oxygen consumption and cardiac output. In addition to the electrocardiograph, the athlete is connected to a device that measures the difference between a known amount of inhaled oxygen and the carbon dioxide exhaled. The computed difference shows how effectively the athlete's body is using the available oxygen in the bloodstream (see **Figure 21.5**).

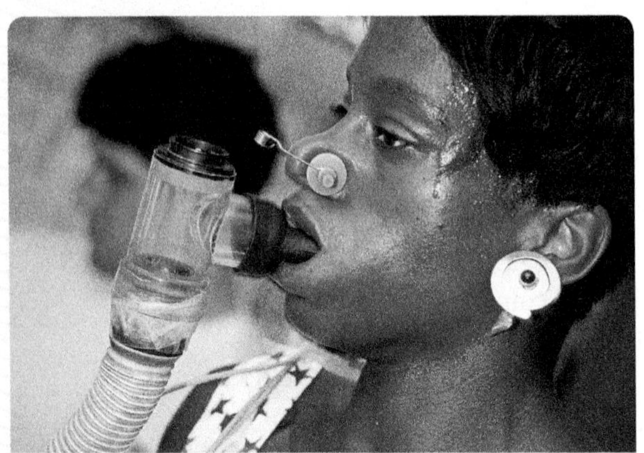

Fig. 21.5 VO2 Max Test During a VO2 max test, the client breathes through a tube while exercising on a treadmill or stationary bike. Usually the nostrils are clamped. *When should this test not be used?*

Photo: Sean Aidan/Eye Ubiquitous/Alamy

READING CHECK

List some topics researched by exercise physiologists.

Sports Physical Therapist

How can a therapist reduce the amount of pain experienced by an injured athlete?

An injured athlete may need rehabilitation before he or she can compete again. A physician must first diagnose the problem. He or she may then prescribe therapy.

The goal is to use the least amount of time to recover with the best results. Sports physical therapists focus on using the correct exercises to reach this goal. They are often certified in other areas. They may be CPTs or CSCSs, or may hold exercise physiology degrees. This helps bolster their grasp of the body's response to exercise in injured and noninjured states.

The program of study for the sports physical therapist is the same for the general physical therapist. See Chapter 20, Rehabilitation, for a discussion of physical therapy. Sometimes, a program will have a specialization track in sports medicine, which includes one or more courses in exercise science. It may benefit the student to complete an undergraduate degree in exercise science prior to enrolling in a physical therapy graduate program.

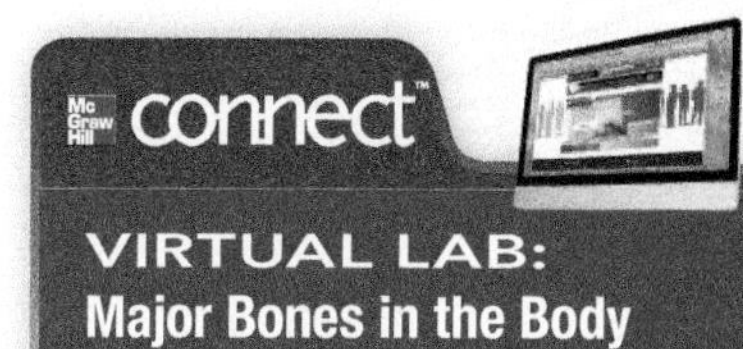

VIRTUAL LAB: Major Bones in the Body

The adult human body is made up of 206 bones, forming the skeleton that gives the body its shape, protects internal organs, and helps muscles move. Bones store minerals, such as calcium, and produce red blood cells.

This lab will help you identify the major bones of the body, as well as place them in correct anatomical position.

connect
Go online to view the virtual lab and complete the assignment.

The Job of the Sports Physical Therapist

Once therapy is prescribed, the physical therapist performs an evaluation to determine the athlete's physical limitations. The first part is subjective—the athlete will describe the injury and how it happened. The therapist finds out the athlete's medical history, any currently prescribed or over-the-counter medications that are being taken, and evaluates the athlete's psychological, or mental, state.

The second part of the evaluation is objective. The therapist evaluates the client using manual techniques and measuring devices. Instruments used during this portion of the evaluation include a goniometer to measure joint angles and a tape measure to determine whether there is swelling in an area or muscle atrophy (see **Figure 21.6**).

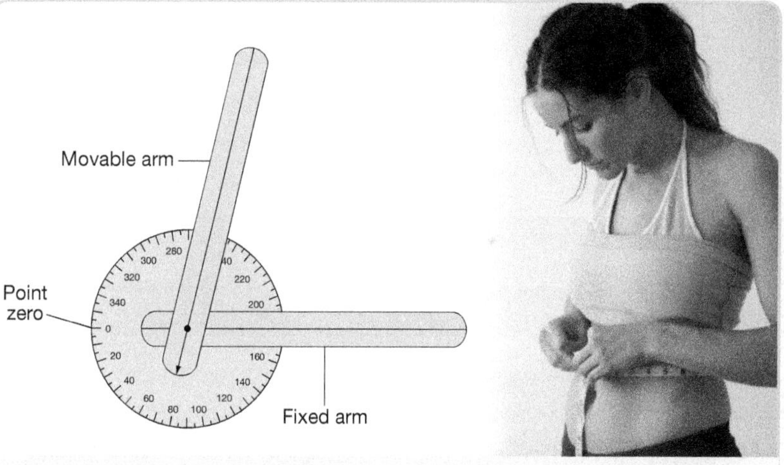

Fig. 21.6 Objective Evaluation A goniometer and a tape measure are used during a sports physical therapist's evaluation. *What is the purpose of the goniometer and the tape measure during evaluation?*

Evaluation may reveal deficits or problems in the following areas:

- Range of motion
- Strength
- Balance
- Neuromuscular coordination
- **Proprioception,** or awareness of posture, movement, and change in the equilibrium of the body

After the data has been collected, the physical therapist will determine what goals need to be set to return the athlete to a competitive condition. This is known as the assessment portion of the evaluation.

Short- and long-term goals will need to be achieved before the athlete can return to competition. The sports physical therapist creates a plan of exercises and modalities to reach the short- and long-term goals in the briefest and safest amount of time.

Photo: Peter Dressel/Getty Images

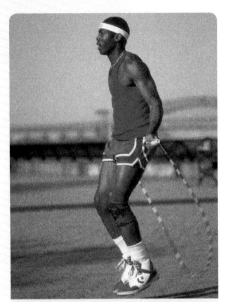

Fig. 21.7 Agility This athlete is performing an agility exercise. *What stage of rehabilitation do you think this athlete has reached?*

A simple way to remember the process of the evaluation is by using the acronym SOAP.

Subjective: Gather subjective data from the athlete (what they tell you).

Objective: Gather objective or measurable data (such as body measurements).

Assessment: Identify deficits (potential problems) and set short- and long-term goals.

Plan: Determine the course of action to reach the goals.

Depending on the severity of the injury, therapy may be scheduled daily or only one or two times a week.

Generally, the physical therapist treats the athlete's deficit by helping to decrease the pain level, using manual techniques such as massage or modalities such as electrical stimulation. They also work to improve the range of motion in an affected area with techniques such as massage; with **passive range of motion,** which is exercise performed by the healthcare employee that moves the joints through their available range; or with modalities such as ultrasound. Increasing the athlete's strength through the use of weight machines, free weights, and resistance also helps. The ultimate goal is to improve agility, reaction time, speed, and proprioception so the athlete can return to his or her sport. (see **Figure 21.7**).

READING CHECK

Recall what data is needed to create an appropriate therapy plan for an injured athlete.

SECTION 21.1 Careers in Sports Medicine Review

AFTER YOU READ

1. **Select** two activities a sports medicine technician will perform at the beginning of the working day, during the working day, and at the end of the working day.
2. **Contrast** a strain and a sprain.
3. **Indicate** three job duties an ATC may perform on the athletic field.
4. **List** four measurements a personal trainer may use to set a client's goals.
5. **Distinguish** aerobic from anaerobic exercise.
6. **Compare** the jobs of a CSCS and a CPT.
7. **Indicate** two common tests an exercise physiologist may perform.
8. **Choose** at least four areas a sports physical therapist may evaluate for deficits.
9. **Define** each part of the SOAP acronym.

Technology ONLINE EXPLORATIONS

Athletic Trainers versus Personal Trainers

Go online to research the differences between an athletic trainer and a personal trainer. Create a table that gives a description of each career, the requirements to practice, and the daily duties. When you have completed your table, determine which career you would prefer and explain why.

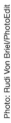

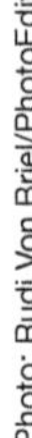

Photo: Rudi Von Briel/PhotoEdit

SECTION **21.2 Sports Medicine Procedures**

Calculating Body Fat Percentages

How can a healthcare professional determine whether or not a person is obese?

One important part of a healthy lifestyle is maintaining a low percentage of body fat. The American Heart Association says a high percentage of body fat is linked to an increased risk of coronary heart disease, stroke, and diabetes. Fitness professionals will often use body fat percentage measurements as a baseline for goal setting and gauging progress.

There are several ways to estimate body fat percentages.

- In **near-infrared interactance testing,** a beam of infrared light is transmitted into the biceps. It is reflected from the underlying muscle and absorbed by the fat. This is a safe, noninvasive, rapid, and easy-to-use test (see **Figure 21.8**). It may be found in fitness centers.
- In **hydrostatic testing,** the client is weighed, submersed in a large tub of water, and weighed again in the water. Since fat is less dense than water, it will create a buoyant effect, and thus lower weight in water. Hydrostatic testing is very expensive, and it can be difficult to account for the volume of air in the lungs when assessing buoyancy.
- In **electrical impedance testing,** a low electrical current passes through the body. The amount of resistance to the current equals a certain percentage of body fat. Electrical impedance can be affected by a client's hydration level at the time of the test.

READING CHECK

Name the simplest way to determine body fat percentage.

Vocabulary

Content Vocabulary

You will learn these content vocabulary terms in this section.

- **near-infrared interactance testing**
- **hydrostatic testing**
- **electrical impedance testing**

Academic Vocabulary

You will see this word in your reading and on your tests. Find its meaning in the Glossary in the back of the book.

- **estimate**

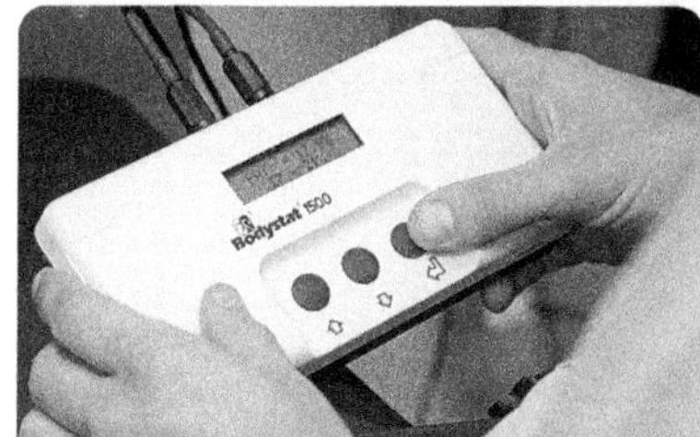

Fig. 21.8 Estimating Body Fat Percentages A near-infrared interactance body fat tester. *What are some advantages of this method?*

Mc Graw Hill connect™ ONLINE PROCEDURES

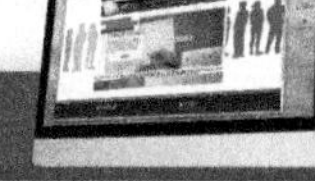

PROCEDURE 21-1

Applying a Hot Pack

Heat is applied to the body to promote relaxation and ease pain. Heat can be applied locally or generally. Local applications target a specific area of the body. Generalized applications are for the whole body. Applying heat locally to the skin increases blood flow to that area of the body. This means that more oxygen and nutrients are available to the cells and tissues for healing. At the same time, toxins and excess fluids can leave the inflamed area more rapidly.

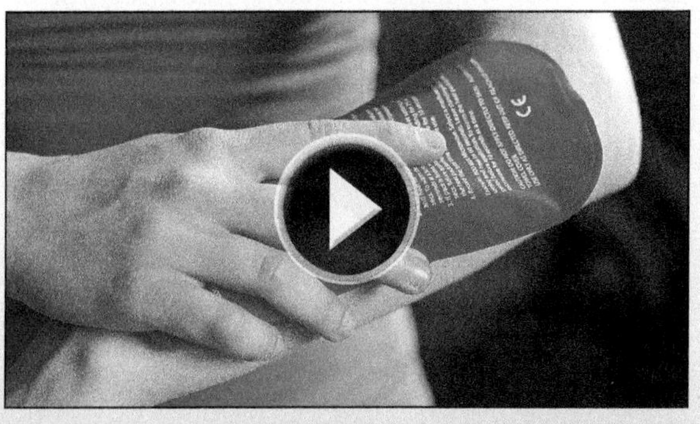

Photos: (t)Antonia Reeve/Photo Researchers, Inc., (b)Jeffrey Blackler/Alamy

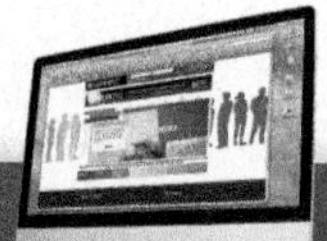

connect ONLINE PROCEDURES

PROCEDURE 21-2

Applying an Ice Pack

Cold modalities are used when swelling reduction is the primary focus. Ice packs are sometimes used to help decrease muscle spasms and swelling.

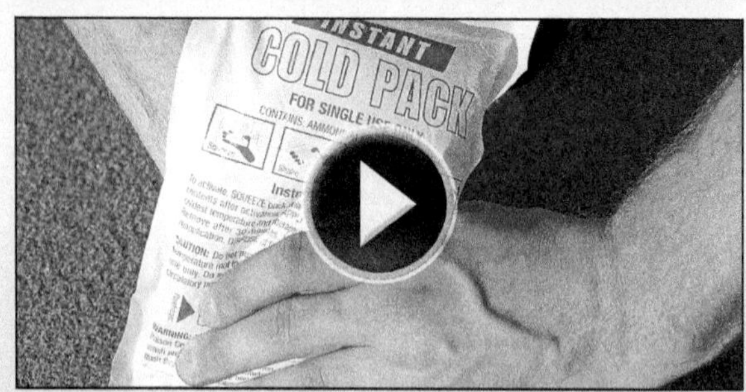

PROCEDURE 21-3

Using a Cold Whirlpool

A cold whirlpool may be used if cold therapy is needed for a large or irregularly shaped area. The whirlpool provides massage action to the injured area. Some clients may not tolerate this much cold. On rare occasions, cold therapy may have an adverse effect. If the client reports feeling lightheaded or looks pale, immediately help the client out of the whirlpool, stop the treatment, and tell your supervisor.

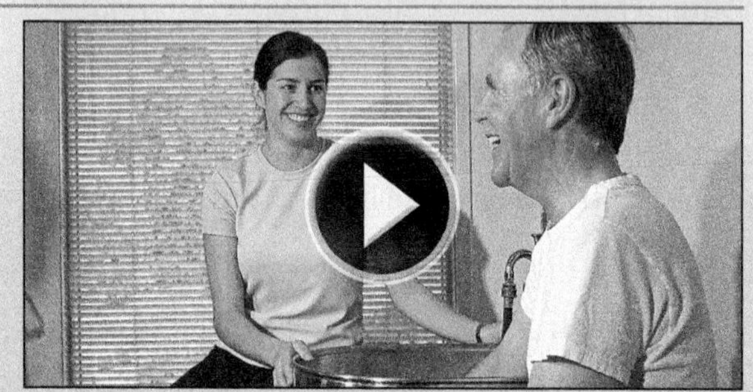

PROCEDURE 21-4

Calculating Body Fat Percentages

One way to determine body fat percentages is with the use of a body fat caliper. More fat collects in certain areas on men and women; measuring the width of these areas will help calculate the percentage of fat.

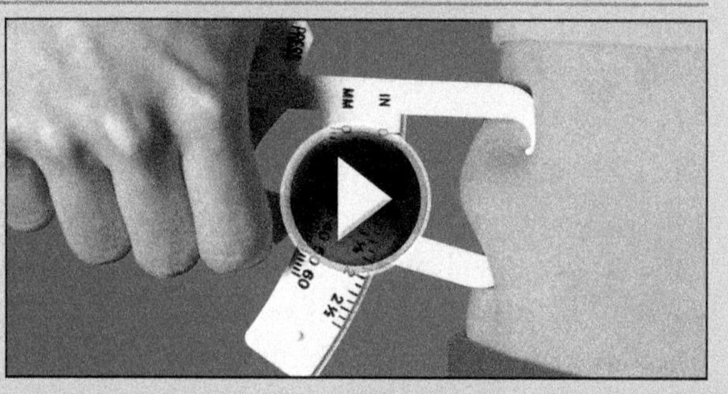

Photos: (t)Charles D. Winters/Photo Researchers, Inc., (c)PhotoSpin, Inc./Alamy, (b)Comstock Images/Getty Images

SECTION 21.2 Sports Medicine Procedures Review

AFTER YOU READ

1. **Explain** why it is important to test the client's sensitivity to a light touch before performing a hot or cold treatment.
2. **Describe** what the sports medicine technician should do if a client has an adverse effect from a treatment or test.
3. **Identify** the appropriate temperature for a hydrocollator.
4. **Choose** three reasons not to use a heat treatment.
5. **Indicate** two reasons not to use a cold treatment.
6. **Explain** why you would use heat instead of cold when treating a client.

Technology ONLINE EXPLORATIONS

Body Fat Estimation

Go online to research a method of body fat estimation that requires only the use of a tape measure and a formula. Once you have found the method, determine your own body fat estimations using the instructions and formula provided.

CHAPTER 21 Review

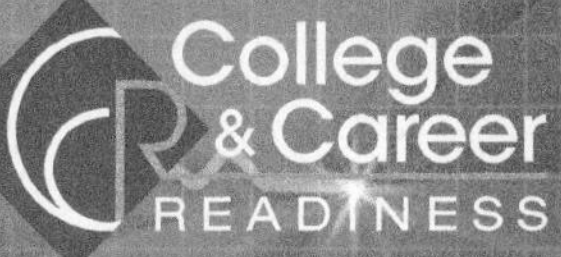

Chapter Summary

SECTION 21.1

- Sports medicine technicians perform job duties that increase the quality of care by allowing therapists to spend more time with clients. **(pg. 526)**
- Proper diet and regular exercise promote a healthy lifestyle. **(pg. 529)**
- Athletic trainers primarily evaluate on-the-field injuries at scholastic and professional levels. They also work in rehabilitation facilities and industrial settings. **(pg. 530)**
- Certified strength and conditioning specialists study athletes' performance, looking for weak points, in order to suggest changes in their training programs. **(pg. 532)**
- Personal trainers and strength and conditioning specialists have similar job duties but may focus on different outcomes for their clients. **(pg. 532)**
- Exercise physiologists study the effects that exercise, nature, and human-made adverse conditions have on the body. They perform research that assists in the development of recovery aids, such as supplements and proper conditioning for athletes and cardiac care patients. **(pg. 533)**
- Sports physical therapists, with assistance from technicians, use their expertise to facilitate safe and timely recovery from injuries through the use of manual techniques, therapeutic exercise, various other modalities, and sport-specific drills and conditioning. **(pg. 534)**

SECTION 21.2

- Practice safety when applying heat or cold modalities to a client. Check the client frequently for comfort. **(pg. 537)**
- Body fat percentage is a fairly good indicator of overall fitness. Body fat must be measured with consistency and accuracy. **(pg. 537)**

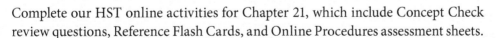

Mc Graw Hill connect™ ONLINE ACTIVITIES

Complete our HST online activities for Chapter 21, which include Concept Check review questions, Reference Flash Cards, and Online Procedures assessment sheets.

- **Concept Check** review questions
- **Reference Flash Cards** medical terminology practice
- **Online Procedures** assessment sheets

CHAPTER

21 Assessment

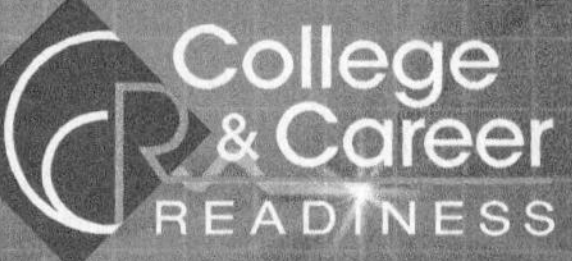

Critical Thinking/Problem Solving

1. Imagine you are an athlete trying to improve your performance. Choose a sport and then describe which sports medicine professionals you would ask for help. State several ways in which they would assist you. You should choose more than one professional.
2. An athlete is injured on the field during a game. Discuss how various sports medicine disciplines work in cooperation to help the athlete return to his or her playing condition.
3. What are some types of emotional difficulties that an injured athlete might have to overcome?
4. How might a trainer use ergonomics to help a person who works sitting at a computer all day?
5. Prepare a hot pack and apply it to the top of your arm or leg. Leave it in place for about 15 minutes if possible, but remove it if you experience any discomfort. Describe the sensations that you felt during and after treatment. Reheat the pack and apply it to your neck or the inside of your arm. Did you experience any differences? Summarize your findings.
6. Using a watch, an ice cube, and a paper towel or cloth, measure how long you can tolerate a cold application. Hold the ice cube with a cloth to the back of your arm and start timing. Keep it there until you feel uncomfortable. How long were you able to apply the ice? What did it feel like when it became uncomfortable? Describe the appearance of the skin when you removed the ice.

21ST CENTURY SKILLS

7. **Teamwork** Referring to the STEM Connection Box "Target Heart Rate," determine the target heart rate for a partner. Have your partner run or walk in place until he or she reaches this range. At intervals during the exercise, count your partner's pulse for six seconds and multiply by ten to determine the pulse rate. Continue the exercise until the target range has been reached. Describe how it felt to be at the target rate.
8. **Information Literacy** Contact five to ten agencies that certify personal trainers and list their certification requirements. Based upon those requirements, determine which association you would most likely contact if you were hiring a personal trainer.
9. **Information Literacy** Search the Internet for sports medicine educational programs that interest you. Find out what is required to enter the program of your choice, including courses and the amount and type of volunteer experience.

CHAPTER

22 Complementary and Alternative Medicine

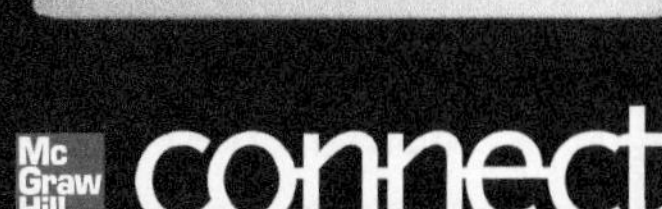

Essential Question:

What are some reasons to visit a chiropractor or massage therapist?

People turn to complementary and alternative treatments for many reasons. Chiropractic adjustments, massage, acupuncture, herbal therapies, and aromatherapy are popular methods that some healthcare professionals use to address a wide range of patient conditions and problems. This chapter will introduce you to the basic theory and procedures related to these fields of treatment.

Mc Graw Hill connect™

It's Online!

- Online Procedures
- STEM Connection
- Medical Science
- Medical Terms
- Medical Math
- Ethics in Action
- Virtual Lab

Photo: Shoosh/Form Advertising/Alamy

READING GUIDE

OBJECTIVES

After completing this chapter, you will be able to:

- **Explain** the chiropractor's general theory of health.
- **Describe** the responsibilities and practice of a chiropractor.
- **Identify** the effects of massage on the body.
- **Describe** the responsibilities and practice of a massage therapist.
- **Explain** the general theory of acupuncture.
- **Describe** the responsibilities and practice of an acupuncturist.
- **Discuss** information about the study and use of herbs in healing.
- **Describe** the responsibilities and practices of an herbalist.
- **Explain** the general theory of aromatherapy.
- **Demonstrate** one alternative medicine procedure.

BEFORE YOU READ

Connect Have you ever considered using non-traditional therapy such as chiropractic or acupuncture for pain management?

Main Idea

Chiropractors, acupuncturists, massage therapists, aromatherapists, and herbalists provide alternatives to conventional healthcare.

Note-Taking Activity

Draw this table. Write key terms and phrases under **Cues**. Write main ideas under **Note Taking**. Summarize the section under **Summary**.

Cues	Note Taking
o o	o o
Summary	

Graphic Organizer

Before you read the chapter, draw a diagram like the one below. As you read, write different careers from the chapter into the diagram.

Complementary and Alternative Medicine Careers				

connect Downloadable graphic organizers can be accessed online.

STANDARDS

HEALTH SCIENCE

NCHSE 1.13 Analyze the basic structure and function of the human body.

NCHSE 9.13 Discuss complementary (alternative) health practices as they relate to wellness and disease prevention.

SCIENCE

NSES B Develop an understanding of the structure of atoms, structure and properties of matter, chemical reactions, motions and forces, conservation of energy and increase in disorder, and interactions of energy and matter.

NCHSE *National Consortium for Health Science Education*

NSES *National Science Education Standards*

COMMON CORE STATE STANDARDS

MATHEMATICS

Number and Quantity

Quantities N-Q Reason quantitatively and use units to solve problems.

ENGLISH LANGUAGE ARTS

Reading

Key Ideas and Details R-3 Follow a complex multistep procedure when carrying out experiments, taking measurements, or performing technical tasks; analyze specific results based on text explanations.

Speaking and Listening

Comprehension and Collaboration SL-2 Integrate multiple sources of information presented in diverse media or formats (e.g., visually, quantitatively, orally) evaluating the credibility and accuracy of each source.

SECTION 22.1
Careers in Alternative Medicine

Careers in Complementary and Alternative Medicine

Do you practice any type of complementary or alternative medicine?

Complementary and alternative medicine (CAM) is a group of practices and products that are not necessarily considered to be part of conventional or standard medicine, which is medicine as most of us know it. Although the term "complementary and alternative medicine" groups these two kinds of medicine together, they do differ.

Complementary medicine is used along with conventional medicine. One example of a complementary therapy is the use of aromatherapy to help lessen a patient's discomfort following surgery. Complementary medicine offers something in addition to standard or conventional medicine.

Alternative medicine is used in place of conventional medicine. It consists of approaches to diagnoses and therapy that may not result from the application of scientific methods. Alternative medicine, then, offers people something different from conventional medicine. Conventional treatments and drugs can be costly and may cause side effects. Their use may be futile or only partly useful. For these reasons, patients sometimes choose other options. They may also choose alternative medicine to promote overall wellness. This chapter will cover five of the better-known careers in the field of complementary and alternative medicine (see **Table 22.1** on page 544 for more information). The five careers are:

- Chiropractor
- Acupuncturist
- Aromatherapist
- Massage therapist
- Herbalist

READING CHECK

Recall why some patients turn to alternative medicine.

The Chiropractor

Chiropractors treat patients without drugs or surgery because they believe the body has a natural power to heal itself. They use manual and physical therapy treatments, and exercise programs to correct problems. Manual treatments are called **adjustments.** They also offer nutritional advice and suggest lifestyle changes.

Vocabulary

Content Vocabulary

You will learn these content vocabulary terms in this section.

- **complementary medicine**
- **alternative medicine**
- **chiropractors**
- **adjustments**
- **subluxated**
- **massage therapist**
- ***qi***
- **meridians**
- ***yin***
- ***yang***
- **acupuncturist**
- **embolus**
- **herbalists**
- **aromatherapists**
- **essential oils**

Academic Vocabulary

You will see this word in your reading and on your tests. Find its meaning in the Glossary in the back of the book.

- **alternative**

Treatment is focused on the patient's spine. Spinal nerves relay messages from the brain and spinal cord to the rest of the body. They then return messages to the brain. The spine is made up of bony segments called vertebrae. When the vertebrae are **subluxated,** or out of place, the function of the spinal nerve is restricted as it passes through the foramen, which is the passage inside the bone. One or more vertebrae could be subluxated for months or years before symptoms are felt and the patient goes for treatment. **Figure 22.1** shows the spinal nerves. **Figure 22.2** shows how the vertebrae, disks, and spinal nerves work together.

An adjustment is a treatment to realign the vertebrae. The goal is to restore the function of the spinal nerves. Patients may sometimes hear a popping sound during the treatment. Some chiropractors use a mechanical tool, such as an activator, while others adjust with gentle pressure. They try to relax muscles so the vertebra realigns without force.

Table 22.1 Overview of Complementary and Alternative Medicine (CAM) Occupations

OCCUPATION	EDUCATIONAL REQUIREMENTS	CERTIFICATION OR LICENSING AGENCY	JOB OUTLOOK
Chiropractor	Two to four years of related university or college courses. Successful completion of a four-year course at a chiropractic college.	Certification from the National Board of Chiropractic Examiners. Licensed in each state by the Board of Chiropractic Examiners	Faster than average growth as consumer demand for CAM grows and insurance reimbursement and payment for these therapies increases.
Massage therapist	For national certification, 500 hours of training. Some states require additional training, while others require no formal training at all.	Certification from National Certification Board for Therapeutic Massage and Bodywork	Faster than average growth as consumer demand for CAM grows.
Acupuncturist	For licensure or certification in some states, 1300 to 2600 hours of training. In some states acupuncture is illegal unless performed by a licensed physician.	National Certification Commission for Acupuncture and Oriental Medicine	About average but may improve because consumer demand for CAM is increasing.
Herbalist	No national or state system of licensure or certification. May be licensed as another alternative medicine provider and use herbs in that capacity.	Professional membership in the American Herbalists Guild	About average but may improve because of expected consumer growth in demand for knowledgeable herbalists.
Aromatherapist	May take classes or work with herbalists.	There currently is no separate certification required to practice aromatherapy.	Unknown demand because aromatherapy can be practiced along with other forms of CAM.

Often, people who go to a chiropractor have pain due to a musculoskeletal condition. They may have back, arm, neck, shoulder, or leg pain, or they may have frequent headaches. Spinal adjustments, exercise, early return to activities, and over-the-counter pain medications have been very effective for treating these conditions. Chiropractic care has also been effective in treating other problems that may occur as a result of spinal subluxation, which include respiratory problems and digestive disorders.

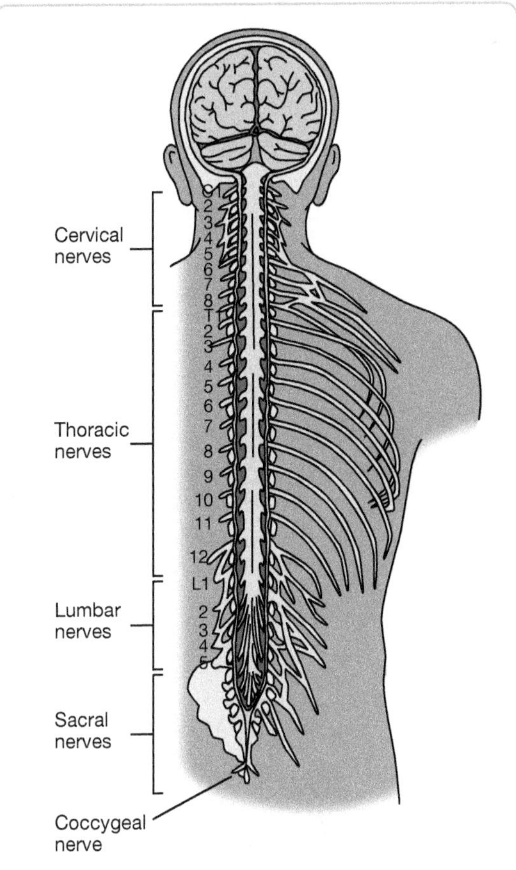

Fig. 22.1 Spine Vertebrae, disks, and spinal nerves work together. *If pressure was on a spinal nerve at cervical nerve number 5, where do you expect a patient would have pain?*

Types of Chiropractic Practices

Many chiropractors work in a single-physician office. Others work in a clinic setting where several chiropractors or other healthcare professionals share office space. Most of them have staff to assist in caring for patients.

As chiropractors and other medical professionals have learned more about each other's methods and results, a cooperative working relationship has developed. Some chiropractors work as a partner with a medical doctor and a physical therapist or massage therapist. Chiropractors and medical physicians refer patients to one another for treatment. Chiropractors may work in general practice, family practice, occupational health, or rehabilitation. Some specialize in sports injuries, automobile accident injuries, or in X-ray interpretation for other physicians.

The Job of a Chiropractor

The chiropractor does an examination and takes a history of illnesses, surgeries, and current symptoms when a patient visits for the first time. The chiropractor asks many of the same questions about health problems that a medical doctor asks. The chiropractor also asks about lifestyle, nutrition, stress, and exercise. Possible trauma to the neck and spine is considered, whether or not it occurred recently. Trauma may occur from falls, car accidents, or sports injuries.

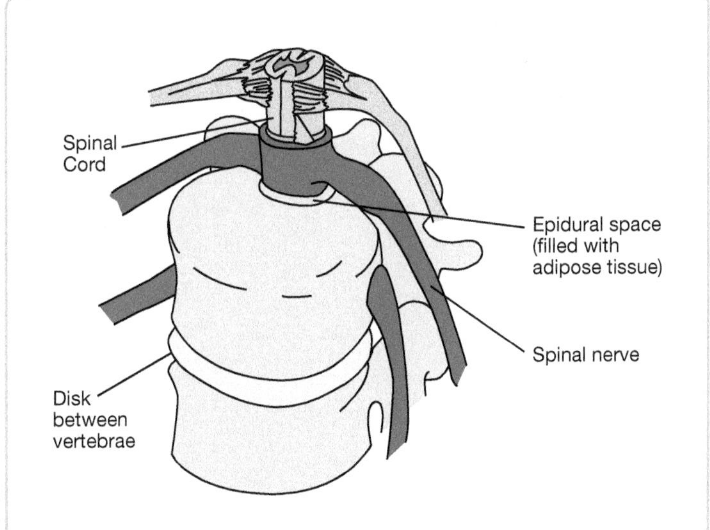

Fig. 22.2 The Spinal Nerves Spinal nerves provide communication between the brain and the spinal cord. *What are the bones that make up the spine called?*

Chiropractors take X-rays, perform muscle testing, and analyze posture to make their diagnoses. Unlike medical doctors, chiropractors base their diagnoses on which vertebrae are subluxated and in which direction they have tilted or rotated. The chiropractor then develops a treatment plan, which generally requires several visits per week for several weeks or months. Because this treatment does not involve drugs or surgery, the body may need longer to correct itself.

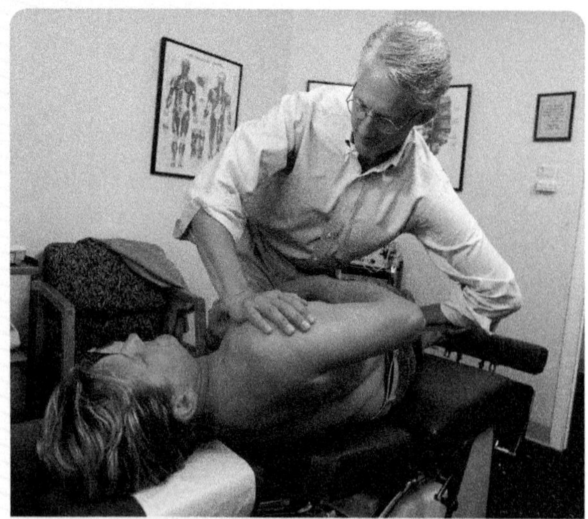

Fig. 22.3 Chiropractor Shown is a chiropractic adjustment. *What other types of therapy would a chiropractor perform to relieve subluxation?*

When the patient returns for follow-up visits, the chiropractor adjusts the areas of the spine that are subluxated (see **Figure 22.3**). Some chiropractors apply heat, ultrasound, gentle traction, or massage therapy prior to the adjustment. These therapies help relax the tight muscles around the spine, so that the vertebra will move more easily and the adjustment will last longer.

Chiropractors may also see patients who are not ill or in pain at the time. After an acute condition has been successfully treated, patients may return for maintenance care. Since a subluxation can be present without causing any symptoms, the chiropractor can check for problems before they cause pain. After treating a patient with an acute problem, the chiropractor may see that same patient for years of maintenance care. They often know their patients well and have a close relationship with them.

Job Responsibilities of a Chiropractor

Chiropractors deal with people who are in pain or experiencing discomfort. They must be patient and kind, and must communicate effectively. They must also be able to run a business efficiently, managing revenue and overhead expenses. Chiropractors also interview, hire, and train their assistants and physical or massage therapists.

The job of a chiropractor requires a great deal of knowledge, skill, and responsibility. Successful chiropractors must:

- Obtain accurate and thorough medical histories from patients
- Perform diagnostic tests using X-rays and muscle testing
- Analyze the symptoms and diagnostic tests to determine a plan of care for the patient
- Determine the frequency and duration of treatment
- Provide appropriate therapy and adjustments at the scheduled frequency and duration
- Evaluate the effectiveness of the therapy and adjustments, making changes as needed to increase response
- Communicate effectively with patients regarding symptoms and progress
- Counsel and teach patients regarding lifestyle changes to improve health
- Implement plans to attract new patients and retain existing patients
- Handle money responsibly, paying bills, taxes, and employee salaries and benefits in a timely manner
- Reinvest money in the practice to improve equipment and the premises
- Be available to patients during established office hours and in case of emergency

READING CHECK

Explain why a chiropractor might see a patient who is not ill or in pain.

The Massage Therapist

What are the medical benefits of massage?

A **massage therapist** uses pressure, kneading, stroking, vibration, and tapping to positively affect the health and well-being of clients. They may also apply warm and cold treatments during massage therapy.

Therapeutic massage helps the client relax and counteracts the effects of stress. During the massage, the heart rate and blood pressure are lowered, and blood circulation and lymph flow increase. Massage helps reduce pain caused by tight muscles and helps relax muscle spasms. Massage benefits the mind by improving concentration and promoting restful sleep. It relaxes the mind. Many clients find that they handle daily stress better when they have regular massage.

People who get regular massage often find that they do not get as sick as they did before. They feel less stressed and tense. When they notice that their muscles are beginning to tighten, they know that massage will ease that muscle tension before it becomes severe.

Types of Massage

Massage therapists study a number of types of massage. Types of massage vary greatly. Several types are based on Eastern philosophy and the Asian theory of ***qi***, which is pronounced "chi" and is defined as the life force within the body. *Qi* energy flows through 12 **meridians**, or channels (see **Figure 22.4**). Some types of massage are based on removing blockages of *qi* or restoring the flow of *qi*. Western style massage is based on somatic therapies or therapies that demonstrate a physical response from the body.

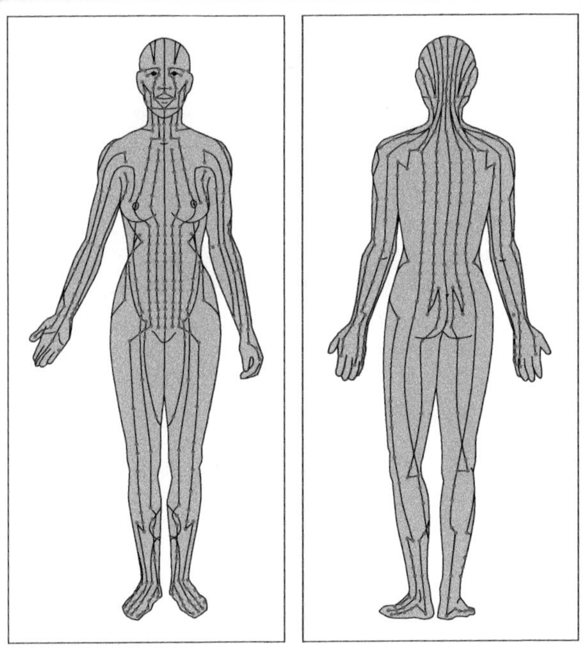

Fig. 22.4 Meridians The meridians are the channels in the body through which the life forces of qi flow. *What is the meridians' relationship to* qi?

Western Styles of Massage The three types of Western massage are Swedish massage, neuromuscular massage, and seated massage.

- **Swedish massage** is one of the best-known and most frequently taught massage techniques. It stimulates circulation and lymph flow with five basic strokes used to manipulate the soft tissues of the body. The strokes are kneading, rolling, vibration, percussion, and tapping. Oil is used to reduce friction on the client's skin. One type of Swedish massage is done immediately after exercise.

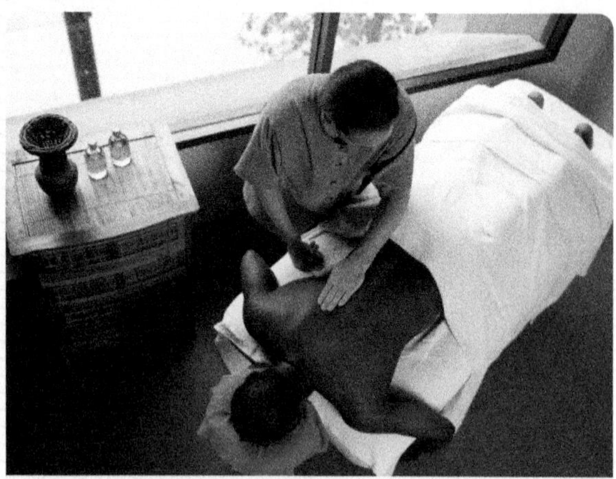

Fig. 22.5 Massage There are several different types of massage. *Which would you prefer?*

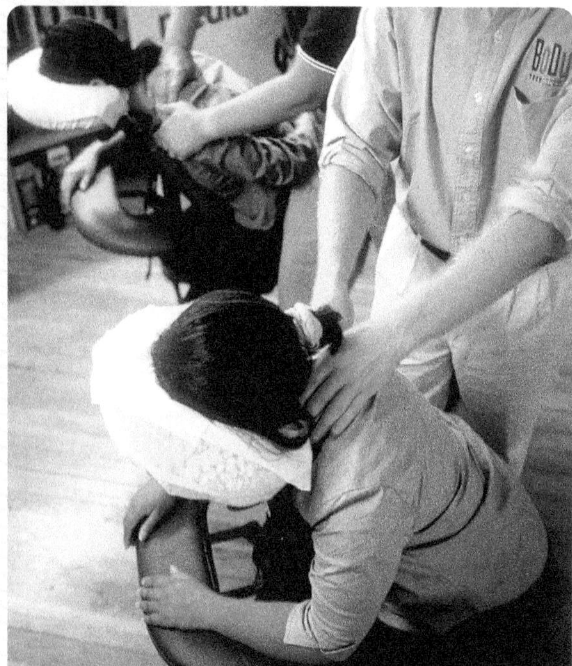

Fig. 22.6 Seated Massage This massage is especially common in a business or commercial setting. *What special equipment would be needed for this type of massage?*

Another type is stress-reduction massage. This is done on clients who have not been exercising. **Figure 22.5** shows a typical massage.

- **Neuromuscular massage** This massage type is applied to specific muscles to relieve tension and knots, pain and pressure on nerves, and increase blood flow. Trigger-point therapy is a type of neuromuscular massage in which finger pressure is applied to trigger points in the muscles.
- **Seated massage** Shiatsu and Swedish techniques may be used to massage to a fully clothed client who is seated in a massage chair. It is popular for short massages focused on the back and the neck. This massage is common in business settings (see **Figure 22.6**).

Eastern Styles of Massage Here are two of the many kinds of Eastern massage.

- **Shiatsu and acupressure** Finger pressure is used with these types of massage. Both are based on removing the blockages from the 12 meridians so that *qi* can flow. Practitioners of this type of massage believe that blocked meridians cause physical discomfort. The finger pressure of shiatsu applied to specific meridian points releases the blockage and balances energy flow. Shiatsu is generally done on a mat on the floor rather than on a massage table.
- **Reiki** This is also based on the principle of *qi*. Reiki is believed to have Tibetan and Buddhist origins. Reiki practitioners use visualization and touch to balance the client's energy flow and to bring healing energy to specific organs and glands. The practitioner serves as a channel for the life energy, which promotes emotional and physical healing.

Types of Massage Therapist Practices

As a massage therapist, you might have an office. If you worked independently, you would need an office with a private area for clients to dress and undress, a bathroom, and possibly a washer and dryer for linens. Some massage therapists do not have an office. Instead, they take their massage table to clients' homes or businesses. This works well for some clients, but others have difficulty relaxing in their regular environment. The massage should take place in a quiet, relaxed setting without distractions.

Massage therapists also work in day spas or resorts. These therapists may see the same clients on a regular basis. They may also see people who are temporarily staying in the area. These therapists are sometimes paid a salary by the facility, but more often they are paid a percentage of the money the facility gets for the massage.

Massage therapists may also work in beauty salons, allowing clients to have beauty treatments and massage at the same location. In some settings, the clients pay the therapist directly and the therapist pays rent to the salon owner. In other settings, the salon owner pays the therapist a percentage of the price of the massage.

Some massage therapists work in a chiropractor's office or in a clinic setting along with physical therapists and physicians. Massage therapists may also refer clients to a chiropractor or medical doctor for pain or muscle spasm that is not responding to massage.

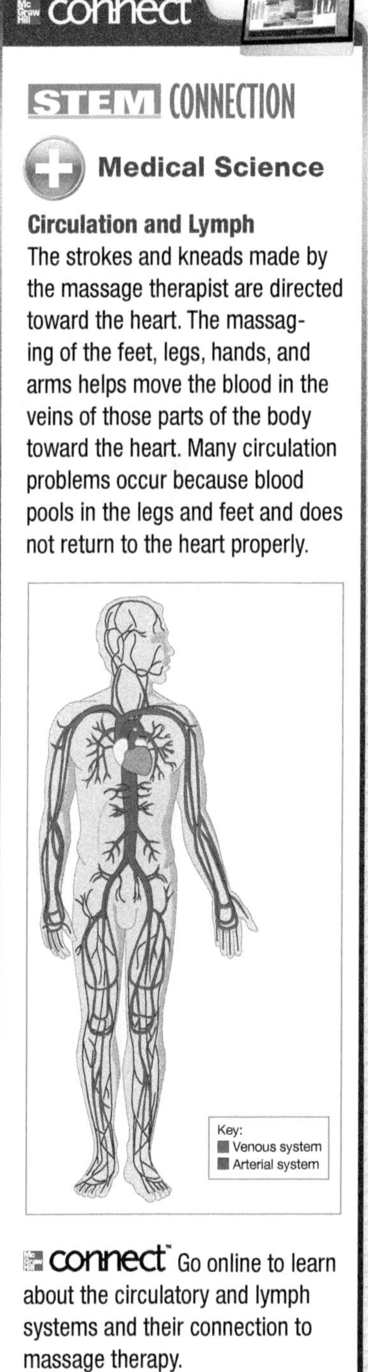

connect
STEM CONNECTION
Medical Science
Circulation and Lymph
The strokes and kneads made by the massage therapist are directed toward the heart. The massaging of the feet, legs, hands, and arms helps move the blood in the veins of those parts of the body toward the heart. Many circulation problems occur because blood pools in the legs and feet and does not return to the heart properly.
Key:
Venous system
Arterial system
connect Go online to learn about the circulatory and lymph systems and their connection to massage therapy.

It is important that a massage therapist be able to select the most appropriate modality to address the problem and to customize the treatment to meet each client's needs. Some insurance companies will pay for massage therapy when a chiropractor or medical doctor orders it.

The Job of a Massage Therapist

When a client visits a massage therapist, the therapist takes a brief medical history. He or she must be sure that the client does not have any conditions that could be made worse by massage. Many therapists avoid performing massage on a client who has a cancerous tumor that has not been surgically removed. The concern is that massage might cause the tumor to spread. Recent research, however, seems to suggest that this may not be so. Some clients who have severe osteoporosis or blood clots may not be candidates for the more vigorous types of massage.

The massage therapist must always maintain a high level of professionalism by explaining the procedure clearly before it begins and maintaining the client's privacy at all times. Just as a patient disrobes in a doctor's office to be examined, so the client must disrobe for some types of massage.

The therapist leaves the room to allow the client to remove the necessary clothing. A large towel or lightweight blanket is provided for the client to use as a covering. Only the area of the body being massaged is exposed. The rest of the body is kept covered.

When the massage therapist reenters the room, he or she dims the lights and plays soothing, relaxing music. Some massage therapists use candles or other aromatherapy techniques to involve all the senses in the massage experience.

Job Responsibilities of the Massage Therapist

Massage therapists must have the ability to detect subtle changes in muscle tension. They must be sensitive to the client and aware of any embarrassment and discomfort. They must take steps to relieve these problems.

On the business side, massage therapists make appointments, keep schedules, manage their businesses, and attract clients.

Some of the most important responsibilities of a massage therapist are the following:

- Take a brief medical history of each client
- Explain what the client needs to do to prepare for the massage
- Communicate what will take place during the massage so that the client knows what to expect
- Create a restful, relaxing atmosphere during the massage
- Assess the types of strokes or methods to use when muscle resistance is encountered
- Communicate with the client regarding any discomfort
- Use effective body mechanics to prevent injury to himself or herself
- Preserve the client's privacy at all times
- Judge when to refer clients to another massage therapist or healthcare provider
- Implement plans to attract new clients and retain existing clients
- Handle money responsibly, by paying bills, taxes, and rent in a timely manner

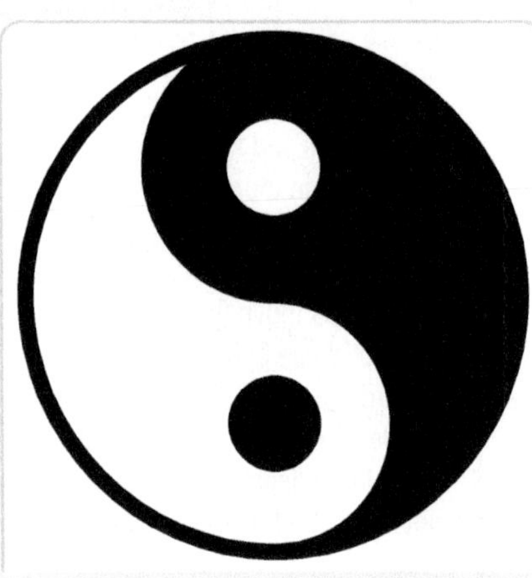

Fig. 22.7 Yin and Yang *Qi* is made up of *yin* and *yang*. *Why should* yin *and* yang *be perfectly balanced?*

READING CHECK

List some methods massage therapists use to ensure the comfort and relaxation of their clients.

The Acupuncturist

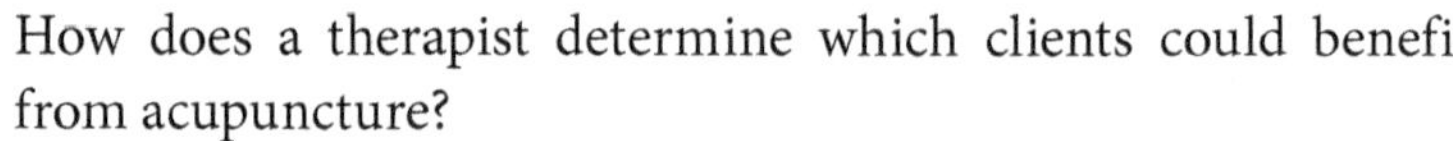

Which types of clients could benefit from acupuncture?

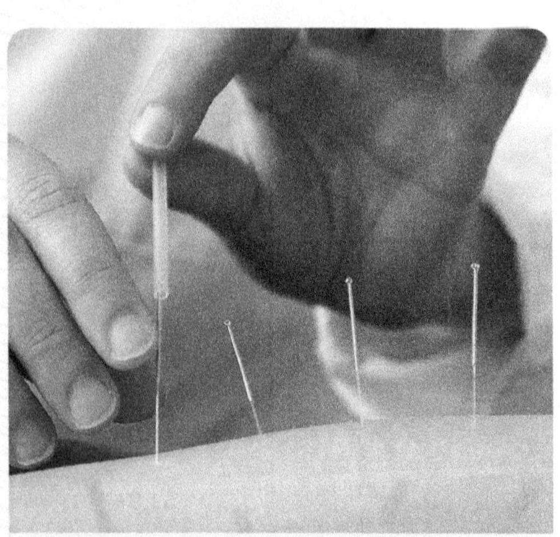

Fig. 22.8 Acupuncture Needles Acupuncture needles have a thin end that is inserted into the skin and a thicker end to make them easy to handle. *Is acupuncture painful?*

How does a therapist determine which clients could benefit from acupuncture?

The theory of acupuncture is based on Chinese beliefs about *qi*, ***yin***, and ***yang***. Remember that *qi* is the name for the "life energy" of the body. It is made up of two opposite forces called *yin* and *yang*. The acupuncturist works to bring these two forces into perfect harmony. This is based on the Chinese theory of health and illness, which holds that emotional, spiritual, mental, and physical aspects of life are affected if the flow of *qi* is not balanced. Insufficient or interrupted *qi* will have the same negative effect as imbalance. **Figure 22.7** shows perfectly balanced *yin* and *yang*.

Hollow needles like those in **Figure 22.8** are used by an **acupuncturist.** The acupuncturist inserts the needles under the skin to balance the flow of *qi* in the body. The needles are inserted in exact locations where the meridians come to the skin's surface. Refer again to **Figure 22.4** on page 547, which shows the meridians. The acupuncturist may twirl, raise, rotate, thrust, or vibrate the needles to achieve desired effects.

Acupuncture Treatment Types

The acupuncturist may use a variety of treatments. Some of these are described here.

- **Electro-acupuncture** This method is generally used to relieve or prevent pain. A very small amount of electrical current at varying frequencies is applied through the acupuncture needles. The amount is so small as to present no danger of electrical shock to the client. High-frequency electrical current has been used successfully to block the pain of surgery without the use of anesthesia.
- **Moxibustion** In this method, the acupuncturist applies heat to the points where the needles are inserted, to increase the effectiveness of the treatment. Moxibustion is used to treat conditions such as arthritis, bronchial asthma, bronchitis, and certain kinds of paralysis.
- **Acupressure** This type of acupuncture is performed without needles. Instead, the points along the meridians are stimulated using an instrument or finger pressure.
- **Reflexology** This type of acupressure is performed only on the feet and hands.

The Chinese, Korean, and Japanese versions of acupuncture differ slightly from one another. No matter which version is practiced, though, the acupuncturist focuses on the client's medical history, nutritional habits, and environmental factors.

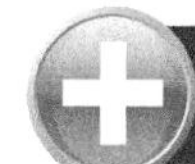

Safety

Embolus

Clients who have a history of blood clots may not be good candidates for massage, especially to their legs. If a clot is forming, the massage might cause it to break loose and travel through the bloodstream. A traveling clot, known as an **embolus**, can lodge in the blood vessels of other organs and decrease circulation. Decreased circulation to the heart, brain, or lungs can cause serious complications such as a myocardial infarction (heart attack), cerebrovascular accident (stroke), or pulmonary embolus (lung blood clot).

Types of Acupuncturist Practices

An acupuncturist may have his or her own office, which includes a private room for treating clients. Some acupuncturists work in a clinic setting with other healthcare practitioners. Acupuncture is often offered at a pain management clinic. Sometimes doctors learn acupuncture techniques and offer it as a part of their practice. Some chiropractors or medical doctors employ an acupuncturist to provide treatment for their clients. In some states, an acupuncturist must be a licensed medical doctor.

The Job of the Acupuncturist

When a client arrives for an acupuncture treatment, the acupuncturist first takes a detailed medical history, which includes information about nutrition and environment. Unlike Western doctors, the acupuncturist also inspects the tongue for shape and color variation. He or she may take a pulse in as many as 50 sites as part of the physical exam. The acupuncturist also asks detailed questions about the type of problem the client is having.

Clients with certain conditions may not be good candidates for acupuncture. For example, a client who has a cardiac pacemaker should not have electro-acupuncture, because the electrical current could interfere with the pacemaker's function. Clients who have hemophilia or clients who bruise very easily should not have acupuncture, because there could be bleeding or bruising at the insertion sites.

21ST CENTURY SKILLS

Cultural Differences in Perceptions of Health and Illness

Different cultures perceive health and illness in different ways. In ancient China, doctors were paid to keep their clients well. If a client became ill, the doctor was not paid. Chinese doctors thus concentrated on treating clients in order to prevent them from becoming ill. In the West, however, many people do not go to the doctor until they cannot manage the symptoms of illness on their own.

Eastern medicine and Western medicine also differ in their approach to what causes illness. In the Eastern approach, the body is able to remain healthy as long as *yin* and *yang* are balanced and sufficient *qi* flows without blockages. The doctor of Eastern medicine focuses his or her efforts on restoring balance and energy flow.

Western medicine focuses on finding a cause for illness. Western doctors look for an injury, infection, malignancy, or allergen that is causing symptoms and discomfort. Treatment plans include developing and administering a medication to kill the pathogen or treat allergic reactions, performing surgery to treat some injuries and remove cancers, and using laboratory tests to diagnose disorders and follow patient progress.

Most acupuncture treatments take from 20 minutes to 1 hour. The acupuncturist determines the type of treatment needed and the location for insertion of the needles. Six types of acupuncture needles are commonly used. Needles are disposable and used only once. They are discarded according to regulations on biohazardous materials.

The acupuncturist inserts the needles at 15- to 90-degree angles, depending upon the treatment needed. As the needles are inserted, the client feels a sensation similar to a mosquito bite. As electrical stimulation, twirling, vibration, or rotation is applied to the needle, the client may experience a sensation that ranges from a mild tingling to a mild ache. This sensation is desirable and is referred to as *de qi*.

The acupuncturist knows how far to insert the needles, from a fraction of an inch to an inch. The acupuncturist also determines how long to leave the needles in place. This may range from a few seconds to 30 minutes, depending on the treatment needed.

The acupuncturist may complement the treatment by using moxibustion, burning different types of herbs to create heat at the site of the needle insertion.

Another type of treatment used to enhance the effects of acupuncture is called cupping. The acupuncturist applies suction using a heated metal, wood, or glass jar to create a partial vacuum. Cupping causes blood to pool at the site to increase the effects of the acupuncture.

Job Responsibilities of the Acupuncturist

An acupuncturist is responsible for diagnosing clients and providing treatment. Acupuncturists must be knowledgeable about the client's problems and the appropriate meridians to access. They must be aware of which points along the meridians to insert needles. They must know how far the needles should be inserted and how long the needles should remain in place. In addition, acupuncturists must choose appropriate complementary therapies as indicated by the client's problems.

Other job responsibilities of the acupuncturist include

- making an accurate diagnosis of the client's problems based on acupuncture theory.
- determining appropriate treatment based on the diagnosis.
- communicating with clients about what will be done and what to expect.
- communicating with the client about discomfort.
- implementing plans to attract clients and retain existing clients.
- handling money responsibly, by paying bills, taxes, and rent .

READING CHECK

Recall what types of therapy an acupuncturist might perform that do not involve needles.

The Herbalist

Is an herb a medicine?

Herbalists use the leaves, flowers, berries, stems, and roots of herbs to make treatments. The purpose is to prevent, relieve, or treat illnesses. Herbalists may also grow or farm herbs, or gather herbs that grow in nature (this is known as wildcrafting). They may teach or write about herbs. Many herbalists do all of these things.

Ethnobotany is the university-level study of how plants are used as medicines in various countries. The work and writings of ethnobotanists help herbalists around the world preserve the traditional uses of herbs as medicine.

The herbalist knows where and how different plants grow, and which parts of the plant are most potent. He or she determines what herbs are used to treat specific conditions or illnesses. Sometimes combinations of herbs, or compounds, are used to treat or prevent certain conditions. The herbalist must know which herbs should be mixed together. He or she understands the ratio of the various ingredients that will effectively prevent or treat a problem.

Herbs are medicines and can have powerful effects. Herbalists know about those effects, and they know when a preparation is too strong or too weak for a client. Natural herbs are less likely to cause the drastic side effects that synthesized chemicals can cause. Even with herbs, however, some side effects can occur. The herbalist must explain these possible side effects to the client.

Types of Herbalist Practices

The herbalist may practice in his or her own office. Many herbalists have small offices in or near health food stores. Some herbalists may work in clinics with acupuncturists and other alternative healthcare practitioners.

Some herbalists run small manufacturing companies where they make herbal products and grow herbs for sale to manufacturers or the public. Herbalists may own retail stores where they sell herbs and counsel clients about herbal products. Herbalists are often excellent teachers and may teach at a college or university. They may also give seminars to the general public about herbs and their uses.

The Job of the Herbalist

When a client visits the herbalist, the herbalist assesses the client using a variety of techniques. The herbalist takes a medical history, takes a pulse at a variety of points, may examine the tongue, and may palpate the abdomen. The herbalist may also examine the iris of the eyes, a practice called iridology. The minute markings on the iris of the eye are believed to correlate with specific parts of the body. The markings indicate disease or illness in those areas. These diagnostic techniques

21ST CENTURY SKILLS

Science and CAM Therapy

The National Center for Complementary and Alternative Medicine (NCCAM) is the Federal Government's agency for scientific research on complementary and alternative medicine (CAM). NCCAM is a division of the National Institutes of Health.

NCCAM uses rigorous scientific investigation to determine the usefulness and safety of CAM treatments and their roles in improving health and healthcare. For example, NCCAM recognizes that acupuncture is effective in treating some types of pain and in counteracting nausea and vomiting caused by pregnancy, anesthesia, or chemotherapy. Other scientific studies identifying positive and negative aspects of CAM therapy are currently underway, as CAM therapies become increasingly popular.

Preventive Care & Wellness

Herbal Treatments

Do not use herbal remedies or supplements casually. Although they are readily available, you should do some research before you consider taking one. Consult a health professional or other reliable source to find out:

- Why the remedy or supplement is used
- The correct dosage and the dangers of overdose
- How and when the remedy or supplement should be taken

are similar to those used by acupuncturists. Acupuncturists may also be educated as herbalists.

After evaluating the client, the herbalist suggests individual herbs or herbal compounds to treat the conditions. The herbs are given to treat symptoms and to strengthen the affected body system. The herbalist also instructs the client on what effects to expect.

The herbalist must consider any prescription medications and over-the-counter medications a client is taking when recommending herbal medicine, since herbal preparations may interact with other types of medications and cause undesirable reactions. The herbalist must also be aware if a client is pregnant. Some herbs can cause problems if taken during pregnancy.

The herbalist communicates with clients, telling them when to expect improvement in their condition. Since herbs are less concentrated than synthetic medicines, their effects are more gradual. It may take several days to weeks to see results.

Job Responsibilities of the Herbalist

The herbalist's job requires a great deal of study and knowledge about different herbs and their effects on health. He or she must know about both the adverse and positive effects of herbs and their combinations. Knowledge about the interactions between herbs and conventional medications is also essential. Herbalists who grow their own herbs are careful about location and soil, so that their herbs will be pure and unspoiled by air or water pollution.

The herbalist's job includes

- making an accurate diagnosis of the client's problems based on a history and examination.
- determining the appropriate herbal treatment for client's diagnosis (single herbs or compounds).
- explaining to clients which herbs to take and how to take them.
- communicating with clients regarding which effects are expected and which should be reported to the herbalist.
- growing or selecting the purest herbs for use in treatments.
- keeping track of the shelf life of herbs and replacing herbs as necessary.
- implementing plans to attract new clients and retain existing clients.
- handling money responsibly, by paying bills, taxes, and rent in a timely manner.

READING CHECK

Identify some reasons why an herbalist might grow his or her own herbs.

The Aromatherapist

How can a background in chemistry lead to a career as an aromatherapist?

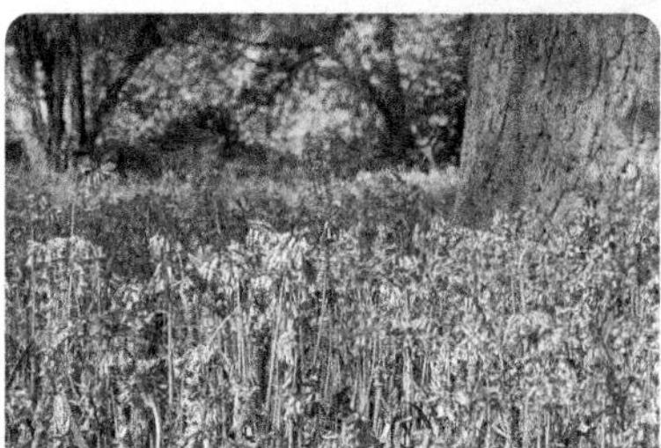

Fig. 22.9 Lavender Lavender is one of the most common plants used to make essential oils. *What is one use of an essential oil?*

Aromatherapy is the art and science of matching scents to symptoms. **Aromatherapists** use **essential oils** derived from plants (see **Figure 22.9**). They may teach or write about aromatherapy. Healthcare professionals such as massage therapists may also use aromatherapy as part of their treatment plan.

The aromatherapist knows how to select the appropriate scent or combination of scents for treating specific disorders. He or she determines which essential oils are used to treat specific conditions or illnesses. The aromatherapist understands what combination of scents will be effective and how to mix essential oils with a carrier oil if a client wants to use it on the skin, as during massage therapy.

Essential oils are concentrated and have powerful effects. Aromatherapists are aware of those effects and are responsible for determining the correct type and amount of essential oil needed. Some essential oils can have very serious side effects. The aromatherapist must explain these possible side effects to the client.

The olfactory system centers on the part of the brain that picks up smells introduced through the nasal passage (see **Figure 22.10**). That area of the brain is stimulated by scents released from essential oils. A signal is then sent to the part of the brain that controls emotions and retrieves learned memories. Certain chemicals (endorphins) are released, and the person may then feel relaxed, calm, energized, or stimulated. If the aromatherapy is used with massage therapy, the effects may be greater than if the two treatments are applied separately.

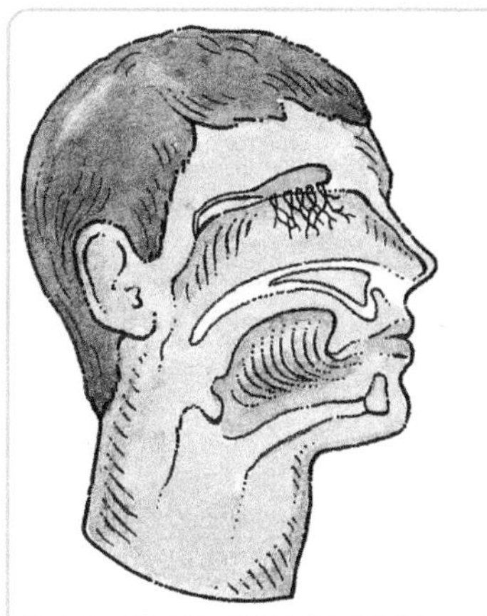

Fig. 22.10 The Olfactory System Scents travel through the nasal passage and are detected by the olfactory lobe, which sends signals directly to the brain. *What is one type of chemical that is released from these scents?*

Aromatherapy is both an art and a science. It is not a matter of burning scented candles to make the room smell good. Particular scents are used to address specific problems. For example, the scent of peppermint can relieve digestive problems and orange flower oil can help reduce depression. Essential oils are used with knowledge and skill.

The Job of the Aromatherapist

When a client arrives for an aromatherapy treatment, the aromatherapist first takes a detailed medical history, which includes information on the types of problems the client is having. The aromatherapist then determines which scent or combination of scents may best address most of the client's problems. He or she selects and mixes the essential oils for the client to use in an infuser (see **Figure 22.11** on page 556). These essential oils can be mixed with a carrier oil if the client wants to use the essential oils on the skin, because the essential oil may be too toxic to use on the skin without a "buffer." If the aromatherapist is also a massage therapist, he or she may use the oil mixture during a massage therapy treatment.

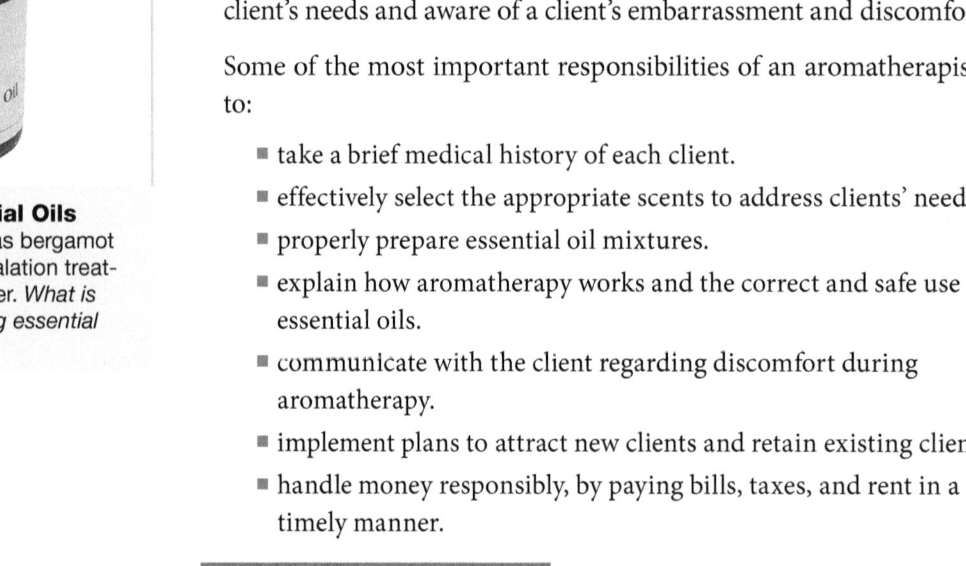

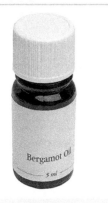

Fig. 22.11 Essential Oils Essential oils such as bergamot can be used for inhalation treatments with an infuser. *What is another way of using essential oils?*

Job Responsibilities of the Aromatherapist

Aromatherapists must have an understanding of the chemistry of essential oils and their toxicity. They make appointments, keep schedules, manage their businesses, and attract clients. Aromatherapists may couple aromatherapy with massage therapy and must be sensitive to the client's needs and aware of a client's embarrassment and discomfort.

Some of the most important responsibilities of an aromatherapist are to:

- take a brief medical history of each client.
- effectively select the appropriate scents to address clients' needs.
- properly prepare essential oil mixtures.
- explain how aromatherapy works and the correct and safe use of essential oils.
- communicate with the client regarding discomfort during aromatherapy.
- implement plans to attract new clients and retain existing clients.
- handle money responsibly, by paying bills, taxes, and rent in a timely manner.

READING CHECK

Summarize how the aromatherapist prepares a treatment plan for a client.

SECTION 22.1 Careers in Alternative Medicine Review

AFTER YOU READ

1. **Explain** why chiropractors focus treatment on the patient's spine.
2. **Identify** the job responsibility of a chiropractor that you think would be the most difficult.
3. **Indicate** the parts of the body other than the muscles that are affected by massage.
4. **Assess** which of the five types of massage would you most like to receive and why.
5. **Illustrate** how acupuncture affects *qi*, *yin*, and *yang*.
6. **Describe** two ways in which the acupuncturist enhances the effects of the treatment.
7. **Identify** what an herbalist needs to teach patients when suggesting herbal treatment.
8. **List** what the herbalist must consider when recommending herbal medicines.
9. **Explain** how aromatherapy goes beyond simply burning scented candles.
10. **Analyze** how aromatherapy can be used with complementary and alternative medicines.

Technology ONLINE EXPLORATIONS

Herbs

Go online to research three or four herbs. Review the information about each herb. Prepare a report about use, interactions, and precautions for each.

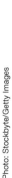

Photo: Stockbyte/Getty Images

SECTION
22.2 Complementary and Alternative Medicine Procedures

The Back Massage

Have you ever had a massage?

Massage can range from a simple back rub to a full body massage. Below you will learn how to do a back massage and a foot massage. Although these procedures are not as comprehensive as a full body massage, they will give you a good introduction to massage techniques. A back or foot rub is often performed as part of daily care for hospitalized patients.

Massage is generally performed on a **massage table** or in a **massage chair,** both of which are made to comfortably accommodate clients in optimal positions for massage. If you do not have access to a massage table, it can be done with the client on a bed in a prone position.

As with any healthcare procedure, it is important to apply infection control skills and good body mechanics in massage. The massage table or bed should be positioned at the correct working height. As you stand next to the table or bed, the palms of your hands should rest comfortably on the top, with your elbows straight. Adjust the height of a massage table by changing the placement of the pegs on the table legs. Adjust the height of a bed using the electronic or manual controls.

Massage oil is used to prevent friction on the skin during a massage. Lotion is not as effective for massage because it soaks into the skin. Oil remains on the skin, allowing your hands to glide easily over the surface. Use lotions only if no oil is available.

Various types of oil are used in massage, such as grapeseed, coconut, almond and other nut oils. Coconut oil washes out of linens more easily than most other types of oil, and it can be warmed to a liquid state by placing the bottle in a sink or basin filled with warm water.

It is not a good idea to heat oils in a microwave because the oil could catch fire if overheated. To avoid an undesired reaction, always check that your client is not allergic to any ingredient in the oil or oil combination. Massage therapists may also use scented oils for their aromatherapy qualities. However, essential oils (made from plant materials such as flowers, herbs, and fruits) designed for aromatherapy can be toxic and should be used with caution.

READING CHECK

Explain how to choose the correct oil for a massage.

Vocabulary

Content Vocabulary

You will learn these content vocabulary terms in this section.

- **massage table**
- **massage chair**
- **massage oil**

Academic Vocabulary

You will see this word in your reading and on your tests. Find its meaning in the Glossary in the back of the book.

- **adjust**

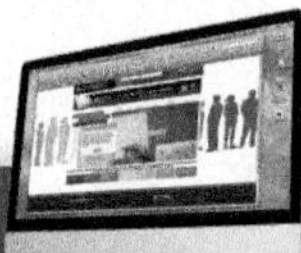

connect ONLINE PROCEDURES

PROCEDURE 22-1

Performing a Back Massage

Massage can range from a simple back rub to a full body massage. A back rub is often performed as part of daily care for hospitalized patients. If you do not have access to a massage table, it can be done with the client lying on a bed in a prone position. As with any healthcare procedure, it is important to apply infection control skills and good body mechanics in massage.

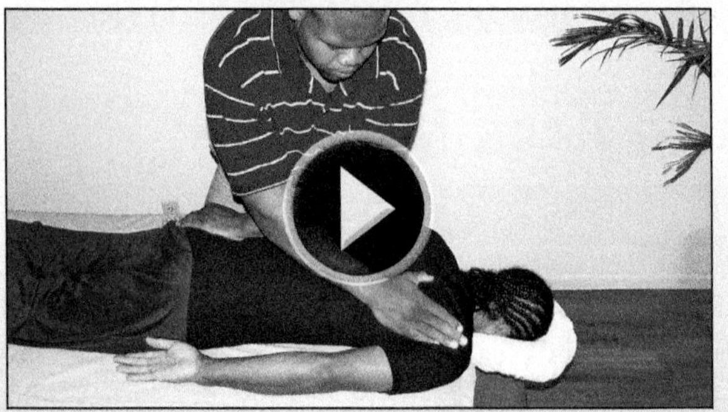

PROCEDURE 22-2

Performing a Foot Massage

Many people enjoy having their feet massaged. Even people who have ticklish feet can enjoy massage when the correct amount of pressure is used. The foot massage you will learn is the massage of the foot to relieve tension in the muscles and improve circulation. It would be included in a total body massage.

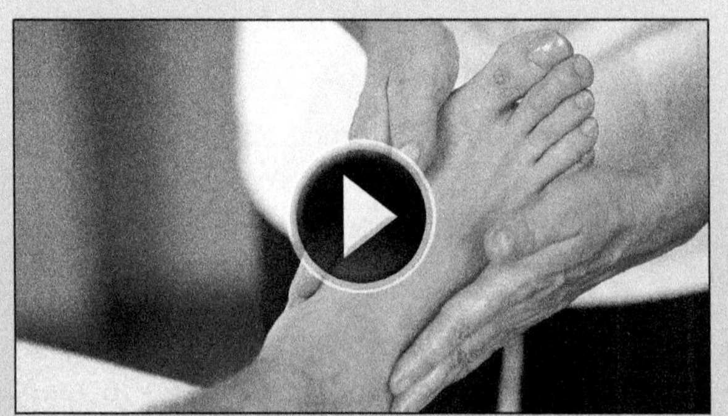

Photos: (t)The McGraw-Hill Companies, Inc./Shaana Pritchard, photographer, (b)Image Source/Jupiterimages

SECTION 22.2 Complementary and Alternative Medicine Procedures Review

AFTER YOU READ

1. **Identify** the correct height for a massage table or bed.
2. **Explain** how oil differs from lotion in its effectiveness for massage.
3. **List** some of the oils frequently used for massage and explain why they should be used with caution.
4. **Describe** what you should do if a massage client has a rash on his or her back.
5. **Identify** the part of your fingers that you should use when performing a massage.

Technology ONLINE EXPLORATIONS

Massage Therapy

Go online to research the job of a massage therapist. Find out more about possible places of employment. Compare the type of massage used and learn more about each technique. Share the information with your classmates in the form of an oral or written report.

CHAPTER
22 Review

Chapter Summary

SECTION 22.1

- Chiropractic adjustments focus on the spine. When the spinal vertebrae are subluxated, the function of the spinal nerves is restricted. A chiropractic adjustment is a manual treatment to realign the vertebrae and restore the function of the spinal nerves. **(pg. 544)**
- Chiropractors perform physical exams and take medical histories. Chiropractors may work in general practice, family practice, occupational health, or rehabilitation. They may specialize in sports injuries or automobile accident injuries. **(pg. 545)**
- Therapeutic massage promotes relaxation and counteracts the effects of stress. It also lowers blood pressure and heart rate during the massage and increases blood circulation and lymph flow. It helps reduce pain caused by tight muscles, promotes restful sleep, and helps the mind relax. **(pg. 547)**
- Massage therapists may work in their own offices, clients' homes or businesses, day spas, resorts, beauty salons, or a clinic setting such as a chiropractor's office. **(pg. 548)**
- Acupuncture is based on restoring balance between *yin* and *yang*, opposite forces that make up *qi*, the life energy of the body. **(pg. 550)**
- Acupuncturists must know how far to insert needles, how long to leave them in place, and what complementary therapies are appropriate. Acupuncturists may work in their own offices, in clinics with other healthcare practitioners, or in a pain management center. **(pg. 550)**
- Herbs are medicines and have powerful effects. Herbs are used to treat specific conditions or illnesses. Herbs may be combined to treat or prevent certain conditions. **(pg. 553)**
- Herbalists may have offices in or near health food stores, run small herbal manufacturing companies, own retail stores, and/or teach about herbs. **(pg. 553)**
- Herbalists must know how herbs interact with each other and interact with prescription and over-the-counter medicines that the client is also taking. **(pg. 554)**
- Aromatherapy is based on the effect that scents have on the brain. **(pg. 555)**
- Aromatherapists must know how to select the best essential oil or oils to meet a client's needs. Aromatherapists may also be massage therapists or practice other forms of complementary and alternative medicine. **(pg. 556)**

SECTION 22.2

- Good body mechanics and infection control techniques must be practiced during all types of therapeutic massage. **(pg. 558)**
- A back massage may be a simple back rub. A back rub is often part of the care given to hospitalized patients. **(pg. 558)**

CHAPTER 22 Assessment

Critical Thinking/Problem Solving

1. Explain reasons why you would need to go to a chiropractor for several visits over a period of time when you may only go once to a medical doctor when you are ill.
2. A friend of yours asks you to press on his back along his spine while he lies on the floor. He says that he wants you to "pop his back" because he has pain between his shoulder blades. What should you say and do?
3. Several friends at your school tell you they are taking an herb called *ma huang* to lose weight. They tell you that it is all natural, so it cannot possibly do any harm or have any side effects. What should you say?

21ST CENTURY SKILLS

4. **Teamwork** Locate a partner's spinal column and the regions of the vertebrae. Your partner may need to bend forward slightly. Find the cervical, thoracic, lumbar, and sacral regions by counting each space between the vertebrae. Review **Figure. 22.1** in this chapter for the anatomy of the spine if you need to do so.
5. **Teamwork** Gently massage a partner's hand. Be sure to remove your rings, bracelets, and watch. Use lotion or oil if it is available. Use a variety of strokes and pressure levels. Ask your partner which strokes felt the best. Pay attention to the changes, if any, in skin color. Share this information about the massage experience with the class.
6. **Information Literacy** Are you interested in alternative medicine? Go online to learn more about other alternative medicine careers. Look for topics such as reflexology, iridology, and homeopathy. Choose one that interests you and write a brief report covering purpose, training, and potential job opportunities.

McGraw-Hill connect™ ONLINE ACTIVITIES

Complete our HST online activities for Chapter 22, which include Concept Check review questions, Reference Flash Cards, and Online Procedures assessment sheets.

- **Concept Check** review questions
- **Reference Flash Cards** medical terminology practice
- **Online Procedures** assessment sheets

CHAPTER **23** # Dental Care

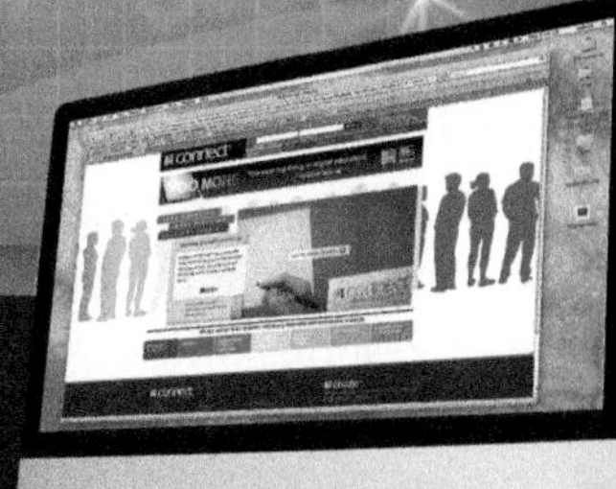

Essential Question:

What aspects of a career in dentistry would appeal to you?

Dentistry is a healthcare field familiar to nearly all of us as patients. It deals primarily with the diagnosis, prevention, and treatment of diseases and disorders of the teeth and oral tissues. Dental professionals such as the dental assistant, dental laboratory technician, dental hygienist, and dentist work in a variety of fields, including dental public health, endodontics, oral and maxillofacial pathology, oral and maxillofacial radiography, oral and maxillofacial surgery, orthodontics and dentofacial orthopedics, pediatric dentistry, periodontics, and prosthodontics. Careers in dentistry offer job security, personal satisfaction, variety, and opportunities to use advanced technology.

McGraw Hill connect™

It's Online!

- **Online Procedures**
- **STEM Connection**
- **Medical Science**
- **Medical Terms**
- **Medical Math**
- **Ethics in Action**
- **Virtual Lab**

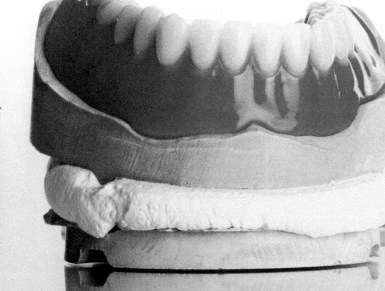

Photo: blickwinkel/McPHOTO/KPA/Alamy

READING GUIDE

OBJECTIVES

After completing this chapter, you will be able to:

- **Identify** the members of the dental team and their responsibilities, education, and credentials.
- **Describe** the dental specialty areas.
- **Recall** the teeth in the primary and the permanent dentition.
- **Recognize** surfaces, tissues, and anatomical features of the teeth and related structures.
- **Demonstrate** universal and Palmer's notation.
- **Examine** the factors that may cause dental diseases.
- **Demonstrate** aseptic techniques and maintenance of equipment in the dental treatment room.
- **Evaluate** conditions of teeth and record the treatment given.
- **Demonstrate** four dental care procedures.

BEFORE YOU READ

Connect What career options might you have in the field of dental care?

Main Idea

Dentists, dental assistants, dental hygienists, and dental technicians provide valuable services to ensure the growth of healthy teeth and to prevent and treat dental diseases.

Note-Taking Activity

Draw this table. Write key terms and phrases under **Cues**. Write main ideas under **Note Taking**. Summarize the section under **Summary**.

Cues	Note Taking
○	○
○	○
Summary	

Graphic Organizer

Before you read the chapter, draw a diagram like the one below. As you read, write the dental careers covered in the chapter into the diagram.

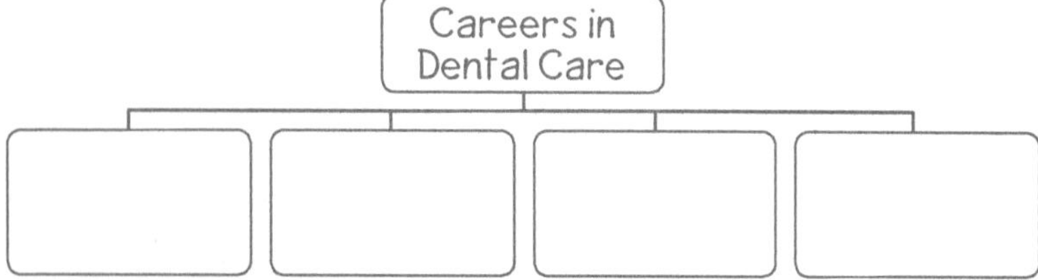

connect™ Downloadable graphic organizers can be accessed online.

STANDARDS

HEALTH SCIENCE

NCHSE 1.32 Analyze diagrams, charts, graphs, and tables to interpret healthcare results.

NCHSE 9.12 Describe strategies for the prevention of diseases including health screenings and examinations.

SCIENCE

NSES E Develop abilities of technological design, understandings about science and technology

NCHSE *National Consortium for Health Science Education*

NSES *National Science Education Standards*

COMMON CORE STATE STANDARDS

MATHEMATICS

Number and Quantity

The Real Number System

N-Q Reason quantitatively and use units to solve problems.

ENGLISH LANGUAGE ARTS

Speaking and Listening

Presentation of Knowledge and Ideas SL-6 Adapt speech to a variety of contexts and tasks, demonstrating a command of formal English when indicated or appropriate.

Language

Vocabulary Acquisition and Use

L-4c Consult general and specialized reference materials (e.g., dictionaries, glossaries, thesauruses), both print and digital, to find the pronunciation of a word or determine or clarify its precise meaning, its part of speech, or its etymology.

SECTION
23.1 Careers in Dental Care

The Dental Assistant

How many dental assistants work with one dentist?

When you visit the dentist, the person working with the dentist is the dental assistant. He or she has one of the most interesting jobs in the dental office. This career requires versatility, knowledge, clinical skills, and interpersonal skills. Dental assistants increase the efficiency of the dentist as he or she provides oral healthcare. They are valuable members of the dental team. **Figure 23.1** shows a dental assistant.

The types of settings in which dental assistants work include:

- Dental offices of general dentists and dental specialists
- Dental school clinics
- Private and government hospitals and clinics
- Public health clinics
- Insurance companies
- Dental laboratories
- Dental suppliers

Employment opportunities are excellent. Although state regulations vary, dental assistants may

- expose and process radiographs (X-rays).
- provide clients with instructions on oral care following surgery or other treatment procedures.
- teach clients how to brush and floss properly.
- make impressions of teeth for study models.
- assist the dentist in a variety of treatment procedures in general and specialty practices.
- polish coronal surfaces of teeth.
- manipulate dental materials.
- make dental appliances and temporary crowns.
- develop infection control protocol.
- prepare and sterilize instruments and equipment.
- perform office management tasks.

READING CHECK

Identify five tasks that may be performed by a dental assistant.

Vocabulary

Content Vocabulary

You will learn these content vocabulary terms in this section.

- **prosthesis**
- **crown**
- **bridge**
- **periapical tissue**
- **maxillofacial region**
- **malocclusion**
- **periodontal disease**

Academic Vocabulary

You will see this word in your reading and on your tests. Find its meaning in the Glossary in the back of the book.

- **assist**

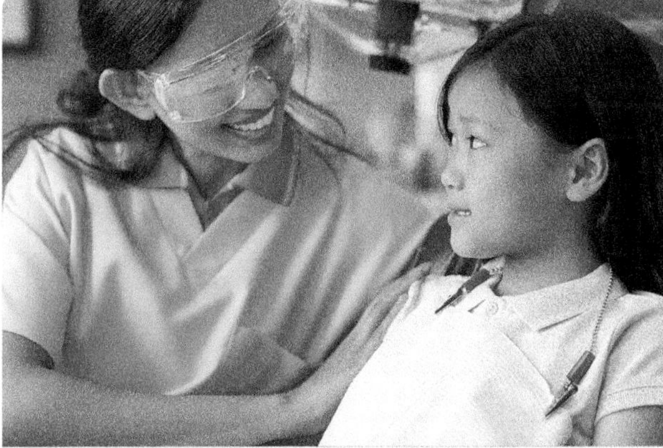

Fig. 23.1 Dental Visit Dental professional working with patient in a dental office. *Can you name the dental professional in this photo?*

Photo: Karin Dreyer/Blend Images LLC

Table 23.1 Careers in Dentistry

OCCUPATION	EDUCATIONAL REQUIREMENTS	CERTIFICATION OR LICENSING REQUIREMENTS	JOB OUTLOOK
Dental assistant	One- or two-year program in a community college or postsecondary vocational-technical school. On-the-job training is also available.	Certification or registration requirements vary according to state. Certification is available through the Dental Assisting National Board, Inc. Some states require an additional state registration.	Growth is expected to be much faster than average. As dentists' workloads increase, they are expected to hire more assistants to perform routine tasks.
Dental laboratory technician	On-the-job training is the most common path for an entry-level technician. To become a fully trained technician requires an average of three to four years. Formal educational programs are also available through community and postsecondary vocational-technical schools, and the armed forces.	Voluntary certification is available through the National Board for Certification in Dental Laboratory Technology in five areas: crowns and bridges, ceramics, partial dentures, complete dentures, and orthodontic appliances.	Growth is expected to be faster than average. An aging population will require more products fabricated by dental lab technicians.
Dental hygienist	Two to four years of college in a program accredited by the Commission on Dental Accreditation of the American Dental Association.	Dental hygienists must be licensed by the state in which they practice. To qualify for licensure, a candidate must graduate from an accredited dental hygiene school and pass both a written and a clinical examination.	Growth is expected to be much faster than average in response to an increasing demand for preventive dental care and the greater use of hygienists for services previously performed by dentists.
Dentist	Two to four years of college-level pre-dental education plus four years of dental school are required to become a general dentist. An additional two to four years of postgraduate education is needed to enter a specialized area of dentistry.	Dentists must graduate from a dental school accredited by the American Dental Association's Commission on Dental Accreditation and pass a written and practical examination given by an individual state or regional testing agency.	Faster than average employment growth. Job prospects are good as a result of the need to replace the large number of dentists expected to retire. The demand for dental services is expected to continue to grow as the population, especially the number of older people, increases.

The Dental Laboratory Technician

What items does a dental laboratory technician make?

Dental laboratory technicians are important members of the dental care team. Unlike the dental assistant, they seldom work with clients. The dental lab tech follows the written instructions of a licensed dentist to create dental **prostheses** (artificial devices), replacements for natural teeth, and dental appliances (see **Figure 23.2**). He or she needs artistic skills, fine hand dexterity, and good vision to recognize very fine color shadings and variations in shape. Most dental laboratory technicians are trained on the job in dental labs or dental offices, or in special programs beyond high school. Most work in commercial dental labs that employ five to ten technicians. Employment opportunities are also available in some private dental offices, dental schools, hospitals, and companies that manufacture dental prosthetic materials.

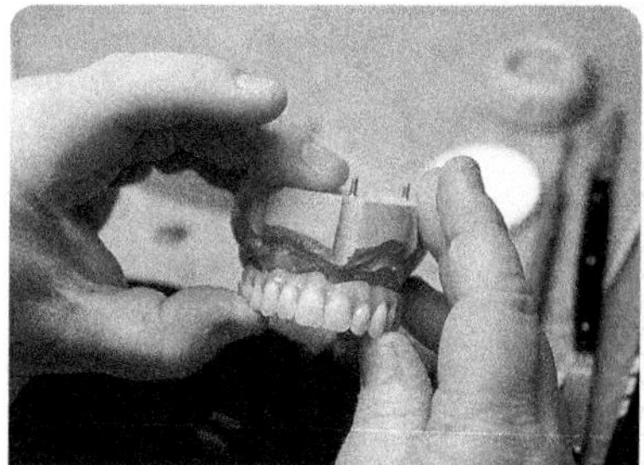

Fig. 23.2 Dentures Working on dentures. *What type of dental professional would be responsible for creating these dentures?*

Dental technicians use a variety of materials—waxes, plastics, precious and nonprecious metals, porcelains, and composites—to fabricate

- full or partial dentures.
- artificial **crowns** and **bridges.** A crown restores the anatomy and function of all or part of the natural crown of the tooth. A bridge is a fixed prosthesis that replaces a missing tooth or teeth.
- veneers.
- orthodontic appliances and splints.

READING CHECK

Summarize the skill set of a dental laboratory technician.

The Dental Hygienist

What tasks do dental hygienists perform?

Dental hygienists provide oral hygiene care and dental health education to the client. They need good communication skills and clinical skills. Dental hygienists must have at least two years of college education, classroom and clinical. Many programs require at least one year of college prerequisites for admission. Once licensed, graduates find jobs in private dental offices, nursing homes, public health clinics, and educational institutions. Employment opportunities are excellent.

Although specific responsibilities are governed by state regulations, dental hygienists may

- chart conditions and review the client's health and dental history.
- expose and process dental radiographs (X-rays).

- instruct clients in oral hygiene techniques.
- provide nutritional counseling in relation to dental health.
- remove calculus and plaque.
- apply preventive materials such as fluoride and sealants to the teeth.

READING CHECK

List some settings in which a dental hygienist may work.

21ST CENTURY SKILLS

Teeth and Technology

Dental implants are a dramatic advancement in dentistry that gives some people a second chance for their teeth. Implants consist of a synthetic crown, the top portion of the tooth, and a metallic cylinder as the root. The metallic cylinder is placed in the jawbone where the original tooth used to be. Implants can also be used to tighten loose teeth and make them last longer. The future looks good for advanced techniques in tooth replacement, although keeping your own teeth is the best idea of all!

The Dentist

What are some advantages of a career as a dentist?

A career as a dentist may be a good choice if you have scientific ability and interest, and enjoy helping people. It may also be a good choice if you want a career in which you can be your own boss. To prepare for dental school while you are in high school and college, you should develop a solid foundation in math and science.

Dentists usually have eight years of education beyond high school. They complete a bachelor's degree and then continue on to four years of dental school. After completing dental school, dentists receive a doctor of dental surgery (DDS) or doctor of dental medicine (DMD) degree. Both degrees allow the dentist to practice general dentistry.

A dentist has the education and training to

- diagnose and treat diseases of the teeth and their supporting tissues, the tongue, lips, and jaws.
- restore teeth damaged by decay or trauma.
- replace missing teeth with artificial materials.
- straighten teeth and perform cosmetic procedures to improve a client's appearance.
- perform corrective surgery on the jaws and supporting tissues.
- perform oral hygiene procedures and give instructions to clients.

Some dentists choose to focus their practice in one of the specialty areas of dentistry. An additional postgraduate education of two to four years is required to become a dental specialist.

READING CHECK

Name the two types of degrees held by dentists.

Specialty Areas of Dental Practice

Which dental fields involve research?

Dentists may choose to specialize in one of the following areas:

- Dental public health: Dental disease prevention, dental health education, and dental treatment programs at the community level

- Endodontics: Treatment of diseases of the pulp and **periapical tissues,** the tissues surrounding the apex of the root of the tooth
- Oral and maxillofacial pathology: Research, identification, and management of diseases affecting the oral structures
- Oral and maxillofacial radiology: Interpretation of radiographic images for diagnosis of conditions of the head and neck
- Oral and maxillofacial surgery: Surgical treatment of diseases, injuries, and defects of the oral and **maxillofacial region**
- Orthodontics and dentofacial orthopedics: Correction of tooth alignment and **malocclusions,** which is an abnormal relationship of the teeth when biting or closing
- Pediatric dentistry: Comprehensive dental care of infants and children though adolescence, including clients with special needs
- Periodontics: Prevention and treatment of **periodontal diseases,** diseases of the supporting and surrounding tissues of the teeth
- Prosthodontics: Replacement of missing teeth and oral structures

Most dentists own their own practices, but some have partners or are employed by other dentists. There are employment opportunities in hospitals, clinics, government agencies, research facilities, and educational institutions. Dentists employ dental hygienists, dental assistants, and dental laboratory technicians.

READING CHECK

Recall the area of dental practice that involves the treatment of diseases affecting the oral structures.

SECTION 23.1 Careers in Dental Care Review

AFTER YOU READ

1. **Compare** the length of education and training of the dental assistant, dental laboratory technician, dental hygienist, and dentist.
2. **Name** the two types of degrees that a dentist may have earned.
3. **Identify** three types of procedures that a dentist is trained to perform.
4. **Describe** four dental specialty areas.
5. **Compare and contrast** the job responsibilities of the dental assistant and dental hygienist.

Compare Programs

Choose one member of the dental team and research two educational programs that would prepare you for that specific job. Compare the programs in terms of their cost, length, prerequisites for admission, and accreditation. Locate the website of a school, college, or university that offers one of those programs and download or request a program brochure or application, if available. Otherwise, write a letter or e-mail your request.

SECTION

23.2 Dental Care Procedures

Vocabulary

Content Vocabulary

You will learn these content vocabulary terms in this section.

- deciduous dentition
- maxilla
- mandible
- midline
- resorb
- mixed dentition period
- distal
- permanent dentition
- anterior
- posterior
- crown
- root
- apex
- cervical line
- mesial
- facial
- buccal
- labial
- incisal
- occlusal
- lingual
- proximal surface
- contact area
- cusp
- interproximal space
- marginal ridge
- developmental groove
- fissure
- pit
- fossa
- enamel
- cementum
- dentin
- pulp
- pulp chamber
- pulp canal
- gingiva
- caries
- plaque
- cavity
- The Palmer System
- supragingival calculus
- impression
- amalgam

Basic Dental Anatomy

What parts make up a tooth?

During their lifetime, human beings have two sets of teeth, the primary teeth and the permanent teeth.

The Primary Teeth

The first set of teeth, the primary or **deciduous dentition,** consists of 20 teeth. These erupt, or emerge, at about six months of age. All primary teeth have erupted by the time a child is two to $2\frac{1}{2}$ years of age. The teeth are positioned in the **maxilla** (upper jawbone) and **mandible** (lower jawbone) in a U-shaped pattern. There are ten teeth in the maxillary arch and ten teeth in the mandibular arch.

Each arch is divided by the **midline** (midsagittal plane), which separates the oral cavity into quadrants. These are named according to location: maxillary right quadrant, maxillary left quadrant, mandibular left quadrant, and mandibular right quadrant (see **Figure 23.4**).

Each quadrant has the same type and number of teeth. Starting at the midline and moving posteriorly, the primary teeth are: central incisor, lateral incisor, canine, first primary molar, and second primary molar (see **Figure 23.5**).

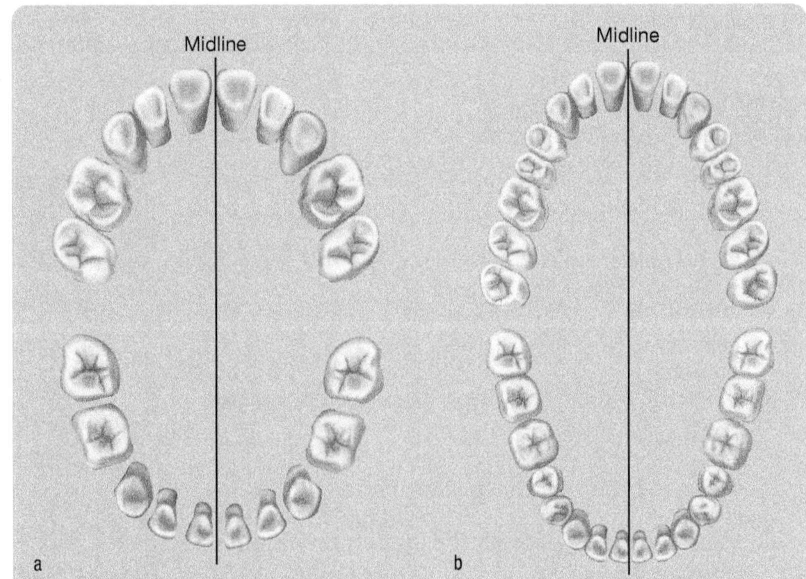

Fig. 23.4 Quadrants (a) Primary dental arches divided by midline into four quadrants. (b) Permanent dental arches divided by midline into four quadrants. *By what age have most of the permanent teeth replaced the primary teeth?*

The Permanent Teeth

Between the ages of six and 12, the primary teeth become loose, fall out, and are replaced with permanent teeth. Primary teeth become loose when the roots **resorb,** or dissolve, from the pressure of the developing permanent teeth directly below them in the jawbone.

During this time, both primary and permanent teeth are present. This is known as the **mixed dentition period** and is illustrated in **Figure 23.6.** The permanent molars erupt **distal** to the primary molars and therefore do not replace the primary teeth. As the child grows, the jaws become longer and larger, creating more space for additional teeth. All permanent teeth, except for the permanent molars, replace primary teeth.

The **permanent dentition** (see **Figure 23.7**) consists of 32 teeth that begin to erupt at age six. With the exception of the third molars, all permanent teeth have erupted by age 12 to 14. Starting at the midline and moving posteriorly, the permanent teeth of one quadrant are: central incisor, lateral incisor, canine, first premolar, second premolar, first permanent molar, second permanent molar, and third molar (wisdom tooth). Teeth are classified as either **anterior,** at the front of the mouth, or **posterior,** at the back of the mouth (see **Figure 23.8**). Anterior teeth are covered by the lips. Posterior teeth are covered by the cheeks.

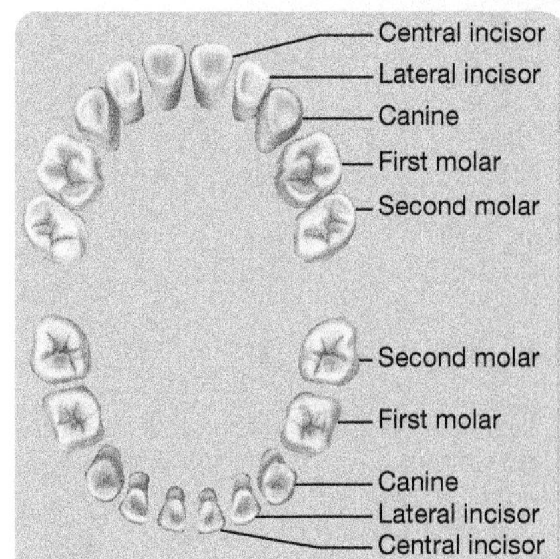

Fig. 23.5 Primary Teeth Names of the primary teeth. *How many primary teeth are there?*

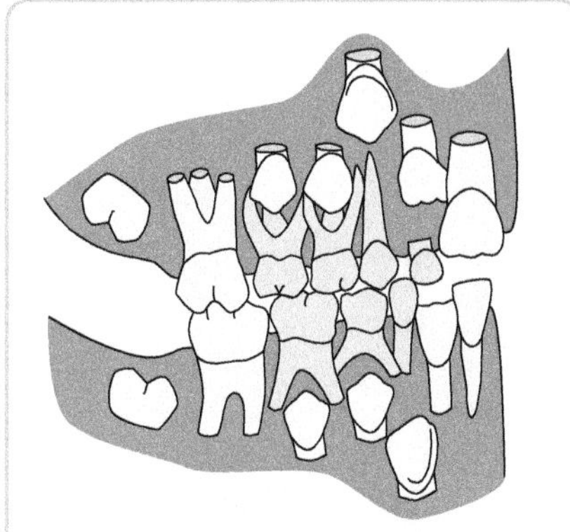

Fig. 23.6 Mixed Dentition Period Both primary and permanent teeth are present. *When does the mixed dentition period occur?*

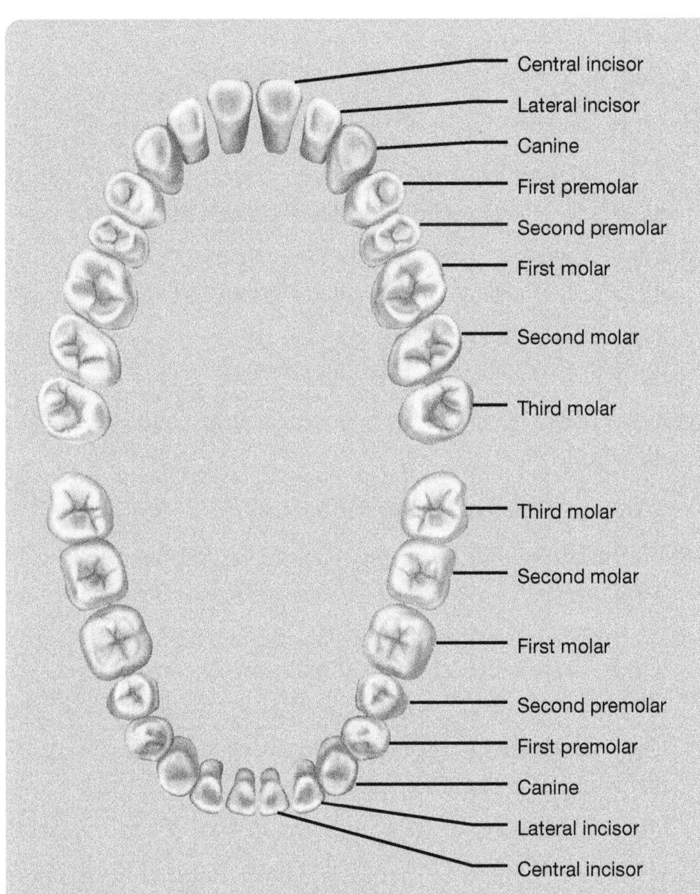

Fig. 23.7 Permanent Teeth Names of the permanent teeth. *How many permanent teeth are there?*

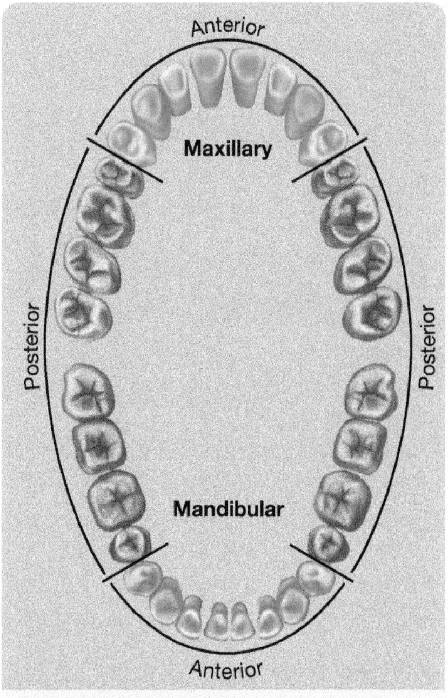

Fig. 23.8. Anterior and Posterior Anterior and posterior teeth. *How many anterior teeth are there?*

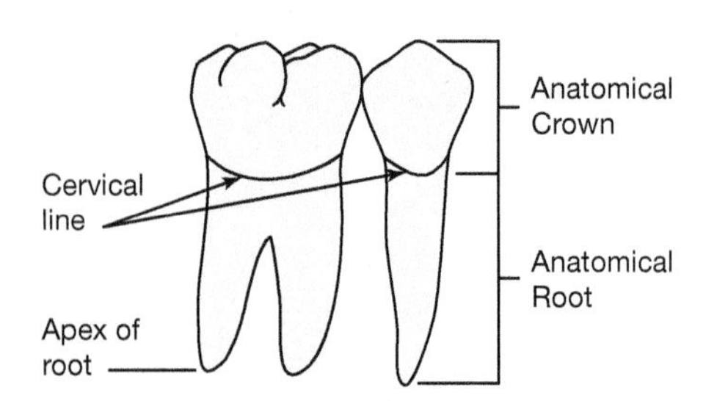

Fig. 23.9 Tooth Parts Parts of a tooth include the crown and the root. *What is another name for the cervical line?*

Tooth Divisions

Each tooth has two main parts, the **crown** and the **root,** as shown in **Figure 23.9.** The crown is the portion of the tooth normally visible in the oral cavity. The root is embedded in the bone. The root holds the tooth in its position in the oral cavity. The **apex** is the end of the root located farthest away from the crown. The **cervical line** is the line formed by the junction of the crown and the root. The cervical line is also known as the cementoenamel junction or the "neck" of the tooth.

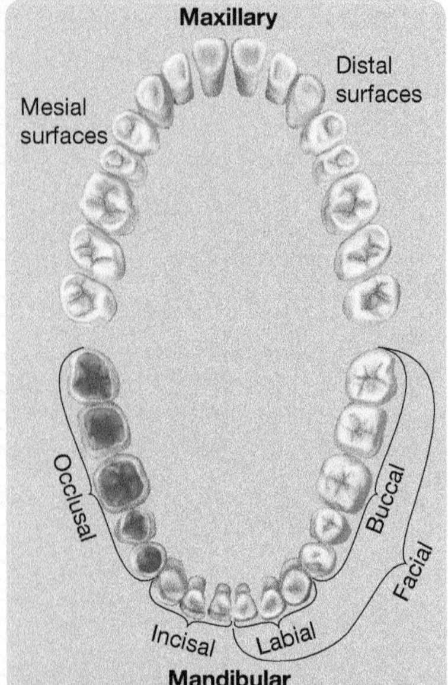

Fig. 23.10 Tooth Surfaces Surfaces of the tooth include the mesial, distal, facial, incisal, and occlusal. *How can the facial surfaces of the teeth be distinguished?*

Surfaces of the Tooth

Every tooth crown has six surfaces that are named according to their location. These surfaces are shown in **Figure 23.10** and are:

- **Mesial:** Surface of the tooth closest to the midline
- **Distal:** Surface of the tooth farthest away from the midline
- **Facial:** Surface of the tooth closest to the face; it may also be called the buccal or labial surface
- **Buccal:** Surface of a posterior tooth closest to the cheek
- **Labial:** Surface of an anterior tooth closest to the lips
- **Incisal:** Cutting edge of an anterior tooth (incisors and canines)
- **Occlusal:** Chewing surface of a posterior tooth (premolars and molars).
- **Lingual:** Surface of the tooth next to the tongue.

Other terms related to the surfaces of the tooth are

- **Proximal surface:** Tooth surface next to an adjacent tooth; a general term that includes both mesial and distal surfaces.
- **Contact area:** A small area on the proximal surfaces where two adjacent teeth touch one another. **Figure 23.11** shows this area.
- **Interproximal space:** Triangle-shaped space between adjacent teeth, normally filled with gingival tissue.

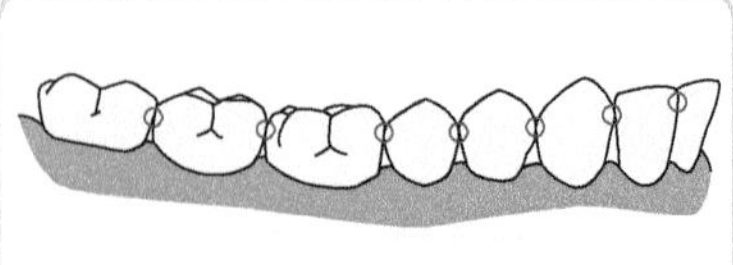
Fig. 23.11 Contact Areas Interproximal contact areas. *What is between the interproximal spaces?*

Structural features of the occlusal surface are shown in **Figure 23.12** and are as follows:

- **Cusp:** A pointed elevation on the surface of a tooth.
- **Marginal ridges:** The boundaries or edges of the occlusal surface.
- **Developmental grooves:** Lines on the occlusal surface that mark the junction of the developmental lobes. Each tooth develops from four or more centers of formation known as developmental lobes. These centers fuse together to form the crown portion of the tooth.
- **Fissures:** Deep developmental grooves resulting from incomplete fusion of the developmental lobes.
- **Pit:** A small, deep depression on the surface of a tooth, usually found at the end of a developmental groove or at the junction of two or more grooves.
- **Fossa:** A rounded depression on the surface of a tooth.

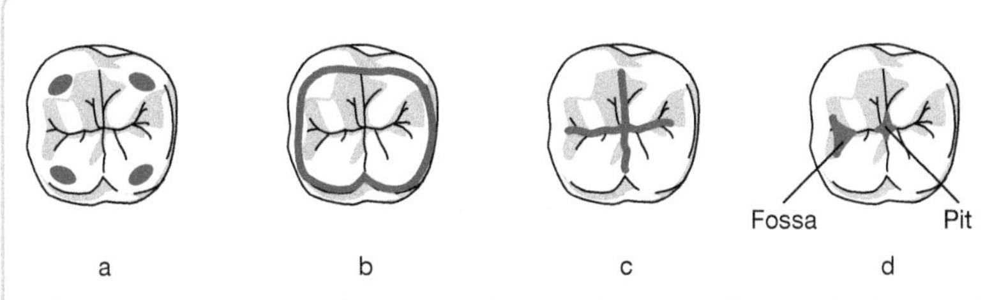

Fig. 23.12 Occlusal Surface Structural features of the occlusal surface: (a) Cusps (b) Marginal ridges (c) Developmental grooves (d) Fossa and pit. *What are the occlusal surfaces used for?*

Tooth Tissues

As shown in **Figure 23.13,** a tooth is made up of four tissues: enamel, cementum, dentin, and pulp.

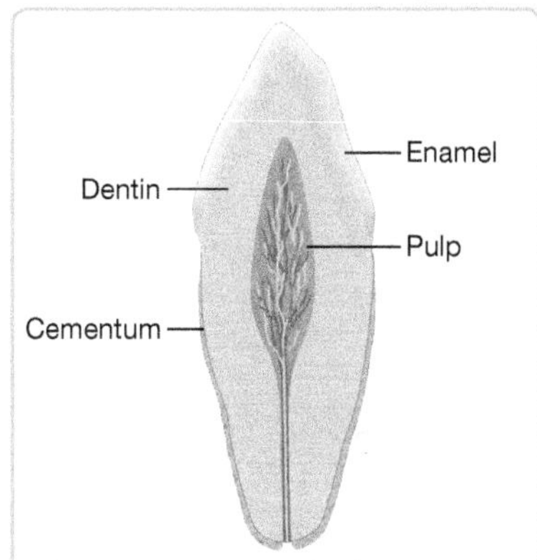

Fig. 23.13 Tooth Tissues The four tissues of a tooth. *How can tooth enamel be damaged?*

Enamel The outer layer of the crown of the tooth is **enamel.** This is the hardest tissue in the body and is white in color. It is harder than bone, but the body cannot repair or add to it. Enamel can be damaged by decay or worn away by chewing forces, abrasion, and chemical erosion.

Cementum The thin outer layer of the root of the tooth is the **cementum.** This tissue is similar in hardness to bone and is not as white as the enamel. The junction of the cementum and the enamel at the neck of the tooth is called the cementoenamel junction (CEJ), or cervical line.

Dentin The **dentin** lies just below the enamel of the crown and the cementum of the root. Dentin makes up the bulk of the tooth and provides support for the enamel. Dentin is not as dense as enamel and is yellower in color than enamel and cementum.

Pulp The **pulp** is the innermost tissue of the tooth. This soft tissue is composed of blood vessels, nerves, lymphatics, and connective tissue. This tissue nourishes the tooth, produces dentin, and acts as a defense system. It registers thermal and chemical changes in, and injury to, the enamel and dentin. The pulp is large in newly erupted teeth, making them more sensitive to thermal changes. As the tooth ages, the amount the pulp becomes smaller. The pulp within the crown of the tooth is the **pulp chamber.** The pulp in the roots of the tooth is the **pulp canal.** The number of pulp canals usually corresponds to the number of roots.

Adjacent Tissues A fibrous membrane known as the periodontal ligament surrounds the cementum of the root. The periodontal ligament contains fibers that attach to the cementum on the tooth side and to the alveolar bone on the other side. This ligament suspends the tooth in the tooth socket. It acts as a shock absorber for the tremendous amount of pressure generated by the cutting, grinding, and chewing of food. **Figure 23.14** shows the supporting tissues of the teeth.

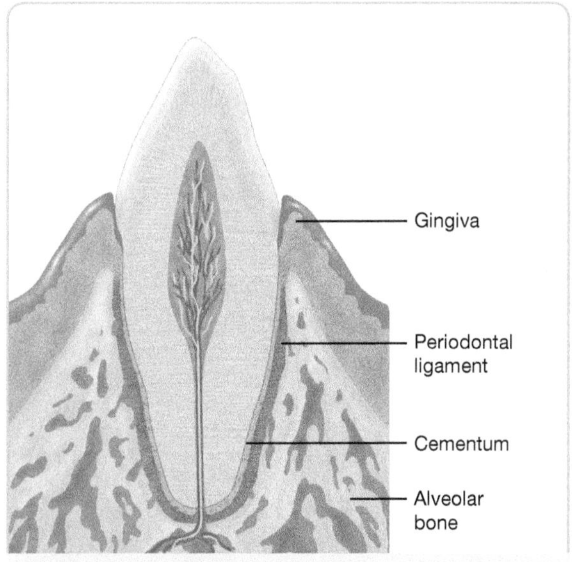

Fig. 23.14 Supporting Tissues Cross-sectional view of the supporting tissues of the teeth. *What is the purpose of the periodontal ligament?*

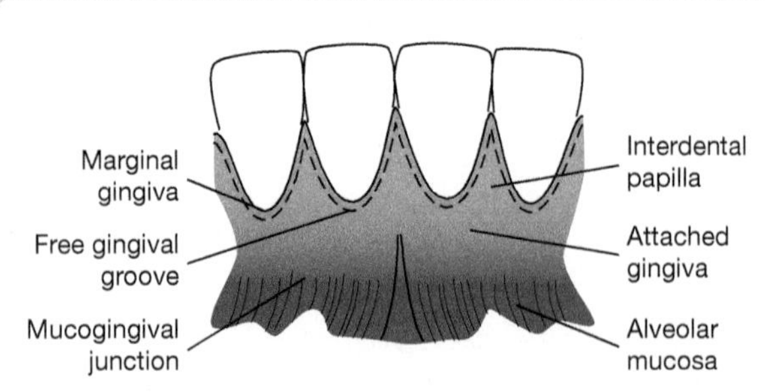

Fig. 23.15 Soft Tissue Cross sectional view of the soft tissues surrounding the teeth. *In a healthy mouth, how large is the space between the free gingiva and the tooth?*

Gingiva is the soft tissue that surrounds the neck of the tooth, fills the interproximal spaces, and covers the underlying alveolar bone. **Figure 23.15** shows the soft tissues surrounding the teeth. The free gingiva immediately surrounds the neck of the tooth and is not actually attached to the tooth or underlying bone. The space between the free gingiva and the tooth is known as the gingival sulcus. In a healthy mouth, this space is no deeper than three millimeters (mm).

Measuring the depth of the gingival sulcus is one of the most accurate methods available to determine a person's periodontal health. The attached gingiva, which is firmly bound to the underlying bone, extends apically from the base of the free gingiva. This means the gingiva extends toward the root of the tooth.

The attached gingiva then merges with the alveolar mucosa, which covers the remaining alveolar bone, the interior of the cheek, and the floor of the mouth. The interdental papilla is the V-shaped gingiva that lies between teeth and fills the interproximal space.

Healthy gingiva is pink and firm to the touch. There are sharp margins at the gingival edge. The texture of healthy gingiva is stippled like an orange peel. Gingiva is darker in color in people who have greater skin pigmentation.

Types of Teeth

The main job of the teeth is to cut, chew, and grind food. This process, which is the first stage in digestion, is known as mastication.

In the permanent dentition, teeth are classified according to their form and function into four types.

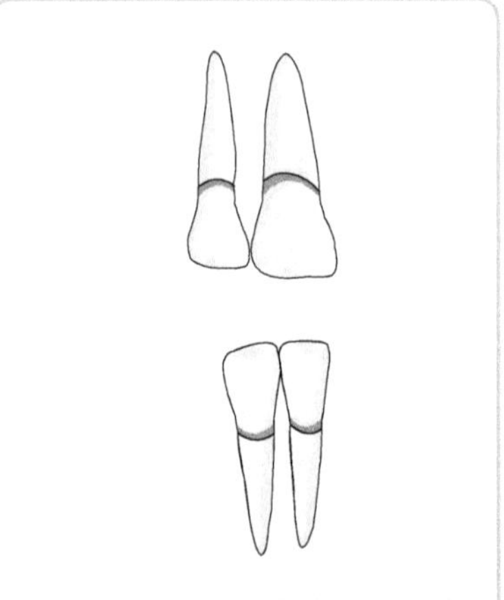

Fig. 23.16 Incisors Facial view of maxillary and mandibular right central incisor and lateral incisor. *What purpose do the incisors serve?*

- Incisors (central incisors and lateral incisors) have a relatively sharp edge used to cut, or "incise," food. **Figure 23.16** shows the incisors. Incisors have one root. The maxillary incisors are larger than the mandibular incisors. The mandibular central incisor is the smallest tooth in the mouth.
- Canines, also known as cuspids, have one pointed cusp used for holding and tearing food. **Figure 23.17** shows the canines. Canines generally have one root. The maxillary cuspid is the longest tooth in the mouth.
- Premolars, also known as bicuspids, generally have two cusps: one on the buccal surface, and one on the lingual surface. They have a broad occlusal surface that is used for chewing food. **Figure 23.18** shows the premolars. Premolars have one root except for the maxillary first premolar, which has two roots—one buccal and one lingual.

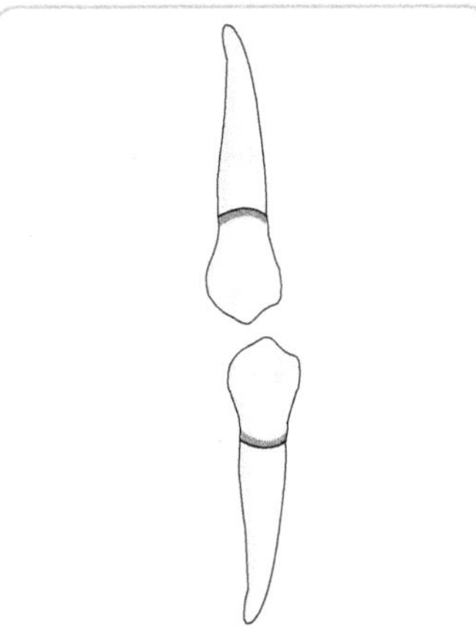

Fig. 23.17 Canines Facial view of maxillary and mandibular right canines (cuspids) *What is the function of the canine teeth?*

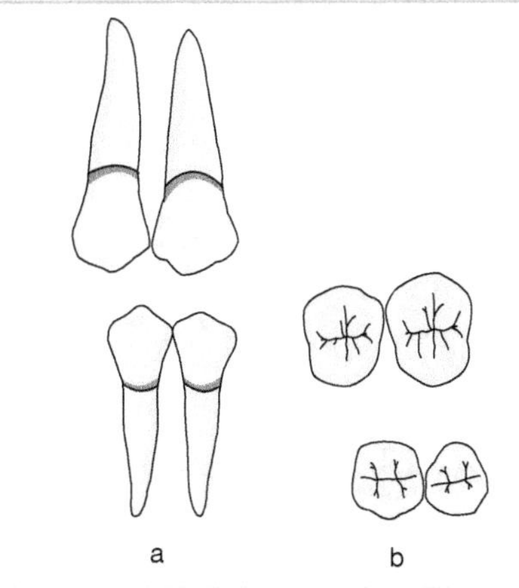

Fig. 23.18 Premolars (a) Facial views of maxillary and mandibular premolars. (b) Occlusal views of maxillary and mandibular premolars. *What is the function of the premolars?*

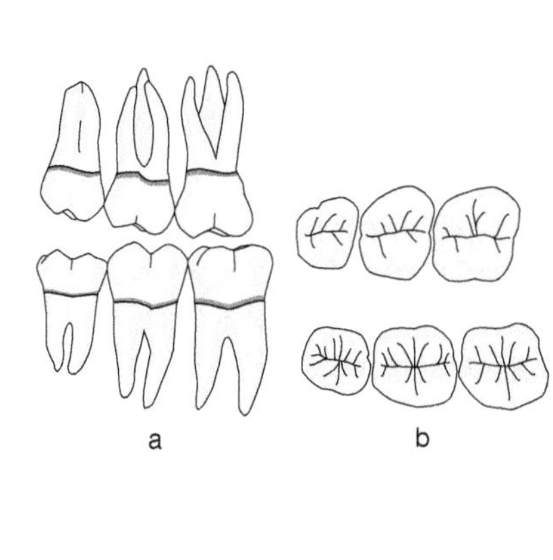

Fig. 23.19 Molars (a) Facial view of maxillary and mandibular right molars. (b) Occlusal view of maxillary and mandibular right molars. *What purpose do the molars serve?*

- Molars generally have four cusps and a very broad occlusal surface used for chewing, crushing, and grinding food. **Figure 23.19** shows the molars. Molars have four functional cusps, except for the mandibular first molar, which has five cusps. Maxillary molars have three roots: the mesiobuccal, distobuccal, and lingual.
- Mandibular molars have two roots: the mesial and distal. The third molars, or wisdom teeth, are often the smallest of the molars. They may have fused roots and resemble either the first or the second molar in the same arch.

READING CHECK

Recall when the mixed dentition period occurs.

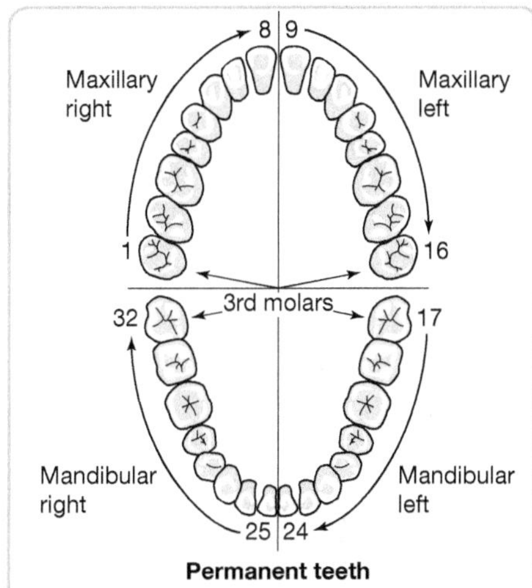

Fig. 23.20 Numbering Permanent Teeth Universal numbering system—permanent dentition. *Why is it necessary to have tooth numbering systems?*

Tooth Numbering Systems

Do you know how to identify each of your teeth?

Tooth numbering systems are used to identify and communicate information about specific teeth. Two such systems are the Universal System and the Palmer System.

The Universal System

The universal system is approved by the American Dental Association. It is the most commonly used system in the United States. Every permanent tooth is given a number from 1 to 32. Numbering proceeds, as shown in **Figure 23.20,** beginning with the maxillary right third molar.

The universal system uses the letters A to T to identify individual primary teeth. This is shown in **Figure 23.21.**

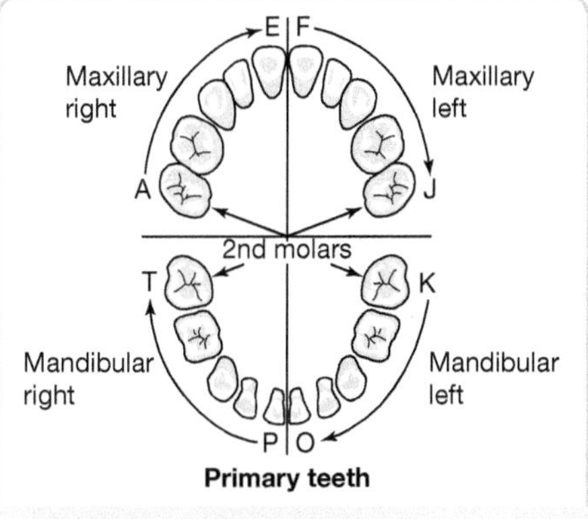

Fig. 23.21 Numbering Primary Teeth Universal numbering system—primary dentition. *How are the deciduous teeth identified in the universal numbering system?*

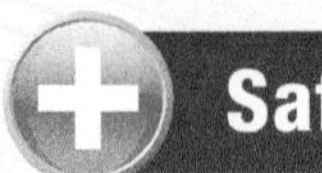

Safety

Barriers

All tubing in a dental office may be covered with plastic barriers to reduce the amount of chemical disinfection required after each patient. The barriers can simply be removed and replaced after use. Barriers are also used to cover the headrest of the dental chair, light handles, and any switches handled during treatment procedures.

The Palmer System

The Palmer System is used mostly in orthodontic and pediatric practices. In this system, permanent teeth are numbered from 1 to 8 in each quadrant beginning at the midline, with the central incisor numbered 1, and ending at the third molar, which is 8. A right-angle symbol is used with the number to identify the quadrant, and the tooth number is written in the angle. The quadrants are identified as follows.

- Mandibular right quadrant #|
- Mandibular left quadrant |#
- Maxillary left quadrant |#
- Maxillary right quadrant #|

The tooth number is written in the angle. For example, the maxillary left permanent canine is |3.

In the Palmer system, the primary teeth are lettered from A to E in each quadrant, beginning at the midline, with A as the primary central incisor and ending with E as the primary second molar. Once again, the right-angle symbol must be added to identify the quadrant. For example, the mandibular left lateral incisor is designated as |B.

READING CHECK

Identify the tooth numbering system that is most commonly used in the United States.

The Dental Treatment Area

How is a dentist's office furnished?

Most dental offices have a number of rooms in which dental treatment is provided. Each room is equipped with a dental chair, a dental assistant's chair, an operator's chair, a dental unit, an operating light, fixed and mobile cabinets, a sink, and an X-ray unit. **Figure 23.22** shows a dental treatment room.

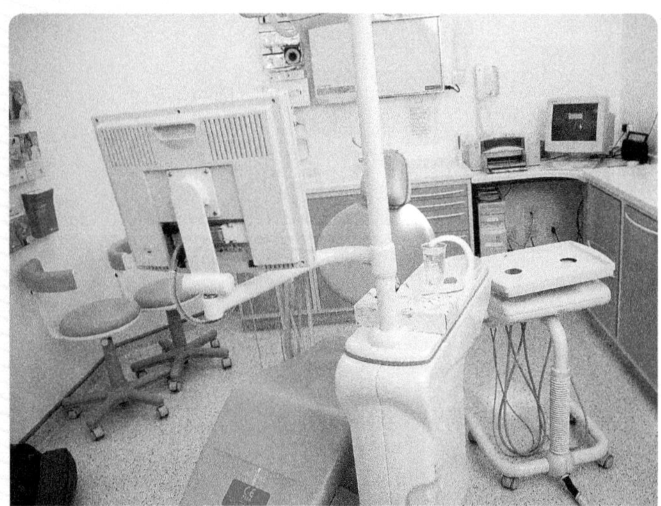

Fig. 23.22 Dental Treatment Room Note that the dental chair is in an upright position. *How can the position of the dental chair be adjusted?*

Photo: Michael Donne/Photo Researchers, Inc.

The dental chair is a contour chair that supports the patient's head, neck, and back in a number of positions. During most dental procedures, the patient is in the supine position, on his or her back, with the head and knees at the same level. Control buttons to adjust the back position and height of the chair may be located on either side of the backrest, on a keypad on the dental unit, or on a foot switch unit on the floor. The keypad and the foot switch are becoming more popular, because they reduce or eliminate the possibility of contamination and the need for post-treatment disinfection.

Dental units may be wall-mounted, mounted on the base of the dental chair, or placed on mobile cabinets. The dental unit (see **Figure 23.23**) is supplied with electricity, water, compressed air, and suction. The unit contains

- An on-off switch for the electricity, water, and compressed air.
- Handpiece tubing to carry the compressed air that powers the slow- and high-speed dental handpiece. This tubing also carries water for the high-speed handpiece.
- A rheostat, a foot control that regulates the speed of the handpiece.
- An air-water syringe with buttons that control the supply of air and water, or combination spray. Syringe tips are removed after use with each patient. They are sterilized in an autoclave or disposed of if they are plastic.
- Suction tubing for the oral evacuator (high-volume evacuator, aspirator, or suction device), which provides high-volume suction to quickly remove saliva, blood, and any debris from the oral cavity. These fluids pass through a disposable plastic trap that filters out any debris. Then the fluids are carried to the wastewater system. The oral evacuator is manipulated and held in place by the dental assistant. Oral evacuator tips are removed after use and sterilized or disposed of if they are plastic. The collection trap is checked at the end of the day. If debris is present, it must be either emptied or discarded and replaced. A sanitizing solution is sucked through all the suction tubing at the end of each day.
- Suction tubing for the saliva ejector, which provides lower-level suction. Saliva ejector tips are removed and discarded after use. The small filter trap in this tubing must be checked at the end of the day. If debris is present, it must be emptied or discarded and replaced.

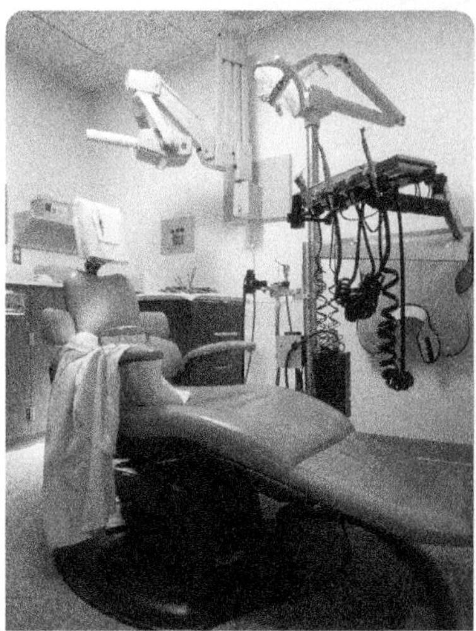

Fig. 23.23 Dental Unit The operator's portion of the unit is mounted on the chair base. *Why are plastic barriers used to cover parts of the dental chair and other equipment?*

READING CHECK

List the components of a dental unit.

Other important features of the dental treatment room are:

- An operating light, used to illuminate the oral cavity. This light is on a movable arm that is mounted to the ceiling or to the base of the chair. Since the light gets very hot during use, disinfectant solutions should not be sprayed on the light unless it is cool. Between patients, it is enough to replace the light handle barriers and light switch barriers. The light can be cleaned thoroughly at the end of the day when it is cool.
- The operator's and assistant's chairs, which are designed to provide support and comfort during long procedures. Both are height-adjustable. The operator's stool has a backrest that provides lumbar support. The assistant's stool, shown in **Figure 23.24,** has an arm in the front that provides support when the assistant leans forward. The assistant needs to be at a higher level than the dentist. Thus, the assistant's stool is equipped with an adjustable foot platform to position the assistant's legs properly and prevent back strain.

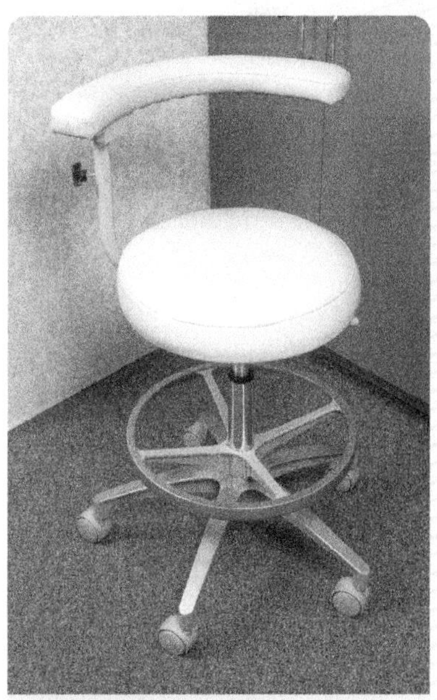

Fig. 23.24 Assistant's Stool Special seats are used for the tasks the dental care workers perform. *What is the purpose of the bar attached to the top of this stool?*

Photos: (t)Will & Deni McIntyre/Photo Researchers, (b)Aaron Haupt Photography

The dental treatment room is equipped with fixed and mobile cabinets. Often the dental assistant uses a mobile cart with a movable top. The instrument tray is placed on this during procedures. This arrangement keeps instruments and materials within easy reach.

A dental office also has a central air compressor and a central vacuum unit. They are often located in a supply room or basement but have an on-off switch in a more accessible location. If this equipment is not working correctly, the following should be checked:

- The manufacturer's care instructions.
- The connection, to be sure the equipment is properly plugged in and turned on.
- The fuse box and air compressor.

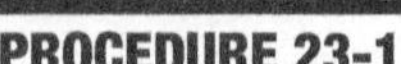

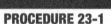

ONLINE PROCEDURES

PROCEDURE 23-1
Demonstrating the Bass Toothbrushing Technique

To prevent dental disease, plaque must be removed at least once every 24 hours. It is preferable to brush after each meal. It is especially important to remove plaque before bedtime. Brushing removes plaque from the facial, lingual, and occlusal surfaces of the teeth.

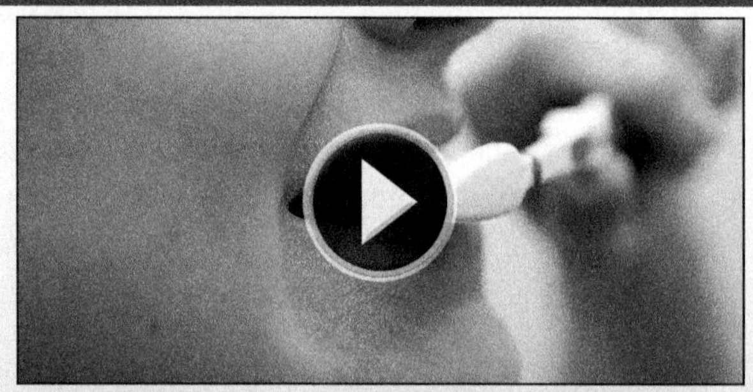

PROCEDURE 23-2
Demonstrating Correct Flossing Technique

Flossing should be done at least once a day. Flossing removes plaque from between the teeth on mesial and distal surfaces. Wrap the length of the floss around the middle finger, leaving two to three inches of working space between the fingers. You will also need to curve the floss tightly around the proximal side of one tooth while flossing.

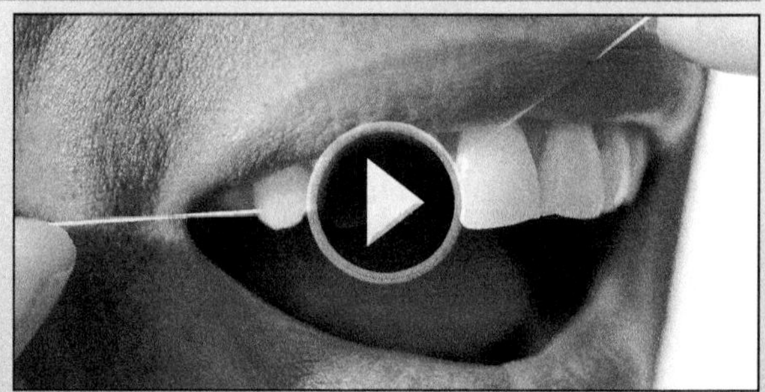

PROCEDURE 23-3
Preparing and Maintaining the Dental Treatment Area

Most dental offices have a number of rooms where dental treatment is provided. Each room is equipped with a dental chair, a dental assistant's chair, an operator's chair, a dental unit, an operating light, fixed and mobile cabinets, a sink, and an X-ray unit. These treatment areas must be maintained.

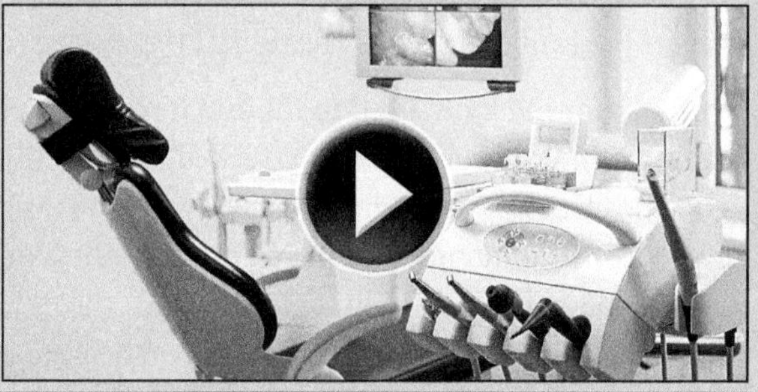

PROCEDURE 23-4
Positioning the Client and the Dental Assistant

One of the basic duties of the dental assistant is to position the client in the dental chair. Proper positioning is necessary to maintain client comfort and provide efficient dental treatment. The client is usually placed in a supine position and at a height at which both the dentist and dental assistant can easily view the oral cavity.

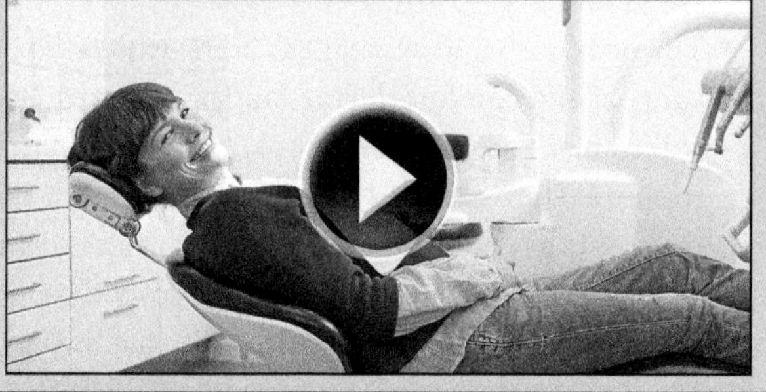

Photos: (t to b)Ingram Publishing/SuperStock, image100/Getty Images, Image Source/Getty Images, Hengleir and Steets/Cultura/Getty Images

Stress and the Dental Patient

Have you ever been afraid to go to the dentist?

Having dental work done is stressful for many people. Follow the steps below to build a trusting relationship with a patient.

- Wear a name tag, introduce yourself, and smile.
- Listen to the patient. Look at the patient as you are listening so that you will also "hear" the patient's nonverbal messages.
- Take an interest in the patient. Use the patient's name frequently in conversation. Try to remember information about the patient's family, hobbies, and special events in his or her life.
- Patiently explain procedures to the patient. Place the patient in an upright position to improve communication.
- Respect individual differences. Treat each patient with respect.
- Always maintain patient privacy and confidentiality.

READING CHECK

Recall some ways in which a dental professional can establish a patient's trust in the dental team.

Dental Instruments and Tray Setups

Which instruments are used in common dental procedures?

Here you will learn about some of the most common dental instruments used in general dentistry. Instruments vary based on the preferences of the individual dentist or hygienist. Dental instruments may be classified as either hand instruments or rotary instruments, which are mechanically driven.

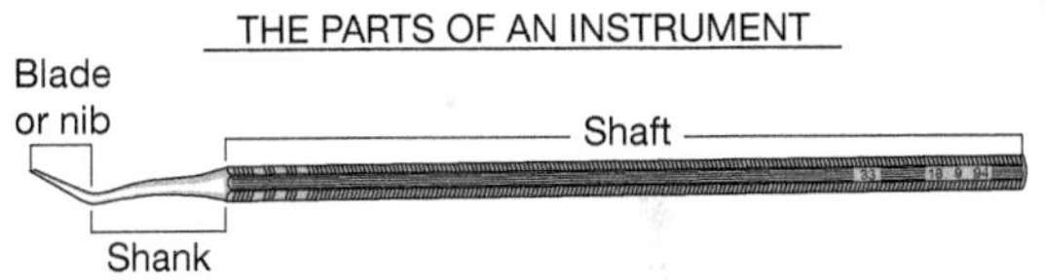

THE PARTS OF AN INSTRUMENT

Blade or nib

Shaft

Shank

Fig. 23.25 Hand Instrument Three parts of a hand instrument. *Why is the shank often angled?*

Hand Instruments

Most hand instruments are made of a stainless steel alloy. Some are composed of a plastic resin material. A hand instrument has three parts (see **Figure 23.25**).

- Handle or shaft: This is the part held by the operator. It may be round or hexagonal.
- Blade or nib: This is the working end. It may have a cutting edge or a blunt surface. It may be single- or double-ended.
- Shank: This connects the handle to the working end. It is often angled to allow better accessibility to all areas of the oral cavity.

The hand instruments described below are included in the basic tray setup that is used for an examination procedure. The basic setup also forms the basis of more complex tray setups.

Table 23.2 Common Hand Instruments

INSTRUMENT	DESCRIPTION/USE
mouth mirror	The **mouth mirror** is used to view tissues of the oral cavity and reflect light for better visibility.
cotton pliers	**Cotton pliers** are used to place small objects in, and remove them from, the oral cavity.
explorer	The **explorer** is used to examine, by touch, tooth surfaces for caries, calculus, or defects.
periodontal probe	The **periodontal probe** is used to measure the depth of the gingival sulcus.
saliva ejector tip	The **saliva ejector tip** is used to remove saliva and maintain a dry working field with low-volume evacuation.
oral evacuator tip	The **oral evacuator tip** is used to maintain a dry working field by removing saliva, blood, and debris with high-volume evacuation.
aspirating anesthetic syringe	The **aspirating anesthetic syringe** is used to deliver local anesthesia to an intraoral site. Anesthesia is a loss of sensation. Local anesthesia means that only a particular site loses sensation.

Restorative Instruments Restorative instruments are included in the composite resin tray setup and the **amalgam** tray setup. Composite resin and amalgam (a mixture of silver alloy and mercury) are common materials used for a dental restoration. These are discussed later in this chapter. During dental restoration, decay is removed and a filling material is placed and shaped.

Cavity Preparation Instruments These instruments may be used in addition to the high speed handpiece for removing decay and shaping the enamel and dentin to hold a restoration.

Table 23.3 Common Cavity Preparation Instruments

INSTRUMENT	DESCRIPTION/USE
spoon excavator	The spoon excavator is used to remove soft decay and other materials from the tooth.
straight, (a) binangle (b) and Wedelstaedt (c) chisels a b c	Straight, binangle and Wedelstaedt chisels are used to remove decay and refine the **cavity** preparation.
enamel hatchet	The enamel hatchet is used to remove decay and refine the cavity preparation.
gingival margin trimmer	The gingival margin trimmer is used to remove decay and refine the cavity preparation. It is similar to the enamel hatchet but has a curved blade.

Amalgam Instruments. The following instruments are used in the amalgam tray setup.

Table 23.4 Common Amalgam Instruments

INSTRUMENT	DESCRIPTION/USE
amalgam carrier	The amalgam carrier is used to carry and place amalgam in the cavity preparation.
amalgam condenser	The amalgam condenser is used to compact amalgam in the cavity preparation.
amalgam carvers a b	The amalgam carver is used to remove excess material and carve anatomy in amalgam. Discoid-cleoid (a) and Hollenback (b) carvers are commonly used.
burnisher	The burnisher is used to smooth and shape amalgam.
matrix band and retainer	The matrix band and retainer are used to hold and shape the restoration material when a mesial or distal surface is missing.

Composite Instruments The following instruments are included in the composite tray setup.

- The composite placement instrument is used to place composite restorative material in a cavity preparation. It is essentially a plastic instrument coated with Teflon®.
- The matrix strip is a plastic strip used during placement of a composite material to hold and shape the material when a mesial or distal surface is missing.

Other Instruments Other commonly-used hand instruments are the following.

Table 23.5 Other Instruments

INSTRUMENT	DESCRIPTION/USE
scaler	The scaler is used to remove **supragingival calculus** and cement.
plastic instruments	Plastic instruments are used to place moldable ("plastic") restorative materials and cements in the cavity preparation.
cement spatula	The cement spatula is used to mix dental cements on a glass slab or mixing pad.
alginate spatula	The alginate spatula is used to mix alginate impression material in a flexible bowl.
impression paste spatula	The impression paste spatula is used to mix elastomeric impression materials.
impression material syringe	The impression material syringe is used to carry elastomeric impression materials to the mouth and to eject the material around the prepared tooth.

Surgical Instruments There are numerous surgical instruments. The following are instruments used for simple extraction procedures.

Table 23.6 Surgical Instruments

INSTRUMENT	DESCRIPTION/USE
periosteal elevator	The periosteal elevator is used to detach tissue from bone following an incision or to detach the gingival tissues prior to the placement of the extraction forceps.
root elevator	The root elevator is used to loosen a tooth or root from a bony socket prior to the placement of the extraction forceps.
surgical curette	The surgical curette is used to remove tissue or debris from bony sockets.
scalpel and scalpel blade	The scalpel is a surgical knife used to cut soft tissue.
hemostat	The hemostat is used to hold small items securely or to remove small pieces of tooth or bone.
extraction forceps	Extraction forceps are used to remove a tooth from its socket.
surgical tissue scissors	The surgical tissue scissors are used to trim soft tissue and cut sutures.

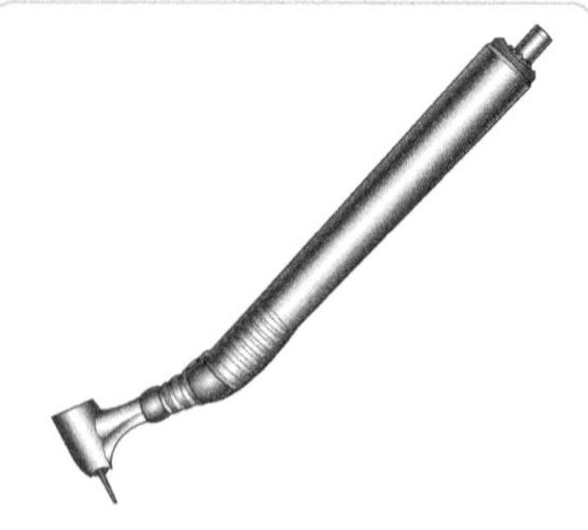

Fig. 23.26 Dental Handpiece
High speed handpiece. *Why is a water coolant necessary when using a high speed handpiece?*

High-Speed Dental Handpieces and Rotary Instruments

Handpieces are mechanical instruments. They can be powered by compressed air or by electricity. A foot pedal or rheostat controls the speed of the handpiece. Dentists have available for use both high-speed and low-speed handpieces, chosen depending on the type of procedure.

A high-speed handpiece (see **Figure 23.26**), the instrument colloqially known to patients as the dental drill, is used to remove decay and shape the tooth to accept a filling material or a crown. Some models have top speeds of up to 500,000 rpm. This handpiece has its own water line. Water is needed to help cool the tooth during the use of the high-speed handpiece; this is needed because friction creates heat when a tooth structure is cut at high speeds.

The low-speed handpiece, also known as the straight handpiece, is used to polish teeth and restorations, make the final refinement to a cavity preparation, and adjust appliances. A contra-angle attachment and a right-angle attachment are used with the straight handpiece, to provide better accessibility to all areas of the oral cavity. **Figure 23.27** shows the straight handpiece, along with two high-speed handpieces.

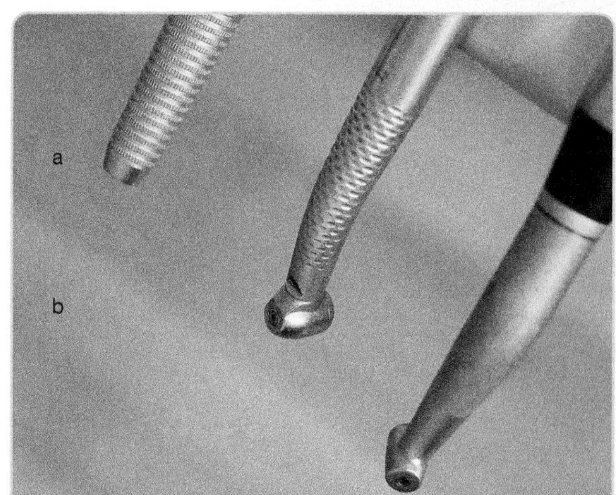

Fig. 23.27 Handpieces The low-speed handpiece is also known as a straight handpiece. (a) Straight handpiece (b) high-speed handpiece *When is the straight handpiece used?*

Burs and diamonds (shown in **Figure 23.28**) are used with the handpieces. They are the instruments that shape teeth, smooth restorations, and adjust appliances. Diamonds are used to remove large amounts of tooth structure, which is necessary when a tooth is being prepared for a crown. Burs are used to remove decay and prepare a cavity for the filling material, to smooth restorations, and to adjust appliances.

Burs have three parts: the head, the neck, and the shank. The head is the working end, the neck connects the head to the shank, and the shank is designed to fit into the handpiece. Different shanks are required for different handpieces. **Figure 23.29** shows the parts of a bur and different bur shank types. Shank types are

- Straight or handpiece shank, used in straight handpieces
- Latch-type shank, used in contra-angle attachments
- Friction-grip shank, used in high-speed handpieces

Rotary instruments with a screw-type base are used with the right-angle attachment. Common rotary instruments are the prophylaxis cup and brush (**Figure 23.30**). In this case, prophylaxis refers to the removal of plaque (microorganisms) and stain from tooth surfaces.

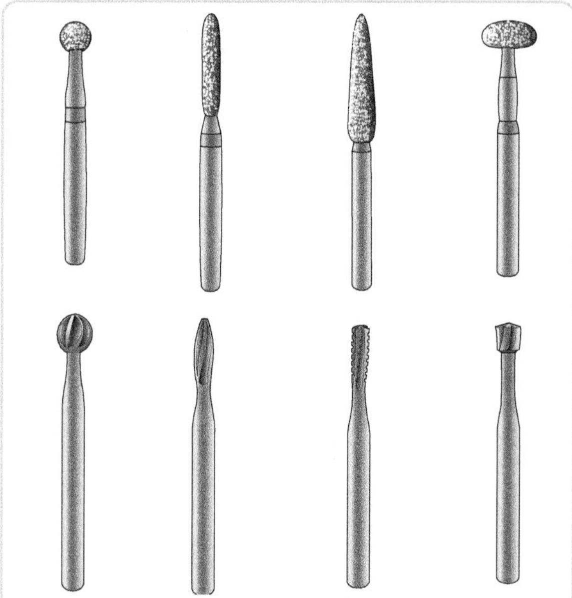

Fig. 23.28 Burs and Diamonds Burs and diamonds are the attachments that are used with the handpieces. *When would diamonds be used instead of burs?*

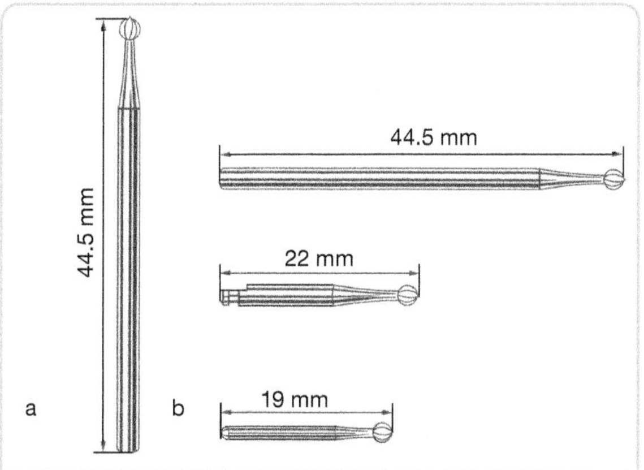

Fig. 23.29 Bur Parts (a) Parts of a bur. (b) Bur shank types. *What is the purpose of having different types of shanks?*

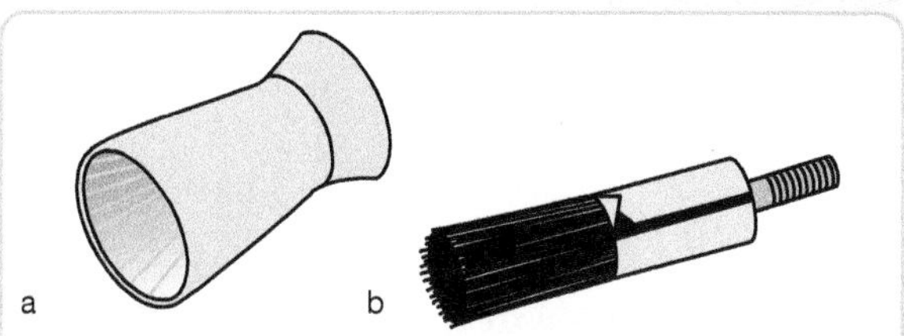

Fig. 23.30 Prophylaxis Instruments (a) Prophy cup. (b) Prophy brush with screw type base for use with the right angle handpiece attachment. *What does the term "prophy" mean?*

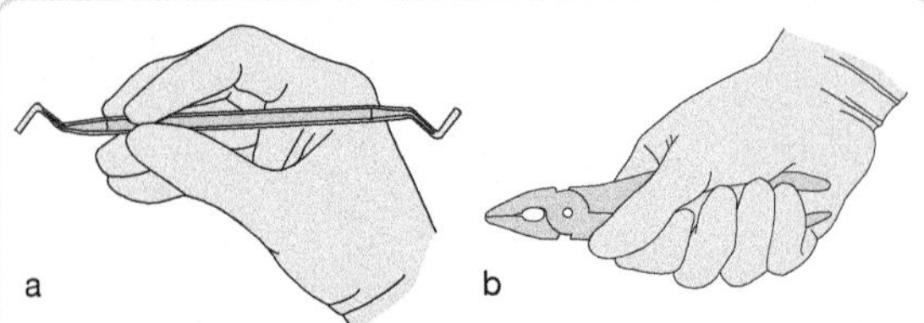

Fig. 23.31 Grasping Holds (a) The operator using a pen grasp. (b) The operator using a palm grasp. *For what procedure would you use a palm grasp?*

Instrument Transfer and Oral Evacuation

"Four-handed dentistry" is the term used to describe the method of dental care when the dentist and dental assistant are both seated at chairside and working as a coordinated team. By employing a trained dental assistant, the dentist is able to remain focused on the treatment area, reduce movements of the eyes and hands, and increase productivity. The dental assistant prepares materials and instruments, transfers them to the dentist, and maintains a clear working area with effective oral evacuation and tissue retraction.

Instrument Grasps The way an instrument is held depends on how the instrument will be used and the design of the instrument. The pen grasp and the palm grasp, shown in **Figure 23.31**, are the two most often used instrument grasps.

The pen grasp is used with most instruments. As the name indicates, the instrument is held as if you were holding a pen or pencil.

The palm grasp is used with instruments that have two handles, such as the extraction forceps. The handles fit in the palm of the hand with the working end pointing toward the operator's fingers.

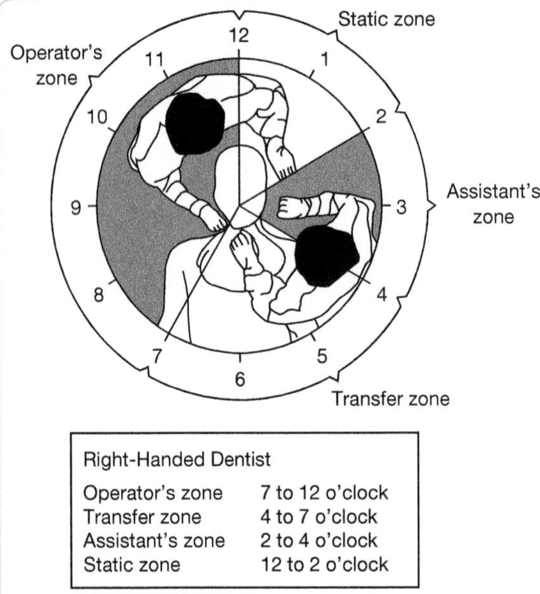

Right-Handed Dentist	
Operator's zone	7 to 12 o'clock
Transfer zone	4 to 7 o'clock
Assistant's zone	2 to 4 o'clock
Static zone	12 to 2 o'clock

Fig. 23.32 Clock Concept Working positions using the clock concept. *What is necessary for an efficient instrument transfer?*

Instrument Transfer Instrument transfer occurs in the transfer zone, which is over the patient's chest in the "4 to 7 o'clock" area. The "clock" concept is shown in **Figure 23.32**. For efficient instrument transfer, the assistant must be able to anticipate the next instrument needed and have it already in the transfer zone when the dentist wants it. The assistant brings the instrument to the dentist so that the dentist does not have to reach for the instrument.

The dentist signals for the next instrument by moving the current instrument away from the tooth being treated and toward the transfer zone. **Figure 23.33** shows how the signal for the next instrument is given.

When transferring pen grasp instruments, the assistant

- uses the left hand to transfer when working with a right-handed dentist.
- picks up the instrument from the dental tray between the thumb and index and middle fingers.
- grasps the instrument at the end farthest away from the working end.
- holds the instrument parallel to the instrument the dentist is currently using.

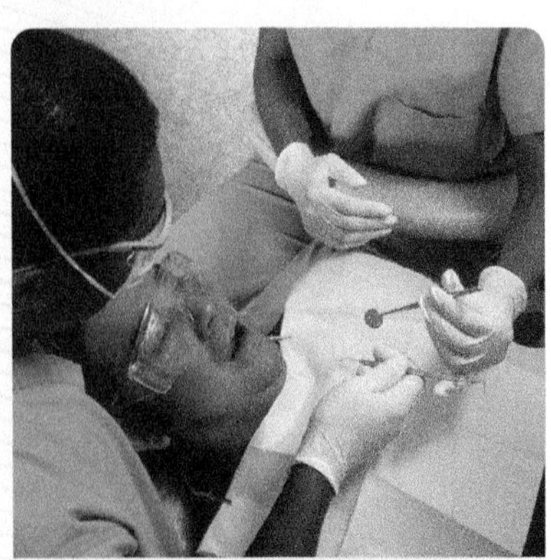

Fig. 23.33 Instrument Transfer The dentist signals an instrument transfer. The assistant retrieves the used instrument and transfers the next one. *How does the dentist signal for the next instrument?*

Photo: Aaron Haupt Photography

- Directs the working end toward the arch being treated.
- Picks up the used instrument from the dentist's grasp, using the little finger.
- Places the next instrument firmly in the dentist's hand.
- Returns the used instrument to its original position on the dental tray. At a glance, most instruments look very similar. If instruments are out of position on the tray, it is very difficult to locate a needed instrument quickly.

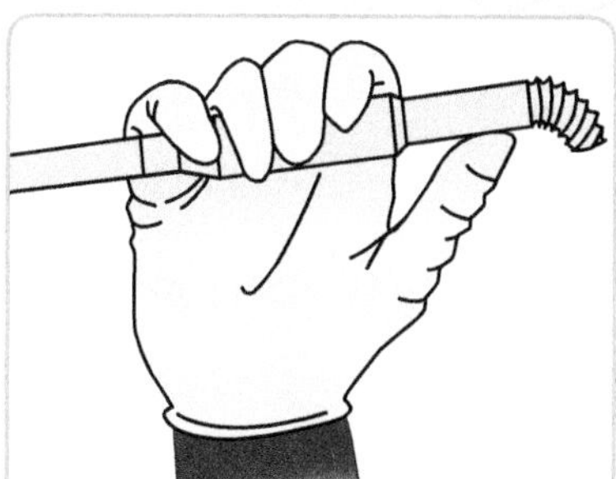

Fig. 23.34 Oral Evacuator Holding the oral evacuator in a thumb-to-nose grasp. *What is the advantage of using an oral evacuator?*

Oral Evacuation Effective use of the oral evacuator removes fluids and retracts tissue during treatment procedures. This improves visibility and accessibility of the treatment area. It also reduces the amount of airborne microbes, prevents swallowing of debris by the patient, and ensures that dental materials will not be adversely affected by moisture. In general, the oral evacuator is

- held in the right hand using a thumb-to-nose grasp (see **Figure 23.34**).
- placed slightly posterior to the tooth under treatment.
- placed parallel (the tip opening) to the facial or lingual surface.
- rotated slightly toward and beyond the incisal or occlusal surface.
- placed before the dentist positions the handpiece.
- for posterior teeth, placed on the surface closest to the assistant. For example, if the dentist is preparing a tooth in the patient's maxillary or mandibular right posterior area, the assistant places the tip on the lingual surface. If the dentist is preparing a tooth in the patient's maxillary or mandibular left posterior area, the assistant places the tip on the facial surface (See **Figure 23.35**).
- for anterior teeth, placed on the surface opposite the tooth surface being treated. For example, if the dentist is preparing the lingual surface, the assistant places the tip on the facial surface. If the dentist is preparing the facial surface, the tip is placed on the lingual surface (see **Figure 23.36**).

The assistant must never place the evacuator tip on the soft palate, the center of the back of the tongue, or the soft tissue on the floor of the mouth.

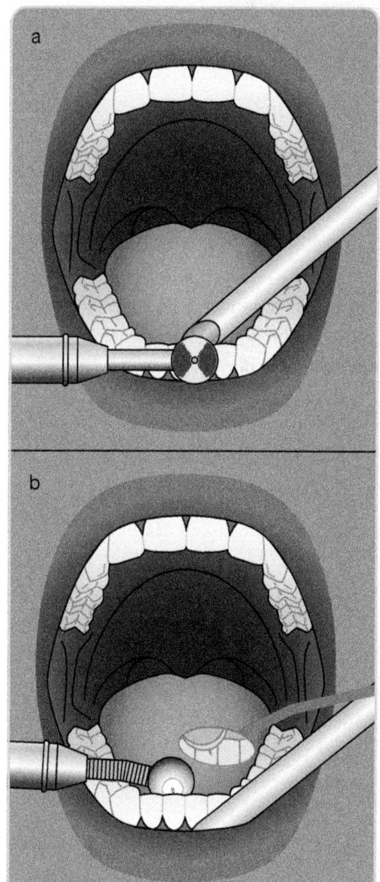

Fig. 23.36 Placement of the Oral Evacuator Tip in the Anterior Area (a) Placed on the lingual if the dentist is working on the facial (b) Placed on the facial if the dentist is working on the lingual. *Which teeth are in the anterior area?*

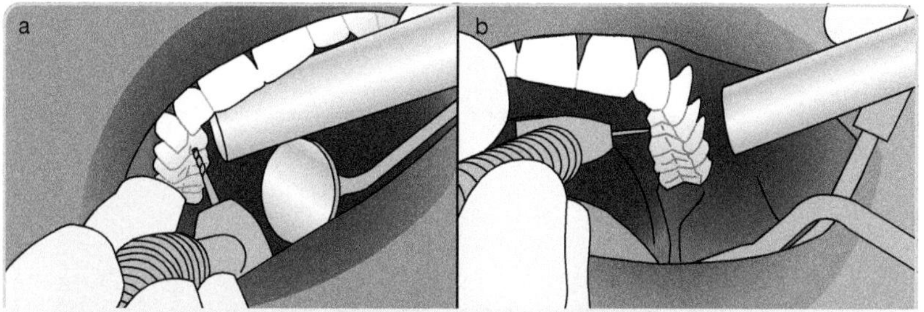

Fig. 23.35 Placement of the Oral Evacuator in the Posterior Area (a) When the dentist is treating the patient's right side, the assistant places the oral evacuator on the lingual. (b) When the dentist is treating the patient's left side, the assistant places the oral evacuator on the facial. *Which teeth are in the posterior area?*

If the dentist is using a mouth mirror to view the treatment area, the mirror must be kept clear of moisture and debris. This is accomplished by holding the air-water syringe at the edge of the mirror and blowing air across the surface.

READING CHECK

Describe the purpose of a high-speed and a low-speed handpiece.

Dental Anesthesia

When would a dentist use topical anesthesia rather than local anesthesia?

"Anesthesia" means the loss of feeling or sensation. Local anesthesia is loss of feeling in a small area. Topical anesthesia is loss of sensation

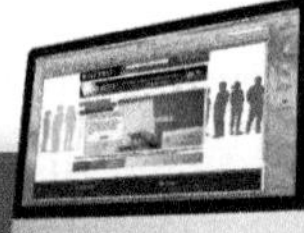

connect ONLINE PROCEDURES

PROCEDURE 23-5

Dental Tray Setups

One of the primary duties of the dental assistant is to assemble the instruments and materials for a given procedure. Instruments and materials are arranged on the dental tray from left to right in their order of use. Consumable supplies and materials such as cotton rolls, saliva ejector tips, and restorative materials can be placed with the sterilized instruments on plastic or metal trays of various designs for transport and use in the treatment room.

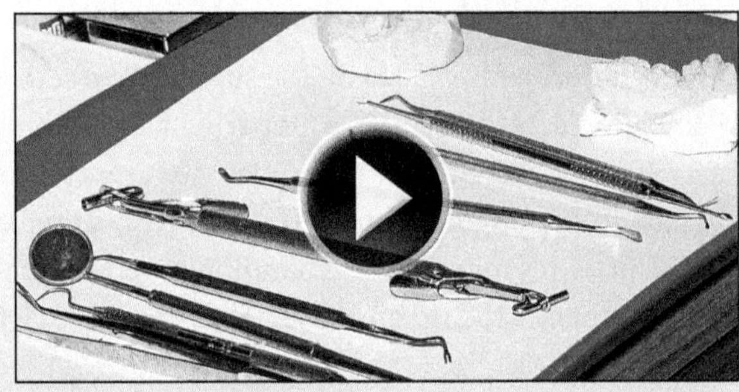

PROCEDURE 23-6

One Handed Instrument Transfer

The dental assistant prepares materials and instruments, transfers them to the dentist, and maintains a clear working area with effective oral evacuation and tissue retraction. For efficient instrument transfer, the assistant must be able to anticipate the next instrument needed and have it in the transfer zone when the dentist wants it. The assistant brings the instrument to the dentist so that the dentist does not have to reach for the instrument.

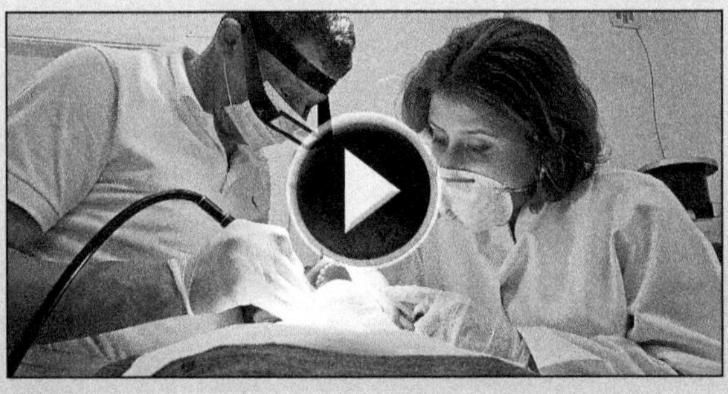

PROCEDURE 23-7

Using the Oral Evacuator

Effective use of the oral evacuator removes fluids and retracts tissue during treatment procedures. This improves the visibility and accessibility of the treatment area. It reduces the amount of airborne microbes, prevents the swallowing of debris by the patient, and ensures that dental materials will not be adversely affected by moisture.

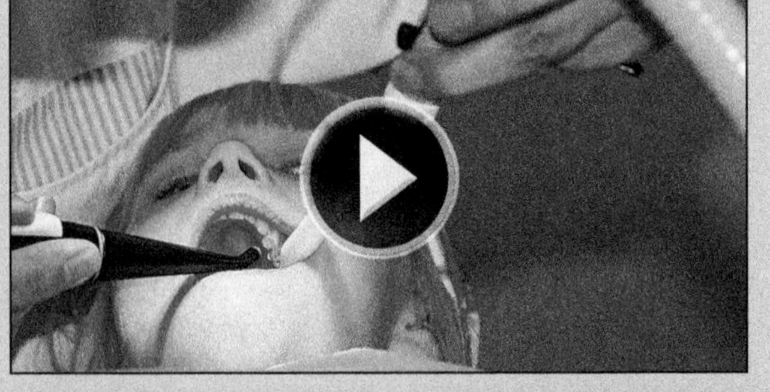

Photos: (t)C. Sherburne/PhotoLink/Getty Images, (c)B. O'Kane/Alamy, (b)Johann Helgason/Alamy

on the surface of soft tissues. Both types of anesthesia are commonly used in dentistry to achieve a pain-free experience for the patient.

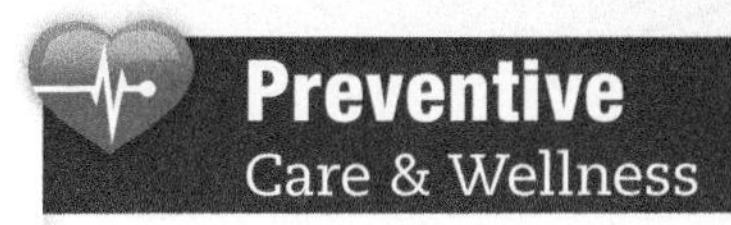

Maintain Your Teeth and Gums

Healthy teeth and gums are essential to good health. In addition to brushing at least twice a day and flossing once a day, there are other ways to maintain dental health.

- Appliances such as water irrigation or other devices can supplement, but not replace, brushing and flossing.
- Fluoride or anti-plaque toothpastes or mouth rinses may be recommended.
- Regular tooth cleaning is important to remove plaque and calculus that may develop even with brushing and flossing.
- Most dentists recommend routine examination of the teeth every year, which may include dental X-rays.

Local Anesthesia

Local anesthesia is administered by injecting an anesthetic agent near the nerves that supply the area to be treated. This blocks the conduction of nervous impulses to the central nervous system and makes the area supplied by that nerve insensitive to pain.

Many such agents are available. The dentist selects the agent based on the medical history of the patient and the duration of anesthesia required. Anesthetic agents may be short, intermediate, or long-acting. A vasoconstrictor is often added to local anesthetics to decrease bleeding during surgical procedures and to prolong the duration of the anesthesia. Vasoconstrictors, or agents that cause constriction or the narrowing of blood vessels, can interact with some medications that the patient may be taking. They also may increase heart rate and blood pressure. Before preparing the local anesthetic syringe, make sure that the patient's medical history is updated. Check with the dentist for the type of local anesthetic to use.

Local anesthetic is supplied in glass cartridges, or carpules. The cartridges have a rubber stopper at one end and an aluminum cap at the other. Never use a cartridge that is cracked or damaged, contains discolored or cloudy solution, or has an expired "Use by" date or a loose rubber stopper.

The disposable injection needle is available in two lengths, 1 inch and $1\frac{5}{8}$ inch. The 1-inch length is generally used for maxillary injections, and the $1\frac{5}{8}$-inch length for mandibular injections.

Topical Anesthesia

Topical anesthesia is applied to the surface tissue of the injection site, to minimize the discomfort caused by the insertion of the anesthesia needle. Topical anesthesia is available as an ointment, liquid, or spray.

READING CHECK

Explain how a dentist chooses a local anesthesia agent.

Materials for Impressions, Models, and Restoration

What material is used for making the most precise impression?

Dental models are positive reproductions or three-dimensional duplicates of a patient's teeth and surrounding tissues (see **Figure 23.37** on page 586). Dentists use models to record information for study and

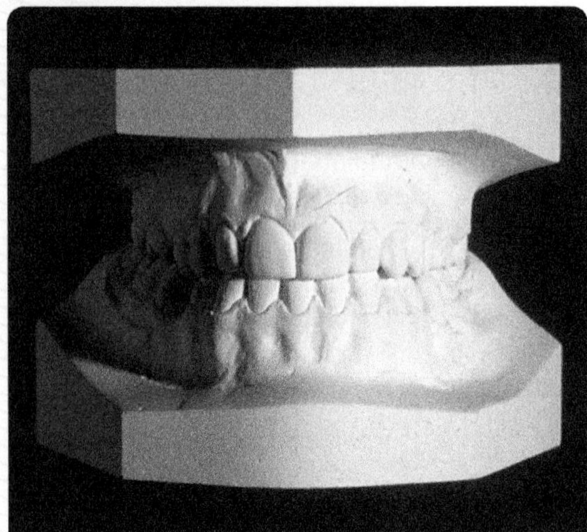

Fig. 23.37 Dental Model Dental models are positive reproductions or three-dimensional duplicates of a patient's teeth and surrounding tissues. *Why are models used?*

diagnosis in orthodontic and prosthodontic cases. The dental lab technician uses models as he or she makes crowns, dentures, retainers, night guards, bleaching trays, and other appliances. The first step in making a model is to make an **impression,** or negative reproduction, of the patient's teeth and surrounding tissues. Then a positive model is made using the negative impression as a mold.

Impression Materials

The two classifications of the most commonly used impression materials are

- An irreversible hydrocolloid commonly known as alginate
- Elastomeric materials, which include vinylpolysiloxane (VPS), polysulfide (rubber-base), polyether, and silicone

Impression materials are chosen on the basis of how the resulting model is to be used and how precise that model needs to be.

Alginate Alginate is a powder that is mixed with water (see **Figure 23.38**). The mixture is then inserted into a perforated impression tray and placed in the patient's mouth until it sets to a firm, gel-like consistency (see **Figure 23.39**). Alginate does not produce as accurate a reproduction as elastomeric material, but alginate impressions are economical, easy to manipulate, and quick-setting. These impressions are used for study models and models for making mouth guards, custom impression trays, bleaching trays, and orthodontic appliances. Other materials are used for impressions used to build models for devices in which a greater amount of precision is required.

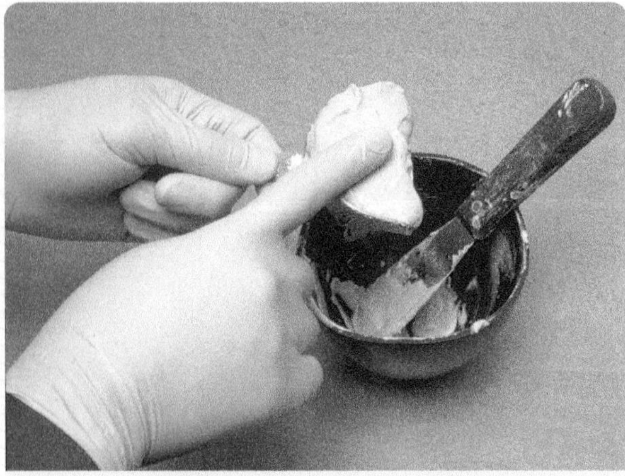

Fig. 23.38 Alginate Loading and smoothing the alginate in a maxillary tray. *What are the advantages of using alginate?*

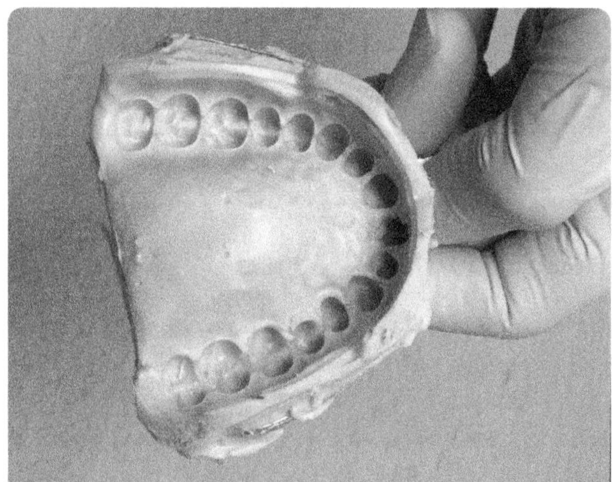

Fig. 23.39 Impression An alginate impression. *What can this impression be used for?*

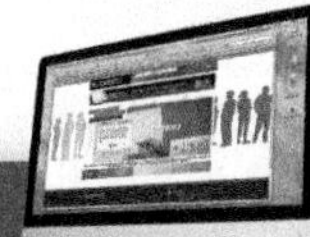

connect ONLINE PROCEDURES

PROCEDURE 23-8

Preparing the Anesthetic Syringe and Assisting with the Administration

Local anesthesia is administered by injecting an anesthetic agent near the nerves that supply the area to be treated. This blocks the conduction of nervous impulses to the central nervous system and makes the area supplied by the nerve insensitive to pain.

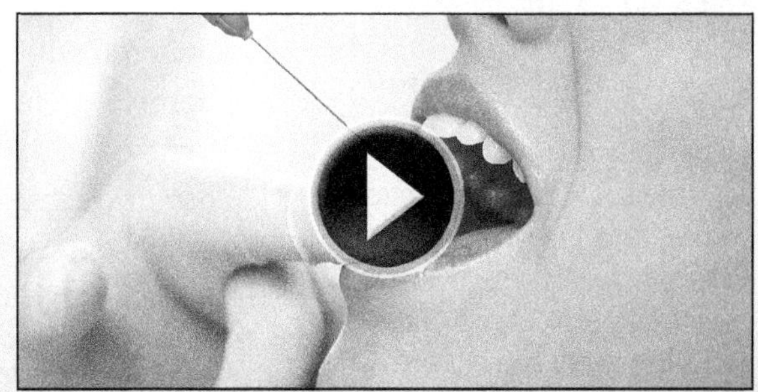

PROCEDURE 23-9

Preparing Alginate and Assisting with an Alginate Impression

Alginate is a powder that is mixed with water. After it is mixed, it is inserted into a perforated impression tray and placed in the mouth to set to a firm, gel-like consistency. These impressions are used routinely for study models and models for making mouth guards, custom impression trays, bleaching trays, and orthodontic appliances.

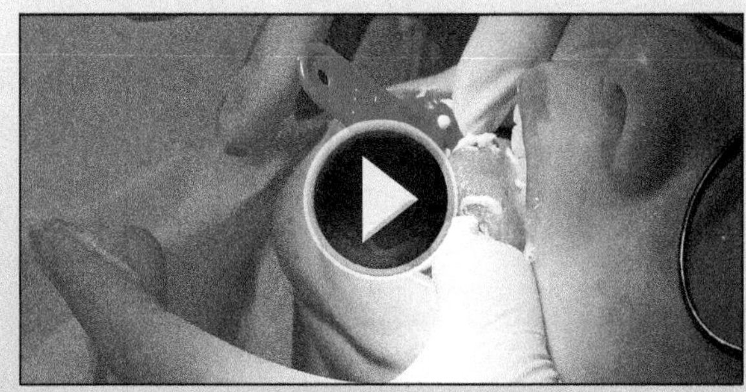

PROCEDURE 23-10

Mixing and Assisting with an Elastomeric Impression

Elastomeric materials are required for very precise procedures, such as fabricating crowns, bridges, and dentures. Elastomeric materials are generally supplied in two pastes, an accelerator and a base, and chemically change to an elastic, rubberlike material when mixed and allowed to set in the client's mouth.

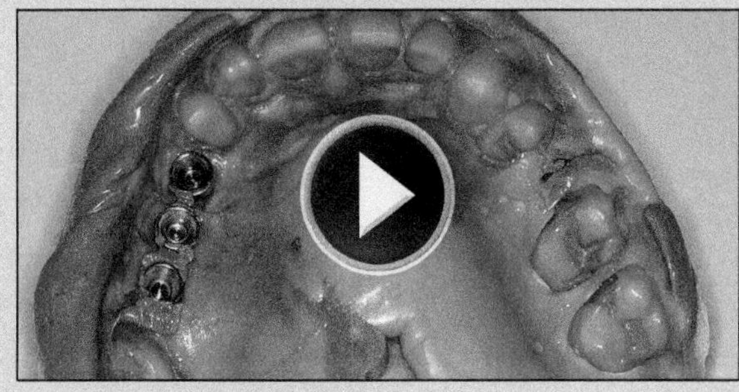

PROCEDURE 23-11

Mixing Dental Plaster and Stone and Fabricating a Model

Impressions are made from dental plaster to fabricate crowns, bridges, and dentures. A stone model is created using the impression.

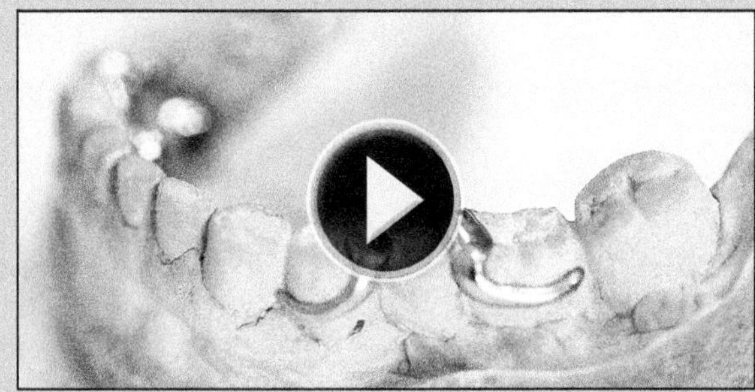

PROCEDURE 23-12

Preparing Amalgam and Assisting with an Amalgam Restoration

Amalgam is a metal material made up mainly of silver, tin, and mercury. It is a common material for direct restoration of cavities.

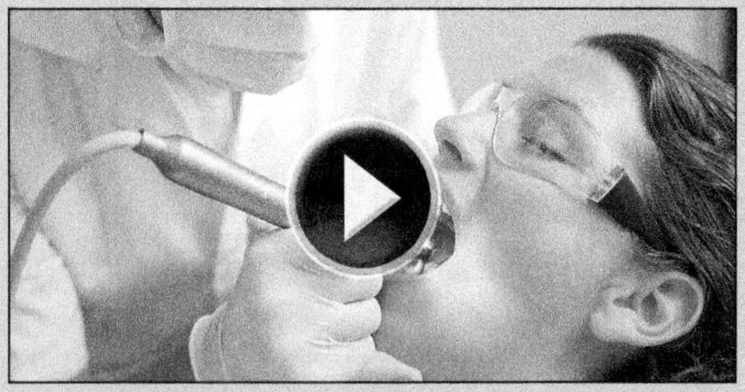

Photos: (t to b)Ingram Publishing, Tony McConnell/Photo Researchers/Photo Researchers, Inc., AJPhoto/Photo Researchers, Inc., Creatas/SuperStock, Robert Daly/Alamy

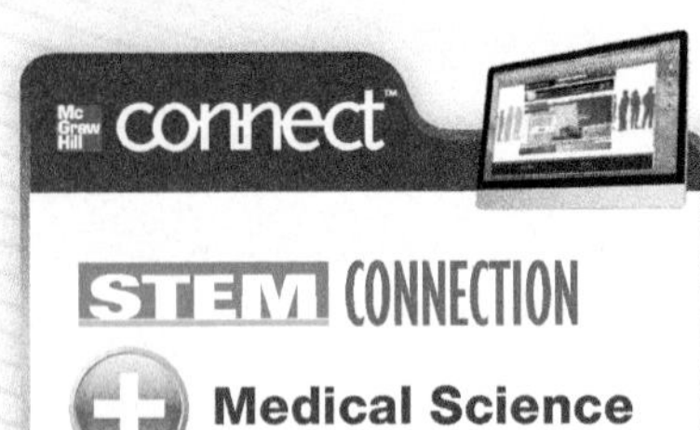

STEM CONNECTION

Medical Science

Dental Disease
Dental decay, or **caries,** creates the need for a great number of dental procedures. Caries is a major cause of tooth loss, and preventing decay is one of the primary goals in dentistry. If you are going to provide patient education, you will need to understand the decay process.

connect™ Go online to learn about plaque, bacteria, and periodontal disease.

Elastomeric Materials Elastomeric materials are required for very precise procedures such as fabricating crowns, bridges, and dentures.

Elastomeric materials are generally supplied in two pastes, an accelerator and a base, which chemically change to an elastic, rubberlike material when mixed and allowed to set in the patient's mouth. Some dentists prefer to use elastomeric materials that are available in both a light-bodied form, for use in the syringe, and a heavy-bodied form, for use in the impression tray. If this is the case, two mixes are required. Other dentists prefer to use the regular form, which can be used as both syringe and tray material.

When impressions are needed for fabricating crowns and bridges, the dentist prepares the teeth prior to taking the impression. After the impression has been made, temporary coverage for the prepared teeth is provided. Temporary coverage is necessary to protect the prepared tooth from oral fluids and temperature changes, to allow the patient to bite and chew, and to keep the patient's mouth looking and feeling relatively normal while the permanent crown or bridge is being made. When the dental laboratory has fabricated the crown or bridge, usually in one to three weeks, the patient will return for final fitting and cementing or bonding of the permanent crown or bridge.

Amalgam and Resin Restorative Materials

Restorations, also called fillings, are needed when tooth tissues are damaged by decay. The dentist removes the decay and shapes the remaining tooth structure to hold a restoration. This is known as a cavity preparation. Cavity preparation and placement of restorative material remove disease and restore tooth function and appearance.

Amalgam and composite resin are the two most commonly used materials for direct restoration of cavities. Amalgam is a metal material made up mainly of silver, tin, and mercury.

Composite is a tooth-colored restorative material composed of plastic resin, with glass fillers added for strength. Composite can be bonded to the tooth through acid etching, in which

- Acid is applied to the enamel surface after the cavity is prepared.
- A liquid resin that bonds with the rough enamel surface is applied.
- Composite material that bonds with the bonding resin is added.

Dental Cements

Dental cements are used in dentistry for many purposes. Most cements are mixed by hand on a paper pad or glass slab. They are supplied in a two-paste or a powder-and-liquid form. Mixing techniques and required ratios for each component vary based on the material, its intended use, and the manufacturer. The manufacturer's instructions must be followed carefully. Cements may be set (hardened) by a chemical reaction called self-curing or by exposure to a curing light.

Cements are classified both according to their use and according to their chemical properties. Each cement has unique characteristics. Dentists choose a cement based on the characteristic required for a given procedure. **Table 23.7** lists the various types of dental cements.

Dental cements are used as

- Bases and liners. These are placed on the pulpal wall of the cavity preparation prior to the placement of the restorative material. They protect the pulp from thermal changes. They also help the tooth recover from the trauma of decay and the irritation of the cavity preparation procedure.
- Luting agents. Luting means "cementing or bonding." Luting agents help materials such as crowns, bridges, orthodontic bands, and brackets adhere to tooth structures. There are different cements for permanent and temporary luting.
- Temporary restorations. These are soothing short-term restorations that are relatively inexpensive and easy to place. They are often used to restore the tooth just until the dentist is sure of the best treatment for the patient. They relieve discomfort until the time is available to place a permanent restoration.

Varnishes and dentin sealants are liquid agents also used to seal the dentin and protect the pulp from chemical irritation. They do not require mixing. They are applied to cavity walls with a disposable plastic brush or with a small cotton pellet.

21ST CENTURY SKILLS

Digital Impressions

New three-dimensional (3D) intraoral scanners are now an alternative to the messy impression-taking procedure. The intraoral scanner can capture detailed, accurate images of the teeth and bite relationship. Those images can then be transmitted to the dental laboratory. In the dental lab, a prototyping technology is used to make a model for use in fabrication of dental restorations. Or the dentist or dental lab can use a computer-aided design and manufacturing (CAD/CAM) system to create a virtual model and design and fabricate, or "mill," the dental restoration from a ceramic block.

READING CHECK

Recall when it would not be appropriate to use an alginate impression.

Table 23.7 Types of Dental Cements

TYPE OF CEMENT	USES	BRAND NAMES
Zinc oxide eugenol	Sedative base or liner Temporary restoration Temporary luting	IRM®, Cavitec™, ZONE
Calcium hydroxide	Liner, especially useful with pulp exposures	Dycal®, Life™, Hydrox™
Glass ionomer	Permanent luting Base and liner Permanent restoration	Fuji™, Ketac™, Vitrebond™, Vitremer™
Polycarboxylate	Permanent luting Insulating base	Durelon™, Tylok® Plus
Zinc phosphate	Permanent luting Insulating base	Fleck's Zinc Cement®
Resin cement	Permanent luting	PanaviaF2.0, Infinity®, RelyX™, Calibra®

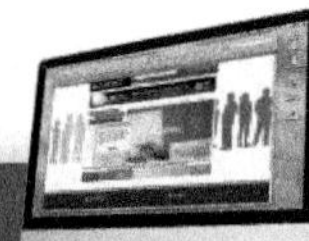

connect ONLINE PROCEDURES

PROCEDURE 23-13

Preparing Composite and Assisting with a Composite Restoration

Composite is a tooth-colored restorative material composed of plastic resin, with glass fillers added for strength. Composite can be bonded to the tooth by the process of acid etching.

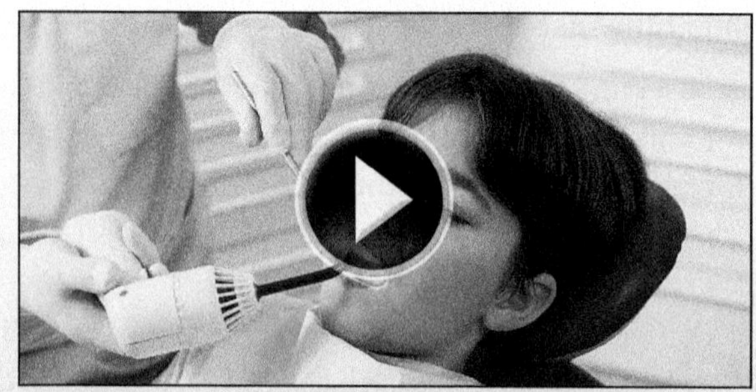

PROCEDURE 23-14

Mixing Zinc Oxide Eugenol Cement

Zinc oxide eugenol cement is used for permanent luting and insulating base.

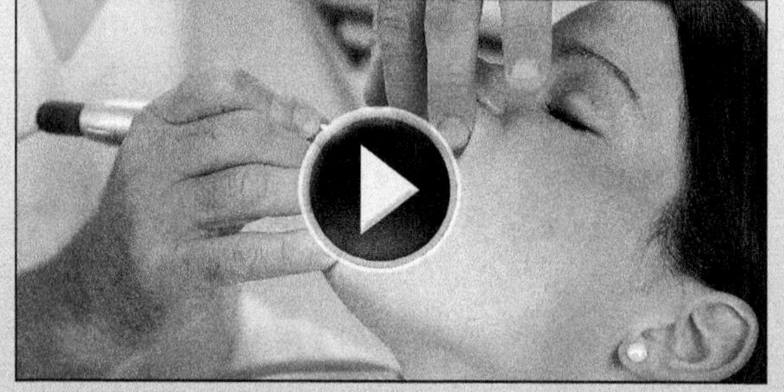

PROCEDURE 23-15

Mixing Calcium Hydroxide Cement

Calcium hydroxide is used as a liner. It is especially useful with pulp exposures.

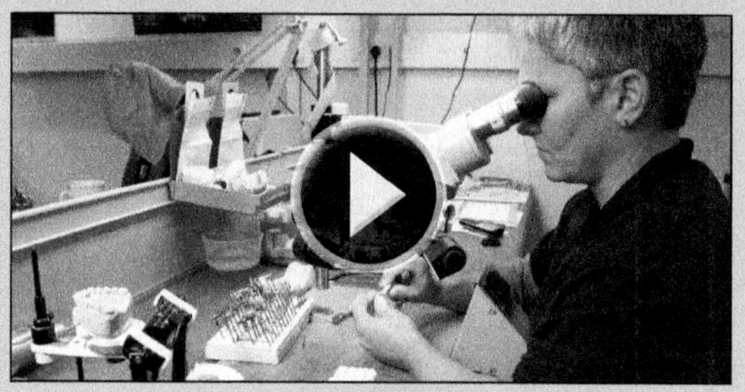

PROCEDURE 23-16

Mixing Polycarboxylate Cement

Polycarboxylate cement is used for permanent luting and insulating base.

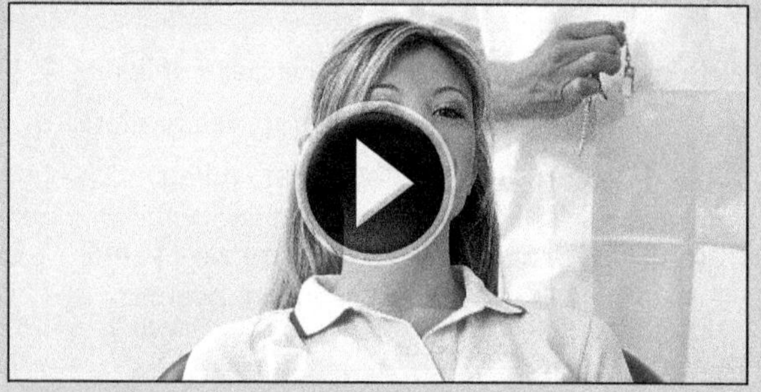

PROCEDURE 23-17

Mixing Glass Ionomer Cement

Glass ionomer cement is used for permanent luting, base and line, and permanent restorations.

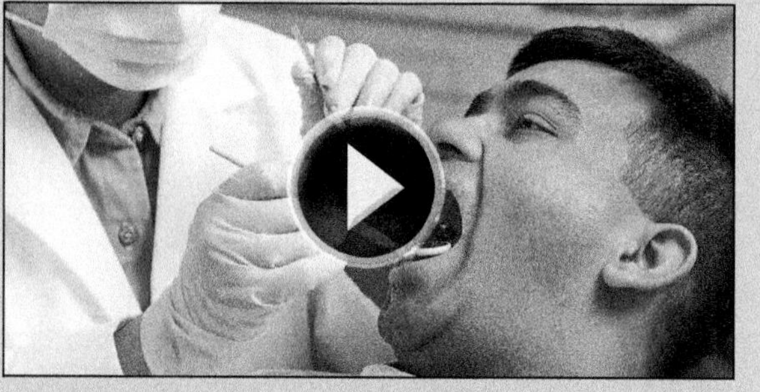

Dental Records

What do red and blue marks on a tooth diagram signify?

A dental record or chart is kept on all patients. A chart is usually a folder that contains a patient registration form, a medical history, an exam and treatment form, and radiographs (X-rays). This record is a legal document, so all entries must be legible and accurate. Many offices are now using computerized dental records (see **Figure 23.40**).

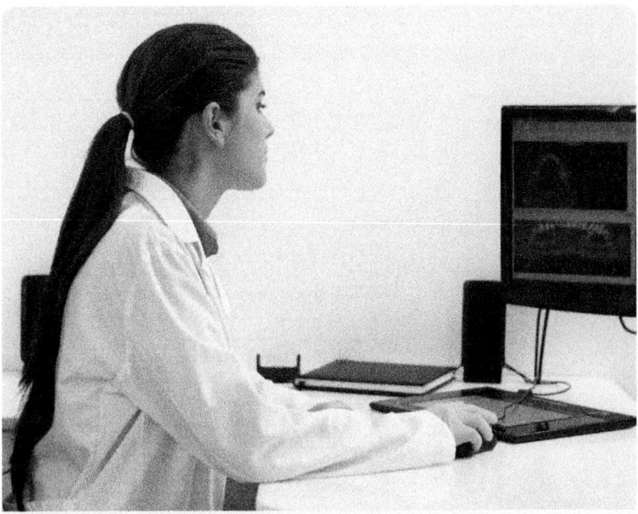

Fig. 23.40 Electronic Records A computerized dental record. *What is an advantage of a computerized dental record?*

The dental assistant is often responsible for recording all treatment provided to the patient. To speed up this process, many standard abbreviations are used to document dental conditions and treatment given.

Tooth diagrams, as shown in **Figure 23.41** on page 592, are used to record information during an examination. The rest of the form is used to record the treatment performed (see **Figure 23.42** on page 592). Red and blue pencils may be used on tooth diagrams. Red indicates disease or treatment needed. Blue indicates existing restorations or treatment completed. Electronic charting may follow the same color coding.

Tooth diagrams may be anatomic or geometric, depending on the dentist's preference. You should study both anatomic and geometric diagrams to become familiar with the location of the maxillary and mandibular teeth and all tooth surfaces on these diagrams (see **Figure 23.43**).

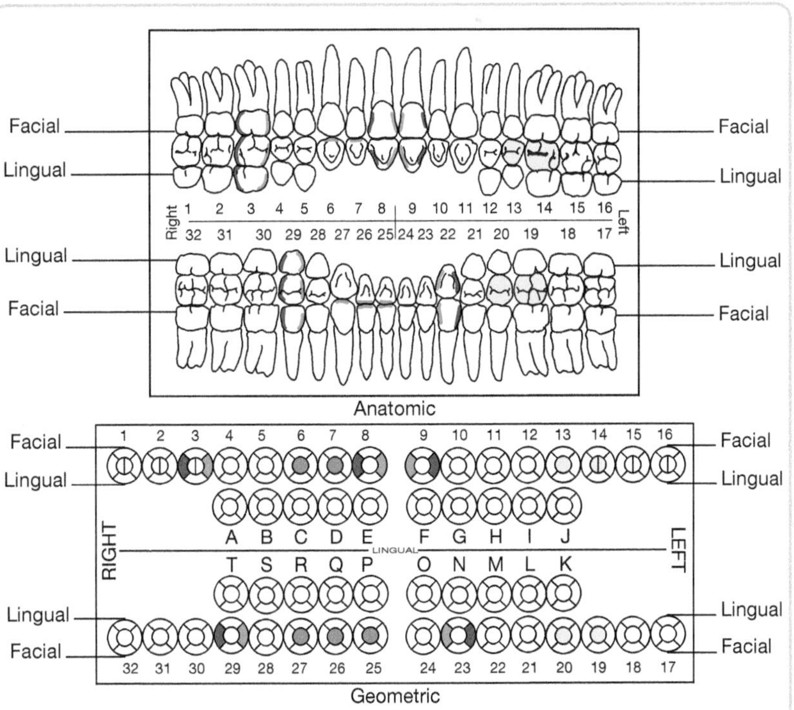

Fig. 23.43 Examples of Surfaces on Dental Charts Color codes are the following: incisal is green, occlusal is yellow, mesial is blue, and distal is red. *Which is preferred, anatomic or geometric diagrams?*

Common charting symbols and abbreviations are discussed below. Individual dentists may use slightly different charting symbols and abbreviations. It is important to learn the meanings of the ones used in each office. Some examples of commonly used charting symbols are shown in **Figure 23.44** on page 593. They are also listed below.

- Caries: Outline the surfaces involved.

NAME ____________________ **DENTIST** ____________________

PATIENT NO. __________

ADDRESS ____________________ PHONE NO. __________

CITY ____________________ OFFICE PHONE NO. __________

OCCUPATION __________ PHYSICIAN __________ RECOMMENDED BY __________

BIRTH DATE __________ AGE __________

1. Do you now have a sore throat or cold?	NO	YES
2. Are you sensitive to any drugs or medicines?	NO	YES
What?		
3. Have you had severe pain or bleeding after extractions?	NO	YES
4. Do your gums bleed when you brush your teeth?	NO	YES
5. Has a doctor told you that you have heart trouble?	NO	YES
6. Are your ankles often swollen?	NO	YES
7. Do you get short of breath easily?	NO	YES
8. Do you faint easily?	NO	YES
9. Do you suffer from stomach trouble?	NO	YES
10. Do you easily get overly tired?	NO	YES
11. Has a doctor said you have kidney or bladder trouble?	NO	YES
12. Do you have to get up every night to urinate? (Pass water)	NO	YES
13. Do you suffer from frequent loose bowl movements?	NO	YES
14. As a child did you have growing pains or twitching of limbs?	NO	YES
Or were you confined to bed for a long time?	NO	YES
15. Have you gained or lost much weight recently?	NO	YES
16. Have you been under a doctor's care within the past year?	NO	YES
17. Are you taking medicine at the present time?	NO	YES
What?		

18. Have you had?

Asthma	NO	YES	Heart Trouble	NO	YES	Kidney Trouble	NO	YES
Rheumatic Fever	NO	YES	High Blood			Allergies	NO	YES
Scarlet Fever	NO	YES	Pressure	NO	YES	Penicillin	NO	YES
Pneumonia	NO	YES	Anemia	NO	YES	Any Others		
Tuberculosis	NO	YES	Diabetes	NO	YES			

PERMIT FOR OPERATIONS

This is to certify that I, undersigned, consent to the performing of the dental and oral surgery procedures agreed to be necessary or advisable, including the use of local or general anesthesia as indicated.

Patient's (Parents) Signature __________ Date __________

UPPER FACIAL

UPPER PALATAL

8 7 6 5 4 3 2 1 | 1 2 3 4 5 6 7 8

RIGHT E D C B A | A B C D E LEFT

8 7 6 5 4 3 2 1 | 1 2 3 4 5 6 7 8

LOWER LINGUAL

LOWER FACIAL

R L

88-15-0226

PARTIALS UPPER	TYPE	HOW LONG
LOWER	TYPE	HOW LONG
X-RAYS F M	B W	AREA
STUDY MODELS		AGE
PHOTOS BEFORE	AFTER	
OCCLUSION		
ABNORMALITIES		
GENERAL CONDITION OF TEETH & GUMS		

TOOTH	MOULD UPPER	MOULD LOWER	SHADE UPPER	SHADE LOWER
CENT				
LAT				
CUSP				
POST				

ORAL FINDINGS				
HYGIENE	1	2	3	4
DEPOSITS	1	2	3	4
PERIODONT	1	2	3	4

Fig. 23.41 Tooth Diagrams Sample treatment and exam form (front). *What will be recorded on the tooth diagram shown above?*

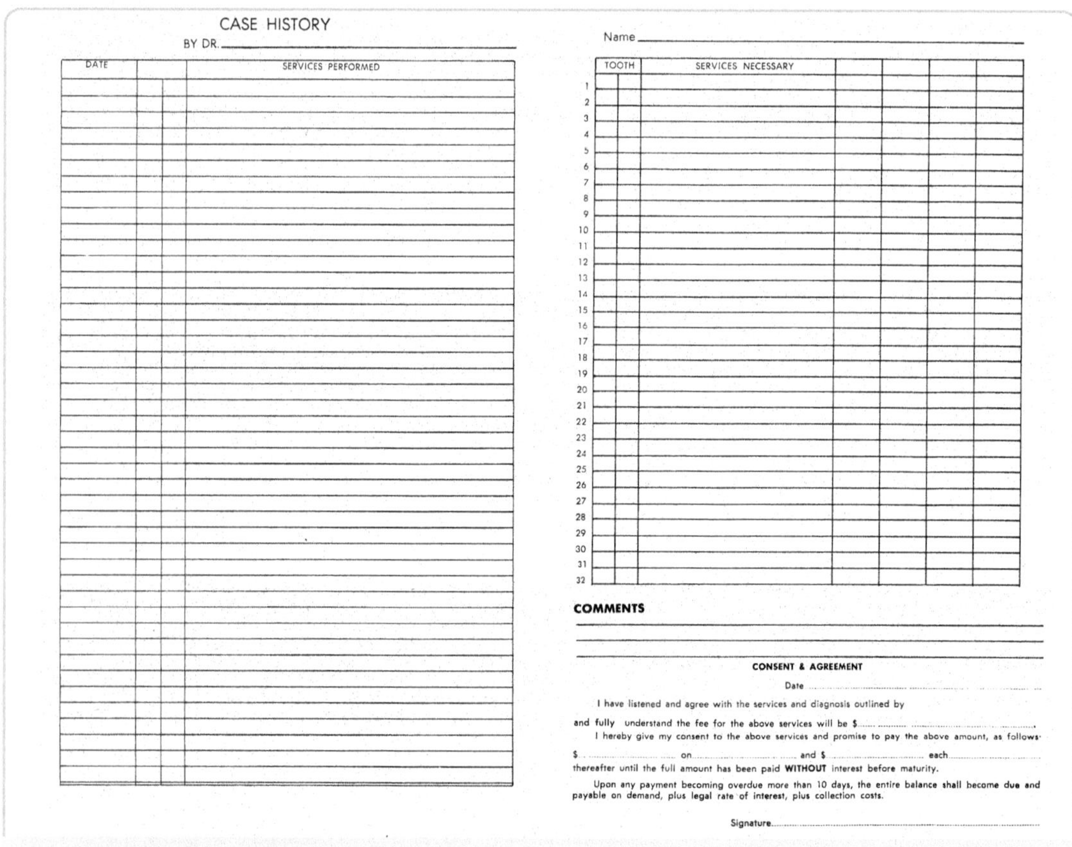

CASE HISTORY

BY DR. ____________________

DATE			SERVICES PERFORMED

Name ____________________

	TOOTH	SERVICES NECESSARY
1		
2		
3		
4		
5		
6		
7		
8		
9		
10		
11		
12		
13		
14		
15		
16		
17		
18		
19		
20		
21		
22		
23		
24		
25		
26		
27		
28		
29		
30		
31		
32		

COMMENTS

CONSENT & AGREEMENT

Date __________

I have listened and agree with the services and diagnosis outlined by __________ and fully understand the fee for the above services will be $ __________.

I hereby give my consent to the above services and promise to pay the above amount, as follows: $ __________ on __________ and $ __________ each __________ thereafter until the full amount has been paid **WITHOUT** interest before maturity.

Upon any payment becoming overdue more than 10 days, the entire balance shall become due and payable on demand, plus legal rate of interest, plus collection costs.

Signature __________

Fig. 23.42 Treatment Chart Sample treatment and exam form (back). *What does red pencil indicate on a dental exam and treatment form?*

- Amalgam: Outline and shade in the surfaces involved.
- Composite: Outline and dot the surfaces involved.
- Missing tooth: Cross out the missing tooth.
- To be extracted: Draw a diagonal line through the tooth.
- Impacted tooth: Draw a circle around the entire tooth.
- Gold crown: Outline the crown surfaces. Draw diagonal lines through the outlined area.
- Porcelain crown: Outline the crown surfaces.
- Root canal: Draw a line through the root of the tooth.
- Periapical abscess: Place a circle at the apex of the root.
- Fracture: Draw a zigzag line across the affected area.

All treatment provided, any medications administered or prescribed, and any complications experienced must be thoroughly documented.

Tooth surfaces are abbreviated by using the first letter of the surface. For example, MO stands for mesial occlusal, and DI stands for distal incisal. The following abbreviations may also be used.

Adj: adjustment

Amal: amalgam

Anes: anesthesia

BWX: bitewing radiographs (X-rays)

Cr: crown

Ext: extraction

Imp: impression

PA: periapical radiograph

Pro, prophy: prophylaxis

RCT: root canal therapy

TX: Treatment

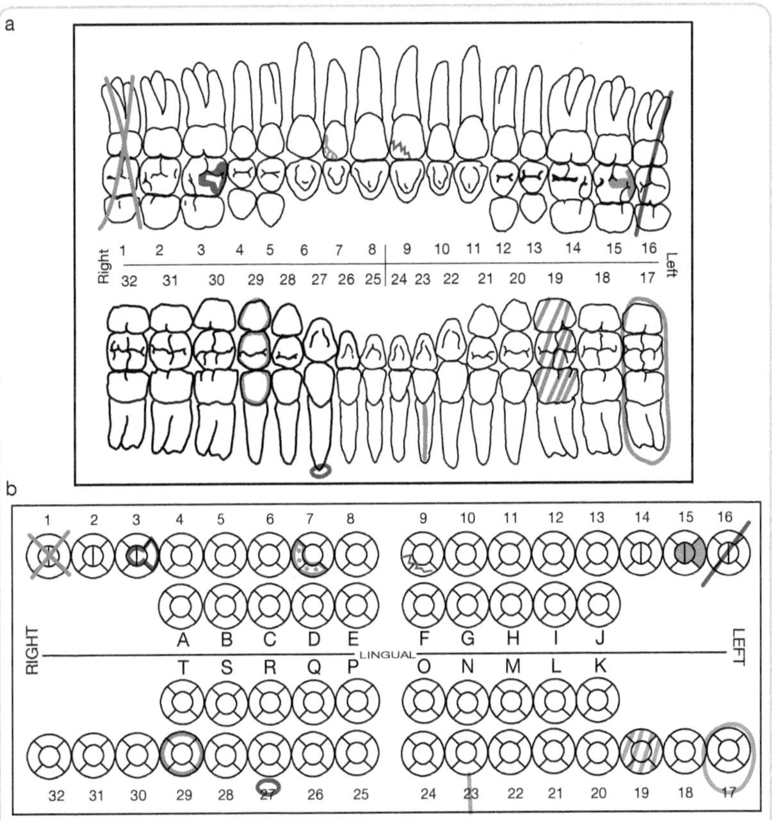

Fig. 23.44 Examples of Charting Symbols (a) On the anatomic chart (b) On the geometric chart *What does the red diagonal line indicate? What do the blue diagonal stripes indicate?*

Dental Radiographs

Dental radiographs are images of the teeth and oral structures used to diagnose disease and to monitor growth and development. X-rays are used to create these images on a special film. Since radiation has the potential to damage living tissue, producing radiographs requires a high level of skill. Only trained personnel are allowed to expose radiographs. Many states require such personnel to be licensed or credentialed.

When X-rays pass through oral structures and strike the film, an invisible image is created on the film. That image becomes visible

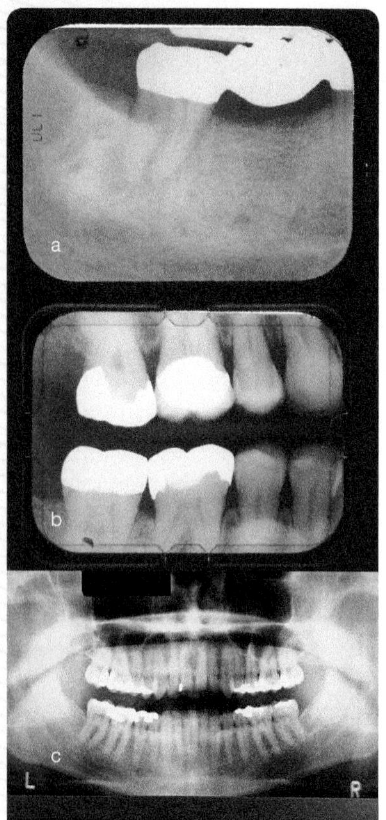

Fig. 23.45 Dental Radiographs (a) Periapical radiograph of mandibular premolar area; (b) Premolar bitewing radiograph; (c) Panoramic radiograph. *Why are dental radiographs used?*

after processing. "Radiolucent" and "radiopaque" are terms used to describe the darkness or lightness of an image on the film.

- "Radiolucent" refers to darker areas on the film. X-rays more easily penetrate structures that are less dense, creating a darker image.
- "Radiopaque" refers to lighter or white areas on the film. Denser tissues stop or absorb X-rays. This results in lighter images.

The film is then processed to create an image of the oral structures.

Types of Dental Radiographs The main types include:

- Periapical: Includes the entire length of the tooth and the tissues surrounding the apex of the root (see **Figure 23.45a**).
- Bitewing: Includes the crowns of the maxillary and the mandibular teeth on one film (see **Figure 23.45b**).
- Occlusal: Includes the maxillary or mandibular arch on one film.
- Panoramic: Positioned outside the mouth in a special cassette. This shows all the maxillary and mandibular teeth and supporting structures (see **Figure 23.45c**).

A full series of radiographs (FMX) for an adult often consists of 14 periapical films and four bitewing films, although the number will depend on the dentist's specifications.

Intraoral Dental Film Intraoral film is supplied in different sizes.

- Size 0, the smallest film, is used for children up to age 5
- Size 1 is used for children age 5 to 10 and for narrow anterior areas in adults
- Size 2 is used for adults
- Size 4 is occlusal film

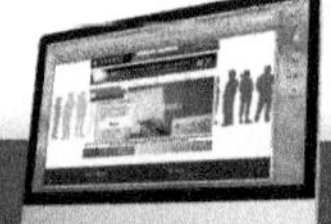

Mc Graw Hill connect™ ONLINE PROCEDURES

PROCEDURE 23-18
Manual Processing of Dental Radiographs

Dental radiographs are images of the teeth and oral structures used by the dentist to diagnose disease and to monitor growth and development. X-rays (a type of radiation) are used to create these images on a special film. Radiation has the potential to damage living tissue. Producing quality radiographs requires a high level of skill. Only trained personnel are allowed to expose radiographs.

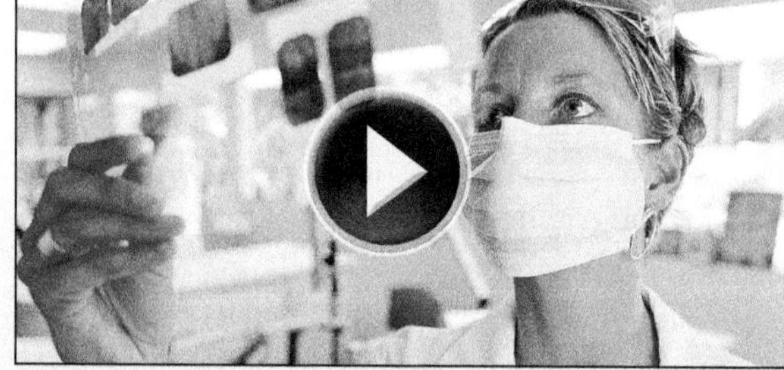

PROCEDURE 23-19
Mounting Dental Radiographs

The dental film has a small raised bump, or dot, in one corner, and the bump is also on the front of the film packet. After films are processed, the dot is used to identify the front side of the film. It is needed for the correct mounting of radiographs.

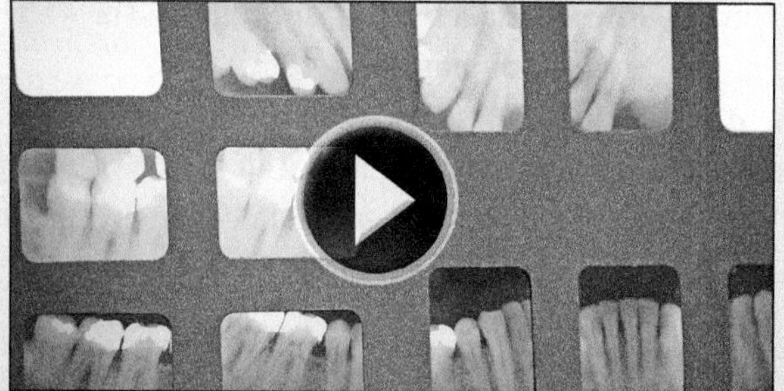

Photos: (t to b)Spencer Grant/PhotoEdit, Spencer Grant/PhotoEdit, Keith Brofsky/Getty Images, Andersen Ross/Digital Vision/Getty Images, C. Sherburne/PhotoLink/Getty Images

The film packet consists of a plastic outer wrap, an inner black paper wrapped around the film, and a sheet of lead foil, as shown in **Figure 23.46**. The film has a small raised bump, or dot, in one corner and also on the front of the film packet. The front side is always placed next to the teeth and toward the X-ray tube. After films are processed, the dot is used to identify the front side of the film. It is needed for the correct mounting of radiographs.

Digital Imaging New technology is available that replaces conventional dental radiography. Instead of placing a dental film in the patient's mouth to record the image, a sensor is used to digitally record the image. The images are electronically sent to a computer and viewed on the computer monitor. This process is quicker, produces images with less radiation, and eliminates the use of processing chemicals.

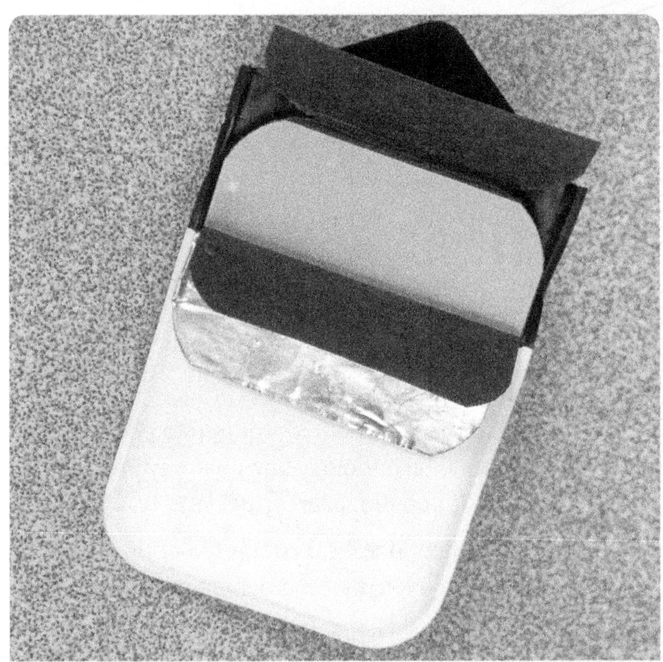

Fig. 23.46 Intraoral Film Intraoral dental film packet. *How many sizes of dental film are available?*

READING CHECK

Name the two types of tooth diagrams used by dentists.

SECTION 23.2 Dental Care Procedures Review

AFTER YOU READ

1. **Define** the following anatomical terms: deciduous, posterior, anterior, mesial, distal, incisal, occlusal, facial, lingual, buccal, labial, contact area, cusp, developmental groove, and pit.
2. **Name** and describe the four tissues of a tooth.
3. **Identify** the type of symbol that designates permanent teeth in both the Universal and the Palmer notation.
4. **Describe** the correct seated position of a dental assistant at chairside.
5. **List** the instruments in the basic tray setup.
6. **Recall** the instruments used for the removal of decay and preparation of a cavity.
7. **Name** and describe the two instrument grasps.
8. **Indicate** which impression material is typically used to make study models.
9. **Name** an impression material that is used when a tooth has been prepared for a crown.
10. **List** the two types of film exposures used in a full mouth survey.

Technology ONLINE EXPLORATIONS

Dental Technology

Technology has changed the field of dentistry, especially when it comes to charting, images, and impressions. Choose one of these topics and then search the Internet for the latest technology including electronic charting, digital imaging, and 3D scanners. Write a summary of your findings.

CHAPTER

23 Review

Chapter Summary

SECTION 23.1

- A dental assistant is required to perform many different duties. A basic knowledge of dental terminology and anatomy provides a foundation for learning more complex skills and procedures. **(pg. 563)**
- The dental team is composed of the dental assistant, dental laboratory technician, dental hygienist, and dentist. **(pg. 564)**
- The dental laboratory technician uses a variety of materials to create dental prostheses, replacement teeth, and dental appliances. **(pg. 565)**
- Dental hygienists provide oral hygiene care and dental health education to the patient. **(pg. 565)**
- The specialty areas of dentistry are dental public health, endodontics, oral and maxillofacial pathology, oral and maxillofacial radiography, oral and maxillofacial surgery, orthodontics and dentofacial orthopedics, pediatric dentistry, periodontics, and prosthodontics. **(pg. 566)**

SECTION 23.2

- During their lifetime, human beings have two sets of teeth, the primary teeth and the permanent teeth. **(pg. 568)**
- The Universal and Palmer numbering systems are used to efficiently communicate about and record information on dental conditions and treatment. **(pg. 573)**
- Dental treatment is provided in areas equipped with a dental unit, dental chair, operator and assistant's stools, operating lights, cabinets, sinks, and X-ray units. Specific procedures are necessary to decontaminate this equipment after use and to maintain all equipment in good operating condition. **(pg. 574)**
- Having dental work done is stressful for many people. Dental professionals should work to build a trusting relationship with each patient.. **(pg. 577)**
- Instruments and materials required for a procedure are grouped together in a tray setup. **(pg. 577)**
- There are many dental instruments designed for many different purposes. The handpiece is a rotary instrument used to remove decay, shape teeth, and adjust appliances. **(pg. 580)**
- Delivery of dental care with a dentist and dental assistant working as a team is known as "four-handed dentistry." The assistant transfers instruments, mixes materials, and uses the oral evacuator to maintain a clear working area. **(pg. 582)**
- During an exam, oral conditions are noted, or charted, on the treatment and exam form. When a procedure is completed, information is recorded regarding the treatment provided, specific materials and anesthetic used, and instructions given. **(pg. 591)**

CHAPTER

23 Assessment

Critical Thinking/Problem Solving

1. A patient needs an MO restoration on tooth number 5. The dentist has given the patient the options of restoring the tooth with either composite or amalgam. The patient asks you for help in making the decision. What should you do?

2. Using an anatomical diagram of the permanent dentition, chart the conditions listed below. Use a red pencil to chart the disease or treatment needed and a blue pencil to chart existing restorations or treatment that has already been completed.

Tooth	Chart
1, 16, and 17	missing
3	gold crown
8	porcelain crown
10	MI fracture
13	abscessed; needs a root canal
19	MO decay
24	D composite
30	DO amalgam
32	impacted; needs to be extracted

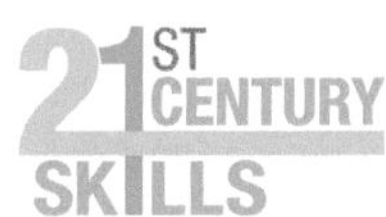

3. **Information Literacy** Go online to learn more about wisdom teeth, tooth decay, mouth guards, temporomandibular joint (TMJ) disorders, braces, or a related topic. Summarize what you have learned in a brief information sheet.

McGraw Hill connect™ ONLINE ACTIVITIES

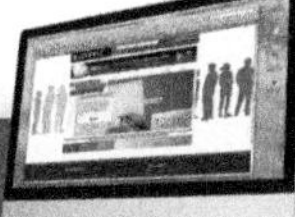

Complete our HST online activities for Chapter 23, which include Concept Check review questions, Reference Flash Cards, and Online Procedures assessment sheets.

- **Concept Check** review questions
- **Reference Flash Cards** medical terminology practice
- **Online Procedures** assessment sheets

CHAPTER

24 Animal Healthcare

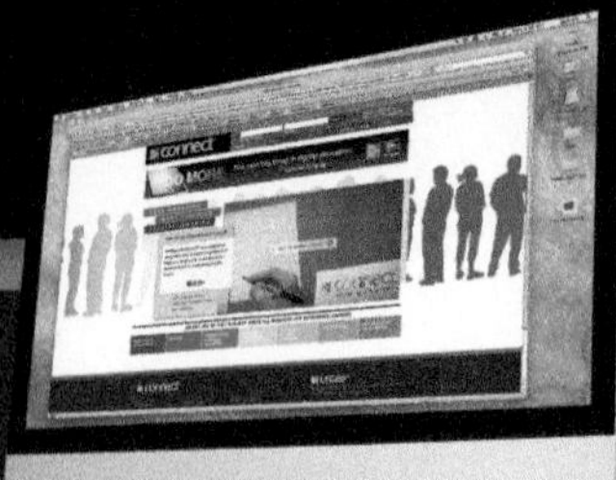

McGraw Hill connect™

It's Online!

- Online Procedures
- STEM Connection
- Medical Science
- Medical Terms
- Medical Math
- Ethics in Action
- Virtual Lab

Essential Question:

What are some healthcare career options for people who enjoy working with animals?

The animal healthcare field mirrors human medicine in many ways. Many of the procedures that are used in hospitals to treat humans are also used in veterinary hospitals. Animal healthcare training is very broad. There are many specialties to choose from, such as internal medicine and surgery. The three most common careers in the animal health field, which are discussed in this chapter, are veterinarian, veterinary technician (also known as a veterinary technologist or animal health technician), and veterinary assistant.

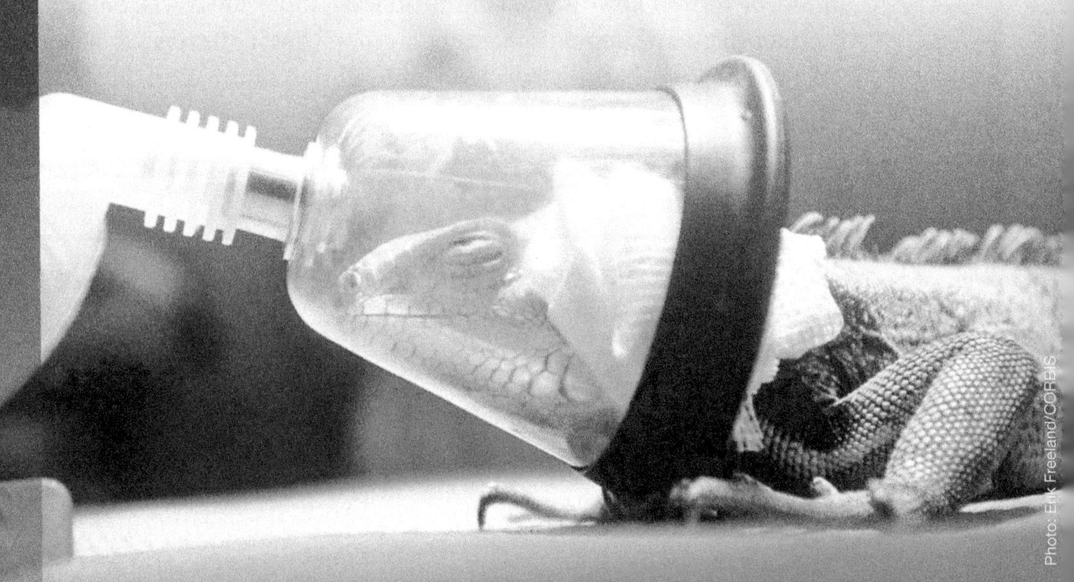

Photo: Erik Freeland/CORBIS

READING GUIDE

OBJECTIVES

After completing this chapter, you will be able to:

- **Illustrate** the role and responsibilities of the veterinarian.
- **Describe** the role and responsibilities of the veterinary technician.
- **Examine** career opportunities available to veterinarians and veterinary technicians.
- **Identify** the role and responsibilities of the veterinary assistant.
- **Demonstrate** five animal health procedures.

BEFORE YOU READ

Connect Have you ever had to take an animal to the vet? What happened during your visit?

Main Idea

Careers in animal veterinary care provide opportunities to improve the health and well-being of animals.

Note-Taking Activity

Draw this table. Write key terms and phrases under **Cues**. Write main ideas under **Note Taking**. Summarize the section under **Summary**.

Cues	Note Taking
○ ○	○ ○
Summary	

Graphic Organizer

Before you read the chapter, draw a diagram like the one below. As you read, write the animal healthcare careers covered in the chapter into the diagram.

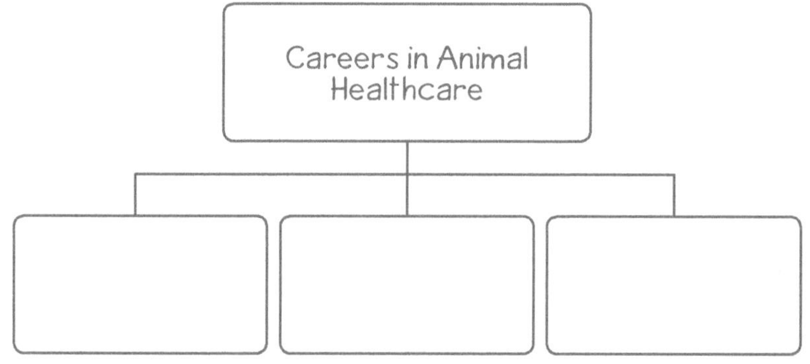

connect
Downloadable graphic organizers can be accessed online.

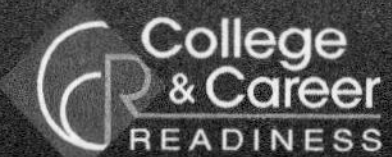

STANDARDS

HEALTH SCIENCE

NCHSE 1.22 Recognize emerging diseases and disorders.

NCHSE 2.11 Interpret verbal and nonverbal communication.

NCHSE 7.31 Apply safety techniques in the work environment.

SCIENCE

NSES F Develop understanding of personal and community health; population growth; natural resources; environmental quality; natural and human-induced hazards; science and technology in local, national, and global challenges.

NCHSE *National Consortium for Health Science Education*

NSES *National Science Education Standards*

COMMON CORE STATE STANDARDS

MATHEMATICS

Number and Quantity

Quantities N-Q Reason quantitatively and use units to solve problems.

ENGLISH LANGUAGE ARTS

Speaking and Listening

Presentation of Knowledge and Ideas SL-6 Adapt speech to a variety of contexts and tasks, demonstrating a command of formal English when indicated or appropriate.

Writing

Research to Build and Present Knowledge W-7 Conduct short as well as more sustained research projects to answer a question (including a self-generated question) or solve a problem; narrow or broaden the inquiry when appropriate; synthesize multiple sources on the subject, demonstrating understanding of the subject under investigation.

SECTION

24.1 Careers in Animal Healthcare

Vocabulary

Content Vocabulary

You will learn these content vocabulary terms in this section.

- **American Veterinary Medical Association (AVMA)**
- **Veterinary Technician National Examination (VTNE)**
- **National Board examination**
- **diagnostic radiograph**
- **zoonosis**

Academic Vocabulary

You will see this word in your reading and on your tests. Find its meaning in the Glossary in the back of the book.

- **injure**

The Veterinarian

How difficult is it to gain admission to veterinary school?

In human medicine, physicians study one species, the human being. Veterinarians study at least five species. Most schools train future vets to treat common domesticated animals, such as dogs, cats, horses, cows, and sheep. **Figure 24.1** shows a veterinarian caring for a cow. Some schools focus on the treatment of particular species such as poultry, swine (pigs), and goats. Others emphasize the care of pet birds, reptiles, zoo animals, fish, or native wildlife. Yet other courses deal with small pets, such as hamsters, gerbils, and guinea pigs.

The course of study in the veterinary field is very broad and includes courses such as anatomy, hematology, and pathology. Students usually begin working in clinics in the third or fourth year of study. Many schools give students opportunities to work in private practices, laboratories, and zoos.

Most veterinary school graduates work in private clinical practice. The majority of them work with companion animals, or pets, such as dogs and cats. Veterinarians also work in a variety of other areas. Veterinarians may specialize in areas such as research, laboratory animal medicine, poultry medicine, pathology, public health, zoo, or wildlife work. They may also work in education, military service, food inspection, private industry, and government. **Figure 24.2** on page 601 draws your attention to how technology has affected veterinary medicine.

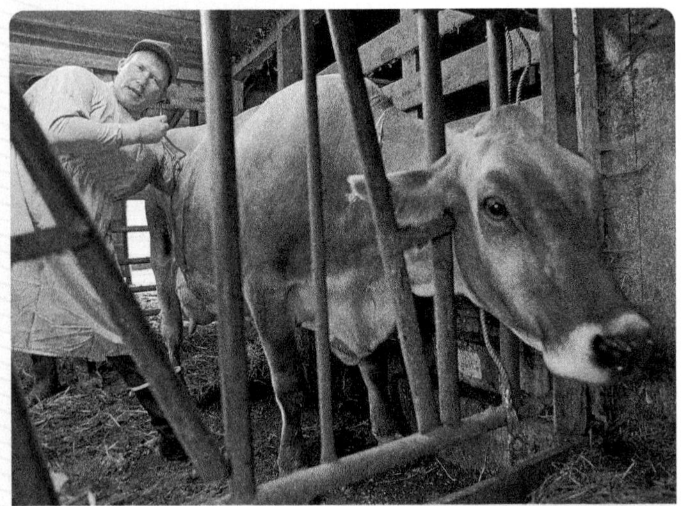

Fig. 24.1 Veterinarian This veterinarian is treating a cow. *What could be the specialty area of this veterinarian?*

Photo: Andy Sacks/The Image Bank/Getty Images

Admission requirements vary from one veterinary school to another. The minimum requirements are two years of college-level courses. It is difficult to gain admission to a veterinary school. Only one out of every five to ten qualified applicants is accepted. Since most veterinary schools are located at state institutions, preference is given to residents of the state in which the school is located or to applicants from other states that have contracts with the school.

Unlike people studying to be medical doctors, most veterinary students do not enter internship programs after they graduate. However, there

Table 24.1 Occupations in Animal Healthcare

OCCUPATION	EDUCATIONAL REQUIREMENTS	CERTIFICATION OR LICENSING AGENCY	JOB OUTLOOK
Veterinarian	At least two years of college and a diploma from a veterinary school. Most veterinary schools have a four-year course of study.	Graduates of veterinary schools accredited by the American Veterinary Medical Association are eligible to take the National Board examination. Some states require additional examinations given by the state board of veterinary medicine.	Better than average. An increased demand for veterinary services has resulted in an increase in the number and size of veterinary hospitals. Pet owners are willing to commit to advanced care for their animals.
Veterinary technician, veterinary technologist, or animal health technician	Two to four years of education in a program accredited by the American Veterinary Medical Association. Veterinary technicians receive an associate in applied science (AAS) degree. Veterinary technologists receive a BS degree in veterinary technology.	Credentialing varies from state to state. The terminology used includes "certified," "registered," or "licensed." Usually the state Board of Veterinary Medicine is the responsible agency. Most states require the National Veterinary Technician Examination; some states require additional testing.	Better than average due to affluent pet owners who are willing pay for advanced veterinary care
Veterinary assistant	On-the-job training; certificate programs also available	None	Better than average due to affluent pet owners who are willing to pay for advanced veterinary care

are more than 20 veterinarian specialties that do require an internship or residency after graduation.

Job Responsibilities of the Veterinarian

A veterinarian is a medical professional who is responsible for protecting the health and welfare of animals and people. Some of the responsibilities are to do the following:

- Treat sick and injured animals
- Diagnose and control animal diseases
- Prevent the transmission of animal diseases to people
- Advise owners on the proper care of companion animals and livestock
- Ensure a safe food supply, by performing thorough food inspections at plants
- Help in conserving and preserving wildlife

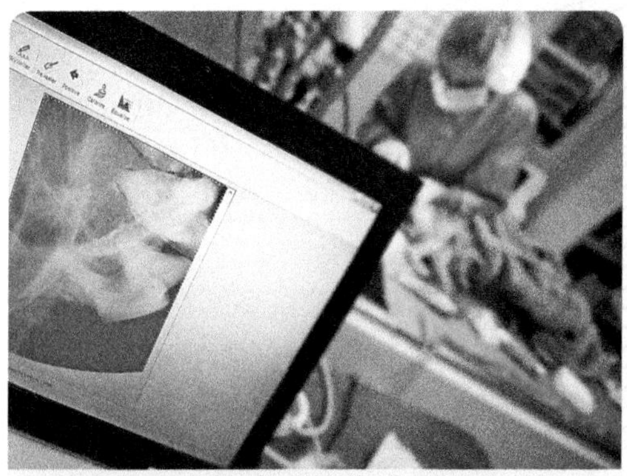

Fig. 24.2 Technology Like regular hospitals, most veterinary practices are computerized. *Can you think of how a computer may be used in this setting?*

READING CHECK

List some settings, other than private clinical practice, in which veterinarians may work.

Safety

Watch Out!

Dog and cat bites are the major injuries suffered by the staff in a veterinary clinic or hospital. Back injury is also very common. Other potential sources of injury or harm are

- Anesthesia
- Excessive noise
- Medical waste
- Radiation
- Darkroom chemicals
- Animal bathing and dipping
- Compressed gas cylinders
- Zoonotic diseases, also known as **zoonosis**. These are animal diseases that can be passed from an animal to a human.
- Chemicals
- Drugs

The animal health practice owner is responsible for operating a safe workplace. Individuals should monitor their own safety, however. Employees must receive training regarding potential hazards and safe work practices. Animal healthcare workers should observe safety precautions at all times.

The Veterinary Technician

How can a person prepare for a career as a veterinary technician?

Veterinary technicians are also called veterinary technologists or animal health technicians. They perform many healthcare procedures while working under the direction of veterinarians. However, they do not diagnose, prescribe drugs, or perform surgery.

This field began in the 1960s in response to a growing need for trained veterinary helpers. Many states require these workers to be certified, registered, or to hold a license. In order to be called a veterinary technician or technologist:

- You must be a graduate of a school of veterinary technology accredited by the **American Veterinary Medical Association (AVMA),** or
- You must complete educational requirements and have a required number of hours of clinical experience, and
- In most states, you must also pass a comprehensive examination known as the **Veterinary Technician National Examination (VTNE).** This is often referred to as the **National Board examination.**

There are now more than 170 AVMA-approved programs in the U.S. There are also distance learning programs that do not require students to travel daily to campus for class. Program entry guidelines range from open-door to highly competitive. Either way, programs are very strict and call for a strong knowledge base. Students must have good study skills for the many science courses that are required. **Table 24.2** gives you some idea of the curriculum in a veterinary technologist program.

Table 24.2 Typical Courses Offered in a Veterinary Technology Curriculum

Animal anatomy and physiology	Laboratory and zoo animal medicine
Animal anesthesiology	Large animal procedures
Animal behavior	Medical math
Animal diseases	Medical terminology
Animal hematology and urinalysis	Microbiology
Animal nursing	Parasitology
Animal science	Radiology
Chemistry	Surgical assisting
Clinical procedures	Veterinary pharmacology
Computer science	Veterinary practice management

Job Opportunities and Specialties for the Veterinary Technician

Most graduates of a veterinary technician program enter private clinical practice. Many veterinary practice experts suggest a ratio of two technicians for every veterinarian. These experts believe that the success of a veterinary practice is directly related to having a well trained staff. There are many career opportunities for veterinary technicians. These include biomedical research, diagnostic laboratories, zoos, animal production facilities, wildlife rehabilitation, private industry, and education.

Job Responsibilities of the Veterinary Technician

More than 350 recommended and essential tasks are listed in the accreditation manual for veterinary technician programs. Job responsibilities of a veterinary technician vary from practice to practice. A veterinary technician is almost like a nurse for animals. Just as nurses work with medical doctors and care for patients, veterinary technicians work with veterinarians and care for animals. **Figure 24.3** illustrates one of the tasks performed by a veterinary technician: cleaning animal teeth. Job responsibilities may include any or all of the following.

- Communicate with animal owners
- Obtain and record information about cases
- Perform physical examination of animals
- Collect blood, urine, tissues, and feces for diagnostic testing
- Perform various diagnostic tests on blood, urine, tissues, and feces
- Administer medications
- Prepare animals, instruments, and equipment for surgery

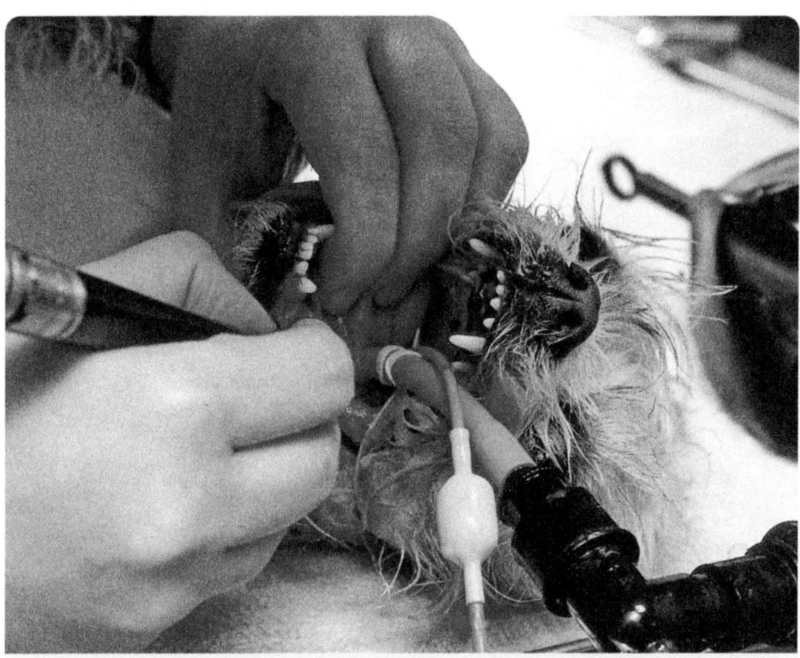

Photo: INTERFOTO/Zoology/Alamy

Fig. 24.3 Dentistry One important duty of a veterinary technician is cleaning teeth. *Can you name at least three other duties?*

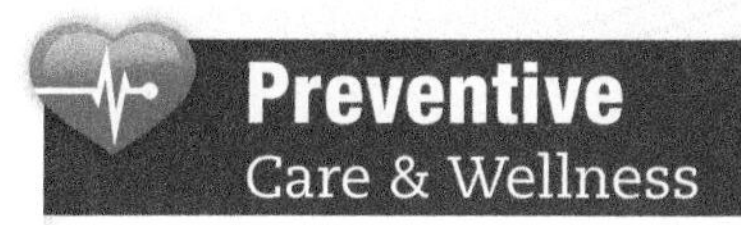

Preventive Care & Wellness

Zoonoses

A zoonosis is a disease that humans may acquire from animals. While animals may appear healthy, they may be carrying a disease that can be transmitted through everyday contact with the animal.

Some of the more common zoonotic diseases may result from being scratched or bitten by an animal. These diseases are caused by bacteria, viruses, fungi, or parasites. Animal sources for zoonosis include cattle, sheep, horses, pigs, chickens, turkeys, dogs, cats, rodents, and some wild animals. Steps to minimize the risk of contacting a zoonotic disease include wearing gloves for certain activities, a well-managed animal vaccination program, good sanitation, and care with personal hygiene.

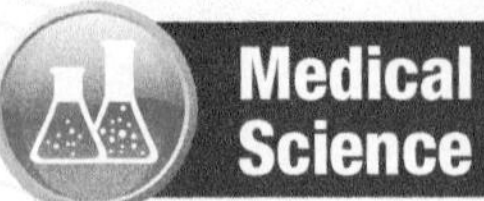

Medical Science

Parasites

Parasites are organisms that live within, upon, or at the expense of another organism. They do not contribute in any way to the organism's survival. Like human beings, animals can have parasites in their digestive tracts. These parasites are dangerous to the health of their hosts.

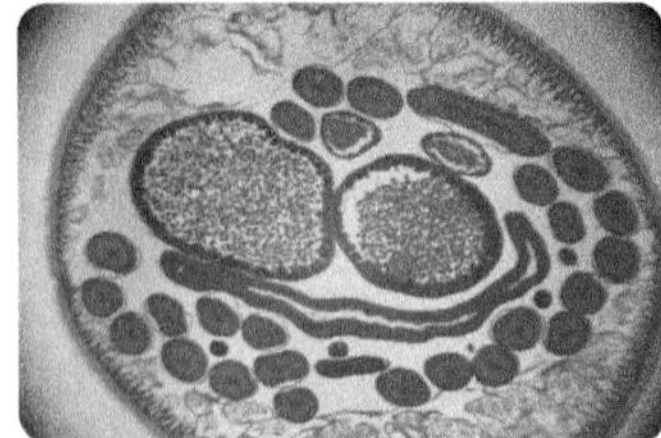

A roundworm egg, magnified 500 times. Roundworm is a common parasite found in dogs and cats.

connect Go online to learn about the parasites that are a threat to the health of animals.

- Induce and maintain anesthesia
- Clean teeth while animals are under anesthesia
- Clean and bandage wounds
- Assist in diagnostic, medical, and surgical procedures
- Position and prepare animals for **diagnostic radiographs**
- Expose and develop diagnostic radiographs
- Supervise veterinary assistants

READING CHECK

Recall how many veterinary technicians should work with each veterinarian.

The Veterinary Assistant

What is the career path of many veterinary assistants?

The term "veterinary assistant" is used to describe a person who works in an animal hospital (see **Figure 24.4**). These workers assist veterinarians or technicians and act under their direct control. The job of a veterinary assistant is much like that of a nursing assistant. Both work under the supervision of a doctor (veterinarian) or nurse (veterinary technician) and give direct care to patients, either human or animal.

This entry-level job is often filled by persons who aspire to a more skilled, higher-level career in animal healthcare. State regulations do not generally apply to workers at this level. However, state laws do define the specific actions that may only be performed by licensed workers.

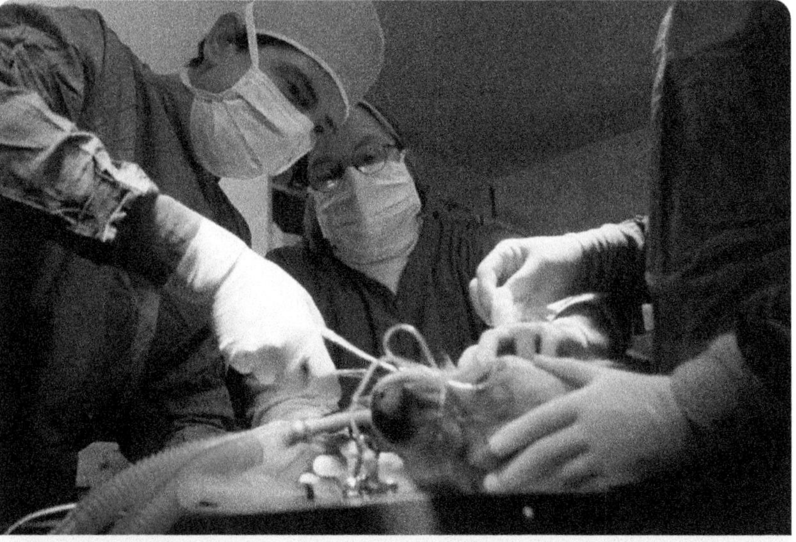

Fig. 24.4 Surgery A veterinarian and veterinary assistant perform surgery. *What safety precautions are being used during this procedure?*

Photos: (t)Duncan Smith/Getty Images, (b)Tom Stewart/CORBIS

Job Responsibilities of the Veterinary Assistant

Veterinary assistants perform a wide range of duties. **Figure 24.5** shows an assistant performing one of these job tasks. An assistant may work directly with the animals, or may work at the reception desk and perform any of the duties listed below.

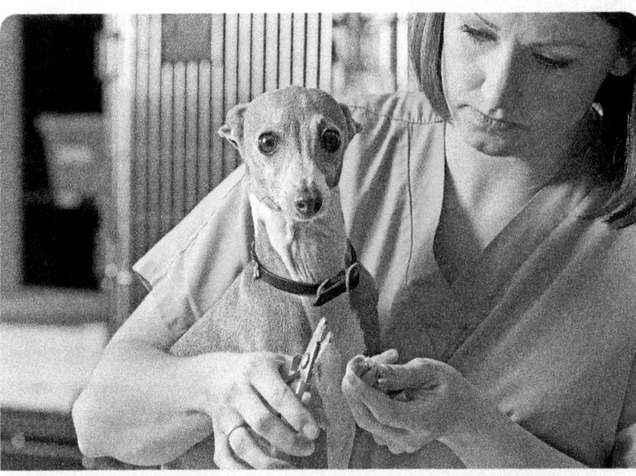

Fig. 24.5 Assistant An assistant working with a patient. *Can you name three other duties an assistant may perform?*

- Greet clients
- Answer phones
- Clean cages
- Exercise animals
- Feed animals
- Bathe animals
- Restrain animals so that various procedures can be performed
- Collect samples for diagnostic testing
- Maintain animal records
- Send reminders
- Collect payment for services

READING CHECK

Identify how state laws affect the responsibilities of veterinary assistants.

SECTION 24.1 Careers in Animal Healthcare Review

AFTER YOU READ

1. **Compare and contrast** the required education for a veterinarian and a veterinary technician.
2. **Explain** how the role of a veterinary technician differs from that of a veterinary assistant.
3. **List** eight areas of employment other than private clinical practice available to veterinarians.
4. **List** six positions other than in private clinical practice that are available to veterinary technicians.
5. **Identify** 3 potential hazards in a veterinary office.

Technology ONLINE EXPLORATIONS

Educational Options

Go online to find the closest schools in your area for veterinary medicine. Find out the qualifications for acceptance into these schools and determine how many students are accepted each year. Present your findings in a report to the class.

Photo: Malcolm MacGregor/Flickr/Getty Images

SECTION
24.2 Animal Healthcare Procedures

Vocabulary

Content Vocabulary

You will learn these content vocabulary terms in this section.

- **fecal examination**
- **centrifuge**
- **urinalysis**

Academic Vocabulary

You will see this word in your reading and on your tests. Find its meaning in the Glossary in the back of the book.

- **restrain**

Animal Care Procedures

What are some of the procedures performed in a veterinary office?

The procedures described below are performed on all animals, but vary slightly based upon the animal. This section will focus on procedures related to dogs. With minor changes, if any, these procedures can apply to cats and other animals. This is a sample of skills you would learn as an animal healthcare employee. Check the policies and procedures at your clinical location for specific information.

Mc Graw Hill connect™ ONLINE PROCEDURES

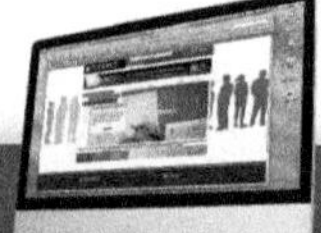

PROCEDURE 24-1

Bathing a Dog

Dogs are bathed for many reasons. Bathing is used to remove offensive odors, to treat various skin diseases, and to kill external parasites. The type of product used determines how long the product must remain on the skin before it is rinsed away. Review the directions on the product before you begin the bath procedure.

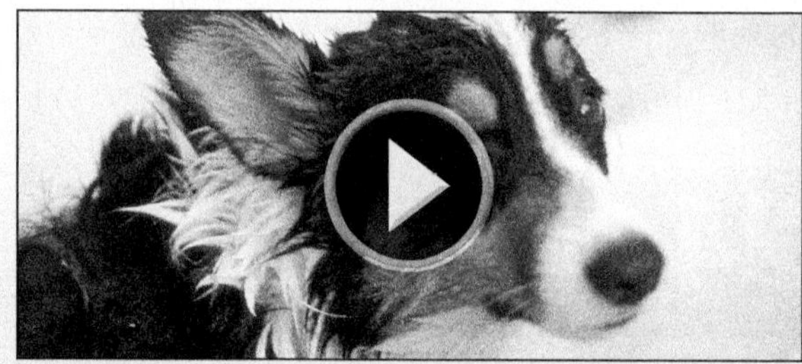

PROCEDURE 24-2

Giving a Pill to a Dog

Dogs do not necessarily like to take pills. It may be necessary to place the pill in the dog's mouth and force the dog to swallow it. When giving a pill to a dog, you should use a special technique to restrain and muzzle the animal. Practice on smaller and gentler dog breeds while you are learning this procedure.

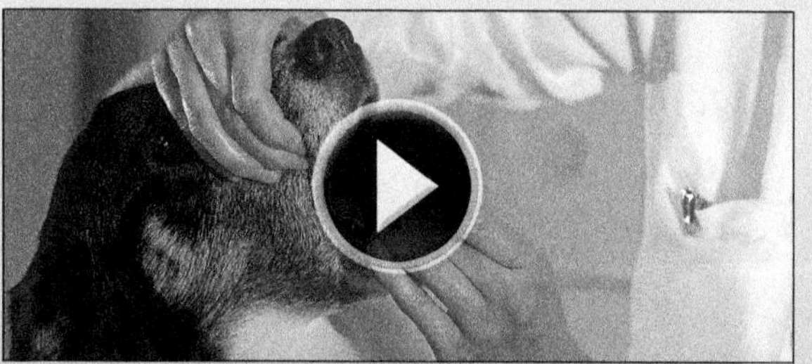

PROCEDURE 24-3

Performing a Fecal Examination

A **fecal examination** is commonly performed in veterinary hospitals as a diagnostic test for parasites. Parasites found in the stool of an animal indicate that an organism is living in the animal's intestines. This can be very harmful to the animal's health. The fecal specimen is tested using a **centrifuge** and a microscope.

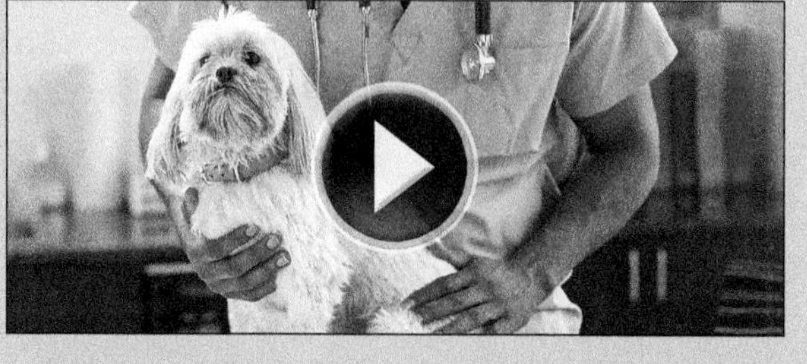

Photos: (t)Vicky Kasala/Photodisc/Getty Images, (c)Juniors Bildarchiv/Alamy, (b)Royalty-Free/CORBIS

connect ONLINE PROCEDURES

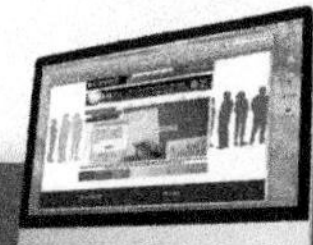

PROCEDURE 24-4

Performing a Urinalysis on a Dog

A **urinalysis** is a series of tests performed on urine. Results help the veterinarian determine whether the animal has a urinary tract infection or another disease that causes changes in the urine. It is a quick and easy procedure but demands close attention to detail.

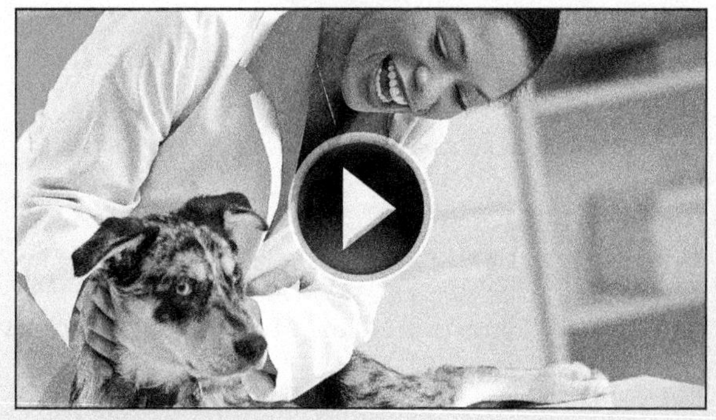

PROCEDURE 24-5

Administering a Medication by Subcutaneous Injection

Vaccinations and other medications are administered to animals by the subcutaneous route. You will remember that subcutaneous means "under the skin." Only sterile medications and equipment should be used for this procedure.

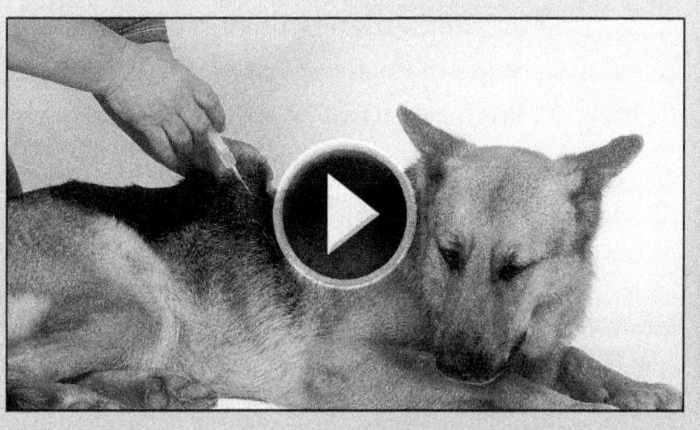

SECTION 24.2 Animal Healthcare Procedures Review

AFTER YOU READ

1. **Identify** what to look for in a fecal exam.
2. **Name** the protective precautions to take when bathing an animal.
3. **List** three reasons why a dog may need to be bathed.
4. **Recall** what must always be done after medicating an animal.
5. **Describe** where in a dog's mouth a pill should be placed.
6. **Identify** what a refractometer can tell about a urine sample.

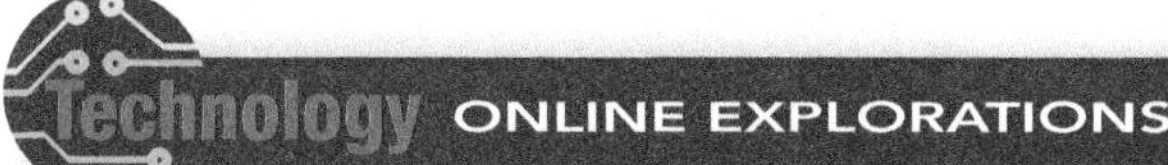

Examining Samples

Go online to learn more about what to expect when you examine urine or fecal samples from an animal. Search for terms such as "parasites," "urinalysis," "fecal sample," or "urine cells and casts." Write a brief report describing one abnormality that might be found and how it might affect the animal.

Photos: (t)JUPITERIMAGES/Comstock Premium/Alamy, (b)Juniors Bildarchiv/Alamy

CHAPTER

24 Review

Chapter Summary

SECTION 24.1

- Veterinarians study at least five species. Most schools train future vets to treat common domesticated and farm animals, such as dogs, cats, horses, cows, and sheep. **(pg. 600)**
- The course of study in the veterinary field is very broad and includes courses such as anatomy, hematology, and pathology. **(pg. 600)**
- A veterinarian is an animal healthcare professional who has completed at least six years of post-secondary education, graduated from a veterinary school, passed a comprehensive examination, and been licensed by his or her state. **(pg. 600)**
- Many professional opportunities are available to both veterinarians and veterinary technicians in addition to private clinical practice. **(pg. 601)**
- A veterinary technician has completed at least two years of post-secondary education, graduated from an appropriate program, and been certified, licensed, or registered by his or her state. **(pg. 602)**
- A veterinary assistant works in a veterinary practice and assists the veterinarian or veterinary technician. **(pg. 604)**

SECTION 24.2

- An animal needs to be bathed for a number of different reasons, and some of the products used may be hazardous to the bather. **(pg. 606)**
- Fecal exams and urinalysis procedures are common screening procedures used for animals in a veterinary hospital or clinic. **(pg. 606)**
- Vaccinations and other medications are administered to animals by subcutaneous injection. **(pg. 607)**

McGraw Hill connect™ **ONLINE ACTIVITIES**

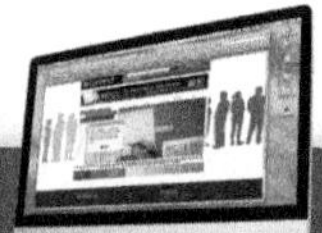

Complete our HST online activities for Chapter 24, which include Concept Check review questions, Reference Flash Cards, and Online Procedures assessment sheets.

- **Concept Check** review questions
- **Reference Flash Cards** medical terminology practice
- **Online Procedures** assessment sheets

CHAPTER 24 Assessment

Critical Thinking / Problem Solving

1. What would happen to an animal if intestinal parasites were not detected or were not identified correctly? How might this occur?
2. If an animal's urine test showed a high specific gravity, would this mean that the urine was concentrated or diluted?
3. A client has brought her 140-pound dog to your practice for its medicated bath. The dog is very aggressive and hates getting wet, and is already somewhat agitated upon arriving at the veterinarian's office. Describe the steps you would take to bathe this animal safely.
4. You are asked to perform a urinalysis on a dog's urine specimen. What precautions must you keep in mind in order to prevent the spread of infection during this procedure?
5. Practice giving a pill to a small, gentle dog. You may use your own pet and a dog treat or other small edible item when practicing. Follow the steps in **Procedure 24-2**, Giving a Pill to a Dog.

21ST CENTURY SKILLS

6. **Teamwork** With a partner or in a group, practice analyzing various specimens under a microscope.
7. **Critical Thinking** Research online or by contacting nearby veterinary schools to learn about the care and treatment of "exotic" animals not covered in this chapter. Prepare a report about the types of animals that are kept as pets but have needs that fall outside of the scope of traditional pet care. Include information about your community's laws or regulations regarding the types of animals that are allowed to be kept as pets. These may include small animals such as reptiles, large mammals, or other animals.
8. **Information Literacy** Using the American Veterinary Medical Association website, research at least two veterinary technology programs and a veterinary school located in your state or closest to your state. Determine the admission requirements for each of the programs and schools that you find. Write a brief report or be prepared to share your findings with the class.
9. **Information Literacy** Research online to find out more about the differences between giving an injection to an animal and to a human. Create a diagram, table, or report identifying these differences.

UNIT 3

Careers in Diagnostic Services

Photo: Ocean/CORBIS

CHAPTER 25

Medical Laboratory

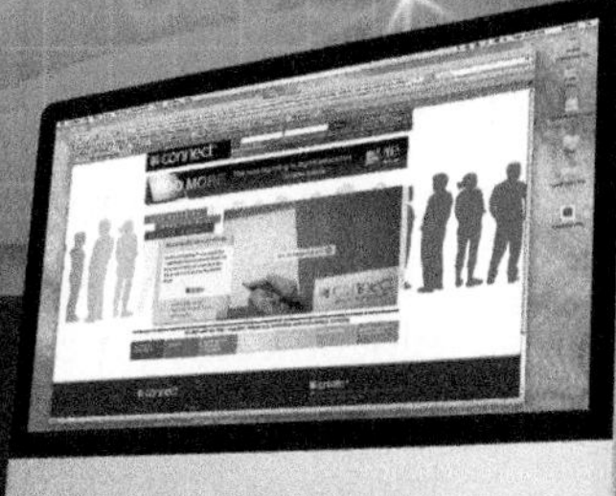

Essential Question:

Have you ever needed a lab test?

The medical laboratory is the site for a number of important diagnostic procedures. These are carried out by the phlebotomy technician, medical laboratory assistant, medical laboratory technician, medical laboratory scientist, histotechnician, histotechnologist, and cytotechnologist. These professionals work in clinical offices or clinic laboratories in physician group practices, hospitals, nursing homes, and other healthcare facilities. In this chapter, you will learn the role of each of these healthcare professionals, as well as the importance of aseptic technique and the classification of microorganisms and blood.

McGraw Hill connect™

It's Online!

- Online Procedures
- STEM Connection
- Medical Science
- Medical Terms
- Medical Math
- Ethics in Action
- Virtual Lab

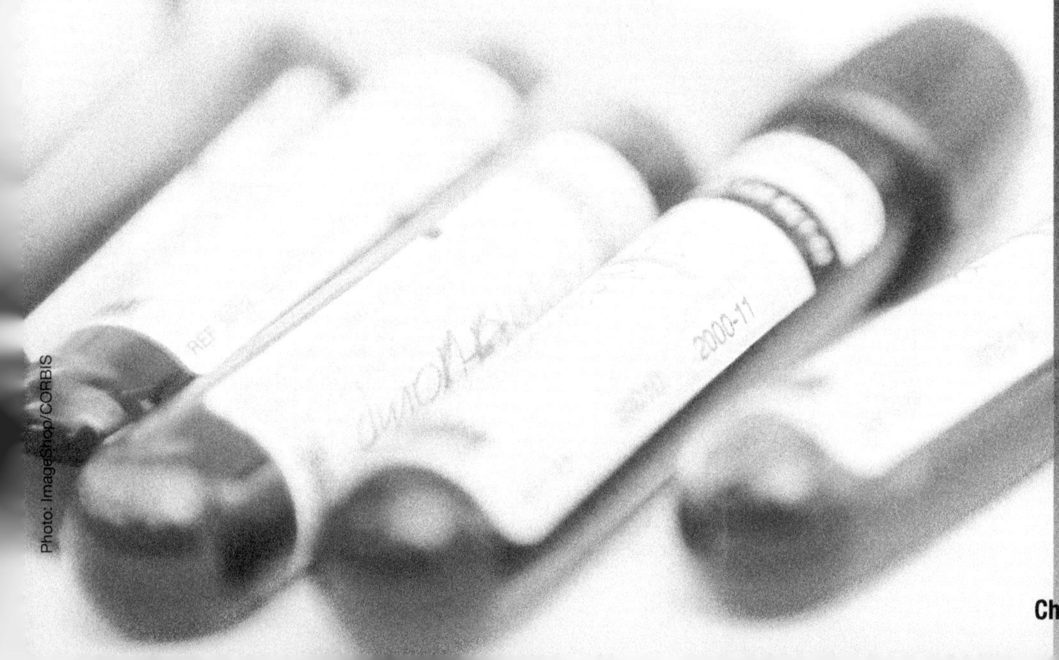

Photo: ImageShop/CORBIS

READING GUIDE

OBJECTIVES

After completing this chapter, you will be able to:

- **Compare** the roles and responsibilities of a phlebotomist, medical laboratory assistant, medical laboratory technician, medical laboratory scientist, histotechnician, histotechnologist, and cytologist.
- **Indicate** the various places where a medical laboratory worker can be employed.
- **Describe** phlebotomy.
- **Identify** various methods used to draw blood.
- **Explain** the importance of aseptic techniques during laboratory procedures.
- **Demonstrate** twenty-one medical laboratory procedures.

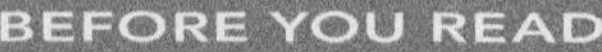

BEFORE YOU READ

Connect Have you ever wondered what happens to a specimen after the client leaves the doctor's office?

Main Idea

The medical laboratory is where healthcare professionals perform a wide range of important diagnostic procedures.

Note-Taking Activity

Draw this table. Write key terms and phrases under **Cues**. Write main ideas under **Note Taking**. Summarize the section under **Summary**.

Cues	Note Taking
o o	o o
Summary	

Graphic Organizer

Before you read the chapter, draw a diagram like the one to the right. As you read, write the careers covered in the chapter into the diagram.

Medical Laboratory Careers

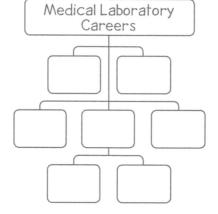

connect
Downloadable graphic organizers can be accessed online.

STANDARDS

HEALTH SCIENCE

NCHSE 1.31 Apply mathematical computations related to healthcare procedures (metric and household, conversions and measurements).

NCHSE 7.12 Describe methods of controlling the spread and growth of microorganisms.

SCIENCE

NSES F Develop understanding of personal and community health; population growth; natural resources; environmental quality; natural and human-induced hazards; science and technology in local, national, and global challenges.

NCHSE *National Consortium for Health Science Education*

NSES *National Science Education Standards*

COMMON CORE STATE STANDARDS

MATHEMATICS

Statistics and Probability

Making Inferences and Justifying Conclusions S-IC Make inferences and justify conclusions from sample surveys, experiments, and observational studies.

ENGLISH LANGUAGE ARTS

Speaking and Listening

Presentation of Knowledge and Ideas SL-4 Present information, findings, and supporting evidence clearly, concisely, and logically such that listeners can follow the line of reasoning and the organization, development, substance, and style are appropriate to purpose, audience, and task.

SECTION 25.1 Careers in Medical Laboratories

The Phlebotomy Technician

What methods do phlebotomy technicians use to collect blood samples?

Phlebotomy is the term for tests and procedures involving an incision, or cut, that is made into a vein or capillary in order to draw blood. Many diagnostic tests require a blood sample; these samples are collected by a phlebotomy technician, or phlebotomist. These professionals may be trained either on the job or in a formal training program. As recently as 2010, the vacancy rate for phlebotomists was 8%, making this a career with numerous opportunities.

Phlebotomy technicians use any number of methods to obtain blood samples. One of the two most commonly used methods is **venipuncture** (see **Figure 25.1**). This is the puncturing of a vein with a needle that is specially designed for blood collection. These needles have a threaded end connected to a holder that encloses special tubes for blood collection.

Phlebotomists also perform capillary punctures. This involves puncturing the skin and collecting blood samples from the smallest blood vessels, called capillaries. Most of the time, the capillary method is used for small samples. This method is frequently performed on infants and children.

Some phlebotomy technicians may be cross-trained in other areas. They may collect specimens for other types of tests, such as urine samples or throat cultures, and perform simple tests themselves on urine or blood samples. They may also assist laboratory personnel in other functions.

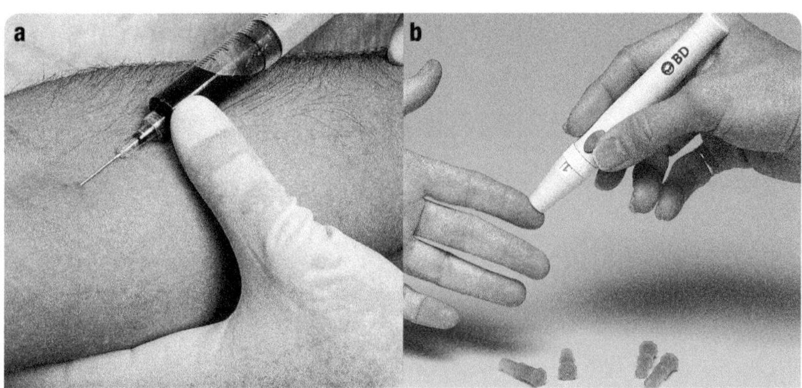

Fig. 25.1 Drawing Blood The phlebotomist commonly draws blood with venipuncture (a) or capillary puncture (b). *What is the difference between the two methods?*

Photos: (l)Kim Steele/Photodisc/Getty Images, (r)McGraw-Hill Companies, Inc./Kevin May, photographer

Vocabulary

Content Vocabulary

You will learn these content vocabulary terms in this section.

- **phlebotomy**
- **venipuncture**
- **waived tests**
- **quality control**

Academic Vocabulary

You will see this word in your reading and on your tests. Find its meaning in the Glossary in the back of the book.

- **accurately**

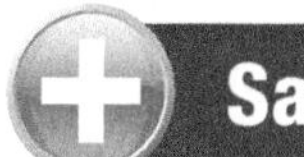

Safety

Invasive Laboratory Procedures

Capillary blood collection is considered an invasive surgical procedure because the skin is penetrated with a sterile lancet. For that reason, this type of blood collection is regulated by specific rules and regulations. Strict standard precautions should be followed at all times. Before performing this or any other invasive procedure, first make sure that it is within your scope of practice.

Table 25.1 Overview of Medical Laboratory Careers

OCCUPATION	EDUCATIONAL REQUIREMENTS	CERTIFICATION OR LICENSING AGENCY	JOB OUTLOOK
Phlebotomy technician	High school diploma. Graduation from an approved phlebotomy program or on-the-job training. Various routes of certification include clinical practice.	American Medical Technologists American Society of Clinical Pathologists American Society of Phlebotomy Technicians National Phlebotomy Association	Average growth
Medical laboratory assistant (MLA)	Graduation from an accredited program or institution. Various routes of certification and registration including passing a national examination.	American Association of Medical Assistants American Medical Technologists American Society of Clinical Pathologists	Above average growth
Medical laboratory technician (MLT)	Minimum two-year degree or certificate from hospital, or postsecondary vocational-technical or Armed Forces school. National certification examination must be passed.	American Medical Technologists American Society of Clinical Pathologists	Average, with greater growth in workplaces other than the inpatient hospital
Medical laboratory scientist (MLS)	Minimum four-year degree in medical technology or life sciences. Passing a national certification examination.	American Medical Technologists American Society of Clinical Pathologists International Society for Clinical Laboratory Technology	Above average growth
Histotechnician (HT)	Graduation from an accredited program or institution. Various routes of certification and registration, including passing a national examination.	American Society of Clinical Pathologists	Above average growth
Histotechnologist (HTL)	Minimum four-year degree in an accredited program or institution. National certification examination must be passed.	American Society of Clinical Pathologists	Average growth
Cytotechnologist (CT)	Minimum four-year degree in an accredited program or institution. National certification examination must be passed.	American Society of Clinical Pathologists	Above average growth

Usually, phlebotomy technicians work in a hospital or large clinic. Other job opportunities are in smaller clinics, clinical offices, large group practices, laboratories, nursing homes, blood banks, and health departments. In a smaller clinic or clinical office, the phlebotomist is likely to be responsible for more patient interaction than in a larger facility.

Some phlebotomists are employed by insurance companies to perform routine testing for insurance. These technicians are also usually cross-trained to perform other procedures, such as urine collection, electrocardiograms (ECGs or EKGs), and vital signs. They may also complete insurance questionnaires.

Phlebotomy technicians are valuable members of the healthcare team. They are responsible for ensuring that specimens collected are properly identified. The results given to the physician are only as good as the phlebotomist's accuracy and attention to detail while collecting the sample.

The Job of the Phlebotomy Technician

The primary job of the phlebotomy technician involves patient interaction during the process of obtaining blood samples. A phlebotomist must of course have the required knowledge and expertise, but also must have a professional appearance and a personality suited to dealing with patients who are nervous or frightened. The phlebotomy technician is the main person patients interact with in the clinical setting. It is challenging to reassure or comfort a patient while at the same time obtaining the required specimen. Patients often feel comfortable enough with the phlebotomist to ask questions concerning their healthcare, so the phlebotomy technician must recognize the importance of patient confidentiality.

Job Responsibilities of the Phlebotomy Technician

The most important job responsibility of the phlebotomy technician is the correct identification of the blood sample that has been collected for testing. This is the responsibility of any professional who performs phlebotomy, regardless of his or her job title.

Other responsibilities of the phlebotomy technician are:

- Explaining the procedure to patients
- Obtaining the correct specimen in the correct manner
- Treating all samples correctly
- Transporting the specimen in the proper manner to the designated location
- Accurately labeling all samples
- Maintaining patient confidentiality

READING CHECK

Name some tasks that phlebotomy technicians may perform in addition to collecting blood samples.

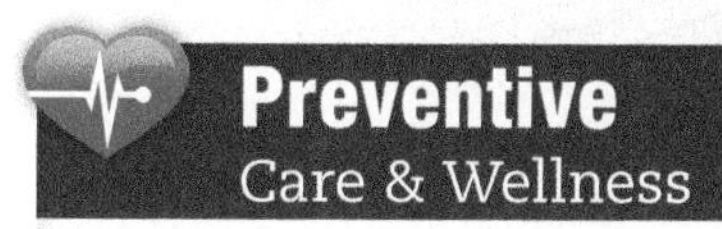

Maintain your Cholesterol

Cholesterol is a waxy, fat-like substance that occurs naturally in all parts of the body. It is needed in a small amount for the body to function normally. There are two types of cholesterol: low-density lipoprotein (LDL, or "bad" cholesterol) and high-density lipoprotein (HDL, or "good," useful cholesterol). If you have too much LDL cholesterol, the excess is deposited in arteries, including the coronary arteries. These deposits contribute to narrowing and blockages that cause the signs and symptoms of heart disease.

Heredity, age, and gender all contribute to high cholesterol. These are factors you cannot control. But there are other factors that you can control.

- Reduce your intake of fats.
- Maintain your weight at a normal level.
- Exercise regularly.
- Avoid excessive alcohol and stress.

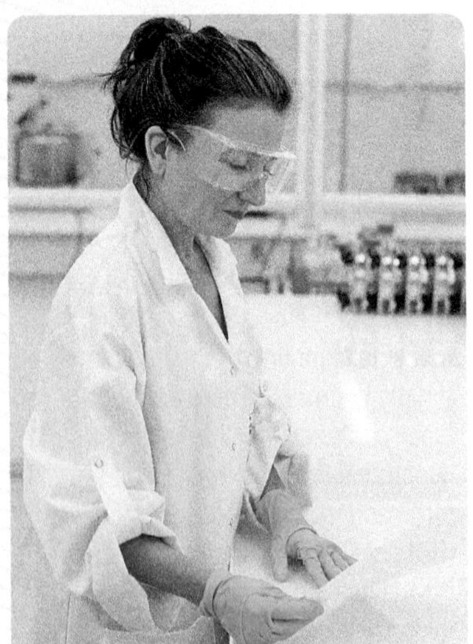

Fig. 25.2 Face Shield It is important to use a face shield or eye protection while performing laboratory tests. *Why are face and eye protection so important?*

Medical Laboratory Assistant

What is a waived test?

Medical laboratory assistants (MLA) often start at the phlebotomy technician level. They are then trained to perform low-complexity tests. In the lab, they may work under the supervision of a medical laboratory scientist. In a clinic or clinical office, a nurse or physician may direct the MLA.

The Job of the Medical Laboratory Assistant

The MLA performs many lab tests to help the physician diagnose diseases (see **Figure 25.2**). He or she may collect specimens, prepare them for testing, analyze the samples, and report the results.

Many lab tests performed by MLAs are called **waived tests.** This means that lab workers, with the training of an MLA and other healthcare personnel, can perform the analysis. Waived tests are subject to the same **quality control** requirements as other more complex tests. They are regulated by personnel who have a higher level of education and training than the MLA.

Waived tests are defined by the Clinical Laboratory Improvement Amendments of 1988 (CLIA). Although laboratories must register to perform these tests, there are no specific personnel, quality control, quality assurance, or proficiency testing requirements. But laboratory personnel who perform these tests must follow carefully the manufacturer's instructions on use of the testing equipment.

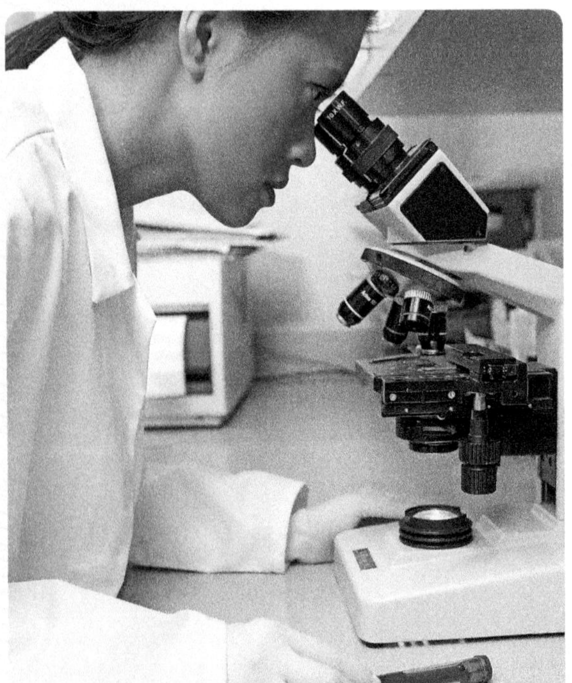

Fig. 25.3 Laboratories A clinical office laboratory may be large or small. *What would be the advantages of working in a small laboratory? A large laboratory?*

Medical laboratory assistants use sophisticated laboratory equipment. They must measure fluids with accuracy, follow instructions fully, and be responsible for patient and specimen identification. In a clinic or clinical office, the medical laboratory assistant performs ECGs or EKGs, calculates and gives injections, and conducts breathing tests along with his or her phlebotomy and specimen-testing duties. **Figure 25.3** shows an MLA assisting in a clinical office.

MLAs in clinical offices may remove sutures or change wound dressings. Often they are responsible for sterilizing medical instruments and documenting daily quality control. Many MLAs are also responsible for patient education. For example, they instruct patients about collection techniques or diet restrictions in preparation for a medical test.

MLAs may also be responsible for taking and accurately recording vital signs and medical histories. In addition, MLAs may also be trained to perform administrative or front office responsibilities. In this capacity they may assist the office manager (see **Figure 25.4**).

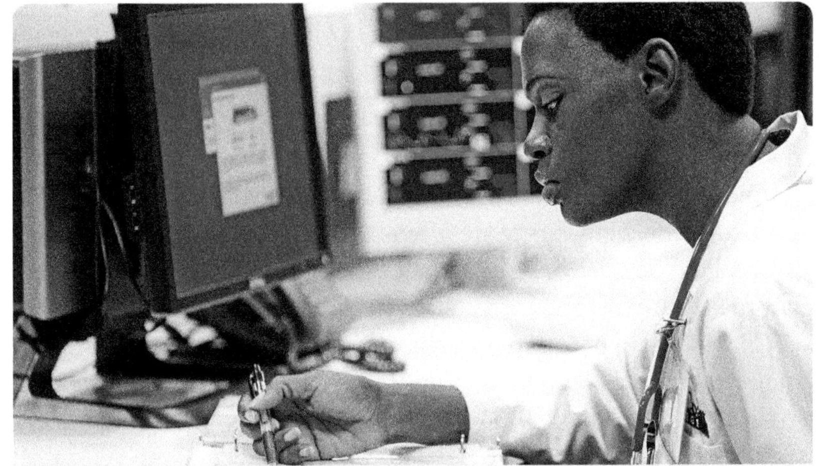

Fig. 25.4 Documentation Electronic health record documentation is performed by medical laboratory professionals. *How is unauthorized access to patient records prevented?*

Of the medical laboratory careers in this chapter, the job of the MLA has the greatest growth potential. One reason for this is the increase in preventive testing. MLAs often perform those tests.

Job Responsibilities of the Medical Laboratory Assistant

The MLA is responsible for the following:

- Identifying the patient
- Identifying the proper procedure for specimen collection
- Collecting the specimen properly
- Accurately labeling the specimen
- Properly transporting the specimen
- Performing waived lab tests
- Transmitting accurate and timely reports to the physician
- Maintaining patient confidentiality

Some tests that a medical laboratory assistant does in addition to regular sample collection are:

- Collecting throat specimens for culture of organisms
- Preparing bacteriological smears
- Staining culture smears with Gram's stain for use in organism identification
- Testing urine with chemical reagent strips
- Testing urine for glucose using copper reduction
- Collecting capillary blood samples
- Performing blood glucose and cholesterol tests

Several of these tests will be explained in Section 25.2.

READING CHECK

Explain the job outlook for medical laboratory assistants.

21ST CENTURY SKILLS

Recording Information

Recording information accurately, whether in writing or electronically, is an essential part of the MLA's duties. Documentation in a patient's medical record is important from a legal as well as a medical perspective. The physician's appointment book and the patient's chart are considered legal documents. Great care must be taken to ensure the accuracy and strict confidentiality of the information entered. According to the American Association of Medical Assistants, the following areas are essential in applying legal concepts to communication.

- Maintain confidentiality.
- Properly prepare and maintain medical records.
- Document accurately.
- Follow appropriate guidelines when releasing information.
- Follow employer's established policies dealing with the healthcare contract.
- Follow legal guidelines and keep informed about healthcare legislation and regulations.

Follow-up

Why is it important to keep the appointment schedule and medical records confidential? What could happen if you did not?

Medical Laboratory Technician

What types of tests are performed by medical laboratory technicians?

The medical laboratory technician (MLT) prepares specimens and runs automatic analyzers more often than he or she collects samples. MLTs follow detailed instructions when they perform manual tests. They make sure that the correct data is conveyed to the physician. The MLT may work in one of many areas in a clinical lab, under the supervision of a medical laboratory scientist. However, when they work in a physician's office lab or clinic, they may be the person in charge.

The Job of the Medical Laboratory Technician

Medical laboratory technicians perform routine tests on blood, tissue, cells, and other body fluids, which help in the diagnosis and treatment of diseases. MLTs perform less complex tests and lab procedures than medical laboratory scientists. For example, they may prepare specimens and operate automated analyzers. They may also perform manual tests following detailed instructions.

MLTs may work in several areas of the clinical laboratory or specialize in just one. They may choose to work only in blood banks, chemistry, hematology, immunology, or microbiology. They usually work under the supervision of medical laboratory scientists or laboratory managers (see **Figure 25.5**).

Job Responsibilities of the Medical Laboratory Technician

The MLT will perform a variety of duties. Here are some common responsibilities:

- Operate automated instruments
- Troubleshoot problems with the equipment
- Prepare chemical solutions

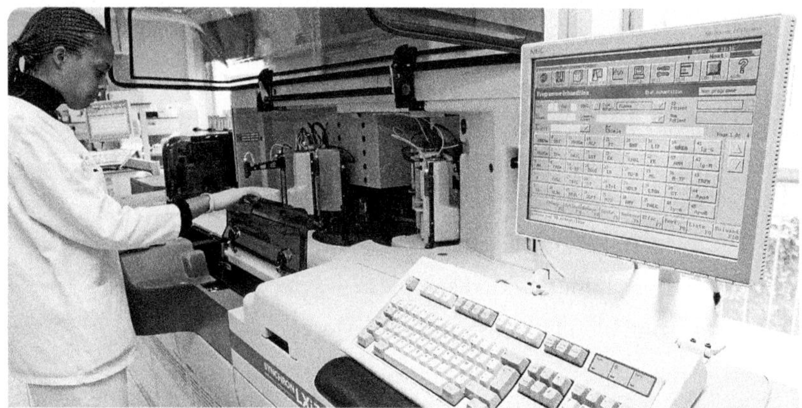

Fig. 25.5 Automation Automated instruments are used by medical laboratory technicians. *Do you think that automated or manual laboratory equipment would be easier to use?*

- Perform moderate complexity tests
- Maintain quality control for the tests being performed
- Keep accurate records

READING CHECK

List some medical facilities that employ medical laboratory technicians.

Medical Laboratory Scientist

How does a medical laboratory scientist help operate a laboratory?

Medical laboratory scientists (MLS), formerly called medical technologists or clinical laboratory scientists, are highly trained, highly skilled scientists. Most MLSs need little or no supervision. They are able to perform a range of tests from the routine to the highly complex. Given their background and education, MLSs may also be teachers, supervisors, laboratory managers, or researchers. In 2010, the average vacancy rate for all jobs (MLT and MLS) in blood banks, chemistry, hematology, immunology, and microbiology combined was 8%, with blood banks showing the greatest shortage at nearly 12%.

The Job of the Medical Laboratory Scientist

Medical laboratory scientists perform many types of tests that may be very complex. They look for fungi, bacteria, parasites, and other microorganisms (microbiology). They analyze the chemical content of blood and body fluids, and test for therapeutic levels of drugs in the blood, to determine how well a patient is responding to treatment (chemistry). They cross-match blood for transfusions (immunohematology/blood bank). They perform tests to detect bleeding and clotting disorders, count cells, and look for abnormal cells in order to detect anemia, leukemia, and other diseases of the blood (hematology). They can also perform many DNA-based tests to detect infectious diseases or genetic mutations (molecular diagnostics).

Laboratory scientists use automated equipment and instruments capable of performing a number of tests simultaneously. Some chemistry analyzers can test for several chemicals at the same time. Laboratory scientists evaluate test results and relay them to physicians. With increasing automation and the use of computer technology, the work of medical laboratory scientists has become more analytical. The complexity of tests performed, the degree of judgment needed, and the levels of responsibility workers assume depend largely on the amount of education and experience they have. The laboratory scientist can also supervise laboratory sections or manage the entire laboratory, research and validate new tests and procedures, and maintain the laboratory's information systems.

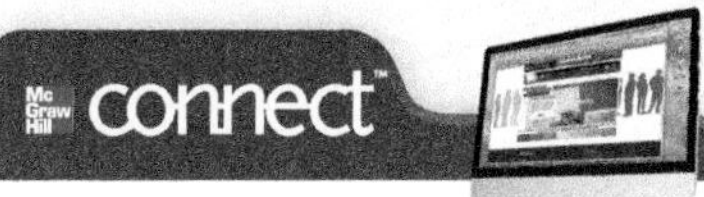

STEM CONNECTION

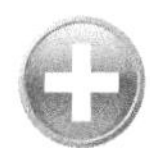

Medical Math

Laboratory Solutions

Medical laboratory tests often involve the use of reagents, which are solutions made up of mixtures of chemicals that react in known ways with a tested substance such as blood or other body fluids. Reagents can be mixed using weight-to-weight ratios and weight-to-volume ratios.

connect Go online to learn how to calculate weight-to-weight ratios and weight-to-volume ratios.

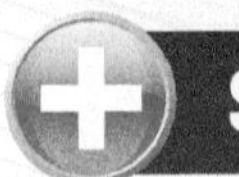

Safety

Disinfection

Medical lab professionals must keep equipment and lab areas clean through disinfection at all times. Disinfection greatly reduces the number of pathogenic (disease-producing) microorganisms. Commercially prepared solutions are available, but you may also use a solution of household bleach and tap water. If you do this, a fresh solution of disinfectant must be prepared each working day. Label the solution with the name, date, and the initials of the person who prepared it. When cleaning, make sure the item is completely soaked and then dried to ensure that pathogens are killed.

The Centers for Disease Control and Prevention (CDC) recommends two concentrations of bleach solution:

- 1:10 bleach solution is a strong solution used to disinfect bodies and items contaminated with body waste. Mix 1 part household bleach with 9 parts of tap water.
- 1:100 bleach solution is used to disinfect surfaces and equipment, patient bedding, and reusable protective clothing before it is laundered. Mix 1 part of the 1:10 solution with 9 parts of tap water.

Job Responsibilities of the Medical Laboratory Scientist

The medical laboratory scientist performs many complex tasks, including:

- Identifying fungi, parasites, or bacteria
- Examining and analyzing body fluids including blood, tissues, and cells
- Performing therapeutic drug tests
- Preparing and cross-matching blood for transfusion
- Detecting the presence of leukemia, anemia, clotting disorders, and other blood disorders
- Analyzing the chemical content of blood and body fluids
- Testing for genetic mutation
- Determining antibiotic susceptibility of microorganisms
- Detecting the presence of infectious disease
- Reporting patient sensitivity to antibiotics or identified microorganisms
- Interpreting results to assist physicians in the diagnosis of disease
- Operating and maintaining complex precision equipment
- Developing procedures, quality control, and quality assurance
- Maintaining the integrity of the laboratory information system
- Supervising laboratory personnel
- Teaching laboratory students

READING CHECK

Recall some types of tests performed by medical laboratory scientists.

Histotechnician

How do histotechnicians assist pathologists?

The histotechnician (HT) prepares tiny sections of body tissues that have been removed from patients during surgical procedures. The preparations, sometimes called specimens, are examined by pathologists (doctors who work in the lab). These prepared tissues help to diagnosis diseases and determine the best treatment for patients.

The Job of the Histotechnician

Histotechnicians receive specimens and may assist pathologists during dissection of tissue. The HT treats the tissues with various chemicals and embeds the tissues in wax. He or she then slices tiny sections from the wax block that contains the tissue and places them on slides. The slides are then stained, to make them ready to show the pathologist.

Histotechnologist

Why do histotechnologists need management skills?

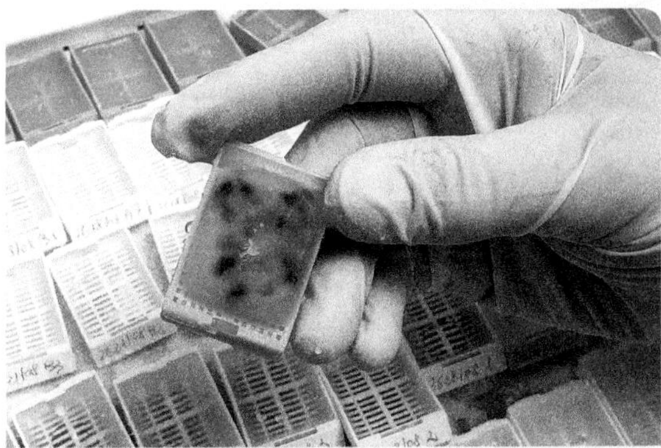

Fig. 25.6 Specimen This tissue specimen is a wax preparation. *Which laboratory professionals would work with a specimen like this one?*

The histotechnologist (HTL) performs many of the same functions as the histotechnician. However, additional education and training (See **Table 25.1** on page 614) is required for the HTL. This education and training provides the histotechnologist with a better understanding of specimen collection, handling, and preparation processes. In 2010, the vacancy rate for histotechnologists was 10%.

The Job of the Histotechnologist

Histotechnologists are responsible for managing the histology laboratory. For this reason, they must have management and leadership skills. Also needed are critical thinking skills to troubleshoot technical issues and instrument problems. They must understand how underlying disease may cause unusual results during processing of tissues. HTLs can also evaluate new stains and procedures for use in the histology laboratory.

Job Responsibilities of the Histotechnician and Histotechnologist

Histotechnicians and histotechnologists perform simple to complex tasks, including:

- Assisting in the sampling of body tissue specimens (see **Figure 25.6**)
- Using various chemicals to preserve tissues
- Working with delicate instruments and sharp knives
- Carrying out detailed staining procedures
- Working closely with a pathologist

READING CHECK

Summarize the job outlook for histotechnologists in the near future.

Cytotechnologist

What do cytotechnologists look for in human cells?

The cytotechnologist (CT) performs microscopic analysis of cells to determine the presence of cancer or other diseases. The CT must be familiar with normal and abnormal anatomy and histology, and must understand how diseases cause changes in body tissues. In 2010, the vacancy rate for cytotechnologists was 5%.

The Job of the Cytotechnologist

Cytotechnologists are responsible for judging whether human cells are normal or abnormal. If cells are abnormal, the CT works closely with the pathologist to determine the presence of cancer or other diseases. CTs need very little supervision. They must have excellent eyesight and enjoy detail work, because they spend many hours a day examining cells under a microscope.

Job Responsibilities of the Cytotechnologist

The CT may perform many of the following tasks:

- Prepare and stain slides
- Use the microscope to examine cells
- Troubleshoot staining problems
- Determine if cells are normal or cancerous, or display signs of another disease
- Work closely with a pathologist

READING CHECK

Analyze why good eyesight would be important to the cytotechnologist.

SECTION 25.1 Careers in Medical Laboratories Review

AFTER YOU READ

1. **Name** the medical laboratory career that shows greater growth in areas outside the inpatient hospital.
2. **Identify** the career in the medical laboratory field that requires the most education.
3. **List** the main job responsibilities of the medical laboratory assistant.
4. **Define** phlebotomy.
5. **Assess** the importance of patient confidentiality in the healthcare field.
6. **Compare** and **contrast** the jobs of a cytotechnologist and a histotechnologist.

Technology ONLINE EXPLORATIONS

Opportunities in Your Location

Research online or in other sources to find a school or an on-the-job training program in your area for one of the careers discussed in this chapter. If possible, interview someone currently working in that area of healthcare. From the information you obtain, write a report explaining why you would or would not choose this career field. Give specific reasons for your decision.

SECTION 25.2 Medical Laboratory Procedures

Collecting Specimens

How must specimens be labeled?

When collecting specimens, the medical laboratory professional must

- practice aseptic technique, including disinfecting the work area.
- assemble the correct collection methods, containers, and transport systems.
- know how to obtain the specimen without causing harm, discomfort, or embarrassment to the patient.
- ask the patient about any allergies or current medications that might affect the results of the test being performed.
- give clear, complete information and instructions to the patient regarding the collection method.
- collect the specimen in the proper manner and at the correct time.
- collect the proper quantity of the specimen so that the procedure does not have to be repeated.
- label all specimens with the patient's name, date, and time of collection. Include other required information such as the time and site of the specimen, the physician's name, your initials, and the patient's identification number, age, birth date, gender, or address.

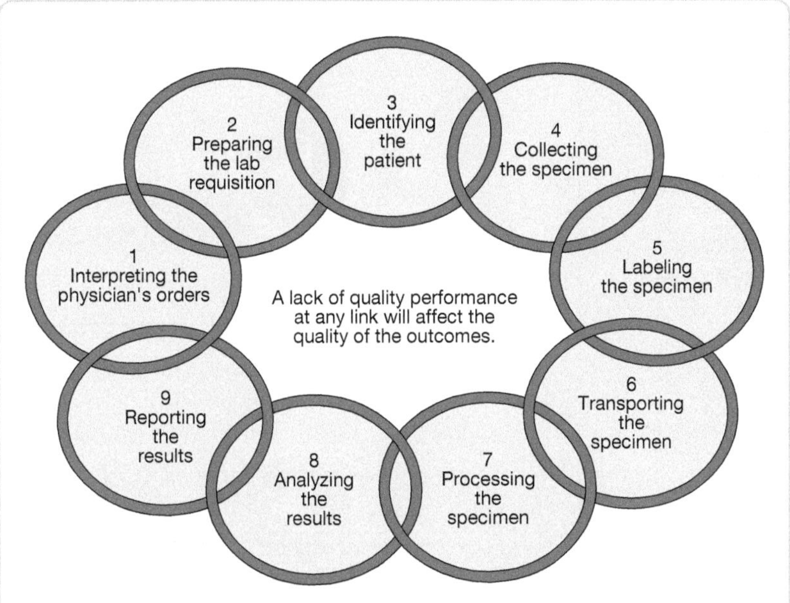

Fig. 25.7 Communication Several communication skills are involved in collecting a laboratory specimen. *What are those communication skills?*

Vocabulary

Content Vocabulary

You will learn these content vocabulary terms in this section.

- **Gram's stain**
- **hematocrit**
- **hemoglobin**
- **reagent**
- **point-of-care testing**

Academic Vocabulary

You will see this word in your reading and on your tests. Find its meaning in the Glossary in the back of this book.

- **identify**

21st CENTURY SKILLS

Communication in the Medical Laboratory Setting

Medical laboratory personnel must perform various procedures. In order for these procedures to have the most accurate results and be of the highest quality, the laboratory communication process must be smooth and efficient. **Figure 25.7** shows the steps in this process. It is essential to practice good communication skills and follow these steps for accurate and successful laboratory practice.

- establish that it is lawful and within the laboratory regulations to perform a diagnostic laboratory test before you perform it. These regulations have been established for quality assurance purposes.

READING CHECK

Summarize what medical laboratory personnel must consider before collecting a specimen.

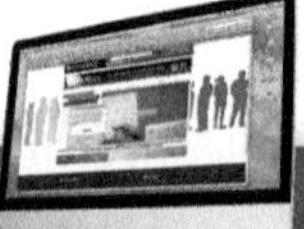

connect ONLINE PROCEDURES

PROCEDURE 25-1

Preparing Bacteriological Smears

Infections happen when microorganisms invade and multiply within the body. This causes disease. An infection may be in one part of the body, or it may involve the entire body. The MLA collects the specimen. If the assistant is trained to do so, he or she may also perform the required microbiological procedure. When the microorganism is identified, the physician can treat the patient.

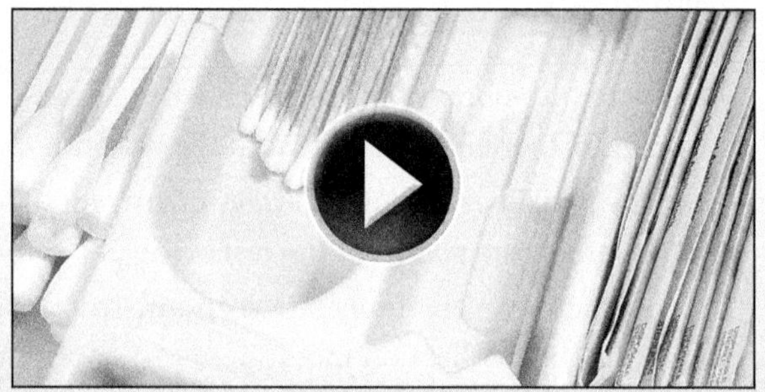

PROCEDURE 25-2

Inoculating an Agar Plate

Agar is a seaweed extract made of different types of algae and is used to grow bacteria and other microorganisms. Agar supplies nutrients so that the microorganisms can grow. It is contained in tubes or plates, called petri dishes. Sheep's blood agar is the choice for growing organisms suspected of causing strep throat. The agar plate is inoculated in a specific pattern using a culture swab and an inoculating loop.

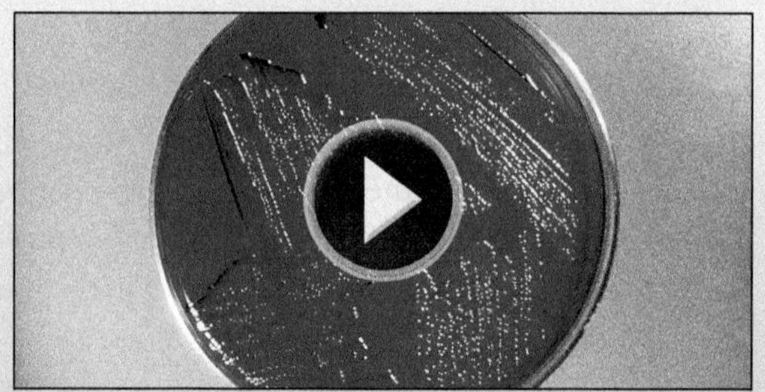

PROCEDURE 25-3

Staining Culture Smears with Gram's Stain

Various stains are applied to a culture smear. These help **identify** the microorganisms present in the specimen. Proper identification helps a physician diagnose and treat infections. **Gram's stain** is the most frequently used stain. The degree to which bacterial walls hold the violet color of Gram's stain is used to classify them as gram-positive or gram-negative bacteria, which assists in their identification.

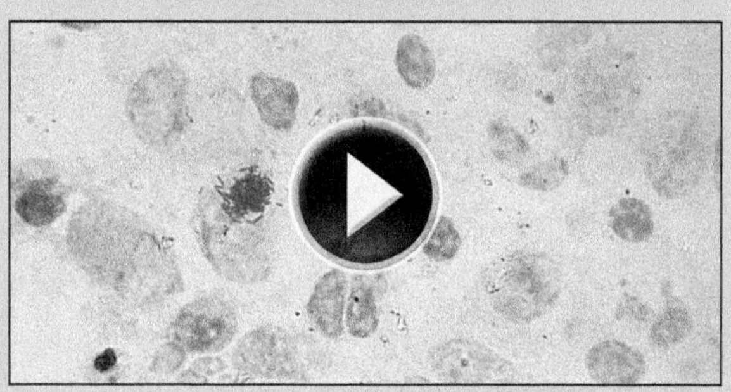

PROCEDURE 25-4

Performing a Rapid Strep Test

If a patient has a sore throat, the organism that the physician most likely wants to identify is *Streptococcus pyogenes* (strep). A rapid strep test is an example of a **point-of-care test,** which provides quick, reliable results in about 15 minutes. Prior to the rapid strep test, at least 24 hours were needed for an organism to be cultured, incubated, and examined. Quick identification allows for a fast treatment.

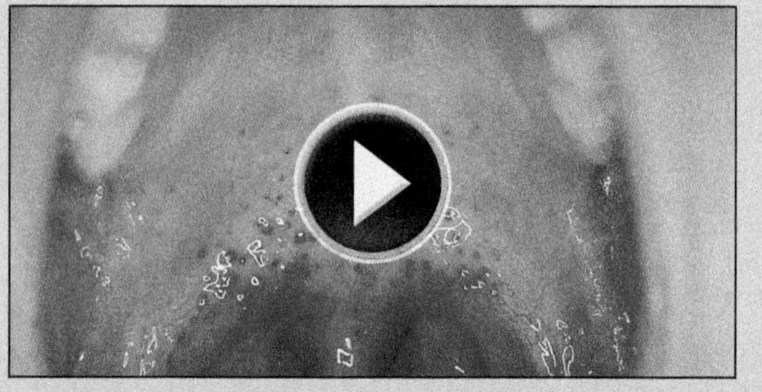

Photos: (t to b)Image Source/Jupiterimages, CDC, CDC, CDC

Performing Tests on Urine

What information can be gained from a urine analysis?

One of the oldest—yet still useful—tests for the rapid screening of many diseases is a urine analysis, or urinalysis. The test gives information about carbohydrate metabolism and liver or kidney function. It also shows the acid-base balance. It can reveal that the patient has a urinary tract infection (UTI).

Urine can be tested with chemical strips or tablets. Larger labs and hospitals have automated equipment that performs many tests in a short amount of time. If an MLA is working with this equipment, he or she may perform confirmatory or other screening tests under the supervision of an MLS.

READING CHECK

Name the ways in which urine can be tested.

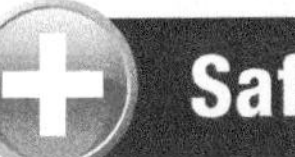

Safety

Handling Body Fluids

As a medical laboratory professional, you will handle many body fluids including blood, culture specimens, and urine. You may also deal with patients who are hospitalized. You must observe standard precautions when you come into contact with patients and their body fluids, so that you will not be contaminated or infected or become a source of contamination. Review Chapter 3, Safety and Infection Control Practices, and follow standard precautions at all times.

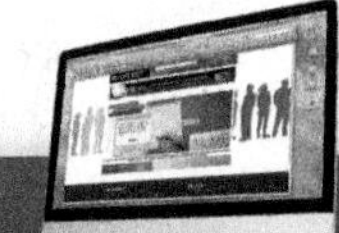

Mc Graw Hill connect™ ONLINE PROCEDURES

PROCEDURE 25-5

Assessing Urine for Color and Turbidity

Examining the urine for color and turbidity (cloudiness) can give the physician an indication of the concentration or the presence of bacteria. Other characteristics of urine, such as clarity, odor, and amount are also significant.

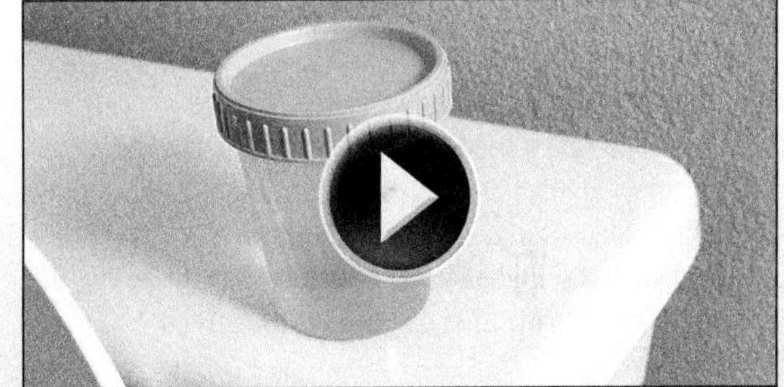

PROCEDURE 25-6

Measuring Specific Gravity Using a Urinometer

The specific gravity test measures the concentration of urine. Substances dissolved in urine increase the specific gravity of urine. These substances include proteins, sugars, and salts. The specific gravity measurement is based on the specific gravity of distilled water being equal to 1.000. Substances dissolved in urine will cause the specific gravity of urine to be greater than that of distilled water.

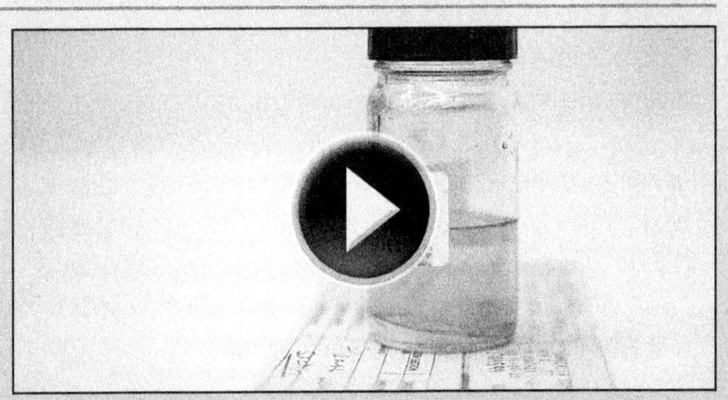

PROCEDURE 25-7

Testing Urine with Chemical Reagent Strips

Medical laboratory assistants usually test urine with plastic strips treated with various **reagents** that react to substances in the urine. These strips, called reagent strips or dipsticks, are the most widely used method of detecting chemicals in the urine. When an area on a dipstick reacts with a substance in the patient's urine, it changes color. This change helps physicians diagnose and treat the patient.

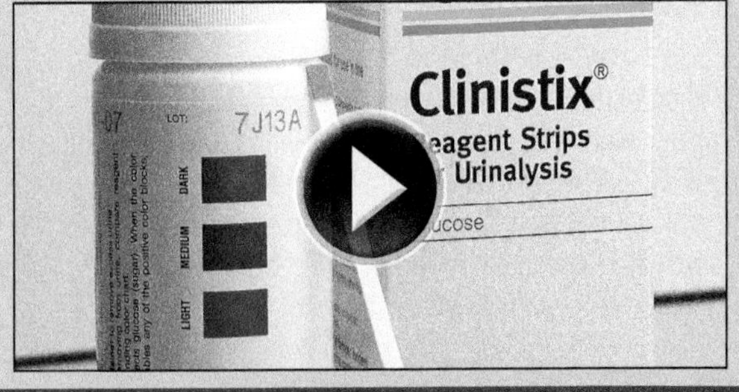

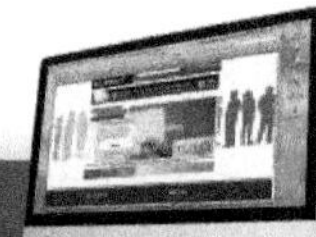

Mc Graw Hill connect™ ONLINE PROCEDURES

PROCEDURE 25-8

Microscopic Urine Analysis

The microscope is used to evaluate urine after it is centrifuged. By spinning the urine at high speed, a centrifuge concentrates the solids present in the urine at the bottom of the tube. The sediment is then examined for cells, casts, crystals, yeast, bacteria, and parasites. It is important that all healthcare personnel in a laboratory use the same counting and reporting system so that urine evaluation is consistent.

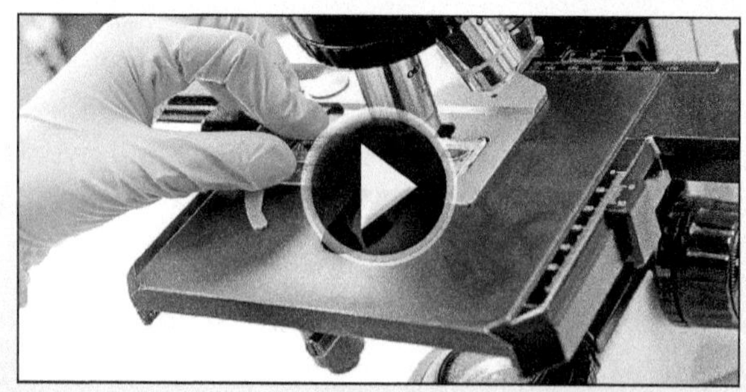

PROCEDURE 25-9

Performing Tests for Infectious Mononucleosis

A rapid test exists for infectious mononucleosis, an acute disease caused by the Epstein-Barr virus or cytomegalovirus. The disease is characterized by fever, weakness, lymphadenopathy, hepatosplenomegaly, and atypical lymphocytes that resemble monocytes. The patient exhibits unexplained fever, fatigue, and sore throat. A rapid test, which can be done in about 15 minutes, helps the physician diagnose the disease.

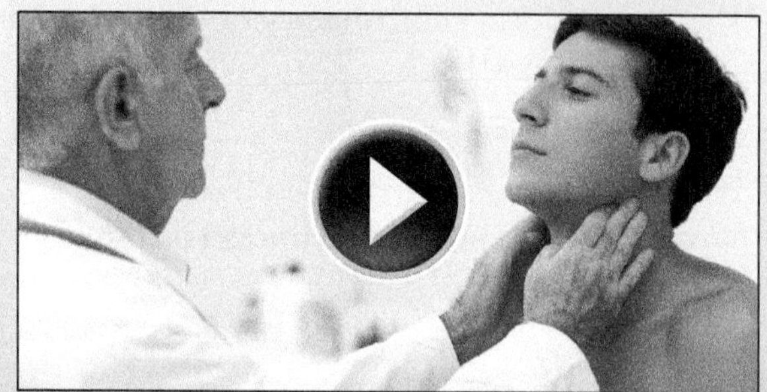

PROCEDURE 25-10

Testing Urine for Glucose Using Copper Reduction

Results obtained from chemical reagent strips are very specific and rarely need to be double checked by a different method. When the glucose test on the reagent strip is positive, it indicates the presence of glucose but no other sugars. A screening test that detects other sugars, such as lactose, galactose, and glucose is called the copper reduction test.

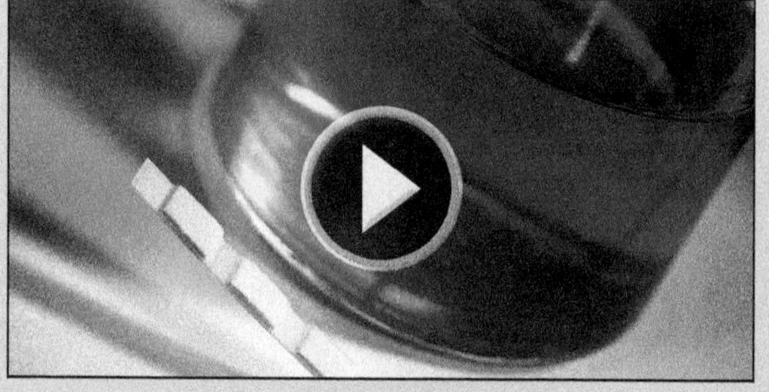

PROCEDURE 25-11

Performing a Pregnancy Test

This test detects the presence or absence of human chorionic gonadotropin (HCG) in the urine. HCG is found in the urine during pregnancy. A first morning urine specimen is the best for pregnancy testing. This is when the concentration of HCG is the highest. These tests are often used in physician office laboratories, but they have a high rate of false positives and false negatives because of problems with technique.

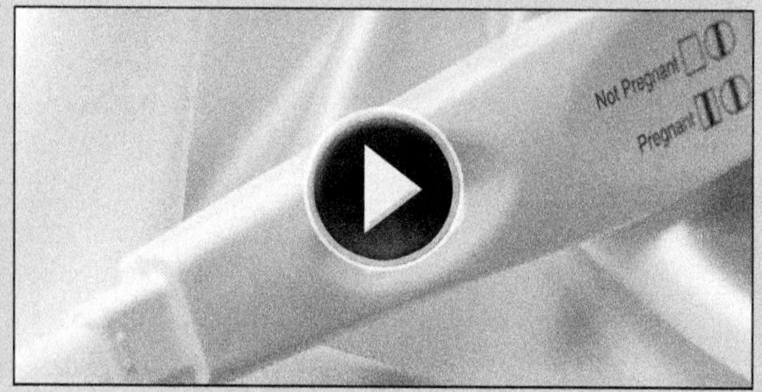

PROCEDURE 25-12

Collecting a Venous Blood Sample

If permitted by state law, medical laboratory assistants may draw blood samples from patients who require a venous sample. A venous blood sample requires a technique called phlebotomy (see **Section 25.1**). The accuracy of the test results relies on the accuracy of the lab assistant in choosing the correct method and treatment of the specimen.

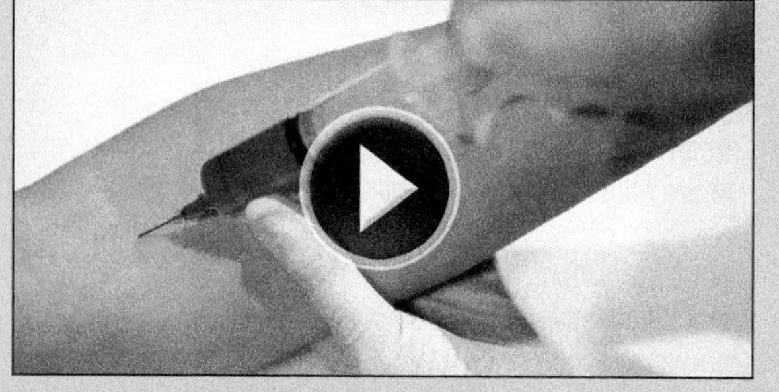

Photos: (t to b)BSIP/Photo Researchers, Inc., PhotoAlto sas/Alamy, C. Sherburne/PhotoLink/Getty Images, Don Farrall/Photodisc/Getty Images, Stockbyte/PunchStock

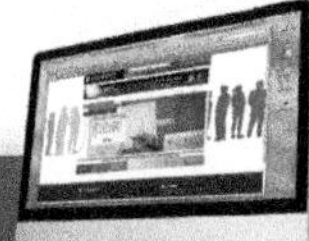

connect ONLINE PROCEDURES

PROCEDURE 25-13

Performing a Butterfly Blood Collection

A butterfly collection set, also known as a winged infusion set, is used for older patients and children who have small and/or fragile veins. The butterfly set is attached to an evacuated tube or, less commonly, a syringe. Butterfly collection makes possible a lower needle-insertion angle. The procedure is done using a surgical or sterile technique.

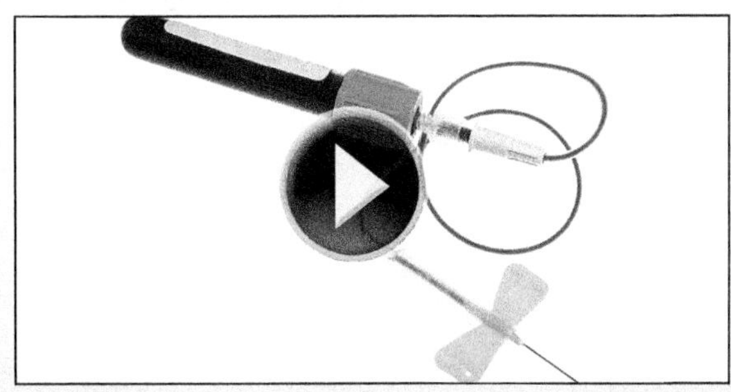

PROCEDURE 25-14

Collecting a Capillary Sample

Capillaries are tiny blood vessels that connect small arteries and veins. Capillary collection is an easy way to obtain a small amount of blood. This method is used most commonly for patients, such as young children, whose veins are too small for a phlebotomy. This technique requires a puncture of the skin with a lancet. Capillary samples are obtained most often for glucose, hematocrit, and hemoglobin tests.

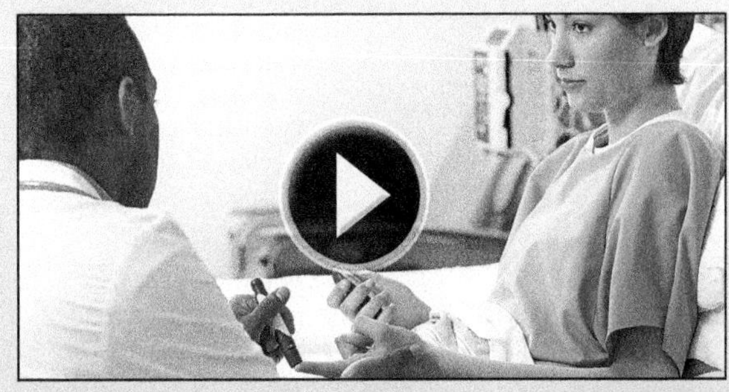

PROCEDURE 25-15

Performing a Hematocrit

A **hematocrit** is a screening test that determines the presence of anemia. Here a small tube of blood is placed in a centrifuge and spun for several minutes. This separates the blood into plasma, buffy coat, and packed red blood cells. The buffy coat is a thin, white layer consisting of white blood cells and platelets. The packed red blood cells are used to determine the percentage of red blood cells.

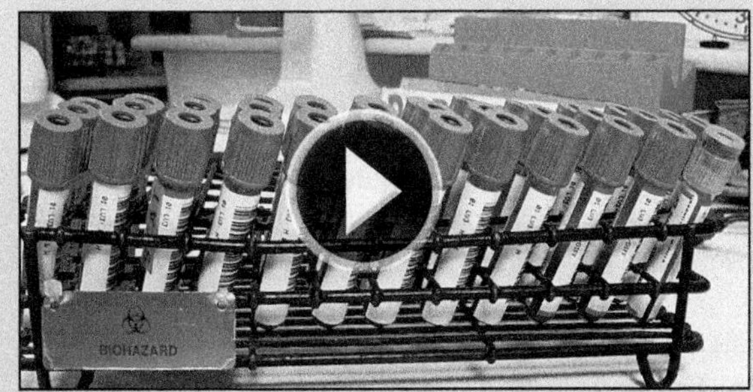

PROCEDURE 25-16

Performing a Hemoglobin Test

A hemoglobin test determines the oxygen-carrying ability of the red blood cells. **Hemoglobin** means blood protein. This protein has the ability to combine with and transport oxygen to body cells. Hemoglobin also assists in carrying carbon dioxide from the body cells to the lungs. The normal amounts of hemoglobin vary with age, sex, diet, altitude, and disease. A hemoglobinometer is used to measure hemoglobin.

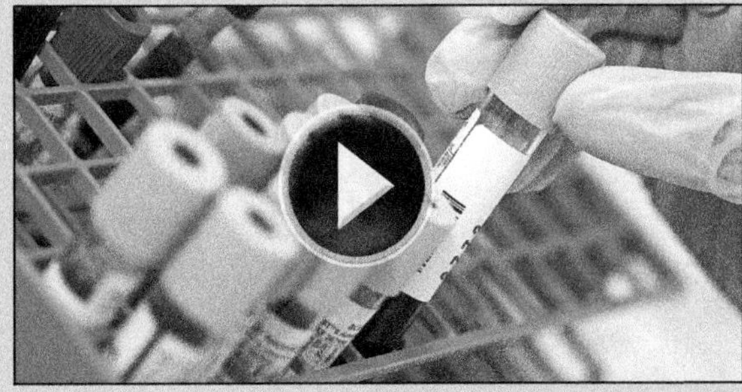

PROCEDURE 25-17

Manual Method for Counting Cells

A complete blood count (CBC) is a diagnostic test that requires the counting of red and white blood cells. If a physician needs to immediately know a patient's red or white blood cell count, a manual count can be performed in the office laboratory. The same basic procedure can be used to count platelets and sperm cells.

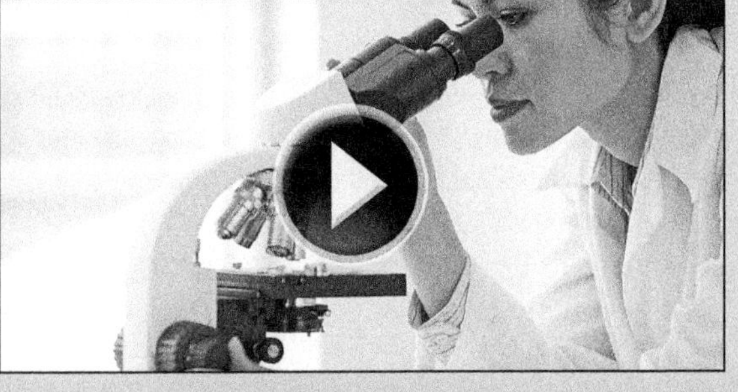

Photos: (t to b)Carlos Davila/Alamy, Purestock/Getty Images, Royalty-Free/CORBIS, Medic Image/Universal Images Group/Getty Images, Digital Vision/Getty Images

Blood Types

Why is it important to know your blood type?

Blood type determines the blood that may be received by a patient. Medical laboratory scientists must carefully and correctly identify blood types to prevent deadly consequences during blood transfusions. For example, type A+ blood has antigens for Group A and the Rh factor. Blood cells transfused into a person with type A+ blood

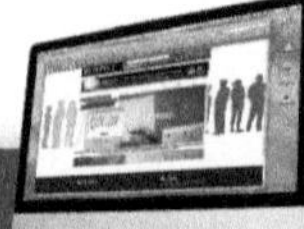

connect ONLINE PROCEDURES

PROCEDURE 25-18

Making a Blood Smear

A complete blood count (CBC) usually requires a differential, the determination of the types of white blood cells present and an evaluation of the way that red blood cells look. A blood smear must be made in order to perform the differential. In a differential count, the number and percentage of each of five different types of white blood cells are determined.

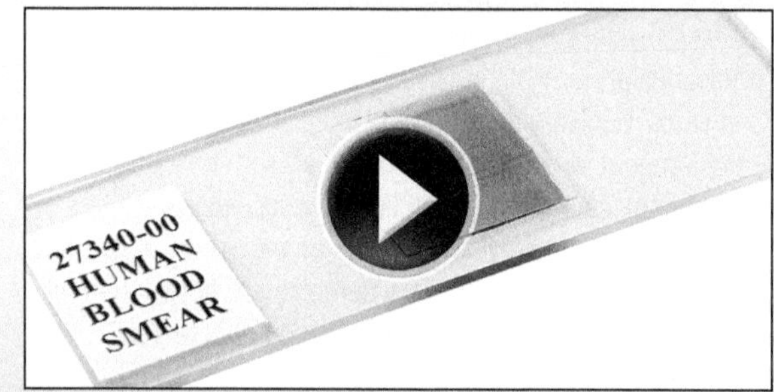

PROCEDURE 25-19

Performing an Erythrocyte Sedimentation Rate Test

An erythrocyte sedimentation rate test measures the rate at which erythrocytes, or red blood cells, separate from plasma and settle to the bottom of a calibrated tube. This test is a good indicator of inflammation and helps in diagnosing infections, arthritis, tuberculosis, hepatitis, cancer, multiple myeloma, and lupus erythematosus.

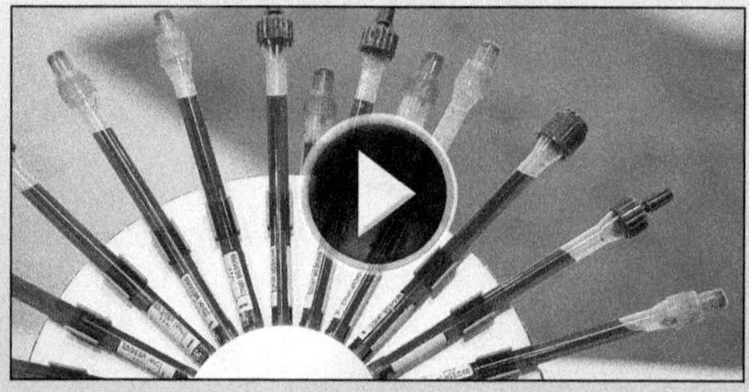

PROCEDURE 25-20

Determining ABO Group

The determination of a patient's ABO group, or blood type, is rarely done outside a blood bank. This test determines the presence of A or B antigens on red blood cells. Testing with a known antiserum and observing for the presence or absence of **agglutination** confirms the patient's blood type. Agglutination occurs when the antigen on the patient's red blood cells corresponds to the antibody.

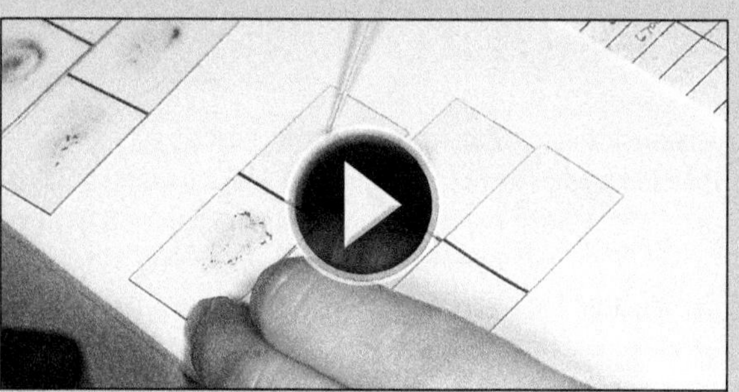

PROCEDURE 25-21

Determining Rh Factor

A patient's Rh factor, rarely determined outside of a blood bank, determines the presence of D antigens on the surface of red blood cells. This is based on the presence or absence of agglutination with anti-D antiserum. D antigens represent the Rh factor in the blood. The Rh factor is also referred to alone as "positive or negative."

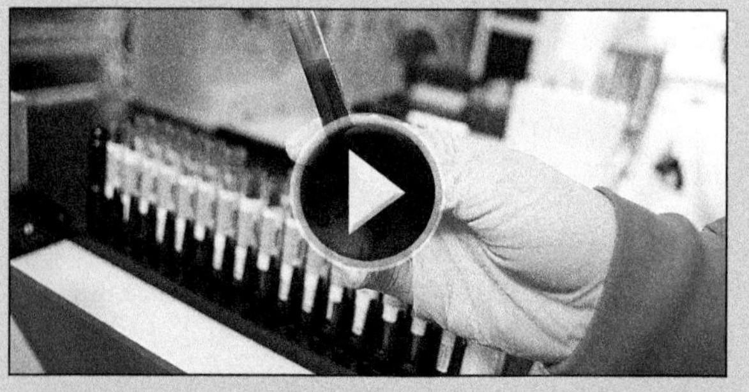

from persons with blood types that are not compatible with type A+ will try to destroy the type A+ cells. This is very dangerous or even fatal. **Table 25.2** shows the antigens that make up the various blood types. To determine the blood type, you must first determine the ABO group and the Rh antigen.

Table 25.2 Blood Types and Antigens

BLOOD TYPE	ABO GROUP ANTIGENS	RH ANTIGEN
A+	A	positive
A–	A	negative
B+	B	positive
B–	B	negative
AB+	A and B	positive
AB–	A and B	negative
O+	no A or B	positive
O–	no A or B	negative

READING CHECK

Identify the two components of a person's blood type.

connect

STEM CONNECTION

Medical Science

Bacteria Streptococci

Streptococci ("strep") are one type of bacteria. They are gram-positive organisms that grow in chains. These groups of streptococci may cause serious illnesses such as subacute bacterial endocarditis, strep throat, respiratory distress, septicemia, meningitis, peritonitis, wound infections, urinary tract infections, and gangrenous lesions. "Flesh-eating" bacteria are an especially dangerous example of strep infection.

connect Go online to learn more about streptococci and the risks they pose to health.

SECTION 25.2 Medical Laboratory Procedures Review

AFTER YOU READ

1. **Recall** how often a fresh solution of disinfectant should be made.
2. **Identify** the type of infection that the abbreviation UTI stands for.
3. **Name** the stain that is commonly used to identify microorganisms.
4. **Explain** the purpose of the copper reduction and sulfosalicylic acid precipitation urine tests.
5. **Name** three methods used for performing phlebotomy.

Technology ONLINE EXPLORATIONS

Strep Throat

The bacterial infection strep throat can be very serious in school-aged patients. Using the Internet or other sources, determine the complications caused by this infection. Report on these complications in written or oral form. In your report, discuss how the complications can be prevented and how they are treated.

CHAPTER 25 Review

Chapter Summary

SECTION 25.1

- Phlebotomy technicians may receive formal training from an approved program; they also may be trained on the job. Their main responsibility is to draw blood for testing. **(pg. 613)**
- Medical laboratory assistants must graduate from an accredited program and pass a national certification exam to earn their credentials. Their main responsibilities include collecting specimens and performing waived tests. **(pg. 614)**
- Medical laboratory technicians perform routine tests on blood, tissue, cells, and other body fluids, which help in the diagnosis and treatment of diseases. MLTs prepare specimens and operate automatic analyzers in addition to performing their sample collection responsibilities. **(pg. 618)**
- Medical laboratory scientists are highly trained, highly skilled scientists who use automated equipment and instruments capable of performing a number of tests simultaneously. In addition to performing many types of complex tests, medical laboratory scientists can also be teachers, supervisors, or researchers. **(pg. 619)**
- Histotechnicians and histotechnologists assist the pathologist with tissue dissection and prepare tissue samples for examination by the pathologist to detect diseases. **(pg. 621)**
- Cytotechnologists perform microscopic analysis of cells with a microscope to determine the presence of cancer or other diseases. **(pg. 621)**

SECTION 25.2

- Aseptic technique is practiced by all medical laboratory personnel to ensure that pathogens are absent or controlled. **(pg. 623)**
- All work areas should be disinfected with prepared solutions or solutions prepared in the lab. **(pg. 623)**
- Microorganisms can be classified as gram-positive or gram-negative. The classification helps to determine the type of infection. **(pg. 624)**
- Body fluids should be handled using standard precautions. **(pg. 625)**
- For the sake of accuracy, it is important that all healthcare personnel in the laboratory use the same counting and reporting system. **(pg. 626)**
- Blood type determines the blood that may be received by a patient. Medical laboratory scientists must carefully and correctly identify blood types to prevent deadly consequences during blood transfusions. **(pg. 628)**

CHAPTER
25 Assessment

Critical Thinking/Problem Solving

1. Which of the medical laboratory careers would be the best fit for you? Why?
2. You have just performed a capillary puncture on a patient to collect blood for a glucose test. The patient is present when you complete the glucose test and asks you to share with her the result. You explain that the physician will discuss the result with her in private during her exam. The patient then asks you to change the value if it is above normal range because "the doctor will be angry with me." How do you respond?
3. While pouring urine into a centrifuge tube, you spill urine on the lab counter and floor. What steps will you follow to ensure your safety and that of your patients?
4. You are collecting urine from a patient for a pre-employment drug screen. Immediately after collection, the urine is 80° F. Is this important? Why or why not?

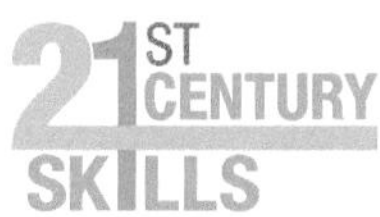

5. **Teamwork** With a partner, role-play drawing blood, communicating with the patient, proper labeling of specimens, and infection prevention.
6. **Information Literacy** Visit the Kidney Foundation's website to obtain information on the types and causes of renal disease. Then visit a dialysis center or interview someone who works in a dialysis center. Prepare an oral presentation or written report.
7. **Problem Solving** Research the proper disposal of hazardous biological wastes that result from laboratory activities. Give a visual demonstration of these procedures.
8. **Information Literacy** Go to the following websites to learn more about the medical laboratory field: ASCP.org, labsarevitalglobal.com, nationalphlebotomy.org, and phlebotomy.com. Research topics such as microorganisms, streptococci, components of the blood, urinalysis, cholesterol, tumor cells, anemia, and leukemia. Prepare a brief oral presentation to your class or prepare a written report for your instructor.

Mc Graw Hill connect™ ONLINE ACTIVITIES

Complete our HST online activities for Chapter 25, which include Concept Check review questions, Reference Flash Cards, and Online Procedures assessment sheets.

- **Concept Check** review questions
- **Reference Flash Cards** medical terminology practice
- **Online Procedures** assessment sheets

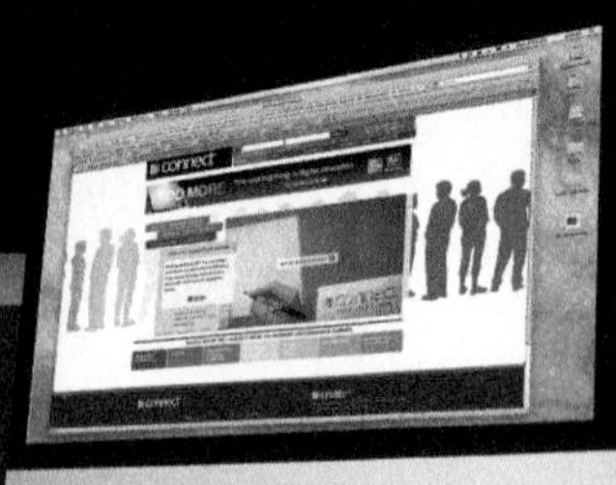

CHAPTER 26 Medical Testing

Connect

It's Online!

- Online Procedures
- STEM Connection
- Medical Science
- Medical Terms
- Medical Math
- Ethics in Action
- Virtual Lab

Essential Question:

What are the biggest responsibilities of medical testing technologists?

There are several medical testing career opportunities in the areas of cardiovascular technology and neurology. This chapter discusses the four most common occupations in this field: the electrocardiography (ECG) technician, cardiovascular technologist, electroencephalography (EEG) technologist, and electroneurodiagnostic (END) technologist. In addition, the chapter reviews the procedures and equipment that these professionals use.

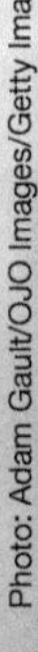

Photo: Adam Gault/OJO Images/Getty Images

READING GUIDE

OBJECTIVES

After completing this chapter, you will be able to:

- **Compare and contrast** the responsibilities of the ECG technician and the cardiovascular technologist.
- **Define** cardiac catheterization and balloon angioplasty.
- **Illustrate** how EEG and END technologists diagnose nervous system disorders using an EEG.
- **Demonstrate** the purpose and process of an EEG.
- **Describe** the ECG machine, its conduction system, and its leads and electrodes.

BEFORE YOU READ

Connect What medical tests, other than laboratory tests, have you had?

Main Idea

Medical professionals use a number of devices to diagnose and monitor body systems and the conditions that affect them.

Note-Taking Activity

Draw this table. Write key terms and phrases under **Cues**. Write main ideas under **Note Taking**. Summarize the section under **Summary**.

Cues	Note Taking
◦	◦
◦	◦
Summary	

Graphic Organizer

Before you read the chapter, draw a diagram like the one to the right. As you read, write the testing techniques covered by the chapter into the diagram.

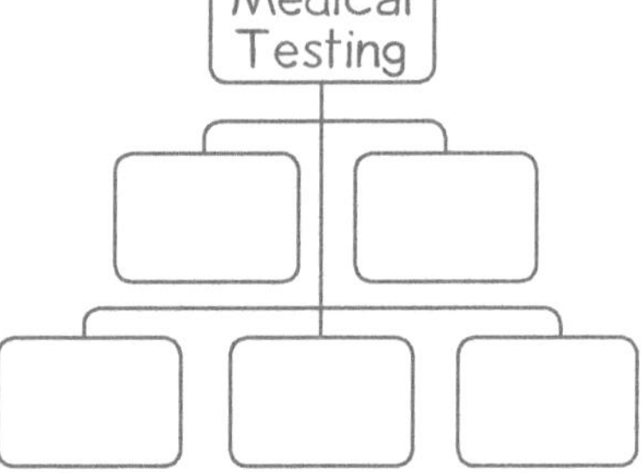

connect
Downloadable graphic organizers can be accessed online.

STANDARDS

HEALTH SCIENCE

NCHSE 1.32 Analyze diagrams, charts, graphs, and tables to interpret healthcare results.

NCHSE 10.11 Apply procedures for measuring and recording vital signs including the normal ranges.

SCIENCE

NSES E Develop abilities of technological design, understandings about science and technology.

NCHSE *National Consortium for Health Science Education*

NSES *National Science Education Standards*

COMMON CORE STATE STANDARDS

MATHEMATICS

Number and Quantity

Quantities N-Q1 Use units as a way to understand problems and to guide the solution of multi-step problems; choose and interpret units consistently in formulas; choose and interpret the scale and the origin in graphs and data displays.

Algebra

Seeing Structure in Expressions A-SSE1 Interpret expressions that represent a quantity in terms of its context.

ENGLISH LANGUAGE ARTS

Speaking and Listening

Comprehension and Collaboration SL-2 Integrate multiple sources of information presented in diverse media or formats (e.g., visually, quantitatively, orally) evaluating the credibility and accuracy of each source.

SECTION 26.1 Careers in Medical Testing

Vocabulary

Content Vocabulary

You will learn these content vocabulary terms in this section.

- **tracing**
- **electrocardiography**
- **exercise electrocardiography**
- **ambulatory monitoring**
- **Holter monitor**
- **echocardiogram**
- **invasive**
- **cardiac catheterization**
- **balloon angioplasty**
- **stent**
- **electroencephalography**
- **electroneurodiagnostic**

Academic Vocabulary

You will see this word in your reading and on your tests. Find its meaning in the Glossary in the back of the book.

- **indicate**

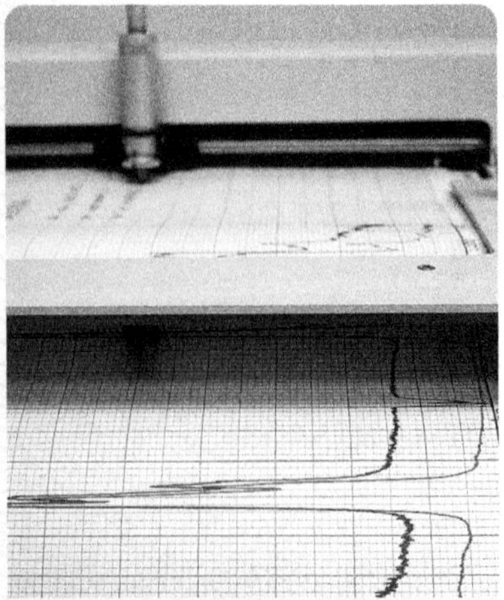

Fig. 26.1 ECG A twelve-lead ECG machine records the electrical activity of the heart. *What is this record called?*

Electrocardiography Technician

Has anyone ever recorded the electrical activity of your heart?

There are excellent career opportunities in medical testing in cardiovascular technology and neurology. To qualify as a cardiovascular technician or technologist or an electroneurodiagnostic technologist, you will need to be able to use complex equipment to evaluate the condition of organs and systems of the body. See **Table 26.1** for an overview of medical testing occupations.

The electrocardiograph machine records the electrical activity of the heart. **Figure 26.1** shows a 12-lead electrocardiograph machine tracing. This kind of machine is discussed in more detail in Section 26.2.

ECG is a commonly used abbreviation for the terms electrocardiograph, electrocardiography, and electrocardiogram. However, you may often also see the abbreviation EKG used in the medical context. That abbreviation is from "Elektrokardiogramm," which is the German spelling of the word electrocardiogram. In this chapter, the form ECG is used.

The ECG machine produces a series of waveforms which are a reflection of the electrical activity within the heart. This activity seen on the screen or as a printout is called an electrocardiogram. This printed record is called a **tracing.** The electrocardiogram helps the physician diagnose and evaluate the presence and extent of cardiovascular disease.

The **electrocardiography** (ECG) technician operates the ECG machine. Once the electrocardiogram is complete, the ECG technician determines whether the tracing is accurate and prepares a report for the physician. ECG technicians are trained to recognize abnormalities in the tracing caused by non-heart related electrical interference or other problems that come up during the recording procedure.

The Job of the Electrocardiography Technician

Most ECG technicians work in hospitals. They may also work in clinical offices, cardiac rehabilitation centers, and other healthcare facilities. Sometimes ECG technicians are employed by a home healthcare agency. When an ECG technician has to perform an ECG in a patient's home, he or she takes the ECG machine there.

Table 26.1 Overview of Medical Testing Occupations

OCCUPATION	EDUCATIONAL REQUIREMENTS	CERTIFICATION OR LICENSING AGENCY	JOB OUTLOOK
Electrocardiography Technician	On-the-job training from eight to 24 weeks. One-year certification programs are also available.	Certification from Cardiovascular Credentialing International, National Board of Cardiovascular Testing or American Certification Agency, National Center for Competency Testing	Faster than average growth. However, more job openings will be available for individuals who are trained to perform cardiovascular tests in addition to the ECG.
Cardiovascular Technologist	Two to four years of education and training in a program approved by the Joint Review Committee on Education in Cardiovascular Technology	Register with Cardiovascular Credentialing International or American Registry of Diagnostic Medical Sonographers	Faster than average growth because of an aging of population and the increase in cases of heart disease
Electroencephalography Technologist and Electroneurodiagnostic Technologist	One to two years of formal education necessary for registration and advancement	Register with American Board of Registration of Electroencephalographic and Evoked Potential Technologists	Faster than average growth, due to advances in diagnostic technologies

After recording the ECG, the ECG technician gives the report to the physician for interpretation. Depending upon the level of technology used, the ECG results may be transmitted by telephone directly to the physician (see **Figure 26.2**). Some 12-lead ECG machines weigh as little as six ounces and can transmit the tracing over a cell phone (see **Figure 26.3**).

The ECG technician must be able to perform a safe and accurate ECG. The tracing of the electrical current of the heart must be accurate

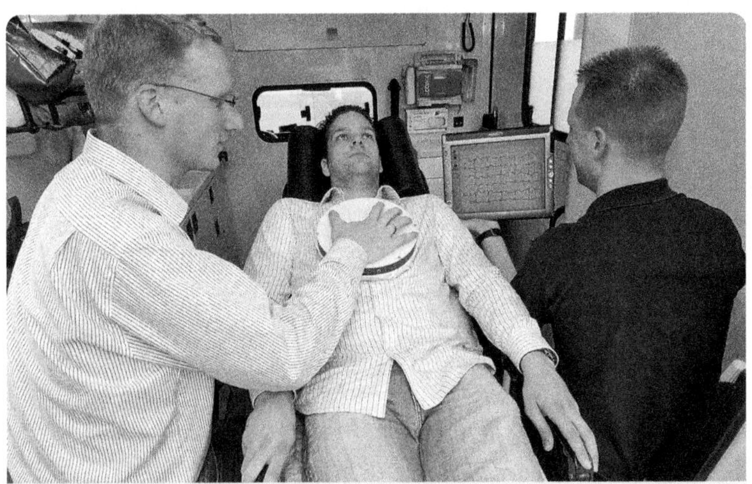

Fig. 26.2 Wireless Technology This is an example of wireless technology in which results are transmitted to a physician. *What is one benefit of using such technology to transmit ECG readings?*

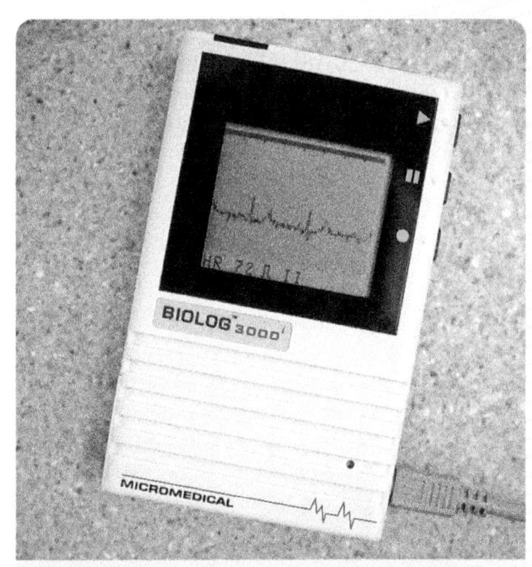

Fig. 26.3 Twelve-Lead ECG This is a transtelephonic twelve-lead ECG. *What is one benefit of a 12-lead ECG?*

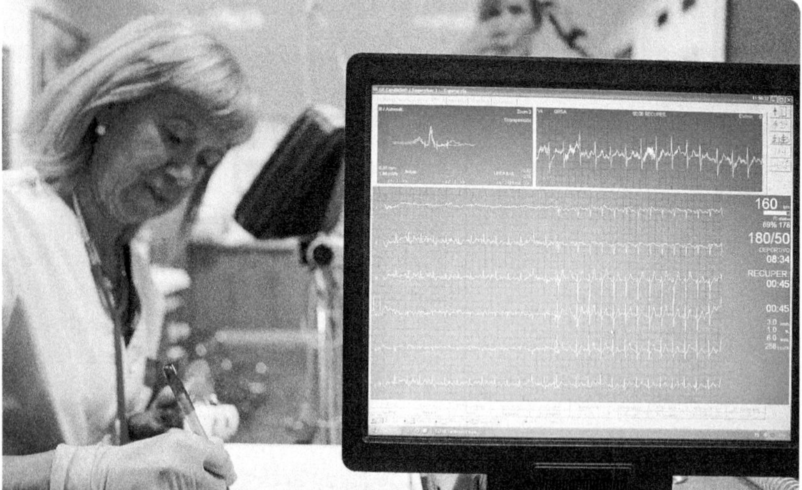

Fig. 26.4 ECG Monitor The ECG technician views tracings of the heart on a monitor. *What should the technician do if an abnormal heart rhythm is seen?*

because it is used to make decisions about a patient's care. An inaccurate tracing could result in a wrong decision on the patient's state of health, medication or treatment. A bad decision could have a serious negative outcome for the patient.

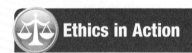

Ethics in Action

Using Discretion

You are working for a gynecologist. A new patient has left her urine sample in the designated area and then has blood drawn for analysis. You run a quick test on the urine sample, and it reveals a problem. While waiting for the doctor to attend to her, you take her blood pressure. She asks you about the urine analysis and rattles off some of her symptoms. What do you tell her?

connect Go online to read more about this ethical challenge and complete the activity.

Some ECG technicians may view and evaluate the electrical tracings of a patient's heart on a monitor (see **Figure 26.4**). An ECG technician whose main responsibility is to examine the ECG tracings will usually work in a hospital or other facility where patients are attached to heart monitors 24 hours a day. This ECG technician, called a monitor technician, may also be asked to perform other duties, such as maintaining patient records. If an abnormal heart rhythm is seen, the ECG technician must promptly alert a supervisor or the patient's physician.

Exercise Electrocardiography

Exercise electrocardiography, used since the 1950s, is known by many names, but it is usually called a stress test or a treadmill stress test. This is because the exercise part of the test is often performed on a treadmill (see **Figure 26.5**). The patient may also pedal an exercise bike or move the handlebars of an exercise machine in a circular motion. The degree of exercise difficulty is increased as the test progresses.

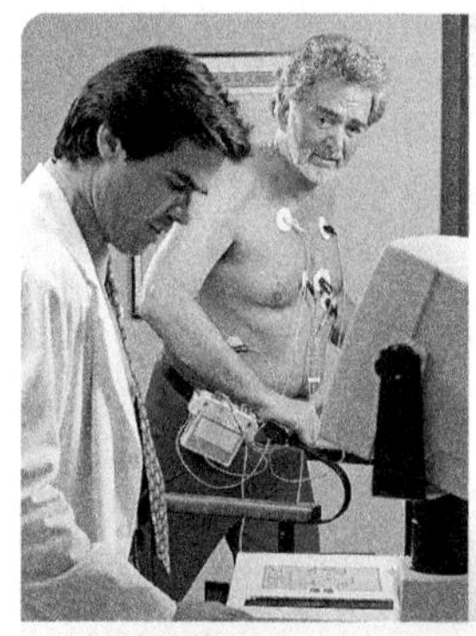

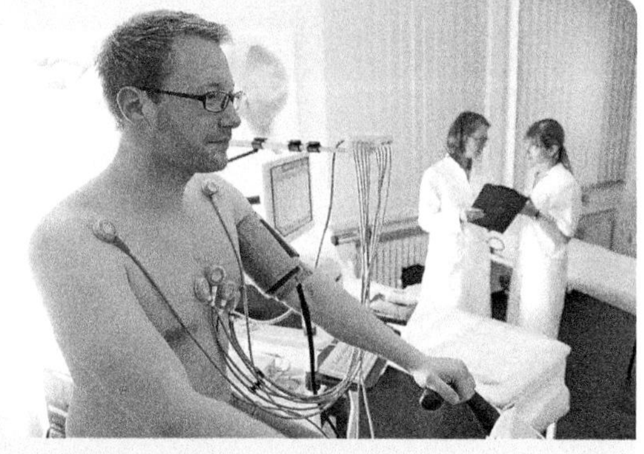

Fig. 26.5 Exercise Electrocardiography In exercise electrocardiography, the heart may be monitored while the patient walks on a treadmill. *Why should the patient be carefully monitored during this test?*

A physician is normally present when this test is performed because the patient must be carefully monitored. The patient's blood pressure, heart rate, skin temperature, oxygen level, and physical appearance are continuously checked. The patient is asked to report chest pain, other discomfort, dizziness, fatigue, difficulty breathing, or other physical changes. Any physical changes or patient complaints could indicate a problem with the blood flow to the heart. Problems or complications could indicate the need for a special procedure called a balloon angioplasty (discussed later in this chapter) or even open heart surgery.

ECG technicians who perform additional tests to evaluate the heart can increase their chances of advancing their careers. Two such tests are exercise electrocardiography and ambulatory monitoring.

Exercise Electrocardiography During exercise electrocardiography, the ECG technician provides patient safety and handles emergencies. In addition, he or she is responsible for

- giving instructions to the patient.
- applying and removing the electrodes.
- helping the physician monitor the patient during the procedure by taking blood pressure and other vital signs, and by watching the heart monitor closely.
- observing for chest pain, other discomfort, dizziness, fatigue, difficulty breathing, or other physical changes.

Ambulatory Monitoring

With **ambulatory monitoring,** an ECG tracing is recorded over an extended period on patients who are able to ambulate, or walk. These patients are not bedridden and can carry out their normal everyday activities. A typical ambulatory monitor is a small box strapped to the waist or shoulder of the patient. Inside is a device that can record an ECG for up to 48 hours. It usually weighs less than a pound. The most common devices used are digital recorders, which weigh only a few ounces. One widely used type of ambulatory monitor is the **Holter monitor** (see **Figure 26.6**). It is named after its inventor, Norman Holter. Ambulatory monitoring is also called Holter monitoring.

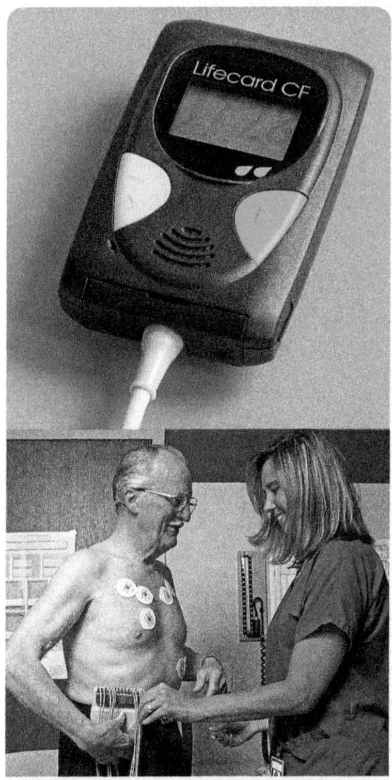

Fig. 26.6 Holter Monitoring During Holter monitoring, the patient is attached to a small box that monitors the heart during normal daily activities. *Who evaluates the ECG tracing produced by Holter monitoring?*

For ambulatory monitoring, three to five leads are attached to a patient's chest. A lead is an insulated electrical cable connected to an electrocardiograph or other monitor. The patient performs his or her daily activities and keeps a diary of activities. The patient also notes any symptoms or abnormal sensations, such as chest pain, indigestion, palpitations (irregular sensations in the chest), or dizziness. The patient will note the date and time and describe what he or she was doing prior to and during the time it took place.

When the monitoring is completed, the information from the monitor and diary is reviewed and interpreted. The ECG tracing can be viewed via a special computer program. The results can be subjected to computer analysis, but a cardiologist must perform the final evaluation.

Photos: (t)Chris Harris/Alamy, (b)Alvis Upitis/Brand X Pictures/Getty Images

21ST CENTURY SKILLS

Written Communication

Skills in written communication are important in medical testing. When a patient comes to your facility for an echocardiogram or other diagnostic test, you must take the patient's medical history. To do this, you will ask questions and record the data on a form or in the electronic medical record. For a test that evaluates the heart, you should find out whether the patient is taking any medications that may have an effect on the heart. You must record each of the medications accurately. You will need to spell the name of the medication correctly and, if possible, write the amount (dosage) and frequency taken.

Follow-up
Why is it important to take a patient's medical history? What could happen if you did not?

Ambulatory Monitoring Responsibilities During ambulatory monitoring, the ECG technician is responsible for these tasks:

- Attaching and removing the ambulatory monitor
- Giving instructions to the patient
- Ensuring that the results are placed in the patient's chart
- Maintaining the equipment

READING CHECK

Summarize the process of ambulatory monitoring.

Cardiovascular Technologist

What types of testing can be performed by a cardiovascular technologist?

If you enjoy the field of cardiology and are willing to obtain advanced skills and education, you may choose to be a cardiovascular technologist. You may need from two to four years of schooling and training. You will work directly with cardiologists in hospitals, clinics, clinical offices, medical centers, and mobile diagnostic units. Have you ever been to a health fair or other public event and seen a large van with a sign offering heart-screening tests? Chances are that the people doing those tests were cardiovascular technologists (see **Figure 26.7**).

The Job of the Cardiovascular Technologist

In general, the cardiovascular technologist needs

- a thorough understanding of the anatomy and physiology of the cardiovascular system.
- the ability to communicate and work well with others.
- the ability to work with computers and other technical equipment.

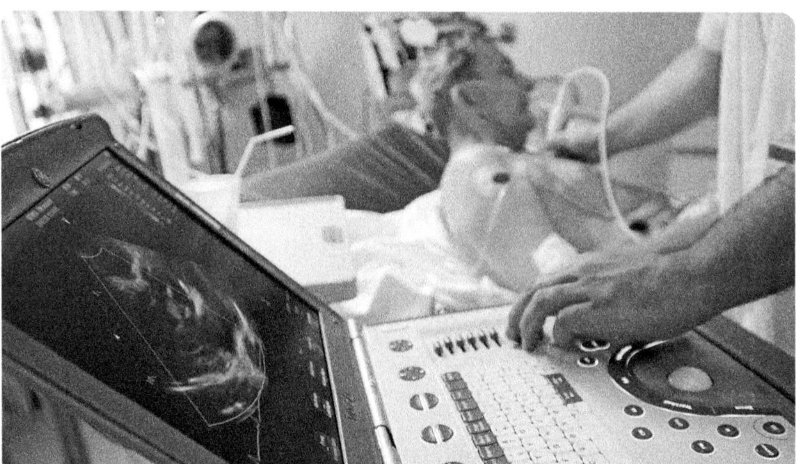

Fig. 26.7 Echocardiogram The cardiovascular technologist performs an echocardiogram, which uses sound waves to produce images of the heart. *Why might an echocardiogram be performed?*

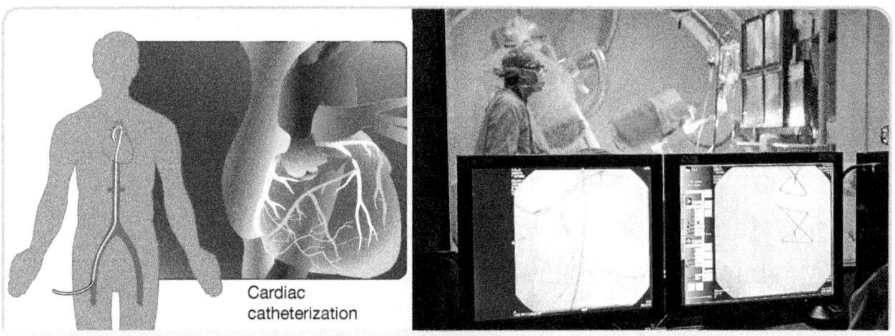

Fig. 26.8 Cardiac Catheterization During cardiac catheterization, a tube is inserted through the blood vessels to the heart and a dye is injected to check the blood vessels for blockages. *How might the cardiovascular technologist prepare a patient for this procedure?*

Some cardiovascular technologists specialize in performing ultrasound tests on the heart and blood vessels. Ultrasound equipment picks up sound waves produced by organs in the body that cannot be heard by the human ear. The ultrasound equipment converts the echoes produced by those sound waves to create an image on a screen. An ultrasound of the heart is known as an **echocardiogram.**

A cardiovascular technologist specializing in ultrasound tests of the heart is known as an echocardiographer. Cardiovascular technologists who specialize in performing ultrasound tests on the vascular system or the blood vessels are known as vascular technologists.

In addition to carrying out tests such as the ECG, a cardiovascular technologist may also assist with **invasive** tests or procedures that require entry into the body. Cardiovascular technologists who assist with those procedures are often called invasive cardiovascular technologists. Examples of invasive procedures are cardiac catheterization, balloon angioplasty and stent placement, the implantation of pacemakers, and heart surgery.

Cardiac Catheterization **Cardiac catheterization** is a test that looks at the structures of the heart (see **Figure 26.8**). It is a very accurate way to diagnose coronary artery disease (CAD), which is caused by blockage of the blood vessels of the heart. A small tube is wound through the patient's blood vessels to the heart, usually beginning from a site on the patient's leg. The pressure inside the heart chambers is measured and dye is injected through the tube. The dye allows a picture to be made of the inside of the blood vessels.

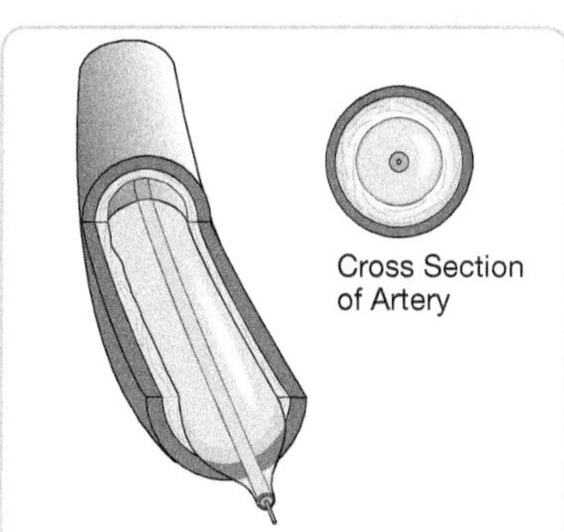

Fig. 26.9 Angioplasty A balloon angioplasty expands the blocked vessel, which is then fitted with a stent. *What should the cardiovascular technologist monitor during this procedure?*

Balloon Angioplasty and Stent Placement If a patient has blockages in the coronary arteries, the cardiovascular technologist may assist the physician with a procedure called **balloon angioplasty.** During this procedure, a catheter with a balloon on its end is inserted into a blood vessel (see **Figure 26.9**). The balloon is then blown up to expand the blocked vessel. Next, a **stent** is placed inside the blocked blood vessel to act as a bridge. After insertion, it expands outward when the balloon on the catheter is inflated. This keeps the blood vessel open and improves blood flow to the heart muscle. To prepare for this procedure, the cardiovascular technologist may clean and shave the site where the catheter will be inserted.

Job Responsibilities of the Invasive Cardiovascular Technologist

The invasive cardiovascular technologist is responsible for

- reviewing and recording the patient's history.
- performing diagnostic tests.
- providing accurate and complete data to the physician.
- informing the physician if something appears wrong.
- monitoring heart rate, blood pressure, and the ECG.
- directly assisting the physician during the invasive procedure.

EEG and END Technologists

How much do you know about the brain?

As an electroencephalography (EEG) or electroneurodiagnostic (END) technologist, you will need to know about the nervous system—how it works and some of its disorders. The principal responsibility of the EEG or END technologist is to perform electroencephalograms (EEGs), which measure the electrical activity of the brain. These tests are done with an electroencephalograph. The title END technologist is used more often now because it describes the occupation best.

Other terms in this area of healthcare are **electroencephalography,** which refers to recording the electrical activity in the brain, and **electroneurodiagnostic,** which refers to evaluating the electrical activity of the nervous system.

21ST CENTURY SKILLS

Technology and Heart Disease Diagnosis

Exciting research is taking place in the field of cardiology. Two new methods of diagnosing heart disease allow almost immediate evaluation of an ECG tracing.

- In transtelephonic monitoring, patients carry or wear a small monitor to record the electrical impulses of the heart (see **Figure 26.10**). The monitor is about the size of a credit card, even small enough to be worn on the wrist. The ECG tracing is stored in the monitor's memory, and the patient transmits it by landline or via cell phone to a diagnostic center.
- In wireless monitoring, the physician uses a handheld computer (see **Figure 25.11**). These computers allow physicians to view and evaluate ECG tracings.

READING CHECK

Identify the types of invasive procedures that a cardiovascular technologist may assist with.

The Job of the EEG or END Technologist

In addition to performing EEGs, the EEG or END technologist may perform tests that evaluate the spinal cord, the nervous system, and

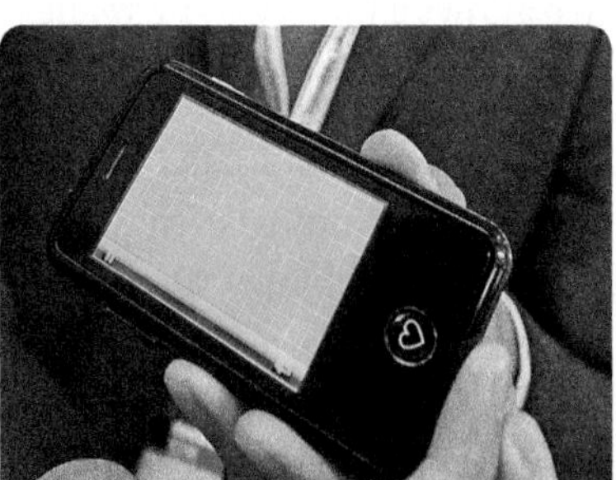

Fig. 26.10 Monitor A small monitor records the heart's electrical activity. The patient then transmits the recording for evaluation. *What is this method of monitoring called?*

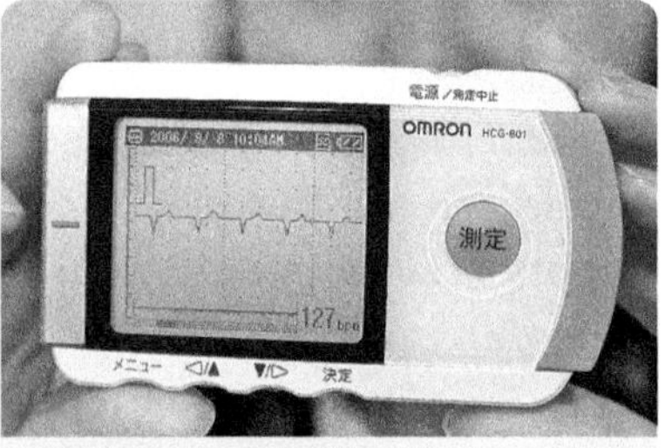

Fig. 26.11 Handheld Computer Physicians can use a handheld computer to receive wireless transmission of the ECG tracing. *In what situations would wireless technology be especially helpful?*

Table 26.2 Tests Performed by EEG and END Technologists

TEST	PURPOSE	USES
Electroencephalogram	To record the electrical activity of the brain	To diagnose brain disorders and evaluate the effect of infectious disease and injury on the brain
Evoked Potential	To record the electrical activity of the brain, spinal cord, and nerves in response to stimulation	To make sure that nerves have not been damaged during surgery on the spine
Nerve conduction studies	Measuring the electrical activity of the peripheral nerves, which cause muscles to contract	To evaluate how long it takes nerves to cause muscles to contract
Polysomnogram	Monitoring of the electrical activity of the brain, the heart, and respiratory rates	To evaluate sleep and sleep disorders

sleep. These tests help physicians diagnose brain tumors, strokes, epilepsy, and sleep disorders. **Table 26.2** describes some of the tests performed by EEG and END technologists. END technologists are usually employed in acute care hospitals, neurologists' offices, and some ambulatory care facilities. They also work in newborn nurseries, sleep-study laboratories, operating rooms, and epilepsy research centers.

The Electroencephalogram

It is hard to imagine, but the brain contains about 15 trillion cells. Each cell can generate an electrical signal, and each cell is linked to all the other brain cells. It is said that every second the brain receives, analyzes, and stores 100 trillion bits of information.

The electroencephalograph (EEG) machine records the electrical impulses of the brain, producing a record called the electroencephalogram (see **Figure 26.12**). To produce the tracing, electrodes are applied to the scalp or just under the skin of the scalp.

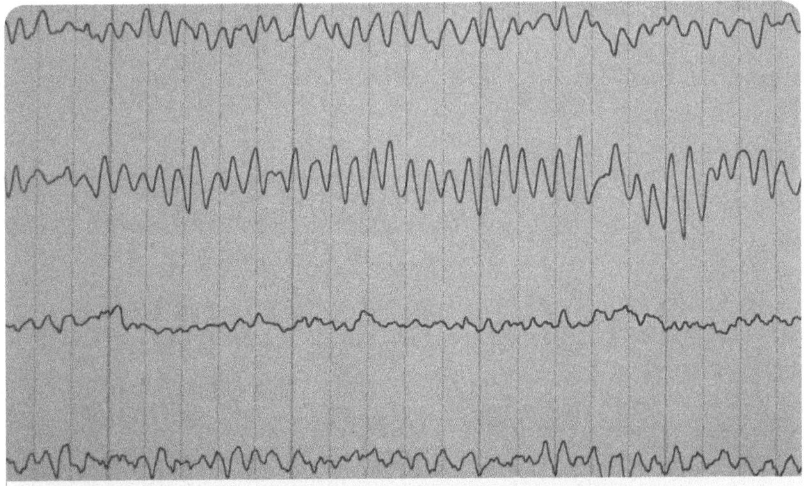

Fig. 26.12 EEG Tracing Electrodes applied to the scalp produce the tracing. *What electrical activity is being traced in this figure?*

Changes in the electrical impulses of the brain may be caused by trauma (injury), brain tumors, stroke, epilepsy, and other neurological problems.

Prior to performing the EEG, the EEG or END technologist obtains the patient's medical history. Then the technologist applies electrodes to specified spots on the head. While the EEG is being performed, the technologist corrects errors on the tracing caused by interference and makes notes about the patient's activity during the procedure.

Job Responsibilities of the EEG or END Technologist

EEG and END technologists have a rewarding job because they are personally involved with patients. Their job involves the use of a variety of techniques and equipment, including computers.

The EEG or END technologist is responsible for

- placing the electrodes.
- adjusting the machine.
- monitoring the patient.
- recording the outcome on the patient's chart.

READING CHECK

Name some tests other than EEGs that the EEG or END technologist may perform.

SECTION 26.1 Careers in Medical Testing Review

AFTER YOU READ

1. **Describe** the main responsibility of the ECG technician.
2. **Name** the two tests other than the ECG that an ECG technician should learn to help ensure employment and career advancement.
3. **Identify** the additional education required to become a cardiovascular technologist. Explain why it is necessary.
4. **Describe** the purpose of cardiac catheterization, balloon angioplasty, and stent insertion.
5. **Define** the terms electroencephalography and electroneurodiagnostic.
6. **Describe** the diagnostic test most often performed by an EEG or END technologist.

Technology ONLINE EXPLORATIONS

Medical Testing Opportunities

Research the Internet for job opportunities in Medical Testing. Remember to search using the specific name of the job you are interested in. Review the job qualifications, salary, and responsibilities, and then prepare a letter of application for the position you choose.

SECTION 26.2 Medical Testing Procedures

The Anatomy and Physiology of the Heart

What is the Purkinje network?

The normal heart is a strong, muscular pump that is a little larger than a fist. It pumps blood continuously through the circulatory system. Each day the average heart beats 100,000 times and pumps 2,000 gallons of blood.

Electrical impulses control the pumping cycle of the heart muscle. These electrical impulses normally begin in very specific locations within the heart and travel throughout the heart. The special tissues in the heart that produce electrical impulses form the cardiac electrical conduction system.

The cardiac electrical conduction system consists of the following elements:

- Sinoatrial (SA) node
- Atrioventricular (AV) node
- Bundle of His (AV bundle)
- Bundle branches
- Purkinje fibers (network)

The heart, with these parts labeled, is shown in **Figure 26.13**. Each part of the cardiac conduction system is described on page 644.

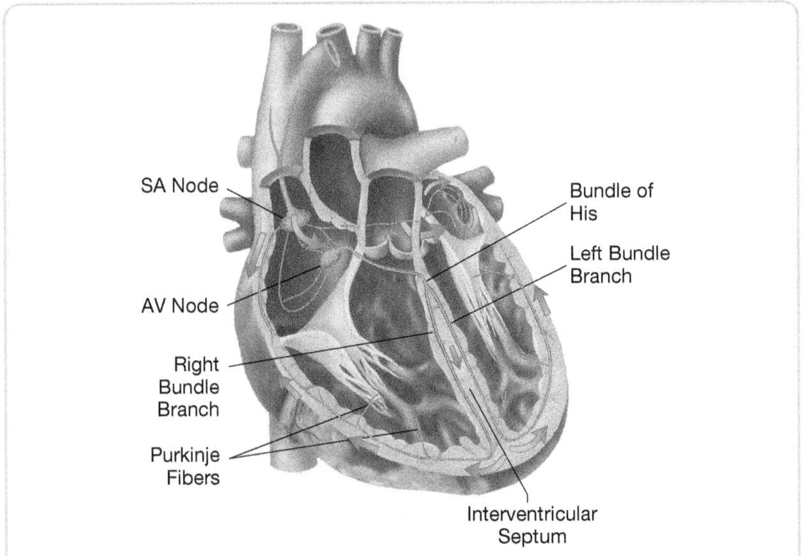

Fig. 26.13 The Cardiac Conduction System The heart's conduction system plays a vital role in carrying the electrical impulses that cause the heart to pump blood throughout the body. *Why is it important to understand the cardiac conduction system in order to perform an ECG?*

Vocabulary

Content Vocabulary

You will learn these content vocabulary terms in this section.

- **atrium**
- **isoelectric**
- **artifact**

Academic Vocabulary

You will see this word in your reading and on your tests. Find its meaning in the Glossary in the back of the book.

- **transmits**

The Sinoatrial (SA) Node The SA node is a small round structure. It is located in the upper part of the right **atrium**, or chamber in the heart. (The plural of atrium is "atria.") You have probably heard of pacemakers, which are electrical devices that help make the heartbeat steady. The SA node is a natural pacemaker. The SA node **transmits** an electrical impulse, or "fires" about 60 to 100 times per minute. Since conduction begins in the SA node each heartbeat also begins there.

The Atrioventricular (AV) Node The AV node is also a small round structure. It is located on the floor of the right atrium. Special electrical conduction pathways (like roads) carry the electrical impulse to the AV node. When the impulse arrive at the AV node, the node delays or slows down the electrical impulse. If the SA node is not working, the AV node can act as an emergency or "backup" pacemaker. This is a good feature to have, but it does not "fire" as fast the SA node. It fires at a slower rate of 40 to 60 times per minute, which results in the heart pumping more slowly.

The Bundle of His The bundle of His (the AV bundle) is located next to the AV node. It transfers the electrical impulse from the atria to the ventricles. When the impulse reaches the ventricles, it is divided into the bundle branches.

The Bundle Branches The bundle branches are located along the left and right side of the interventricular septum, or the division between the two ventricles. Electrical impulses travel through the right and left bundle branches to the right and left ventricles. You might think of the right and left bundle branches as a fork in the road. Some electrical impulses travel to the right ventricle, and some travel to the left. The bundle branches act as pathways down the interventricular septum.

The Purkinje Network The Purkinje network spreads the impulses throughout the ventricles, through a system of fibers called the Purkinje fibers. These fibers provide an electrical pathway for each of the cardiac cells. At this point, the electrical impulses speed up. They activate the right and left ventricles simultaneously, causing the ventricles to contract. The electrical impulses produce an electrical wave, which can be recorded on the ECG as a waveform.

READING CHECK

List the elements of the cardiac conduction system.

Recording an Electrocardiogram

In what situations are ECGs performed?

Let's investigate more about how the heart works and about the basic equipment needed to perform an ECG. Then we will review the step-by-step procedure for recording an ECG.

The ECG Tracing

The ECG tracing (see **Figure 26.14**) provides information about the patient's heart rate and rhythm. The tracing can show abnormal heart changes or reveal damage to the heart. An ECG may be performed to

- determine heart rate and rhythm.
- check for any problems with the flow of electricity through the heart.
- diagnose changes in the heart rhythm.
- show abnormal heart changes.
- reveal damage to the heart.
- check before surgery for abnormal heart changes.
- help evaluate a person's overall health during a complete physical exam.
- monitor or evaluate individuals who have been diagnosed with heart conditions.

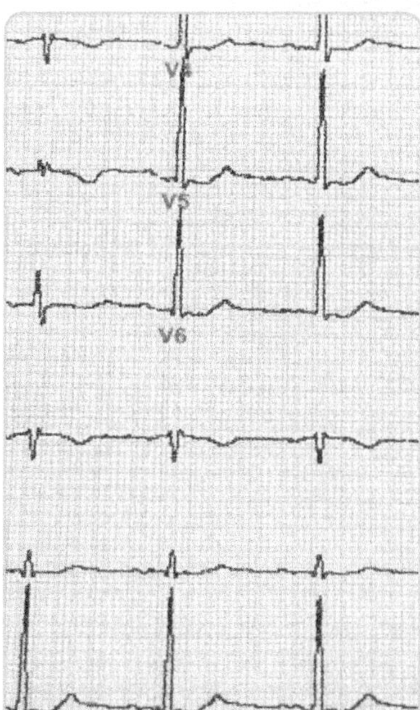

Fig. 26.14 Tracing ECG tracing provides information about the heart rate and rhythm. *Who would perform tests on this machine?*

The ECG Waveform

An ECG waveform on an electrocardiogram is a series of up-and-down deflections, or waves. These waves rise above or fall below a straight line—known as an **isoelectric** line—that is also called the baseline.

The ECG machine measures the electrical impulses produced by the heart's conduction system. Then it translates the signal and produces the waveform that shows how the heart is working. Each wave represents specific activity in the patient's heart. Positive deflections go up, while negative ones go down. The waves are labeled P, Q, R, S, and T (see **Figure 26.15**). If there is no activity in the heart, only the line appears.

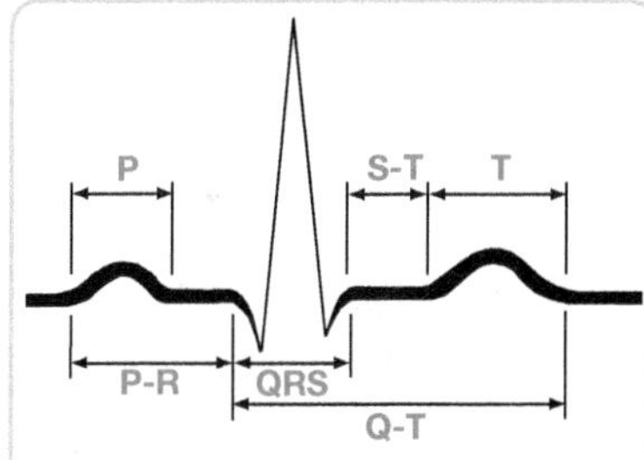

Fig. 26.15 Waveforms The heart's electrical activity produces an ECG waveform; each wave indicates activity within the heart. *What are the labels for the waves?*

READING CHECK

Recall the information about a patient's heart that an ECG tracing provides.

The Twelve-Lead ECG Machine

Why should an electrode be called a "sensor" when talking to patients?

In order to get a good look at a three-dimensional object such as the heart, you need to view it from all sides. The heart's electrical impulses must therefore be viewed from different sides. A type of test called the 12-lead ECG allows physicians to view a heart's electrical activity from 12 different angles. The 12 views provide important information about how the electrical impulses travel through various parts of the heart.

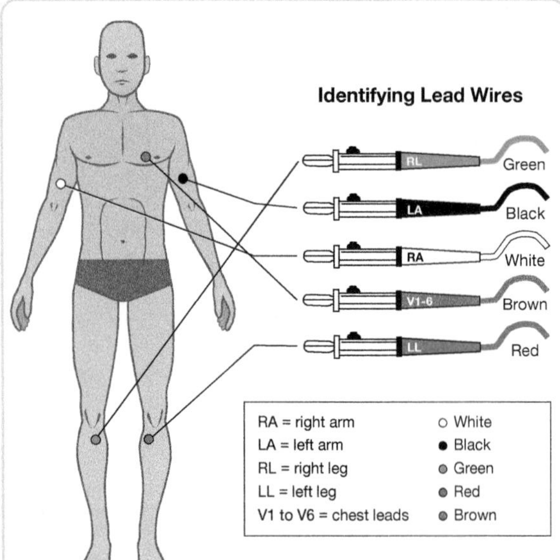

Fig. 26.16 Lead Wires Lead wires are colored and labeled to indicate their placement when recording an ECG. *How many leads are attached to chest electrodes? How many are attached to arm and leg electrodes?*

Attaching the Leads and Electrodes

Electrodes are sensors that are placed on the patient to pick up the electrical activity of the heart and conduct it to the ECG machine. Ten lead wires are used to perform a twelve-lead ECG. Six leads are attached to chest electrodes, and four are attached to the electrodes on the arms and legs. (Electrodes are discussed in more detail below.) For easy identification, the lead wires are color-coded. The lead wires are also labeled with letters that indicate where to place the leads on the patient's body. **Figure 26.16** shows the color coding and labels used on lead wires.

Each lead wire consists of one or more wires leading from the electrodes to the ECG machine. The 10 lead wires produce 12 different lead circuits. The 12 circuits produce 12 different tracings, or views of the heart. The electrodes, or a combination of electrodes, identify each of the 12 lead circuits, as shown in **Table 26.3** and **Figure 26.17.**

Safety

Inaccurate Tracing

You should never mix two different types of electrodes. This could cause an inaccurate tracing, which could result in incorrect treatment for the patient.

Table 26.3 Lead Tracings

LEAD TRACING NAME	LOCATION OF ELECTRODE(S) CREATING LEAD TRACING
Lead I	Right arm negative to left arm positive
Lead II	Right arm negative to the left leg positive
Lead III	Left arm negative to left leg positive
aVR	Heart to right arm
aVL	Heart to the left arm
aVF	Heart to left leg
V1	Fourth intercostal space, right sternal border
V2	Fourth intercostal space, left sternal border
V3	Halfway between V2 and V4
V4	Fifth intercostal space, at the midclavicular line
V5	Same horizontal level with V4, at the anterior axillary line
V6	Same horizontal level with V4 and V5, at the midaxillary line

Working with Electrodes

Each of the 10 lead wires used to perform the 12-lead ECG is connected to the patient with an electrode. Electrodes are available in a variety of types. They can be single-use or disposable. If an electrode ever has to be moved before or during an ECG, it should be discarded and a new one put in its place.

In an effort to reduce patient anxiety, it is advisable to use the term "sensor," rather than "electrode" when speaking with your patient. Many patients may be afraid that a machine with "electrodes" is going to give them a painful electric shock.

Disposable Electrodes Disposable electrodes (see **Figure 26.18**) are most commonly used because they reduce the possibility of contamination. After being removed, they are simply discarded, which makes cleanup easier. The self-adhesive disposable electrodes adhere easily to the patient's body. The gel is already applied, so the electrodes will properly conduct the electrical impulses. Disposable electrodes are normally designed for one-time use only. The only exception is when a second ECG is performed on the same patient immediately after the first ECG and the electrodes have not been moved or disturbed in any way. However, if the electrodes stay on the patient's skin for any length of time, the gel will dry out, resulting in inaccurate ECG tracings.

Handling and Storage of Electrodes Electrodes must be handled and stored properly. If a package contains more electrodes than needed at a particular time, keep the remaining electrodes in a sealed plastic bag so that the gel will not dry out. Check the expiration date on the package before using the electrodes, and make sure the gel has not dried out. Always check electrodes fresh out of the package before you use them.

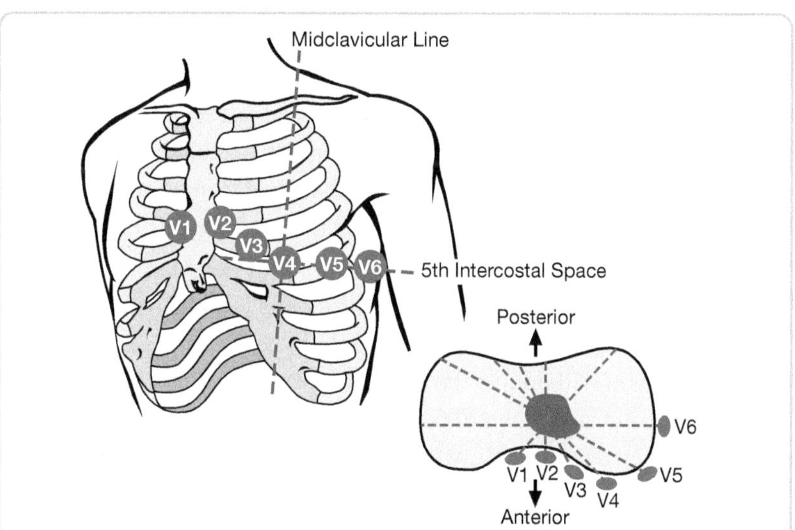

Fig. 26.17 Twelve-Lead ECG The twelve-lead ECG measures 12 different views of the heart. *Why is it important to have 12 different views?*

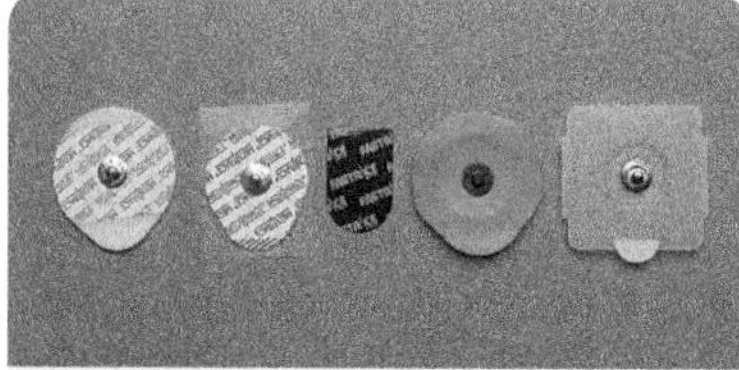

Fig. 26.18 Electrodes Disposable electrodes should be used once and discarded immediately after use. *Why is it important to discard disposable electrodes immediately?*

READING CHECK

Explain how an ECG machine's 10 lead wires produce 12 different tracings.

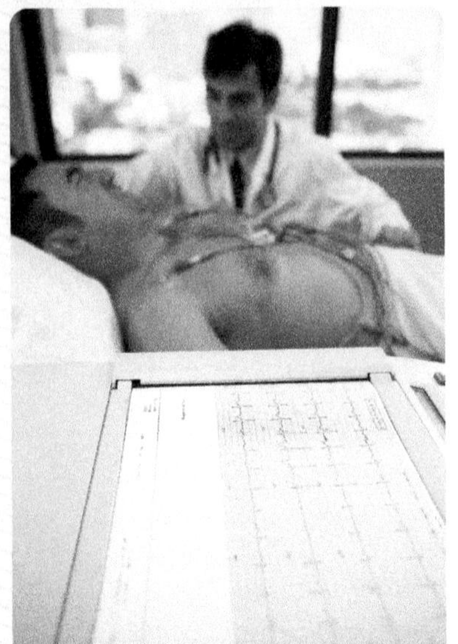

Fig. 26.19 Multichannel ECG Machine The multichannel ECG machine records three ECG tracings at one time on special graph paper. *What is the recording time for this multichannel ECG machine?*

The Multichannel ECG Machine

What features are unique to multichannel ECG machines?

The multichannel ECG machine (see **Figure 26.19**) produces 12 lead tracings on a single sheet of paper by recording three leads simultaneously and switching automatically. The recording time is approximately 15 to 20 seconds. This tracing does not usually need to be mounted, so you may need to attach it to a thicker backing if filing it permanently. There are machines that can record up to six lead tracings at one time.

Some ECG machines perform functions other than those described above, such as computerized measurement and analysis, storage, and communication. Computerized measurement and analysis provide an ECG reading that can quickly distinguish between a normal and abnormal tracing. It is not meant, however, to replace a physician's reading. Some machines can store results that can be called up and printed later. Most machines are also equipped for digital transmission.

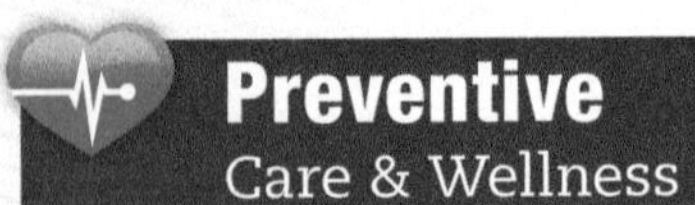

Preventive Care & Wellness

Caring for Your Heart

As a healthcare professional who evaluates the heart for disease and disorder, you will have a special responsibility to yourself and your profession. Consider how you can be a good role model for patients with heart problems and make sure you are taking care of your own heart. Exercise regularly, keep your weight in check, avoid saturated fats and refined sugar in your diet, do not smoke, and learn how to manage your stress.

ECG Machine Controls

What is artifact?

You should become familiar with the variety of ECG machine controls. In order to perform an ECG, you should be aware of the machine controls described in the following paragraphs.

- **Speed** The speed control regulates how fast or slow the paper runs during the ECG procedure. The normal rate is 25 millimeters per second (mm/sec). The physician may ask for the speed to be increased or decreased. If you change the speed from the standard 25 mm/sec, however, you must note this on the tracing.
- **Gain** The gain control regulates the output or height of the ECG waveform, which is measured in millimeters per millivolt (mm/mV). The normal setting is 10 mm/mV. By setting the gain to 20 mm/mV, you will double the size of the waveform; by setting the gain to 5 mm/mV, you will reduce the size by half. If you change the gain setting during any lead tracing, you must record this change on the tracing.
- **Artifact Filter** The ECG machine may have an artifact filter setting. In this context, an **artifact** is an abnormal mark on an ECG tracing caused by things such as muscle tremor or patient movement. The usual setting of the artifact filter is between 40 and 150 hertz (Hz). Forty hertz is normally used to reduce artifacts.
- **Computerized Controls** Computerized controls allow you to program the ECG machine to provide specific information. For example, you can enter information about the patient that will be included on the printout along with the ECG results. Some machines

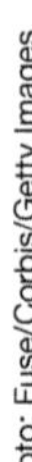

can also detect if the arm leads or chest leads are reversed and will display this information on the display panel. With some cardiac monitors, you may be able to set the heart rate limits. This means that you can set a heart rate that the machine will interpret as bradycardic (too slow) or tachycardic (too fast). If the heart rate is above or below the set heart rate limit, the machine will sound an alarm and mark the tracing.

- **Lead Selector** Most 12-lead ECG machines record each lead automatically. A lead selector can be used to run each lead individually, in case one or more lead tracings need to be repeated.

READING CHECK

List the ways in which ECG results can be transmitted.

connect ONLINE PROCEDURES

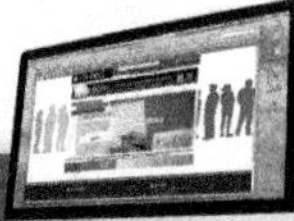

PROCEDURE 26-1

Recording an Electrocardiogram

There is more to recording an ECG than just turning on the machine. The technician must also understand the heart's electrical conduction system. Each contraction of the heart muscles is controlled by electrical impulses. This is the pattern that the ECG machine records.

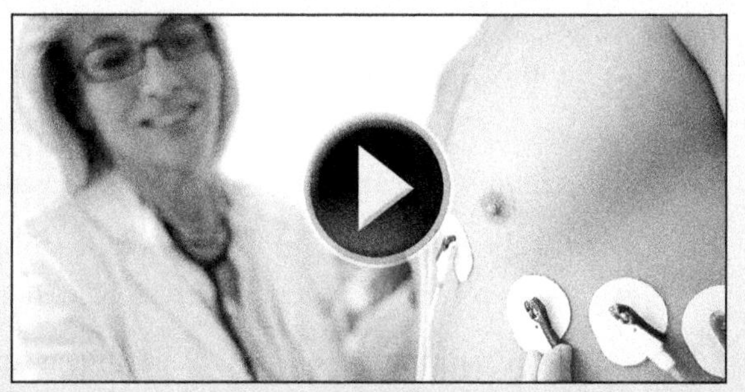

SECTION 26.2 Medical Testing Procedures Review

AFTER YOU READ

1. **Name** the parts of the cardiac conduction system.
2. **Explain** why you need to understand how the parts of the cardiac conduction system work when you perform an ECG.
3. **Identify** three or more important steps to follow when applying electrodes and lead wires.
4. **Recall** what document you should use if questions arise during the recording of an ECG.
5. **Summarize** how to handle the electrodes of an ECG machine correctly.

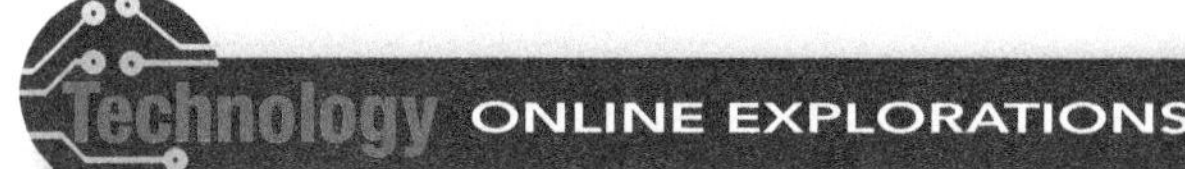

ECG Equipment

Search the Internet for companies that manufacture ECG equipment. Write an email to a company to obtain more information about the latest equipment. Determine the kind of training the ECG equipment manufacturer offers for its product. Compile your findings into a written report.

Photo: Science Photo Library/Alamy

CHAPTER **26 Review**

Chapter Summary

SECTION 26.1

- ECG technicians perform noninvasive tests on the heart. They learn their profession from on-the-job training or in a training program of one year or less. Their main responsibility is to record an ECG safely and accurately. **(pg. 634)**
- ECG technicians may work in hospitals, clinical offices, cardiac rehabilitation centers, or in a patient's home. **(pg. 634)**
- Exercise electrocardiography, also called a stress test or a treadmill stress test, monitors a patient's response to exercise that increases in difficulty. **(pg. 636)**
- The most important responsibility of the ECG technician is to provide patient safety and to handle emergencies. **(pg. 637)**
- With ambulatory monitoring, an ECG tracing is recorded over an extended period on patients who are able to ambulate, or walk. **(pg. 637)**
- Cardiovascular technologists require more education than ECG technicians. They assist physicians with tests that evaluate the heart and blood vessels. **(pg. 638)**
- Two important tests that the cardiovascular technologist assists with are cardiac catheterization and balloon angioplasty. Cardiac catheterization determines whether a patient has coronary artery disease (CAD). Balloon angioplasty with the insertion of a stent corrects CAD. **(pg. 639)**
- EEG and END technologists perform EEGs and other tests that involve diagnosis of nervous system disorders. The term END technologist is the more accurate description of the profession. **(pg. 640)**
- The main test an EEG and END technologist performs is an EEG. This test measures the electrical activity of the brain. This measurement helps in diagnosing various disorders. **(pg. 641)**

SECTION 26.2

- The cardiac electrical conduction system consists of the following elements: sinoatrial (SA) node, atrioventricular (AV) node, bundle of His (AV bundle), bundle branches, and Purkinje fibers (network). **(pg. 643)**
- To perform an ECG safely and accurately, you must have a basic understanding of the conduction system, the leads and electrodes, and the ECG machine. You must follow safety guidelines and troubleshoot the tracing during the procedure. **(pg. 645)**
- Electrodes are sensors that are placed on the patient to pick up the electrical activity of the heart and conduct it to the ECG machine. **(p. 646)**
- ECG machine controls include speed, gain, artifact filter, computerized controls, and lead selector. **(p. 648)**

CHAPTER
26 Assessment

Critical Thinking/Problem Solving

1. A patient with a history of heart disease has arrived at the cardiology department. She is scheduled for an ECG and is taking the medications listed below. You are responsible for listing all medications on the ECG history, but you are not familiar with all these. The ECG must be done in the next 15 minutes. What should you do?
   - Cartrol 10 mg PO bid
   - Vioxx 12.5 mg qd
   - Valium 5 mg PO tid
   - Claritin syrup 10 mg PO qd
   - Isoptin SR 180 mg q12 h
   - Cimetidine 400 mg PO qid hs
2. While you are preparing to perform an ECG on a child, he screams, "Don't put those wires on me! The electricity will hurt me." What should you say or do?
3. Become familiar with an ECG machine. Using the manufacturer's directions and this textbook ("ECG Machine Controls" on pg. 648), locate the parts of the machine and the machine controls.
4. As an END technologist, you will frequently perform EEGs on patients who have epilepsy. Research the Internet for this neurological disorder. What should you do if a patient has a seizure while you are performing an EEG?

21ST CENTURY SKILLS

5. **Teamwork** Discuss how exercise affects the cardiovascular system. With a partner, take each other's pulse and record the rates. Next, calculate the target heart rate (THR). Walk in place for five to ten minutes and recheck the pulse. What happened to the pulse and THR? How can exercise benefit the cardiovascular system?
6. **Information Literacy** As an ECG technician or a cardiovascular technologist, you should be well informed about heart disease. Go online to learn more about the risks of heart disease and how it can be prevented.

McGraw Hill connect™ ONLINE ACTIVITIES

Complete our HST online activities for Chapter 26, which include Concept Check review questions, Reference Flash Cards, and Online Procedures assessment sheets.

- **Concept Check** review questions
- **Reference Flash Cards** medical terminology practice
- **Online Procedures** assessment sheets

CHAPTER 27

Radiology

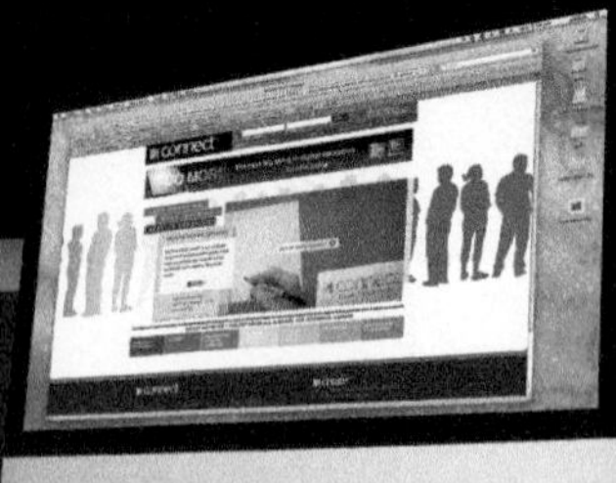

McGraw Hill connect™

It's Online!

- **Online Procedures**
- **STEM Connection**
- **Medical Science**
- **Medical Terms**
- **Medical Math**
- **Ethics in Action**
- **Virtual Lab**

Essential Question:

What is the role of radiology professionals in the fight against cancer and other life-threatening diseases?

Excellent career opportunities exist in radiology and radiologic technology. To qualify for a position, you will need to learn to use sophisticated diagnostic imaging or radiation therapy equipment. This equipment is used for the diagnosis and treatment of patient disease or injury. There are numerous careers available in the field of radiology or radiologic technology, including radiologist, nuclear medicine technologist, dosimetrist, and several others described in this chapter.

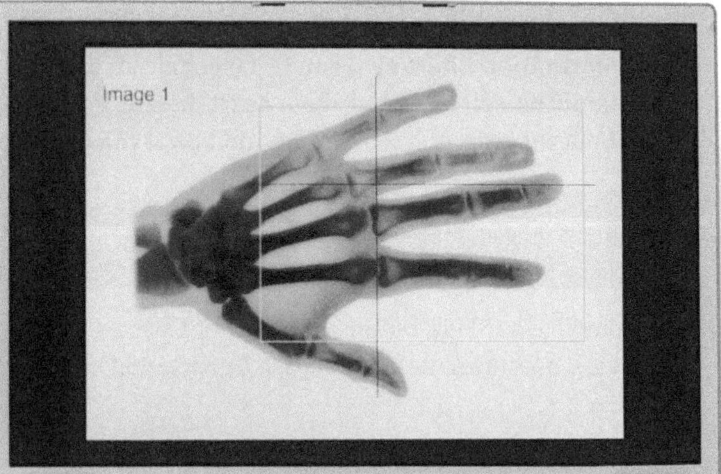

Photo: Fuse/Getty Images

READING GUIDE

OBJECTIVES

After completing this chapter, you will be able to:

- **Indicate** two primary roles of the radiologist.
- **Name** three primary roles of the radiologic technologist.
- **Identify** the advanced practice roles of the radiologic technologist.
- **Illustrate** settings in which radiologists and radiologic technologists work.
- **Differentiate** between invasive and noninvasive diagnostic imaging procedures.
- **Indicate** the steps required to protect the patient and radiologic healthcare professionals from unnecessary exposure to radiation.
- **Explain** the importance of the inverse square law.
- **Demonstrate** two radiologic procedures.

STANDARDS

HEALTH SCIENCE

NCHSE 1.21 Describe common diseases and disorders of each body system (prevention, pathology, diagnosis, and treatment).

NCHSE 2.11 Interpret verbal and nonverbal communication.

SCIENCE

NSES C Develop understanding of the cell; molecular basis of heredity; biological evolution; interdependence of organisms; matter, energy, and organization in living systems; and behavior of organisms.

NCHSE *National Consortium for Health Science Education*

NSES *National Science Education Standards*

COMMON CORE STATE STANDARDS

MATHEMATICS

Algebra

Creating Equations A-CED 2 Create equations in two or more variables to represent relationships between quantities; graph equations on coordinate axes with labels and scales.

ENGLISH LANGUAGE ARTS

Speaking and Listening

Presentation of Knowledge and Ideas SL-4 Present information, findings, and supporting evidence, conveying a clear and distinct perspective, such that listeners can follow the line of reasoning, alternative or opposing perspectives are addressed, and the organization, development, substance, and style are appropriate to purpose, audience, and a range of formal and informal tasks.

BEFORE YOU READ

Connect Have you ever had a disease or injury that was diagnosed by a radiology team? What was that experience like?

Main Idea

Radiology professionals use advanced medical technology to diagnose and treat many diseases and injuries.

Note-Taking Activity

Draw this table. Write key terms and phrases under **Cues**. Write main ideas under **Note Taking**. Summarize the section under **Summary**.

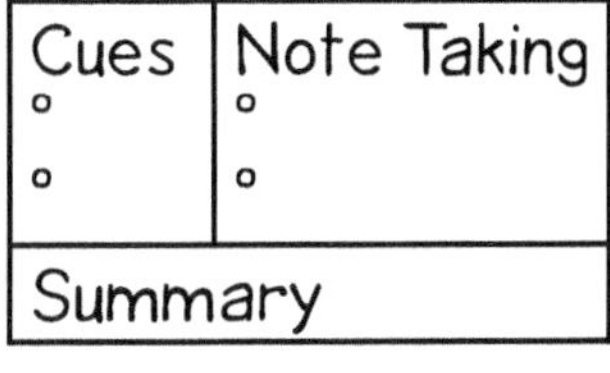

Graphic Organizer

Before you read the chapter, draw a diagram like the one to the right. As you read, write the main radiology careers covered in section one into the diagram.

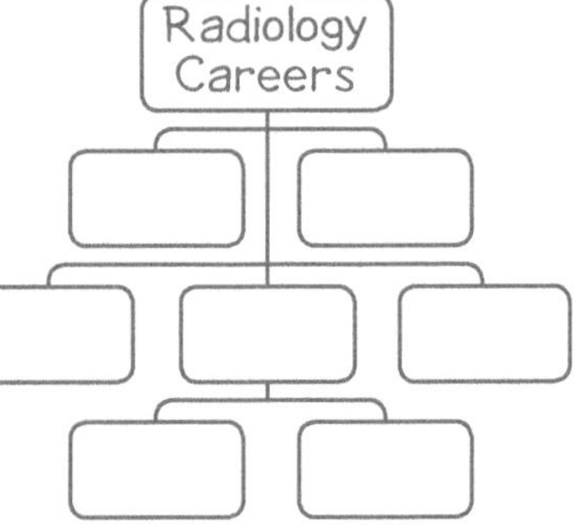

connect

Downloadable graphic organizers can be accessed online.

SECTION 27.1 Careers in Radiology and Radiologic Technology

Vocabulary

Content Vocabulary

You will learn these content vocabulary terms in this section.

- **noninvasive imaging**
- **invasive imaging**
- **contrast media**
- **angiogram**
- **arteriogram**
- **fluoroscopy**
- **atheroma**
- **external beam therapy**
- **brachytherapy**
- **radiograph**
- **X-ray**
- **radiopaque**
- **radiolucent**
- **As Low As Reasonably Achievable (ALARA)**

Academic Vocabulary

You will see this word in your reading and on your tests. Find its meaning in the Glossary in the back of the book.

- **energy**

Overview

What are X-rays?

Dr. Wilhelm Conrad Roentgen discovered the X-ray on November 8, 1895 and started the field of radiology. He named the ray after the symbol "X," the mathematical symbol for "unknown." The first recognized radiograph using photographic glass plates generated by Dr. Roentgen was of the hand of his wife, Bertha. It shows her hand with a ring on her finger (see **Figure 27.1**). This famous image was taken the same day as the discovery of the X-ray. Sometimes X-rays are referred to as Roentgen rays in honor of Dr. Roentgen.

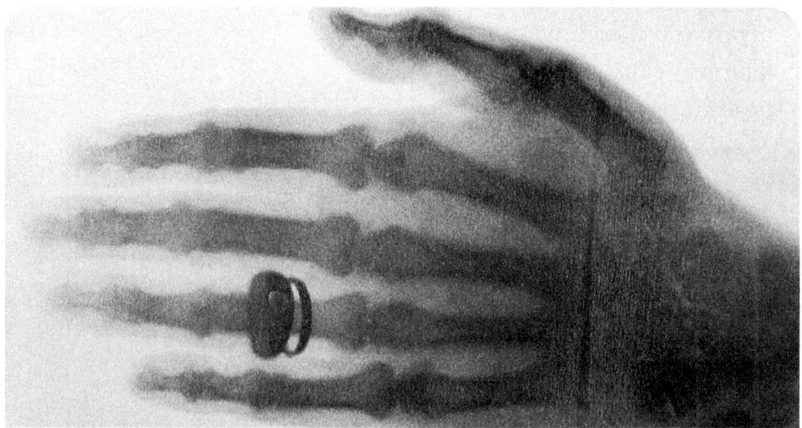

Fig. 27.1 Radiograph Image taken by Dr. Wilhelm Roentgen. *Why is this image of the hand of Dr. Roentgen's wife, Bertha, so famous?*

READING CHECK

Identify what the letter "X" in X-ray represents.

Table 27.1 Overview of Radiology and Radiologic Technology Occupations

OCCUPATION	EDUCATIONAL REQUIREMENTS	CERTIFICATION OR LICENSING AGENCY	JOB OUTLOOK
Diagnostic Radiologist	Four-year residency in radiology beyond medical school and internship	American Board of Radiology, American Osteopathic Board of Radiology	Faster than average growth with increased use of diagnostic imaging
Medical Dosimetrist	AS, BA or BS in physical or biological sciences or Registered Radiation Therapist qualification and two to four years on-the-job training under a Certified Medical Dosimetrist or Medical Physicist	Medical Dosimetrist Certification Board (state license may also be required)	Above average growth

Photo: Bettmann/CORBIS

Table 27.1 Overview of Radiology and Radiologic Technology Occupations continued

OCCUPATION	EDUCATIONAL REQUIREMENTS	CERTIFICATION OR LICENSING AGENCY	JOB OUTLOOK
Radiologic Technologist	One to four years of training in an approved Joint Review Committee on Education in Radiologic Technology (JRCERT) postsecondary program leading to a certificate or two- or four year degree	American Registry of Radiologic Technologists (state license may also be required)	Average growth
Nuclear Medicine Technologist	One to four years training in a JRCERT-approved postsecondary program leading to a certificate or two- or four-year degree	American Registry of Radiologic Technologists and/or Nuclear Medicine Technology Certification Board (NMTCB). States may require licensure.	Average growth
Radiation Therapist	One to four years of training in a JRCERT-approved postsecondary program leading to a certificate or 2- or 4-year degree	American Registry of Radiologic Technologists (state license may also be required)	Average growth
Cardiovascular-Interventional Technologist	American Registry of Radiologic Technologists (ARRT) registered technologist Certification and ARRT-specified clinical experience	American Registry of Radiologic Technologists (state license may also be required)	Average growth
Computed Tomography Technologist	ARRT Certification as a registered technologist and ARRT-specified clinical experience	American Registry of Radiologic Technologists (state license may be required)	Average growth
Magnetic Resonance Technologist	ARRT Certification as a registered technologist and ARRT-specified clinical experience	American Registry of Radiologic Technologists (state license may be required)	Average growth
Mammographer	ARRT Certification as a registered technologist and ARRT-specified clinical experience	American Registry of Radiologic Technologists (state license may be required)	Average growth
Sonographer	Certification as a registered technologist with ARRT and documentation of ARRT-specified clinical experience or completion of one- to four-year JRCERT-approved program	American Registry of Radiologic Technologists, American Registry of Diagnostic Medical Sonographers (state license may also be required)	Average growth
Bone Densitometry Technologist	ARRT Certification as a registered technologist and ARRT-specified clinical experience	American Registry of Radiologic Technologists (state license may be required)	Average growth
Quality Management Technologist	ARRT Certification as a registered technologist and ARRT-specified clinical experience	American Registry of Radiologic Technologists	Average growth
PACS Administrator	Education requirements vary from facility to facility, but in a majority of cases PACS administration is performed by an RT	American Board of Imaging Informatics or PACS Administrator Registry and Certification Association	Above average growth
Radiology Aide	On-the-job or vocational training of two to four weeks	None	Average growth

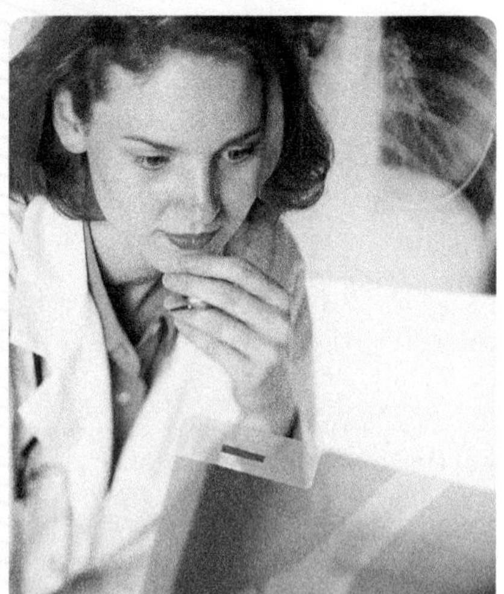

Fig. 27.2 Diagnostic Radiologist Diagnostic radiology helps doctors to diagnose a patient's disease or injury *What does this kind of doctor use to diagnose disease and injury?*

The Radiologist

How does radiation fight cancer?

Radiologists specialize in the use of radiant energy to diagnose and treat disease. Most of them work in hospitals, but they may also work in private practice and at diagnostic imaging or radiation therapy centers (see **Figure 27.2**). Doctors in this field may specialize in diagnostic radiology or radiation oncology.

The Diagnostic Radiologist

What is coronary angiography?

Diagnostic radiology creates images using X-rays, magnetic fields, sonar, and radioactivity. These images allow the doctor to make a diagnosis of a patient's disease or injury. Radiologists may specialize further in areas such as angiography or nuclear medicine.

The Job of the Diagnostic Radiologist

The diagnostic radiologist conducts general and specialized imaging examinations of the human body. **Noninvasive imaging** studies are taken from outside the body and do not require the use of a contrast medium. These examinations may use radiography, magnetic resonance imaging, computed tomography, mammography, or sonography (see **Figure 27.3**). Most radiologists delegate responsibility for these images to radiologic technologists.

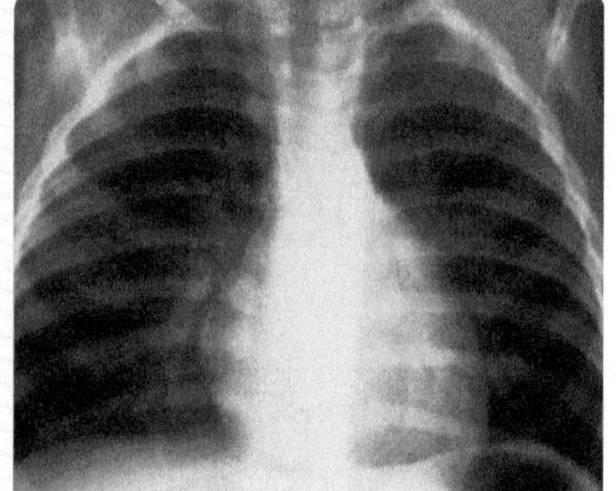

Fig. 27.3 Chest Radiograph Posterior-anterior (PA) chest radiograph. *Is this color-enhanced posterior-anterior (PA) chest radiograph an example of a noninvasive or invasive imaging procedure?*

Invasive imaging studies are taken by introducing a contrast agent into the body. Virtually every internal organ can be imaged in this way. **Contrast media** are substances that allow internal structures to be viewed. Risk to the patient is increased for these examinations, in which the diagnostic radiologist may insert catheters and inject drugs or contrast agents. Invasive examinations include angiograms, upper gastrointestinal exams, barium enemas, and nuclear medicine scans.

Diagnostic radiologists must have extensive knowledge and skill in both medicine and radiology. The importance of their expertise is clear, especially when invasive imaging tests like angiography must be performed on patients.

Job Responsibilities of the Diagnostic Radiologist

The diagnostic radiologist is responsible for

- maintaining aseptic and sterile techniques, and following standard precautions when dealing with patients and coworkers.
- using various imaging modalities. Examples of modalities in diagnostic radiology are general and digital radiography, fluoroscopy, computed tomography, ultrasound, magnetic resonance, and nuclear medicine.

- administering contrast agents, such as barium, iodine-based solutions or air into the patient's digestive tract, joints, and circulatory system to enhance imaging results.
- responding to emergencies and administering drugs to counteract adverse reactions to contrast media, such as anaphylactic shock.
- using a fluoroscope to inspect internal structures of the body and guide catheters through arteries and veins.
- taking spot films that identify suspicious and routine findings.
- studying the findings for all images produced.
- generating a written report for the patient's attending physician.
- supervising a diagnostic imaging team of radiographers, nuclear medicine technologists, advanced practice specialists, and aides.

Coronary Angiography Coronary angiography is an invasive imaging procedure designed to determine where a coronary artery is narrowed or blocked. The radiologist injects contrast media into the coronary artery of the heart through a catheter inserted through the femoral artery of the groin. Sometimes the brachial artery of the arm is used to advance the catheter into the heart's coronary artery.

There is also a similar procedure called arteriography. The images from this procedure are called angiograms or arteriograms. An **angiogram** is an image showing both arteries and veins filled with contrast media. An **arteriogram** is an image that shows only arteries filled with contrast media.

Patients are sedated but conscious during both procedures. Because they are awake, they can respond to instructions from the radiologist during the procedure. These procedures must be performed under sterile conditions.

Fluoroscopy **Fluoroscopy** is an imaging process that is used to advance the catheter through the artery, into the heart, and then into the coronary artery. In fluoroscopy, the X-ray image is projected onto a fluorescent screen. This allows real-time visual examination of the anatomy. Contrast media is injected through the catheter using a pressure injector machine. A series of rapid radiographic pictures of the coronary artery and its branches are recorded digitally or on X-ray films. Depending on the type of system that is used, the images will display an outline of the heart showing white, black, or color-enhanced lines filling with contrast media and reveal the coronary artery and its branches.

The diagnostic radiologist looks for lines that are narrower than normal. This indicates the presence of plaque. The abrupt stopping of a line

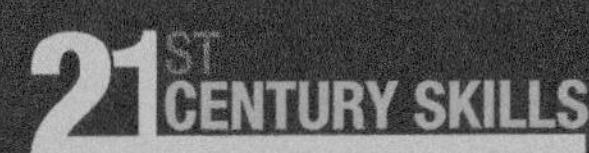

Provide Reassurance but Be Prudent

Patients about to undergo a radiology procedure are under considerable stress because of their illness or injury. Consequently, radiologic technologists must interact with them in a reassuring and confident manner. Patients will often ask the technologist for a prediction or explanation of their status. Although technologists must be sensitive to the patient's need for reassurance, they also must be prudent. It is important to explain to the patient that they are performing the procedure so that a physician can make a diagnosis and produce a treatment plan.

The Health Insurance Portability and Accountability Act (HIPAA) was enacted in 1996 by the U.S. Congress to protect the security and privacy of patient information. Always be mindful of what patient information you discuss and where you discuss it.

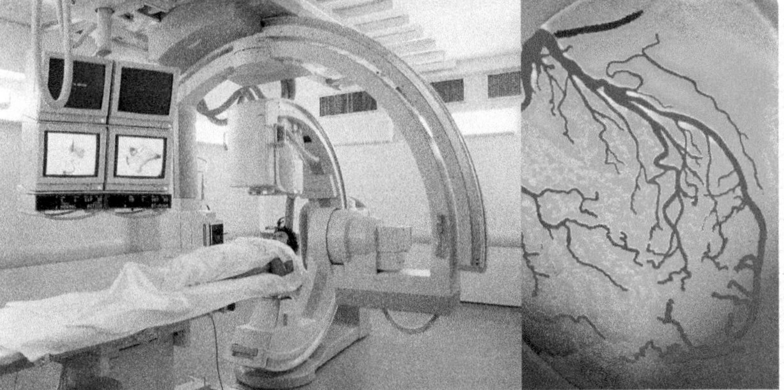

Fig. 27.4 Angiography Color-enhanced coronary angiography. *Why is coronary angiography considered an invasive imaging procedure?*

Photos: (l)Laurent/Photo Researchers, (r)CGA/CNRI/Phototake

indicates that a branch of the main coronary artery is blocked by a blood clot or by **atheroma,** which is a fat deposit on the inside of the arterial wall (see **Figure 27.4**).

READING CHECK

Recall some examples of non-invasive procedures performed by diagnostic radiologists.

The Radiation Oncologist

What types of therapy are used by radiation oncologists?

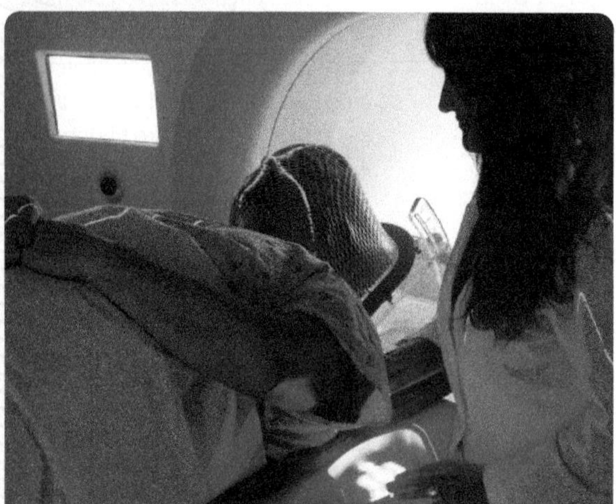

Fig. 27.5 Radiation Oncologist The radiation oncologist determines the tumor treatment plan. *How does this kind of doctor use radiation in the treatment of cancer?*

Radiation oncology deals with the use of radiation in the treatment of cancer (see **Figure 27.5**). When radiation strikes cancer cells, cell growth stops or slows down. This decreases the rate of cell division or impairs DNA synthesis.

The Job of the Radiation Oncologist

The radiation oncologist determines a tumor treatment plan for a patient. The goals of the plan are to cure a cancer, relieve pain and distress, enhance the action of drugs, or establish local tumor control (see **Figure 27.6**). The radiation oncologist must have knowledge of and skill in medicine, osteopathy, and radiology.

Job Responsibilities of the Radiation Oncologist

The radiation oncologist will

- maintain aseptic and sterile techniques and follow standard precautions with patients and coworkers.
- use radiation treatments to destroy or inhibit the reproductive ability of cancerous cells or tumors.
- identify the volume of the patient's body to be treated; the entry and exit points for the radiation beam; the radiation source; the amount and number of doses to be delivered; the total tumor dose; and the prescription point, or isodose.
- explain the treatment plan to the patient and obtain informed consent.
- use positioning and immobilizing devices, and normal tissue shielding.
- assess the patient's tumor response after radiation therapy treatments so that serious problems can be avoided.
- supervise a team of radiation therapists, medical physicists, medical dosimetrists, and radiology aides.

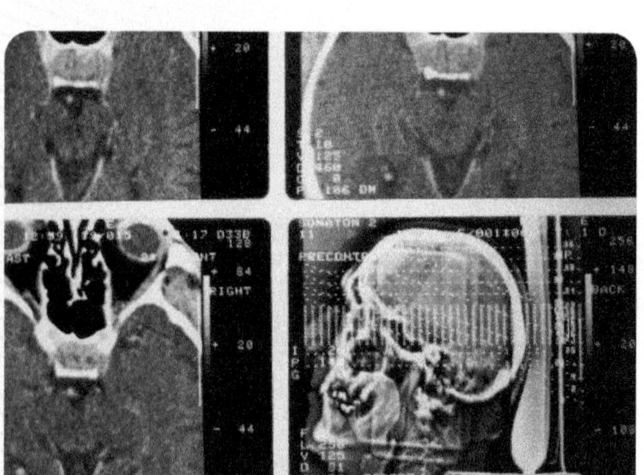

Fig. 27.6 CT Scan A CT scan is used to guide radiation therapy. *What are some reasons why a patient may have radiation therapy treatment?*

Radiation Therapies Performed by the Radiation Oncologist

Two types of radiation therapies are performed by radiation oncologists.

External beam therapy External beam therapy is usually delivered in daily doses over several weeks. Cobalt 60 may be used in this treatment (see **Figure 27.7**). Treatments are given by the radiation therapist, but the prescription and treatment plans are designed by the radiation oncologist. The radiation oncologist monitors the patient's progress and informs the referring physician as needed. One version of **external beam therapy** involves the use of a linear accelerator.

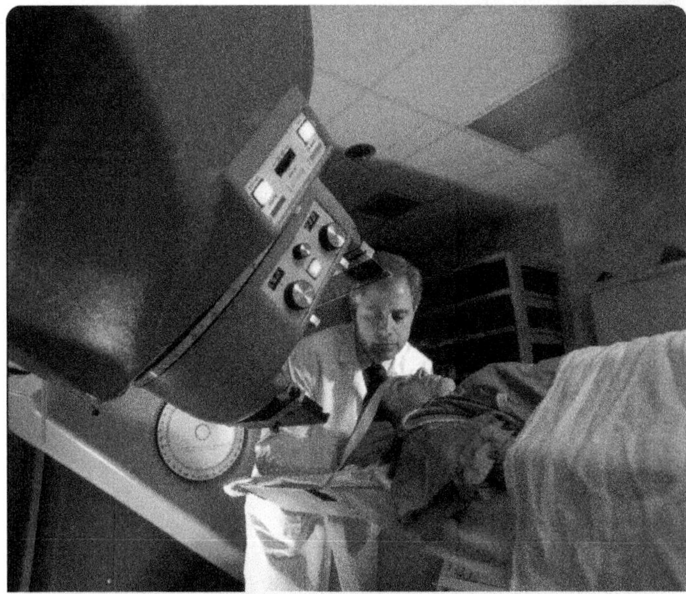

Fig. 27.7 External Beam Therapy A cobalt 60 teletherapy unit. *What are the two types of radiation therapies performed by radiation oncologists?*

Linear Accelerator A linear accelerator (LINAC) uses microwave technology to accelerate electrons to incredible speeds in order to collide them into a heavy-metal target. This collision produces powerful X-rays. The radiation therapist focuses the X-rays closely on the patient's tumor, to destroy cancer cells without damaging normal surrounding tissue. External beam therapy using a LINAC is common. Depending on the patient's disease and general condition, radiation therapy treatments are administered each day for five days per week for up to eight weeks. Daily treatments take less than 15 minutes. The X-ray beam is turned on for about a minute and exposes the patient's tumor in two or more directions (see **Figure 27.8**).

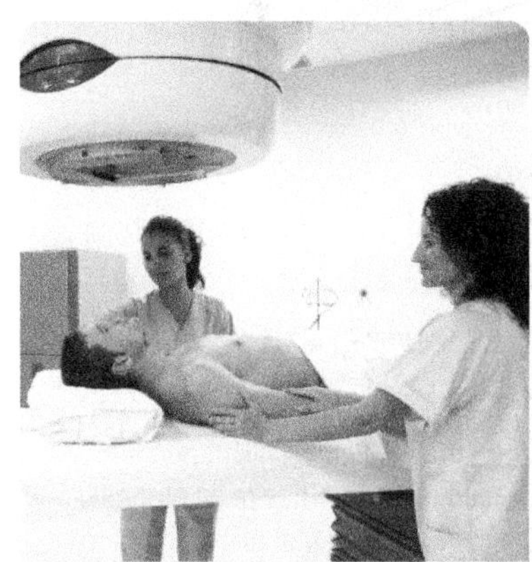

Fig. 27.8 LINAC A LINAC uses microwave technology. *How does a LINAC generate radiation to treat cancer?*

Brachytherapy The other main form of radiation therapy, **brachytherapy,** involves using radionuclide sources to treat tumors inside the body. For example, the radiology oncologist may insert radioactive seeds into the prostate gland to treat prostate cancer (see **Figure 27.9**).

Other treatment types can be combined with external beam radiation and brachytherapy to reduce tumors and decrease the effect of the radiation on surrounding normal tissues.

READING CHECK

Recall how the radiation oncologist determines the frequency and number of radiation treatments.

Medical Dosimetrist

How does a medical dosimetrist design a treatment plan for cancer patients?

The medical dosimetrist is a member of the radiation oncology team who has knowledge of the characteristics and relevance of radiation oncology treatment machines and equipment. The medical

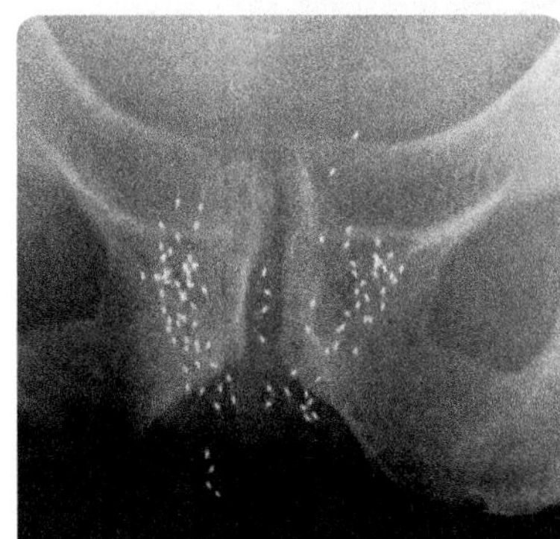

Fig. 27.9 Brachytherapy Radionuclide seeds are placed inside the prostate gland to treat prostate cancer. *What kind of radiation therapy is this?*

Photos: (t-b)Yoav Levy/Phototake,Pixtal/age fotostock, B.Bates, MD/Custom Medical Stock Photography

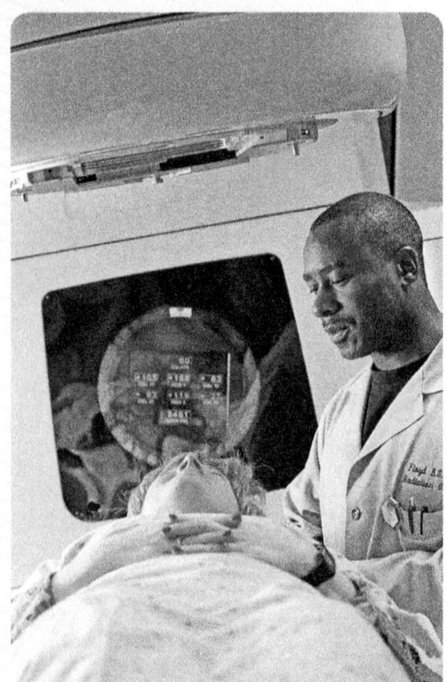

Fig. 27.10 Dosimetrist The amount of radiation given during radiation therapy is determined by the medical dosimetrist. *Why does a patient receive radiation therapy?*

dosimetrist is familiar with brachytherapy procedures. He or she has the expertise necessary to generate radiation dose distributions and dose calculations in collaboration with the medical physicist and radiation oncologist. Working under the supervision of a medical physicist, the dosimetrist will design a treatment plan that will deliver the prescribed radiation dose and specify the placement technique (see **Figure 27.10**).

READING CHECK

Explain the difference between noninvasive imaging and invasive imaging.

Radiologic Technologist

How do radiologic technologists support the work of radiologists?

Radiologic technologist is the preferred title for the healthcare professional who assists the radiologist. The term "technologist" indicates the degree of responsibility associated with the job. It implies that this individual is capable of independent thought and judgment, and has the skill to carry out professional actions. Radiologic technologists can pursue a number of occupations. Registered radiologic technologists (RT) are certified and supported by the American Registry of Radiologic Technologists (see **Figure 27.11**).

The Job of the Radiologic Technologist

Radiologic technology includes the fields of radiography, nuclear medicine technology, and radiation therapy technology. Registered radiologic technologists can also document specific clinical experience and test for advanced practice certification in areas such as cardiovascular-interventional technology, computed tomography, magnetic resonance imaging, mammography, sonography, bone densitometry, and quality management technology.

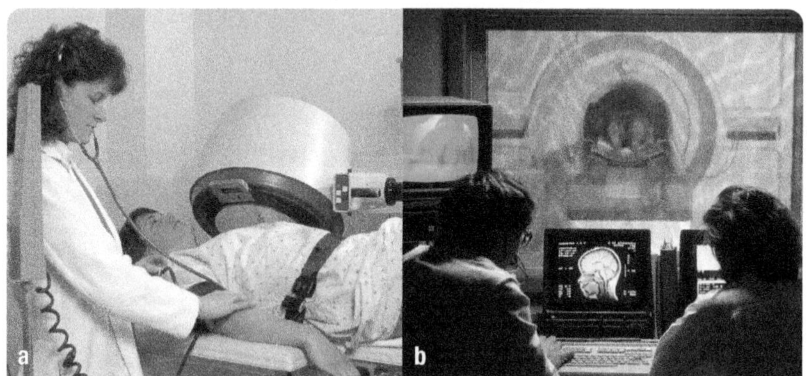

Fig. 27.11 Radiologic Technologists (a) A radiologic technologist assists the radiologist. **(b)**The blurry image shown here illustrates the protection that is built into the screen to shield the MRI scanner from radio frequency interference. *What professional organization supports radiologic technologists in the performance of their duties? What does the abbreviation MRI stand for?*

21ST CENTURY SKILLS

Leadership Skills

Radiologists and radiology managers must have excellent human relation skills. They need empathy toward others that allows them to identify with a variety of patients and situations. They need to understand the importance of body language as nonverbal communication. They must know how to listen, how to give verbal and nonverbal feedback, and how to judge the effectiveness of their communications. In leading the radiology team, radiologists and radiology managers delegate responsibilities, provide performance feedback, and monitor the outcomes of treatment. They also make sure that patient-flow in the radiology department is handled efficiently. A great sense of humor also helps.

Most radiologic technologists work in hospital radiology departments. They may also work in private physician offices, diagnostic-imaging centers, radiation treatment centers, and emergency care clinics. After receiving advanced education, some become educators in hospital- or college-based programs. Some become radiology administrators at facilities that offer diagnostic imaging or radiation treatment services. RTs may also be employed in the medical industry as sales, marketing and service representatives, product managers, or equipment application specialists. Some RTs start their own businesses, as authors, publishers, consultants, corporate trainers, providers of mobile imaging services, and owners of imaging manufacturing and supply agencies.

Continuing Education for the Radiologic Technologist To remain a registered radiologic technologist (RT) in good standing with the ARRT, RTs must receive a minimum of 24 approved continuing education units in a 24-month period. If certification expires, the RT will have to complete additional education and training. The purpose of ARRT's mandatory continuing education policy is to ensure that all RTs remain current in their areas of specialization, because rapid technological advances in equipment and procedures are constantly altering standards of patient care.

Radiographer About two thirds of radiologic technologists are employed as radiographers, and are in high demand because of the use of radiographs in medical diagnosis. **Radiographs** are two-dimensional images on X-ray film. The patient's anatomy is visible as light and dark shadows. The images can also be generated in digital and analog form for recording on computer disk or videotape (see **Figure 27.12**). Radiographers also perform fluoroscopy and use contrast media to produce images. **Table 27.2** on page 662 shows a list of procedures that radiographers perform.

Note: The term "X-ray" is often incorrectly used to describe what is actually a radiograph. An **X-ray** is an electromagnetic wave that has a wavelength much shorter than that of visible light. This shorter wavelength allows X-rays to penetrate objects and generate radiographs.

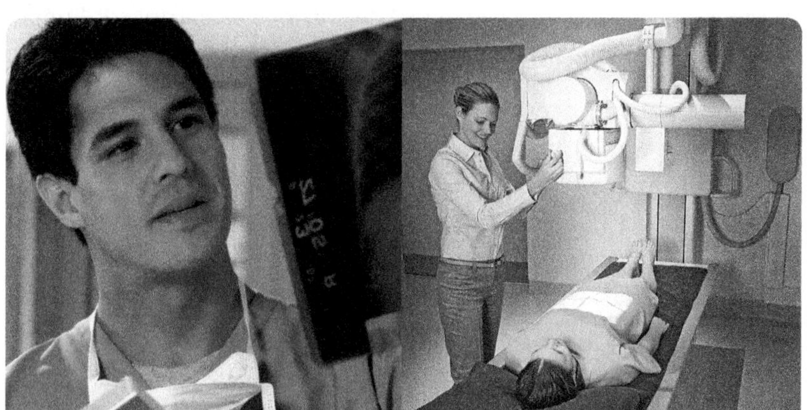

Fig. 27.12 Radiography Radiographers are in high demand because of the use of radiography in medical diagnoses. *How can a fluoroscopic image be stored?*

Photos: (l)Paul Barton/CORBIS, (r)OJO Images/Getty Images

21ST CENTURY SKILLS

Communicating with Voice Recording

Radiologists rely on medical transcriptionists or computer technology to create written diagnostic and treatment reports from their dictation. While dictating into a voice recorder, the radiologist speaks precisely and uses correct medical terminology. Clarity is essential so that all members of the healthcare team will understand all parts of the report. Radiologists often spell out a complex term, to make sure it is transcribed correctly. They may identify exactly where they want the punctuation marks—periods, commas, colons, semicolons, and so on—to be placed.

Follow-up
Why do radiologists take the time to spell certain words and include punctuation marks when they dictate findings?

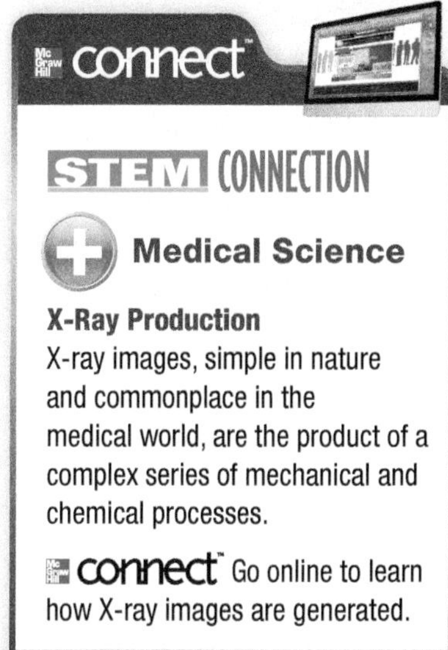

connect

STEM CONNECTION

Medical Science

X-Ray Production
X-ray images, simple in nature and commonplace in the medical world, are the product of a complex series of mechanical and chemical processes.

connect Go online to learn how X-ray images are generated.

Table 27.2 Procedures Performed by Radiographers

INVASIVE RADIOGRAPHIC PROCEDURES (REQUIRING CONTRAST MEDIA)	NONINVASIVE RADIOGRAPHIC PROCEDURES (NOT REQUIRING CONTRAST MEDIA)
Angiogram	Acromion Process
Arteriogram	Cervical Spine
Arthrogram	Chest
Barium Enema	Clavicle
Bronchogram	Facial Bones
Cholecystogram	Lumbar Spine
Cystogram	Mastoids
Esophogram	Nasal Bones
Hysterosalpingogram	Pelvis
Intravenous Cholangiogram	Sacrum/Coccyx
Intravenous Pyelogram	Shoulder
Lower Bowel Examination	Skull
Lymphangiogram	Thoracic Spine
Myelogram	Lower Extremities: femur, knee, tibia/fibula, ankle, foot, toes
Sialogram	Upper Extremities: humerus, elbow, radius/ulna, wrist, hand, fingers
Upper Gastrointestinal Examination	
Venogram	
Ventriculogram	

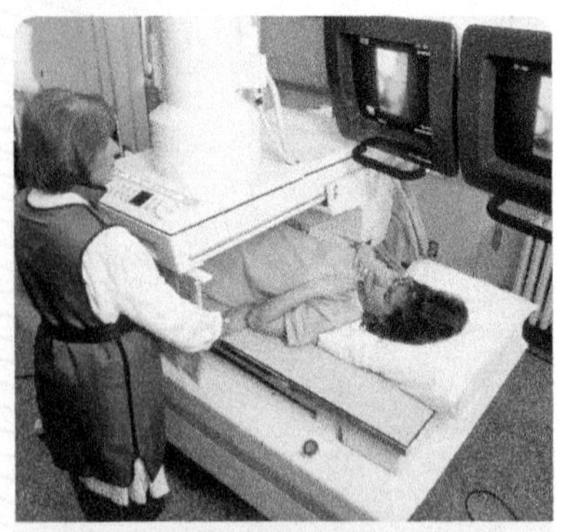

Fig. 27.13 Fluoroscopy Radiographers also perform fluoroscopy. *What kind of output is created by this type of X-ray imaging process?*

Radiographers also may perform fluoroscopy. These X-ray images of a patient's anatomy can be displayed on a monitor and stored on videotape or computer. Radiographic and fluoroscopic images use film emulsion or fluorescent screens to record decreasing differences of the X-rays as they pass through the various structures of human anatomy (see **Figure 27.13**).

The radiographic densities (blacks and grays) between two body parts are so similar that it is difficult to view them. Contrast media are used to make viewing easier. These are **radiopaque** or **radiolucent** substances that alter the passage of X-rays to the film emulsion or digital imaging plate. They are injected into the body to assist in imaging internal structures of the body. Iodine-based contrast media are injected into blood vessels; barium, often with air, may be swallowed or inserted into the rectum. After ingesting barium for upper gastrointestinal examinations, patients are advised to drink plenty of water since water prevents barium from hardening in the intestinal tract. (See **Figure 27.14** on page 663.)

Table 27.3 Procedures Performed by Nuclear Medicine Technologists

PROCEDURE	TO DIAGNOSE
Gallium Scan	Lymphomas and metastatic tumors
Gastroesophageal Reflux Scan	Heartburn, regurgitation of stomach contents, and difficulty swallowing
Multigated Acquisition Scan	Heart disease
Positron Emission Tomography (PET) often performed in conjunction with a CT scan	Blood flow, heart metabolism, brain biochemical activity, and various cancers
Radioactive Iodine Uptake	Thyroid function
Single Photon Emission Computed Tomography (SPECT)	Blood flow and liver function
Thallium Exercise Test	Heart disease

Nuclear Medicine Technologist

Nuclear medicine technologists use radioisotopes, often chemically bound to other chemicals, to obtain information about how well human anatomy functions. Radioactive drugs are used to help produce images. After radioisotopes are injected into the body, special multi-detector cameras detect radioactivity and translate the signals into images of the anatomy on a computer. **Table 27.3** shows examples of procedures produced by nuclear medicine technologists.

Radiation Therapist

Radiation therapists assist radiation oncologists by administering targeted radiation doses to cancer cells in the patient's body. Radiation therapists work with other staff members to ensure comprehensive treatment of cancer patients. They must be good team players.

Advanced Practice Roles of the Radiologic Technologist With additional education, training, and experience, a radiologic technologist can perform advanced techniques and procedures in the careers listed below.

Cardiovascular-interventional technologists use special radiographic and fluoroscopic imaging equipment. They work with radiologists and other specialists, such as cardiologists and neurologists. The physicians guide catheters into a patient's body and inject contrast media to visualize veins and arteries. Cardiovascular-interventional technologists take sophisticated images of the circulatory systems.

Computed tomography technologists use a kind of X-ray machine called a computed axial tomography (CT or CAT) scanner. This equipment obtains transverse cross-sectional anatomical images of the body called CT or CAT scans (see **Figure 27.15** on page 664). Those images view the body in slices, like slices of bread in a loaf. Each image is one "slice." The newest technologies use multiple detectors and continuous (spiral) imaging, which provides more information in less time.

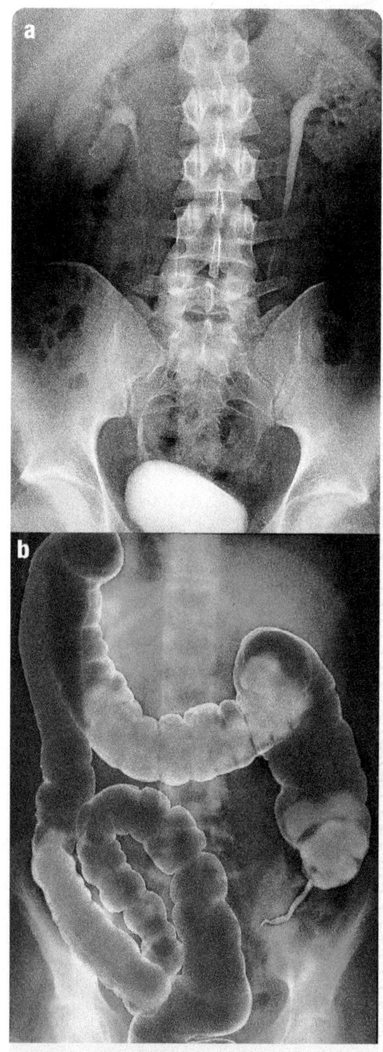

Fig. 27.14 Contrast Contrast media make viewing easier. **(a)** *What kind of contrast medium is used to visualize kidneys, ureters, and bladders?* **(b)** *What kind of contrast medium is used to visualize a patient's colon?*

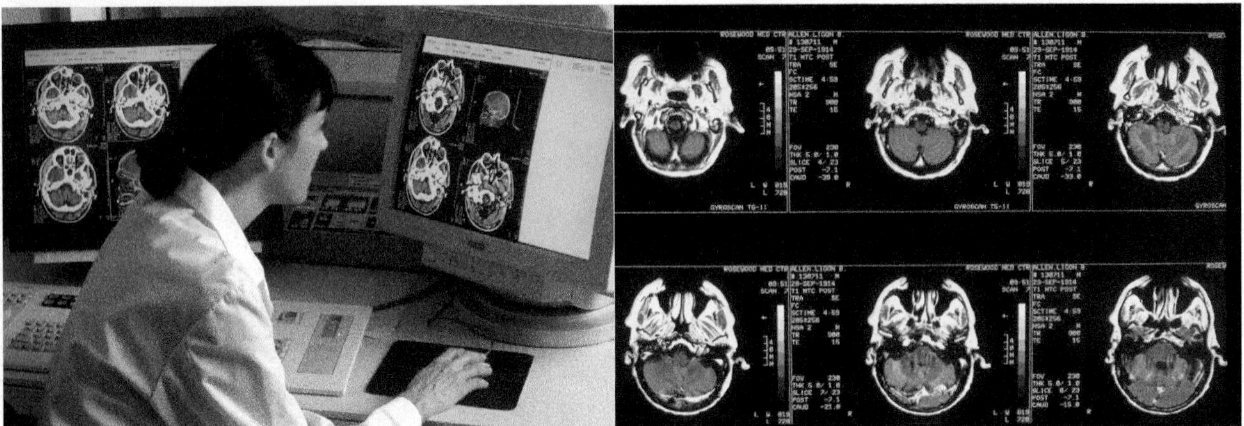

Fig. 27.15 CT Scan In a CT scan, the images appear on monitors and are transferred to film. *What kind of RT obtains special X-ray–generated cross-sectional images like this CAT scan of the brain?*

The images may be viewed and manipulated on a computer, even allowing 3D reconstruction.

Magnetic resonance technologists use a special machine to take longitudinal (vertical) and transverse (horizontal) cross-sectional anatomical images of the body. These images may be viewed on a computer monitor and transferred to film.

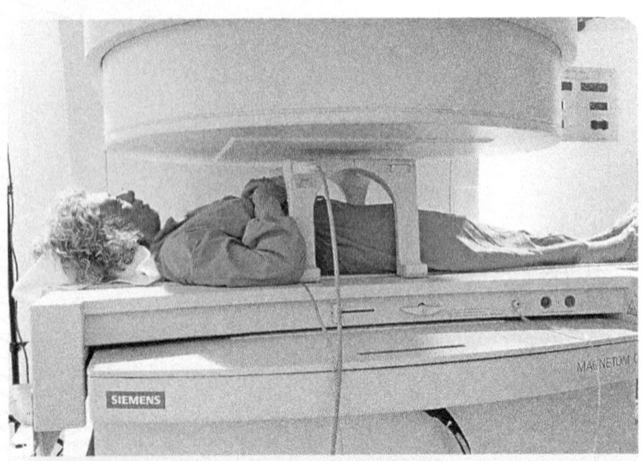

Fig. 27.16 MRI An open MRI unit. *What patient problem does this type of unit help solve?*

A magnetic resonance imaging (MRI) unit contains a large electromagnet that subjects the body to a strong magnetic field. The field aligns the hydrogen atoms in the body. When a pulse of radio waves is directed at the tissues to be imaged, the hydrogen atoms change the alignment of their nuclei. When the radio waves are turned off, the nuclei realign and give off energy that is converted to an electrical signal. The signal is clearer than most images produced by radiography or computed tomography.

Magnetic resonance technologists have two major concerns when they perform MRI examinations. Patients must be questioned about the presence of metal objects in their body, such as metal plates, pins, or sutures. The strong magnetic field can cause these metal objects to move in the body or even emerge through the skin, causing injury. For this reason, the room where MRIs take place must be magnet-free. Although an MRI does not expose the patient to ionizing radiation, patients who are claustrophobic find it difficult to remain in the gantry, or tube, for extended periods. The recent development of open MRI units has helped to solve this problem (see **Figure 27.16**).

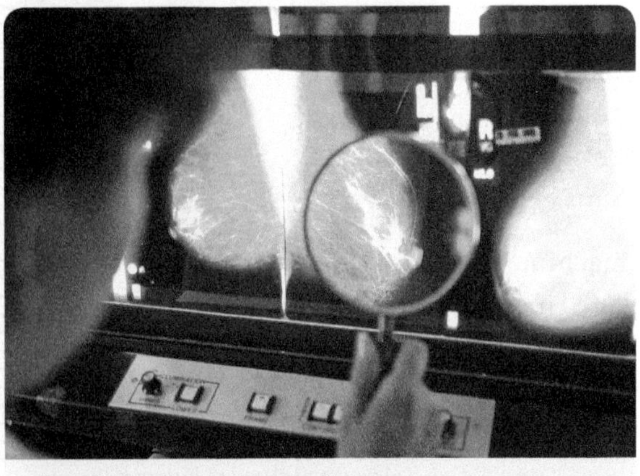

Fig. 27.17 Mammography Breast-cancer screening. *What kind of RT works with special X-ray equipment to take images of patient breast tissue?*

Mammographers produce diagnostic images of breast tissue with special mammography machines (see **Figure 27.17**).

They work in facilities certified by the U.S. Food and Drug Administration. This certification indicates that the facility is in compliance with the Mammography Quality Standards Act. Mammograms are used to assist in the early detection and treatment of breast cancer. An estimated 40,000 women died of breast cancer and an estimated 207,000 new cases were diagnosed in the United States in 2010. Early treatment increases the patient's chances of survival. MRIs are even more sensitive than mammograms, and their use in breast imaging is increasing.

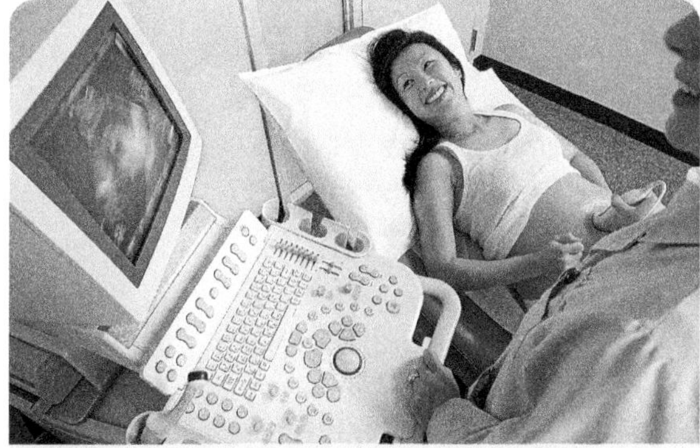

Fig. 27.18 Sound Waves Viewing an unborn child. *What kind of RT works with high-frequency sound waves to produce images of a fetus?*

Sonographers use a transducer to pass harmless high-frequency sound waves through the body. Sound waves are then returned from internal organs and tissues. These sound waves are converted into images displayed on a computer screen (see **Figure 27.18**). The images can be stored digitally in PACS and/or printed to be viewed by a radiologist. The American Registry of Diagnostic Medical Sonographers (ARDMS) certifies most sonographers.

Bone Densitometry Technologists use a special X-ray machine to measure the density of bone mineral at specific locations of the body. This test is used to check for osteoporosis and to estimate the risk of bone fracture.

Quality Management Technologists perform tests on imaging equipment and ancillary components. The purpose is to keep the equipment properly calibrated (see **Figure 27.19**).

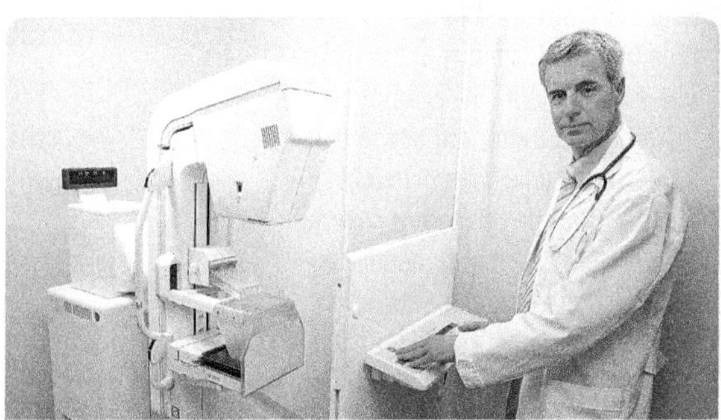

Fig. 27.19 Calibration Testing imaging equipment. *What kind of RT calibrates imaging equipment using special quality management tools?*

Job Responsibilities of the Radiologic Technologist

Regardless of their area of certification or advanced practice, all radiologic technologists

- follow the **As Low As Reasonably Achievable (ALARA)** guideline. It is the responsibility of all imaging technologists to practice radiation safety using all reasonable methods to minimize radiation doses.
- maintain aseptic and sterile techniques and follow standard precautions when dealing with patients and coworkers.
- identify the patient.
- transport patients from the waiting room or patient's room to the radiology department or suite.
- explain the procedure to the patient in a courteous and professional manner.
- assist patients onto and off of examination tables as necessary.
- position patients for the desired anatomy to be imaged or irradiated. Use alternative positioning methods as the patient's condition dictates. Use positioning aids and sponges to minimize patient motion and discomfort.

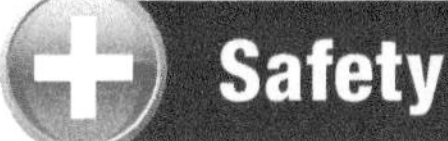

Dangerous Allergies

Shellfish contain iodine. Patients who are allergic to shellfish may find it difficult to tolerate iodine-based contrast media used for certain procedures. Frequently, they develop an allergic reaction to the contrast media. In some cases that reaction can be life-threatening. It is important to ask the patient about any allergies to food or medications before using contrast media.

21ST CENTURY SKILLS

Create a Comforting Environment

The radiology environment can be intimidating to patients who are under the stress of illness or injury. Large pieces of equipment and technical personnel in lab coats can paint a cold and sterile picture in the patient's mind. This may be interpreted as dehumanizing. RTs can help prevent this by making sure that patients are treated like people and not just a number or a body part. This involves making sure that all aspects of the patient's needs are attended to during the time he or she spends in the radiology environment. For example, imaging and treatment tables can be hard and cold. Attentive RTs will see that the tables are covered with sheets and that patients have access to pillows, blankets, and cushions for support and warmth. They also will ensure that their patients have access to bathrooms, drinking water, and other comforts.

- use proper shielding and radiation protection to ensure the safety of patient and healthcare personnel.
- calculate and set proper imaging exposure and radiation treatment factors. The result must be high-quality images or effective radiation treatments based on a proper assessment of the patient's age, body type, physical condition, and suspected pathology.
- assist the radiologist during procedures by changing films, positioning patients, and preparing contrast media and drugs.
- use aseptic and sterile technique when assisting radiologists in needle, guide wire, and catheter insertions, and tissue biopsies.
- perform image-processing procedures such as film development, reloading cassettes, radiographic film duplication and image subtraction, reloading of film bins, and cleaning cassettes and screens.
- maintain a clean and orderly work environment that is properly supplied for all diagnostic procedures. Ensure that sterile packaged supplies are on hand and are not damaged or outdated.
- use all equipment and accessories in a hygienic and efficient manner.
- perform office tasks, such as film and report filing, scheduling examinations, answering phones and relaying information, completing examination requisitions, retrieving previous films, and ensuring files and records are properly completed. Understand departmental policies and procedures, including examination routines, examination scheduling, and patient preparation. Instruct patients and nursing personnel as required.
- work after-hours "on-call" shifts.
- perform quality assurance analysis and document quality control.
- maintain employee-patient professionalism in all aspects of patient care by appearing professional and hygienic at all times.

READING CHECK

List some technologies other than X-ray technology that a radiologic technologist might use.

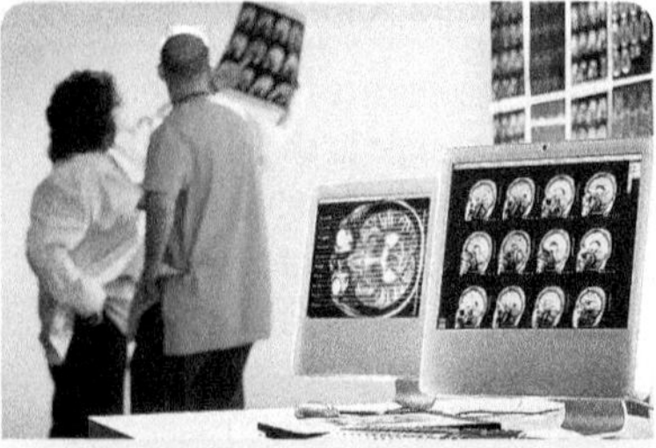

Fig. 27.20 PACS Administrator Managing archived images. *What is the name of computer system called that allows RTs to capture, manipulate, transmit, archive, and retrieve a patient imaging report within a network or over the Internet?*

Photo: Ron Levine/Photodisc/Getty Images

Picture Archival and Communications Systems (PACS) Administrator

What role does image management play in the field of radiology?

The use of Picture Archival and Communications Systems (PACS) is common. Diagnostic images that are digitized can be viewed on computers and archived electronically. Some radiologic technologists are making a career change to become information management experts. In that capacity, they capture, manipulate, transmit, archive, and retrieve images within a computer network or over the Internet.

When a patient's file is archived on the Internet, healthcare professionals can retrieve reports from practically anywhere (see **Figure 27.20**). The PACS Administrator is the person who oversees the PACS system planning, implementation, and maintenance.

READING CHECK

Explain the benefit of having patient files archived on the Internet.

Radiology Aide

How does the radiology aide help a radiology department function?

Most busy radiology departments employ one or more radiology aides to provide assistance to members of the radiology team. Aides may take over some of the radiologic technician's functions listed above, such as transporting patients to and from the radiology department, keeping equipment and rooms clean, answering phones, filing, and developing films (see **Figure 27.21**).

READING CHECK

List some of the job duties of the radiology aide.

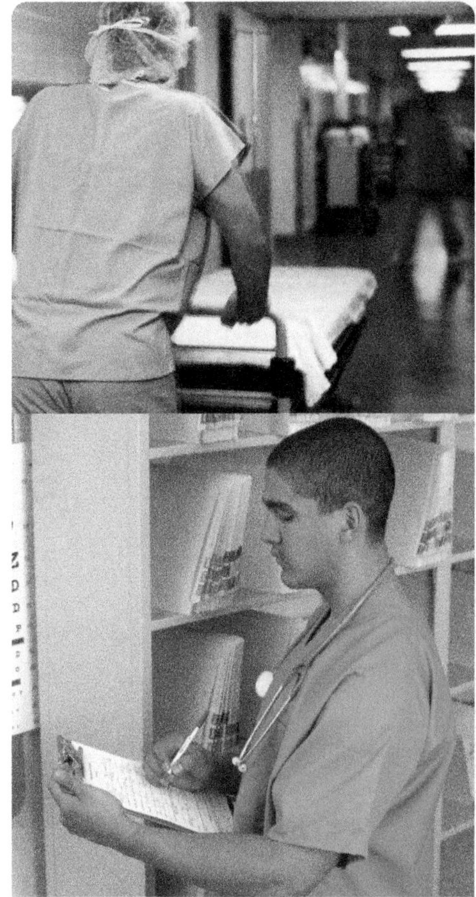

Fig. 27.21 Radiology Aide Managing radiology files. *Which individuals are hired by busy radiology departments to help transport patients and file radiology reports?*

SECTION 27.1 Careers in Radiology and Radiologic Technology Review

AFTER YOU READ

1. **Explain** the two primary roles of a radiologist.
2. **Identify** two primary roles of the radiologic technologist.
3. **List** the radiologic technologist's advanced practice roles.
4. **Describe** the settings in which radiologists and radiologic technologists may work.
5. **Contrast** invasive and noninvasive diagnostic imaging procedures.
6. **Explain** how the medical dosimetrist and the PACS administrator work to assist the radiology team.

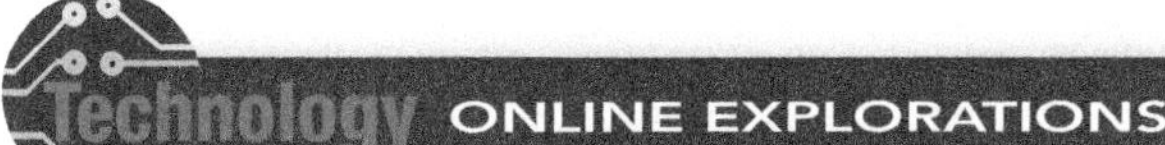

Entry Requirements

Research online to determine the requirements for a radiologic technology school in your area. Assess your career interests and current level of preparation. Write a short paragraph outlining what you would need to accomplish to enter this field.

Photos: (t)Photodisc, (b)David Crow

SECTION 27.2

Procedures in Radiology and Radiologic Technology

Vocabulary

Content Vocabulary

You will learn these content vocabulary terms in this section.

- **collimator**
- **inverse square law**

Academic Vocabulary

You will see this word in your reading and on your tests. Find its meaning in the Glossary in the back of the book.

- **register**

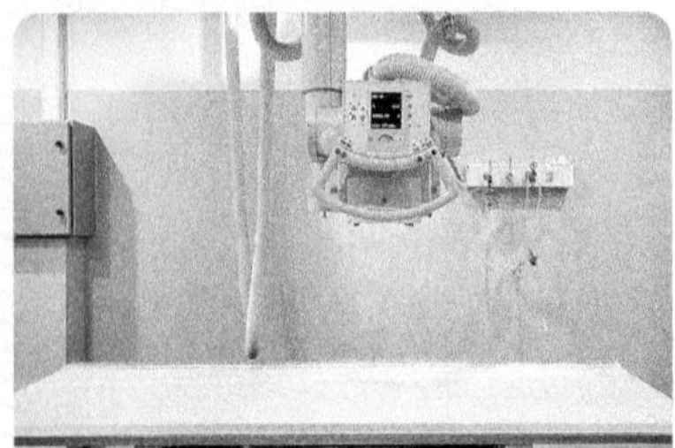

Fig. 27.22 X-rays A typical X-ray setup. *What is the box-like device that is hanging below the X-ray tube housing called? What is its purpose?*

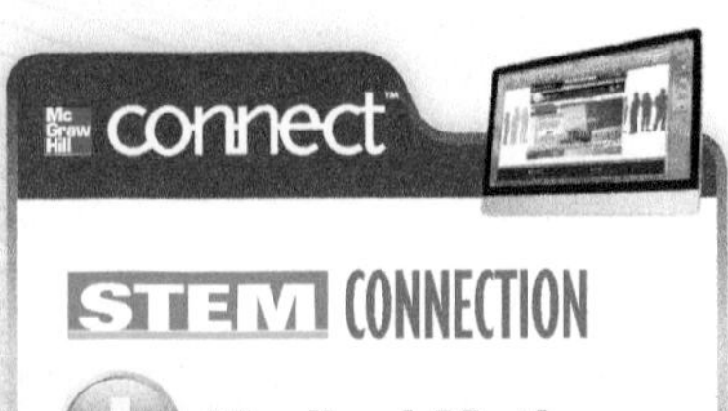

STEM CONNECTION

Medical Math

The Inverse Square Law

The **inverse square law** is used to determine a safe distance from the source of radiation while performing radiographs.

connect Go online to learn how to establish the radiation intensity of a given distance from its source.

Radiation Protection

What methods are used to guard the body against overexposure to radiation?

Exposure to radiation causes cell damage. While some body tissue cells can recover fully from normal levels of radiation, others cannot. The damage can be permanent. Radiation can build up to a level that will cause damage to body cells. Before you perform any procedure, be aware of the dangers of radiation to protect yourself and your patients.

Safety is a key issue in the field of radiology. A career in radiology means working around radiation for many years. Members of the radiology team must protect patients as well as themselves from needless exposure. These precautions will help reduce unnecessary exposure.

- Perform the procedure correctly the first time to eliminate retakes.
- Use the correct film size and be familiar with X-ray film processing techniques that rely on the time, temperature, and specific chemistry methods. Replenish X-ray film processing chemistry regularly.
- Use lead shielding, such as lead-lined aprons, gloves, walls, and blocks, during examinations. These shields should cover the reproductive organs unless that is the site to be imaged. However, do not rely on shielding as the only method of radiation protection. Any body part outside of the shielding may not be protected. Also, a lead-lined wall or partition is not necessarily safe for persons on the other side. Radiation can bounce or scatter.
- Collimate to the part of the body requiring exposure. A **collimator** is a beam-restricting device mounted under the X-ray tube housing. This beam allows you to be precise when performing the radiograph (see **Figure 27.22**). Use the screen-film combination that provides adequate detail at the lowest exposure possible.
- Maintain a distance of at least six feet from the source of radiation.
- Wear a radiation badge that monitors and registers the amount of exposure; maximum allowed exposure is dependent upon age.
- Work within established guidelines. For example, individuals under 18 years of age are not permitted to work around radiation, because their tissue is more susceptible to radiation injury.

READING CHECK

Explain why it is important to limit exposure to radiation.

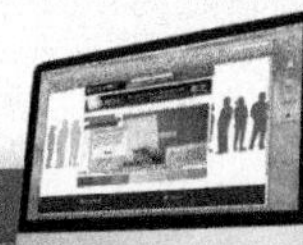

Mc Graw Hill connect™ ONLINE PROCEDURES

PROCEDURE 27-1

Adult Posterior-Anterior (PA) Chest Radiographic

The purpose of this procedure is for you to experience the steps involved in one of the simplest and most frequently performed radiographic procedures, the adult posterior-anterior (PA) chest radiograph. The goal is to generate a PA chest radiograph of the highest quality, so that the radiologist can develop an accurate diagnosis for the patient's physician.

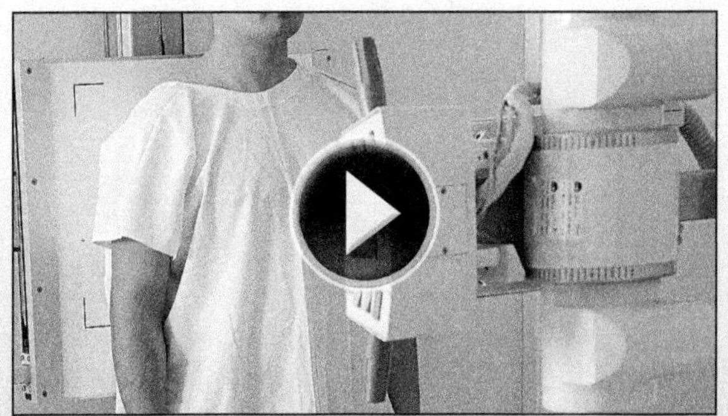

PROCEDURE 27-2

Adult PA Chest Radiographic Film Evaluation

A radiographer must troubleshoot problems. The time, temperature, and specific activity of the X-ray film processing play critical roles in getting the right contrast and density on the radiograph. These affect image quality just as the X-ray exposure settings and scatter radiation can affect image contrast and density. Automatic film processors are monitored and maintained by quality management technologists.

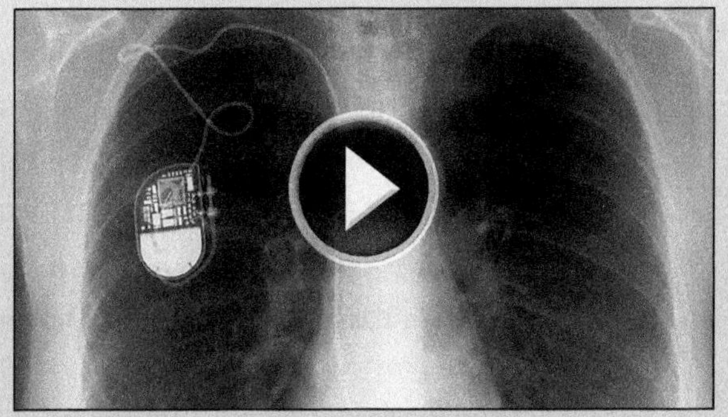

SECTION 27.2 Procedures in Radiology and Radiologic Technology Review

AFTER YOU READ

1. **Identify** an important way of protecting the patient from unnecessary radiation exposure.
2. **Summarize** how to protect the radiologic technologist from radiation exposure.
3. **State** the inverse square law.
4. **Name** the anatomy seen on a chest radiograph.
5. **Recall** why a patient must remove all clothing and objects from the chest prior to a chest radiograph.
6. **Explain** why it is important for a patient not to move during the radiographic exposure.
7. **Analyze** why it is preferable not to repeat a radiographic procedure.

Technology ONLINE EXPLORATIONS

PACS

Go online to learn more about PACS. What are the advantages of PACS? What skills must a healthcare professional have to use the PACS system? Write a brief report on your findings, including an illustration.

Photos: (t)Image Source/Getty Images, (b)Jim Wehtje/Photodisc/Getty Images

CHAPTER 27 Review

Chapter Summary

SECTION 27.1

- Diagnostic radiologists use the imaging modalities of radiography, fluoroscopy, computed tomography, ultrasound, magnetic resonance, and nuclear medicine in the diagnosis of disease and trauma. **(pg. 656)**
- Radiation oncologists use radiation generated from external beam therapy or radioisotopes to treat cancer. **(pg. 658)**
- Radiologic technologists are healthcare professionals who support radiologists in the performance of their duties. They perform the diagnostic procedures for the diagnostic radiologist or administer treatment plans for the radiation oncologist. **(pg. 660)**
- Radiologic technologists in one of the primary fields can qualify to become cardiovascular-interventional technologists, computed tomography technologists, magnetic resonance technologists, mammographers, sonographers, bone densitometry technologists, and quality management technologists. **(pg. 663)**
- Invasive imaging examinations, such as coronary angiography, require the introduction of contrast media into various systems of the body to assist with visualization. Noninvasive procedures, such as a PA chest radiograph, do not. **(pg. 663)**

SECTION 27.2

- An important precaution that a radiographer can take to help protect the patient from unnecessary radiation exposure is to perform the procedure correctly the first time to eliminate the need for retakes. **(pg. 668)**
- An important precaution that helps to protect radiologic technologists from unnecessary radiation exposure is the placement of a protective barrier between themselves and the source of radiation that is strong enough to stop the primary beam. **(pg. 668)**
- The inverse square law states that radiation intensity is inversely proportional to the square of the distance. **(pg. 668)**

McGraw Hill connect™ ONLINE ACTIVITIES

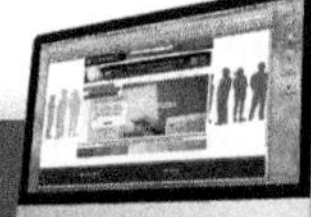

Complete our HST online activities for Chapter 27, which include Concept Check review questions, Reference Flash Cards, and Online Procedures assessment sheets.

- **Concept Check** review questions
- **Reference Flash Cards** medical terminology practice
- **Online Procedures** assessment sheets

CHAPTER 27 Assessment

Critical Thinking/Problem Solving

1. Radiation is used to help diagnose disease and treat cancers. What factors might distinguish the relatively safe use of radiation to diagnose disease from the relatively risky use of radiation to treat cancer? Is there any risk involved in using radiation as a diagnostic tool?
2. Explain why pregnant women should take extra precautions to avoid exposure to radiation. (Hint: fetal cells develop rapidly, as do cancer cells.)
3. You are about to undergo a radiographic procedure. The radiographic technologist gets everything ready, and you notice that he or she has not provided lead shielding to protect your reproductive organs from exposure to X-rays. What should you do? Why is that protection necessary?
4. As the "on-call" radiographer for a hospital, you are awakened at 2 A.M. You learn that there has been a major automobile accident, and that several patients are on the way to the emergency room. Many radiographs will be taken. At the hospital radiology department, you discover that all of the patients are bleeding and that body fluids are everywhere. How will you protect yourself from contracting blood-borne diseases? Should you just assume that your patients have no communicable diseases?
5. Determine all of the infection control practices that are needed to deal with the patients in Question 4. Make a list and give it to your instructor.

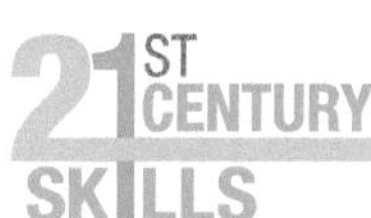

6. **Teamwork** With a partner, practice placing each other in the position necessary to perform a chest radiograph. The patient should stand upright with his or her feet spread slightly apart and weight evenly distributed, then raise the chin and rest it on the film holder. The hands should be on the lower hips, palms out, elbows partially flexed and shoulders rotated against the film holder. Shoulder rotation is important to move the shadow of the shoulder blade out of the lung fields.
7. **Teamwork** Your partner is going to have an abdominal radiograph. Have him or her lie on a bed or treatment table in anatomical position. Using a towel or towels as a "shield," place it on the correct area or areas to protect your partner during the procedure. Pretend that you are going to take the radiograph. Step away from your partner and give him or her the necessary instructions. Click the button to produce the radiograph at the correct moment in your partner's breathing process. Give your partner post procedure instructions.

CHAPTER

28 Ophthalmic Care

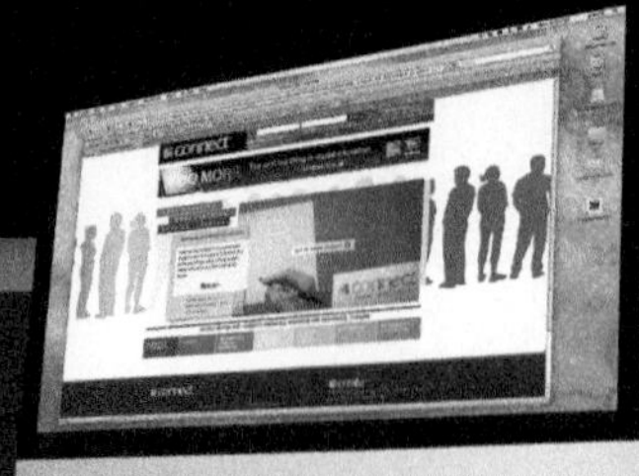

Mc Graw Hill connect™

It's Online!

- Online Procedures
- STEM Connection
- Medical Science
- Medical Terms
- Medical Math
- Ethics in Action
- Virtual Lab

Essential Question:

Would you rather be an optometrist or an opthalmologist?

Without vision, you could not read this book or do many things that you take for granted. More than half of the people in the United States wear glasses or contact lenses to correct their vision. Corrective lenses are obtained from people working in the ophthalmic field. Ophthalmic simply means "pertaining to the eye." People working in this field provide care for the eyes, including the prevention and treatment of eye and vision disorders. This chapter discusses careers including ophthalmologist, optometrist, orthoptist, dispensing optician, ophthalmic technologist, technician, assistant, and laboratory technician.

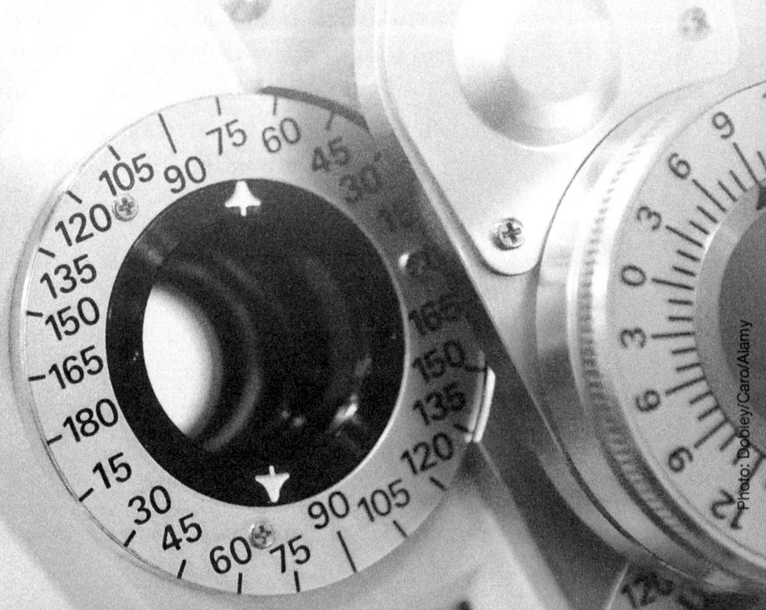

Photo: Dooley/Caro/Alamy

READING GUIDE

OBJECTIVES

After completing this chapter, you will be able to:

- **Compare** the roles and responsibilities of the optometrist and ophthalmologist.
- **Illustrate** the role and responsibilities of an orthoptist.
- **Describe** the roles and responsibilities of ophthalmic medical personnel.
- **Examine** ophthalmic career opportunities related to the preparation and fitting of corrective lenses.
- **Demonstrate** four ophthalmic procedures.

BEFORE YOU READ

Connect Have you ever been examined or treated by an ophthalmic professional? What was the experience like?

Main Idea

Individuals in the opthalmic profession test vision, provide corrective lenses, and perform eye surgery to help prevent or correct vision problems.

Note-Taking Activity

Draw this table. Write key terms and phrases under **Cues**. Write main ideas under **Note Taking**. Summarize the section under **Summary**.

Cues	Note Taking
o o	o o
Summary	

Graphic Organizer

Before you read the chapter, draw a diagram like the one to the right. As you read, write the careers covered in this chapter into the diagram.

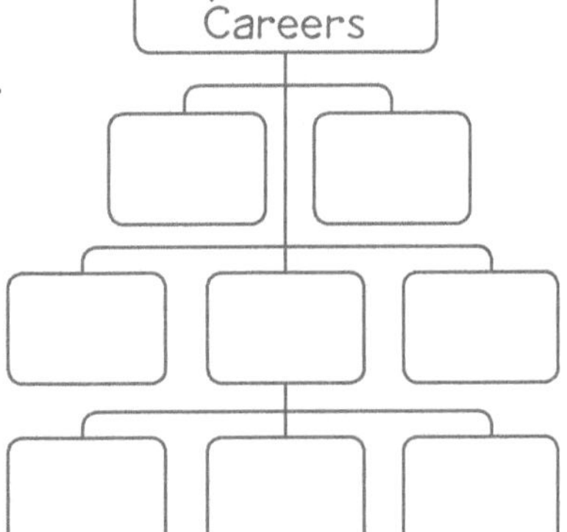

connect Downloadable graphic organizers can be accessed online.

STANDARDS

HEALTH SCIENCE

NCHSE 1.22 Recognize emerging diseases and disorders.

NCHSE 9.12 Describe strategies for the prevention of diseases including health screenings and examinations.

SCIENCE

NSES E Develop abilities of technological design, understandings about science and technology.

NCHSE *National Consortium for Health Science Education*

NSES *National Science Education Standards*

COMMON CORE STATE STANDARDS

MATHEMATICS

Number and Quantity

Quantities N-Q Reason quantitatively and use units to solve problems.

ENGLISH LANGUAGE ARTS

Reading

Integration of Knowledge and Ideas R-9 Synthesize information from a range of sources (e.g., texts, experiments, simulations) into a coherent understanding of a process, phenomenon, or concept, resolving conflicting information when possible.

Writing

Text Types and Purposes W-3d Use precise words and phrases, telling details, and sensory language to convey a vivid picture of the experiences, events, setting, and/or characters.

SECTION 28.1 Careers in Ophthalmology

Vocabulary

Content Vocabulary

You will learn these content vocabulary terms in this section.

- **cataract**
- **myopia**
- **retina**
- **hyperopia**
- **astigmatism**
- **presbyopia**
- **cornea**
- **amblyopia**
- **strabismus**

Academic Vocabulary

You will see this word in your reading and on your tests. Find its meaning in the Glossary in the back of this book.

- **focus**

The Optometrist and the Ophthalmologist

What types of eye doctor are there?

Two types of doctors can examine eyes and prescribe glasses. They are the ophthalmologist and the optometrist (see **Figure 28.1**). Although they are both eye doctors, their training and practice are not the same. The ophthalmologist is a medical doctor, who diagnoses and treats diseases, injuries, and disorders of the eye. He or she may perform eye surgery as well. An optometrist is a doctor of optometry. The doctor of optometry has the title of doctor but is not a medical doctor. He or she examines the eyes to diagnose vision problems and eye diseases. For an overview of all ophthalmic careers, see **Table 28.1**.

The Job of the Ophthalmologist

An ophthalmologist is an MD who is licensed to practice medicine and surgery. About two to three percent of physicians become ophthalmologists. They may perform any or all of the same duties as an optometrist but they can also treat eye injuries and perform surgery on the eye.

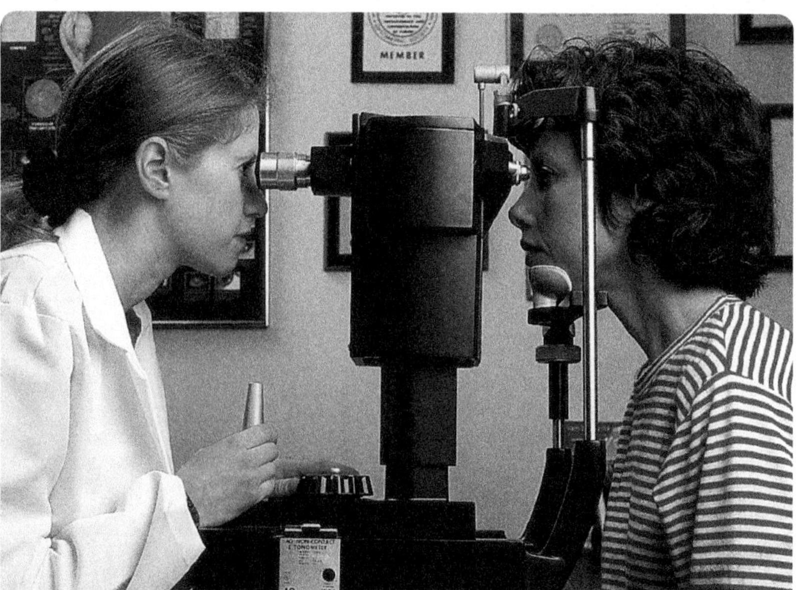

Fig. 28.1 Testing for Glaucoma *Which two types of doctors are qualified to perform this test?*

Photo: Terry Wild Studio

Table 28.1 Overview of Ophthalmic Careers

OCCUPATION	EDUCATIONAL REQUIREMENTS	CERTIFICATION OR LICENSING AGENCY	JOB OUTLOOK
Ophthalmologist	Four years undergraduate education, four years graduate education, three years minimum specialization in ophthalmology	Individual state boards of medical examiners, additional board examinations specific to ophthalmology as administered by the state medical board	Average growth as healthcare industry expands
Optometrist	At least three years of preoptometric study, a four-year doctor of optometry degree from an accredited optometry school	State board of optometry, American Optometric Association	Much faster than average due to an aging population and increased attention to vision care
Orthoptist	Completion of a 24-month accredited program	Certificate of proficiency from the American Orthoptic Council	Above average growth
Ophthalmic Technologist	Completion of an ophthalmic medical technologist training program accredited by the Commission on Accreditation of Allied Health Education Programs (CAAHEP)	Certification from the Joint Commission on Allied Health Personnel in Ophthalmology (JCAHPO), demonstration of ability required for certification	Above average growth as the need for qualified clinical support personnel increases
Ophthalmic Technician	Completion of an ophthalmic medical technician training program accredited by CAAHEP	Certification from the Joint Commission on Allied Health Personnel in Ophthalmology (JCAHPO), demonstration of ability required for certification	Above average growth as the need for qualified clinical support personnel increases
Ophthalmic Assistant	Completion of a clinical ophthalmic medical assisting training program approved by the Committee on Accreditation for Ophthalmic Medical Personnel (CoA-OMP) or on-the-job training. Independent study courses are also available	Certification not required but can be obtained through the Joint Commission on Allied Health Personnel in Ophthalmology (JCAHPO)	Above average growth as the need for qualified clinical support personnel increases
Ophthalmic Laboratory Technician	On-the-job training	None	Slower than average growth as automated methods of preparing lenses progress
Dispensing Optician	On-the-job training, sometimes as an apprenticeship; a two-year degree is also available	About half the states require a license through a state licensing group. The American Board of Opticianry (ABO) and the National Contact Lens Examiners (NCLE) also provide certification for skills acquired	Above average growth as the population ages and the demand for stylish glasses increases

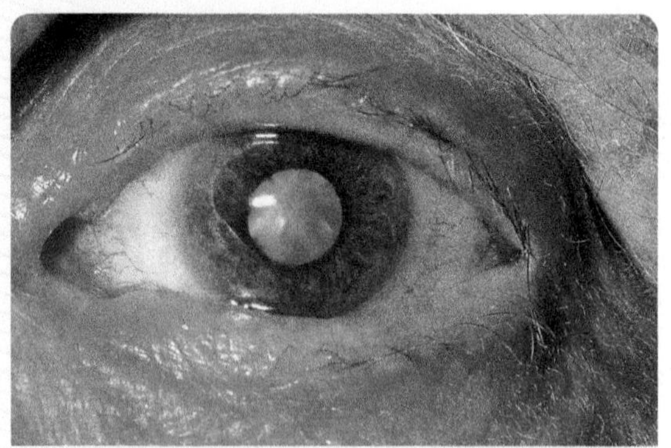

Fig. 28.2 Cataract Cataracts are cloudy areas. *What can be done to correct this cloudy lens?*

Eye Surgery

A common type of surgery is performed to remove **cataracts** (see **Figure 28.2**). Cataracts are cloudy areas on a normally clear eye lens. They interfere with the entrance of light into the eye and cause loss of vision. The surgery removes the cloudy lens and replaces it with an artificial one.

Another common type of surgery is corrective eye surgery, which corrects visual acuity or the ability to see. The objective of the surgery is to reduce or eliminate the need for glasses and contacts. Corrective eye surgery can help visual disorders such as:

- Nearsightedness is also called **myopia.** This is a condition in which visual images come to a focus in front of the **retina**. The result is defective vision of distant objects.
- Farsightedness is also called **hyperopia.** This is a condition in which images come to a focus behind the retina. Near objects are blurry, but far objects are in focus.

Surgical techniques have also been developed (and continue to be developed) to correct the following disorders:

- **Astigmatism** is a condition caused by an irregularly shaped cornea. It results in blurred vision.
- **Presbyopia** is the inability of the eye lens to focus incoming light. This results in blurred vision at a reading distance and eyestrain. Most people develop presbyopia in their 40s.

LASIK, or "laser-assisted in situ keratomileusis," is one type of corrective eye surgery. During this surgery an instrument is used to create a thin, circular flap in the **cornea.** The cornea is the transparent anterior portion of the outer layer of the eyeball. It is important in the correct focus of light. The surgeon folds the flap created out of the way, and removes some corneal tissue with a laser. The laser uses a cool ultraviolet light beam to remove precisely very tiny bits of tissue from the cornea to reshape it. When you reshape the cornea in the right way, it works better to focus light into the eye and onto the retina. It provides clearer vision than before. The flap is then laid back in place, covering the area where the corneal tissue was removed. The actual procedure takes less than one minute for each eye (see **Figure 28.3**).

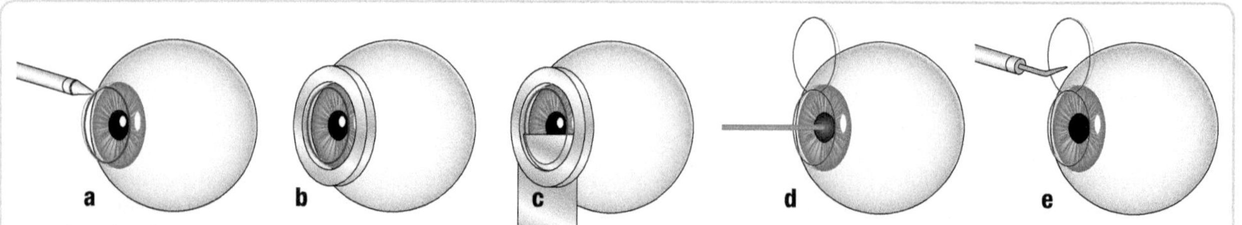

Fig. 28.3 LASIK LASIK is one type of corrective eye surgery. **(a)** After administering drops to numb the eye, the ophthalmologist marks the eye where the flap will be cut and then replaced. **(b)** A suction ring holds the eye still and pressurizes it until it is firm enough to cut. **(c)** A tiny flap is sliced in the cornea. **(d)** The flap is moved out of the way but remains attached. **(e)** A laser is used to remove tissue to reshape the cornea and the flap is replaced. *How is a laser used to correct vision?*

Photo: Dr. P Marazzi/Science Photo Library/Photo Researchers

There are various other types of corrective eye surgery. Photorefractive keratectomy (PRK), corneal implants, and radial keratotomy are examples. In general, these procedures all aim to correct the shape of the cornea. The shape of the cornea affects the way light focuses onto the retina and therefore changing its shape improves and corrects vision. These corrective procedures involve using a laser to remove tissue, inserting implants, and related needs.

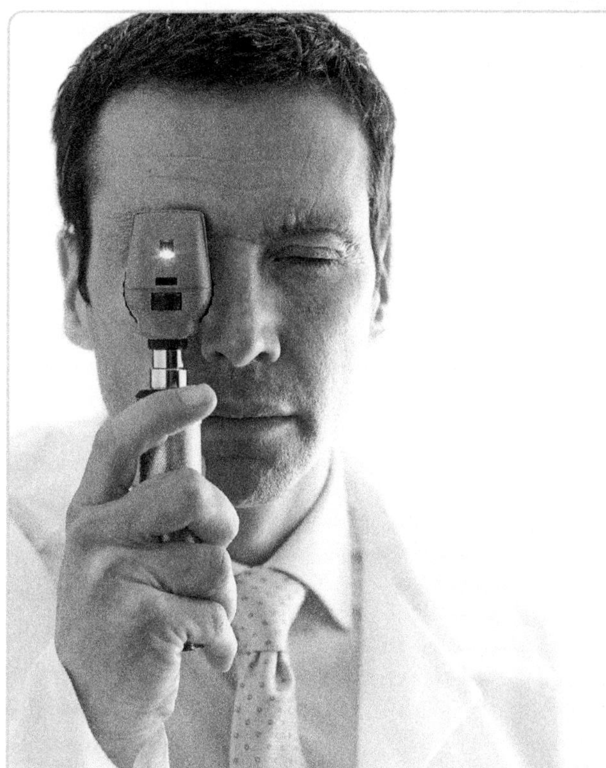

Fig. 28.4 Ophthalmoscope The ophthalmoscope is a common instrument used to view the interior eye structures including the retina, optic nerve, and the blood vessels. *Which vision disorders can occur if light is focused in front of the retina or behind the retina?*

The Job of the Optometrist

Most optometrists work in a private practice. They have their own offices and hire workers to assist them. Operating a professional office requires some knowledge of business practices. The owner must have the skills to develop a patient base; hire, train, and manage employees; keep records; order equipment and supplies; and oversee the finances of the business.

The optometrist

- uses instruments and observation to determine eye health. The ophthalmoscope (see **Figure 28.4**) is one type of instrument commonly used.
- tests patients' visual acuity, depth and color perception, and ability to coordinate and focus the eye.
- prescribes eyeglasses and contact lenses.
- provides vision therapy and rehabilitation.
- administers drugs to aid in the diagnosis of vision problems.
- prescribes drugs to treat some eye diseases.
- diagnoses eye conditions due to diseases such as diabetes and high blood pressure.
- refers patients to other healthcare practitioners.

Optometrists may choose to specialize in any of the following areas:

- Working with the elderly, children, or partially sighted patients to develop specialized visual devices
- Developing and implementing ways of protecting workers' eyes from on-the-job strain or injury
- Providing contact lenses
- Providing sports vision care and/or vision therapy
- Working with ophthalmologists to provide preoperative and postoperative care to patients whose vision has been corrected by laser surgery or have had cataract or other eye surgery
- Working as a consultant for industrial safety programs, insurance companies, and manufacturers of ophthalmic products

Photo: Juice Images/Alamy

- Teaching optometry
- Conducting research

READING CHECK

Compare and contrast the job responsibilities of the ophthalmologist and the optometrist.

Orthoptist

What conditions are the result of problems with eye muscles?

When a patient has a condition of the eyes that involves the eye muscles, they may seek treatment from an orthoptist. Orthoptists diagnose and treat patients with **amblyopia, strabismus,** and defects in their eye movements or their binocular vision. Amblyopia, which is poor vision in one eye, is also known as "lazy eye." Strabismus occurs when one eye focuses properly, but the other eye strays. This creates a cross-eyed appearance. Orthoptists teach patients or their parents how to perform corrective exercises at home.

The number of people in the profession is small, but their services are very important. Most patients are children who suffer from strabismus or other visual disabilities. Children with faulty vision often lack self-esteem. A visual disability can also slow the learning process and make the child feel that he or she is a slow learner. Helping children improve their vision may also help them acquire self-confidence.

An orthoptist usually works with an ophthalmologist, performing any or all of the following tasks:

- Evaluating vision and ocular alignment using special examination techniques
- Measuring visual acuity, ability to focus, and movement of the eyes
- Checking near vision and depth perception
- Estimating the eyeglass correction
- Performing glaucoma tests
- Evaluating color vision
- Assisting in ophthalmic surgery
- Teaching patients and parents exercises to strengthen eye muscles
- Performing research to evaluate current methods of treatment, devise new modes of exercises, and increase the understanding of binocular vision
- Teach orthoptics in hospitals or clinics

READING CHECK

Recall some ways in which an orthoptist can help a child.

Ophthalmic Medical Personnel

How does a career as an ophthalmic assistant begin?

The ophthalmic technologist, ophthalmic technician, and ophthalmic assistant are all classified as ophthalmic medical personnel (OMP). Most work in private clinics or offices under the direction of an ophthalmologist or optometrist. The main OMP function is to assist the ophthalmologist or optometrist, collect data, dispense treatments ordered, and supervise patients. OMPs may also assist with ophthalmic surgery.

Ophthalmic technologists are also trained to perform numerous other duties. They may take ophthalmic photographs or use ultrasound imaging equipment. They may provide instruction and supervise other workers. They are expected to perform at a higher skill level than ophthalmic technicians and assistants and to use clinical technical judgment. However, they do not work on their own. They cannot diagnose or treat eye disorders or prescribe medications.

The tasks of the ophthalmic technician overlap in many ways with those of the ophthalmic technologist. However, the technologist has completed more advanced training than the technician, and has assumed a larger number of advanced responsibilities as a result of that training.

Many ophthalmic medical personnel start with little or no training. They may begin as receptionists in an ophthalmic medical office. With motivation and training, these workers may move up to a more technical position and perform additional duties. Some individuals become medical assistants, and then specialize to become certified in ophthalmic care.

The Job of Ophthalmic Medical Personnel

Depending upon the type of practice and the level of training and certification, OMP may perform any or all of the following tasks:

- Take medical history and perform diagnostic tests
- Take measurements of the eye and surrounding tissue
- Test visual acuity and ocular fields
- Perform all the ophthalmologic tests necessary for both preliminary and highly specific eye exams
- Administer topical ophthalmic and oral medications
- Instruct the patient in the care and use of contact lenses
- Maintain and sterilize surgical instruments
- Assist with ophthalmic surgery
- Assist with fitting contact lenses
- Provide supervision and instruction to other OMP

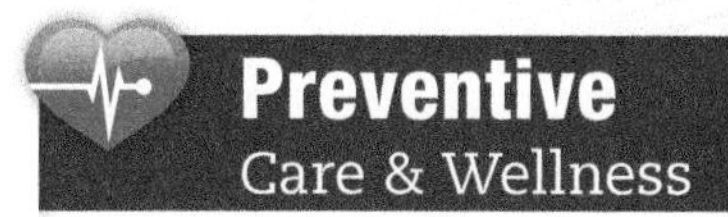

Protect Your Vision

To protect your eyes and vision, follow these simple guidelines:

- Have an eye examination at least every one to two years.
- Have regular health examinations. Your general health can affect your vision.
- Report any abnormalities such as blurred vision, double vision, eye pain, increased sensitivity to light, flashes of light, regular headaches, loss of vision, excessive tearing or dryness, loss of color perception, or halos around lights.
- Wear sunglasses or prescription glasses with ultraviolet (UV) light protection when in the sun, even during winter.
- Wear protective eye equipment when working with chemicals, during sports, when cutting grass and weeds, or in any other situation in which material may fly into your eyes.

The Ophthalmic Laboratory Technician

How are prescription eyeglasses made?

The ophthalmic laboratory technician works with the dispensing optician to prepare corrective lenses. Ophthalmic laboratory technicians are also known as manufacturing opticians, optical mechanics, or optical goods workers. They prepare prescription eyeglasses or contact lenses, and some make lenses for other optical instruments, such as telescopes and binoculars. They cut, grind, edge, and finish lenses according to specifications given by dispensing opticians, optometrists, or ophthalmologists. They may also insert lenses into frames to produce finished glasses. Although some lenses are produced by hand, technicians increasingly use automated equipment to make lenses. In addition, many dispensing opticians grind and insert lenses themselves. For these two reasons the profession of ophthalmic laboratory technician is expected to grow very slowly.

The Dispensing Optician

How do dispensing opticians assist ophthalmologists or optometrists?

Dispensing opticians fit eyeglasses and contact lenses (see **Figure 28.5**), following prescriptions written by ophthalmologists or optometrists. Unlike the job of the ophthalmic laboratory technician, this occupation is expected to grow faster than average. Many dispensing opticians are trained on the job. Frequently, employers hire individuals with experience as ophthalmic laboratory personnel and then provide training. Formal education programs lasting up to two years are also available.

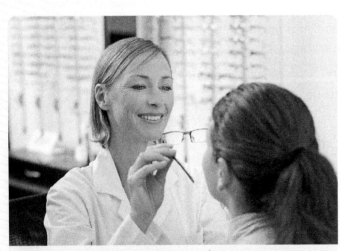

Fig. 28.5 Dispensing Optician A dispensing optician fits glasses and contact lenses. *In what settings could this optician choose to be employed?*

Photo: Chris Ryan/OJO Images/Getty Images

Both ophthalmologists and optometrists may employ dispensing opticians. A dispensing optician may also choose a career in the optical department of a retail store or pharmacy. They may work for themselves or for someone else in a privately owned optical shop. Whatever their place of employment, dispensing opticians always work directly with patients. They may perform any or all of the following duties:

- Examine written prescriptions to determine lens specifications.
- Recommend eyeglass frames, lenses, and lens coatings after considering the prescription and the patient's occupation, habits, and facial features.

- Measure patients' eyes, including the distance between the centers of the pupils and the distance between the eye surface and each lens.
- Prepare work orders that give ophthalmic laboratory technicians the information needed to grind and insert lenses into their frames.
- Verify that the lenses have been ground to specifications. (Or they may grind and insert the lenses themselves.)
- Reshape or bend the frame so that the eyeglasses fit the patient properly.
- Regrind lenses that have been slightly scratched.
- Fix, adjust, and refit broken frames.
- Instruct patients about adapting to, wearing, or caring for eyeglasses.
- Teach insertion, removal and care of contact lenses.
- Keep records on customer prescriptions, work orders, and payments.
- Track inventory and sales, and perform other administrative duties.

READING CHECK

Name several tasks that go into the making of eyeglasses.

SECTION 28.1 Careers in Ophthalmology Review

AFTER YOU READ

1. **Explain** the purpose of LASIK surgery.
2. **Identify** two eye conditions that are treated by an orthoptist.
3. **List** at least three duties of ophthalmic medical personnel.
4. **Assess** how the job of an ophthalmic technologist differs from that of an ophthalmic assistant.
5. **Compare** the responsibilities of an ophthalmic laboratory technician and a dispensing optician.
6. **Contrast** an MD and an OD.

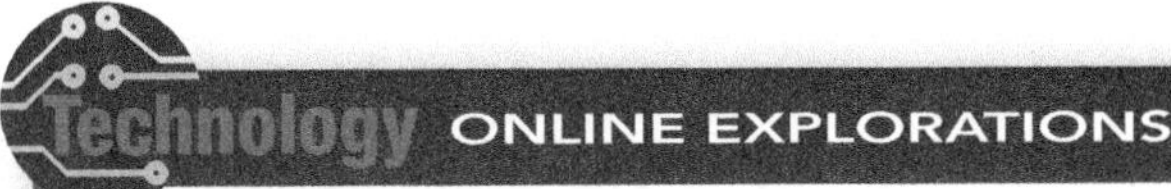

Eye Surgery

Search online for information about new types of eye surgery available to correct vision. Choose one type of surgery and write a brief report describing the procedure, its purpose, and possible complications.

SECTION
28.2 Procedures in Ophthalmic Care

Vocabulary

Content Vocabulary

You will learn these content vocabulary terms in this section.

- **visual acuity**
- **glaucoma**

Academic Vocabulary

You will see this word in your reading and on your tests. Find its meaning in the Glossary in the back of this book.

- **vision**

Ophthalmology Career Skills

How can you assess another person's vision?

The procedures in this section involve some of the career skills that are performed by optometrists, ophthalmologists, and other eye-care professionals. Correctly assessing the vision of patients (both their ability to see objects at different distances and their perception of color) is a skill central to these professions.

Helping patients care for eyeglasses and administering eye drops are additional tasks that you may perform, depending on your chosen career path and the environment in which you work. Eye drops are often used before the optometrist or ophthalmologist performs an examination. They may also be used for reasons including pain management, antibiotic treatment, antihistamine treatment, or eye lubrication.

Mc Graw Hill connect™ ONLINE PROCEDURES

PROCEDURE 28-1

Measuring Visual Acuity

Visual acuity, or the ability to see, is tested as part of a physical or visual exam. Routine vision screening tests near and far **vision**. The Snellen eye chart is most commonly used to test far vision. Variations of the Snellen eye chart are used for young children and others who are unable to read.

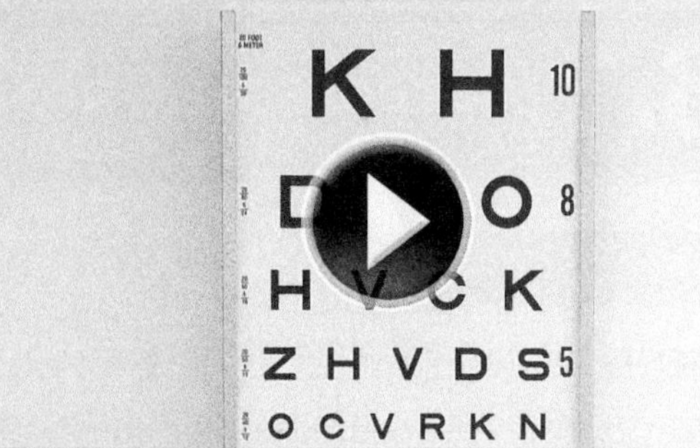

PROCEDURE 28-2

Testing Color Vision

The ability to perceive color is based upon seeing red, green, and blue. Most people with color deficiency have difficulty seeing one or two of those colors, not all three. It is uncommon for someone to see no color at all.

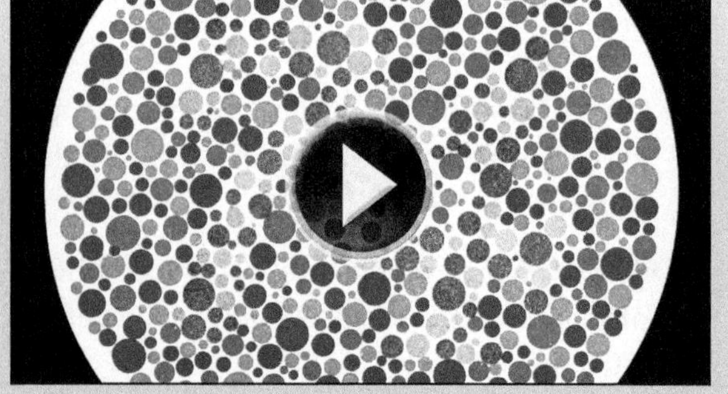

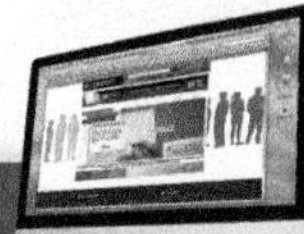

connect ONLINE PROCEDURES

PROCEDURE 28-3

Caring for Eyeglasses

Eyewear is an important investment and must be cared for properly. Glasses can easily be broken or scratched. Replacing an expensive pair of glasses is a hardship for many patients.

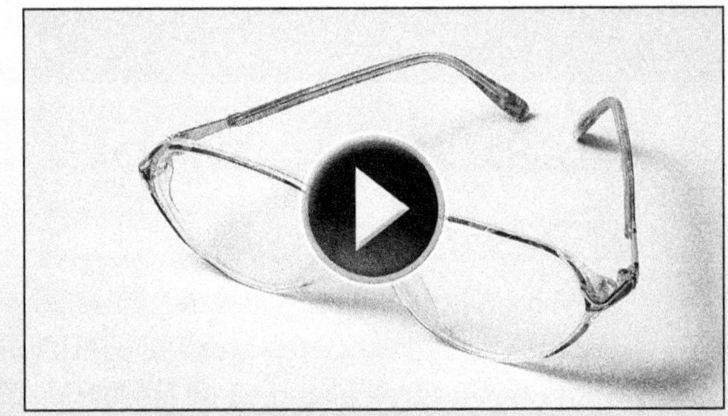

PROCEDURE 28-4

Administering Eye Drops

Eye drops may be used for a variety of reasons, some of which are pain management, antibiotic treatment, antihistamine treatment, or eye lubrication. They are also used to treat certain conditions such as infections and **glaucoma,** a group of diseases involving pressure in the eye. Eye drops are often used before the optometrist or ophthalmologist performs an examination.

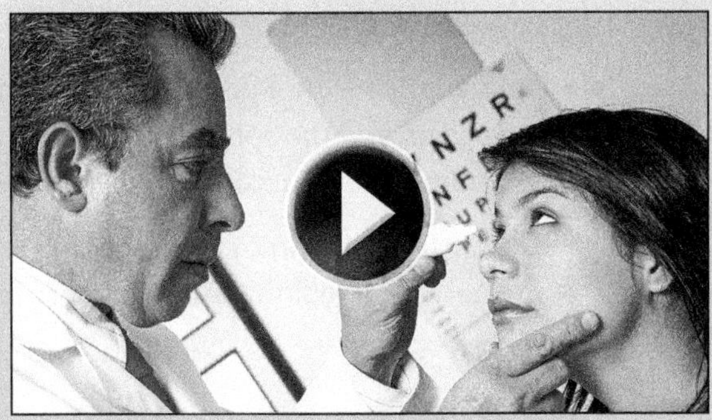

SECTION 28.2 Procedures in Ophthalmic Care Review

AFTER YOU READ

1. **Determine** how far the vision chart should be from the patient when testing far vision or when testing near vision.
2. **Indicate** three ways that you may be able to tell a patient is having difficulty when screening for visual acuity.
3. **Describe** what it means to have the vision problem known as color deficiency.
4. **Name** at least two ways to prevent scratching and breaking eyeglasses when cleaning or caring for them.
5. **Identify** three reasons why a patient would need eye drops.

Technology ONLINE EXPLORATIONS

Visual Acuity

Search for an online visual acuity or color vision-screening test. Read the directions carefully and test your own or a partner's vision or color vision. Compile the results into a written report.

Photos: (t)PIXTAL/PunchStock, (b)GlowImages/Alamy

CHAPTER
28 Review

Chapter Summary

SECTION 28.1

- The ophthalmologist and the optometrist are both doctors who examine eyes and prescribe glasses. However, the ophthalmologist is a medical doctor and can also perform surgery on the eye. **(pg. 674)**
- The orthoptist works with patients who have visual problems that require eye exercises and other visual therapies. **(pg. 678)**
- Ophthalmic medical personnel include the ophthalmic technologist, ophthalmic technician, and the ophthalmic assistant. These individuals assist the ophthalmologist or optometrist with care and treatment of the eye and vision. **(pg. 679)**
- Careers in ophthalmic care that involve the preparation and fitting of corrective lenses are those of the ophthalmic laboratory technician and the dispensing optician. **(pg. 680)**

SECTION 28.2

- When performing vision screening, you will test for near and far vision using specially designed charts. These determine the vision based upon the size of the letter and the distance from the patient. **(pg. 682)**
- Color deficiency is the inability to see one or more of the primary colors of red, green, or blue. Color vision must be tested in children and in individuals who require perfect color perception as part of their job. **(pg. 682)**
- Keeping the patient's glasses clean will prevent accidents. Care must be taken to ensure the glasses are not broken or scratched during the cleaning process. **(pg. 683)**
- Eye drops are administered during eye examinations to treat disease, infection, and pain. Eye drops may be administered by various levels of ophthalmic personnel depending upon the type of medication. **(pg. 683)**

Mc Graw Hill connect™ ONLINE ACTIVITIES

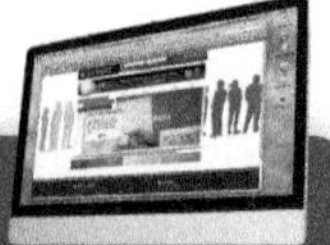

Complete our HST online activities for Chapter 28, which include Concept Check review questions, Reference Flash Cards, and Online Procedures assessment sheets.

- **Concept Check** review questions
- **Reference Flash Cards** medical terminology practice
- **Online Procedures** assessment sheets

CHAPTER 28 Assessment

Critical Thinking/Problem Solving

1. As an ophthalmic assistant, you are performing a vision screening. The patient starts reading the letters on the 20/20 line in order. Once you start randomly pointing at the letters on that line, you notice the patient is squinting and leaning forward. After not being able to read the line in a random fashion, the patient becomes angry and says, "I've already read that line. You don't have to test me anymore." What should you do?
2. You are administering a color vision test and come to a plate with a number to be identified. The patient says, "There's no number there! Why are you asking me about a number?" What should you say or do?
3. Explain what it would be like to practice as an ophthalmologist as compared to other medical specialties such as internal medicine, general surgery, gastroenterology, or emergency medicine.
4. How would you handle setting up an eye examination for a person who is confused or impaired because of Alzheimer's disease or dementia? Which testing tools could you use?
5. The patient has had eye drops administered to dilate his pupil. After a few minutes, he becomes agitated and says, "I can't see! I'm going blind!" What should you say or do in response?
6. Get a pair of old glasses or goggles and coat the lenses with Vaseline or semi-transparent tape. Put on the glasses and try to do some of your normal activities, including eating lunch, talking with friends, or changing classes. Write a brief report or tell the class how it felt to have limited vision. Explain what techniques you used to cope with your limited vision.

21ST CENTURY SKILLS

7. **Teamwork** In pairs, practice caring for eyeglasses. Remember to follow the guidelines given in **Procedure 28-3**.
8. **Information Literacy** Go online to research an ophthalmic care career. Learn more about the career you choose and its education requirements. Find the website of a school in your area and determine the requirements for entry. If possible, contact a member of the administrative staff at that facility and conduct an interview to learn more about the qualifications for employment. Prepare a brief report to share with the class.

UNIT 4

Careers in Health Informatics

- **CHAPTER 29** Administrative Office
- **CHAPTER 30** Health Information

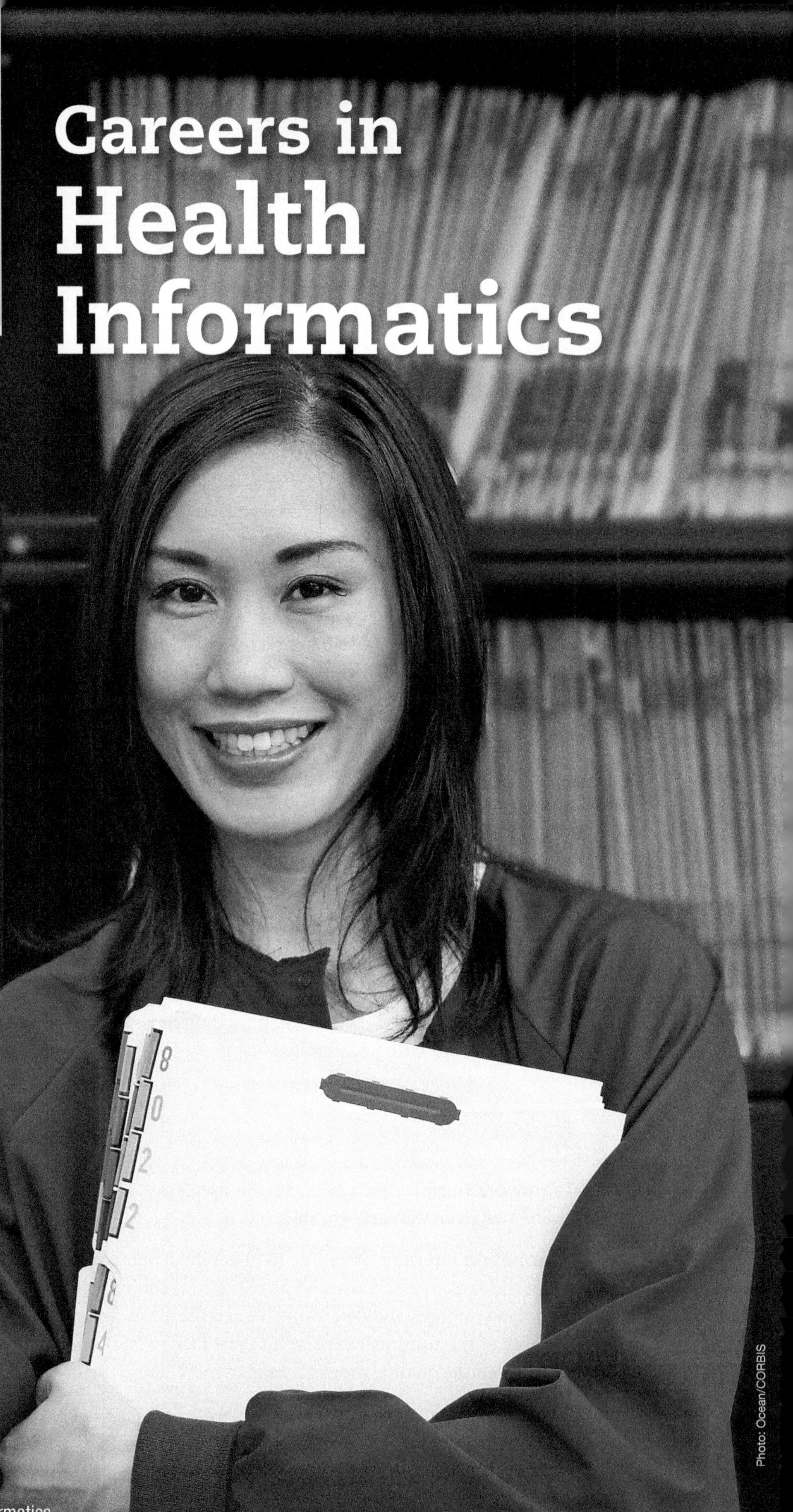

Photo: Ocean/CORBIS

CHAPTER 29 Administrative Office

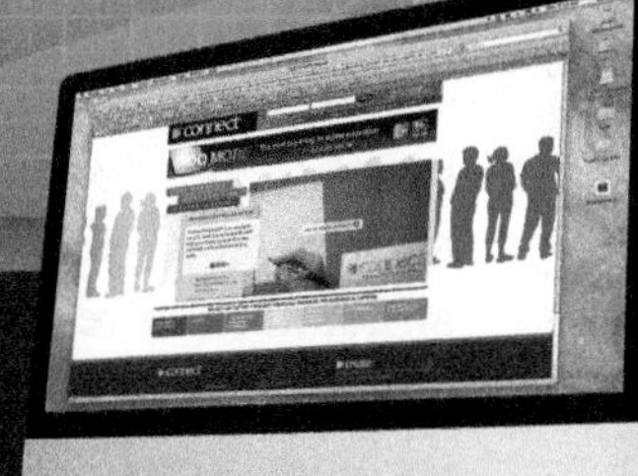

Essential Question:

Why does a medical office visit often begin with completing insurance or patient information forms?

Every medical facility, from the small clinic to the large hospital, needs administrative professionals—people to handle records and finances, manage employees, and interact with patients. These varied jobs are vital to the success of the office, clinic, or other healthcare facility. This chapter discusses four administrative career opportunities in healthcare: administrative medical assistant, medical insurance specialist, medical office manager, and medical billing and reimbursement specialist.

McGraw Hill connect™

It's Online!

- Online Procedures
- STEM Connection
- Medical Science
- Medical Terms
- Medical Math
- Ethics in Action
- Virtual Lab

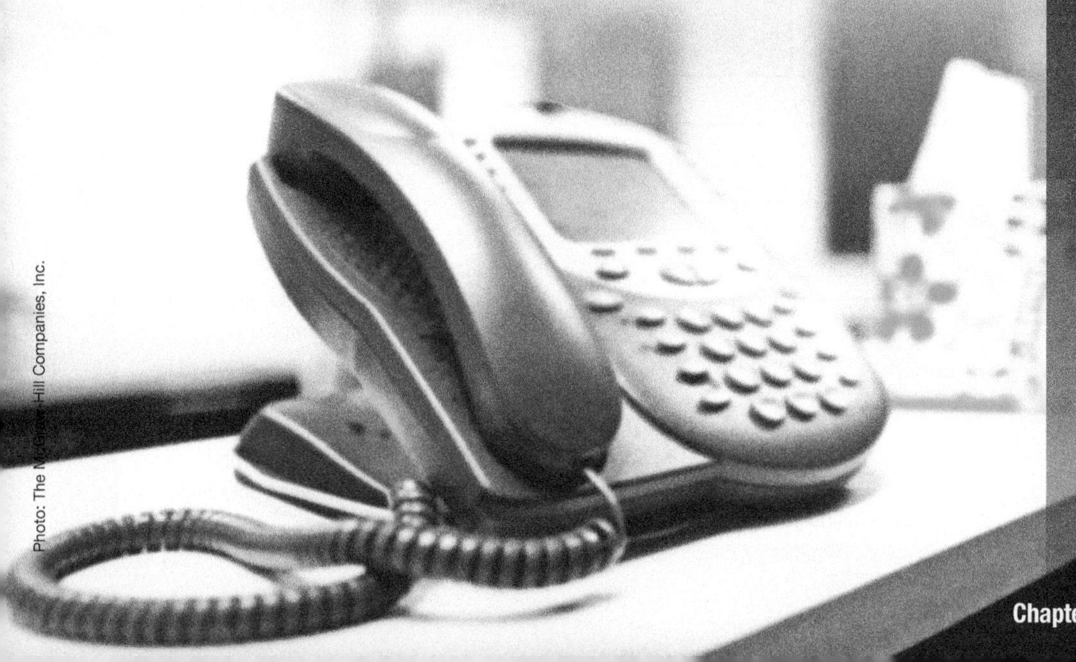

READING GUIDE

OBJECTIVES

After completing this chapter, you will be able to:

- **Identify** the education and training required to become an administrative medical assistant, a medical insurance specialist, a medical office manager, and a medical billing and reimbursement specialist.
- **Distinguish** the job responsibilities of the administrative medical assistant from those of the medical office manager.
- **Illustrate** the specific duties of the medical insurance specialist and the billing and reimbursement specialist.
- **Explain** the legal and ethical issues involved in working with patient information in the medical office.
- **Identify** the various types of technology and office equipment that may be used to perform administrative tasks in the medical office.
- **Define** the interpersonal skills necessary for working in a medical office.
- **Demonstrate** six medical office procedures.

BEFORE YOU READ

Connect How does the first greeting you hear in a medical office set the tone for your entire visit?

Main Idea

Administrative medical assistant, medical insurance specialist, medical office manager, and billing and reimbursement specialist are healthcare careers for those who enjoy working with computers and information as well as working with people.

Note-Taking Activity

Draw this table. Write key terms and phrases under **Cues**. Write main ideas under **Note Taking**. Summarize the section under **Summary**.

Cues	Note Taking
∘ ∘	∘ ∘
Summary	

Graphic Organizer

Before you read the chapter, draw a diagram like the one to the right. As you read, write the medical office careers covered by the chapter into the diagram.

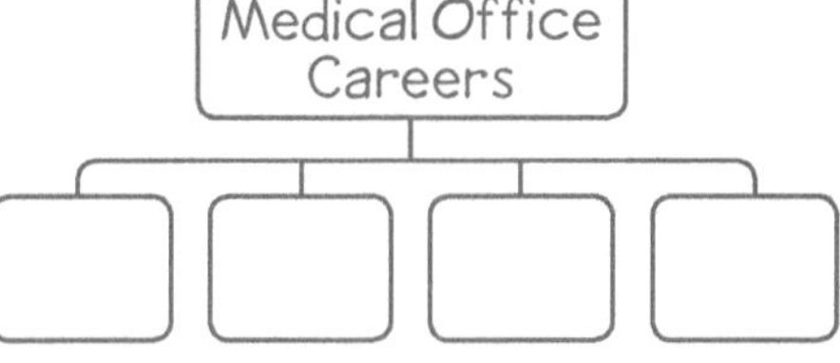

connect

Downloadable graphic organizers can be accessed online.

STANDARDS

HEALTH SCIENCE

NCHSE 2.22 Use medical abbreviations to communicate information.

NCHSE 3.15 Discuss common methods of payment for healthcare.

NCHSE 11.11 Identify records and files common to the healthcare setting.

SCIENCE

NSES F Develop understanding of personal and community health; population growth; natural resources; environmental quality; natural and human-induced hazards; science and technology in local, national, and global challenges.

NCHSE *National Consortium for Health Science Education*

NSES *National Science Education Standards*

COMMON CORE STATE STANDARDS

MATHEMATICS

Number and Quantity

Quantities N-Q1 Use units as a way to understand problems and to guide the solution of multi-step problems; choose and interpret units consistently in formulas; choose and interpret the scale and the origin in graphs and data displays.

ENGLISH LANGUAGE ARTS

Reading

Integration of Knowledge and Ideas R-9 Synthesize information from a range of sources (e.g., texts, experiments, simulations) into a coherent understanding of a process, phenomenon, or concept, resolving conflicting information when possible.

SECTION **29.1** # Administrative Office Careers

The Administrative Medical Assistant

Why are communication skills essential for administrative medical assistants?

Some administrative medical assistants may be high school graduates with basic office skills. Others may have completed one or more programs beyond high school. A person who is hired for this entry-level job should have taken classes in keyboarding, computer skills, records management, and general office skills.

Many post-secondary technical or vocational schools offer training programs for administrative assisting. As a rule, students who complete these programs receive a certificate at the end of the program. Certification for entry-level office skills is also offered through the International Association of Administrative Professionals (IAAP).

Some administrative medical assistants complete formal programs in medical assisting, where they are specially trained to perform clinical and administrative duties in the medical office. Those duties are discussed in Chapter 16, The Clinical Office. Medical assisting programs may take one to two years to complete and may qualify the student to take a certification exam offered by the American Association of Medical Assistants (AAMA) or the American Medical Technologists (AMT).

The Job of the Administrative Medical Assistant

Job titles for the administrative medical assistant vary. Some of these are medical secretary, medical assistant, and medical administrative assistant. Some employees begin their careers in the medical office as medical receptionists, answering phones and taking messages.

With additional training, most front office personnel can schedule appointments and create and maintain patient financial and medical records. In addition, the administrative medical assistant should be skilled in using various types of office equipment. Such equipment includes computers multiple-line phone and intercom systems, facsimile (fax) machines, photocopiers, and personal paging devices.

Computer skills are essential in order to be successful as an administrative medical assistant. The administrative assistant should be competent in creating documents and emails, producing spreadsheets, maintaining databases, and managing billing and

Vocabulary

Content Vocabulary

You will learn these content vocabulary terms in this section.

- **empathy**
- **encounter form**
- **superbill**
- **beneficiary**
- **insured**
- **dependent**
- **explanation of benefits (EOB)**
- **benefits**
- **appeal**
- **subscriber**
- **policyholder**
- **fraud**
- **human relations**
- **budget**
- **reimbursement**
- **copayments**
- **deductibles**
- **insurance carriers**
- **ledger**
- **balance**
- **statement**
- **tickler report**
- **collection agency**

Academic Vocabulary

You will see this word in your reading and on your tests. Find its meaning in the Glossary in the back of the book.

- **schedule**

Table 29.1 Overview of Administrative Office Occupations

OCCUPATION	EDUCATIONAL REQUIREMENTS	CERTIFYING OR LICENSING AGENCY	JOB OUTLOOK
Administrative Medical Assistant	On-the-job training, short-term programs (less than one year), and two-year associate degree programs are available.	Students of either CAAHEP or ABHES approved medical assistant programs take either the American Association of Medical Assistants (AAMA) or American Medical Technologist (AMT) certification exam. Those who pass the AAMA exam receive a CMA (certified medical assistant) credential. Students passing the AMT exam receive a RMA (registered medical assistant) credential. AMT also offers a Medical Administrative Specialist certificate. Certified or registered administrative assistants can obtain additional certification and training in areas such as coding, billing, insurance or health information.	Faster than average growth is expected because of the increase in numbers of ambulatory and outpatient healthcare facilities.
Medical Insurance Specialist	Short-term programs (less than one year) and two-year associate degree programs in medical assisting or health information are available. Continuing education through workshops and seminars can lead to certification.	Students graduating from an accredited program who pass a written examination offered by the American Health Information Management Association (AHIMA) can become registered health information technicians.	Much faster than average growth is expected. A large part of this growth will occur in clinical offices and outpatient surgery centers.
Medical Office Manager	Short-term medical assistant programs (less than one year) and two-year associate degree programs in medical assisting. Larger healthcare facilities will require a degree in business administration or healthcare administration.	A bachelor's or master's degree is the standard credential. Clinical offices and smaller facilities may offer on-the-job experience that substitutes for formal education after becoming certified or registered as an administrative office or medical assistant.	Growth will be faster than average because of the increase in number of healthcare facilities.
Medical Billing and Reimbursement Specialist	Short-term programs (less than one year) and two-year associate degree programs are available. Individuals who have an education with a background in either area are qualified to work in billing and collections. A high school diploma and experience in medical billing allows you to sit for the certification exam.	Formal training and certification are often required. Certification through the Certifying Board of the American Medical Billing Association (CBAMBA) is obtained by examination. After successfully completing the examination you have the CMRS certification and must obtain yearly continuing education.	Growth will be much faster than average because of the rapid growth in health-care service areas. Specialists with a strong background in insurance coding will be in especially high demand.

scheduling software. He or she must also be comfortable working with electronic health records (see **Figure 29.1**).

Fig. 29.1 Administrative Assistant The administrative medical assistant will use several types of communication equipment. *What equipment, in addition to the telephone, is shown here?*

The administrative medical assistant is often the first person the patient or visitor sees upon entering the medical office. Therefore, a professional appearance and good interpersonal communication skills are a must at all times.

In some offices, the administrative medical assistant wears a uniform. In other offices, they wear business attire and, perhaps, a lab coat. Regardless of the office dress requirement, the administrative medical assistant should always be clean and neat. Conservative makeup, jewelry, and other accessories are appropriate. Fingernails should be short and clean. Professionalism also means no gum chewing, food, or beverages at the front desk (see **Figure 29.2**).

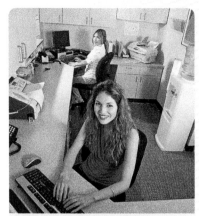

Fig. 29.2 Professional Appearance Visitors to the medical office include patients and medical sales representatives. *What personal and professional traits should the administrative medical assistant display?*

The assistant must be professional in his or her interactions with patients, other staff, and visitors. The first area of interaction in the medical office is often the waiting room. The administrative assistant should create a safe, clean, comfortable, and appealing reception area. The reception area shown in **Figure 29.3** is inviting to patients.

Administrative assistants must have good verbal and nonverbal communication skills. They should treat all patients and visitors with respect, dignity, and courtesy. This can be challenging when dealing with an emotional, upset, or angry patient, or an impatient or aggressive sales representative. In such situations, the assistant who demonstrates **empathy** and professionalism can often reverse, or at least defuse, emotional reactions expressed by an angry or upset visitor.

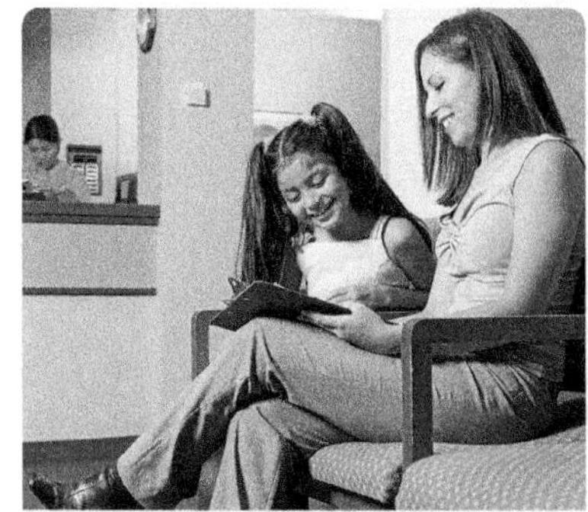

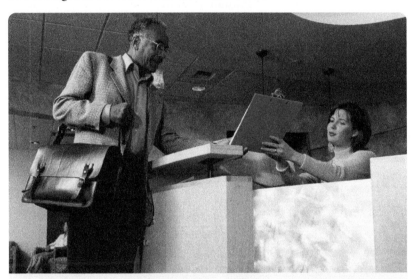

Fig. 29.3 Waiting Room The waiting room should be inviting. *What details in this picture convey a warm, comforting feeling to patients waiting to see the physician?*

READING CHECK

Describe the range of education required for a career as an administrative medical assistant.

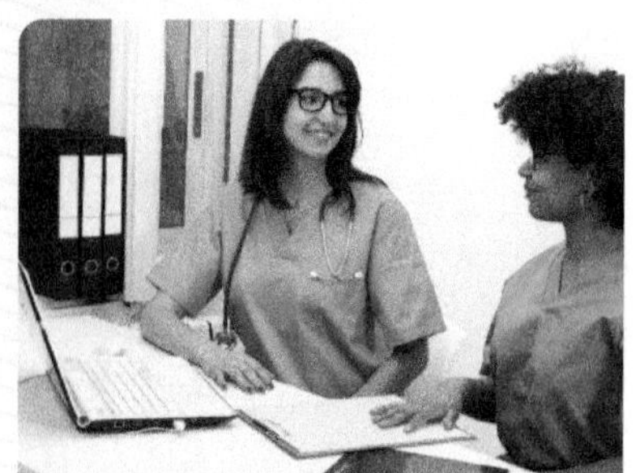

Fig. 29.4 Medical Insurance Specialist The medical insurance specialist typically completes forms electronically, using a computer and specialized software. *Why should a medical insurance specialist be familiar with medical terminology?*

The Medical Insurance Specialist

Why does a medical insurance specialist need to understand medical terminology?

Large practices may hire an outside company to manage the paperwork involved in filing insurance claims. Many medical offices, though, hire in-house staff to manage patient financial records such insurance claims. The person shown in **Figure 29.4** is working on an insurance claim. These specialists may have a range of titles. However, the duties of all healthcare workers who manage health information and insurance claims are nearly the same.

Medical insurance specialists should know medical terminology and have a basic knowledge of human anatomy and physiology. In addition, this specialist must have excellent reading and comprehension skills. These skills are particularly important.

The insurance specialist must also develop skills in recording a client's illness or condition and the physician's treatment using the medical record and an **encounter form.** An encounter form,

Lakeridge Medical Group
262 East Pine Street, Suite 100
Lakeridge, NJ07500

☐ **PRIVATE** ☐ **BLUECROSS** ☐ **IND.** ☐ **MEDICARE** ☐ **MEDI-CAL** ☐ **HMO** ☐ **PPO**

PATIENT'S LAST NAME	FIRST	ACCOUNT #	BIRTHDATE / /	SEX ☐ MALE ☐ FEMALE	TODAY'S DATE / /
INSURANCE COMPANY	SUBSCRIBER		PLAN #	SUB. #	GROUP

ASSIGNMENT: I hereby assign my insurance benefits to be paid directly to the undersigned physician. I am financially responsible for non-covered services. SIGNED: (Patient, or Parent, if Minor) DATE: / /

RELEASE: I hereby authorize the physician to release to my insurance carrers any information required to process this claim. SIGNED: (Patient, or Parent, if Minor) DATE: / /

✓	DESCRIPTION	M/Care	CPT/Mod	DxRe	FEE
	OFFICE CARE				
	NEW PATIENT				
	Brief		99201		
	Limited		99202		
	Intermediate		99203		
	Extended		99204		
	Comprehensive		99205		
	ESTABLISHED PATIENT				
	Minimal		99211		
	Brief		99212		
	Limited		99213		
	Intermediate		99214		
	Extended		99215		
	Comprehensive		99215		
	CONSULTATION-OFFICE				
	Focused		99241		
	Expanded		99242		
	Detailed		99243		
	Comprehensive 1		99244		
	Comprehensive 2		99245		
	Dr.				
	Case Management		98900		
	Post-op Exam		99024		

✓	DESCRIPTION	M/Care	CPT/Mod	DxRe	FEE
	PROCEDURES				
	Tread Mill (In Office)		93015		
	24 Huur Hulter		93224		
	If Medicare (Set up Fec)		93225		
	Physician Interpret		93227		
	EKG w/Interpretation		93000		
	EKG (Medicare)		93005		
	Sigmoidoscopy		45300		
	Sigmoidoscopy, Flexible		45330		
	Sigmoidos., Flex. w/Bx.		45331		
	Spirometry, FEV/FVC		94010		
	Spirometry, Post-Dilator		94060		
	LABORATORY				
	Blood Draw Fee		36415		
	Urinalysis, Chemical		81005		
	Throat Culture		87081		
	Occult Blood		82270		
	Pap Handling Charge		99000		
	Pap Life Guard		88150-90		
	Gram Stain		87205		
	Hanging Drop		87210		
	Urine Drug Screen		99000		
	SUPPLIES				

✓	DESCRIPTION	M/Care	CPT/Mod	DxRe	FEE
	INJECTIONS/IMMUNIZATIONS				
	Tetanus		90718		
	Hypertet	J1670	90782		
	Pneumococcal		90732		
	Influenza		90724		
	TB Skin Test (PPD)		86585		
	Antigen Injection-Single		95115		
	Multiple		95117		
	B12 Injection	J3420	90782		
	Injection, IM		90782		
	Compazine	J0780	90782		
	Demerol	J2175	90782		
	Vistaril	J3410	90782		
	Susphrine	J0170	90782		
	Decadron	J0890	90782		
	Estradiol	J1000	90782		
	Testosterone	J1080	90782		
	Lidocaine	J2000	90782		
	Solumedrol	J2920	90782		
	Solucortef	J1720	90782		
	Hydeltra	J1690	90782		
	Pen Procaine	J2510	90788		
	INJECTIONS - JOINT/BURSA				
	Small Joints		20600		
	Intermediate		20605		
	Large Joints		20610		
	Trigger Point		20550		
	MISCELLANEOUS				

DIAGNOSIS:	ICD-9										
Abdominal Pain	789.0	Gout	274.0	C.V.A. - Acute	436.	Electrolyte Dis.	276.9	Herpes Simplex	054.9		
Abscess (Site)	682.9	Asthma	493.90	Cere. Vas. Accid. (Old)	438	Fatigue	780.7	Herpes Zoster	053.9		
Adverse Drug Rx	995.2	Asthmatic Bronchitis	493.90	Cerumen	380.4	Fibrocys. Br. Dis	610.1	Hydrocele	603.9		
Alcohol Detox	291.8	Atrial Fib.	427.31	Chestwall Pain	786.59	Fracture (Site)	829.0	Hyperlipidemia	272.4		
Alcoholism	303.90	Atrial Tachi.	427.0	Cholecystitis	575.0	Open/Close		Hypertension	401.9		
Allergic Rhinitis	477	Bowel Obstruct.	560.9	Cholelithiasis	574.00	Fungal Infect. (Site)	110.8	Hyperthyroidism	242.9		
Allergy	995.3	Breast Mass	611.72	COPD	492.8	Gastric Ulcer	531.90	Hypothyroidism	244.9		
Alzheimer's Dis.	290.1	Bronchitis	490	Cirrhosis	571.5	Gastritis	535.0	Labyrinthitis	386.30		
Anemia	285.9	Bursitis	727.3	Cong. Heart Fail.	428.9	Gastroenteritis	558.9	Lipoma (Site)	214.9		
Anemia - Pernicious	281.0	Cancer, Breast (Site)	174.9	Conjunctivitis	372.30	G.I. Bleeding	578.9	Lymphoma	202.8		
Angina	413.9	Metastatic (Site)	199.1	Contusion (Site)	924.9	Glomerulonephritis	583.9	Mit. Valve Prolapse	424.0		
Anxiety Synd.	300.00	Colon	153.9	Costochondritis	733.99	Headache	784.0	Myocard. Infarction (Area)	410.9		
Appendicitis	541	Cancer, Rectal	154.1	Depression	311.	Headache, Tension	307.81	M.I., Old	412		
Arterioscl. H.D.	414.0	Lung (Site)	162.9	Dermatitis	692.9	Migraine (Type)	346.9	Myositis	729.1		
Arthritis, Osteo.	715.90	Skin (Site)	173.9	Diabetes Mellitus	250.00	Hemorrhoids	455.6	Nausea/Vomiting	787.0		
Rheumatoid	714.0	Card. Arrhythmia (Type)	427.9	Diabetic Ketosis	250.1	Hernia, Hiatal	553.3	Neuralgia	729.2		
Lupus	710.0	Cardiomyopathy	425.4	Diverticulitis	562.11	Inguinal	550.9	Nevus (Site)	216.9		
		Cellulitis (Site)	682.9	Diverticulosis	562.10	Hepatitis	573.3	Obesity	278.0		

DIAGNOSIS: (IF NOT CHECKED ABOVE)

SERVICES PERFORMED AT: ☐ Office ☐ E.R. ☐ ☐ | ☐ CLAIM CONTAINS NO ORDERED REFERRING SERVICE | REFERRING PHYSICIAN & I.D. NUMBER

RETURN APPOINTMENT INFORMATION: 5 - 10 - 15 - 20 - 30 - 40 - 60 [DAYS] [WKS.] [MOS.] [PRN] | NEXT APPOINTMENT M - T - W - TH - F - S DATE / / TIME: AM PM | ACCEPT ASSIGNMENT? ☐ YES ☐ NO | DOCTOR'S SIGNATURE

INSTRUCTIONS TO PATIENT FOR FILING INSURANCE CLAIMS:

1. Complete upper portion of this form, sign and date.
2. Attach this form to your own insurance company's form for direct reimbursement.

MEDICARE PATIENTS - DO NOT SEND THIS TO MEDICARE.
WE WILL SUBMIT THE CLAIM FOR YOU.

☐ CASH ☐ CHECK # ______ ☐ VISA ☐ MC ☐ CO-PAY

TOTAL TODAY'S FEE	
OLD BALANCE	
TOTAL DUE	
AMOUNT REC'D. TODAY	

INSUR-A-BILL ® BIBBERO SYSTEMS, INC. • PETALUMA, CA • UP. SUPER. © 6/94 (BIBB/STOCK)

Fig. 29.5 Superbill The encounter form, or superbill, is printed for each patient at each visit. A copy can be also given to the patient as a receipt of services. *Why would this form be useful to the insurance specialist?*

also called a **superbill,** is shown in **Figure 29.5.** The medical record contains the patient's insurance and personal information, as well as his or her medical history. The encounter form is used to record the patient's illness or condition, the diagnosis, and the procedure received during each office visit. Standard coding systems are used for both the diagnosis and the procedure. These coding systems are described in Chapter 30, Health Information.

The medical insurance specialist also needs a basic knowledge of medical law and ethics. Dealing with patients' medical and financial records and submitting insurance claim forms means having access to confidential patient information. The insurance specialist must use patient information appropriately, following all federal and state laws regarding the insurance claims process, and staying current with medical insurance rules and regulations.

The Job of the Medical Insurance Specialist

A medical insurance specialist working in a physician's office retrieves information from the patient's medical and financial records as well as the encounter form. He or she then fills out the insurance claim form. **Figure 29.6** shows a universal insurance claim form.

When this form is used, the diagnosis and treatment ordered for the patient must be coded and correctly written on the bottom of the insurance claim form. The top section of the form must also be completely filled out with information on the **beneficiary** receiving services as well as the **insured.** The insured is not always the same person as the beneficiary. For example, a minor child may be insured under a parent's plan. In this case, the child is the **dependent** or beneficiary of services, and the parent is the insured.

The form must be filled out accurately and completely, so that the medical office will receive payment, as quickly as possible and in the correct amount. Once the form is filled out, the medical insurance specialist must submit the form to the insurance provider. The form is submitted electronically or in some cases by mail.

Once the insurance company has determined the amount of payment to be made to the medical office based on the completed insurance form, that payment and an **explanation of benefits (EOB)** form are sent back. The EOB indicates how much, if any, payment is enclosed based on the **benefits,** or agreed-upon services, available to the insured. If errors were made on the claim form or if the form was filled out incompletely, a partial payment will be sent or the claim will be denied. The problem will be explained on the EOB.

21ST CENTURY SKILLS

Completing Forms

To maintain accurate patient records, always keep the six Cs of charting in mind:

- **Client's words** Be sure to record the patient's exact words, rather than your interpretation.
- **Clarity** Use precise descriptions and accepted terminology.
- **Completeness** Make sure that all forms are filled out completely.
- **Conciseness** Keep it brief and to the point.
- **Chronological order** Make all entries in chronological order.
- **Confidentiality** Protect patient confidentiality at all times.

Follow-up

Can you name any other ways to ensure accuracy when completing patient forms?

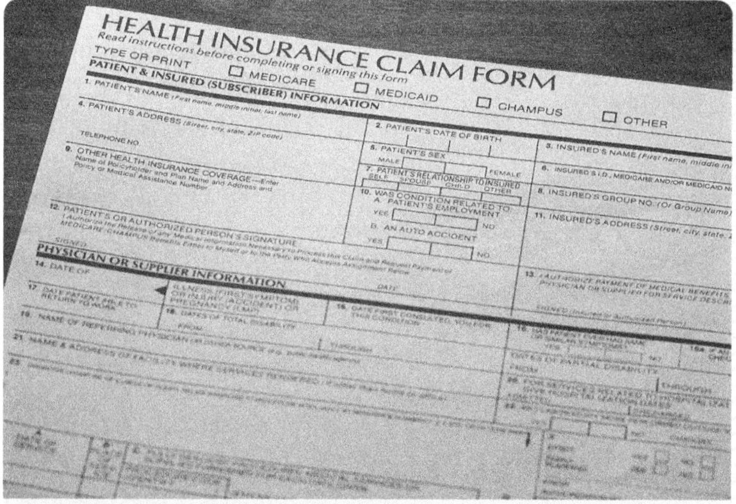

Fig. 29.6 Medical Forms A CMS-1500 form is a universal health insurance claim form for clinical office billings. *Who is responsible for completing this form?*

Photo: K.Knudson/PhotoLink/Photodisc/Getty Images

The medical billing and reimbursement specialist, whose job is explained on page 697, is responsible for reviewing and filing the EOB forms. If there is a problem, the insurance specialist makes corrections on the health claim form and resubmits it to the insurance company. In the case of a denial, the insurance specialist may **appeal** the decision based on the guidelines of the insurance company and with the patient's consent.

The duties of the medical insurance specialist are far from simple. There are many different types of private and government-sponsored insurance. In addition, each insurance carrier may offer numerous policy plans and benefits to the **subscriber** or **policyholder** (the insured).

The insurance specialist must know the details of policies for each plan offered and each provider's rules and procedures for filing claim forms. Some examples of private insurance companies are Blue Cross and Blue Shield, Anthem, and various health maintenance organizations (HMOs). Government providers include Medicare, Medicaid, and Tricare, a plan available to military personnel and their families.

Efficient medical insurance specialists must use many resources, including policy manuals for each insurance plan accepted by the medical office and the phone number and name of individual insurance representatives. An electronic database is valuable to the insurance specialist for this purpose. Also, most private and government-sponsored insurance plans send out periodic electronic or paper newsletters updating the specialist on new laws, rules, or regulations. The specialist is responsible for reading these newsletters and noting any changes in plans or procedures.

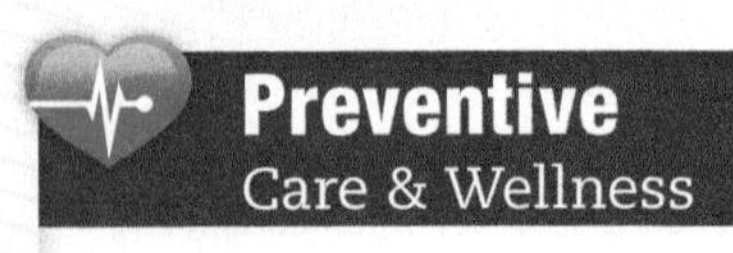

Practicing Proper Posture

Sitting at a desk all day can be tiring if you do not have correct posture. Here are some guidelines.

- The keyboard should be below elbow height when the user is seated.
- The keyboard base should be gently sloped away from the user so that the key tops are accessible to the hands in a neutral posture.
- The user should sit in a slightly reclined position, with the lower back resting against the lumbar support of the chair.
- The elbow angle should be open, to promote blood circulation to the lower arm and hand.
- The knee angle should be slightly open, to promote blood circulation in the lower legs.
- The user's feet should rest firmly on the floor.

Insurance Fraud and Compliance

One area of particular concern to the medical insurance specialist is fraud. **Fraud** can be defined as the intentional misrepresentation of facts in order to mislead or deceive another person or entity, such as a business or government organization. Insurance specialists must carefully review the diagnostic and procedural information on claims. These must be correctly linked. For each procedure code noted on the insurance claim form, there must be a corresponding diagnosis code, which should be relevant and supported by complete documentation in the patient's medical record.

An example of an incorrect linkage would be a procedural code for mammography linked to a diagnostic code for pneumonia. In this scenario, the insurance carrier would not see a relationship between a mammography and pneumonia.

An example of an error that might constitute fraud would be the use of a code that results in a higher payment, rather than a code for a procedure that is paid at a lower rate. Although the specialist may simply have made an error when recording codes, the insurance carrier might assume that a deliberate attempt was made to collect more money for payment and may investigate.

Individual medical offices should have an established plan or procedure to follow. This helps ensure that insurance claims are completed correctly and consistently. Claims could also be reviewed by another employee in the office before being submitted to the insurance company.

READING CHECK

Summarize the content and purpose of the encounter form.

The Medical Office Manager

What organizational skills are important for a medical office manager to have?

In the medical office, the person who is in charge of the operation of equipment, supplies, and staff is often known as the office manager. In a small office, that staff member reports to the physician. In turn, the office manager may oversee one or more other office workers. Offices that have more than one physician may have a human resources department. In this case, the medical office manager would report to a human resources manager. The office manager has a great deal of responsibility as well as the prospect of a higher income than that of other office workers.

In many offices, the office manager is a medical assistant who has been trained in the administrative and clinical duties of the medical office. The medical assistant who has received formal training is likely to have taken specific courses in office management and organization, medical law and ethics, therapeutic communication, and **human relations**. The office manager may also be a clinician, such as a registered nurse.

The office manager is often expected to provide evidence of formal training and to have several years of experience working in a clinical office before being hired or promoted. The office manager who is a trained medical assistant can further contribute to the efficiency of the office by performing clinical or administrative tasks and by being available to fill in if a staff emergency or problem arises.

The Job of the Medical Office Manager

The responsibilities of the office manager include the supervision of employees and other duties associated with running a busy medical practice. The office manager should strive to be a positive role model for all employees while motivating them to do their best. It is often the office manager who arranges staff meetings, schedules training on new equipment, and meets with visitors such as medical sales representatives on the physician's behalf.

21ST CENTURY SKILLS

Protected Health Information and E-mail

HIPAA law requires that all transactions containing protected health information be kept secure. Consider the following guidelines when sending e-mail within a healthcare facility.

- Do not send e-mail containing protected health information without specific written authorization from the patient.
- Always check the patient's medical record and the computer records for any special instructions on contacting the patient through e-mail. Follow all patient requests. When in doubt, do not send an e-mail and discuss what to do next with your office manager or supervisor.
- Make sure that the computer system's virus protection is up to date, to guard your computer system against viruses, which commonly infect systems through e-mail.

Follow up:
How would you be certain that an e-mail with patient information can be sent?

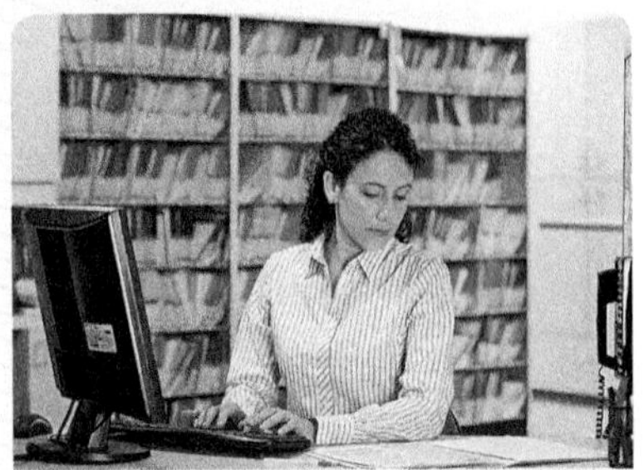

Fig. 29.7 Office Manager The medical office manager should be professional in appearance and attitude. *What are the medical office manager's most important duties?*

Some knowledge of the business aspects of the practice is also required. Some office managers review financial reports with the physician. They need to understand how these relate to office revenue.

Organizational skills required of the office manager include being able to manage the priorities of the office and appropriately assign tasks to other employees. These duties require excellent communication skills. Management and organization of the staff involve creating and maintaining the office work schedule, performing employee evaluations, and dealing with staff or patient problems throughout the workday. In addition, the effective office manager must be able to solve problems quickly and accurately, and set personal and professional goals for the office staff. He or she may also design and implement an employee recognition program to motivate employees.

The office manager often sets the general atmosphere or tone of the office (see **Figure 29.7**). When the office manager sets a positive overall tone, employees are more likely to be satisfied and to strive for excellence every day. Such an atmosphere promotes a caring attitude toward patients. Patients, in turn, express their appreciation by remaining loyal to the physician and the medical practice.

In addition to the tasks already mentioned, the medical office manager may manage the office **budget**, handle business aspects such as public relations and marketing, and hire new employees. The job description may also include handling patients' financial records, preparing and maintaining the office policy and procedures manual, and training new employees.

21ST CENTURY SKILLS

Leadership

An office manager is the leader of the personnel in an office. To be a leader, the office manager must have a good grounding in human relations. Human relations may be defined as the ability to understand human behavior and to use this knowledge in interacting with colleagues and creating a positive and productive work environment. The office manager must know how to motivate employees to achieve personal and professional goals. To do this, the manager must lead, influence, and reward performance or behavior appropriately. Knowledge of human development, psychology, and behavior is especially helpful.

READING CHECK

Name some ways in which the medical office manager can improve the atmosphere of a medical office and boost the staff morale.

The Medical Billing and Reimbursement Specialist

What is a tickler report?

The physician and other healthcare office workers enjoy their work and get pleasure from helping patients get well and feel better. The truth, however, is that the rent for the building or space must be paid, equipment must be bought and maintained, and employees must receive wages in order to provide for themselves and their families. The medical practice is a business, and if it is to stay in business, it must receive payment, or **reimbursement,** for the services it provides to patients. A person may be hired to handle these duties, or these duties may be assigned to the administrative assistant, the insurance specialist, or the office manager.

As a rule, collecting **co-payments** or **deductibles** from patients is one of the tasks of the front office staff. Some physicians in larger offices

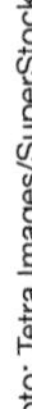
Photo: Tetra Images/SuperStock

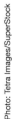

may hire outside companies to manage the paperwork involved in billing and collecting payments for the medical office.

The medical billing and reimbursement specialist who is responsible for billing and collecting payments from patients or **insurance carriers** may have formal training in a medical assistant program, or may have a background in medical coding, billing, or insurance. Careers in these areas are discussed in more detail in Chapter 30, Health Information.

The Job of the Medical Billing and Reimbursement Specialist

The person responsible for the billing and reimbursement operations of the medical office has frequent contact with the medical insurance specialist. Most insurance companies do not cover 100 percent of all services. This means that the patient must pay any additional or uncovered costs. Also, some patients are "self-pay," which means that they do not have insurance and are responsible for the entire cost of any medical care they receive. These patients ideally pay at the time they receive service. In either case, the billing and reimbursement specialist deals with the patient or other responsible party in determining a schedule or process for payment.

One duty of the billing and reimbursement specialist is to develop and maintain records on patient third-party payers. Each patient's account is recorded in a **ledger,** which is a financial record that shows a history of charges and payments. Computerized software typically maintains these account files. Patients' financial records are always kept separate from their medical records, although it may be necessary to refer to medical records for financial purposes. Practice management software that interfaces the patient financial record and electronic health record (EHR) is useful for all medical financial specialists.

The billing and reimbursement specialist creates tickler reports and a billing schedule. For patients who have a **balance,** or an unpaid amount, **statements** are sent out on a regular basis. Statements detail for the patient the service provided and the amount he or she owes for that service.

The **tickler report** is organized according to the calendar. It may be checked every day to allow the billing and reimbursement specialist to keep track of when to ask the insurance specialist about an overdue account or when to contact a patient who agreed to make a payment but did not do so.

The billing schedule is a method of billing patients monthly based upon certain criteria. For example, on one type of billing schedule, the billing and reimbursement specialist bills patients whose last name begins with the letters A through F during the first week of the month. The remainder of the month is further divided according to the patients' last names. This system distributes the workload of the billing and reimbursement specialist throughout the month.

21ST CENTURY SKILLS

The Headset

The wireless headset, also called a hands-free headset, is popular in healthcare offices. It allows the user to speak on the phone while using his or her hands to do other work. Also, it reduces office-related neck, back, and shoulder pain.

If you must move about the office while on the line with a patient, always keep HIPAA and patient confidentiality in mind. Anything you say can easily be heard by anyone within listening range.

Follow up:
Explain why a wireless headset is more efficient yet increases the risk of violating HIPAA.

21ST CENTURY SKILLS

Answering Emergency Calls

Many people think to dial 911 before calling the doctor to respond to a life-threatening situation. However, if a patient calls with any of the following problems or symptoms, consider it an emergency situation: severe bleeding, electrical shock, allergic reactions causing breathing difficulties, seizures, injuries to the head, neck, or back, chest pain including other symptoms of a heart attack, snake bites, injuries caused by violence, and poisoning. The list is not comprehensive, but covers the most common emergencies.

Follow-up
Why should you remain calm while handling a telephone call for any of the above situations? Can you name any other potential emergency situations?

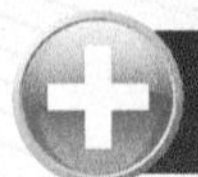

Safety

Preventing Infection

Although as an administrative professional you may have minimal contact with patients in a medical office, you can still pass on or acquire an infection. To prevent transmission of infection you should

- wash your hands frequently, especially before eating.
- not touch any objects that may be contaminated, and then touch your nose, mouth, or face.
- use a tissue to cover your nose and mouth when sneezing and coughing.
- wash your hands after sneezing and coughing.
- use a hand sanitizer often during the day.

The billing and reimbursement specialist must monitor patient accounts and follow up on collecting payments. To assist in this process, the specialist should have a plan of action to collect overdue accounts. This plan should be outlined in the medical office policy and procedures manual and should include a time frame for completing each step of the plan.

For example, the patient may receive a bill or statement within 30 days of receiving treatment, a reminder statement and phone call after 60 days, and a formal letter after 90 days. After 150 days, the office may turn over the account to a **collection agency,** which is a company that specializes in collecting delinquent, or badly overdue, accounts. But the collection agency may charge the practice a fee as high as 40 percent of the amount due to the practice. For that reason, the billing and reimbursement specialist's persistent follow-up from the beginning is essential if the office is to avoid this loss of revenue. In some cases, a patient may be taken to small claims court in order to collect the overdue account without involving a collection agency.

READING CHECK

Explain how the billing and reimbursement specialist goes about collecting patient payments.

SECTION 29.1 Administrative Office Careers Review

AFTER YOU READ

1. **Name** the educational requirements for an administrative medical assistant, a medical insurance specialist, a medical office manager, and a billing and reimbursement specialist.
2. **Compare and contrast** the duties of the administrative medical assistant and of the office manager.
3. **Distinguish** the duties of the medical insurance specialist from those of the billing and reimbursement specialist.
4. **List** two professional associations that might be of interest to the professional administrative office employee.
5. **Identify** how the confidentiality of patient information is a legal and an ethical concern for an administrator in a medical office.

Technology ONLINE EXPLORATIONS

Professional Organizations

Research online the following professional organizations related to medical office employment: American Association of Medical Billers, American Association of Medical Assistants, Professional Association of Healthcare Office Managers, and American Health Information Management Association. Compare the mission statements of these organizations and the certification offered by each. Write a short summary or develop a fact sheet of your findings.

SECTION 29.2 Medical Office Procedures

Medical Office Career Skills

How are healthcare records managed?

The following procedures provide guidelines for some of the more common administrative tasks performed by administrative healthcare professionals. Some of these procedures are common to offices of many different industries, as all office environments need employees with clerical skills.

However, the healthcare workplace also has its own considerations. Patient confidentiality is foremost among these concerns. Completing and handling the records and forms of clients, including insurance claims and forms, should always be done with HIPAA in mind.

Vocabulary

Content Vocabulary

You will learn these content vocabulary terms in this section.

- **records management system**
- **claim**

Academic Vocabulary

You will see this word in your reading and on your tests. Find its meaning in the Glossary in the back of the book.

- **tasks**

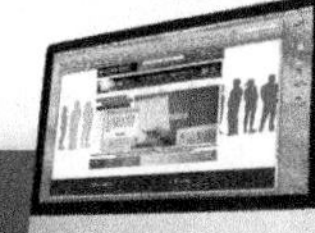

connect ONLINE PROCEDURES

PROCEDURE 29-1

Using the Telephone

Any healthcare professional should be prepared to answer the telephone. Since this is often the first contact with the patient, it is essential that the medical office employee answer the phone promptly and pleasantly, and assign the correct priority to each call when there are multiple calls to handle.

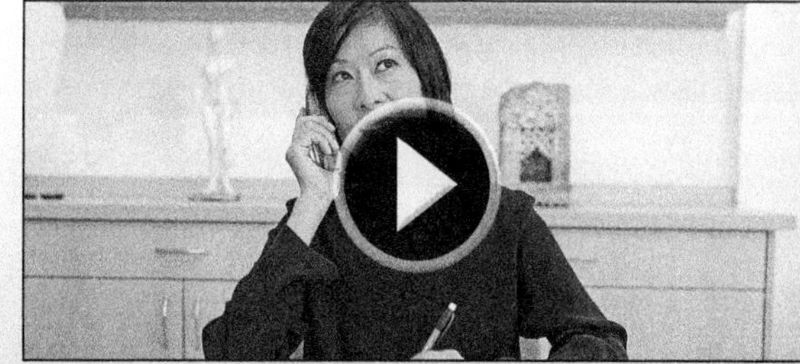

PROCEDURE 29-2

Scheduling Appointments

Most medical offices have specific policies and procedures for scheduling patients throughout the day. Scheduling may be performed in a variety of ways. The type of medical practice and the preference of the physician usually determine the method used to schedule patient appointments.

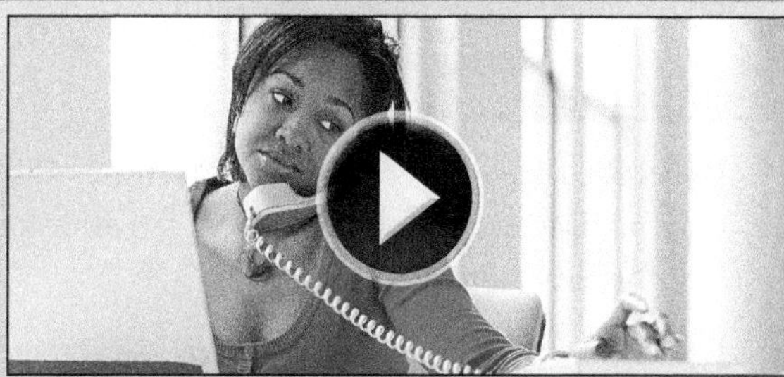

PROCEDURE 29-3

Greeting a Patient

The medical employee who greets the patient may be the medical administrative assistant, the office manager, or a receptionist hired specifically to answer the phone and schedule appointments. The importance of properly greeting the patient should never be underestimated.

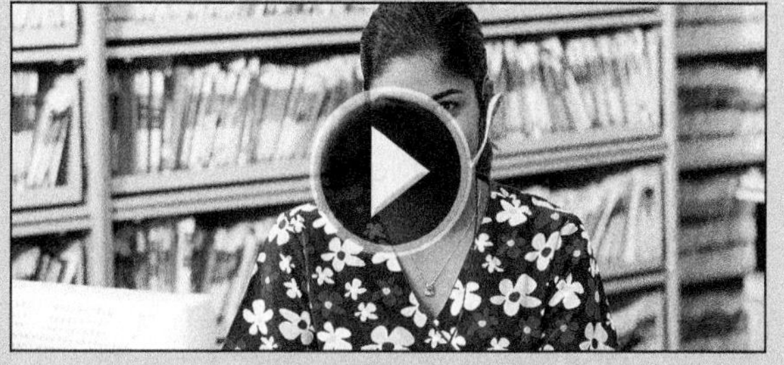

Photos: (t)Ralf Schultheiss/Corbis, (c)Image Source/Getty Images, (b)Stewart Cohen/Pam Ostrow/Getty Images

connect ONLINE PROCEDURES

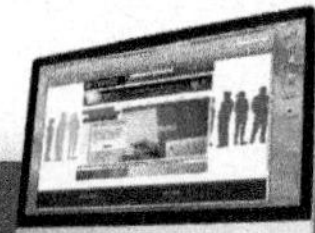

PROCEDURE 29-4

Assembling a Client Record

A medical record is created for each patient seen in a medical practice to record the patient's medical history, document the care and instructions given in the course of treatment, and keep laboratory or radiology reports and other test results in good order. In addition, the medical record may be used as a reference for providing care or in research and education.

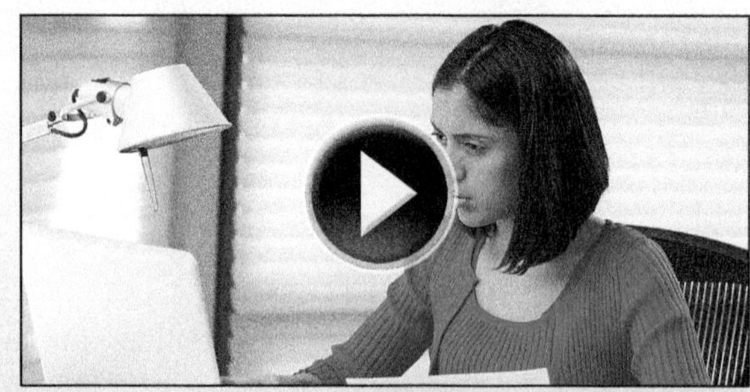

PROCEDURE 29-5

Filing Medical Records

Traditionally, medical records were in kept in hard copy and filed in a folder. Today, medical records are being converted to electronic health records (EHR); this will affect how each medical facility handles its **records management system**.

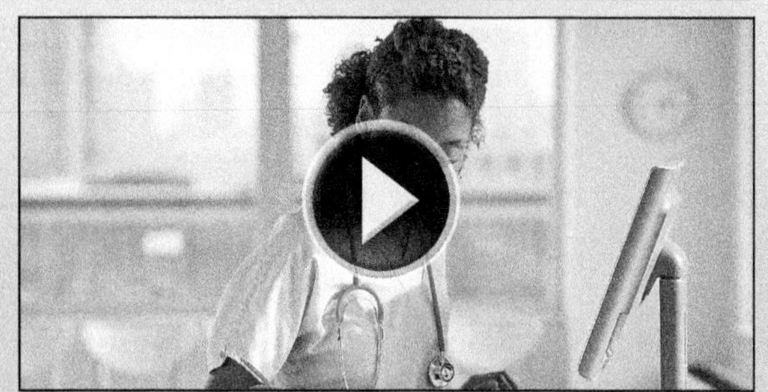

PROCEDURE 29-6

Completing Insurance Forms

An important part of running a medical office involves correctly filling out insurance **claim** forms for the patient. Handling each claim, or request for reimbursement for medical costs, is often the responsibility of the medical insurance specialist. However, the administrative medical assistant or office manager may perform this task in offices that do not have a medical insurance specialist.

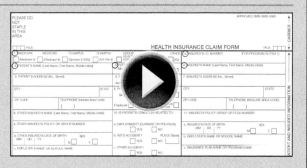

HEALTH INSURANCE CLAIM FORM

SECTION 29.2 Medical Office Procedures Review

AFTER YOU READ

1. **Describe** three types of office machines that may be used to perform administrative tasks. List the function or functions of each.
2. **Explain** why good interpersonal skills are important for administrative employees in medical office.
3. **List** three examples of phone calls that may be received by the medical office.
4. **Name** some types of phone calls that require immediate attention.
5. **Describe** how you would greet a patient.

Technology ONLINE EXPLORATIONS

Electronic Records

Go online to find information on electronic health records systems. Develop a list of the advantages of electronic health records over paper health records. Share the list with your class.

Photos: (t)Ariel Skelley/Blend Images/Getty Images, (b)JGI/Daniel Grill/Blend Images/Getty Images

CHAPTER 29 Review

Chapter Summary

SECTION 29.1

- The administrative medical assistant must have good interpersonal and clerical skills. **(pg. 689)**
- Healthcare jobs that do not involve direct, clinical patient care are the administrative medical assistant, the medical insurance specialist, the medical office manager, and the medical billing and reimbursement specialist. **(pg. 690)**
- The administrative medical assistant, the medical insurance specialist, and the medical billing and reimbursement specialist may receive training in short-term technical or vocational school programs. **(pg. 690)**
- The medical insurance specialist is hired by a medical office to manage patient financial records as well as complete and submit insurance forms. The insurance specialist must know the details of the policies for each plan held by the office's patients. He or she must also be familiar with each provider's rules and procedures for filing claim forms. **(pg. 692)**
- An effective medical office manager supervises employees while managing all of the duties associated with running a busy medical practice. He or she helps all employees achieve their full potential and success. **(pg. 695)**
- The medical billing and reimbursement specialist works closely with the medical insurance specialist. After the insurance payment has been received, the reimbursement specialist determines the balance due from the patient and mails a bill or statement to the patient. **(pg. 697)**

SECTION 29.2

- All patient information, including patient records and insurance claims and forms, needs to remain confidential. **(pg. 699)**

Mc Graw Hill connect™ ONLINE ACTIVITIES

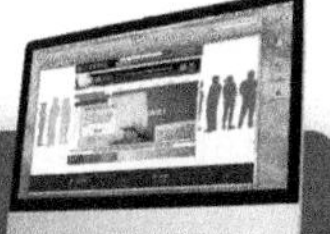

Complete our HST online activities for Chapter 29, which include Concept Check review questions, Reference Flash Cards, and Online Procedures assessment sheets.

- **Concept Check** review questions
- **Reference Flash Cards** medical terminology practice
- **Online Procedures** assessment sheets

Critical Thinking/Problem Solving

1. Two unscheduled patients call the office. One fell, hit his head, was unconscious for several minutes, and is complaining of a severe headache. The other has been stung by a wasp and is short of breath. Only one buffer remains in the appointment book. What would you do?
2. You have been asked to retrieve a patient file. To do so, you access the EHR. You are having difficulty locating the file. Explain the steps that you will take to solve the problem.
3. As a medical insurance specialist, you submit an electronic claim for a patient who received a vitamin B_{12} injection. You realize that the consent forms allowing you to release information to the insurance company and receive payment are more than a year old. However, you indicated on the form you submitted that the consent forms were "on file." The administrative medical assistant is new and did not update the consent forms. How would you handle this situation professionally? Describe the interpersonal skills you should use.
4. Obtain copies of a CMS-1500 form and complete the form as if you were filing a claim. Create information as necessary to ensure that the form can be filled out completely.

21ST CENTURY SKILLS

5. **Problem Solving** With a partner, practice answering the telephone. Role-play different situations. For example, role-play what you would say if you could not spell a patient's name, if the physician were with a patient and the physician's spouse called, or if an angry patient called insisting on speaking with the physician immediately.
6. **Information Literacy** Using online employment resources, find a job opening for an administrative medical office employee. Determine the qualifications and experience necessary to apply to the opening that you have chosen. Then write a summary of what you would need to obtain this job, including education and previous employment experience.
7. **Information Literacy** Using the Internet, find programs of study that can prepare you to enter the administrative medical office field. Locate a school in your area that offers such a program and contact the school, preferably by email, to find out entrance requirements and program of study. Inquire about whether you can apply for certification upon completion of the program.

CHAPTER 30

Health Information

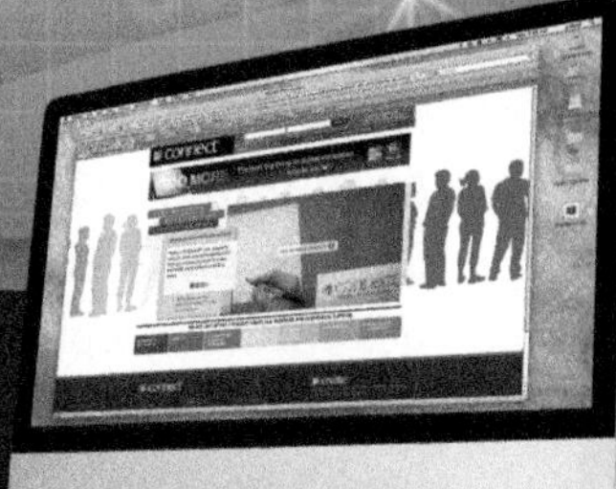

Essential Question:

How would you protect the confidentiality of a patient's healthcare information?

Think about what it would be like to run a hospital or other healthcare facility without any information about the patients. You would not know their names, ages, illnesses, and previous surgeries or treatments. You would not know if they had insurance to pay their bills or how much they owed. You would have no way of telling if patients who had the same illnesses got better or worse when given the same, or different, treatments. You would also be unable to manage the business side of the facility. Because keeping track of all this data is so important, hospitals and other healthcare facilities employ health information professionals.

McGraw Hill connect™

It's Online!

- Online Procedures
- STEM Connection
- Medical Science
- Medical Terms
- Medical Math
- Ethics in Action
- Virtual Lab

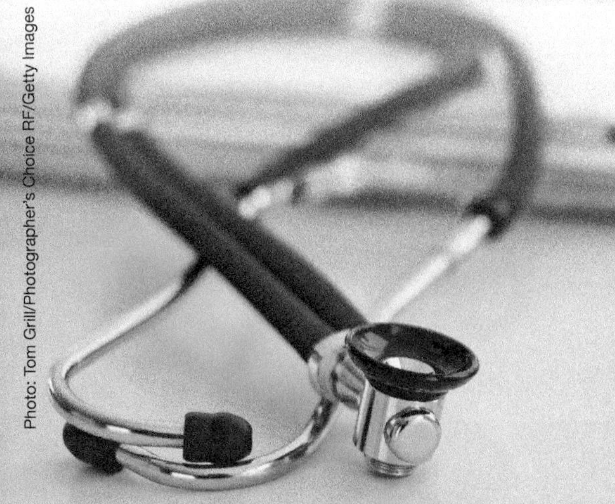

Photo: Tom Grill/Photographer's Choice RF/Getty Images

READING GUIDE

OBJECTIVES

After completing this chapter, you will be able to:

- **Distinguish** the key roles and responsibilities of a healthcare receptionist, health unit coordinator, health information technician, medical biller and coder, medical transcriptionist, compliance officer, and medical chart auditor.
- **List** the various settings in which health information professionals are employed.
- **Explain** the importance of keeping patient healthcare information confidential.
- **Illustrate** the reasons for documentation standards.
- **Identify** the reference books used for coding health records.
- **Categorize** the steps to follow in locating correct diagnosis and procedure codes.
- **Explain** the importance of verifying patients' bills and auditing medical charts.
- **Demonstrate** two health information procedures.

BEFORE YOU READ

Connect Have you ever had to complete any forms before receiving medical treatment or undergoing surgery? What questions were you asked?

Main Idea

Professionals in the rapidly-growing health information industry admit patients, keep track of medical data and healthcare records, and ensure that billing is accurate.

Note-Taking Activity

Draw this table. Write key terms and phrases under **Cues**. Write main ideas under **Note Taking**. Summarize the section under **Summary**.

Cues	Note Taking
o o	o o
Summary	

Graphic Organizer

Before you read the chapter, draw a diagram like the one to the right. As you read, write the careers covered by this chapter into the diagram.

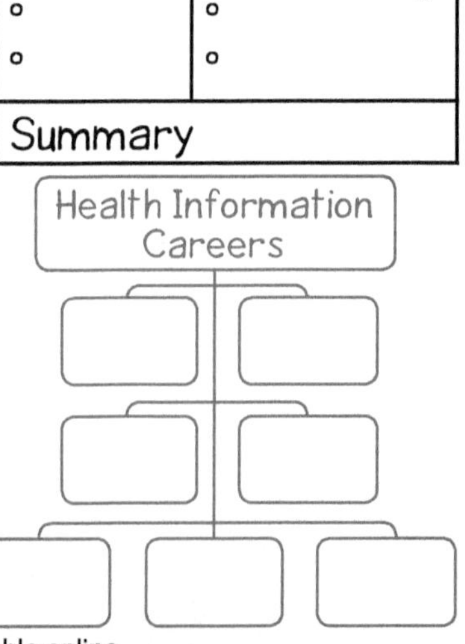

connect
Downloadable graphic organizers are available online.

STANDARDS

HEALTH SCIENCE

NCHSE 5.12 Apply procedures for accurate documentation and record keeping.

NCHSE 6.12 Recognize ethical issues and their implications related to healthcare.

SCIENCE

NSES F Develop understanding of personal and community health; population growth; natural resources; environmental quality; natural and human-induced hazards; science and technology in local, national, and global challenges.

NCHSE *National Consortium for Health Science Education*

NSES *National Science Education Standards*

COMMON CORE STATE STANDARDS

MATHEMATICS

Statistics and Probability

Making Inferences and Justifying Conclusions S-IC 1 Understand statistics as a process for making inferences about population parameters based on a random sample from that population.

ENGLISH LANGUAGE ARTS

Writing

Writing W-6 Use technology, including the Internet, to produce, publish, and update individual or shared writing products, taking advantage of technology's capacity to link to other information and to display information flexibly and dynamically.

SECTION

30.1 Careers in Health Information

Careers in Health Information

How does accurate health information assist medical researchers?

The job of health information professionals is to collect, analyze, and store information and to provide information to physicians and other healthcare providers. Timely, accurate health information also helps researchers improve quality of care, such as new drugs and techniques to treat illnesses. Increasing demand for new services, as well as an aging population, means that opportunities in health information careers will continue to grow. See **Table 30.1** on page 706 for an overview of these opportunities.

The field of health information offers many career paths, from entry-level positions through management of a large facility (see **Figure 30.1**). Some common occupations are:

- Healthcare receptionist
- Health unit coordinator
- Health information technician
- Medical biller and coder
- Medical transcriptionist
- Compliance officer
- Medical chart auditor

READING CHECK

Explain which career in healthcare information may require the most education and training.

Vocabulary

Content Vocabulary

You will learn these content vocabulary terms in this section.

- **inpatient**
- **outpatient**
- **health record**
- **health information management (HIM)**
- **Centers for Medicare and Medicaid Services (CMS)**
- **diagnosis-related group (DRG)**
- **Health Insurance Portability and Accountability Act (HIPAA)**
- **compliance**
- **consent form**

Academic Vocabulary

You will see this word in your reading and on your tests. Find its meaning in the Glossary in the back of the book.

- **discriminate**

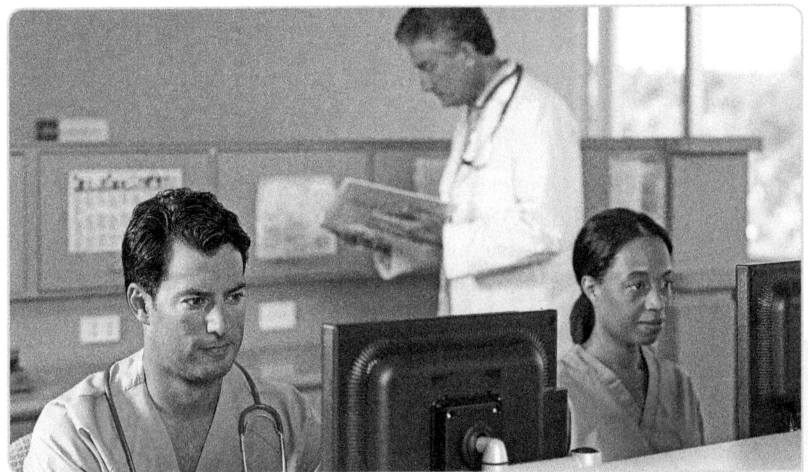

Photo: Brad Wilson/The Image Bank/Getty Images

Fig. 30.1 Information Careers Employees in a hospital. *In what type of medical setting would you prefer to work?*

Table 30.1 Overview of Health Information Occupations

OCCUPATION	EDUCATIONAL REQUIREMENTS	CERTIFICATION OR LICENSING AGENCY	JOB OUTLOOK
Healthcare Receptionist or Hospital Admissions Receptionist	High school diploma	None required	Faster than average growth due to the growing needs of an aging population
Health Unit Coordinator	High school diploma. Community colleges and technical schools may offer programs. Some hospitals and healthcare facilities may offer on-the-job training.	Certification can be obtained by passing an examination given by the National Association of Health Unit Coordinators.	Faster than average growth due to the growing needs of an aging population
Health Information Technician or Medical Records Technician	Associate degree	American Health Information Association national examination for the registered health information technician (RHIT) credential	Rapid growth due to growing healthcare needs of an aging population
Medical Biller and Coder, Health Information Coder or Medical Coder	Associate degree or one-year certificate	National examination given by either the American Health Information Management Association or the American Academy of Professional Coders (for coding credentials)	Rapid growth due to growing healthcare needs of an aging population
Medical Transcriptionist	Associate degree or one-year certificate	National examination given by the American Association for Medical Transcription for the certified medical transcriptionist (CMT) credential	Average growth
Compliance Officer (also called Privacy Officer)	Associate degree and significant experience; bachelor's degree preferred.	Various certifications available, such as the American Health Information Management Association's registered health information administrator (RHIA) credential. The Health Care Compliance Association (HCCA), and the American Academy of Professional Coders (AAPC) also offer credentialing.	Rapid growth
Medical Chart Auditor	Varies	Various certifications. For example the AAPC offers the certified professional medical auditor (CPMA) certificate.	Much faster than average

The Healthcare Receptionist

How can the healthcare receptionist put patients at ease while accurately collecting personal information?

Healthcare receptionists in hospitals and other medical facilities work for patient access departments in the registration or admissions areas. They are sometimes called hospital admissions receptionists. As a front-desk job, this is a very visible position. The healthcare receptionist creates a good first impression by greeting patients promptly and professionally. A warm, friendly greeting sets the right tone. Then he or she collects financial and personal information about the patient's visit. He or she has the patient fill out an identification sheet and other forms, and may give the patient various information sheets and brochures about the facility and its policies and procedures. A hospital patient may be admitted as an **inpatient,** who requires at least an overnight stay, or as an **outpatient,** who will be released on the same day, shortly after a procedure has been performed.

Healthcare receptionists answer many patients' questions, such as directions to a department in the facility. The work pace is often very fast, with patients, visitors, healthcare staff members, and telephones all requiring attention.

Job Responsibilities of the Healthcare Receptionist

The healthcare receptionist may be responsible for:

- Helping patients complete forms
- Checking the information the patient provides for completeness and accuracy
- Entering patient financial and personal data into the facility's information system, to create the patient's **health record** for the visit
- Verifying that patients are eligible for insurance coverage by calling or e-mailing payers such as insurance carriers
- Collecting insurance co-payments from patients and giving them receipts
- Checking facts and records with the patient's primary care physician
- Performing administrative duties such as scheduling appointments and answering and routing incoming calls

Like all health information workers, healthcare receptionists know that the information they gather about patients must be kept confidential. This is both a legal and an ethical requirement. Everyone who works with patients in health services guards the privacy of patient information.

READING CHECK

List several things that might compete for the attention of a healthcare receptionist.

21ST CENTURY SKILLS

Confidentiality

One of the first forms you are likely to sign as a health information professional will be a confidentiality statement. All information that you encounter in the medical environment must remain strictly confidential. For example, computer screens that show patient information must not be visible to the public. You must never discuss confidential patient information in the hospital cafeteria or in any other public setting. You may not share confidential information with anyone unless you need to do so in order to complete the task at hand.

The Health Unit Coordinator

What types of activities are managed by the health unit coordinator?

Health unit coordinators work at nursing stations in hospitals, nursing homes, rehabilitation facilities, and clinics.

Job Responsibilities of the Health Unit Coordinator

The health unit coordinator manages non-nursing patient care activities. He or she works with patients, visitors, and other healthcare professionals. The health unit coordinator may be responsible for

- relaying information to nurses, physicians, and other staff.
- reviewing patients' health records.
- ordering diets, drugs, equipment, supplies, laboratory tests, and X-rays as instructed by a physician or a member of the nursing staff
- checking physicians' orders.
- completing reports and admission forms and discharging them; transferring patients to other facilities; or transferring reports and forms related to the death of a patient.

READING CHECK

Identify the types of facilities in which a health unit coordinator could work.

> **21ST CENTURY SKILLS**
>
> **Working with Electronic Health Records**
>
> Electronic health records (EHRs) are a computerized recording of patient information. They are also called computer records, electronic medical records, electronic charts, and computer health records.
>
> As a healthcare professional working with electronic records, you must:
>
> - Become familiar with the hardware and software used at your facility for record keeping. When you are comfortable with the system, your attention will not be distracted when you are with a patient. If necessary at first, take notes and enter the information in the computer after the patient leaves.
> - Retrieve the patient record carefully, just as you would a paper record. Make sure you have identified the patient with at least two identifiers such as name, date of birth, and/or medical record number.
> - Check your entries carefully before hitting Enter. An EHR is a legal document, just like a paper chart.
> - Keep your password secure. Change the password on a regular basis or as directed by facility policy.
> - Secure the computer on which the EHRs are kept and back up the files.

The Health Information Technician

What types of forms and records are the responsibility of a health information technician?

Health information management (HIM) departments maintain health record systems. Work settings include hospitals, clinics, surgery centers, physician practices, managed care organizations, insurance carriers, long-term and home care organizations, and law firms.

Job Responsibilities of the Health Information Technician

The three major functions of health information technicians are:

- Analyzing patients' health records to ensure that they are complete and accurate
- Assigning codes from medical coding references to the patients' diagnoses and the procedures performed by physicians
- Preparing physicians' reports about the treatments and procedures they performed for patients

In large facilities, a healthcare information professional may specialize in one of those tasks. In smaller facilities, a single professional may handle all three.

The health information technician's job is highly detail oriented, and they will probably be expected to:

- ensure that patients have completed and signed all necessary forms.
- enter data about diagnoses, procedures, and charges into the information system.
- highlight items in the record that are missing or confusing, so that physicians can supply or correct the information.
- check that all hospital departments providing services to a patient have completed their sections of the record.
- prepare census and statistical reports, such as reports on the number of people treated by a hospital for a particular condition and the health outcomes. These reports are prepared for hospital-sponsored or privately-sponsored studies.

READING CHECK

List the three major functions of the health information technician.

The Medical Biller and Coder

What is the main connection between medical billing and medical coding?

The functions of the medical biller and coder go hand in hand. The codes taken from the patient diagnosis or treatment must be assigned to the bill to ensure the bill is paid. Billers and coders work in patient accounting and reimbursement departments.

Medical coders assign codes to patient records using coding procedures and guidelines. They work in the health information management departments of hospitals and other healthcare facilities, including clinical offices, medical billing companies, and commercial insurance companies. In larger facilities, the healthcare information professional may be hired to do only billing or only coding. In smaller facilities, one person will probably do both. Healthcare professionals must have a basic knowledge of both billing and coding, even if they only perform one of those tasks.

Job Responsibilities of the Medical Biller

In a smaller facility, the medical biller's tasks may include the following:

- Making sure that all client charges have been recorded in the billing system
- Entering data such as charges into the client accounts database
- Preparing claims to send to payers such as insurance agencies

- Preparing bills to send to clients
- Tracking payments due from payers and clients.

In a larger facility, the medical biller may specialize in only one of those tasks or in some other area of billing. For example, some medical billers specialize in Medicare, the insurance program for people over age 65. It is run by the **Centers for Medicare and Medicaid Services (CMS),** a government agency that has many rules and regulations about paying for client services. Billers who are familiar with those rules are able to prepare claims properly, thus ensuring prompt payment.

Job Responsibilities of the Medical Coder

Medical coders review each health record to locate the patient's diagnosis. They also look for the procedures that were performed during the visit. Sometimes they need to ask a physician or other healthcare professional to explain an item in the record. Codes are assigned to the diagnosis and the various procedures from standard code sets that have been developed for the healthcare industry. Software programs that make it easier to look up codes are often used as coding aids.

Accurate coding is crucial. The codes assigned determine how much a healthcare facility will be paid for its services to patients or even if it will be paid at all. In hospitals, the payment allowed by Medicare for services to inpatients is based mainly on the patients' diagnoses. The CMS analyzes clinically related groups of patients—for example, heart transplant patients—to decide what hospital services and length of stay each group usually needs. CMS assigns a payment amount for the average hospital stays of patients in each of these **diagnosis-related groups (DRGs).** Most other insurance carriers base their payments on the Medicare payments. A different scale of payments is used for outpatient procedures performed in the hospital outpatient clinic or an ambulatory care center.

READING CHECK

Name some possible specializations for the medical biller.

The Medical Transcriptionist

What special skills does a medical transcriptionist need?

Medical transcriptionists use special software and a computer to listen to a recording made by a physician or other healthcare professional on patient assessment and treatment. They then input in exactly what they hear, to create an electronic copy. The completed work can be viewed in the electronic health record (EHR), sent to other healthcare professionals caring for the patient, or printed out for a hardcopy record. The medical transcriptionist must be detail oriented, highly

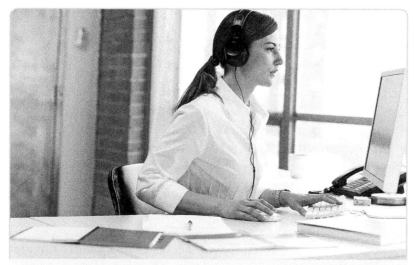

Fig. 30.2 Medical Transcriptionists Transcriptionists should be able to transcribe physicians' dictation quickly and accurately. *What special skills are necessary for this task?*

familiar with medical terminology, and able to edit his or her own work with a critical eye (see **Figure 30.2**).

Transcriptionists work in the health information management department of hospitals, or they may work for a single healthcare practice. They may be employed by a transcription company that provides services to a number of healthcare facilities or physicians. Finally, they may run their own business and have a group of regular clients in the healthcare field.

Job Responsibilities of the Medical Transcriptionist

Medical transcriptionists accurately transcribe medical recordings, such as a physician's report of an operation or an autopsy. Each type of document must follow a specific format for layout and spacing. Transcribed documents are checked and signed by the originator, who is the healthcare professional who made the original recording. They then become a part of the patient's permanent health records.

The medical transcriptionist may also be responsible for the following tasks:

- Logging transcription telephone calls or Internet transmissions
- Sorting and distributing transcribed medical reports
- Placing the transcribed report into the appropriate patient account in the electronic health records system
- Faxing, e-mailing, or uploading transcribed reports to someone other than the originator

READING CHECK

Name some types of documents that are created by medical transcriptionists.

connect

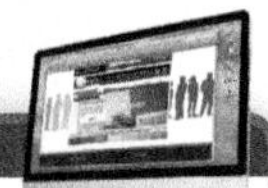

Ethics in Action

Your Personal Health Record
Who owns your health record? It is the physical property of the healthcare practitioner or facility that compiles it. However, you do have the right to access your health record.

Although most healthcare professionals maintain the confidentiality of your health information, breaches can still occur. Health information has been unfairly or illegally used to make decisions about hiring, firing, loan approval, and insurance coverage. Periodically review your medical records to stay informed about what health information is being collected about you, and by whom. To check your health record, contact your doctor or health information management or medical record department at the facility where you received treatment.

Go to connect to read more about this situation and complete the activity.

The Compliance Officer

What is HIPAA?

The compliance officer, also known as the compliance specialist or privacy officer, follows the office compliance program to ensure that the laws and rules of the healthcare industry are followed by all members of the staff. All aspects of healthcare facility procedures, from patient referrals to billing, coding, and other documentation, are coming under increasing scrutiny because of the focus that federal and state regulators have placed on privacy and accuracy in healthcare administration and documentation.

The **Health Insurance Portability and Accountability Act (HIPAA)** is a federal law that provides rules for the use of patient health information. Under this law, health information must be kept private. Facilities that break these rules can be fined. In some cases, they may not be allowed to provide care for Medicare patients.

The misuse of private information can harm patients. Health status can be used to discriminate against people in matters of housing, insurance, and employment. Suppose, for example, that an employer learned about an employee's illness from a hospital or physician and then fired the employee for that reason. This employee's rights to have private information kept secure would have been violated.

Individuals interested in compliance are generally detail oriented with strong, clear values regarding legal, regulatory, and ethical issues. Because of the teaching component inherent in this position, the desire and ability to share knowledge is a plus. The compliance officer frequently works with human resources departments, with potential and new employees, with administrators, and with regulators. This requires excellent communication and interpersonal skills. Highly developed audit, investigatory, and report-writing skills are also necessary.

Job Responsibilities of the Compliance Officer

Compliance officers work to keep their facilities in **compliance** with the law. Compliance with the law means that the individual or facility is abiding by, or obedient to, all rules, regulations, and laws.

The duties of the compliance officer are many and varied but may include:

- Reviewing and updating the office's policies and procedures manual
- Creating and maintaining appropriate coding and billing policies including audit procedures
- Training staff to understand what patient privacy means and to ensure the privacy of patient data

- Creating, conducting, and managing compliance education programs for all staff
- Establishing a process for investigating and taking action on all complaints about privacy policies and procedures
- Recommending disciplinary and remedial action for noncompliance
- Publicizing the reporting system for all providers, staff, vendors, and business associates. Analyzing a facility's risk of releasing information incorrectly, and setting policies and procedures to avoid these risks
- Making sure that the patient's right to inspect, amend, and restrict access to protected health information is observed
- Working with lawyers and managers to make sure that the organization has the appropriate privacy and confidentiality **consent forms,** information notices, and materials. An example of a hospital consent form is shown in **Figure 30.3.** The consent form, signed by the patient, authorizes the physician or facility to release information for certain specific purposes, such as insurance reimbursement.
- Monitoring government sanction lists for excluded individuals/entities when considering potential employees or business associates

CONSENT FOR MEDICAL TREATMENT

I, the undersigned, acknowledge and understand that, in presenting myself for voluntary registration, Inpatient, Outpatient, or Emergency Services at Memorial Hospital, authorize and consent to such diagnostic procedures, tests, or treatments as may be ordered by my physician(s) and/or emergency department physician and carried out by members of the medical staff and hospital associates. I voluntarily consent to such health care, medical and surgical, including anesthesia, X-ray, and lab procedures as may be conduced, requested, directed by delegate, or designated in the judgment of the attending physician or consulting physician. Administrative fluids, blood, and blood products/components, medications, and radiology procedures are included in this consent.

RELEASE OF MEDICAL INFORMATION

I authorize Memorial Hospital to release medical information or copies from my medical record from my date of admission through my date of discharge to insurance companies, third-party payers or authorized paying agent, or claims review organizations in order to process a claim for payment in my behalf. This information may be disseminated to any and all employers, insurance companies, or their designees present in the Hospital by the patient or the patient's representative that may provide coverage for the health care organization's charges, and to comply with the requirement of any Professional Review Organization for Joint Commission on Accreditation of Healthcare Organizations for Utilization Review and Medical Audit. I also authorize release of information to agencies that may be involved in my continuity of care. I authorize any health care provider including my physician and consulting physicians to provide to the hospital or its designee, upon request, information concerning my care, condition, and treatment for quality assurance and risk management purposes.

VALUABLES: RELEASE FROM RESPONSIBILITY

I understand that Memorial Hospital does not assume responsibility for personal possessions unless they are registered in the hospital safe. This opportunity has been offered to me.

ADVANCE DIRECTIVES

Has a living will or health care power of attorney been prepared?	Yes	No	N/A
I have provided Memorial Hospital with the most current copy.	Yes	No	N/A
I have received advance directives information.	Yes	No	N/A
The Patient's Bill of Rights has been presented to me.	Yes	No	N/A

Courtesy of Ilini Hospital, Silvis, Illinois

FINANCIAL AGREEMENT AND ASSIGNMENT OF INSURANCE BENEFITS

I hereby assign, transfer, and convey all my rights, title, and interest to medical reimbursement under by insurance policy(s) to Memorial Hospital. It is understood, whether I sign as agent, patient, or as guarantor that I am directly responsible and will pay for service rendered and not paid by insurance agency. An assignment of benefits by any insurance policy or medical reimbursement plan shall not be deemed a waiver of Memorial Hospital's right to require payment directly from the undersigned or the patient. Memorial Hospital expressly reserves the right to require such payment. Should the account be referred to any agency for collection (collection agency or attorney), the undersigned shall pay all reasonable attorney fees, collection costs, and interest. All delinquent accounts may bear a late payment penalty of not more than 10 1/2% per month thereafter charged from the date of service. I assign payment of all insurance benefits to physicians providing professional services at Memorial Hospital in conjunction with hospital services.

BILLING OF PROFESSIONAL SERVICES

I understand that I am financially responsible for professional services of the radiologist(s), pathologist(s), anesthesiologist(s), emergency department physician, and other physician charges that are not billed by the hospital. I acknowledge that the physicians providing professional services, including consultants and on-call physicians, are an independent medical staff who are not employees or agents of Memorial Hospital. I hereby authorize release of information requested by insurance/billing agencies to the aforementioned parties.

AN IMPORTANT MESSAGE FROM MEDICARE

I acknowledge that I have received a copy of *An Important Message from Medicare* and have been directed to read this brochure.

I have read this form that consists of six important areas and understand its contents. I have had an opportunity to ask questions that have been answered to my satisfaction. I voluntarily sign immediately below.

MR#________ Date of Admission/Service ________

PA# ________ Signature: ________________________

Witness (name and relation) ________________

Hospital Representative: ________________
UCF0004 Rev: 3/97

Fig. 30.3 Consent Form Hospital consent form. *What authorization does the patient give by signing this form?*

READING CHECK

Recall some of the people with whom the compliance officer will need to communicate regularly.

The Medical Chart Auditor

For whom do medical chart auditors work?

Medical chart auditors review medical charts. They are typically medical and coding specialists who, because of the government clampdown on fraudulent billing practices, are in high demand. Insurance carriers, government agencies (such as Centers for Medicare and Medicaid Services), and healthcare facilities and practices all need to comply with all applicable regulations. Healthcare facilities and practices especially want to be sure that medical records meet current documentation guidelines for billing and coding. In that way they will avoid fines and penalties imposed by the government.

Medical chart auditors may be consultants who work in a healthcare facility at the request of the practice. They may also work for an agency outside the medical practice, such as an insurance plan or a government agency like Medicare or Medicaid. Excellent communication skills are extremely helpful for this career path. Medical chart auditors in the private sector must explain to the healthcare facility's administration where and why improvement is needed in medical chart documentation.

Job Responsibilities of the Medical Chart Auditor

Medical chart auditors are typically experienced medical coding specialists. They must have knowledge of medical necessity, coding and compliance regulations, auditing and abstracting, and quality assurance and risk analysis. They review charts to make sure that the healthcare facility's employees are coding, billing, and documenting health information accurately and completely.

READING CHECK

Identify why medical chart auditors are in high demand.

SECTION 30.1 Careers in Health Information Review

AFTER YOU READ

1. **Explain** why health information careers offer a growing employment opportunity.
2. **Describe** the main responsibilities of a healthcare receptionist, a health unit coordinator, and a medical transcriptionist.
3. **Compare** and contrast the various job responsibilities of health information technicians, medical billers and coders, and medical chart auditors.
4. **Analyze** why the confidentiality of patient health information is so important.
5. **Describe** the key responsibilities of a compliance officer.
6. **Explain** why the need for medical chart auditors has increased.

Technology ONLINE EXPLORATIONS

Educational Programs

Search online to learn about educational programs in the field of health information. Choose the program that best fits your current or future needs. Consider the length, cost, and entrance requirements of the program, and the certification that may be offered. Prepare a written summary of your findings, comparing the elements of several programs.

SECTION 30.2 Health Information Procedures

Documenting Healthcare

What is the purpose of documenting healthcare procedures?

In all jobs in health information, you will work with health records. These records contain the **documentation**, or systematic record, of a patient's chronological health status. Health records are the link among physicians and between physicians and other healthcare professionals involved in a patient's care. They are also legal records of treatment. The health information these records contain may also be used in research and for education, but without identifying the particular patient unless that patient has given his or her consent.

Hospital Records

The health information management (HIM) department maintains a health record system that permits you to store and retrieve clinical information by patient name or number, physician, diagnosis, or procedure. Each patient is listed under a unique number. These numbers make up the **master patient index**, which is the main database that identifies patients. This index also contains the patient's name, age, gender, address, admission date, and **attending physician**, who is the doctor responsible for the patient's care while the patient is hospitalized. When a patient is admitted to a hospital, the health record also contains documentation of previous visits to physicians that relate to the reason for admission.

During hospital stays, patients are examined by physicians and receive various treatments or procedures. The following items of hospital documentation may be added to their record:

- History and physical examination, or an H and P, which describes the physician's interview and examination of the patient (see **Figure 30.4** on page 716)
- Surgery report, describing procedures performed
- Anesthesia report, for the anesthesia administered during surgery
- Pathology report, if tissue was removed and examined
- Recovery room record that describes the patient's condition after surgery
- Graphic record, plotting the patient's vital signs
- Discharge summary (see **Figure 30.5** on page 717), including the reason for the admission, test findings, procedures done, the patient's response to treatments, condition at discharge, and follow-up care instructions

Vocabulary

Content Vocabulary

You will learn these content vocabulary terms in this section.

- **documentation**
- **master patient index**
- **attending physician**
- **principal diagnosis**
- **admitting diagnosis**
- ***International Classification of Diseases*, Ninth Revision, *Clinical Modification* (ICD-9-CM)**
- ***Current Procedural Terminology* (CPT)**
- **Healthcare Common Procedural Coding System, Level II (HCPCS)**
- **modifier**
- **chargemaster**

Academic Vocabulary

You will see this word in your reading and on your tests. Find its meaning in the Glossary in the back of the book.

- **principal**

21ST CENTURY SKILLS

Teamwork

For the healthcare delivery system to work smoothly, many professionals must work together as a team. Healthcare receptionists register the patients. Physicians and other healthcare providers evaluate patients, prescribe and implement treatment, and summarize their activities in dictated form. Transcriptionists put this information into document form. Health information technicians and medical coders assemble the various reports in the patient's record, identify the appropriate information, and assign codes. From there, the information flows to the business office, where medical billers submit insurance claims and send bills to patients.

Documentation Standards

Because health records are so important, medical professionals have set standards for documentation. Every face-to-face meeting with a patient should be documented with the following information:

- The patient's name, the date of the visit, and the reason for the visit
- History and physical examination, including vital statistics such as blood pressure
- Review of all tests ordered
- The diagnosis
- The plan of care, or notes on treatments that were given
- The instructions or recommendations given to the patient
- The signature of the provider who saw the patient

You should be aware of the following standards and encourage their use to ensure complete and proper documentation:

- **Records must be complete:** The health record should be complete, and if handwritten must be legible.
- **Entries must be signed:** Whether electronic, written, or transcribed, each entry must have the signature or initials and title of the responsible provider.

Room: 360 Admission Date: 12/23/2003
Patient: BEVILARK, George

HISTORY OF PRESENTILLNESS: Mr. Bevilark is a 56-year-old white male with a diagnosisof emphysema.He presentedto the emergencyroom with shortnessof breath and a partially compensatedrespiratory acidosis.Patient stateshe has been becomingincreasingly short of breath over the last 2-3 days.He has had somepedal edema.At home, he takes someother medicinesthat he doesnot know the name of. He denies any chestpain. He has had nonproductive coughfor 2 days.He denies any fever or chills.

PAST MEDICAL HISTORY: Patient denies any allergies and denies blood transfusions.He is a heavy smoker and continues to smoke. He has been hospitalized in the pastfor his lung diseaseon several occasions.He denies hypertension or diabetes.There is no history of TB or rheumatic fever.

REVIEW OF SYSTEMS:Otherwise unobtainable.

FAMILY HISTORY: Negative.

SOCIALHISTORY: Apparently patient lives alone. On his last discharge from here, he was supposedto have gone to the hospital but I am not exactly sure when he left there.

PHYSICAL EXAMINATION: Patient is a white male looking older than his statedage in moderately severe respiratory distress.Blood pressure is 140/90 with about 25 mm of paradoxical pulse. Heart rate is 120 and regular, respirations 40. He is not jaundiced.

HEENT: Discsare flat. No adenopathy

LUNGS: Decreasedbreath sounds,inspiratory and expiratory rhonchi.

CARDIOVASCULAR: Regular rate and rhythm. Heart soundsare distant. S1 and S2 are normal.

ABDOMEN: Soft.

EXTREMITIES: Trace edema. Pedal pulsesare good.

NEUROLOGIC:Nonfocal.

RECTAL: Deferred.

IMPRESSION: 1) Chronic obstructivepulmonary diseasewith acute exacerbationassociatedwith respiratory failure. 2) Cigarette smoker.

PLAN: Patient to be admitted to the Intensive Care Unit and treated with I.V. aminophylline and aerosolized Metaprel, steroids, and antibiotics. We will monitor blood gasescarefully and it is hoped intubation can be avoided.

DEC:df Duane E. Rabier, MD
D
T

Fig. 30.4 H and P Sample history and physical examination, called a H and P. *Which employee would help to store and retrieve this document?*

Patient: LOPEZ, Gloria

Admission Date: 06/01/2003
Discharge Date: 06/08/2003

FINAL DIAGNOSIS EXPLAINING ADMISSION: Well-differentiated adenocarcinoma of the rectosigmoid colon withtransmural invasion and negative mesenteric lymph nodes.

OTHER DIAGNOSES: Glaucoma by history.

OPERATIONS: Anterior resection of the rectosigmoid colon and incidental appendectomy.

COMPLICATIONS: None.

SUMMARY: The patient is a 62-year-old-woman who was admitted to the hospital after she was found to have a large bulky rectosigmoid tumor that was documented by flexible sigmoidoscopy. She was admitted to the hospital for the purpose of bowel preparation and colon resection. Following both mechanical as well as antibiotic bowel preparation, the patient was taken to the operating room at which time a resection of the rectosigmoid colon was performed with primary anastomosis utilizing Baker's type of procedure. The postoperative course of this patient was uneventful. She was doing well. She remained afebrile throughout her hospital course. At the time of discharge she was on a soft diet, was ambulatory, required no pain medication or any other maintenance medication. Instruction was given as to the extent of her activity as well as her diet and she will be followed up in the office about a week following discharge.

Laboratory studies performed on this patient included an admission CBC with a hemoglobin of 12.5, hematocrit 37.2, white blood count of 8,200 and normal differential. She required no blood transfusion while in the hospital. Repeated CBC done postoperatively showed a hemoglobin of 14.2, hematocrit 41.1, white blood count of 14,200 with a minimal left shift. She had a normal serum electrolytes, normal urinalysis. Prothrombin time and partial thromboplastin time were within normal range. A CEA performed prior to surgery was reported as 2.9 ng. She had a normal liver as well as normal bone scan done prior to surgery. Chest x ray also was found to be within normal limits. Electrocardiogram done prior to surgery was found to be within normal limits. A chemistry profile showed as light increased alkaline phosphatase to 68 and a low serum protein and albumin, and the rest of the tests were much within normal range.

JLB:df Jay L. Bradshaw, MD
D
T ______________________

Fig. 30.5 Discharge Summary Sample discharge summary. *What should this form include?*

- **Changes must be made clearly:** For paper records, a single line should be drawn through the words to be changed, leaving the words legible. The correct information should be entered after the incorrect entry. The date and the initials of the individual making the change should be added. For electronic records, you will typically enter an addendum, or correction. The EHR will record the date, time, and initials of person making the addendum.
- **Diagnostic information must be easy to locate:** Past and present diagnoses should be placed so that they are easy to locate by each physician who uses the health record.
- **Practitioners' entries must be made promptly:** Entries should be made in a timely manner and placed in a consistent chronological order.

READING CHECK

Recall the types of clinical information that can be stored and retrieved.

Diagnostic Coding

How does coding help research?

Scientists and researchers gather data from hospitals about illnesses and causes of death. The goal is to learn more about the disease process. To help in communication and to make sure that the same terms are used, written diagnoses are assigned codes from a standard coding system.

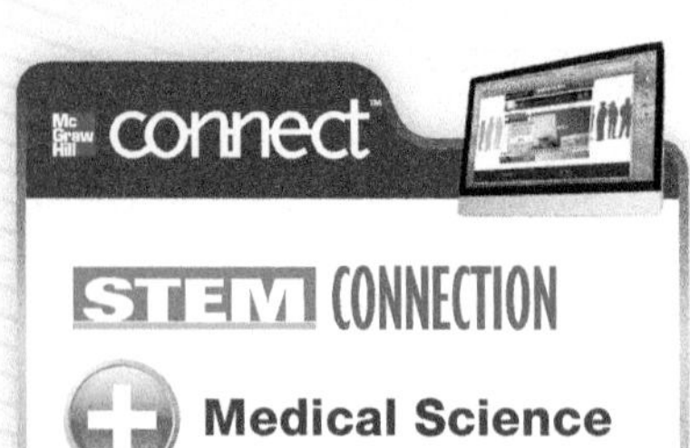

STEM CONNECTION

Medical Science

Anatomy and Health Information
Most health information careers require a basic knowledge of human anatomy. This is especially true for coders. In many cases, the fifth-level diagnosis codes are based on the anatomical part affected by the disease.

connect Go online to learn more about anatomy and codes.

In this system, a code number is assigned to each type of disease. The codes are grouped by disease or by the area of the body that is involved.

The most important diagnosis to be coded is the **principal diagnosis.** This code stands for the condition that is the main, or principal, reason for the patient's hospital visit. The principal diagnosis remains the same even if the patient also has other, more severe conditions, if those conditions are not treated during the hospital stay.

The **admitting diagnosis,** which is the condition identified by the physician at admission to the hospital, may also be coded. This is an example of the difference between the admitting diagnosis and the principal diagnosis. A patient may be admitted to the hospital complaining of strong pains in the belly area. That patient will be given an admitting diagnosis of severe abdominal pain. Tests and surgery may later reveal that the patient had acute appendicitis, which then becomes the principal diagnosis.

Other conditions that have an effect on a patient's hospital stay or course of treatment are also coded. For example, a patient with chronic obstructive pulmonary disease (COPD) with emphysema will need additional care. Likewise, if hypertension (high blood pressure) appears as a postoperative complication, recovery will be more difficult. Coding additional diagnoses is important, because those conditions may increase the healthcare facilities' payment for care.

The ICD-9-CM and ICD-10-CM

The codes assigned to patients' diagnoses are taken from the *International Classification of Diseases,* a standard reference that is revised each year. The ***International Classification of Diseases,* Ninth Revision, *Clinical Modification* (ICD-9-CM)** is the most recent publication. New ICD manuals are available prior to October 1 of each year, the date on which the new diagnosis codes are to be used on claims. ICD-10 is scheduled for release on October 1, 2013. The ICD-10 will work directly with electronic health claims processing.

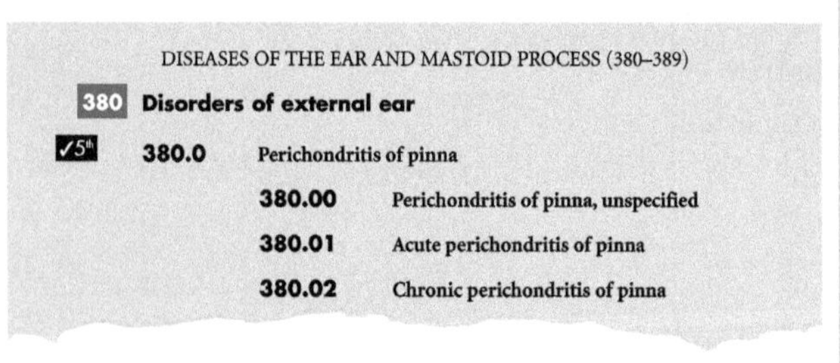

DISEASES OF THE EAR AND MASTOID PROCESS (380–389)

380 Disorders of external ear

✓5th	**380.0**	Perichondritis of pinna	
		380.00	Perichondritis of pinna, unspecified
		380.01	Acute perichondritis of pinna
		380.02	Chronic perichondritis of pinna

Fig. 30.6 ICD-9-CM Codes Example of three levels of ICD-9-CM codes with labels. *Do both acute and chronic perichondritis of the pinna require five-digit codes?*

The ICD-9-CM has three-digit categories for diseases, injuries, and symptoms (see **Figure 30.6**). Most of those categories are divided into four-digit code groups, however many are further divided into five-digit code groups. The use of fourth- and fifth-level diagnosis codes allows assignment of the most specific diagnosis possible. A fifth-level code must be assigned when it applies and is available.

The ICD-9-CM used in hospitals has three sections:

- **Volume 1—Diseases:** Tabular List
- **Volume 2—Diseases:** Alphabetic Index
- **Volume 3—Procedures:** Tabular List and Alphabetic Index

These volumes cover the two major areas of diseases and procedures. Volumes 1 and 2 are used to find the correct code for the patient's principal diagnosis. Volume 3 contains procedure codes that are used for hospital tests and treatments.

ICD-9-CM Codes

In the ICD-9-CM, diagnoses are listed in two different places (see **Figure 30.7**). The Alphabetic Index lists diagnoses in alphabetic order and gives their codes. It is never used alone because it does not contain all the necessary information. The Tabular List provides diagnosis codes in numerical order and gives additional instructions.

READING CHECK

Identify the changes that ICD-10 will bring.

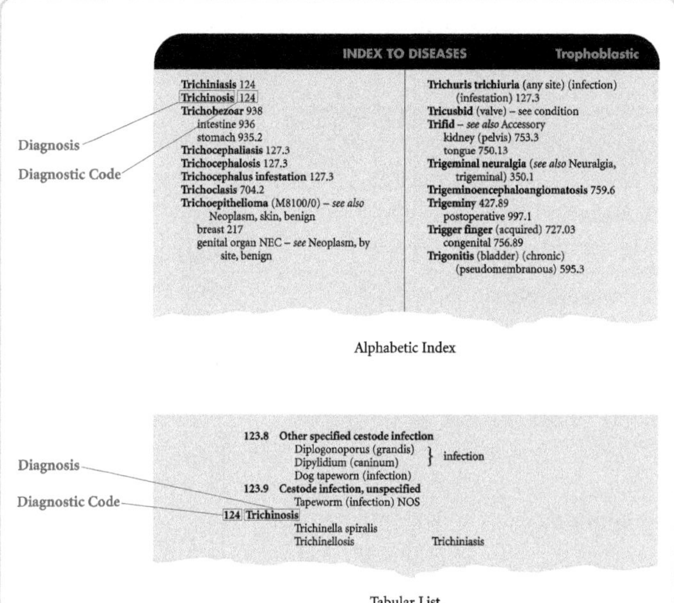

Fig. 30.7 Diagnosis Listings ICD-9-CM alphabetic index and tabular list. *Why is the Alphabetic Index never used alone?*

Procedural Coding

What organization establishes procedural codes?

Procedures that are done by healthcare workers are assigned codes. These codes stand for procedures such as a CT scan or services such as an office visit. In order to be paid for their services by payers other than the patient, healthcare providers must show that the procedures were necessary to examine or treat a patient's condition.

The CPT and HCPCS

Physicians' procedures and services are assigned codes from the ***Current Procedural Terminology,* Fourth Edition (CPT),** published by the American Medical Association (AMA) and updated every year. Hospitals also use codes from the **Healthcare Common Procedural Coding System, Level II (HCPCS),** which is published by the federal government. These codes apply to services not included in CPT codes, such as an ambulance or a wheelchair.

CPT Codes

CPT codes are five-digit numbers, organized into six sections, as shown in **Table 30.2.** Evaluation and management services include patient interviews, examinations, and decision making by physicians to diagnose conditions and plan treatments. Examples are annual physical examinations and physician visits to hospitalized patients.

Each CPT section begins with important guidelines that apply to its procedures. You should always check this material carefully before you choose a procedure code.

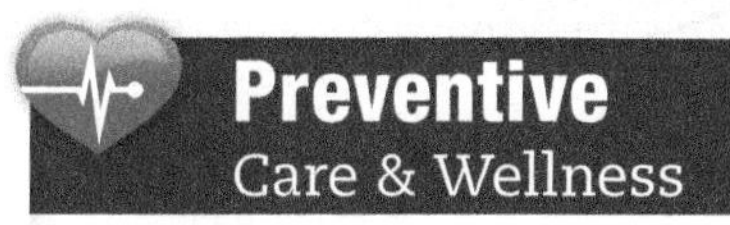

Working at a Computer

Repetitive motion injuries such as carpal tunnel syndrome present risks to health information professionals. Here are some tips to help avoid stress and strain.

- If you can, vary your work duties so that you alternate keyboarding with noncomputer tasks.
- Position the keyboard so that your hands are at the same level as your wrists.
- Use hand and wrist supports.

Table 30.2 Sections and Code Ranges of the CPT

SECTION	RANGE OF CODES
Evaluation and Management	99200 – 99499
Anesthesiology	00100 – 01999, 99100 – 99140
Surgery	10040 – 69979
Radiology	70010 – 79999
Pathology and Laboratory	80002 – 89399
Medicine (except Anesthesiology)	90701 – 99199
Appendix A	All modifiers

In the CPT, some descriptions are indented to show that they include a common entry from above. For example, look at the descriptions for codes 42842, 42844, and 42845 in **Figure 30.8.** Code 42842 is the "parent" code in this list. Its description begins with a capital letter. Codes 42844 and 42845 are indented and begin with a lowercase letter. These indented codes refer to the parent code above. The words in the description of the parent code that precede the semicolon are common to all the indented codes below it. The full description for code 42844 is "Radical resection of tonsil, tonsillar pillars, and/or retromolar trigone; closure with local flap." But if the procedure were described as "closure with other flap," the correct code would be 42845.

Two-digit **modifiers** may also be assigned to the five-digit code. Modifiers follow the five-digit code and are preceded by a hyphen. The use of a modifier shows that some special circumstance applies to the service or procedure the physician provided. For example, in the Surgery section:

- The modifier –62 indicates that two surgeons worked together during an operation, each performing part of the surgical procedure. Each physician will be paid part of the amount normally reimbursed for that procedure code.
- The modifier –80 indicates that the services of a surgical assistant were used and are included in the insurance claim.

READING CHECK

Identify the purpose of two-digit modifiers.

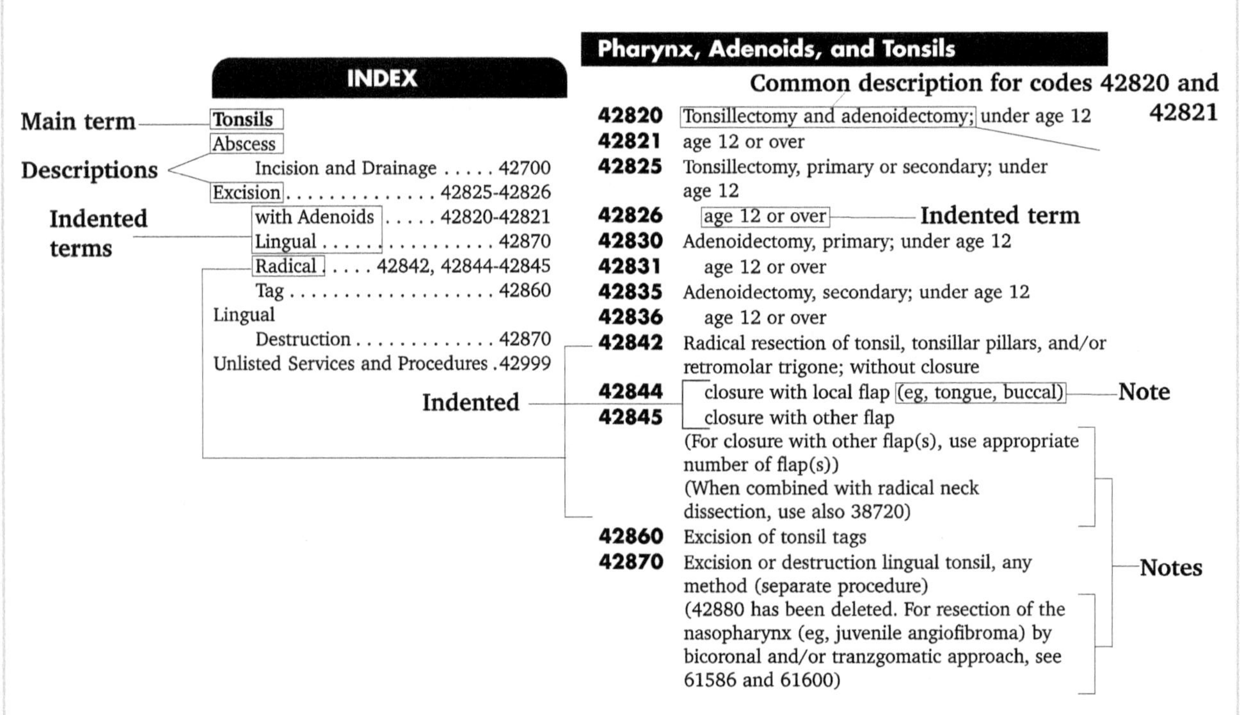

Fig. 30.8 CPT This illustrates the CPT format. *What does the semicolon shown in the definition of code 42820 mean?*

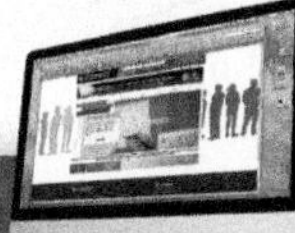

Connect ONLINE PROCEDURES

PROCEDURE 30-1

Diagnostic Coding

Both the Alphabetic Index and the Tabular List are used to find the right code. The Alphabetic Index is never used alone, because it does not contain all the necessary information. After you locate a code in the index, you must always verify it by checking it in the Tabular List.

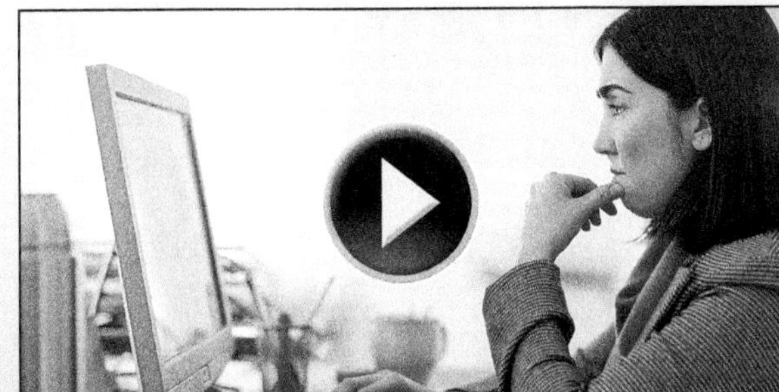

PROCEDURE 30-2

Procedural Coding

Procedural coding begins by identifying the physician's services. Find the procedure code in the CPT index for the specific procedure or service, organ, or condition. Then decide if modifiers are needed.

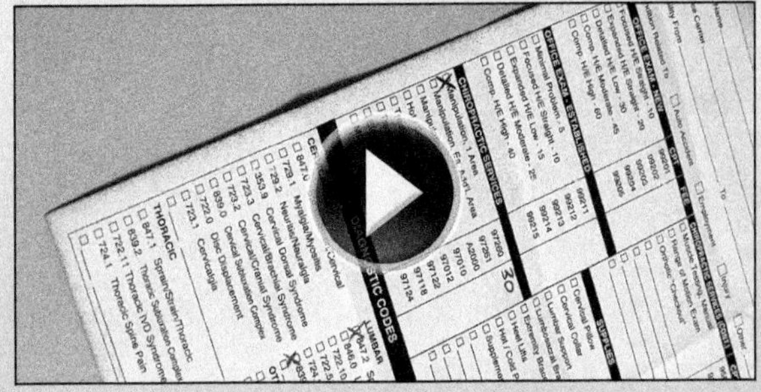

PROCEDURE 30-3

Billing Review

Hospitals and other facilities need to be sure that all patient services appear on the patient's final bill. Each hospital creates a **chargemaster,** which is a document that lists all the services the hospital can provide, along with the procedure code and the charge for each service. The chargemaster is updated when new treatments or services are offered.

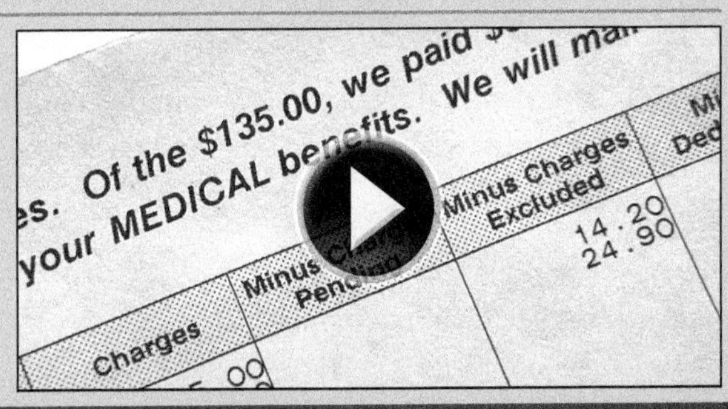

SECTION 30.2 Health Information Procedures Review

AFTER YOU READ

1. **Define** the term "documentation."
2. **Identify** the reference source that contains the codes assigned to diagnoses, and the source that contains the codes assigned to procedures performed by physicians.
3. **Indicate** the two coding lists contained in the ICD-9-CM and explain how each one is arranged.
4. **List** the steps that are followed to assign diagnosis and procedure codes.
5. **Explain** why it is important to verify patients' bills.

Technology ONLINE EXPLORATIONS

Coding Certifications

Visit the websites of the American Health Information Management Association and the American Academy of Professional Coders. Compare the coding certifications that each organization offers for physician coding and hospital coding. Write a report describing the requirements and certifications offered by each organization.

Photos: (t)Ingram Publishing, (c-b)Nancy R. Cohen/Photodisc/Getty Images

CHAPTER **30 Review**

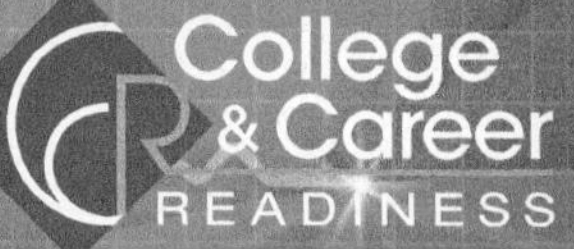

Chapter Summary

SECTION 30.1

- The field of health information offers growing employment opportunities because new drugs and treatments, together with an aging population, are increasing the demand for health services. **(pg. 705)**
- Healthcare receptionists should greet patients promptly and professionally and should also gather accurate financial and personal information about patients' visits to the healthcare facility. **(pg. 707)**
- Health unit coordinators manage non-nursing patient care activities. **(pg. 708)**
- Health information technicians make sure that patients' health records are complete and accurate. **(pg. 708)**
- Medical billers make certain that patients' charges have been gathered. They enter data, prepare claims and bills, and track payments that are due. **(pg. 709)**
- Medical coders assign codes provided in medical coding references to diagnoses and procedures. **(pg. 710)**
- Medical transcriptionists accurately transcribe physicians' reports on treatments and procedures performed for patients. **(pg. 711)**
- Compliance officers keep their facilities in compliance with HIPAA regulations on the confidentiality of patients' health information as well as other laws regulating healthcare. **(pg. 712)**
- The medical chart auditor makes sure that charts comply with current regulations regarding billing and coding, to prevent fraud and to avoid fines and penalties. **(pg. 714)**

SECTION 30.2

- Health records provide continuity and communication among physicians and other healthcare professionals involved in patient care. They are also legal records of treatment. **(pg. 715)**
- The *International Classification of Diseases,* Ninth Revision, *Clinical Modification*, called the ICD-9-CM, is the diagnostic coding reference. ICD-10-CM is expected to be used starting in 2013. The *Current Procedural Terminology,* Fourth Edition, called the CPT, is the procedural coding reference. **(pg. 718)**
- To correctly assign diagnosis codes, first find the main term of the diagnosis in the Alphabetic Index of the ICD-9-CM and then verify the selected code in the Tabular List. **(pg. 718)**
- To correctly assign procedure codes, determine the procedures and services to be coded, look up the procedure code, and decide whether modifiers are needed. **(pg. 719)**
- To verify patients' bills, compare the information about the visit and the claim to be sure that all data is entered and fees are calculated correctly. **(pg. 721)**

CHAPTER 30 Assessment

Critical Thinking/Problem Solving

1. A bank employee calls a health information technician at a hospital. The bank is considering hiring someone who was recently hospitalized. The bank employee wants to know if the applicant has a serious medical problem. The technician explains that the patient was successfully treated for cancer. She adds that she thinks that he would make an excellent employee. Did the technician handle this call correctly? What might result from her answers?
2. While working at a hospital, you observe another employee erasing an entry in a patient's health record and writing in a new one. What should you do?
3. Obtain the ICD-9-CM and the CPT. Look up the diagnoses for Trousseau's syndrome and pink eye, and procedure codes for X-ray of the heel and Mayo procedure.
4. Using the ICD-9-CM and the CPT, locate the diagnosis and procedure codes for a patient admitted to the hospital with peripheral vascular disease. An angiogram and two laboratory tests were performed: (1) a complete blood count (CBC) and (2) an electrolyte panel. Record the codes and submit your work to your instructor.

21ST CENTURY SKILLS

5. **Teamwork** As a group, play the "gossip" game to show the importance of keeping medical information private. Start by whispering a statement that might appear in a medical record, such as "Diagnosis of osteomyelitis secondary to a staph infection in the anterior tibialis." See how the information changes by the end of the game.
6. **Information management** In teams, obtain a list of 20 or 30 codes from a resource manual. Use the codes to find the name of the corresponding diagnosis or procedure. The team finishing first with the highest accuracy wins.

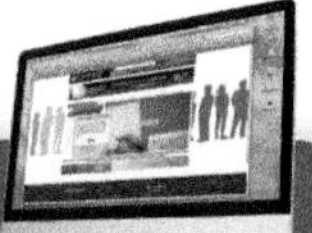

Mc Graw Hill connect™ ONLINE ACTIVITIES

Complete our HST online activities for Chapter 30, which include Concept Check review questions, Reference Flash Cards, and Online Procedures assessment sheets.

- **Concept Check** review questions
- **Reference Flash Cards** medical terminology practice
- **Online Procedures** assessment sheets

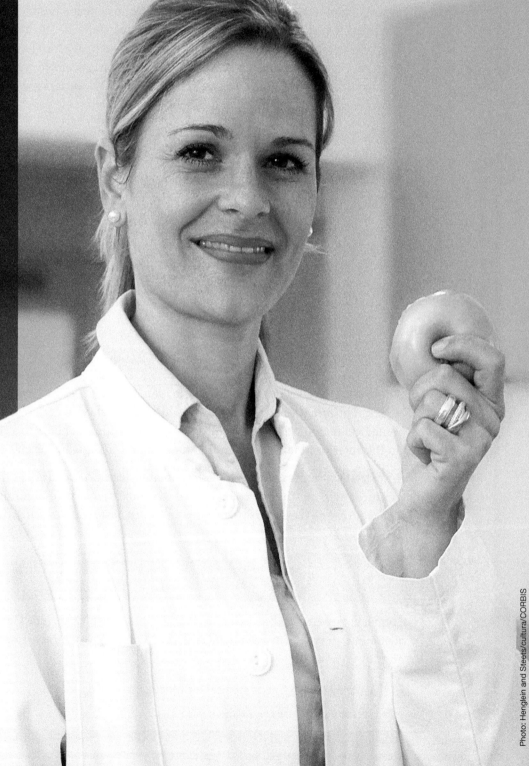

UNIT 5

Careers in Support Services

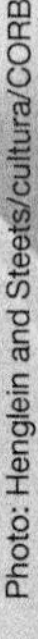

CHAPTER 31 Central Supply and Processing

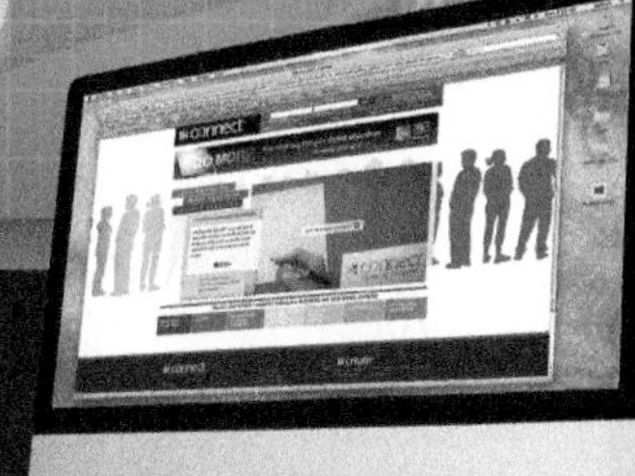

Essential Question:

What procedures are necessary to prevent the spread of germs and disease?

Most medical procedures call for the use of special tools. Any items that are reused must be cleaned, disinfected, or sterilized. The central supply department, also called the sterile processing department, cares for and cleans medical equipment. Workers in this department—central supply assistants, technicians, supervisors, and managers—are responsible for decontaminating, cleaning, processing, assembling, sterilizing, storing, and distributing the sterile medical supplies and equipment needed in the treatment of patients throughout the hospital.

McGraw-Hill connect™

It's Online!

- Online Procedures
- STEM Connection
- Medical Science
- Medical Terms
- Medical Math
- Ethics in Action
- Virtual Lab

READING GUIDE

OBJECTIVES

After completing this chapter, you will be able to:

- **Identify** the areas of the central supply and processing department.
- **Compare** the roles and responsibilities of a central supply technician and a central supply supervisor.
- **Contrast** the education and training of a central supply supervisor and those of a central supply manager.
- **Demonstrate** five central supply and processing department procedures.

BEFORE YOU READ

Connect What would happen if a medical facility were not kept as germ-free as possible?

Main Idea

Central supply personnel ensure that all medical supplies are readily available. It is their responsibility to maintain an aseptic (germ-free) environment in order to prevent the spread of disease.

Note-Taking Activity

Draw this table. Write key terms and phrases under **Cues**. Write main ideas under **Note Taking**. Summarize the section under **Summary**.

Cues	Note Taking
○ ○	○ ○
Summary	

Graphic Organizer

Before you read the chapter, draw a diagram like the one below. As you read, write the careers covered by the chapter into the diagram.

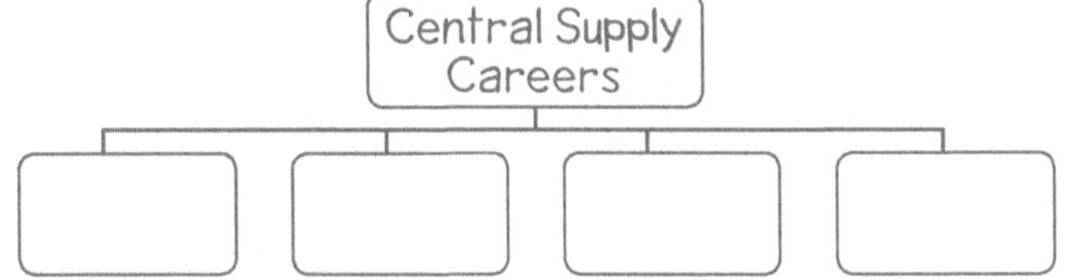

connect

Downloadable graphic organizers can be accessed online.

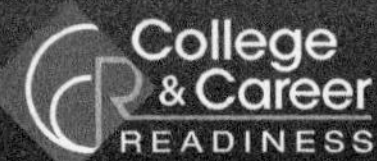

STANDARDS

HEALTH SCIENCE

NCHSE 7.12 Describe methods of controlling the spread and growth of microorganisms.

NCHSE 7.42 Understand implications of hazardous materials.

SCIENCE

NSES F Develop understanding of personal and community health; population growth; natural resources; environmental quality; natural and human-induced hazards; science and technology in local, national, and global challenges.

NCHSE *National Consortium for Health Science Education*

NSES *National Science Education Standards*

COMMON CORE STATE STANDARDS

MATHEMATICS

Number and Quantity

Quantities N-Q Reason quantitatively and use units to solve problems.

ENGLISH LANGUAGE ARTS

Speaking and Listening

Comprehension and Collaboration SL-1 Initiate and participate effectively in a range of collaborative discussions (one-on-one, in groups, and teacher-led) with diverse partners on grades 9–10 topics, texts, and issues, building on others' ideas and expressing their own clearly and persuasively.

SECTION **31.1** # Careers in Central Supply and Processing

The Central Supply or Processing Area

How are soiled or contaminated items handled in a healthcare facility?

Vocabulary

Content Vocabulary

You will learn this content vocabulary term in this section.

- **aseptic technique**

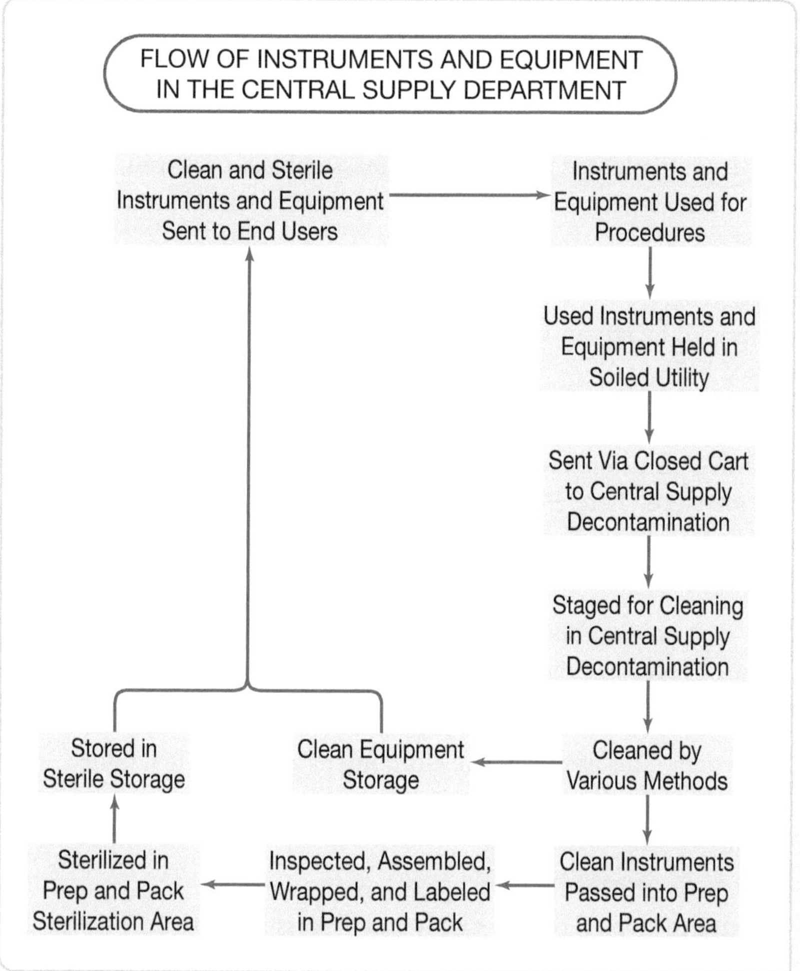

To function as a central supply worker, you will need to know how the department is organized and what its functions are. The department handles dirty, clean, and sterile materials. For that reason, special areas are set up and maintained in order to prevent contamination and cross-contamination. Although central supply departments differ, their basic functions and procedures are similar. The types of functions that take place in the each area of the central supply and processing department are described further on the following pages. **Figure 31.1** shows the flow of materials in the department.

FLOW OF INSTRUMENTS AND EQUIPMENT IN THE CENTRAL SUPPLY DEPARTMENT

Clean and Sterile Instruments and Equipment Sent to End Users → Instruments and Equipment Used for Procedures → Used Instruments and Equipment Held in Soiled Utility → Sent Via Closed Cart to Central Supply Decontamination → Staged for Cleaning in Central Supply Decontamination → Cleaned by Various Methods

Cleaned by Various Methods → Clean Equipment Storage → Clean and Sterile Instruments and Equipment Sent to End Users

Cleaned by Various Methods → Clean Instruments Passed into Prep and Pack Area → Inspected, Assembled, Wrapped, and Labeled in Prep and Pack → Sterilized in Prep and Pack Sterilization Area → Stored in Sterile Storage → Clean and Sterile Instruments and Equipment Sent to End Users

Fig. 31.1 Supply and Processing Equipment and supplies must travel in the correct order through the central supply and processing department. *Why is the correct order important?*

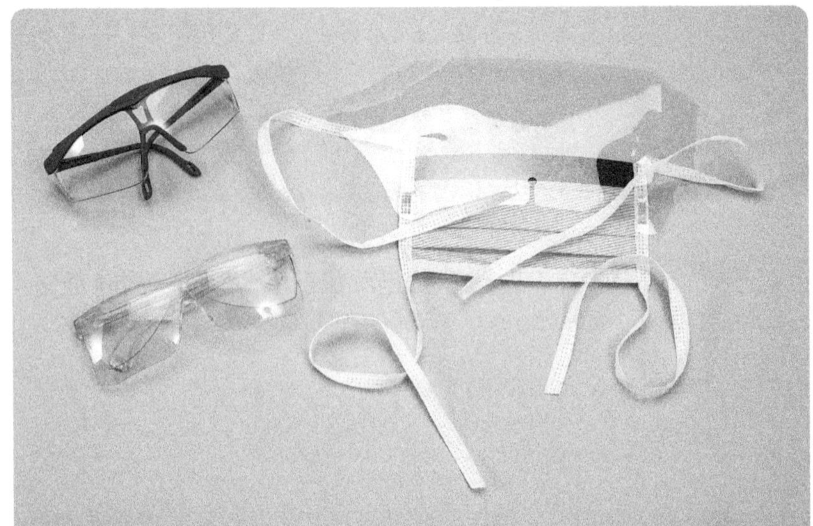

Fig. 31.2 Personal Protective Equipment Shown is some personal protective equipment (PPE). *What other pieces of PPE should be worn in the decontamination section of the central supply department?*

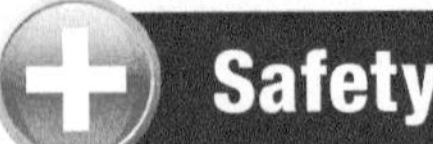

Safety

During Autoclave Sterilization

Practice personal safety during autoclaving by following these rules.

- Check that the pressure gauge is at zero before opening the autoclave door.
- Wear eye protection when opening the autoclave door to prevent the possibility of escaping steam injuring your eyes.
- When closing the autoclave door, pull on it slightly to make sure it is locked before beginning the cycle.
- Handle autoclaved items carefully. Use an oven mitt to protect yourself from burns.
- Do not lean against or touch the outside of the autoclave during sterilization. It may get hot.

Decontamination Soiled carts, instruments, procedure trays, and equipment are brought to the decontamination department from patient care areas. Items are sorted, and the first stage of cleaning takes place. It is highly likely that these items will be contaminated. For that reason, scrub attire is worn to prevent contamination of personal items. Personal protective equipment (PPE) must be worn, including gowns, aprons, goggles, masks, gloves, head coverings, and shoe coverings (see **Figure 31.2**).

Preparation and packaging This is a clean area where items that have been decontaminated are inspected, reassembled, packaged, and sterilized. Scrub attire, along with head and shoe covers, is usually worn.

Clean/sterile storage Clean, disposable supplies and sterilized reprocessed items from the preparation and packaging area must be stored in specified locations. Carts and trays for various procedures are also stocked here.

Equipment storage After decontamination, items such as suction machines, infusion pumps, and emergency and special procedures carts are stored here. Prior to storage, items are checked and reassembled. Some items will need to be plugged in at all times to maintain a charge in their batteries.

Case cart holding/dispatch Linen and supply carts are stored here. This area receives requests from departments for needed items. The staff then retrieves, records, and transports the items.

Linen room This area is where clean linens are inspected, folded, and wrapped for sterilization.

READING CHECK

Name the typical central supply and processing department areas.

Central Supply Career Paths

What is the best way to begin a career in central supply departments?

Everyone who works in the central supply department—from assistants to supervisors and managers—must be able to use medical materials, supplies, and equipment safely. They must follow **aseptic technique** (which means creating a germ-free environment), must keep their work space organized, and must know how to track inventory to prevent waste. The four main occupations in a typical central supply and processing department are listed and explained in **Table 31.1**.

READING CHECK

Summarize the job outlook for central supply technicians, central supply supervisors, and central supply managers.

Table 31.1 Overview of Central Supply and Processing Department Occupations

OCCUPATION	EDUCATIONAL REQUIREMENTS	CERTIFICATION OR LICENSING AGENCY	JOB OUTLOOK
Central Supply Assistant	High school diploma; on-the-job training; some brief college or vocational school programs may be required, depending upon place of employment.	None required	Below average because of increased requirements for certification as a technician
Central Supply Technician	12 months on-the-job training or six months with related education or completion of an approved Central Processing training course leading to certification. Certification Board for Sterile Processing and Distribution credentials may change the job title to Sterile Processing and Distribution Technician.	Credentialing by the Certification Board for Sterile Processing and Distribution or the American Society for Healthcare Central Service Professionals	Above average with employment opportunities in extended care facilities expected to increase
Central Supply Supervisor	18 months full-time experience and certification as a Sterile Processing and Distribution (SPD) Technician, or 18 months full-time SPD experience with six months as SPD supervisor and technician certification; or minimum of six months employment in allied health plus 30 months full-time experience as a SPD Technician (in this case, technician certification is not required).	Credentialing by the Certification Board for Sterile Processing and Distribution	Above average with employment opportunities in extended care facilities expected to increase
Central Supply Manager	Two- or four-year degree and/or experience in inventory management or business administration; may also be cross-trained from another allied healthcare field such as nursing.	Sterile Processing and Distribution Board or American Society for Healthcare Central Service Professionals credentials	Above average with employment opportunities in extended care expected to increase

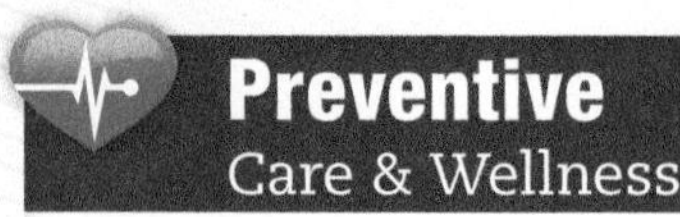

Latex Allergies

Latex gloves have proved effective in preventing transmission of many infectious diseases. You are often required to wear them when working in healthcare. For some people, however, exposure to latex may result in allergic reactions. Mild reactions to latex involve skin redness, rash, hives, or itching. More severe reactions may involve respiratory symptoms such as runny nose, sneezing, itchy eyes, scratchy throat, and asthma. If you have a reaction, report it to your supervisor. If you are allergic to latex, your place of employment is required to provide you with gloves that are not made of latex. Facilities that have eliminated the use of all latex products are known as latex-free facilities.

Central Supply Assistant

How does the central supply assistant help his or her department function?

The duties and tasks of the central supply assistant will vary based upon the assistant's level of knowledge, training, and years of experience. Central supply assistants are, however, becoming a thing of the past because central supply and processing department employees are increasingly required to be certified. Some central supply assistants may work in other areas, such as housekeeping or nursing, before transferring into the central supply and processing department. Their main role is to make sure that supplies and equipment are promptly and accurately provided when requested. The assistant also transports used or contaminated items from various locations in the healthcare facility to the cleansing area of central supply, and then takes clean and fresh items back to each department.

In many facilities, the surgical department has its own area in which to clean and sterilize equipment. If it does not, the central supply assistant must pick up instruments used during surgery and return sterilized instruments back to the surgical department for use the next day. Usually surgery suites are located near central supply to make this job easier.

The central supply assistant may also prepare manual orders for supplies and equipment, using various hardcopy catalogs and order forms. If the inventory system is computerized, the assistant will work with that instead.

READING CHECK

Explain why fewer people will begin central supply careers at the assistant level in the future.

Central Supply Technician

What skills does a central supply technician need?

The central supply technician may also be called a central service technician, a certified instrument specialist, a central sterile supply technician, or a sterile processing and distribution technician. Depending on the place of employment, he or she may perform other duties in addition to those listed above for the central supply assistant. He or she must be attentive to details, reliable, and able to plan work in order of priority.

Training can be obtained on the job or through a formal program. Programs usually range from 12 to 24 weeks, although programs at

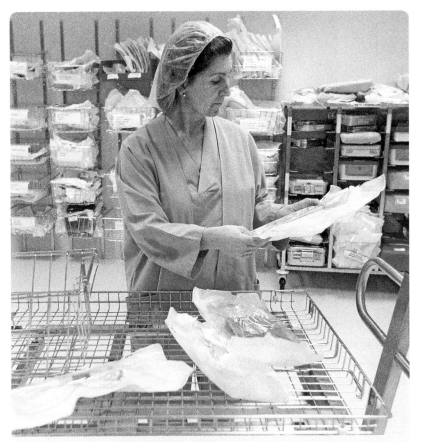

Fig. 31.3 Central Supply Department In the central supply department cental supply technicians may sort and organize supplies and equipment. *What are two other duties of the central supply technician?*

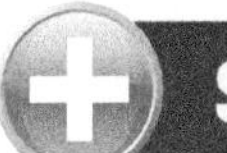

Safety

Practicing Infection Control

A central supply employee will come in contact with equipment and linens that have been contaminated with body substances. It is essential that you always practice infection control techniques including standard precautions and medical asepsis.

community colleges or technical centers may last longer. The programs include courses in anatomy, medical terminology, microbiology, decontamination, sterilization, and human relations. Most programs include a clinical segment during which students study on-site in a medical facility.

Central supply technicians perform a variety of duties under the direct supervision of a supervisor or manager (see **Figure 31.3**). They may be employed in hospitals, clinics, research facilities, blood banks, or clinical offices. The level of the technician's education and the place of employment will determine the extent of the technician's responsibilities.

The responsibilities of a central supply technician working in a research facility, for example, may include the preparation and distribution of laboratory supplies and materials. This includes items such as glassware, surgical instruments, lab coats, scrubs, and gowns. The technician will wash, dry, autoclave, sterilize, bake, and prepare glassware and other devices for continued laboratory use. He or she may also launder lab coats, scrubs, and gowns for the researchers and laboratory technicians. Supply technicians in research facilities maintain an adequate supply of chemicals for distribution and use as needed for various research projects and procedures.

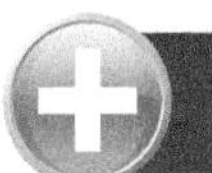

Safety

Handling Linens

For the health and safety of your patients and yourself, special guidelines must be followed when handling linens.

- Wash your hands before handling clean linens and after handling soiled linens.
- Place clean bed linens on a clean surface until they are used in bed making or other procedures.
- Do not allow clean or dirty linens to come in contact with your clothing.
- Do not shake clean or dirty linens in the air. This could contaminate clean linens or spread germs from dirty ones.
- Place dirty linens in a hamper or laundry bag, never on the floor.

21st Century Skills

Technology and Cost Containment

Technology has dramatically improved the ability to track inventories, predict supply usage, and monitor patient charges. Handheld computers enable central supply personnel to maintain accurate and precise inventory records. Computers scan the bar codes of supplies and equipment, and do all the counting. This is far more accurate than hand-counts. Computers are also used to compare prices and order the correct amount of supplies. This in turn assists cost containment in healthcare facilities (see **Figure 31.4**).

Some common tasks of the central supply technician are to

- receive and/or collect needles, syringes, gloves, trays, and other supplies used in the daily operation of a healthcare facility.
- sterilize instruments and supplies by autoclaving and other appropriate methods.
- package and wrap equipment and supplies in accordance with prescribed sterile procedures.
- set up and maintain an adequate supply of various routine and special-purpose trays.
- maintain storage rooms in a neat and orderly manner in keeping with the highest standards of sanitation.
- make recommendations on the purchase of equipment and supplies.
- collect information, keep records, and prepare reports as required.
- supervise central supply assistants and other department employees as instructed.
- help in developing standard operating procedures for the central supply and processing department.

READING CHECK

Identify some of the training routes by which a person can become a central supply technician.

Central Supply Manager

Why does the central supply manager need to communicate with other departments?

The central supply manager is often an RN, LPN, or other healthcare professional. These professionals are cross-trained to take charge of the functions of the central supply and processing department. As a rule, they will have a two- or four-year degree in inventory management or business administration. A central supply technician may work his or her way up to this level through job experience and continuing education.

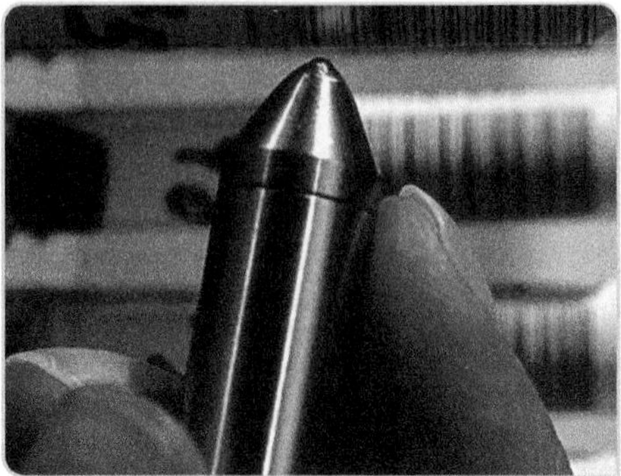

Fig. 31.4 Technology Shown is a bar code scanner. *How does this device help contain costs in a healthcare facility?*

Photo: MedicalRF.com/Getty Images

The central supply manager is the decision-making authority for the department. He or she monitors and coordinates the work of the central supply staff and trains staff members as needed in supply distribution. He or she monitors inventory management procedures and directs the restocking of equipment and supplies. The manager also works with other departments to coordinate the exchange of contaminated and fresh sterile supplies in patient care areas.

Central supply managers need excellent communication and leadership skills. In addition to managing personnel, they may be responsible for directing data collection and data analysis, and for writing reports. A knowledge of computer databases, keyboarding skills, mathematical ability, and good telephone skills are essential. The ability to interact with individuals and with groups of diverse size and composition is also important.

A related position is that of central supply supervisor. The supervisor's responsibilities may overlap with those of the central supply manager. While this position may not require technician certification, it does require a minimum of 18 months of full-time experience in sterile processing and distribution or six months of employment in the field of allied health and 30 months full-time experience as a SPD technician.

READING CHECK

Identify the computer and data management tasks of the central supply manager.

SECTION 31.1 Careers in Central Supply/Processing Review

AFTER YOU READ

1. **Illustrate** the purpose of the decontamination area and the protective garments that must be worn in this area.
2. **Indicate** the main duties of central supply personnel.
3. **List** at least two responsibilities you would have in a typical day as a central supply technician.
4. **Discuss** the education and experience needed to become a central supply technician.
5. **Explain** the job duties of the central supply manager.

Technology ONLINE EXPLORATIONS

Career Planning

Search online to find a school or other facility in your area that provides central supply technician training. Make a list of the requirements for acceptance into that program. Then create a list of facilities in your area where you could be employed if you completed the program.

SECTION 31.2 Central Supply/Processing Procedures

Vocabulary

Content Vocabulary

You will learn these content vocabulary terms in this section.

- **ethylene oxide gas**
- **autoclave**
- **spores**

Academic Vocabulary

You will see this word in your reading and on your tests. Find its meaning in the Glossary in the back of this book.

- **ensure**

Sterilization

What is the difference between disinfection and sterilization?

Any item that penetrates the skin or comes into contact with a normally sterile part of the body should be sterilized. This is also known as surgical asepsis. Sterile technique includes practices used to eliminate microorganisms and spores. In addition to autoclaving, items can be sterilized using dry heat, ethylene oxide gas, or prolonged immersion in a chemical sterilant.

Dry heat sterilization is used on articles that steam will not penetrate. This process minimizes discoloration and retains the sharpness of knives and blades.

Ethylene oxide gas is a sterile technique used on articles that are sensitive to heat such as rubber, leather, delicate fabrics, and sharp instruments. This process requires special equipment, takes longer, and is expensive. Because ethylene oxide gas is potentially dangerous, this process is typically only used in hospitals or large manufacturing environments.

Chemical sterilant immersion is sometimes used in dental offices, outpatient clinics, or clinical offices. The chemicals used in this procedure must be registered with the Environmental Protection Agency. This type of sterilization is generally used on instruments that can be damaged by the prolonged exposure to the high temperatures of an **autoclave**, which is a device that sterilizes by steam pressure for a specified time. The time required for cold chemical sterilization is about ten hours, but the exact amount of time depends upon the chemical used and the manufacturer's directions. A chemical vapor sterilizer may also be used (see **Figure 31.5**).

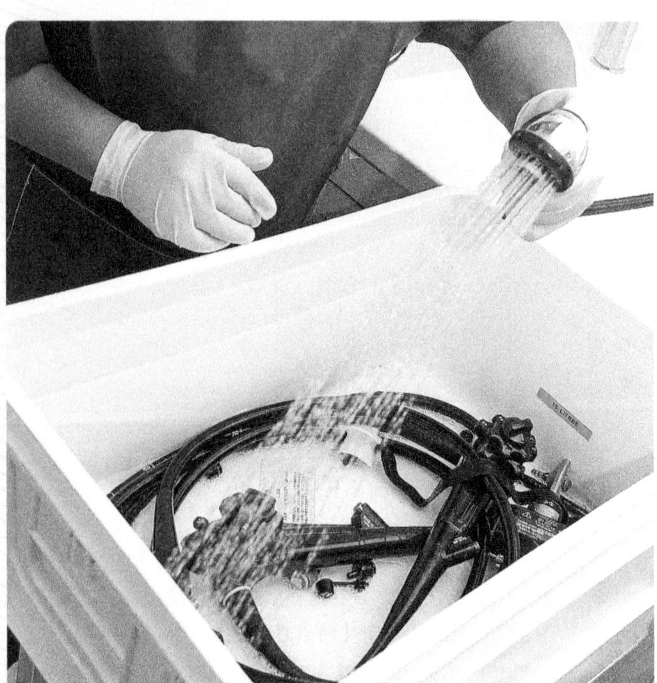

Fig. 31.5 Chemical Vapor Sterilization This unit combines chemical sterilization with steam autoclaving techniques. *What must be done before chemical sterilization?*

READING CHECK

List some sterilization techniques.

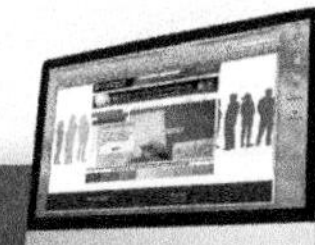

Mc Graw Hill connect™ ONLINE PROCEDURES

PROCEDURE 31-1

Performing Decontamination Cleaning

Every item used on a patient must be decontaminated or sterilized before reuse. Items such as infusion pumps or suction machines will be brought to central supply for sterilization. Reusable instruments from the emergency room or surgery department must be resterilized. This is all part of the practice of medical asepsis, which is used to reduce and prevent the spread of bacteria.

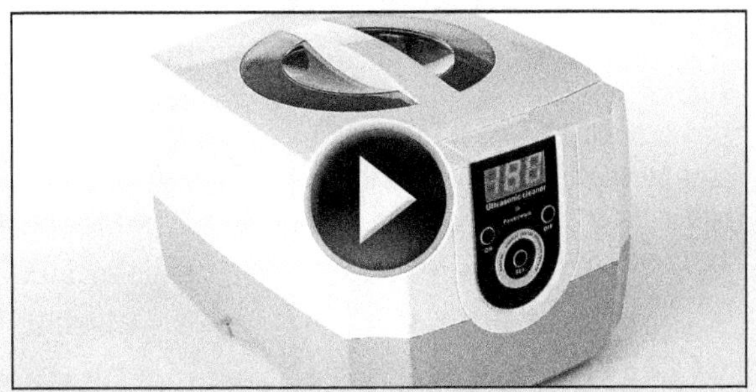

PROCEDURE 31-2

Cleaning Instruments

Doctors and dentists use instruments to perform surgery, suture wounds, and clean teeth. All of the instruments used for these procedures must be cleaned and then sterilized. The cleaning process mechanically removes microorganisms and destroys some of them.

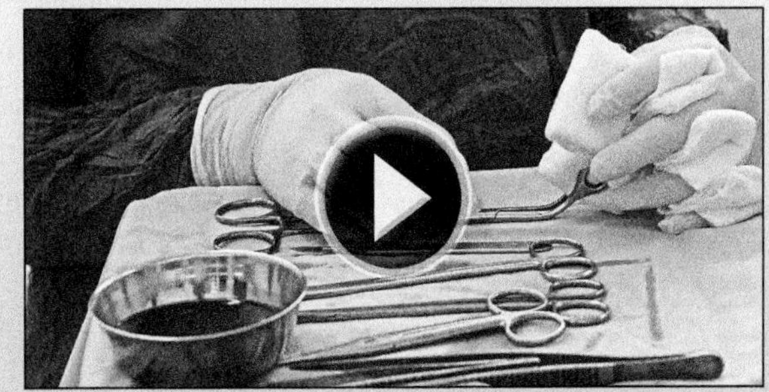

PROCEDURE 31-3

Packaging for Sterilization of Instruments

Sterilization is the process of removing all microorganisms and **spores.** Spores are microorganisms with a thick protective outer wall. Chemical disinfection kills bacteria but does not destroy spores. Sterilization destroys all microorganisms, including spores.

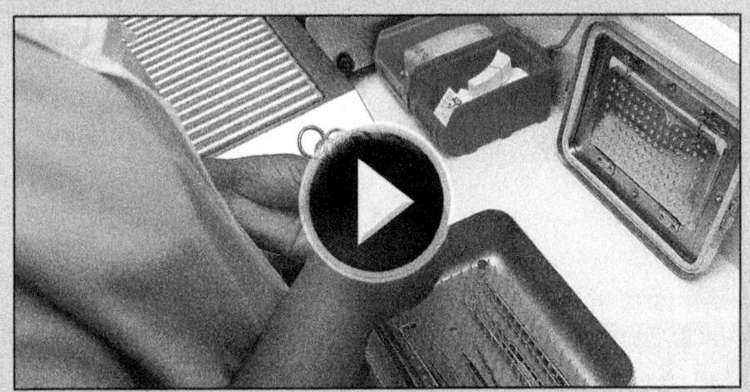

PROCEDURE 31-4

Operating an Autoclave

An autoclave uses steam under pressure to sterilize. The autoclaving process requires high temperatures and high pressures. The combination of steam and pressure brings the temperature to over 270 degrees F. In hospitals and other healthcare facilities, items are usually sterilized in an autoclave.

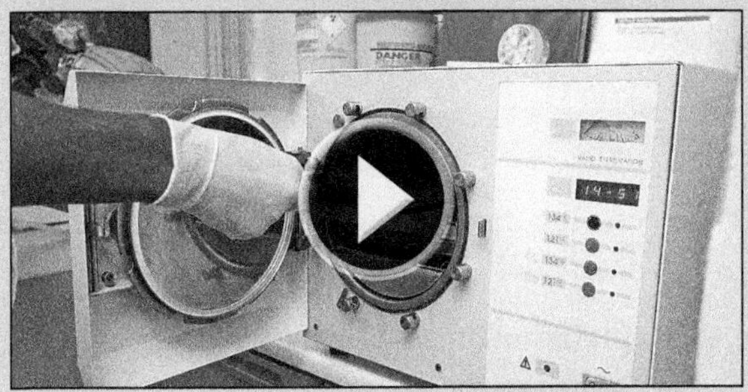

PROCEDURE 31-5

Handling and Preparing Linens

Often the central supply department is responsible for preparing linens for sterilization. Linens are usually washed in the laundry and arrive at the linen room in central supply to be inspected, folded, and wrapped for sterilization.

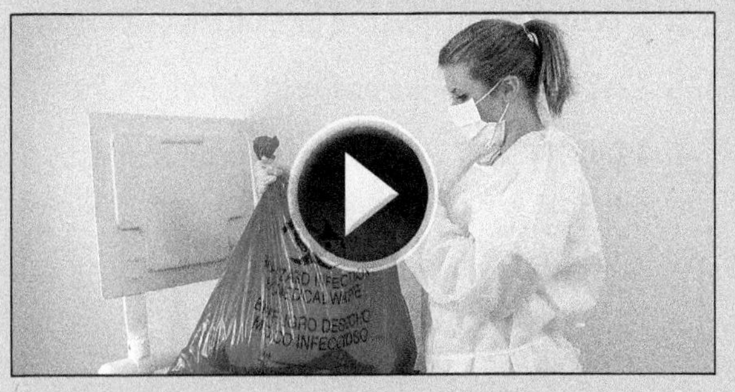

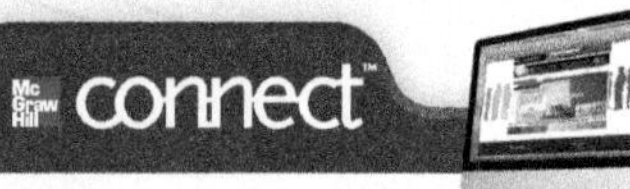

STEM CONNECTION

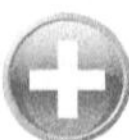

Medical Science

Spores

Spores are thick-walled, resistant cells produced by fungi when they reproduce or by bacteria when they need to withstand harsh environments.

connect Go online to learn about how spores function and transmit disease.

Quality Control Procedures

Why is it important to keep records of the sterilization process?

Quality control procedures are measures that monitor and ensure that the sterilization process is effective. Records of such measures are kept in case of an inspection. These records must be accurately dated and carefully filed. Three quality control methods are commonly used.

- **Mechanical monitoring.** This includes graphing the pressure/vacuum gauge, temperature gauge, and other gauge readings during the sterilization cycle.
- **Chemical monitoring.** Strips of material with chemicals that change color after exposure to enough heat or steam are used to ensure that the sterilization cycle is complete.
- **Biological monitoring.** A small container with live and highly resistant bacteria are placed in the autoclave before the sterilization process has begun. The bacteria are monitored to see if they survive the process. This is indicated by their ability to reproduce when placed in a supportive environment and checked after a specified time. If they did survive, the sterilization was inadequate.

READING CHECK

Name the three methods of monitoring sterilization for quality control.

SECTION 31.2 Central Supply/Processing Procedures Review

AFTER YOU READ

1. **Describe** an ultrasonic cleaner and explain what it does.
2. **Explain** how instruments should be wrapped or placed in the packages for sterilization.
3. **Define** the purpose of an autoclave indicator.
4. **List** four methods of sterilization.
5. **Identify** the monitoring method that uses live bacteria.
6. **Describe** what must be done to linens after they have been washed and dried.

Technology ONLINE EXPLORATIONS

Sterilization

Search online for various methods of equipment sterilization. Gather information and create a report that includes pictures of at least three different types of sterilization.

CHAPTER **31** Review

Chapter Summary

SECTION 31.1

- Each area of the central supply and processing department has a specific function, and materials must flow through the department correctly. The areas usually include decontamination, preparation and packaging, clean/sterile storage, equipment storage, case cart holding/dispatch, and linen room. **(pg. 728)**
- Central supply personnel must use materials, supplies, and equipment safely; follow aseptic technique; track inventory to prevent waste; and maintain an organized work space. **(pg. 729)**
- Central supply technicians perform a variety of duties under the direct supervision of a supervisor or manager. **(pg. 731)**
- The central supply manager is the decision-making authority for the department, directs the restocking of equipment and supplies, and coordinates the work of the central supply staff. **(pg. 733)**

SECTION 31.2

- All items used for patient procedures must be decontaminated prior to reuse. **(pg. 734)**
- Thorough cleaning of all instruments must be performed manually or with an automatic washer or ultrasonic cleaner. **(pg. 735)**
- Wrapping and packaging of instruments and equipment must be completed prior to sterilization if the item will be stored. **(pg. 735)**
- The autoclave uses heat under pressure and creates steam that sterilizes items for use. **(pg. 735)**
- Linens must be cleaned and inspected prior to sterilization. **(pg. 735)**
- Quality control procedures monitor and ensure that the sterilization process is effective. **(pg. 736)**

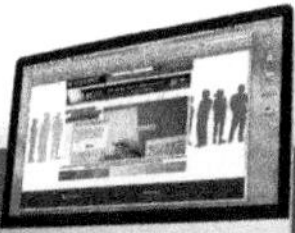

McGraw Hill connect™ **ONLINE ACTIVITIES**

Complete our HST online activities for Chapter 31, which include Concept Check review questions, Reference Flash Cards, and Online Procedures assessment sheets.

- **Concept Check** review questions
- **Reference Flash Cards** medical terminology practice
- **Online Procedures** assessment sheets

CHAPTER 31 Assessment

Critical Thinking/Problem Solving

1. An employee from a patient care unit wheels a cart of used equipment and instruments into the packaging and preparation area of central supply and asks, "What should I do with all of this stuff?" How would you respond?
2. What might happen to a patient if a surgical instrument were not thoroughly decontaminated before it was sterilized and then used during surgery?
3. Obtain several bottles of cleaning solutions or soaps and their Material Safety Data Sheets (MSDS) (see Chapter 3). Read the MSDS and label of each and determine how to use the product and what safety measures to follow. Prepare the substances to perform various cleaning procedures as assigned by your instructor.
4. Practice processing instruments by obtaining various instruments used in surgical or dental procedures. Identify each instrument and practice cleaning, packaging, and sterilizing several of them. Use **Procedures 31-2, 31-3, and 31-4** as reference for practice.

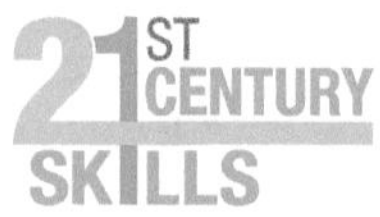

5. **Problem Solving** Practice classifying items in the central processing departments using the following steps.
   a. Create one card each for the following central supply items: linens, scrub attire, personal protective equipment, autoclave, infusion pump, emergency cart, supply carts for various units, and recording equipment.
   b. Form groups of six. One student will represent each area of the central supply and processing department: decontamination, preparation and packaging, clean/sterile storage, equipment storage, case cart holding/dispatch, and linen.
   c. The students then pass the cards around and select the card or cards for the item or items that should be stored and/or used in the area they represent.
6. **Teamwork** Practice wrapping and labeling instruments for sterilization according to the procedure described in **Procedure 31.3**. Substitute pencils, pens, or scissors for instruments if necessary. Use tissue paper, cloth napkins, or towels for wrapping materials. Trade your package with a partner and open the package without "contaminating" the item inside.
7. **Information Literacy** Compare the certification requirements for a central supply technician at the websites of the following two agencies: the Certification Board for Sterile Processing and Distribution, and the American Society for Healthcare Central Service Professionals. Write a summary of the agency you would choose for certification and explain the reasons for your choice.

CHAPTER **32** Dietetics

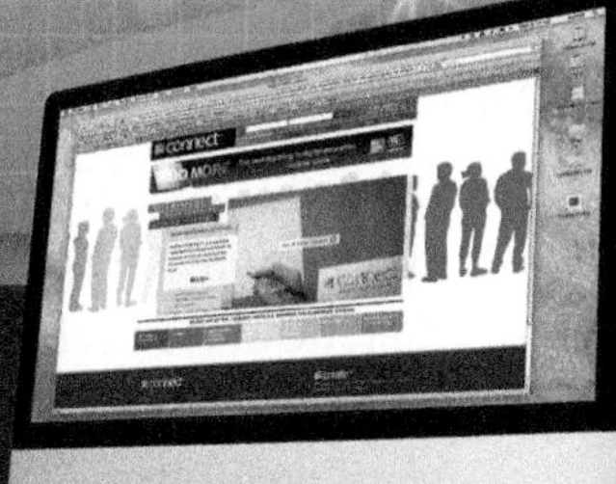

Essential Question:

How do dietetic professionals help people achieve better health?

If you are interested in food and nutrition and enjoy working with people, consider a career in dietetics. Some are support careers, while others are therapeutic careers. The four most common careers in dietetics are dietetic aide; certified dietary manager (CDM); dietetic technician, registered (DTR); and registered dietitian (RD).

The job outlook for careers in dietetics is good, and employment is expected to roughly match the average outlook for all occupations. Job growth in dietetics will be ensured by two main factors: a continued emphasis on using nutrition to help prevent and treat disease, and a growing and aging population.

McGraw Hill connect™

It's Online!

- **Online Procedures**
- **STEM Connection**
- **Medical Science**
- **Medical Terms**
- **Medical Math**
- **Ethics in Action**
- **Virtual Lab**

Photo: Bernard van Berg/Iconica/Getty Images

READING GUIDE

OBJECTIVES

After completing this chapter, you will be able to:

- **Describe** the key roles and responsibilities of a dietetic aide; a certified dietary manager; a dietetic technician, registered; and a registered dietitian.
- **Identify** various settings in which a registered dietitian may be employed.
- **Explain** four steps for preventing food-borne illness.
- **Illustrate** the process of cleaning and sanitizing.
- **Describe** the importance of correct positioning when patients are helped to eat.
- **Demonstrate** how to assist a patient to eat and how to feed a patient safely.
- **Compare** two or more types of therapeutic diets.
- **Demonstrate** three dietetic procedures.

BEFORE YOU READ

Connect Have you ever thought about eating a healthier diet? How does your diet contribute to your overall health and well-being?

Main Idea

Dietetic aides, certified dietary managers, dietetic technicians, and registered dietitians promote health and wellness through better nutrition and proper food handling.

Note-Taking Activity

Draw this table. Write key terms and phrases under **Cues**. Write main ideas under **Note Taking**. Summarize the section under **Summary**.

Cues	Note Taking
o o	o o
Summary	

Graphic Organizer

Before you read the chapter, draw a diagram like the one to the right. As you read, write the types of therapeutic diets covered by the chapter into the diagram.

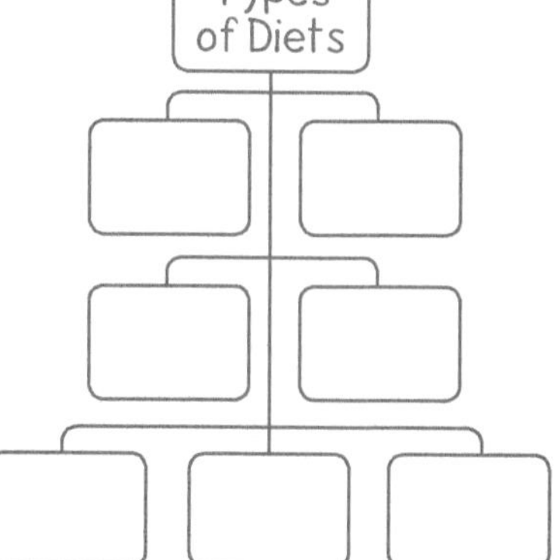

connect

Downloadable graphic organizers can be accessed online.

STANDARDS

HEALTH SCIENCE

NCHSE 6.32 Demonstrate respectful and empathetic treatment of ALL patients/clients (customer service).

NCHSE 7.12 Describe methods of controlling the spread and growth of microorganisms.

NCHSE 9.11 Apply behaviors that promote health and wellness.

SCIENCE

NSES F Develop understanding of personal and community health; population growth; natural resources; environmental quality; natural and human-induced hazards; science and technology in local, national, and global challenges.

NCHSE *National Consortium for Health Science Education*

NSES *National Science Education Standards*

COMMON CORE STATE STANDARDS

MATHEMATICS

Statistics and Probability

Conditional Probability and the Rules of Probability S-IC 6

Evaluate reports based on data.

ENGLISH LANGUAGE ARTS

Speaking and Listening

Speaking and Listening SL-4

Present information, findings, and supporting evidence, conveying a clear and distinct perspective, such that listeners can follow the line of reasoning, alternative or opposing perspectives are addressed, and the organization, development, substance, and style are appropriate to purpose, audience, and a range of formal and informal tasks.

SECTION

32.1 Careers in Dietetics

The Dietetic Aide

What is the main goal of the dietetic aide?

The dietetic aide works in a healthcare facility in which food for specialized diets is prepared and served. Hospitals, extended care facilities, and nursing homes are examples of such facilities. The dietetic aide works with food and people on a daily basis (see **Figure 32.1**). For an overview of careers in dietetics, see **Table 32.1** on page 742.

Job Responsibilities of the Dietetic Aide

If you become a dietetic aide, your main duty will be to ensure that patients receive the correct meals and snacks according to the diet their physician has ordered for them. An aide may work only in the kitchen or may work in the kitchen and also interact with patients.

The dietetic aide may be responsible for

- processing diet orders when a patient is admitted or when a diet order changes.
- distributing appropriate menus to patients.
- helping patients in making food choices, if necessary, and collecting menus after selections are made.
- checking food trays for accuracy, temperature, and appearance.
- delivering food trays and scheduled snacks to patients.

READING CHECK

Name some ways in which the dietetic aide directly assists patients.

Vocabulary

Content Vocabulary

You will learn this content vocabulary term in this section.

- **medical nutrition therapy**

Academic Vocabulary

You will see this word in your reading and on your tests. Find its meaning in the Glossary in the back of the book.

- **expert**

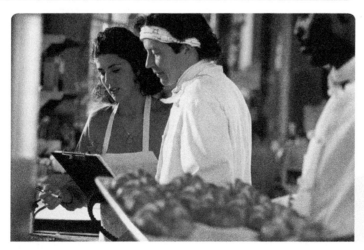

Fig. 32.1 Dietetic Aide Shown are a dietetic aide and a dietary manager. *Where are these two professionals employed?*

Photo: Daniel Bosler/Stone/Getty Images

The Certified Dietary Manager

What functions are managed by a certified dietary manager?

If you like to work with people, do not mind paperwork, and enjoy preparing food, you may choose to be a certified dietary manager (CDM). CDMs are trained to manage food service functions. They may work in hospitals, extended care facilities, nursing homes, schools, and correctional facilities.

Table 32.1 Overview of Careers in Dietetics

OCCUPATION	EDUCATIONAL REQUIREMENTS	CERTIFICATION OR LICENSING	JOB OUTLOOK
Dietetic Aide	High school diploma. Three or four weeks of on-the-job training	None required	Average growth
Certified Dietary Manager (CDM)	High school diploma. Completion of an approved dietary manager training program.	A national certification examination is offered by the Certifying Board for Dietary Managers. Training and examination for credentialing as a Certified Food Protection Professional credential is also available.	Average growth
Dietetic Technician, Registered (DTR)	Two-year associate degree from an accredited program in a community college, postsecondary vocational-technical school, university, or college. Completion of a dietetic technician program approved by the Commission on Accreditation for Dietetics Education (CADE) of the American Dietetic Association (ADA), including 450 hours of supervised practice.	Registration is earned by passing an examination offered by the Commission on Dietetic Registration.	Average growth because of increased emphasis on disease prevention by improved dietary habits
Registered Dietitian (RD)	Four-year degree in dietetics, food science, or a related major at a university or college on a program accredited by the Commission on Accreditation for Dietetics Education of the American Dietetic Association (CADE). Completion of a six- to twelve-month supervised practice program at a healthcare facility, community agency, or food service corporation.	Registration is earned by passing an examination offered by the Commission on Dietetic Registration. Certifications may also be earned in a specialized area of practice, such as pediatric or renal nutrition, nutrition support, oncology nutrition, or gerontological nutrition. There may be additional state licensing requirements.	Average growth because of increased emphasis on disease prevention by improved dietary habits

Job Responsibilities of a Certified Dietary Manager

As a CDM, you will work with registered dietitians (RD) and dietetic technicians, registered (DTR). You will provide food that is safe, tastes good, and meets the nutritional needs of patients. Most CDMs work in food service management, but some may also provide basic nutritional services to patients. The CDM may be in charge of:

- Supervising food preparation and distribution
- Interviewing, hiring, and training food service employees
- Ensuring that regulations for sanitation are followed
- Overseeing the business operations of the dietary department
- Developing and following a budget

READING CHECK

Name some types of facilities that employ certified dietary managers.

The Dietetic Technician, Registered

How does the registered dietetic technician help educate patients?

Dietetic technicians, registered (DTR), work alone or team with registered dietitians. They work in a range of settings, but most often DTRs work in hospitals or nursing homes. They may also work in businesses, government agencies, schools, day care centers, retirement centers, correctional facilities, and fitness centers.

Job Responsibilities of the Dietetic Technician, Registered

As a DTR you may work in a clinical setting, or you may be part of a team that manages food services.

In a clinical setting, such as a hospital, public health agency, or nursing home, the DTR may be in charge of:

- Collecting information from patients about their usual diet, weight, appetite, and food preferences
- Assisting the registered dietitian in creating a nutrition care plan
- Performing basic diet counseling
- Teaching nutrition classes

READING CHECK

Recall three tasks performed by the dietetic technician.

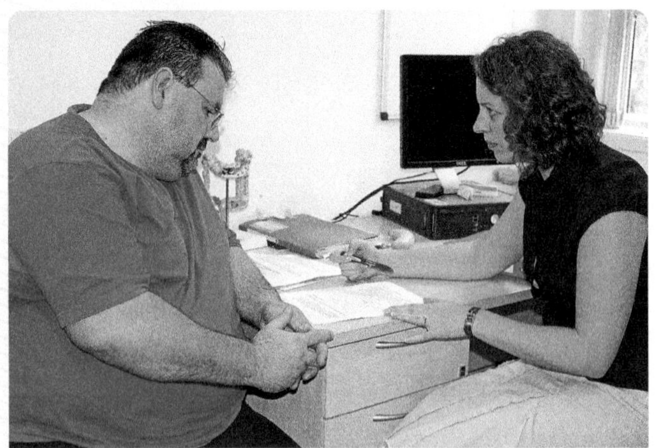

Fig. 32.2 Registered Dietitian A registered dietitian can work in many different settings. *What personal qualities are common traits often found in people who work as registered dietitians?*

The Registered Dietitian

Why is there an increasing need for registered dietitians?

A registered dietitian (RD) is a food and nutrition expert. As seen in **Figure 32.2** the RD works with patients and must have important personal qualities. You may enjoy a career in this field if you:

- Are a motivated "self-starter"
- Have initiative
- Are able to work independently
- Are able to identify and solve problems
- Have a strong interest in food and nutrition

Table 32.2 Places of Employment and Responsibilities of a Registered Dietitian

PLACE OF EMPLOYMENT	JOB RESPONSIBILITIES MAY INCLUDE
Hospital, clinic, nursing home, or other healthcare or extended care facility	• Assessing the nutritional status of patients • Developing specialized nutrition care plans for patients • Communicating nutrition plans to other healthcare professionals in the facility • Educating patients and staff about nutrition and therapeutic diets • Managing food service operations (may include managing staff, food and equipment purchasing, and food preparation)
School, day care center, or correctional facility	• Managing food service operations (may include managing staff, food and equipment purchasing, and food preparation)
Sports nutrition and corporate wellness programs	• Educating patients about the connections between food, fitness, and health
Food and nutrition-related business or industry	• Developing communication, marketing, and public relations plans • Developing new products or recipes • Consulting with chefs in restaurants and culinary schools
Private practice	• Counseling patients on special diets for preventing or treating disease, optimizing health or performance, or managing weight • Providing consulting services to food service or restaurant managers, food vendors, or distributors.
Community or other public health setting	• Teaching, monitoring, and advising the public on the importance of good nutrition • Helping individuals improve their quality of life through healthy eating habits
University or medical center	• Teaching physicians, physician assistants, nurses, dietetic students, dentists, and others about the science of foods and nutrition
Research center in food and pharmaceutical companies, university, or hospital	• Directing or conducting research to answer critical nutrition questions • Developing food and nutrition recommendations based on research results

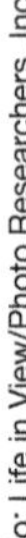

A registered dietitian can work in many settings with different responsibilities (see **Table 32.2**). These include short- and long-term healthcare centers, food service, diabetes education, dialysis centers, public health departments, healthcare sales, and research. A registered dietitian may work for a private practice or a public agency.

The need for **medical nutrition therapy** is growing as a result of the rise in obesity and certain diseases. This type of therapy applies proper nutrition and therapeutic diets to help prevent and treat conditions such as heart disease, diabetes, cancer, and high blood pressure. There is a growing use of nutrition and dietary supplements to improve the way people feel, how they look, and their overall well-being. The increased use of medical nutrition therapy provides increased opportunities for RDs.

Job Responsibilities of the Registered Dietitian

As a registered dietitian, you will have a variety of responsibilities, depending on where you are employed. **Table 32.2** summarizes the responsibilities according to the place of employment.

READING CHECK

Summarize the professional skills you think are needed to be successful as a registered dietitian.

SECTION 32.1 Careers in Dietetics Review

AFTER YOU READ

1. **Explain** why the job outlook for careers in dietetics is good.
2. **Describe** the main responsibilities of the dietetic aide.
3. **Compare and contrast** the education and responsibilities of a certified dietary manager and a dietetic technician, registered.
4. **Describe** the education required to be a registered dietitian.
5. **Identify** the purpose of medical nutrition therapy.
6. **Describe** the key responsibilities of a registered dietitian who works in a hospital setting.

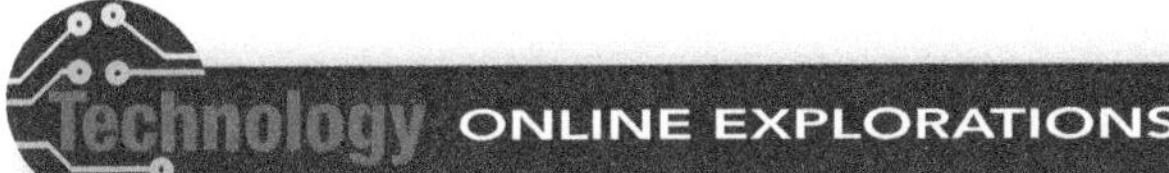

Nutrition

Search the American Dietetic Association website for information on a nutrition topic that interests you. Or you can learn about becoming a DTR or an RD by using search terms such as "careers in dietetics," "nutrition," "specialized diets," "medical nutrition therapy," or "dietary supplements." Prepare a report on one of these subjects.

SECTION 32.2 Procedures in Dietetics

Vocabulary

Content Vocabulary

You will learn these content vocabulary terms in this section.

- food-borne illness
- microorganisms
- cross-contamination
- sanitizing
- therapeutic diet
- diabetes
- diet history
- 24-hour dietary recall

Academic Vocabulary

You will see this word in your reading and on your tests. Find its meaning in the Glossary in the back of the book.

- survive

Observing Food Safety and Sanitation

What makes food safe or unsafe?

To be healthy, food must be safe. To be safe, food must be prepared and served in a sanitary environment.

Sanitary food preparation helps guard against food-borne illness. This means making sure that anything that comes in contact with food, including surfaces, utensils, other foods, and people, is clean. People who are sick, weak, or frail are especially susceptible to becoming ill from eating contaminated foods. Food safety is important in healthcare, as it is in your daily life.

Causes of Food-Borne Illness

A **food-borne illness** is a sickness that results from eating food that is not safe to eat. Tiny living creatures called **microorganisms** cause most cases of food-borne illness. You cannot see, smell, or taste microorganisms (see **Figure 32.3**). They are on your skin, in the air, in the soil, and in the intestines of animals.

Sometimes, they are on food when you buy it. Or they can get into food during storage, preparation, or serving. Many microorganisms are completely harmless or even useful, but others are dangerous and can be deadly.

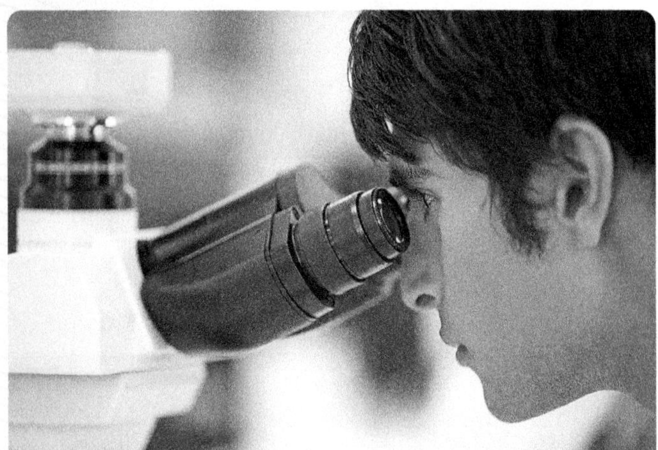

Fig. 32.3 Food-borne Illnesses This scientist uses a microscope to study microorganisms in food. *What is the most common cause of food-borne illness?*

Photo: Adam Gault/OJO Images/Getty Images

Bacteria, parasites, and viruses are examples of microorganisms. The most common causes of food-borne illness are bacteria. Bacteria are everywhere in our environment. When harmful bacteria get into food, they can multiply to dangerous levels if conditions are right. And when ingested in large enough numbers, these harmful bacteria can make people sick.

To survive and multiply, bacteria need:

- **Food to grow on** Bacteria can grow on a variety of foods. The most common foods are raw or undercooked eggs, meat, fish, and poultry, unpasteurized milk or juice, unwashed produce, and prepared foods left too long at room temperature.

- **Moisture** Bacteria need moisture to survive. They cannot survive in foods that have little moisture, such as crackers or breads.
- **Warmth but not heat** Bacteria grow fastest at temperatures in the range of 40° to 140°F. Below 40°F, which is the temperature of a refrigerator, bacteria grow more slowly. The colder the temperature, the more slowly the bacteria grow. At the same time, bacteria cannot multiply at temperatures above 140°F. Most bacteria are destroyed at a cooking temperature that is above 165°F (see **Figure 32.4**).
- **Oxygen** Most bacteria need to be exposed to air in order to multiply. However, a few harmful bacteria can survive and multiply without oxygen.

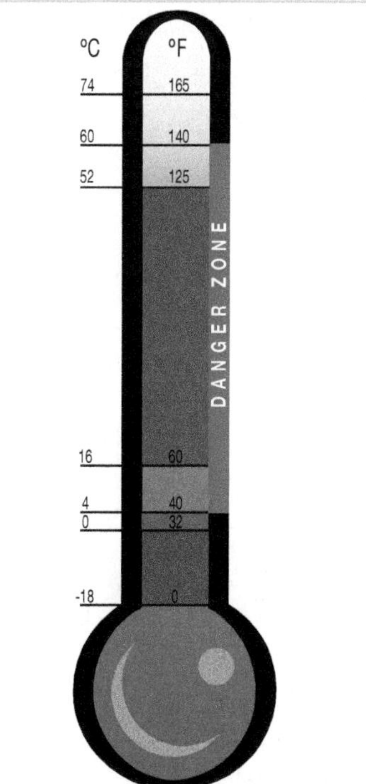

Fig. 32.4 Danger Zone The danger zone for bacteria growth is shown. *At what temperature do bacteria grow the fastest?*

Symptoms of Food-Borne Illness

Food-borne illness can range from mild to very serious or fatal. It can be difficult to diagnose because the symptoms vary and are often similar to those of the flu. Symptoms may include fever, nausea, vomiting, abdominal pain, diarrhea, headache, and muscle pain. These symptoms can occur from 30 minutes to two weeks after eating food containing harmful bacteria. Most often, symptoms appear within four to 48 hours.

Preventing Food-Borne Illness

Food-borne illness can be prevented. How? By taking steps to ensure safe handling, cooking, storage, and preparation of foods.

Keep Raw Meats and Ready-to-Eat Foods Separate **Cross-contamination,** or the transfer of bacteria, can occur if juices from raw meat, poultry, or seafood accidentally touch cooked food or uncooked ready-to-eat foods, such as fruit or salads. Bacteria on utensils, such as knives, or on surfaces, such as cutting boards, can also cross-contaminate food. To prevent cross-contamination:

- Keep raw meat, poultry, and seafood separate from other foods in preparation areas and in the refrigerator, where they should be put on the bottom shelf.
- Wash hands, cutting boards, dishes, and utensils with hot, soapy water after they have been in contact with raw meat, poultry, and seafood. As seen in **Figure 32.5,** you should use specially designated cutting boards, dishes, and utensils for raw meat, poultry, and seafood.
- Never place cooked food on an unwashed plate that previously held raw meat, poultry, or seafood.
- Place washed produce into clean storage containers, not back into the original containers.
- Use clean scissors or blades to open food packages.
- Be especially sure to wear plastic gloves if you have a sore or cut on your hand.

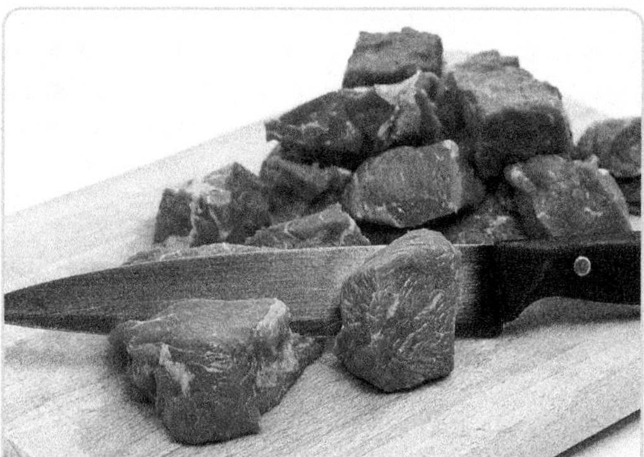

Fig. 32.5 Cross-Contamination Keep raw meats and ready-to-eat foods separate. *What should be done with this cutting board and knife after use?*

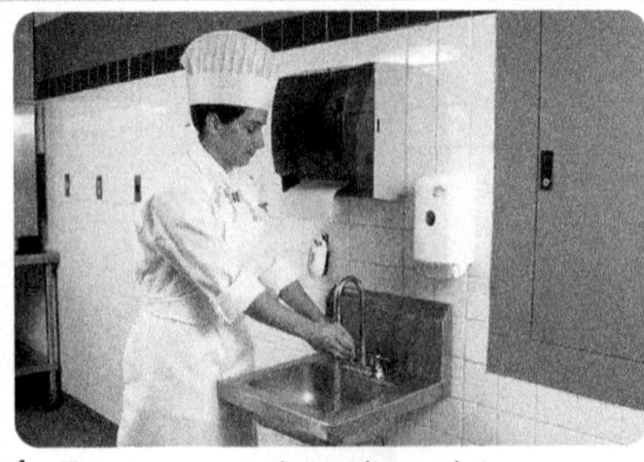

1. Remove any rings, bracelets, or watches. Wet hands and forearms with hot water.

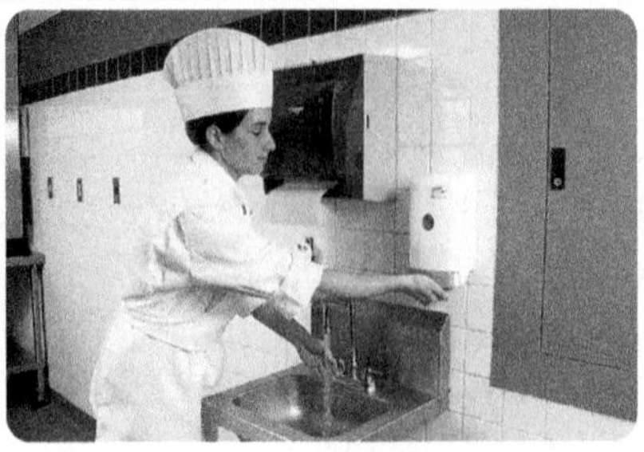

2. Apply enough soap to build up a good lather.

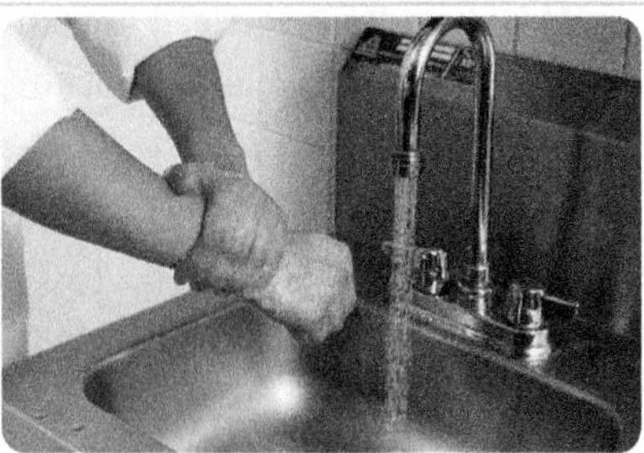

3. Rub hands and arms with the lather for at least 20 seconds.

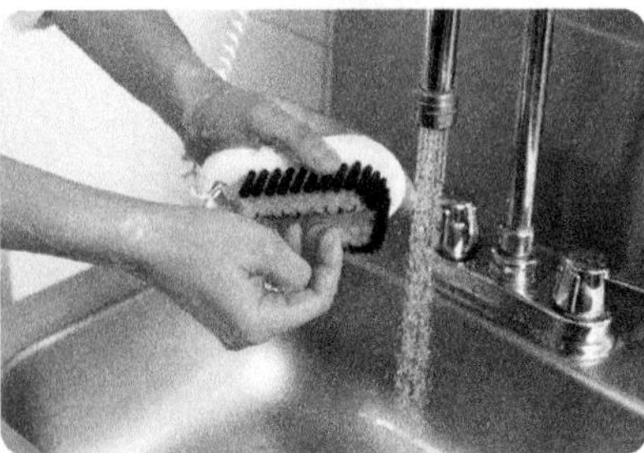

4. Clean fingernails with a brush.

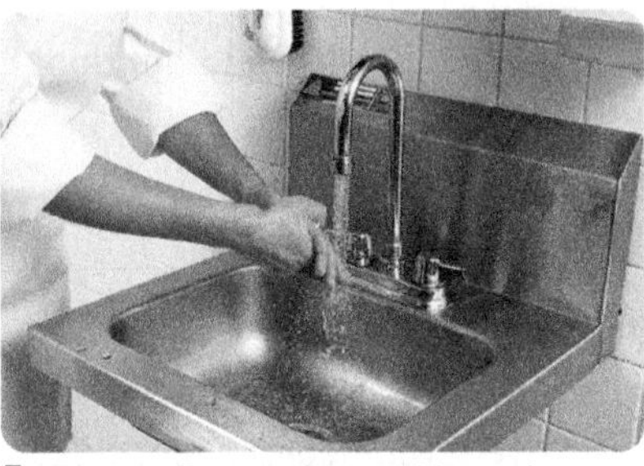

5. Rinse off soap thoroughly under very warm water.

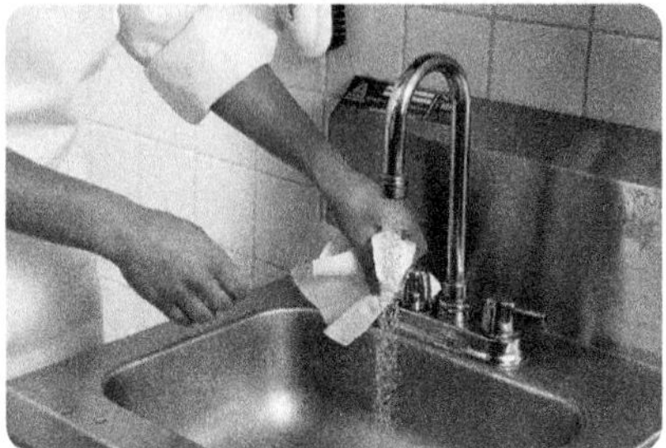

6. Turn off the water faucet using a paper towel.

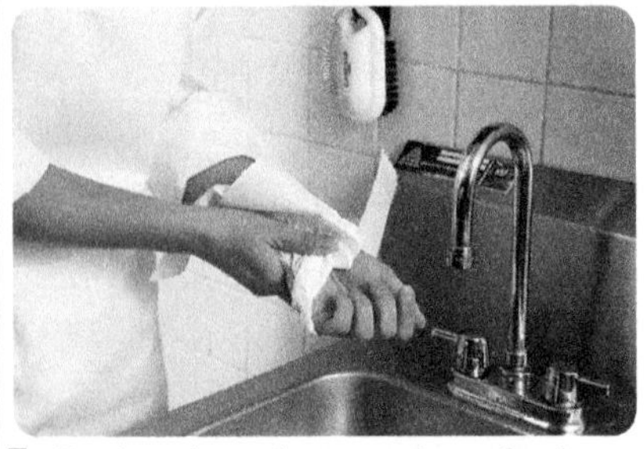

7. Dry hands and arms using a fresh paper towel.

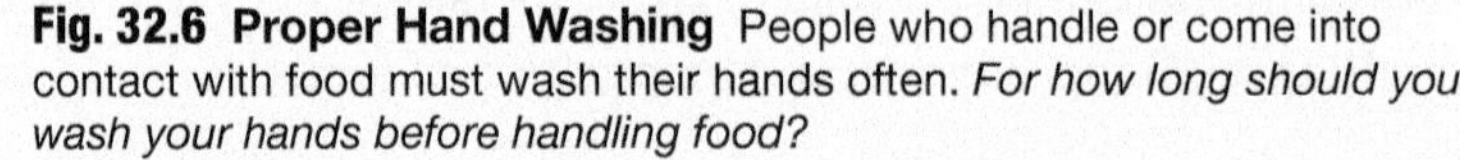

Fig. 32.6 Proper Hand Washing People who handle or come into contact with food must wash their hands often. *For how long should you wash your hands before handling food?*

Photos: Ann Garvin

Wash Hands Often and Well People who come into contact with food—food-service workers as well as patients—can spread harmful bacteria by coughing or sneezing on the food. Bacteria can spread from open sores or from the intestinal tract if people have not washed their hands after using the bathroom. Food handlers should always wash their hands with warm, soapy water for at least 20 seconds before handling food. The handwashing procedure must be performed correctly (see **Figure 32.6**). Food handlers should also wear food handler protection such as non-latex gloves when handling or preparing foods. Hands should be washed and gloves should be changed after doing any of the following actions:

- Using the bathroom
- Using a handkerchief or tissue
- Handling raw foods, such as eggs, meat, fish, poultry, and produce
- Touching or scratching areas of the body, such as ears, mouth, nose, or hair
- Touching unclean equipment, work surfaces, or washcloths
- Clearing away and scraping used dishes and utensils
- Eating or drinking

Cook to the Correct Temperature Harmful bacteria are destroyed when food is heated for a long enough time and at a high enough temperature. The best way to be sure that food has been cooked enough is to use a thermometer to accurately measure the internal temperature of meat, poultry, casseroles, and other cooked foods (see **Figure 32.7**).

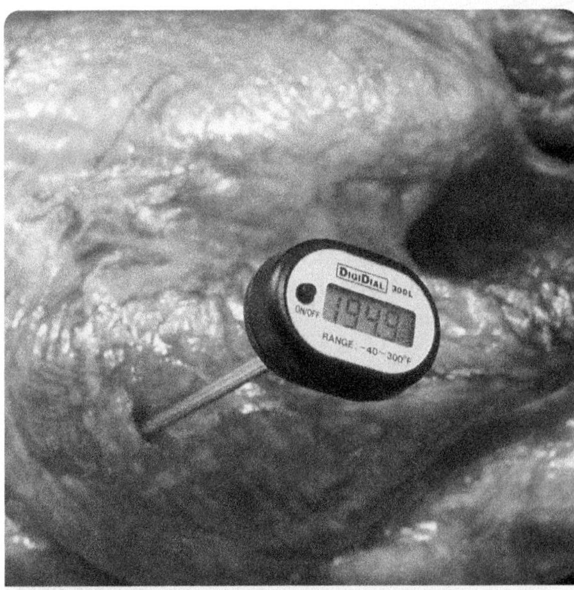

Fig. 32.7 Meat Thermometer Cooking food to the appropriate temperature destroys harmful bacteria. *What is the safe cooking temperature for this whole chicken?*

Follow these guidelines for safe cooking.

- Maintain hot cooked foods at 140°F or higher for no more than two hours.
- Make sure that cooked fish is opaque (not transparent) and flakes easily with a fork.
- Cook eggs until the yolk and white are firm. Egg dishes are done when the internal temperature reaches 160°F.
- When reheating sauces, soups, and gravy, bring them to a boil before serving. Other leftovers should be reheated to 165°F.
- The internal temperature for roasts, beef, veal, and lamb chops, and steaks should reach at least 145°F.
- Whole poultry, such as chicken and turkey, should be cooked to 180°F.
- Ground poultry should be cooked to 165°F.
- Ground beef, ground veal, and pork should always be cooked to at least 160°F.

When meat is ground, bacteria from the grinder's surface are mixed into the meat. That is why it is important to always cook ground meat thoroughly. Do not serve or eat ground meat that is still pink inside.

Chill Promptly to Below 40°F To slow the growth of bacteria, refrigerate or freeze food promptly. This applies to both raw food and leftovers. As seen in **Figure 32.8**, you should check refrigerator temperatures regularly, to be sure that the temperature stays below 40°F. A freezer unit should be set at 0°F.

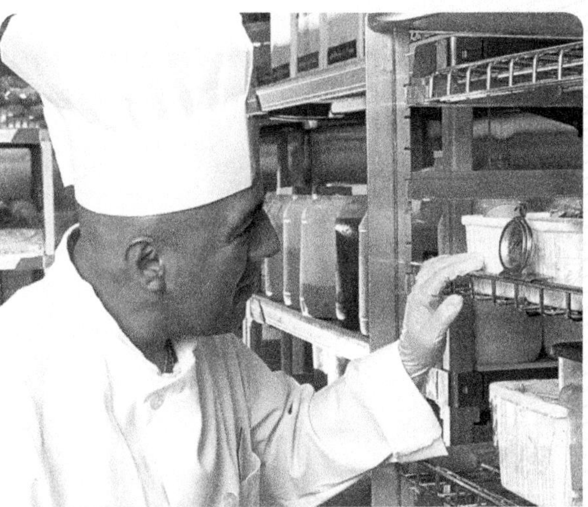

Fig. 32.8 Chill Food Properly Chill food promptly to below 40°F. *At what temperature should the freezer be set?*

Keep the following in mind when chilling food.

- Use the "two-hour rule," which means not letting food sit out at room temperature for more than two hours. Refrigerate or freeze perishable foods, such as milk, prepared foods, raw meats, and leftovers, as soon as possible.
- Never defrost food at room temperature. Thaw food in the refrigerator, under cold running water, or in the microwave.
- If there are large amounts of leftovers, divide the food into small, shallow containers, so that they will cool quickly in the refrigerator.

Photos: (t)Tony Freeman/PhotoEdit, (b)Aaron Haupt Photography

Safety

Transporting Food Safely

Consider these rules for transporting food safely.

- Place perishables in an ice chest if the store-to-home trip is longer than one hour.
- If you buy hot food items, take them home immediately and eat them, refrigerate them as quickly as possible, or hold them for no longer than two hours at 140°F or above.
- Never leave food in a hot car. A good rule of thumb is that if the ice cream is melting, it and the food with it has been too warm for too long.
- Avoid dropping or crushing food packages and cans.
- Make sure perishable foods taken to a picnic are kept cold until eaten.

- Add ice cubes to hot soups, stocks, or broths, plunge the cooking pot into a sink full of cold water and ice cubes, or divide this food into smaller containers to lower the temperature quickly before placing in the refrigerator or freezer. Do not let cooked food sit out to cool before refrigerating or freezing it.
- Make sure that cool air can circulate freely in the refrigerator and freezer.

READING CHECK

Summarize the steps that can be taken to prevent food-borne illness.

Positioning the Patient for Eating

What risks are faced by an improperly-positioned patient when eating?

Correct positioning for eating is important to prevent choking and aspiration.

Choking happens when an object such as food becomes lodged in the airway, blocking a person's ability to breathe. Coughing is the normal reflex to dislodge the object. But when an object such as food or liquid passes beyond the vocal cords and enters the lungs, this is known as aspiration. At this point, the food cannot usually be dislodged by coughing.

Aspiration can cause a serious or even fatal illness called aspiration pneumonia.

The following correct positioning will help to protect a patient's airway when eating.

- Whenever possible, transfer patients from a bed to a dining chair or wheelchair for meals.

McGraw-Hill connect™ ONLINE PROCEDURES

PROCEDURE 32-1

Cleaning and Sanitizing Surfaces, Utensils, and Other Items

If you follow the steps for safe handling, storage, and food preparation, you will greatly reduce the chances of food-borne illness. Any surface that comes into contact with food must be cleaned, rinsed, and sanitized. **Sanitizing** destroys bacteria and viruses that may still be present after the cleaning process. Surfaces can be sanitized with heat or with a sanitizing solution.

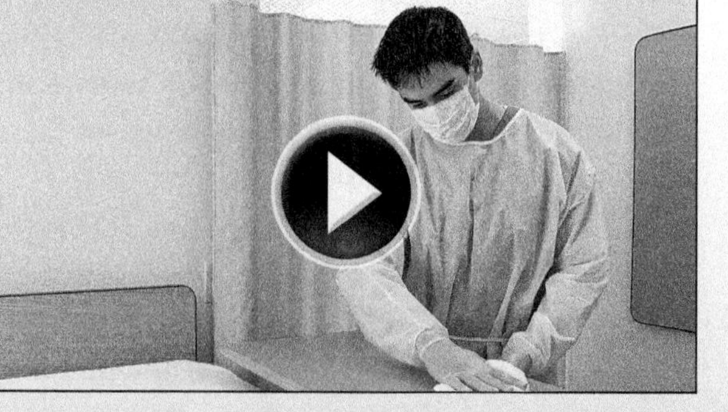

Photo: McGraw-Hill Companies, Inc./Tim Fuller, photographer

- Position the patient as close to upright as possible, at least at a 45-degree angle. The patient's hips, knees, and ankles should be flexed at a 90-degree angle. This helps to maintain the support and balance required for eating (see **Figure 32.9**).
- The position of the patient's head is especially important. Do not allow the patient's head to fall backward during swallowing. When this happens, the airway opens up, and choking or aspiration may occur. The patient's head should be upright, with the chin pointing slightly downward toward the chest.
- If the patient eats in bed, support the head in the upright position with a pillow or a piece of soft foam. After the meal, keep the patient in an upright position at an angle of at least 30 to 45 degrees for at least 30 to 45 minutes. In this position, the patient is less likely to choke on or aspirate any food that is regurgitated.

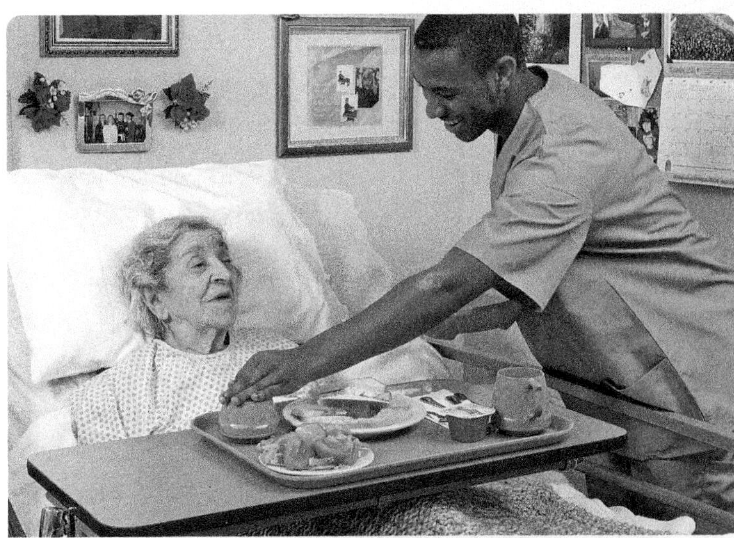

Fig. 32.9 Proper Positioning Position the patient correctly for eating. *What will proper positioning prevent?*

READING CHECK

Recall the meaning of aspiration and why it is dangerous.

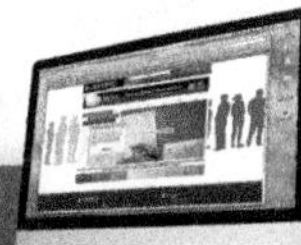

Mc Graw Hill connect™ ONLINE PROCEDURES

PROCEDURE 32-2

Assisting the Patient to Eat

Some patients may be too sick, weak, or injured to feed themselves. Regardless of age or condition, patients who have difficulty feeding themselves need a caring, helping hand. You should expect some frustration from these individuals. Stay calm and positive, keeping in mind that relying on others in matters of personal care can cause great emotional strain.

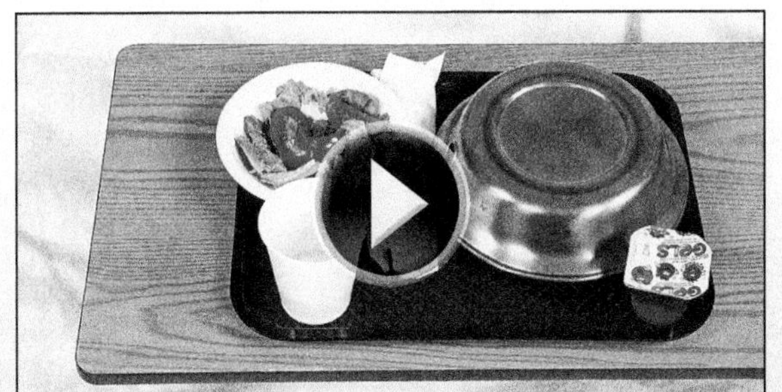

PROCEDURE 32-3

Feeding a Helpless Patient

Some patients may be conscious and alert but unable to feed themselves at all. In this case, the patient will need to be fed in order to ensure that he or she receives the proper nutrition. Correct positioning is very important to protect the patient from choking and aspiration.

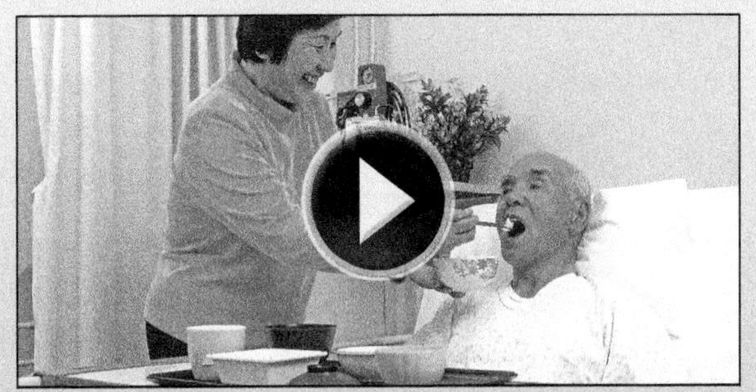

Photos: (t-b)McGraw-Hill Companies, Inc./Tim Fuller, photographer, PhotoLink/Getty Images, Urikiri-Shashin-Kan/Alamy

Therapeutic Diets

Why do some patients need special diets?

A **therapeutic diet** is a special eating plan used to treat or control a condition or disease. A person may need to follow a special diet for a short time or for a lifetime, depending on the condition. Only a doctor or registered dietitian should prescribe a therapeutic diet.

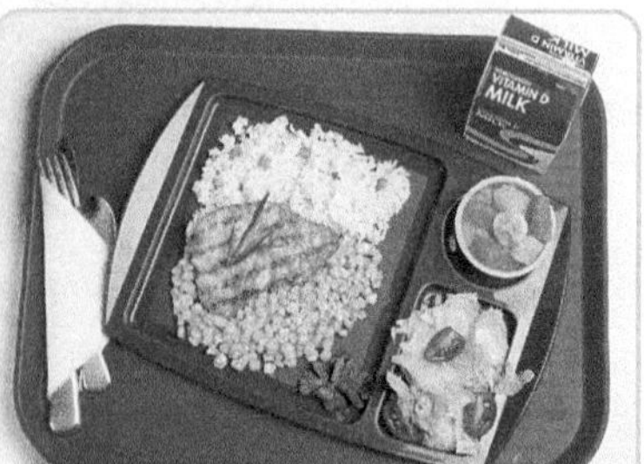

Fig. 32.10 Therapeutic Diets A meal tray would contain only foods that are allowed for the prescribed therapeutic diet. *What are two therapeutic diets?*

Types of Therapeutic Diets

Some types of therapeutic diets require that certain foods be limited or even eliminated. Others may involve choosing foods for their nutrients or for texture. A meal tray would include only the foods allowed in the patient's prescribed diet (see **Figure 32.10**). Some include low-fat, low-cholesterol, low-sodium, diabetic, high-fiber, calcium-rich, modified-consistency, and liquid diets.

Low-Fat, Low-Cholesterol Diet A low-fat, low-cholesterol diet is recommended for people who have high levels of cholesterol in their blood. Along with physical activity and weight loss, if needed, this diet can help to lower blood cholesterol levels and reduce the chances of having a heart attack or stroke.

Patients following this diet must learn to cut back on foods high in fat and cholesterol. Examples are fatty meats, organ meats (liver or kidneys), fried foods, whole-milk dairy products (milk, yogurt, cheese, or eggs), and high-fat desserts. Patients can substitute lower-fat foods, such as lean meats, skinless poultry, baked or broiled seafood, low-fat or fat-free dairy products, egg substitutes, and lower-fat dessert items.

Low-Sodium Diet A low-sodium diet is recommended for people with hypertension, congestive heart failure, or swelling in lower parts of the body or abdomen area. Sodium is a mineral that is part of salt. It adds flavor to foods but can also raise blood pressure and cause other problems when consumed in large amounts.

Following a low-sodium diet of less than 2,000 mg of sodium a day (less than 1 tsp of added sodium) means cutting back on using the salt shaker, both when preparing foods and at the table. Instead, patients can season their foods with herbs, spices, lemon juice, or flavored vinegars. Prepared foods, such as canned vegetables and soups, rice or noodle mixes, frozen meals, and snack foods, are often high in sodium. Patients are encouraged to look for lower-sodium versions of these foods. They may wish to prepare foods from scratch so that they can control the amount of added salt. A low-sodium diet should also include plenty of fruits, vegetables, and low-fat dairy products.

Diabetic Diet Following a diabetic diet is important for people with **diabetes,** a condition in which the body cannot properly regulate levels of glucose in the blood. When foods are digested, especially carbohydrate foods, glucose is formed and enters the blood. A body chemical called

Photo: Elaine Shay

insulin is necessary to move glucose from the blood into the body's cells, where it is used to produce energy. In Type 1 diabetes, the body does not produce insulin. In Type 2 diabetes, the body does not use the insulin it produces. People who are overweight may find that weight loss helps control their blood sugar and prevent the onset of diabetes.

Managing diabetes involves eating regular meals and snacks, making careful food choices, and being physically active. Oral medications or insulin injections may also be necessary, but only for individuals with Type 1 diabetes and those whose Type 2 diabetes cannot be controlled by other means.

A registered dietitian or diabetes educator works closely with a person who has diabetes. A meal plan is created that consists of a variety of foods spaced regularly throughout the day. The plan also provides the right amount of calories to meet the patient's individual needs. A patient who has diabetes can be taught how to include occasional sweets and sugary foods in the meal plan.

High-Fiber Diet A high-fiber diet is used to treat certain digestive problems, such as chronic constipation. It is also recommended as a preventive measure to reduce the risk for some types of cancer. An eating plan with plenty of fiber can also help to lower blood cholesterol levels and control blood sugar levels.

Following a high-fiber diet means choosing foods that are good sources of fiber such as the ones seen in **Figure 32.11**. These foods include fruits, vegetables, legumes (dried beans and peas), whole grain breads and cereals, nuts, and seeds.

Calcium-Rich Diet A calcium-rich diet is recommended as a preventive measure and as part of the treatment for the bone disease osteoporosis, in which bones become brittle and break easily. Calcium is necessary for the development of strong bones and teeth. People who have a small body frame and who do not consume enough calcium while bones are growing (up to about age 35) are at greater risk for developing osteoporosis later in life.

A calcium-rich diet includes a variety of foods high in calcium for meals and snacks such as the ones seen in **Figure 32.12.** The total amount of calcium required depends on the individual's gender and age. Calcium requirements can be met by food choices or by a combination of food choices and a calcium and magnesium plus vitamin D supplement. Good sources of calcium include milk, yogurt, cheese, some types of tofu, salmon and sardines with edible bones, broccoli, bok choy, and pinto beans. Foods that are calcium-fortified such as some soy beverages, juices, breads, and cereals are also beneficial.

Modified-Consistency Diets Diets modified in consistency, or texture, are prescribed for individuals who have problems with chewing or swallowing. The foods in these diets may be pureed, chopped, softened, or mashed. The appropriate consistency is determined by the condition of the patient's teeth and by the patient's ability to swallow

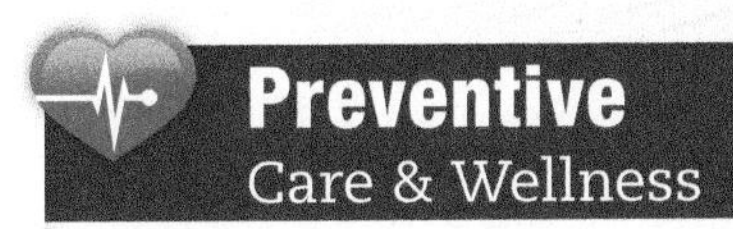

Preventive Care & Wellness

Signs of Poor Nutrition

When caring for patients, especially older adults, you should be alert for the warning signs of poor nutrition listed below. You will see that they spell the word DETERMINE. Anyone who has three or more of these risk factors may need special assistance. Consult a doctor, registered dietitian, or other healthcare professional for help.

Disease

Eating poorly

Tooth loss or mouth pain

Economic hardship

Reduced social contact

Medicines

Involuntary weight loss or gain

Needs assistance in self-care

Elder years above age 80

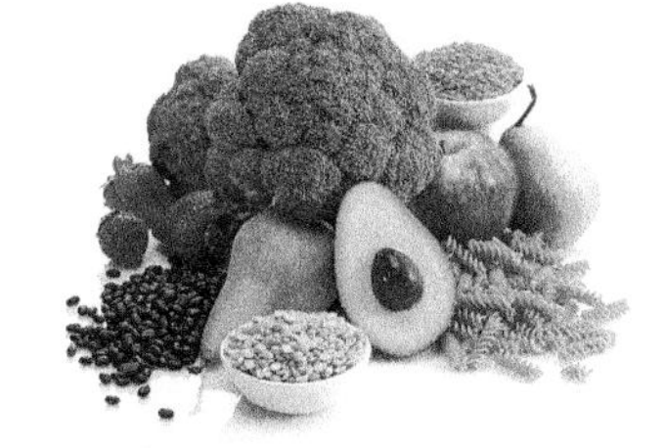

Fig. 32.11 High-Fiber Diet Some ingredients of a high-fiber diet are shown. *What is the benefit of eating high-fiber foods such as these?*

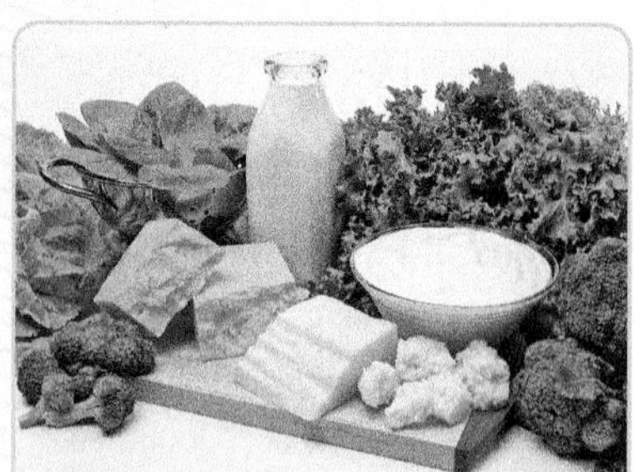

Fig. 32.12 Calcium Foods that contribute calcium are shown. *What is the benefit of eating calcium-rich foods like these?*

foods without risk of choking or aspiration. A physician may have a speech therapist evaluate a patient's chewing or swallowing ability and the risk of aspiration. The speech therapist may recommend the appropriate consistency of food and liquid that is safe for the patient.

The foods in these diets are generally moist and require minimal chewing. Most raw fruits and vegetables are excluded, along with foods containing nuts, seeds, dried fruits, or coconut. Some ripe fruits, such as peaches, pears, and bananas, can be mashed to an appropriate consistency. Soft breads and plain crackers may be softened in a soup or beverage. Meats are usually chopped or pureed and moistened with gravy or broth. Fried foods are not allowed.

Liquid Diets Liquid diets are used before or after surgery or a heart attack, when a patient has an infectious disease or digestive problems, and before certain diagnostic tests.

The most common type is a clear liquid diet, which consists of broth, tea, water, gelatin, clear soft drinks such as ginger ale or lemon-lime soda, and Popsicles®. Since clear liquid diets do not provide balanced nutrition, they should not be used for long periods of time.

Full liquid diets can be liquids or foods that become liquid at room temperature. These diets are prescribed before or after surgery or for patients who are having serious problems with chewing and swallowing. A full liquid diet consists of fruit juices, water, butter, margarine, oil, cream, custard, pudding, honey, syrups, soda, strained soups containing no solids, plain ice cream, frozen yogurt, and sherbet.

Nutrition Counseling for Therapeutic Diets

A RD or a RDR may counsel a patient on therapeutic diets. Nutrition counseling is more than just teaching a patient how to select and prepare foods for a special diet. It also involves

- learning about the patient's usual food choices, portion sizes, and eating habits. This helps determine if a patient's diet is nutritionally adequate and what types of changes may be necessary.
- helping a patient understand why a special diet is important.
- working with the patient to create individualized meal plans and specific goals to help control a disease or condition and achieve better health.
- providing the patient with the knowledge and skills to select and prepare the correct kinds of foods.

Taking a Diet History

What factors influence a person's food choices?

The first step in nutrition counseling is learning about a patient's **diet history,** his or her usual diet, and the factors that influence the patient's eating habits. A RD is the most likely healthcare professional to obtain a diet history.

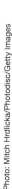

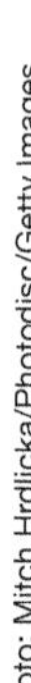

The decisions of what to eat, when to eat, where to eat, and whether or not to eat are very personal choices. Food choices are influenced by many factors, such as a patient's

- food likes and dislikes.
- daily schedule.
- social or cultural influences.
- living conditions.
- economic status.

Taking a diet history involves asking a series of questions. These questions focus on:

- Meal patterns, food preferences, and portion sizes
- Mealtime hours
- Restricted or avoided food items
- Food availability

Taking a diet history may also include asking a patient to recall the amounts of all foods and beverages consumed in a 24-hour period. This is referred to as a **24-hour dietary recall.**

Information obtained from a diet history is useful for estimating whether food intake is adequate or not. It also provides a picture of a patient's food preferences and eating habits. However, patients may have difficulty remembering the kinds and amounts of food eaten. It can be helpful to show the patient food and portion size models and measuring cups and spoons to help them estimate amounts.

connect 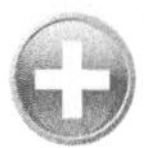

STEM CONNECTION

Medical Math

Understanding and Using Nutrition Facts

Understanding nutrient information is essential for those considering a career in dietetics. It is also vital to you as an individual. The Nutrition Facts panel on food labels can help you make informed food choices for a healthy diet. You can use food label facts to limit those nutrients you want to cut back on and increase those you need to consume in greater quantity.

connect™ Go online to learn more about nutrition information on packaged foods and complete the activity.

READING CHECK

Define a 24-hour dietary recall and its purpose.

SECTION 32.2 Procedures in Dietetics Review

AFTER YOU READ

1. **Describe** the causes of food-borne illness and the conditions needed for bacteria to survive and multiply.
2. **Identify** three or more important steps to follow when handling, storing, and preparing food.
3. **Explain** why it is necessary to sanitize a surface after cleaning it.
4. **Describe** how to sanitize a surface.
5. **Name** at least three safety measures you should follow when positioning a patient for eating.
6. **Describe** the purpose of a therapeutic diet.
7. **Name** two types of therapeutic diets.

Technology ONLINE EXPLORATIONS

Diet Histories

Search the Internet for additional information about a diet history. Find a sample diet history and review its contents. Create a list of questions that would be asked when taking a diet history.

CHAPTER
32 Review

Chapter Summary

SECTION 32.1

- Dietetic aides learn their profession through on-the-job training. Their main responsibility is to ensure that patients receive appropriate meals and snacks. **(pg. 741)**
- Certified dietary managers (CDM) must pass a national certification exam to earn their credentials. Their main responsibility is to manage a food service operation. **(pg. 742)**
- A dietetic technician, registered (DTR) must earn an associate degree and complete an approved training program. Some DTRs work in a clinical setting providing nutrition services to patients. Other DTRs work in a management or food service setting. **(pg. 743)**
- A registered dietitian (RD) must earn a four-year degree and complete an approved training program. A key responsibility of RDs working in a clinical setting is to provide medical nutrition therapy. RDs may also use their knowledge of food and nutrition to work in sales, marketing, public relations, government, food service, fitness centers, food companies, and private practice. **(pg. 744)**

SECTION 32.2

- Food-borne illness may result from eating food that is contaminated with harmful microorganisms. Key steps for preventing food-borne illness are to wash hands often, keep raw meats and ready-to-eat foods separate, cook to proper temperatures, and chill leftovers promptly. **(pg. 747)**
- Surfaces that come in contact with food, such as cutting boards, counters, and utensils, must be cleaned and sanitized often to destroy any harmful bacteria. **(pg. 747)**
- Various categories of patients may need help with eating. Correct positioning is important to prevent choking or aspiration during eating. Hand-over-hand assistance is a technique for helping a patient to eat. **(pg. 750)**
- A therapeutic diet is a special meal plan used to treat or control a condition or a disease. Some types of therapeutic diets require limiting or eliminating certain foods. Others may involve choosing foods for their nutrients or for texture. **(pg. 752)**

Mc Graw Hill connect™ ONLINE ACTIVITIES

Complete our HST online activities for Chapter 32, which include Concept Check review questions, Reference Flash Cards, and Online Procedures assessment sheets.

- **Concept Check** review questions
- **Reference Flash Cards** medical terminology practice
- **Online Procedures** assessment sheets

CHAPTER 32 Assessment

Critical Thinking/Problem Solving

1. An elderly female patient has been admitted to the long-term care facility. You review her chart and find that she is being treated for high blood pressure. You explain that you would like to ask her some questions about what she usually eats. You learn that she has been on a low-sodium diet. You also learn that she has difficulty chewing some foods because of missing several teeth. She also has trouble swallowing dry foods. While you are there, the lunch trays are being delivered. You see that her low-sodium lunch tray includes vegetable soup, a turkey sandwich on a crusty bun, raw carrot sticks, fresh fruit salad, and chocolate chip cookies. She is lying in bed when the tray arrives. What should you do?
2. While preparing trays of food for patients, you notice that an employee who is portioning salad onto plates stops to blow her nose and then continues with her work. What should you do?
3. Obtain a quick-read food thermometer and measure the temperature of various foods in the refrigerator and after cooking or reheating. Compare these temperatures to recommended safe temperatures for refrigerated, cooked, and reheated foods. Explain whether the foods you evaluated would be safe to eat.
4. Examine the nutrition labels from your favorite snack foods. Compare calories, sugar, and sodium content of several snacks. Then compare them to the nutrition facts for healthy snack items such as fruits and vegetables.
5. Using the questions you created for recording a diet history from the Online Activity for Section 32.2 on page 755, take turns completing a diet history with a partner.

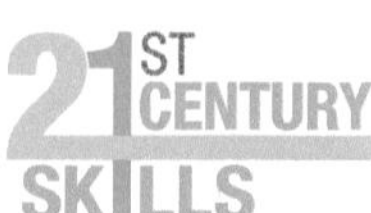

6. **Teamwork** Using the Procedure Troubleshooting in **Procedure 32-2** as a guideline, work with a partner to practice correct positioning for eating and the hand-over-hand assistance technique.
7. **Teamwork/Problem Solving** With a partner, take turns feeding each other lunch or a snack. The partner being fed should be blindfolded and not able to use his or her hands. Write a brief report or describe to your class what it felt like to be fed. What suggestions would you make to improve the way you were fed?
8. **Information Literacy** Search online for information on food-borne illness. Learn about two different types of bacteria that can cause food-borne illness: how these bacteria can contaminate and multiply in food, and specific guidelines for preventing food-borne illnesses caused by these bacteria. Prepare a brief report to share with the class.

UNIT 6

Careers in Biotechnology Research and Development

Photo: Roger Ressmeyer/CORBIS

CHAPTER 33

Biomedical Technology

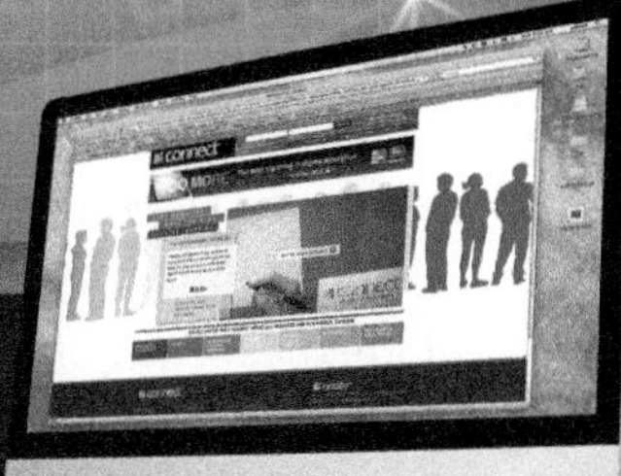

Essential Question:

How can engineering and technology help people with injuries or health problems?

Biomedical engineering and biomedical informatics are branches of biomedical technology, which combines engineering and technology to solve biological or medical problems. Biomedical engineering involves the design, use, and maintenance of devices to diagnose and treat diseases. Biomedical informatics deals with the tracking and measuring of biomedical data. This chapter will introduce you to the key careers in these fields, including the biomedical equipment technician, biomedical engineer, industrial hygienist, bioinformatician, and biostatistician.

Mc Graw Hill **connect**™

It's Online!

- **Online Procedures**
- **STEM Connection**
- **Medical Science**
- **Medical Terms**
- **Medical Math**
- **Ethics in Action**
- **Virtual Lab**

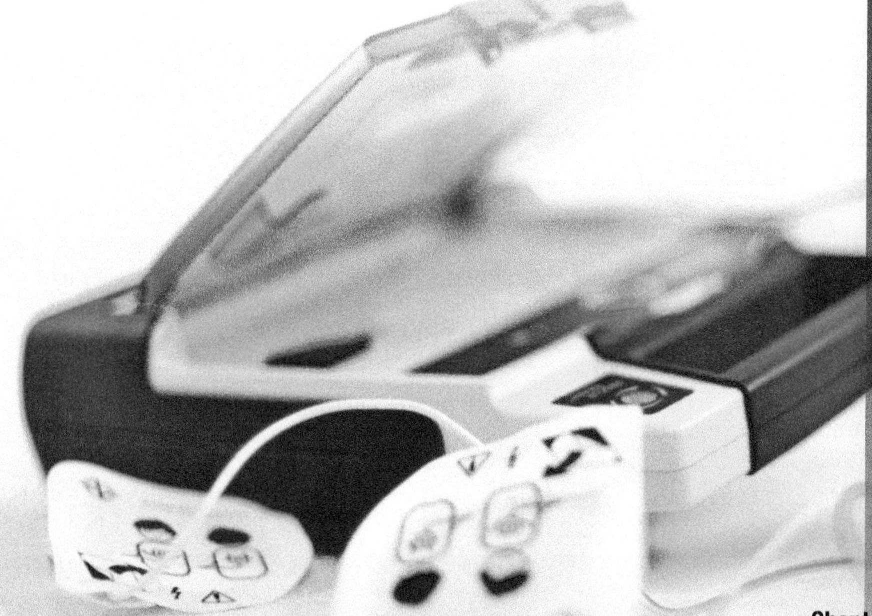

Photo: Gerard Brown/Dorling Kindersley/Getty Images

READING GUIDE

OBJECTIVES

After completing this chapter, you will be able to:

- **Illustrate** the role and responsibilities of a biomedical equipment technician, including at least two safety responsibilities.
- **Compare** the roles and responsibilities of the biomedical engineer and the industrial hygienist.
- **Describe** bioinformatics and the role of the biostatistician.
- **Identify** safe electric current leakage limits for biomedical equipment.
- **Indicate** the two classes of medical equipment that are safety-tested.
- **Recognize** the wire color codes used in hospitals.
- **Explain** the meaning of preventive maintenance, macroshock, and microshock.
- **Demonstrate** one procedure in biomedical technology.

BEFORE YOU READ

Connect Do you enjoy mathematics? Are you interested in engineering? How might those interests lead to a career in healthcare?

Main Idea

Individuals in the field of biomedical technology use advanced technology to help people with diseases or injuries, prevent industrial hazards, and contribute to scientific research in health-related fields.

Note-Taking Activity

Draw this table. Write key terms and phrases under **Cues**. Write main ideas under **Note Taking**. Summarize the section under **Summary**.

Cues	Note Taking
o	o
o	o
Summary	

Graphic Organizer

Before you read the chapter, draw a diagram like the one to the right. As you read, write the careers covered by this chapter into the diagram.

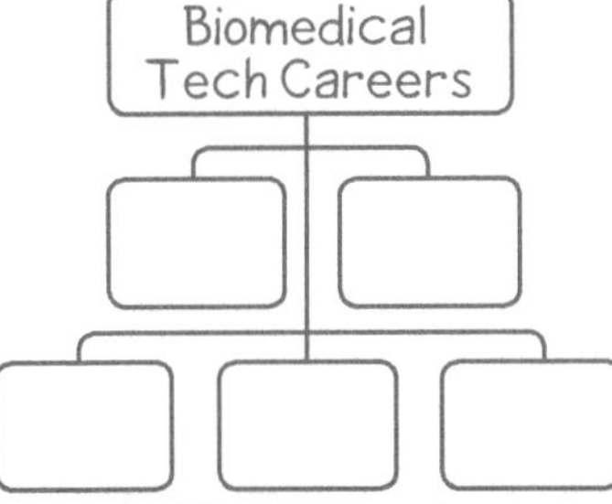

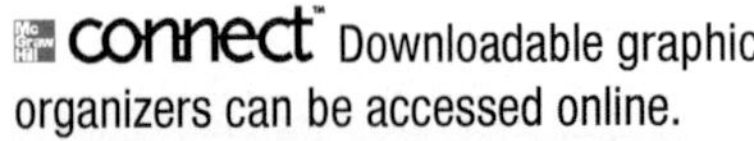

Downloadable graphic organizers can be accessed online.

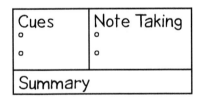

STANDARDS

HEALTH SCIENCE

NCHSE 1.23 Investigate biomedical therapies as they relate to the prevention, pathology, and treatment of disease.

NCHSE 7.31 Apply safety techniques in the work environment.

SCIENCE

NSES E Develop abilities of technological design, understandings about science and technology.

NCHSE *National Consortium for Health Science Education*

NSES *National Science Education Standards*

COMMON CORE STATE STANDARDS

MATHEMATICS

Statistics and Probability

Making Inferences and Justifying Conclusions S-IC Understand and evaluate random processes underlying statistical experiments.

Making Inferences and Justifying Conclusions S-IC 1 Understand statistics as a process for making inferences about population parameters based on a random sample from that population.

ENGLISH LANGUAGE ARTS

Writing

Writing W-7 Conduct short as well as more sustained research projects to answer a question (including a self-generated question) or solve a problem; narrow or broaden the inquiry when appropriate; synthesize multiple sources on the subject, demonstrating understanding of the subject under investigation.

SECTION

33.1 Careers in Biomedical Technology

The Biomedical Equipment Technician

Why must a biomedical equipment technician be both flexible and reassuring?

Do the areas of mechanics and electronics interest you? Are you good with your hands? Would you like to apply your problem-solving skills in the healthcare field? If your answer to these questions is yes, consider a career as a biomedical equipment technician (BMET). The need for specialized technicians in the biomedical equipment area arose when physicians, scientists, and engineers first combined their skills to develop complex equipment to diagnose, prevent, and cure disease and illness.

A biomedical equipment technician is a person who is knowledgeable about the theory and operation of biomedical equipment; the principles behind the operation and maintenance of that equipment; and the safe and efficient use of that equipment in hopsital, clinical, and other settings. The responsibilities of the biomedical equipment technician may include the installation, calibration, inspection, preventive maintenance, and repair of general biomedical and related technical equipment. He or she may also be responsible for the operation or supervision of equipment control, safety, and maintenance programs, as well as for training others in the use of biomedical equipment. **Figure 33.1** shows one type of equipment maintained by BMETs.

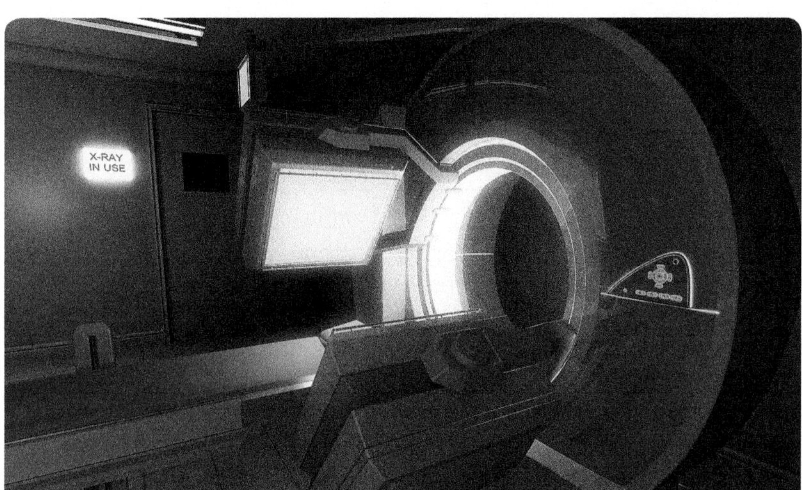

Fig. 33.1 Biomedical Equipment Technician BMETs know about the theory of operation, underlying physiologic principles, and clinical application of biomedical equipment. *What are some duties of the BMET?*

Photo: MedicalRF.com/Getty Images

Vocabulary

Content Vocabulary

You will learn these content vocabulary terms in this section.

- **calibration**
- **National Fire Protection Association (NFPA)**
- **Safe Medical Devices Act (SMDA)**
- **Emergency Care Research Institute (ECRI)**
- **prosthetic device**
- **data mining**
- **algorithm**

Academic Vocabulary

You will see this word in your reading and on your tests. Find its meaning in the Glossary in the back of the book.

- **interact**

A BMET must be flexible because a BMET rarely has an "ordinary" day. For example, you may be performing preventive maintenance on a hospital bed and suddenly be called to one of the operating rooms to stand by during a heart transplant. You may be called to a critical care area of the hospital to repair a faulty respirator while manual artificial respiration is being performed on a patient. Service emergencies caused by faulty equipment may require a BMET to change plans at a moment's notice and handle an urgent situation with a cool head, expertise, and knowledge of the environment.

See **Table 33.1** for an overview of careers in biomedical technology.

It is also important for the BMET to convey confidence during a crisis, when staff and patients may need assurance. Yet regardless of emergencies and urgent requests, BMETs must never let regular schedules and routine maintenance slide.

Table 33.1 Overview of Careers in Biomedical Technology

OCCUPATION	EDUCATIONAL REQUIREMENTS	CERTIFICATION OR LICENSING AGENCY	JOB OUTLOOK
Biomedical Equipment Technician	An associate degree in applied science, specializing in biomedical electronics, is preferred.	Certification from the Association for the Advancement of Medical Instrumentation (AAMI) or the Institute for the Certification of Engineering Technicians (ICET)	Faster than average growth because of the developments in and increased use of complex medical devices
Biomedical Engineer	A four-year degree is required for almost all entry-level jobs. In some cases, an associate degree in biomedical electronics will be accepted.	Degree from a program accredited by the Biomedical Engineering Society	Much faster than average due to aging populations and growing focus on health issues
Industrial Hygienist	A four-year degree in safety or a related field is required.	Certification from the Board of Certified Safety Professionals and the American Board of Industrial Hygiene.	Faster than average growth
Bioinformatician (Bioinformatics Associate, Scientist, or Specialist)	Associate or bachelor's degree is the minimum. A master's degree or doctorate may be required for more advanced positions.	For some positions, additional certification programs are required after completion of a bachelor's degree	Above average growth with more positions available for individuals with post graduate degrees
Biostatistician	Federal government jobs require at least a bachelor's degree. A master's degree in statistics or mathematics is often the minimum educational requirement.	Certification programs may be taken after completion of bachelor's or master's degree	Above average growth

The Job of the Biomedical Equipment Technician

Biomedical equipment technicians inspect, maintain, repair, calibrate, and modify electronic, electrical, mechanical, and other equipment and instruments used in medical therapy, diagnosis, and research. **Calibration** ensures that the instrument is operating at its intended settings. BMETs may be involved in the operation or supervision of equipment and in equipment control.

The job of the BMET involves many different areas, including:

- Ensuring that equipment is operating safely
- Evaluating equipment for servicing
- Repairing equipment
- Maintaining parts inventories
- Carrying out preventive maintenance
- Keeping complete and accurate maintenance and service records
- Making recommendations on replacement equipment
- Training personnel on the use and care of equipment
- Reading professional journals and manufacturers' publications to evaluate and recommend purchase of new, more advanced medical equipment and to keep up with new developments in the field

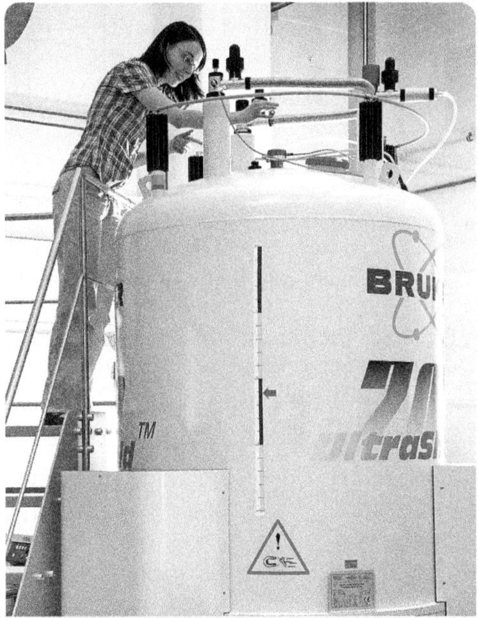

Fig. 33.2 BMETs are Mechanically Inclined As a biomedical equipment technician, you may be called upon to repair complex electrical equipment. *What kinds of skills are called for in equipment repair?*

Photo: Jochen Tack/Alamy

The need for biomedical equipment technicians is universal. Some BMETs work in large hospitals where they maintain diagnostic and lifesaving equipment. Others work for medical equipment manufacturers and distributors, medical supply firms, medical research organizations, and teaching establishments.

As seen in **Figure 33.2**, BMETs should have better than average manual dexterity. They must be mechanically and electronically inclined. The prospective biomedical equipment technician must also be safety-oriented. The work will involve electricity, compressed gas, and radiation—all areas in which safety is of primary concern.

BMETs act as a channel of communication between the disciplines of engineering and the life sciences because of their knowledge of both the technical aspects of a device and the clinical applications of the device. They play a unique dual role. They provide in-service training for the staff that uses the equipment and they modify medical devices based on the needs of the clinician. Much of their time is spent communicating with device manufacturers, users, and nursing educators. Given the frequent need to explain and teach the proper use and care of equipment, a BMET must be able to interact effectively with all levels of hospital staff.

The BMET works closely with physicians, nurses, engineers, and other hospital personnel to keep diagnostic and life-sustaining equipment operating safely and effectively. This may involve explaining the basics of electronic equipment and why it is no longer cost-effective to repair outdated equipment.

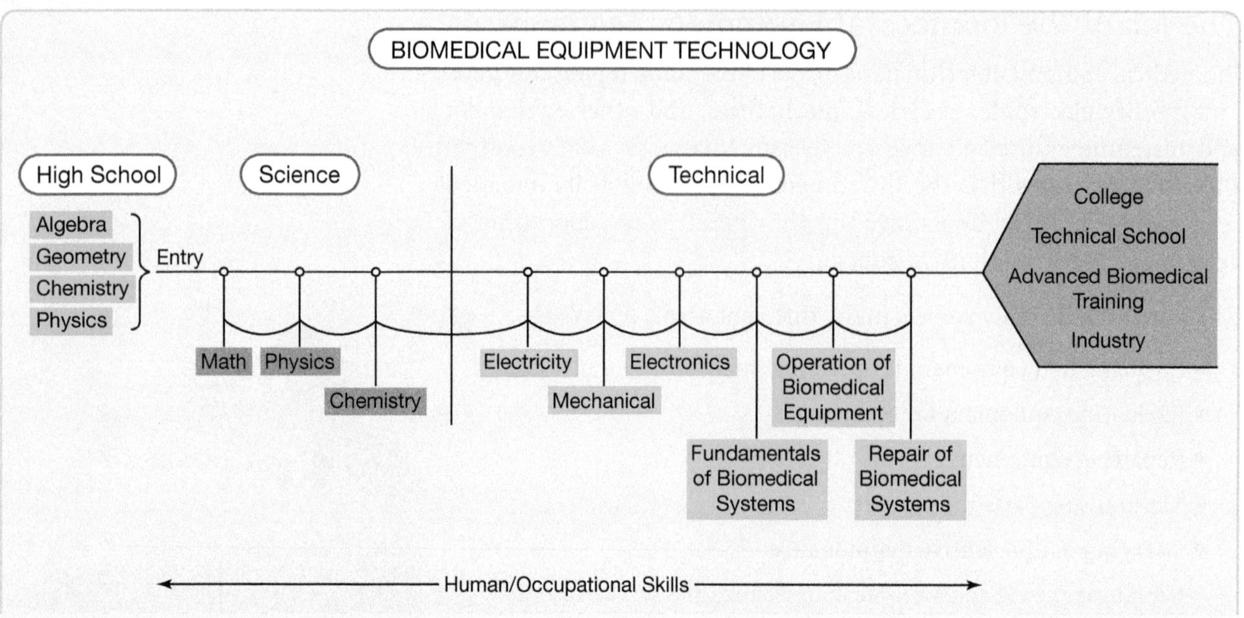

Fig. 33.3 Technician Courses Common biomedical technician courses. *What are two important science classes for a prospective BMET?*

Since BMETs work with physicians, nurses, hospital administrators, purchasing agents, and other personnel, they must be able to positively interact with all kinds of people. You may have direct or indirect contact with ill or injured persons. You must be able to maintain your composure around stressed medical personnel, patients, and family members while assessing and working on equipment.

The BMET must be enthusiastically open to technological change. You must be eager to read professional journals and study technical data, attend manufacturers' equipment seminars, and use all possible resources to keep current on new developments.

Individuals entering biomedical careers frequently train in laboratories and hospitals, where they work with medical instrumentation. You may complete part of your training as an intern for a medical facility while you are taking the courses for an associate of applied science (AAS) degree. **Figure 33.3** shows common courses needed for a biomedical technician degree. After you have earned your degree and are employed, you may have the opportunity to receive additional hospital-sponsored training on specific medical equipment to fill technical gaps in your training. You may become an expert in a particular subject, such as medical imaging, which includes ultrasound and magnetic resonance imaging. Most of these employer-sponsored programs are based on hands-on instruction.

BMETs must know how to install, operate, and troubleshoot a wide variety of diagnostic and therapeutic medical equipment. They use schematic diagrams, precision hand tools, and sophisticated electronic test equipment to install, inspect, test, maintain, calibrate, and repair equipment. Technicians test electronic circuits and components to find faulty circuits or connections and failed components. They use state-of-the-art soldering techniques to replace and repair faulty circuits.

They must be able to diagnose where the problem lies and be able to replace the faulty component. All BMETs should understand how separate equipment components interact with one another. For example, a multifunctional patient-monitoring equipment monitors blood pressure, pulse, respiration, and temperature (see **Figure 33.4**).

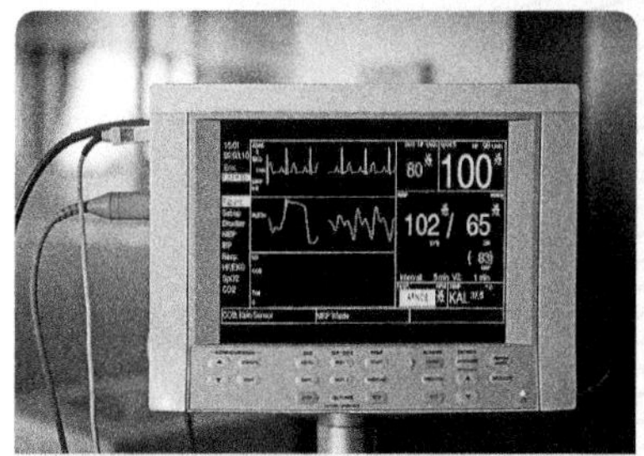

Fig. 33.4 Specialized Equipment A continuous vital sign monitor. *Why would a BMET come in contact with this piece of equipment?*

Safety Concerns of the Biomedical Equipment Technician

The primary concern of the BMET is safety (see **Figure 33.5**). Patients have sometimes been seriously harmed by malfunctioning medical equipment. They have been crushed by electric hospital beds and shocked by improperly maintained equipment.

Under guidelines set forth by the **National Fire Protection Association (NFPA)** and the Association for the Advancement of Medical Instrumentation (AAMI), BMETs conduct safety inspections of electrical equipment in healthcare facilities. However, their training and abilities allow them to go well beyond this function.

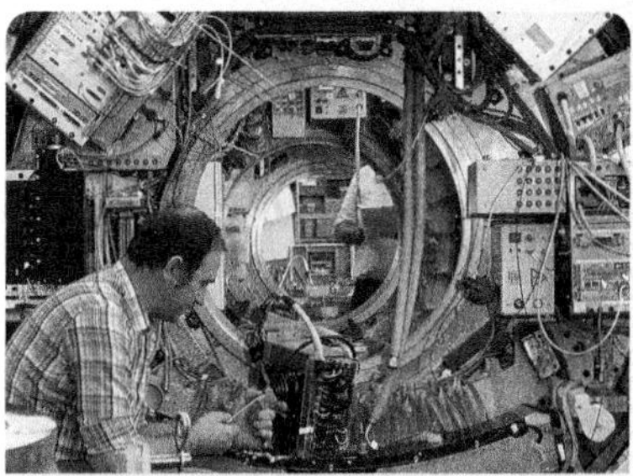

Fig. 33.5 Safety Testing A primary concern of the BMET is safety. *Why must safety tests be performed on biomedical equipment?*

If there is an accident, the BMET can play a role in the incident investigation. The **Safe Medical Devices Act (SMDA)** requires that patient injuries related to medical devices be reported to the device manufacturer and to the Food and Drug Administration (FDA). One section of the SMDA requires the tracking of certain types of medical devices in case such a device has to be recalled. The BMET should be able to coordinate all types of medical device recalls, regardless of whether the FDA, the manufacturer, or a third-party organization such as the **Emergency Care Research Institute (ECRI)** initiates the recall.

READING CHECK

List some types of equipment that the BMET is responsible for testing and maintaining.

The Biomedical Engineer

How has engineering changed healthcare?

Biomedical engineers use their skills to analyze and solve problems in biology and medicine. Since their job involves the design and development of biomedical equipment, this position requires a high level of knowledge and skill in engineering disciplines, a background in physiology and anatomy, and a practical ability in specialized subject matter areas such as computer systems, electronics, or mathematics. Those who choose to work in a hospital environment are sometimes called clinical engineers.

You may consider this field if you want to help people while also applying your technical skills and knowledge. Biomedical engineers are particularly interested in using advanced technology to solve some of the complex problems of healthcare.

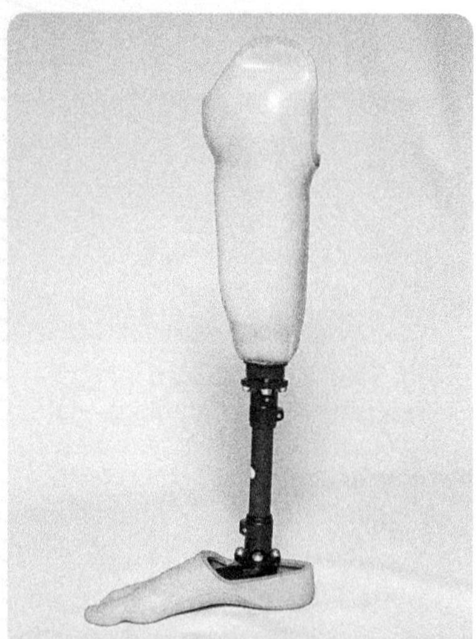

Fig. 33.6 Biomedical Engineering A biomedical engineer might develop a prosthetic leg. *Which specialty of biomedical engineering would develop a prosthetic device such as this one?*

Many schools across the nation offer programs for prospective biomedical engineers. Associate degrees in biomedical engineering technology, as well as bachelor's, master's, and Ph.D. programs in biomedical engineering, are available. These programs add life sciences courses to a basic electronics or mechanical engineering program.

The Job of the Biomedical Engineer

The well-prepared biomedical engineer can work in any one of the many specialized areas of biomedical engineering. Examples of such specialties are biomaterials, biomechanics, medical imaging, rehabilitation, and orthopedic engineering. For example, a biomedical engineer specializing in orthopedic engineering may develop a **prosthetic device** such as an artificial arm or leg (see **Figure 33.6**).

Medical device manufacturers hire biomedical engineers for positions in areas such as marketing, research and development, product design and testing, hardware design, software development, clinical evaluations, production, technical support, bench repair, clinical support, and field service, to name a few.

The biomedical engineer works with other healthcare professionals including physicians, nurses, therapists, and technicians. They may be called upon to perform a wide range of jobs including designing instruments, devices, and software.

The Job Responsibilities of the Biomedical Engineer

The job responsibilities of biomedical engineers depends on their area of specialization and place of employment. They may:

- Develop devices such as hearing aids; cardiac pacemakers; artificial kidneys and hearts; synthetic blood vessels; and prosthetic joints, arms, and legs
- Design computerized blood sample analyzers, cardiac catheters, and other equipment for use in clinical laboratories
- Develop medical imaging systems such as ultrasound, computer assisted tomography (CAT), magnetic resonance imaging (MRI), and positron emission tomography (PET)
- Develop therapeutic and surgical devices, such as laser systems for eye surgery and automated delivery of insulin
- Oversee automated patient monitoring during surgery or in intensive care, and monitoring healthy people in unusual environments such as space
- Advise on sports medicine, rehabilitation, and support devices
- Set up computerized modeling of physiological systems such as cardiovascular, renal, and visual and auditory systems

READING CHECK

Recall some types of devices developed by biomedical engineers.

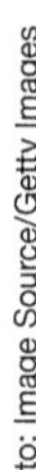
Photo: Image Source/Getty Images

Industrial Hygienist

What workplace environments most benefit from the work of industrial hygienists?

Industrial hygienists, also known as occupational health and safety inspectors, specialists, or technicians, help keep workplaces and workers safe. They promote health and safety by finding safer, healthier, and more efficient ways of working.

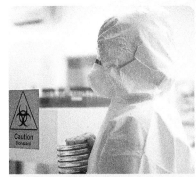

Fig. 33.7 Industrial Hygienist An industrial hygienist is checking the environment. *What type of accident may have occurred here?*

The Job of an Industrial Hygienist

Industrial hygienists look for conditions and practices that are not safe. They may check the environment after a chemical or radiation spill (see **Figure 33.7**). Sometimes they apply the scientific method to develop ways of predicting possible hazards in current or future systems, equipment, products, facilities, or processes. They base those forecasts on experience, historical data, and other sources.

After reviewing causes and effects of a hazard, the industrial hygienist assesses the chances of an accident taking place and estimates how severe that accident might be. For example, he or she might discover patterns in injury data that indicate a specific recurring cause, such as system failure or incomplete or faulty decision making.

Industrial hygienists develop and help enforce plans to eliminate hazards. They conduct training sessions on health and safety practices and regulations. They may check on the progress of the safety plan after it has been implemented. If improvements are not satisfactory, a new plan may be designed and put into practice.

All occupational health and safety specialists and technicians are trained in the applicable laws or inspection procedures through some combination of classroom and on-the-job training. In general, people who want to enter this occupation should have a high sense of responsibility and should be capable of detailed work.

The Job Responsibilities of the Industrial Hygienist

The industrial hygienist analyzes work environments and designs programs to prevent or control disease or injury caused by chemical, physical, biological agents, or ergonomic factors. The industrial hygienist may conduct inspections and enforce adherence to laws, regulations, or employer policies governing worker health and safety.

Their job may include some or all of the following duties:

- Inspect and test machinery and equipment, such as lifting devices, machine shields, and scaffolding, to ensure that they meet appropriate safety regulations.
- Check that personal protective equipment—such as masks, respirators, safety glasses, and safety helmets—are being used in workplaces according to regulations.

Photo: Adam Gault/Getty Images

- Check that dangerous materials are stored correctly.
- Test and identify work areas for potential accident and health hazards, such as toxic fumes and explosive gas-air mixtures, and implement appropriate control measures, such as adjustments to ventilation systems.
- Prepare and calibrate scientific equipment.
- Investigate unsafe working conditions, study possible causes, and recommend remedial action.
- Assist with the rehabilitation of workers after accidents and injuries and make sure that they return to work successfully.
- Prepare reports including observations, analyses of contaminants, and recommendations for control and correction of hazards.

READING CHECK

Name some types of hazards investigated and monitored by industrial hygienists.

Bioinformatics as a Career

What connection can there be between the study of biology and the field of computer science?

Bioinformatics combines health sciences (such as medicine, dentistry, nursing, pharmacy, and allied health) with computer science, management and decision science, biostatistics, engineering, and information technology. Its purpose is to solve problems in healthcare delivery, pharmaceutical, biomedical and health sciences research, health education and clinical or medical decision making. Bioinformatics, also known as biomedical and health informatics, is essential in all aspects of healthcare and biomedicine.

Bioinformatics blends computer science and biology in order to process, sort, analyze, and compare biological data. It applies principles of computer and information science to the advancement of life sciences research, health professions education, public health, and patient care.

Bioinformatics professionals may be associates, scientists, or specialists, depending upon their level of training, experience, and job functions. They use sophisticated computer programs to gather, analyze and track data about specific biological functions or characteristics in order to gain a better understanding of complex biological activities.

Bioinformatics professionals may engage in **data mining.** Data mining is the process of extracting patterns from large data sets by combining methods from statistics and artificial intelligence with database management.

Careers in bioinformatics exist in clinical care and research, personal health management for patients and consumers, public and population health, health policy, and translational science (translating basic genetic discoveries to improve personal healthcare). Bioinformaticians help in the design, implementation, and use of systems that manage increasing amounts of complex information emerging from healthcare research and delivery. For example a bioinformatics scientist may map DNA or study the properties and characteristics of cells.

To enter this field you must have a strong math and science background and interest in mastering advanced computer skills. You should also be detail-oriented and capable of collecting and analyzing large amounts of data. Bioinformatics programs expand on this background by integrating the study of biology with the study of information systems and computer science.

The Job Responsibilities of the Bioinformatician

The following is a list of job responsibilities that a bioinformatics professional may perform.

- Build programs by using computational formulas to determine outcomes based on biological projects or research.
- Develop software, creating query routines and building relational databases.
- Apply problem-solving **algorithms** to data collected. Algorithms are a set of rules used to solve a problem in a finite number of steps.
- Provide information systems support for a laboratory or research project based on knowledge of medical information systems.

READING CHECK

Explain the purpose of data mining.

Biostatistician

With what types of statistics do biostatisticians work?

Biostatisticians develop and apply statistical methods to scientific research in health-related fields, including medicine, epidemiology, and public health. Biostatisticians work in a wide range of industries, including pharmaceuticals, biotechnology, medicine, healthcare, clinical trials, health education, software development, and other specialized fields in science and medicine. Employment opportunities for the biostatistician can be found in hospitals, research centers, universities, pharmaceutical companies, government agencies, or in a number of other organizations that support statistical research in the health sciences.

Biostatisticians work to address medical questions using established statistical methods. In addition, they also develop new statistical techniques. New techniques for analyzing data are being developed as

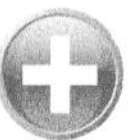 connect 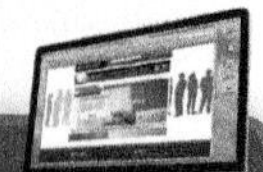

STEM CONNECTION

Medical Science

Scientific Notation

Scientific notation is a way of writing numbers that accommodates values too large or small to be conveniently written in standard decimal format. Scientific notation may be needed when a research study involves a large number of participants. In scientific notation, the numbers are written like this: "$a \times 10^b$" which means "*a* times [ten to the power of *b*]."

connect Go online to learn more about scientific notation and complete the related activity.

quickly as new medical questions arise. Biostatisticians provide information that plays a large role in informing policy makers and the public about health issues. Statistics help in determining risk and protective factors affecting heart and lung disease, in formulating new policies to combat infectious diseases, in assessing environmental protection guidelines, injury risk management, or various cancer treatment outcomes.

The Job Responsibilities of the Biostatistician

The following are some of the biostatistician's possible job responsibilities.

- Assist in formulating medical and health-related questions that can be answered through the use of statistics.
- Develop and apply statistical methods to medical and health-related research.
- Design studies and analyze study data.
- Determine appropriate sampling techniques.
- Coordinate data collection procedures.
- Assist in preparing research material for publication.

READING CHECK

Explain how statistics can help in the development of healthcare practices.

SECTION 33.1 Careers in Biomedical Technology Review

AFTER YOU READ

1. **Describe** the kind of training you would be called upon to provide as a BMET.
2. **Explain** why a BMET must have knowledge of human anatomy and physiology.
3. **Recall** the name of the primary organization for certification of BMETs.
4. **Identify** the BMET's main safety concern.
5. **Name** three types of devices or systems a biomedical engineer might work with.
6. **Describe** the primary responsibility of an industrial hygienist.
7. **Name** the three professional levels in the career of bioinformatician.
8. **Compare** the meaning of the terms "data mining" and "algorithm."

Technology ONLINE EXPLORATIONS

Biomedical Research

Conduct online research on one of the following topics introduced in this Section: algorithms, data mining, bioinformatics, calibration, biomedical engineering, or prosthetic device. Create a brief report or presentation, with illustrations, on the topic you selected.

SECTION 33.2 Biomedical Technology Procedures

Overview of Biomedical Technology Procedures

Who is responsible for maintaining a hospital's biomedical equipment?

The **Association for the Advancement of Medical Instrumentation (AAMI)** brings physicians, equipment manufacturers, and biomedical engineers together to solve common problems arising from the use of medical equipment. The AAMI developed the first standards for the manufacture and safety of medical equipment. If biomedical equipment is not serviced precisely, diagnostic errors can occur and possibly lead to serious medical complications. Also, by performing routine, scheduled service on medical devices, hospitals achieve an improved level of equipment performance and safety, extended life of the equipment, and decreased equipment downtime.

The types of equipment for which a biomedical equipment technology department may be responsible vary widely from hospital to hospital. Among the many types of biomedical equipment are pacemakers, electrocardiographs (ECG), heart-lung bypass equipment, kidney dialysis machines, blood pressure monitors, centrifuges, chemical analyzers, X-ray machines, spectrophotometers, electroencephalographs (EEG), ultrasonic devices, patient-monitoring equipment, electronic laboratory equipment, operating room equipment, hypothermia equipment, electrosurgery units, respirators, and sterilizers (see **Figure 33.8**). Biomedical engineers design this equipment, and industrial hygienists ensure the safety of the environment in which it is used.

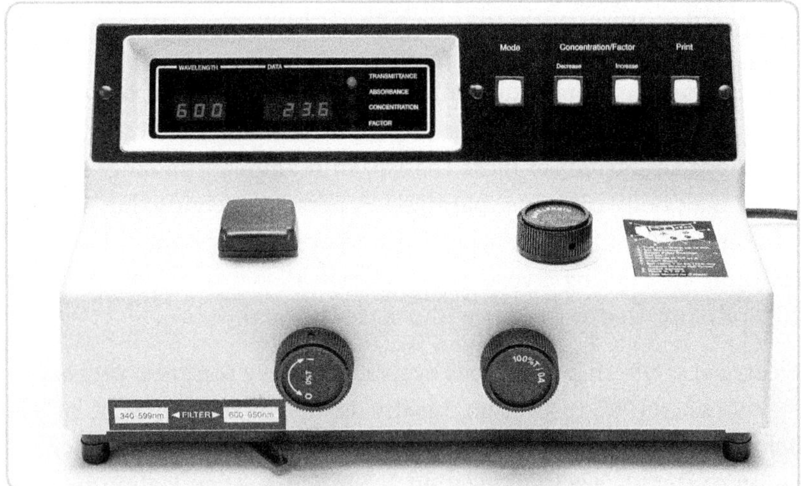

Fig. 33.8 Spectrophotometer Measuring the amount of color in a solution, this spectrophotometer uses two drops of liquid on the palm of the hand to determine a cholesterol level. *Why would it be important to monitor a patient's cholesterol level?*

Vocabulary

Content Vocabulary

You will learn these content vocabulary terms in this section.

- **Association for the Advancement of Medical Instrumentation (AAMI)**
- **telemedicine**
- **teleradiology**
- **asset management**
- **ampere**
- **microampere (μA)**
- **preventive maintenance (PM)**
- **The Joint Commission (TJC)**
- **medical treatment facility (MTF)**
- **electrically sensitive patient location (ESPL)**
- **leakage current**
- **macroshock**
- **microshock**

Academic Vocabulary

You will see this word in your reading and on your tests. Find its meaning in the Glossary in the back of the book.

- cycle

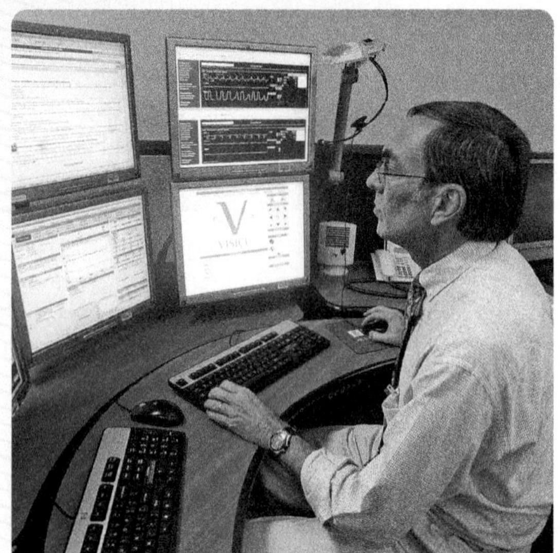

Fig. 33.9 eICU Biomedical equipment allows several patients to be monitored from a single location. *What is this type of medicine called?*

A traditional biomedical technology department may be responsible only for those devices used specifically for diagnosis or therapy. However, many biomedical technology departments have expanded into telecommunications and information systems. A few cutting-edge departments are also working in **telemedicine** and **teleradiology.** In telemedicine, telecommunications equipment transmits the image of, and general information about, a patient to a distant site. Through teleradiology, an X-ray image is transmitted to a distant site, where a specialist will examine the image and develop a diagnosis based on it.

One type of telemedical equipment is an eICU (see **Figure 33.9**), which allows healthcare professionals at one location to monitor patients remotely. Patients are diagnosed and monitored electronically through the Internet or by satellite communication.

Biomedical engineering departments perform many functions. To provide the best service support possible, it is important to be involved in the life cycle of a product from its inception. Evaluations by the biomedical equipment department can help reduce costs by ensuring that proper warranties, service training, repair parts, and other long-term expenses are considered when a purchase is made. By controlling the costs of purchases, maintenance, depreciation, disposition, and other aspects of the life cycle of medical equipment, BMETs provide a service called **asset management.**

READING CHECK

Explain the role telecommunications plays in a biomedical setting.

connect

STEM CONNECTION

Medical Science

Ampere

An **ampere** (A) is a unit of electric current. It is defined as the amount of charge flowing per unit of time. The milliampere (mA) is a rather small amount of electrical current. Smaller still is the **microampere** (μA), which is one-millionth (0.000001) of an ampere.

connect Go online to learn about the measurement of charge in household batteries, a defibrillator, and a bolt of lightning, then complete the related activity..

Safety

How much electricity can the human body safely receive?

One of the most vital duties of the biomedical engineering department is to ensure the safety of equipment. The greatest hazard is electric shock. A current of more than 10 milliamperes passing through the human body can cause paralysis. A person receiving that amount of electricity would not be able to let go of its source and thus would continue conducting a very unsafe electrical charge. If the current is 100 milliamperes or more, the shock can be fatal.

Electrical safety inspection has evolved to a very complete **preventive maintenance (PM)** inspection, mostly due to the requirements of **The Joint Commission (TJC)** (formerly the Joint Commission on Accreditation of Healthcare Organizations). TJC is the organization responsible for accrediting hospitals.

Electrical Safety Testing

Electrical safety principles can be summarized in five words: Keep electricity in its place.

An electrocution hazard exists only when a difference of potential (voltage) exists. The greatest hazard you will encounter if you sit on a 22,000-volt power line is that you might fall off and break something—unless you happen to come into contact with some point that has a different potential, such as the tower, another wire, or a ground. (This is why birds can safely perch on a power line without being electrocuted.) All voltages are referenced to earth ground, which is zero volts. A ground wire will safely eliminate or reduce current leakage by sending it to earth ground.

Electric wires, plugs, and outlets used in a **medical treatment facility (MTF)** are color-coded. **Table 33.2** and **Table 33.3** illustrate the color codes of various electric components. Hospital-grade outlets, which meet additional requirements for durability and grounding, are indicated by a green dot (see **Figure 33.10**).

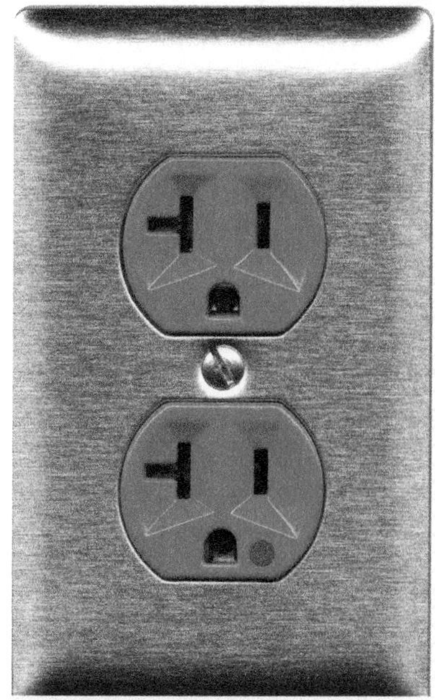

Fig. 33.10 Electrical Safety
This is a typical hospital electrical outlet. *What does the green dot indicate?*

Table 33.2 Coding for Plugs and Receptacles (Outlets)

TYPE OF PLUG OR RECEPTACLE	INDEXED (POLARIZED)	COLOR OF WIRE	COLOR OF SCREW
Large spade shape	Neutral or common	White	Silver
Small spade shape	Hot	Black	Brass
Round lug in the middle	Ground	Green	Green

Table 33.3 Coding for Electric Wire

ELECTRIC WIRE COLOR	TYPE OF WIRE
White	Neutral
Black	Hot (electrically charged)
Green	Ground

In a hospital, patients may be susceptible to electric shock because they are in contact with numerous electric devices, such as blood pressure measurement machines. Electric shock is when an electrical current flows in and through the body. It can cause involuntary muscle tissue contractions, severe burns, paralysis, and death. When blood pressure measurement devices are used in the home or in mass screenings, electric shock is rare, since the user is not normally connected to the device's electric circuit and is not usually attached to other electric devices at the same time.

Electric currents that continue for more than one heart cycle may cause heart fibrillation. The current stops the heart from beating as long as the current flows. The heartbeat and normal circulation may be able to resume when the current ceases. High current can produce respiratory paralysis, which may be reversed with immediate resuscitation.

Table 33.4 Current in Electric Shock

CURRENT IN MILLIAMPERES (MA)	EFFECTS
Less than 1 mA	No sensation and no perceptible effect.
More than 3 mA	Perceptible shock producing the reflex action to jump away. No direct danger from shock, but sudden motion may result in injury.
6 mA	Painful shocks.
9 mA	"Let-go" current for women.
10–15 mA	"Let-go" current for men.
30–50 mA	Local muscle contractions. "Freezing" to the source of electricity for 2.5% of the population.
50–100 mA	Local muscle contractions. "Freezing" to the source of electricity for 50% of the population.
100–200 mA	Prolonged contact may cause collapse and unconsciousness. Death may occur after three minutes of contact because of paralysis of the respiratory muscles.

Severe burns to the skin and internal organs may result in irreparable body damage. **Table 33.4** provides information about the effect of various amounts of electric current on the human body.

Equipment Classes

The two classes of medical equipment are class A and class B.

Class A Equipment is used in critical patient care areas. Typically, the patient has a direct line of electrical conduction to the heart via an infusion line (IV). Operating rooms, emergency rooms, and recovery rooms are all examples of class A areas. Examples of class A equipment are electrosurgical units, defibrillators, pacemakers, intensive care patient monitoring equipment such as cardiac monitors, surgical tables, and intermittent positive pressure breathing (IPPB) apparatus. Areas containing this kind of equipment are classed as **electrically sensitive patient locations (ESPLs)**.

Class B Equipment areas are defined as general patient care and examination areas. Patients in these areas are not usually connected to electronic monitoring equipment and do not have a direct line for electrical conduction to the heart. Examples of class B equipment are examination tables, electric hospital beds, and laboratory equipment.

Leakage Current

Leakage current is naturally occurring current that results from distributed capacitance within equipment or power cords and that leaks from the electronics to the metal chassis of the equipment to ground.

Leakage at certain levels presents an electrical hazard. The acceptable leakage current of equipment in class A or ESPL areas is 10 μA (μ stands for micro, 0.000001, or one-millionth). The acceptable leakage current of class B equipment is 500 μA. If the leakage current in microampheres exceeds that level, the equipment must be immediately removed from service and repaired.

The six main categories of leakage currents are:

- **Loss of instrument ground.** All electric line operated equipment has some leakage current. This leakage is determined by the geometry and construction of the instrument (see **Figure 33.11**). If the electric cord ground is lost, the leakage current may find a return path to ground through the patient or operator.
- **Voltage variations caused by inadequate grounding or improper ground wiring.** Leakage currents flowing through ground wires can produce voltage variations. All equipment should be plugged in as close to the patient as possible as voltage may vary on receptacles located farther away. **Figure 33.12** shows an unintentional current path.
- **Current originating from an instrument during use on a patient.** This conduction can occur if a component in a monitoring device becomes defective. Breakdowns can occur on monitors, for example, during defibrillation or electrosurgery. The patient's monitoring leads can conduct electricity directly to the heart.
- **Inducted current from high-energy sources.** Magnetic fields, radio stations, cell phones, and ultrasound units can accumulate energy and generate enough current into a monitor lead to put a cardiac patient at risk.
- **Self-generating currents or voltage differentials.** Dissimilar metals may generate currents. Static charge may be generated by walking on carpet, moving blankets, and lightning.
- **Other modes of leakage or means of generating current.** These are biological or physical forms of energy conversion. Bioelectricity is generated by the cells of the body. A thermocouple is an example of physical electricity generated by heat.

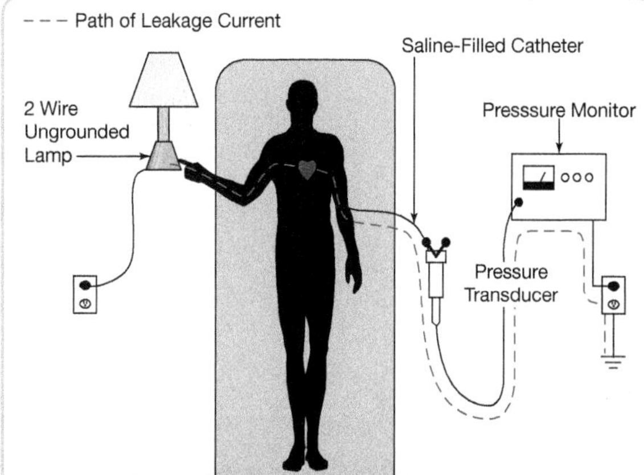

Fig. 33.11 Leakage Current Path The path of leakage current from an ungrounded lamp through a patient to a bedside monitor. *Why is this an electrocution hazard?*

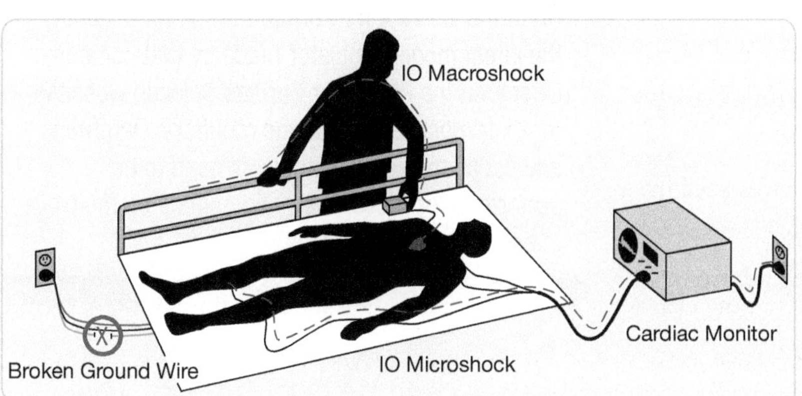

Fig. 33.12 Unintentional Current Path The broken ground wire puts this patient at risk of electrocution. *A cardiac monitor is in which class of medical equipment? What is the acceptable level of leakage for this class?*

Macroshock and Microshock **Macroshock** is a large value of electric current that passes on the skin from one arm to the other. **Microshock** is a small value of electric current that passes directly through the heart. Because electric current is applied directly to the heart via the use of catheters or IVs, microshock is more likely to be fatal than macroshock. This current is measured in microamperes (μA).

READING CHECK

Explain the difference between class A and class B equipment.

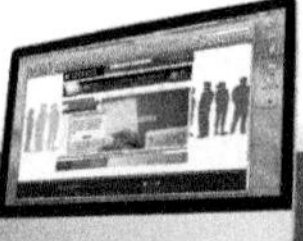

connect ONLINE PROCEDURES

PROCEDURE 33-1

Performing an Electrical Safety Test

An electrical safety test is performed to determine the amount of leakage current produced by a piece of equipment. Electrical safety testing is performed on a routine basis, depending upon the location and type of equipment.

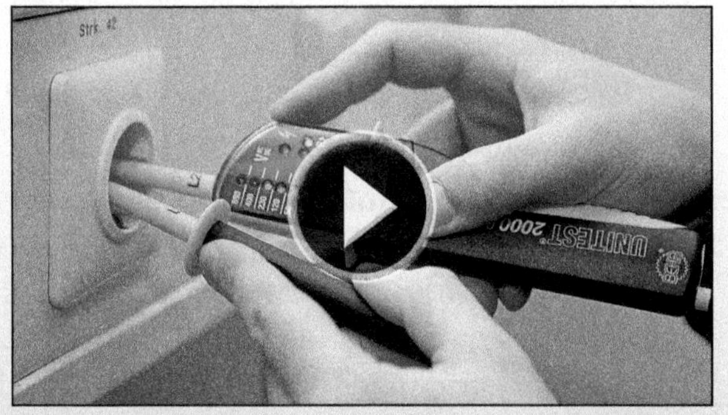

SECTION 33.2 Biomedical Technology Procedures Review

AFTER YOU READ

1. **Name** at least three types of biomedical equipment.
2. **Define** asset management.
3. **Identify** the current leakage limit for a class A area.
4. **Identify** the current leakage limit for a class B area.
5. **List** the color codes for the three wires used in medical equipment cables.
6. **Name** the two ways of identifying a hospital-grade plug.
7. **Define** leakage current.

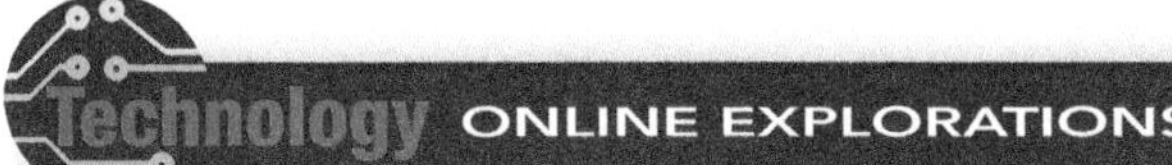

Technology ONLINE EXPLORATIONS

Equipment Maintenance

Go to the website for Puritan Bennett and identify the latest model ventilator made by that company. Or search the Phillips or Cardiac Science websites for their most recent cardiac monitors. Determine and list all the services that will need to be performed for preventive maintenance on the piece of equipment you selected.

Photo: Olaf Doering/Alamy

CHAPTER
33 Review

Chapter Summary

SECTION 33.1

- Biomedical equipment technicians (BMETs) service complex equipment that is used to diagnose, prevent, and cure disease. BMETs are responsible for maintaining the safety of equipment in a medical facility. **(pg. 761)**
- The biomedical engineer designs and develops medical equipment. **(pg. 765)**
- The industrial hygienist evaluates the safety of workplaces. **(pg. 767)**
- The field of bioinformatics combines health sciences with computer science, management and decision science, engineering and information technology. Its purpose is to solve problems in healthcare delivery; pharmaceutical, biomedical and health sciences research; health education; and clinical and medical decision making. **(pg. 768)**
- Biostatisticians develop and apply statistical methods to scientific research in health-related fields using established statistical methods and also by developing new statistical techniques. **(pg. 769)**

SECTION 33.2

- Electrical wires, plugs, and outlets for use in hospital settings are color-coded and designated "hospital grade." **(pg. 773)**
- Electrical safety checks are conducted on a regular basis on all medical equipment. **(pg. 773)**
- Medical equipment is classified as class A and class B, depending on location and usage. **(pg. 774)**
- The acceptable leakage currents of equipment located in class A or ESPL areas is 10 μA. The acceptable leakage current of equipment located in class B areas is 500 μA. **(pg. 774)**
- Macroshock is a large-value electric current that passes from one arm to the other arm, usually across the skin. Microshock is a small-value electric current that passes directly through the heart and may be fatal. **(pg. 776)**

Mc Graw Hill connect™ ONLINE ACTIVITIES

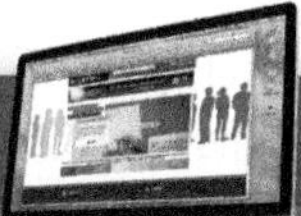

Complete our HST online activities for Chapter 33, which include Concept Check review questions, Reference Flash Cards, and Online Procedures assessment sheets.

- **Concept Check** review questions
- **Reference Flash Cards** medical terminology practice
- **Online Procedures** assessment sheets

CHAPTER 33 Assessment

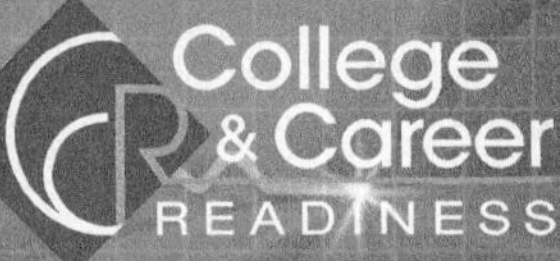

Critical Thinking/Problem Solving

1. As a BMET, you find that 30 pieces of equipment need to be electrically safety tested. However, the safety analyzer is due for calibration, an X-ray machine is not working, and a defibrillator also needs repair. At the same time, you are called to the intensive care unit to check out a monitoring system that continually sets off alarms. Set your priorities and explain your reasons behind those decisions.
2. You have been asked to perform scheduled preventive maintenance on the Puritan Bennett 840 Ventilator System. This is life support equipment. You are not familiar with the equipment's use or requirements. Where do you find this information?
3. Choose one of the following possible safety hazards and develop a plan for correcting it. Explain your plan to the class.
    - Inadequate ventilation
    - Wet locations
    - Inadequate lighting
    - Biological contamination
    - Extension cords with only two conductors
    - Overloaded electrical outlets

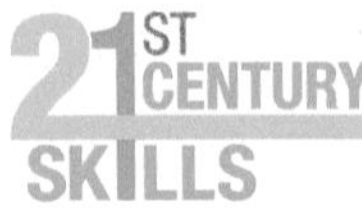

4. **Teamwork** With a partner, choose a piece of biomedical equipment to learn about, or create a design for a new piece of equipment. Draw a diagram and explain how the equipment functions and how it is used. Research online or visit a local biotechnology department. Share the results of your research or the design with the class.
5. **Teamwork** Working with a team or in a group, evaluate the electrical equipment in your classroom or laboratory. Determine if hospital-grade plugs and receptacles are being used. Check the color and shape of the plugs and receptacles. Find out whether there is a ground. Write a one-paragraph report on the level of electrical safety in the classroom or laboratory.
6. **Information Literacy** Search the Internet for a school in your area that offers courses for biomedical equipment technician. Find out the requirements for entrance into the program and for graduation. Visit the websites of the Association for the Advancement of Medical Instrumentation (AAMI) or the Institute for the Certification of Engineering Technicians (ICET) in order to determine how to become certified as a BMET. Write a brief summary of your findings to present to the class.

CHAPTER 34 Biomedical Science

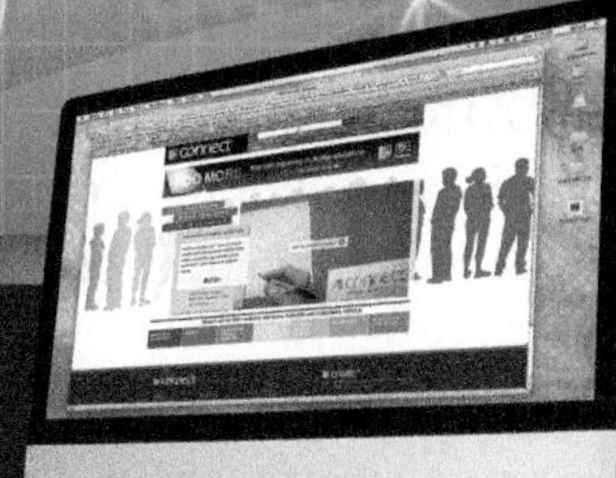

Essential Question:

How can biomedical science improve human health and quality of life?

Biomedical science is the application of chemistry, biology, physics, engineering, and other scientific disciplines to the research and treatment of health issues. The need for researchers, toxicologists, and other scientific professionals is increasing. In this chapter, you will learn about biomedical science careers, including medical scientist, biological technician, geneticist, microbiologist, toxicologist, forensic scientist, laboratory animal technician, and laboratory animal technologist.

McGraw Hill connect™

It's Online!

- **Online Procedures**
- **STEM Connection**
- **Medical Science**
- **Medical Terms**
- **Medical Math**
- **Ethics in Action**
- **Virtual Lab**

READING GUIDE

OBJECTIVES

After completing this chapter, you will be able to:

- **Describe** the role and responsibilities of a medical scientist.
- **Identify** at least three responsibilities of a biological technician.
- **Explain** a geneticist's areas of specialization.
- **Compare** the role of a microbiologist to that of a toxicologist.
- **Relate** how the field of forensics relates to the law.
- **Describe** the careers available in laboratory animal science.
- **Demonstrate** three biomedical science procedures.

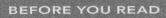

BEFORE YOU READ

Connect What presently incurable diseases do you think biomedical scientists should be working on at this time?

Main Idea

Biomedical scientists work to learn more about diseases and develop new treatments.

Note-Taking Activity

Draw this table. Write key terms and phrases under **Cues**. Write main ideas under **Note Taking**. Summarize the section under **Summary**.

Cues	Note Taking
○ ○	○ ○
Summary	

Graphic Organizer

Before you read the chapter, draw a diagram like the one to the right. As you read, write the biomedical science careers covered by the chapter into the diagram.

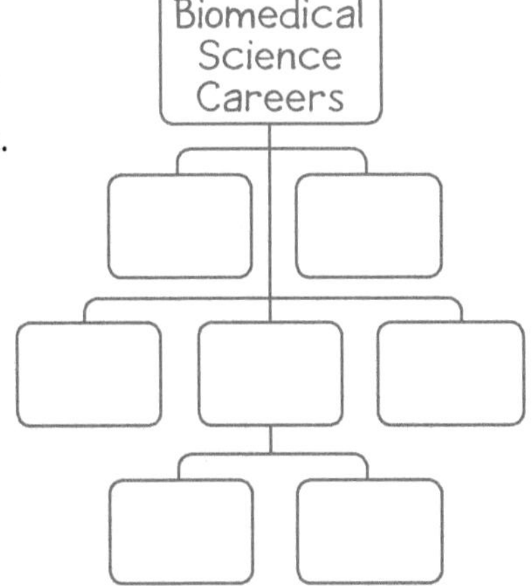

connect

Downloadable graphic organizers can be accessed online.

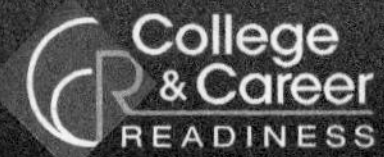

STANDARDS

HEALTH SCIENCE

NCHSE 1.23 Investigate biomedical therapies as they relate to the prevention, pathology, and treatment of disease.

NCHSE 7.12 Describe methods of controlling the spread and growth of microorganisms.

SCIENCE

NSES C Develop understanding of the cell; molecular basis of heredity; biological evolution; interdependence of organisms; matter, energy, and organization in living systems; and behavior of organisms.

NCHSE *National Consortium for Health Science Education*

NSES *National Science Education Standards*

COMMON CORE STATE STANDARDS

MATHEMATICS

Statistics and Probability
Making Inferences and Justifying Conclusions S-IC Understand and evaluate random processes underlying statistical experiments.

Statistics and Probability
Making Inferences and Justifying Conclusions S-IC 6 Use data from a randomized experiment to compare two treatments; use simulations to decide if differences between parameters are significant.

ENGLISH LANGUAGE ARTS

Reading
Integration of Knowledge and Ideas R-8 Evaluate the hypotheses, data, analysis, and conclusions in a science or technical text, verifying the data when possible and corroborating or challenging conclusions with other sources of information.

SECTION 34.1 Careers in Biomedical Science

Medical Scientists

What do medical scientists study?

Medical scientists research human diseases and conditions with the goal of improving human health. Most conduct biomedical research and development to advance knowledge of life processes and living organisms that affect human health. This includes the study of viruses, bacteria, fungi, and other infectious agents. Research has resulted in advances in diagnosis, treatment, and prevention of many diseases.

See **Table 34.1** on page 782 for an overview of biomedical science careers.

Medical scientists work to understand the causes of disease and other health problems. This knowledge is then used to develop treatments for conditions and diseases such as cancer. They may also seek to discover ways to prevent health problems.

The Job of the Medical Scientist

Most medical scientists work in laboratories using a wide variety of equipment. They may also work directly with patients in **clinical trials** (see **Figure 34.1**). Clinical trials are scientific studies to evaluate the effectiveness and safety of medications or devices on large groups of people, with the intention of improving it or proving its fitness for use.

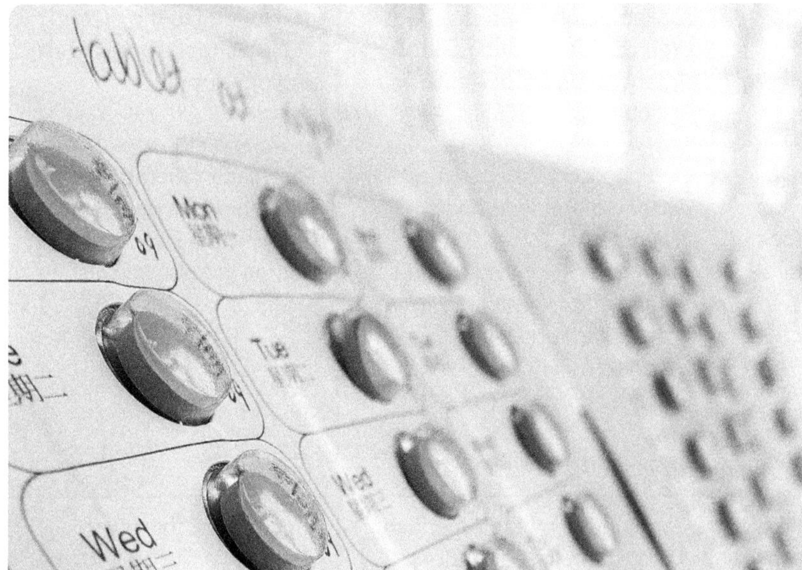

Fig. 34.1 Clinical Trials Clinical trials for new medications are based on a research plan and require a report on the research results. *Which healthcare professional may work in clinical trials?*

Photo: Yon Marsh/Alamy

Vocabulary

Content Vocabulary

You will learn these content vocabulary terms in this section.

- **clinical trials**
- **genetics**
- **risk assessment**
- **forensics**
- **euthanizing**

Academic Vocabulary

You will see this word in your reading and on your tests. Find its meaning in the Glossary in the back of the book.

- **conduct**

Table 34.1 Overview of Biomedical Science Careers

OCCUPATION	EDUCATIONAL REQUIREMENTS	CERTIFICATION OR LICENSING AGENCY	JOB OUTLOOK
Medical Scientist	A doctorate (PhD) in biological science or a medical degree with additional clinical training	Individuals obtaining a medical degree would be licensed through the American Medical Association (AMA).	Much faster than average growth due to advancements in the field of biotechnological research and development
Biological Technician	A bachelor's degree in biology is desired. Associate degree or certificate in applied science or science-related technology may be accepted for some entry-level careers.	Certification is available through the National Accrediting Agency for Clinical Laboratory Science (NAACLS)	Faster than average growth due to increase in biotechnology research and increase in pharmaceutical development
Geneticist	A bachelor's degree in genetics or related subject, such as biological sciences or biochemistry. A master's or PhD in genetics or a medical degree with a certification in medical genetics	Certification is available through the American Board of Medical Genetics for individuals with a medical degree.	Much faster than average growth due to the advancements in the field of biotechnological research and development
Microbiologist	A bachelor's or master's degree in biology. A PhD is required to pursue independent research.	Certification through the American College of Microbiology and the American Society for Clinical Pathology (ASCP)	Faster than average growth due to the growth of biotechnology research and development
Toxicologist	Associate through doctoral degrees. The higher the degree, the more opportunities there will be.	Multiple certifications are available from various organizations including the American Board of Applied Toxicology (ABAT).	Much faster than average growth due to the growth of biotechnology research and development
Forensic Scientist	A bachelor's degree in forensic science or another natural science. An advanced degree is needed in many cases.	Certification through American College of Forensic Examiners International is available for many professionals, in addition to their education and current license. Examples include Certified Forensic Nurse (CFN), Certified Forensic Physician (CFM), and Certified Medical Investigator (CMI).	Faster than average with job opportunities best for those with a bachelor's degree in forensic science
Laboratory Animal Technician/ Technologist	Varies with job title; most often, an associate or bachelor's degree	Certification by the American Association for Laboratory Animal Science	Much faster than average due to the growth of biomedical science and research

Medical scientists may perform the following tasks:

- Administer drugs to patients in clinical trials, monitor their reactions, and observe the results
- Adjust the dosage levels of the drug being studied in a clinical trial, to reduce negative side effects or to produce better results
- Draw blood, excise tissue, or perform other invasive procedures
- Explain research results orally or in written reports
- Develop research plans and write grant proposals

READING CHECK

Explain the purpose of a clinical trial.

The Biological Technician

What kinds of technical support do biological technicians provide?

A biological technician studies living organisms and assists scientists conducting medical research. That research could be directed toward any of several vital areas, such as finding a cure for cancer or AIDS. Biological technicians may work in various areas such as

- pharmaceutical companies, to help develop and manufacture medicinal and pharmaceutical preparations.
- microbiology laboratories, where, as assistants, they study living organisms and infectious agents and analyze organic substances, such as blood, food, and drugs.
- biotechnology laboratories, where the knowledge and techniques gained from basic research are used in new product development.

The Job of the Biological Technician

The following is a list of tasks that may be performed by a biological technician. Tasks vary depending upon the place of employment, and the biological technician will not necessarily perform all the tasks listed.

- Analyze experimental data and interpret results to write reports and summaries of findings
- Clean, maintain, and prepare supplies and work areas
- Conduct, or assist in conducting, research, including the collection of information and samples, such as blood, water, soil, plants, and animals
- Conduct standardized biological, microbiological, and biochemical tests and laboratory analyses
- Examine specimens to detect the presence of disease or other problems
- Measure or weigh compounds and solutions for use in testing

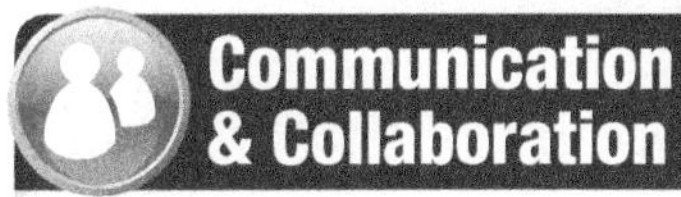

Clinical Trials

Clinical trials are used to evaluate the medication or device effectiveness and safety by monitoring its effects on large groups of people.

People often volunteer to take part in a trial, although sometimes they are paid. For some, clinical research trials offer new therapies that are otherwise not available. Patients with difficult to treat or currently incurable diseases may consider participating in clinical research trials because they are sometimes lifesaving for participants.

In many cases, government agencies approve treatments based on clinical trial results. These trials are effective in preventing harmful treatments from coming to market but do not always reveal all side effects or long-term drawbacks.

There are four possible outcomes from a clinical trial:

- **Positive:** The new treatment has a large beneficial effect and is superior to standard treatment.
- **Non-inferior:** The new treatment is equivalent to standard treatment.
- **Inconclusive:** The new treatment is shown to be neither superior nor inferior to standard treatment.
- **Negative:** The new treatment is inferior to standard treatment.

Follow-Up

1. What do you consider the positive and negative effects of a clinical trial?
2. If you had an incurable disease, would you consider participating in a clinical trial?

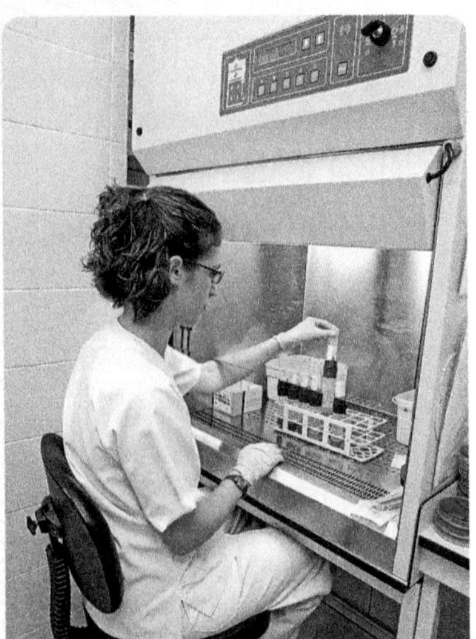

Fig. 34.2 Biological Technicians Biological technicians study living organisms and help with research. *What are the responsibilities of the biological technician in the laboratory?*

- Monitor and observe experiments, recording production and test data for evaluation by research personnel
- Provide technical support and services for scientists and engineers working in fields such as agriculture, environmental science, resource management, biology, and health sciences
- Set up, adjust, calibrate, clean, maintain, and troubleshoot laboratory and field equipment

READING CHECK

List several tasks performed by biological technicians.

The Geneticist

How are genes related to disease?

Genetics is the science of genes, heredity, and variation in living organisms (see **Figure 34.3**). Genetics helps us understand the inheritance of genetic diseases, such as cystic fibrosis. Biologists use genetics to identify the genes that function in the life of the cell and those that control the development of a complex organism from a fertilized egg. The biotechnology field uses genetics to produce a range of products from pharmaceuticals to microchips.

A geneticist may also perform investigations to understand the basis of genetic diseases so that treatments may be developed. They also provide counseling to individuals or families at risk for developing genetic diseases. In criminal cases, they perform sensitive tests to identify individuals from a drop of blood or tiny amounts of other body tissue.

Geneticists may specialize in any of the following:

- Biochemical genetics, studying chemical influences on genes
- Clinical genetics, investigating the importance of genetics in health and disease, including in birth defects
- Molecular genetics, studying genes at the molecular level, including the DNA and RNA molecules

READING CHECK

Explain how genetics can assist in criminal investigations.

The Microbiologist

What do medical microbiologists study?

Microbiologists investigate the growth, structure, development, and other characteristics of microscopic organisms, such as bacteria, algae, viruses, or fungi. Medical microbiologists study the relationship

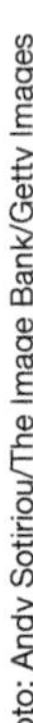

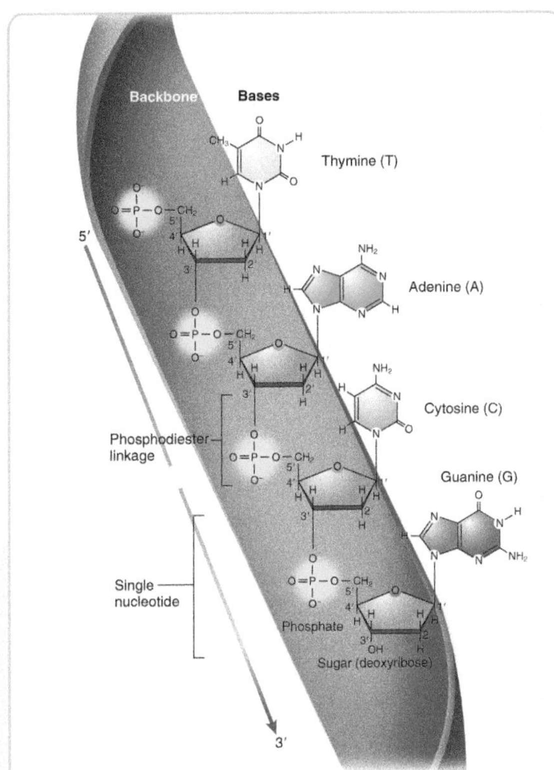

Fig. 34.3 Molecular Genetics Molecular geneticists study DNA molecules. *What are the four bases in DNA?*

between organisms and diseases or the effects of antibiotics on microorganisms. Other types of microbiologists include veterinary microbiology, environmental microbiology, food microbiology, and pharmaceutical microbiology. All of these careers relate to the way in which microbes and other microorganisms affect animals, the environment, the food supply, and healthcare.

Specialty careers within microbiology include:

- Bacteriologist: studies bacteria and how they can help and hurts us
- Virologist: studies viruses and how they infect cells
- Epidemiologist: tracks down outbreaks of disease and learns what caused them
- Immunologist: studies how the body defends itself against microbes

READING CHECK

Identify the specialty areas of microbiology.

The Toxicologist

What substances around us can pose risks to our safety?

A toxicologist studies the effects of chemicals, drugs, environmental contaminants, and naturally occurring substances found in food, water, air, and soil. These substances make up everything around us. Toxicologists help to answer questions such as: Which substances are really dangerous? How much does it take to cause harm? What are

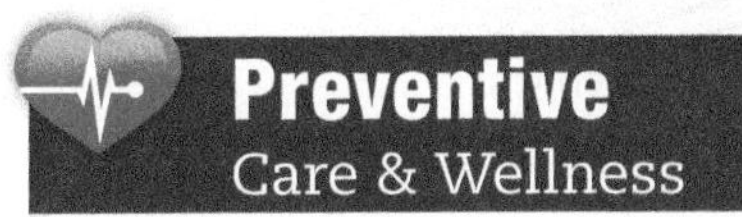

Acetaminophen and Alcohol Poisoning

Just about everything you eat or drink must travel through your liver to be metabolized. The liver breaks down the substance for use by the body and prepares it for elimination from your body. Medications, such as acetaminophen (Tylenol®), are also processed through your liver. Taking too much acetaminophen, taking acetaminophen in combination with alcohol or other medications, or taking it when you have certain infections can overload your liver, causing acetaminophen poisoning. After taking too much acetaminophen, you may have no symptoms for 24 hours. Then you may develop nausea, vomiting, a poor appetite, a general bad feeling, or abdominal pain. Damage to the liver may occur, and a liver transplant may be needed.

Adults over 150 pounds should not take more than four grams (4,000 milligrams) of acetaminophen in 24 hours. Check the label of all over-the-counter or prescription drugs, because many contain acetaminophen. Examples are Actifed, Alka-Seltzer® Plus, Benadryl®, Butalbital, Co-Gesic, Contac, Excedrin, Fioricet, Lortab, Midrin, Norco, Percocet, Robitussin®, Sedapap, Sinutab®, Sudafed®, TheraFlu®, Unisom With Pain Relief, Vick's Nyquil and DayQuil, Vicodin, Wygesic, and Zydone. Taking a combination of any of these medications can easily result in ingesting too much acetaminophen.

An excessive intake of alcohol on a regular basis can also damage your liver. Symptoms of alcohol poisoning include confusion, stupor, vomiting, seizures, slow or irregular breathing, or passing out and becoming entirely unresponsive. Never have more than one drink per hour, and always avoid combining alcohol and acetaminophen.

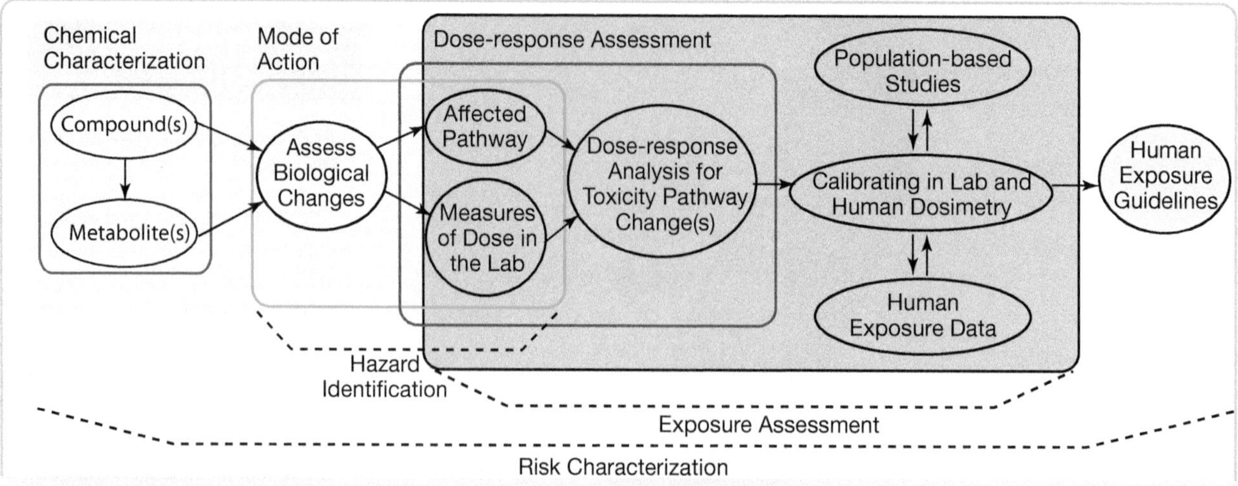

Fig. 34.4 Risk Assessment Toxicologists use the risk assessment process. *What is the purpose of risk assessment?*

the effects of a particular substance? What conditions can these substances cause—cancer, nervous system damage, birth defects?

Toxicologists find answers to these very important questions by applying some highly detailed scientific techniques. The field of toxicology combines the elements of many scientific disciplines, including biology and chemistry, to help us understand the harmful effects of chemicals and other substances on living organisms.

Toxicologists help determine the risk of exposure to a harmful substance. This is called **risk assessment.** A risk assessment determines the likelihood that harmful effects will occur under certain exposure circumstances (see **Fig. 34.4**). If the risks are real, steps must be taken to reduce the exposure.

The Job of the Toxicologist

Research toxicologists search for new knowledge concerning how toxic substances produce their effects. They use laboratory animals, human and animal cells in culture, and other test systems to examine the cellular, biochemical, and molecular processes underlying toxic responses. Industry, scientific, educational institutions, and governments offer opportunities in toxicology research.

Toxicologists may also work in the chemical, pharmaceutical, and many other industries to perform tests and ensure that their products and workplaces are safe. They may also work for local and federal governments to develop and enforce laws to ensure that chemicals are produced, used, and disposed of safely. Toxicologists can also work in academic institutions, teaching others about the safe use of chemicals and training future toxicologists.

READING CHECK

Define risk assessment and identify its purpose in toxicology.

The Forensic Scientist

How do forensic scientists assist law enforcement?

The field of **forensics** is broad and involves many different professionals. But one thing all forensic professionals have in common is they are connected to the law in some way. Their job duties fall into two basic categories: analyzing evidence or acting as an expert witness in a legal proceeding.

Two key scientific careers in forensics are forensic biologist and forensic chemist.

Forensic biologists examine organic substances and perform DNA analysis of samples, such as hair or blood. This career is closely related to forensic pathology and forensic anthropology. Forensic pathologists are medical doctors who perform autopsies or other investigations to help determine a cause of death. Forensic anthropologists specialize in human bones and use this knowledge to study skeletal or other remains and obtain information from them such as age, height, and gender. Forensic anthropologists also help locate and recover remains.

Forensic chemists perform chemical analyses of evidence such as drugs, soil, or shards of glass. A career in forensic chemistry is similar to a career in forensic toxicology. Forensic toxicologists study body fluids and other evidence to help determine if drugs, alcohol, or other toxic substances were involved in a crime or a death. They may also perform drug testing for employers.

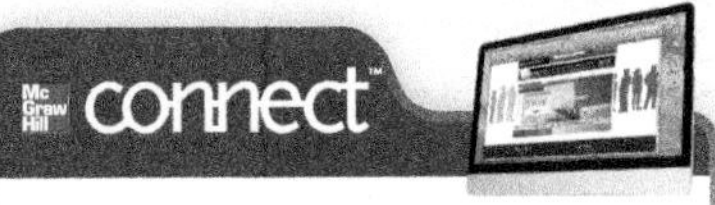

STEM CONNECTION

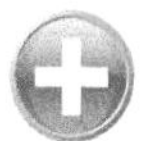

Medical Science

Recombinant DNA
DNA contains all the information needed to recreate an organism. While DNA does not actually make the organism, it does make the proteins that make the organism. The DNA is transcribed into mRNA. Then mRNA is translated into protein, which then forms the organism. If the DNA sequence is changed, the way in which the protein, and the organism, is formed also changes.

connect Go online to learn how biotechnology and healthcare are being changed through scientists' study of rDNA.

The Job of the Forensic Biologist

Forensic biologists examine blood and other body fluids, hair, bones, insects, and plant and animal remains to help identify victims and support criminal investigations. They collect and analyze biological evidence found on clothing, weapons and other surfaces to determine the time and cause of death.

A forensic biologist may perform the following tasks:

- Collect biological evidence from biological materials (see **Figure 34.5**)
- Use microscopes and other equipment to analyze collected evidence
- Photograph, catalog, and test evidence
- Maintain detailed evidence and test logs
- Produce written reports of results

Senior forensic biologists may give expert testimony in court, based on evidence they have studied and analyzed.

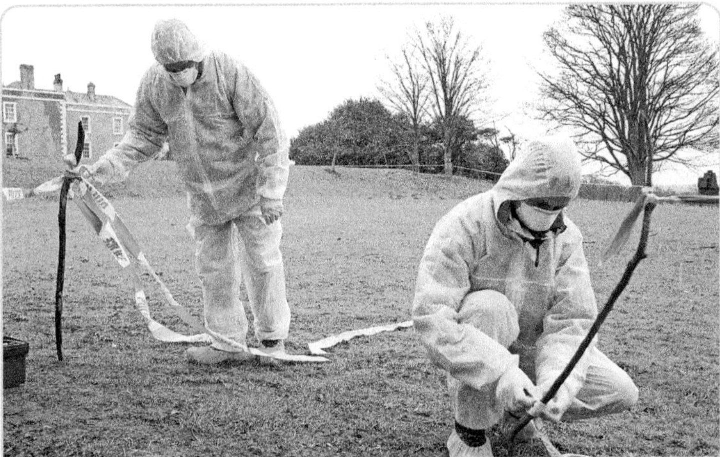

Fig. 34.5 Forensic Biologist Forensic biologists collect biological evidence. *Which forensic specialist is most likely to be involved in collecting evidence?*

The Job of the Forensic Chemist

Forensic chemists apply knowledge from chemistry, biology, science, and genetics to the analysis of evidence found at crime scenes and on or in the bodies of crime suspects and victims. They do not collect evidence. A few of the tasks of the forensic chemist are:

- Testing and analyzing evidence
- Drawing conclusions from tests and analysis
- Providing information to criminal investigators.
- Giving expert testimony based upon the analysis of evidence

READING CHECK

Describe the forensic chemist's responsibilities regarding evidence.

Laboratory Animal Science

Why must some animals be euthanized?

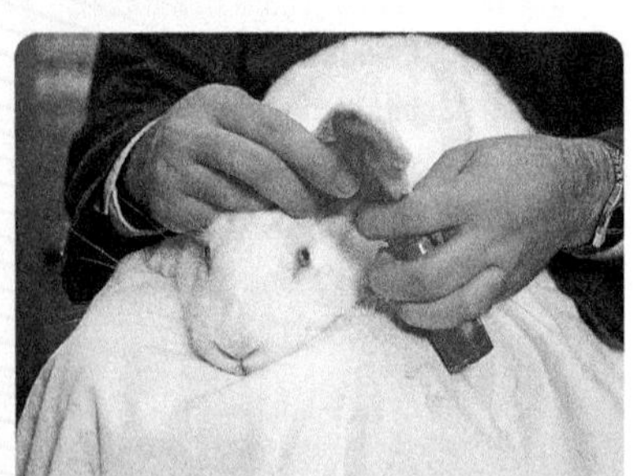

Fig. 34.6 Animal Science Lab Laboratory animal professionals assist in caring for animals that are used for research. *Which organizations regulate laboratory animal research?*

The biomedical research facility is one of the primary settings in which a laboratory animal scientist works (see **Figure 34.6**). Positions in this field include laboratory animal technician and technologist. The career of veterinary technician, also known as veterinary technologist and animal health technician, was discussed in Chapter 24, Animal Healthcare.

Laboratory animal technicians perform a wide range of tasks. They have more responsibility than veterinary technicians in private practice. For instance, they may perform some types of animal surgery. Unlike that of veterinary technicians, their work relates generally to biomedical research.

The general duties of the laboratory animal scientist include:

- Vaccinating newly-admitted animals
- Recording information on an animal's genealogy, weight, medications, diet, food intake, and clinical signs of pain and distress
- Administering medications to lab animals orally or topically
- Preparing samples for laboratory examination
- Performing standardized laboratory tests on animal specimens and reporting findings
- Assisting medical personnel during animal surgery
- Providing routine preoperative and postoperative care to animals
- **Euthanizing** seriously ill, injured, or unwanted animals. To euthanize an animal is to put it to death in a humane way.
- Ordering supplies and instruments and performing minor equipment maintenance
- Maintaining the lab operating room by following established standards of sanitation, including sterilizing laboratory and surgical equipment

The three skill levels in laboratory animal science are:

- Assistant laboratory animal technician (ALAT)
- Laboratory animal technician (LAT)
- Laboratory animal technologist (LATG)

Each level requires a particular amount of education and experience. Graduates of approved programs must complete six months of on-the-job training before they take qualifying examinations. They must then work two more years before they can take the examination on the next level. Some programs provide training in the advanced skills used in research. However, most research methods are taught on the job.

Animal science technicians who work in biomedical research must be certified by the American Association for Laboratory Animal Science (AALAS). These workers care for animals used in research and teaching.

Laboratory animal research is closely regulated. Agencies such as the United States Department of Agriculture (USDA) and the American Association for Laboratory Animal Care (AALAC) regulate biomedical research.

READING CHECK

Explain how laboratory animal science professionals help the lives of both animals and humans.

SECTION 34.1 Careers in Biomedical Science Review

AFTER YOU READ

1. **Describe** the level of education attained by most medical scientists.
2. **Identify** the work locations of most biological technicians.
3. **Indicate** three common tasks of the biological technician.
4. **Describe** three areas of expertise that a geneticist may have.
5. **Name** the professional who would determine if it is safe to go into an area after a hazardous chemical has been spilled.
6. **Explain** what all professionals in the field of forensics have in common.
7. **Indicate** the first level of certification in laboratory animal science.

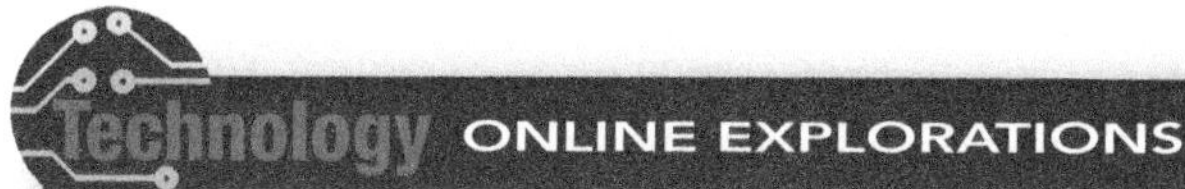

Biomedical Research

Search online for more information on biomedical research. Find out if there is a biomedical research facility near your school. Learn what type of research is performed there and what animals are used in the research. Write a report on your findings to share with the class.

SECTION 34.2 Biomedical Science Procedures

Vocabulary

Content Vocabulary

You will learn these content vocabulary terms in this section.

- **invasive procedures**
- **sterile field**

Quality Assurance and Quality Control in Biomedical Science

How do quality control professionals contribute to product safety?

Quality control and assurance are important to biomedical technology and biomedical science. Quality control is a process to ensure a certain acceptable level of quality in a product or service. Professionals test and inspect products, such as food and drug samples or raw materials, to ensure they are safe and not contaminated. Test data is recorded on graphs and charts, findings are evaluated, and summary reports are written.

When a failure occurs, a quality control professional is expected to make sure that the product does not reach consumers by correcting the error or keeping it off the market. A quality control professional may evaluate medical devices as they are being manufactured and look for defects.

Quality assurance professionals help set up and monitor the quality process. They systematically monitor and evaluate all aspects of a project, service, or facility in order to ensure that applicable quality standards are being met. In the health sciences, a quality assurance professional may monitor or evaluate treatments, medications, or the scientific methods used to develop them. A quality assurance professional may set the standards for testing of a new medication during a clinical trial.

Quality assurance professionals also work to test and improve biomedical software and other types of software. With increasing automation and computer control of many biomedical and related procedures, it is more important than ever before to ensure the safety and effectiveness of advancing technology. Complex machinery such as imaging equipment must be monitored and maintained using quality-control programs or techniques in order to stay compliant with various regulations.

READING CHECK

Name several products or services that are monitored by quality control professionals.

Safety

Sterile Fields

The outer one inch of the sterile field is considered contaminated. So before you add sterile items to the sterile field, carefully plan where you will place the instruments so that they are well within the sterile field.

The sterile field is considered contaminated and must be redone when:

- An unsterile item touches the field
- Someone reaches across the field
- The field becomes wet
- The field is left unattended and uncovered
- You turn your back on the field

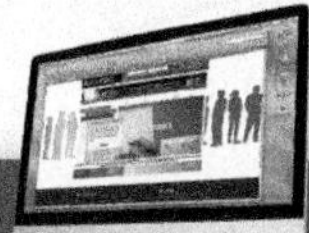

Mc Graw Hill connect™ ONLINE PROCEDURES

PROCEDURE 34-1

Performing a Surgical Scrub

A surgical scrub removes dirt and microorganisms from under the fingernails and the surface of the skin, hair follicles, and oil glands of the hands and forearms. It is different from handwashing, which removes some of the bacteria. A surgical scrub more thoroughly removes bacteria and in deeper skin layers. A surgical scrub makes your hand surgically clean; it does not make your hands sterile.

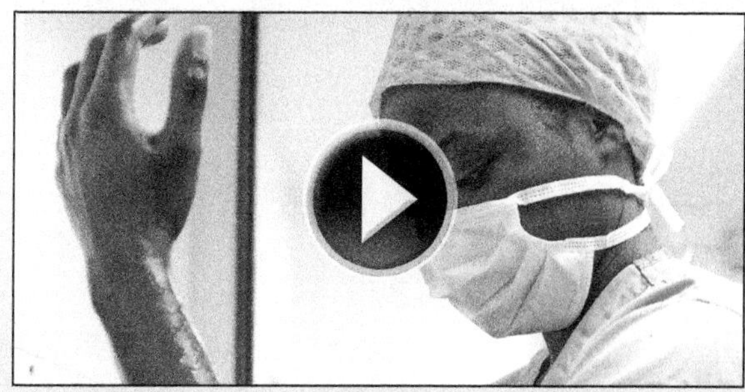

PROCEDURE 34-2

Putting on Sterile Gloves

Sterile gloves are used for **invasive procedures** or any procedure that requires an area to be free from microorganisms (sterile). Invasive procedures occur when there is a break in the skin such as a surgical procedure. Sterile parts of the body are those not exposed to the outside of the body.

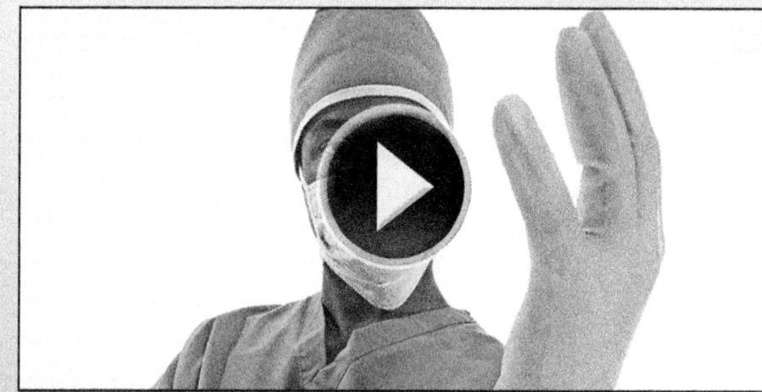

PROCEDURE 34-3

Preparing a Sterile Field and Opening Sterile Packages

A **sterile field** is an area free of microorganisms that will be used as a work area during procedures. Sterile fields are prepared for surgical or other invasive procedures. To maintain sterility throughout this procedure, follow the troubleshooting steps listed in this procedure.

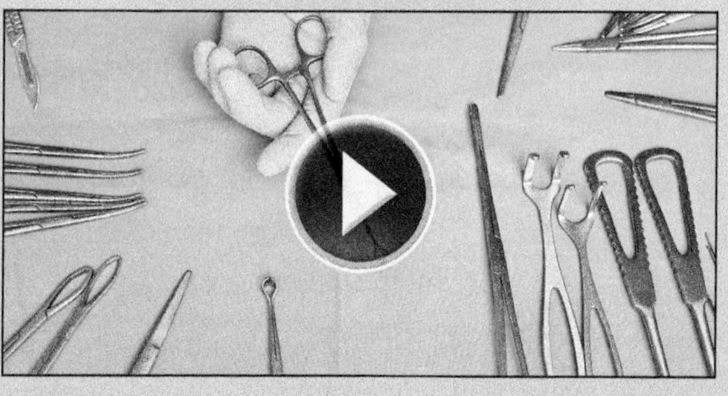

Photos: (t)Ingram Publishing, (c)Creatas Images/Jupiter Images, (b)OJO Images/Getty Images

SECTION 34.2 Procedures in Biomedical Science Review

AFTER YOU READ

1. **Explain** why a surgical scrub is performed.
2. **Indicate** when sterile gloves should be used.
3. **List** at least three steps to follow when preparing a sterile field.
4. **Choose** four things that could occur to make a sterile field contaminated.
5. **Explain** why quality control and quality assurance professionals are important to ensure safety.

Technology ONLINE EXPLORATIONS

Clinical Trials

Search online for information about a current clinical trial. Write a report on the clinical trial including information such as what is being tested, the number of participants, how long the trial is going to last, and the desired results or outcomes.

CHAPTER 34 Review

Chapter Summary

SECTION 34.1

- Medical scientists research human diseases and conditions with the goal of improving human health. Most work in laboratories, or they may also work directly with patients in clinical trials. **(pg. 781)**
- Biological technicians conduct standardized laboratory tests, maintain the laboratory and its equipment, and analyze biological data. **(pg. 783)**
- Biological technicians may work in various areas such as pharmaceutical companies, microbiology laboratories, and biotechnology laboratories. **(pg. 783)**
- Geneticists may study the chemical influences of genes, investigate the importance of genetics in health and disease, or study genes on a molecular level including DNA and RNA. **(pg. 784)**
- Geneticists may specialize in biochemical genetics, clinical genetics, and molecular genetics. **(pg. 784)**
- Microbiologists study the details of microscopic organisms and their relationship to human health. Although toxicologists may study the details of microorganisms they are more interested in how substances affect our health. **(pg. 784)**
- A toxicologist studies the effects of chemicals, drugs, environmental contaminants, and naturally occurring substances found in food, water, air and soil. **(pg. 785)**
- Forensic scientists work in the legal field, analyzing evidence and testifying on their findings in legal proceedings. **(pg. 787)**
- There are three levels of certification for laboratory animal science professionals: assistant laboratory animal technician (ALAT), laboratory animal technician (LAT), and laboratory animal technologist (LATG) **(pg. 789)**

SECTION 34.2

- In the healthcare science fields, a quality assurance professional may monitor or evaluate treatments, medications, or the scientific methods used to develop them. **(pg. 790)**
- Quality assurance professionals also work to test and improve biomedical software and other types of software. **(pg. 790)**
- Surgical scrubbing and sterile gloves are used for procedures that require sterile technique. **(pg. 791)**
- When preparing a sterile field, strict guidelines must be followed to prevent contamination. **(pg. 791)**

CHAPTER

34 Assessment

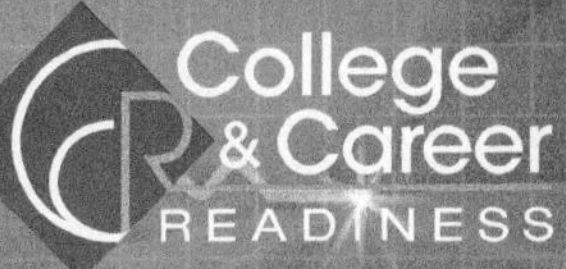

Critical Thinking/Problem Solving

1. Develop a plan for testing new medicines and medical products for side effects without using animals.
2. When performing a surgical scrub, you notice that the sink does not have a knee or foot pedal. What should you do?
3. Select a topic related to biomedical science presented in this chapter, such as animal euthanization, clinical trials, risk assessment, or rDNA. Create a report providing detailed information about that topic, including graphics and images, to present to your class.
4. Debate with a partner the cases for and against using cells from an aborted human fetus for rDNA research.

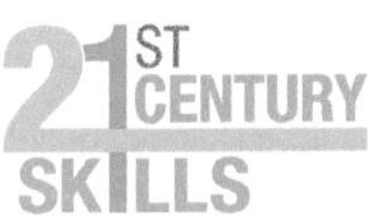

5. **Teamwork** With a partner, practice putting sterile gloves and working with a sterile field. Assemble a group of objects as "surgical instruments" and arrange them correctly in the sterile field. Monitor your partner to see if he or see contaminates the gloves, objects, or sterile field during practice.
6. **Information Literacy** Search online for information about a specific career in biomedical science. Find a school in your area that offers instruction in this field. Determine the entry qualifications, how long the program lasts, and what courses will be included. Identify what specialties within that field are taught at that school. Write a report based on your findings.

Mc Graw Hill connect™ ONLINE ACTIVITIES

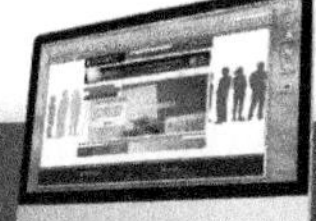

Complete our HST online activities for Chapter 34, which include Concept Check review questions, Reference Flash Cards, and Online Procedures assessment sheets.

- **Concept Check** review questions
- **Reference Flash Cards** medical terminology practice
- **Online Procedures** assessment sheets

Appendix A

Parliamentary Procedure

As part of your responsibility to a professional organization, you will attend or conduct meetings. Parliamentary procedure is a set of rules to follow in order to conduct a meeting in an efficient manner.

General Henry M. Robert wrote *Robert's Rules of Order*, to help protect democratic procedures in organizations. He wanted to ensure the right to present business, discuss issues, and vote. His basic principles are:

1. Take up business one item at a time.
2. The majority rules.
3. Protect the minority's right to speak and to vote.

Organizations using these rules usually follow a fixed order of business. Here is an example:

- Call to order
- Roll call of members present
- Reading and approval of minutes of last meeting
- Officers' reports
- Unfinished business
- New business
- Announcements
- Adjournment

Procedures for Motions

Issues for discussion are presented as "motions," or proposals for action. The membership considers each motion and then votes on it.

1. Obtain the floor.
   - Wait until the last speaker has finished speaking.
   - Rise and address the Chairman by saying, "Mr. (or Madam) Chairman."
   - Wait for the Chairman to recognize you.
2. Make your motion.
   - Speak clearly; be as concise as possible.
   - Always state a motion affirmatively. Say, "I move that we..." not, "I move that we do not..."
   - Avoid personal comments or attacks.
3. Either another member will second your motion, or the Chairman will call for a second.
4. If no one seconds your motion, it is lost.
5. If someone seconds your motion, the Chairman states your motion.
   - The Chairman will say, "It has been moved and seconded that we . . ." This places the motion before the members for consideration and action.
   - Either the membership debates your motion, or the motion moves directly to a vote.
   - Once a motion is presented to members, it cannot be changed without members' consent.
6. Expand on your motion.
   - This is when you speak in favor of your motion.
   - As the mover, you are allowed to speak first.
   - All comments and debate about the motion must be directed to the Chairman.
   - Limit your speaking to the established time.
   - The mover may speak again only after others are finished, unless called by the Chairman.
7. Whether or not to vote is put to the membership.
   - The Chairman asks, "Are you ready to vote?"
   - If there is no more discussion, a vote is taken.
   - On a motion to move, the previous question may be adapted.

Voting on a motion will depend upon the organization or the motion that requires a vote. There are five methods used to vote by most organizations.

1. **Voice:** The Chairman asks those in favor to say "aye" and those opposed to say "no." After a voice vote, a member can move for an exact count.
2. **Roll Call:** The list of members' names is read aloud. Each member answers "aye" or "no" when his or her name is called. In this manner, each person's vote can be noted.
3. **General Consent:** The Chairman can state, "If there is no objection . . ." Agreement is shown by members' silence. If a member says, "I object," the item must be put to a vote.
4. **Division:** Similar to a voice vote, this does not require a count unless the Chairman so desires. Members raise their hands or stand.
5. **Ballot:** Members write their vote on ballots or slips of paper when secrecy is desired.

Table 5.1 Commonly Used Medical Abbreviations *(continued from page 128)*

ABBREVIATION	MEANING
oz.	ounce
P	pulse
p.c.	after meals, ½ hour after a meal
pH	power of hydrogen concentration (degree of alkalinity or acidity)
PM, p.m.	afternoon
PO, po, p.o.	by mouth
PRN, prn	Repeat as needed
q.am.	every morning
q.h.	every hour
q.i.d.	four times a day
QNS	quantity not sufficient
q.s.	quantity sufficient
r, R	rectal
Rx	prescription
$\bar{s}$	without
SIDS	sudden infant death syndrome
Sig	give the following directions
SOB	shortness of breath
ss, ss	one-half
stat	immediately
syr.	syrup
susp.	suspension
sup., supp.	suppository
T	temperature
T & A	tonsillectomy and adenoidectomy
tab.	tablet
tbsp.	tablespoon
TID, t.i.d.	three times a day
TPR	temperature, pulse, and respirations
tsp.	teaspoon
Tx	treatment
VS	vital signs
W/C, w/c	wheelchair

Table 5.2 Commonly Used Symbols

MEDICAL SYMBOLS	MEANING
°	degree
♀	female
↑	higher, up
↓	lower, down
♂	male
#	pound
i̇, or ṫ	one

Glossary

A

abdominal thrusts compressing the abdomen to clear a blocked airway (p. 89)

absorption the process by which a drug enters the blood plasma (p. 321)

access means of getting to (p. 31)

accommodate cope with (p. 442)

accurately correctly, precisely (p. 616)

acquired immunodeficiency syndrome (AIDS) a condition of subjectivity to opportunistic infections, caused by the human immunodeficiency virus (p. 208)

activities of daily living (ADL) routine daily activities (p. 38)

acupuncturist professional who uses needles to balance the flow of *qi* in the body (p. 550)

adapting adjusting to change (p. 30)

adequate sufficient (p. 256)

adjust change (p. 557)

adjustment manual treatment used by chiropractors (p. 543)

administration giving (p. 313)

admitting diagnosis the condition identified by the physician at admission to the hospital (p. 718)

advance directive a legal document that makes known a person's wishes about life-support measures and other medical procedures (p. 347)

advocate someone who tries to ensure that the patient's needs are being met (p. 423)

aerobic exercise cardiovascular activity that focuses on fat loss or muscle toning (p. 529)

aerobic microbes microbes that can live only in the presence of oxygen (p. 61)

affect change or influence (p. 208)

aggressive personality a person who tends to put his or her own needs ahead of the needs of others and to push others out of the way to get to goals (p. 369)

algorithm a set of rules used to solve a problem in a finite number of steps (p. 769)

alternative available as something different (p. 543)

alternative medicine therapy used in place of conventional medicine (p. 543)

alveolar in the lungs (p. 300)

amalgam a mixture of silver alloy and mercury used in dental restoration (p. 578)

amblyopia poor vision in one eye (p. 678)

ambulate walk (p. 417)

ambulatory monitoring recording information over an extended period on clients who are able to walk (p. 637)

American Association for Respiratory Care a professional society for respiratory therapists, managers of respiratory and cardiopulmonary services, and educators who provide respiratory care training (p. 491)

American Sign Language (ASL) precise hand shapes and movements for communication (p. 520)

American Veterinary Medical Association (AVMA) organization that accredits schools of veterinary technology (p. 602)

amino acids compounds that make up proteins (p. 270)

amniotic sac a fluid-filled membrane that surrounds the fetus (p. 230, p. 408)

ampere the amount of electrical charge flowing per unit of time (p. 772)

ampule a small glass container with a narrow neck (p. 450)

anaerobic exercise movement that focuses on increasing muscle mass (p. 529)

anaerobic microbes microbes that grow best in the absence of oxygen (p. 61)

anaphylaxis a type of shock that occurs quickly, with severe life-threatening consequences (p. 99)

angiogram an image showing both arteries and veins filled with contrast media (p. 657)

annually every year (p. 193)

antecubital space the space on the inside of the bend of the elbow (p. 290)

anterior at the front of the mouth (p. 569)

antibodies specialized proteins that fight disease (p. 164)

antioxidants chemicals that protect body cells from damage that can lead to health problems (p. 272)

antiseptics solutions that are applied directly to the skin to prevent or slow the growth of pathogens (p. 62)

apex the end of a tooth root located farthest away from the crown (p. 570)

aphasia an impairment of the ability to communicate through speech, writing, or signs (p. 360)

apical referring to a pulse heard in the chest (p. 290)

appeal request for a reversal of denial of insurance payment (p. 694)

appropriate consistent with the requirements of a situation (p. 87)

aromatherapist practitioner who matches scents to symptoms (p. 555)

arteriogram an image that shows only arteries filled with contrast media (p. 657)

arteries vessels that carry blood away from the heart (p. 159)

artifact an abnormal mark on an ECG tracing (p. 648)

As Low As Reasonably Achievable (ALARA) a guideline for keeping radiation exposure as low as possible (p. 665)

aseptic technique procedures to create a germ-free environment (p. 729)

aspiration inhalation of food or liquid past the vocal cords into the lungs (p. 170)

assertive personality a person who tends to stand up for his or her own rights, but recognizes and respects the rights and needs of others (p. 369)

assess evaluate (p. 387)

assessment evaluation (p. 288)

asset management control of costs of purchases, maintenance, depreciation, disposition, and other aspects of medical equipment (p. 772)

assign designate (p. 427)

assist help (p. 563)

assisted-living centers long-term care facilities that offer separate living quarters while providing meals, housekeeping, and medical supervision (p. 38)

associate's degree two-year degree offered by community colleges and some technical and career schools (p. 13)

Association for the Advancement of Medical Instrumentation (AAMI) an organization that brings professionals together to solve common problems arising from the use of medical equipment (p. 771)

asthma a condition of bronchial airway obstruction causing sudden breathing difficulty accompanied by wheezing and coughing (p. 210)

astigmatism a condition caused by an irregularly shaped cornea that causes blurred vision (p. 676)

atelectasis lung collapse (p. 498)

atheroma a fat deposit on the inside of the arterial wall (p. 658)

atrium a chamber in the heart (p. 644)

attending physician the doctor responsible for the patient's care while the patient is in the hospital (p. 715)

attitude personal view of or feelings toward something (p. 373)

audiogram a graph used to determine the extent of hearing loss (p. 519)

audiometer a device that measures hearing (p. 515)

auscultate listen for sounds (p. 290)

autism a self-centered mental state that can involve inaccessibility, aloneness, rage reactions, and language disturbances (p. 460)

autoclave a device that sterilizes by steam pressure (p. 734)

autoimmune refers to a disease in which the body's immune system attacks the body (p. 190)

automated external defibrillators (AEDs) devices to restore the normal heart rhythm (p. 93)

avoirdupois system measurement system that measures by units such as the fluid ounce and pound (p. 326)

aware able to recognize and respond (p. 89)

axillary in the armpit (p. 288)

B

baby boom the large number of births in the U.S. from 1946 to 1964 (p. 33)

bachelor's degree a degree offered by universities or four-year colleges (p. 13)

bag-valve mask (BVM) a self-inflating bag and a one-way valve attached to a face mask (p. 94)

balance an unpaid amount (p. 697)

balloon angioplasty procedure of inserting a catheter with a balloon on its end into a blood vessel, where the balloon is blown up to expand the blocked vessel (p. 639)

barrier devices devices that prevent the spread of pathogens (p. 94)

Glossary

basal metabolic rate (BMR) the rate at which the body uses energy just for maintaining its own tissue, without doing any voluntary work (p. 275)

basic life support (BLS) skills abilities essential to maintain life (p. 389)

beneficiary the person who receives services (p. 693)

benefits agreed-upon services (p. 693)

benign referring to a tumor that stays localized in the tissue (p. 190)

binding joining together with (p. 310)

biological agents viruses, bacteria, or other microorganisms used to harm others (p. 66)

biotechnology a field of applied biology that involves living organisms and bioprocesses such as engineering, technology, and medicine (p. 12)

bioterrorism the use of microorganisms as weapons (p. 66)

blood pressure (BP) amount of pressure exerted on the arterial walls as blood pulsates through them (p. 296)

BLS (basic life support) skills abilities essential to maintain life (p. 389)

BMI (body mass index) a number indicating the relationship between weight and height (p. 528)

BMR (basal metabolic rate) the rate at which the body uses energy just for maintaining its own tissue, without doing any voluntary work (p. 275)

body mass index (BMI) a number indicating the relationship between weight and height (p. 528)

BP (blood pressure) amount of pressure exerted on the arterial walls as blood pulsates through them (p. 296)

brachial referring to a pulse found in the antecubital space of the arm (p. 290)

brachytherapy therapy using radionuclide sources to treat tumors inside the body (p. 659)

bridge a fixed prosthesis that replaces a missing tooth or teeth (p. 565)

bronchodilate open up the airways (p. 498)

buccal surface of a posterior tooth closest to the cheek (p. 570)

budget itemized summary of intended expenditures (p. 696)

BVM (bag-valve mask) a self-inflating bag and a one-way valve attached to a face mask (p. 94)

C

caduceus a symbol of two snakes entwined around a pole (p. 23)

calibration adjusting an instrument to operate at its intended settings (p. 763)

calorie unit of energy (p. 268)

cancer a malignant growth or tumor (p. 190)

cane a walking aid to help patients who have weakness on one side of the body (p. 518)

carbon dioxide a gas formed during respiration (p. 491)

cardiac arrest sudden stopping of the heart (p. 93)

cardiac catheterization a test that looks at the structures of the heart through a tube threaded through the blood vessels to the heart (p. 639)

cardiopulmonary resuscitation (CPR) a series of ventilations (breaths) and chest compressions used on a person who has stopped breathing or whose heart has stopped (p. 81)

career long-term field of work (p. 16)

career assessment evaluation of needs, interests, personality, and aptitudes related to work (p. 16)

caries dental decay (p. 588)

cataract cloudy area on a normally clear eye lens (p. 676)

cavity a soft area in a decayed tooth (p. 578)

cementum the thin outer layer of the root of a tooth (p. 571)

Centers for Disease Control and Prevention (CDC) a government agency that monitors and prevents disease outbreaks, guards against international disease transmission, maintains health statistics, provides immunization services, supports disease and injury prevention research, and promotes healthy behaviors and environments (pp. 42-43)

Centers for Medicare and Medicaid Services (CMS) a government agency that regulates the payment of client services (p. 710)

centrifuge a device that separates parts of a solution (p. 606)

cephalocaudal development development of the embryo and fetus in a head-to-tail manner (p. 227)

cerebral palsy a condition characterized by various problems such as mental retardation, epilepsy, and motor impairment or paralysis (p. 460)

certificated nursing assistant position requiring at least 75 hours of training and passing of a competency evaluation that includes knowledge and skill tests (p. 416)

certification standing achieved by passing an examination (p. 339)

certified nursing assistant position requiring at least 75 hours of training and passing of a competency evaluation that includes knowledge and skill tests (p. 416)

cervical collar a device to immobilize the neck, back, or spinal injuries (p. 389)

cervical line line formed by the junction of a tooth's crown and its root (p. 570)

chain of infection factors that must be present for an infection to result (p. 69)

channel a path for conveying chemicals (p. 311)

chargemaster a document listing all the services the hospital can provide, along with the procedure code and the charge for each service (p. 721)

chemical relating to the interaction of substances (p. 322)

chief complaint reason that the patient came for treatment (p. 442)

chiropractor professional who uses manual and physical therapy treatments and exercise programs to correct physical problems (p. 543)

cholesterol a waxy substance that is part of every cell in the body (p. 269)

chorion the outer fetal membrane (p. 230)

chronic disease a disease that may progress slowly and not show dramatic change over short periods of time (p. 267)

chronic obstructive pulmonary disease (COPD) a disease of the airways, such as emphysema (p. 496)

cilia small hairs in the nasal cavity (p. 170)

circulation the flow of blood through the blood vessels around the entire body (p. 158)

circumcision the surgical removal of the foreskin of the penis (p. 235)

circumference distance around (p. 261)

civil relating to laws concerned with private rights and remedies (p. 335)

claim request for reimbursement of medical costs (p. 700)

cleft palate a condition in which the two plates that form the roof of the mouth are not completely connected (p. 514)

clinical trials scientific studies to evaluate the effectiveness and safety of medications or devices on large groups of people (p. 781)

closed bed bed that is in readiness for the next patient (p. 427)

cochlear implant a device that partially restores the ability to hear (p. 515)

collection agency a company that specializes in collecting overdue accounts (p. 698)

collimator a beam-restricting device that allows precision when performing a radiograph (p. 668)

combining form (CF) a word root plus a vowel that is used to help pronounce certain medical terms (p. 106)

communicate to read, write, speak, or listen (p. 5)

community an interacting population (p. 83)

complementary medicine therapy used along with conventional medicine (p. 543)

complex composed of many units (p. 268)

compliance obedience to rules, regulations, and laws (p. 712)

component part (p. 359)

compound consisting of several parts (p. 110)

conception penetration of the ovum by a sperm (p. 230)

conduct perform (p. 783)

confidentiality privacy (p. 342)

conscious able to respond to one's surroundings (p. 88)

consensus agreement (p. 368)

consent form authorization for a physician or facility to release information for certain specific purposes (p. 713)

consist made up of (p. 177)

construct build (p. 109)

contact area area on the proximal surfaces where two adjacent teeth touch one another (p. 570)

Glossary

contagious describing infections that can be spread to other living beings (p. 69)

continuing education ongoing education undertaken while working in your career (p. 13)

contracture the permanent shortening of muscles due to lack of use (p. 516)

contrast medium a substance that allows internal structures to be viewed (p. 656)

convert change (p. 261)

copayment a fee paid by the patient at the time of service (p. 696)

cornea the transparent anterior portion of the outer layer of the eyeball (p. 676)

coronary relating to the heart (p. 160)

cover letter a brief written introduction of yourself to a prospective employer (p. 377)

create make (p. 104)

cross-contamination transfer of bacteria from one type of food to another (p. 747)

crown artificial addition that restores the anatomy and function of all or part of the natural crown of a tooth (p. 565); the portion of a tooth normally visible in the oral cavity (p. 570)

crowning the first appearance of a baby's head from the vaginal opening (p. 408)

crutches a walking aid for patients who are unable to use one leg or who need to gain strength in both legs (p. 518)

culture the set of shared attitudes, values, goals, and practices characterizing a group of people (p. 222)

***Current Procedural Terminology* (CPT)** manual of codes for services (p. 719)

cusp a pointed elevation on the surface of a tooth (p. 570)

cycle a single sequence of events (p. 772)

D

data information (p. 345)

data mining the process of extracting patterns from large data sets (p. 768)

decibel (dB) a unit of loudness (p. 520)

deciduous dentition first set of teeth (p. 568)

decubitus ulcer an open sore, sometimes known as a bedsore (p. 426)

deductibles amounts of payment for which the insured is responsible (p. 696)

defibrillation restoration of normal heart rhythm (p. 93)

defibrillator a device that delivers an electrical shock to the heart (p. 402)

degenerative referring to diseases that cause tissue or organs to worsen, or degenerate, over time (p. 200)

deltoid a muscle in the upper arm (p. 451)

dentin part of a tooth that makes up the bulk of the tooth and provides support for the enamel (p. 571)

dependent one who is covered by someone else's insurance (p. 693)

derive take from (p. 127)

dermatology a field of medicine dealing with treatment related to the skin (p. 444)

dermis the layer of skin that contains connective tissue that holds many capillaries, lymph cells, nerve endings, sebaceous and sweat glands, and hair follicles (p. 140)

detect discover (p. 196)

developmental groove lines on the occlusal surface of a tooth that mark the junction of the developmental lobes (p. 570)

developmental milestones markers at each stage of growth and development (p. 227)

developmentally disabled referring to a person with a condition caused by a congenital anomaly, trauma, deprivation, or disease (p. 460)

device a piece of equipment made for a particular purpose (p. 495)

diabetes a condition in which the body cannot properly regulate levels of glucose in the blood (p. 752)

diagnosis-related group (DRG) groups of patients with similar diagnoses (p. 710)

diagnostic radiograph X-ray used in animal procedures (p. 604)

diagnostic services creating "pictures" of clients' health status at one point in time (p. 11)

diastolic blood pressure (DBP) resting pressure on the arteries as the heart relaxes between beats (p. 296)

diet history an account of a patient's meals and eating habits (p. 754)

dietary fiber a plant substance that your body cannot digest (p. 268)

Dietary Guidelines for Americans guidelines that provide advice about food and lifestyle choices that promote wellness for healthy people aged two and older (p. 277)

diluent liquid used to dilute something (p. 450)

diminish make less; reduce (p. 479)

discriminate make decisions or act in a way that is unfair to a person or a group (p. 712)

discrimination decisions based on race, color, religion, national origin, sex, age, or disability (p. 374)

disinfection using strong chemicals to kill pathogens (p. 62)

distal farthest away from a given point (p. 570)

distort change from the original (p. 359)

distribution apportionment of supplies (p. 731) where a drug goes after entering the plasma (p. 322)

diverse consisting of many different elements (p. 476)

diversity differences (p. 371)

Do Not Resuscitate (DNR) an order that no extraordinary measures will be taken to prevent a patient's death (p. 471)

doctorate a degree requiring two to six more years of education beyond a master's degree (p. 13)

document report in writing on conditions, procedures, and findings (p. 397)

documentation systematic record (p. 715)

dorsalis pedis on the lower leg (p. 297)

dorsogluteal a muscle in the buttocks (p. 451)

dosage the amount of a drug to be administered (p. 323)

durable power of attorney a document that gives one person, called the designee, the authority to make a variety of legal decisions on behalf of another person, called the grantor (p. 348)

E

echocardiogram an ultrasound of the heart (p. 639)

edema swelling (p. 261)

electrical impedance testing a test of body fat that passes a low electrical current through the body (p. 537)

electrically sensitive patient location (ESPL) areas containing class A medical equipment (p. 774)

electrocardiography study of the electrical activity of the heart (p. 634)

electroencephalography recording of the electrical activity in the brain (p. 640)

electroneurodiagnostic evaluating the electrical activity of the nervous system (p. 640)

electronic health records (EHRs) computer-based or digital recording of patient information (p. 29)

electrotherapy the use of electrical energy as a medical treatment (p. 510)

eliminate get rid of (p. 172)

elimination the process that removes a drug from the body (p. 322)

embolus a traveling blood clot (p. 551)

embryo a human being growing in the uterus from conception to about the eighth week (p. 227)

Emergency Care Research Institute (ECRI) an organization that can recall unsafe medical devices (p. 765)

empathy the capacity to understand another person's thoughts, feelings, or state (p. 691)

enamel the outer layer of the crown of a tooth (p. 571)

encounter form a form used to record the patient's illness or condition, the diagnosis, and the procedure received during each office visit (p. 692)

energy a property of matter and radiation that is capable of performing work (p. 656)

ensure make certain of (p. 736)

entrepreneur person who organizes, manages, and takes on the responsibilities and risks of a business or enterprise (p. 15)

environment surroundings (p. 60)

enzymes chemicals that convert complex proteins, sugars, and fat molecules into simpler substances that can be used by the body (p. 172)

epidermis the outer layer of skin (p. 140)

equivalent the same as or equal to (p. 280)

ergonomics the design of work areas to accommodate human physical characteristics (p. 531)

error mistake (p. 345)

essential oils oils derived from plants that are used in aromatherapy (p. 555)

estimate roughly calculate (p. 537)

ethics a set of principles that determines what is morally right or wrong (p. 8)

Glossary

ethylene oxide gas a gas used to sterilize articles that are sensitive to heat (p. 734)

euthanize put an animal to death in a humane way (p. 788)

exercise electrocardiography a stress test or a treadmill stress test to evaluate heart activity (p. 636)

exhalation breathing out (p. 169)

expert someone who is extraordinarily knowledgeable or capable (p. 744)

explanation of benefits (EOB) a form indicating how much, if any, insurance payment is to be received (p. 693)

expose make accessible to a microorganism (p. 69)

external outside (p. 121)

external beam therapy radiation therapy delivered in daily doses over several weeks (p. 659)

extremity an arm or a leg (p. 469)

F

facial surface of the tooth closest to the face (p. 570)

factor a substance that functions in or promotes the function of a physiological process (p. 179)

fallopian tube the tube that extends from the uterus to the ovary (p. 230)

febrile referring to a person with a temperature above 100.4°F or 38.0°C (p. 289)

fecal examination a diagnostic test for parasites in animal stool (p. 606)

feedback the verbal or nonverbal response to a sender of information (p. 360)

fertilization penetration of the ovum by a sperm (p. 230)

fetus a human being growing in the uterus from the eighth week until birth (p. 227)

fire triangle three elements necessary for a fire to occur (p. 85)

first aid initial help given to a sick or injured person (p. 81)

fissure deep developmental groove resulting from incomplete fusion of the developmental lobes (p. 570)

flexible able to bend (p. 139)

fluid balance relationship of fluid intake and output (p. 428)

fluoroscopy an imaging process used to advance a catheter through an artery, into the heart and then into the coronary artery (p. 657)

focus the coming together of images (p. 676)

fomites nonliving materials that house microorganisms (p. 69)

Food and Drug Administration (FDA) an agency that ensures that food and cosmetics are safe and that medication and medical devices are safe and useful (p. 43)

food-borne illness sickness that results from eating food that is not safe (p. 746)

forensics the field of analyzing evidence or acting as an expert witness in legal proceedings (p. 787)

fossa a rounded depression on the surface of a tooth (p. 570)

foundation basic knowledge and skills (p. 5)

framework underlying structure (p. 142)

franchise an agreement that allows an individual or a group to use a company's name and sell its goods or services (p. 480)

fraud the intentional misrepresentation of facts in order to mislead or deceive another person or entity (p. 694)

function perform tasks (p. 133)

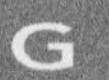

G

gag reflex a reflex causing retching and vomiting when something is placed far back in the mouth (p. 398)

gait (transfer) belt a band of fabric or leather that is positioned around a patient's waist during transfers or ambulation (p. 518)

gastroenterology a field of medicine dealing with disorders of the stomach and intestines (p. 444)

gauge a measurement of the thickness of a needle (p. 319)

genes units of hereditary material contained in a person's cells (p. 228)

genetics the science of genes, heredity, and variation in living organisms (p. 784)

geographic information system (GIS) technology integrating hardware, software, and data for capturing, managing, analyzing, and displaying all forms of geographically referenced information (p. 35)

geriatrics the field of medicine concerned with the problems of aging (p. 257)

germ cells specialized sex cells (p. 182)

geropsychology the study of the mind and behavior of elderly patients (p. 464)

gingiva soft tissue that surrounds the neck of a tooth (p. 572)

GIS (geographic information system) technology integrating hardware, software, and data for capturing, managing, analyzing, and displaying all forms of geographically referenced information (p. 35)

glaucoma condition caused by elevated pressure in the eye (p. 683)

Gram's stain stain applied to a culture smear (p. 624)

group insurance coverage offered by employers to their employees (p. 45)

guidelines procedures to follow (p. 93)

H

health informatics recording of clients' healthcare information (p. 11)

health information management (HIM) maintenance of health record systems (p. 708)

Health Insurance Portability and Accountability Act (HIPAA) a federal law that provides rules for the use of patient health information (p. 712)

Health Maintenance Organization (HMO) organization whose focus is prevention and wellness care (p. 46)

health record all data of a patient's visit (p. 707)

Healthcare Common Procedure Coding System, Level II (HCPCS) codes for services not included in CPT codes (p. 719)

healthcare proxy power of attorney for healthcare (p. 349)

healthcare reform move for major changes in the healthcare system (p. 34)

heart attack a condition caused by the heart muscle being deprived of oxygen-rich blood and nutrients (p. 93)

heat cramps sudden development of cramps in skeletal muscles resulting from exposure to high temperatures (p. 101)

heat exhaustion weakness, nausea, dizziness, and profuse sweating resulting from physical exertion in a hot environment (p. 101)

heat stroke a dangerous condition involving cessation of sweating and very high body temperature (p. 101)

height bar device that measures height (p. 261)

hematocrit a screening test that determines the presence of anemia (p. 627)

hemodynamics blood flow (p. 190)

hemoglobin blood protein (p. 627)

hepatitis B one of the most serious types of hepatitis, which can cause death (p. 66)

herbalist one who makes treatments using leaves, flowers, berries, stems, and roots of herbs (p. 553)

high-efficiency particulate air (HEPA) filter a filter that prevents the airborne spread of pathogens (p. 75)

Hippocrates a medical practitioner in ancient Greece who developed a system of ethics (p. 23)

Holter monitor an ambulatory heart monitor (p. 637)

homeostasis balance in the body (p. 153)

hormones chemicals secreted by glands and other tissues of the endocrine system (p. 179)

host something that is capable of becoming or has been infected (p. 70)

human immunodeficiency virus (HIV) a virus spread by sexual contact, exchange of bodily fluids, receipt of tainted blood, or use of intravenous drugs (p. 208)

human relations administrative activities dealing with employees (p. 695)

hydrocollator a machine that holds and heats gel-filled packs for hot therapy (p. 528)

hydrostatic testing a test of body fat in which the client is weighed, submersed in a large tub of water, and weighed again in the water (p. 537)

hyperglycemia abnormally high amount of sugar in the blood (p. 100)

hyperopia farsightedness (p. 676)

hypertension high blood pressure (p. 205)

hypoglycemia abnormally low amount of sugar in the blood (p. 100)

hypothermia a condition where a patient's entire body is affected by cold (p. 101)

Glossary

I

ICD-9-CM *(International Classification of Diseases,* Ninth Revision, *Clinical Modification)* a manual of diagnosis codes to be used on claims (p. 718)

identify determine or discover (p. 624)

immunity a state of not being susceptible to pathogens (p. 70)

implantation the attachment of the embryo to the uterus wall (p. 230)

implement put into practice (p. 532)

impression a negative reproduction of a patient's teeth (p. 586)

incisal cutting edge of an anterior tooth (p. 570)

incontinent not able to control excretion (p. 432)

indicate be a sign of (p. 637)

individual a single person (p. 42)

individual identifiable health information (IIHI) data that is specific to a particular patient (p. 346)

Industrial Revolution a period in the late eighteenth and early nineteenth centuries characterized by great changes caused by machines (p. 28)

indwelling urinary catheter a tube placed in the urethra to drain urine (p. 434)

inevitable unavoidable (p. 470)

inflammation a vascular response of tissue to an injury, infection, allergy, or autoimmune disease (p. 190)

informed consent agreement to treatment based on communication of full information about the treatment (p. 341)

inhalation breathing in (p. 169)

injure hurt or damage (p. 601)

inpatient a patient who requires at least an overnight hospital stay (p. 707)

insurance carriers companies providing insurance (p. 697)

insured the person who has an insurance policy (p. 693)

intake and output measurement of fluids taken in and excreted (p. 428)

integrate combine into a whole (p. 400)

interact engage with (p. 763)

intercostal space space between two ribs (p. 290)

internal inside (p. 121)

***International Classification of Diseases,* Ninth Revision, *Clinical Modification* (ICD-9-CM)** a manual of diagnosis codes to be used on claims (p. 718)

interproximal space triangle-shaped space between adjacent teeth (p. 570)

intervene interrupt (p. 464)

intradermal (ID) into the superficial layer (dermis) of the skin (p. 450)

intramuscular (IM) into a muscle (p. 450)

invasive requiring entry into the body (p. 639)

invasive imaging studies taken by introducing a contrast agent into the body (p. 656)

invasive procedure any procedure in which an instrument is introduced into the body (p. 791)

inverse square law used to determine a safe distance from a source of radiation while performing radiographs (p. 668)

investigations evaluations and analyses of any event (p. 53)

involve include (p. 190)

isoelectric referring to a straight line on an ECG above and below which the ECG waveform rises and falls (p. 645)

J

jaundice condition caused by excessive bilirubin in the blood that causes a yellow discoloration of the skin (p. 214)

The Joint Commission (TJC) the organization responsible for accrediting hospitals (p. 772)

K

kilogram metric unit of weight (p. 261)

kinesiology the study of body movement (p. 532)

kyphosis curvature of the spine (p. 258)

L

labial surface of an anterior tooth closest to the lips (p. 570)

labor the process of contractions that push the baby out through the vaginal canal (p. 408)

law a rule of conduct or action (p. 335)

law of agency legal liability for acts performed by employees (p. 340)

layer a part of a structure that lies on, under, or between other parts (p. 183)

leakage current a naturally occurring current that leaks from the electronic equipment to the metal chassis of the equipment to ground (p. 774)

ledger a financial record showing a history of charges and payments (p. 697)

legal according to the law (p. 352)

lesions tissues that are altered because of a disease or disorder (p. 192)

liable legally responsible (p. 340)

license legal permission to practice (p. 338)

licensed practical nurse (LPN) performs nursing care for patients under the supervision of a physician or registered nurse (p. 422)

licensed vocational nurse (LVN) performs nursing care for patients under the supervision of a physician or registered nurse (p. 422)

licensure obtaining a license for certain professions within a state (p. 338)

ligaments tissue that attaches bone to bone (p. 147)

lingual surface of a tooth next to the tongue (p. 570)

living will instructions to physicians, hospitals, and other healthcare providers involved in a client's medical treatment (p. 348)

loading dose a large initial dose of a drug, given so that the concentration of the drug in the plasma reaches the therapeutic range more quickly (p. 322)

lock and key principle a principle involving drugs (the key) and the chemicals to which the drugs bind (the lock) (p. 310)

long-term care facility a healthcare facility for patients who do not require acute care but are unable to live alone (p. 417)

lung expansion therapy a treatment to prevent or treat lung collapse (p. 501)

lymph a fluid consisting mainly of white blood cells (p. 164)

M

μA (microampere) one-millionth of an ampere (p. 772)

macroshock a large value of electric current that passes on the skin from one arm to the other (p. 776)

maintain keep up or continue (p. 243)

maintenance dose smaller doses of a drug taken at regular intervals to keep the plasma concentration in the therapeutic range (p. 322)

malignant referring to a tumor that has the ability to spread to distant sites (p. 190)

malnutrition a condition caused by continued lack of nutrients or by the body's inability to absorb or use nutrients properly (p. 281)

malocclusion abnormal relationship of the teeth when biting or closing (p. 567)

managed care organizations that manage, negotiate, and contract for healthcare with the primary goal of keeping healthcare costs down (p. 46)

mandible lower jawbone (p. 568)

marginal ridge boundary or edge of the occlusal surface of a tooth (p. 570)

massage chair a chair that comfortably accommodates clients in optimal positions for massage (p. 557)

massage oil prevents friction on the skin during a massage (p. 557)

massage table a table that comfortably accommodates clients in optimal positions for massage (p. 557)

massage therapist professional who uses pressure, kneading, stroking, vibration, and tapping to positively affect the health and well-being of clients (p. 547)

master patient index the main database that identifies patients (p. 715)

master's degree a degree requiring one or more years of education after a bachelor's degree (p. 13)

mastication chewing food (p. 173)

Material Safety Data Sheets (MSDS) documents that give information on all chemical products sold (p. 53)

mature fully grown or developed (p. 227)

maxilla upper jawbone (p. 568)

maxillofacial region the area of the jaw and face (p. 567)

Mayo stand equipment that holds a sterile drape, with sterile supplies placed on the drape (p. 449)

mechanism of action (MOA) effects produced by interacting with other chemicals in the body (p. 310)

mechanism of injury the force that caused the injury (p. 392)

medical asepsis practices used to reduce and prevent the spread of infection (p. 28)

Glossary

medical malpractice negligence in healthcare (p. 336)

medical nutrition therapy application of proper nutrition and therapeutic diets to help prevent and treat conditions (p. 745)

medical treatment facility (MTF) any facility for treating medical conditions (p. 773)

menarche the first menstruation (p. 183)

meniscus upper surface of a liquid in a glass cylinder (p. 297)

menopause the end of the menstruation cycle (p. 183)

meridian energy channel in the body (p. 547)

mesial surface of the tooth closest to the midline (p. 570)

metabolism the chemical change that takes place in a drug after it has been absorbed by the body (p. 322)

method process by which a task is completed (p. 451)

metric system a decimal system, and the most widely used system of measurement (p. 324)

microampere (µA) one-millionth of an ampere (p. 772)

microbiology the science that studies living organisms that cannot be seen with the naked eye (p. 60)

microorganisms very small living things (p. 746)

microshock a small value of electric current that passes directly through the heart (p. 776)

micturition excreting urine (p. 178)

midline midsagittal plane; imaginary line that divides down the middle (p. 568)

minimal the least amount necessary (p. 416)

minimize make less likely (p. 72)

mixed dentition period time when both primary and permanent teeth are present (p. 569)

MOA (mechanism of action) effects produced by interacting with other chemicals in the body (p. 310)

mobility ability to move (p. 510)

modality method of treatment (p. 530)

mode of transmission the way a disease is passed along (p. 69)

modifier digits showing that some special circumstance applies to a service or procedure (p. 720)

monitoring observing; keeping track of (p. 420)

mononucleosis a highly contagious disease common in teenagers and young adults (p. 208)

morals ideas formed from personal values and reflecting your concept of right and wrong (p. 337)

morula cells of a zygote (p. 230)

myocardial infarction (MI) heart attack (p. 206)

myopia nearsightedness (p. 676)

N

nasal cannula a device that delivers high concentrations of oxygen to a breathing client (p. 400)

nasopharyngeal airway airway through the nostrils (p. 397)

National Board examination a comprehensive examination to become a veterinary technician (p. 602)

National Consortium for Health Science Education an organization that sets National Standards that identify the knowledge and skills that a healthcare worker needs (p. 5)

National Fire Protection Association (NFPA) organization that sets fire safety guidelines (p. 765)

National Formulary (NF) national listing of medications (p. 483)

National Institute for Occupational Safety and Health (NIOSH) a government agency that conducts research and makes recommendations for the prevention of work-related disease and injury (p. 55)

National Institutes of Health (NIH) a government medical research organization (p. 43)

nature of illness symptoms that assist in determining the specific problem (p. 393)

near-infrared interactance testing a test of body fat that transmits a beam of infrared light into the biceps (p. 527)

negligence an unintentional tort (p. 336)

neoplasm tissues that grow out of control (p. 190)

network interconnected system (p. 164)

networking regular communication with personal and professional contacts (p. 374)

neurons nerve cells (p. 150)

neuropsychology a psychological specialty dealing with patients who have neurological disorders (p. 464)

noninvasive imaging studies taken from outside the body, not requiring the use of a contrast medium (p. 656)

nonrebreather mask a device that delivers high concentrations of oxygen to a breathing client (p. 400)

nonverbal communication conveying information through means other than speaking (p. 360)

normal usual and appropriate (p. 250)

nosocomial infection infections unrelated to an illness (p. 70)

nutrient-dense referring to foods that contribute a significant amount of several nutrients relative to the food energy they contain (p. 279)

nutrients substances that nourish your body (p. 267)

nutrition the science of how foods affect your body (p. 267)

O

objective factual (p. 395)

objective comment statement based on facts, not opinions (p. 362)

occlusal chewing surface of a posterior tooth (p. 570)

Occupational Safety and Health Administration (OSHA) a government organization that oversees workplace safety (p. 53)

occupied bed a bed on which linens must be changed while the patient is in the bed (p. 428)

occur happen (p. 210)

olfactory related to the sense of smell (p. 157)

Omnibus Budget Reconciliation Act (OBRA) law that specifies that nursing assistant training include at least 75 hours of education for individuals who work in a long-term care facility (p. 416)

onset of action the time needed before a drug takes effect (p. 317)

open bed bed being used by a patient but unoccupied when it is being made (p. 426)

opportunistic referring to infections that take hold because of a lowered immune response (p. 208)

options choices (p. 425)

oral within the mouth or under the tongue (p. 288)

oropharyngeal airway airway through the mouth (p. 397)

ossification hardening and development process of osteocytes (p. 145)

osteoarthritis joint disease (p. 258)

osteocyte cells of a bone (p. 145)

osteoporosis a condition in which bones become brittle and break easily (p. 274)

otoscope an instrument used to examine inside the ear (p. 519)

outpatient a patient who will be released on the same day of a procedure (p. 707)

overall general (p. 267)

oversecretion the release of too much of a hormone (p. 216)

over-the-counter (OTC) medication medication that can be dispensed without a prescription (p. 484)

oxygen gas that supports life (p. 491)

oxygen toxicity a condition that may occur if too much oxygen is delivered for too long a period of time (p. 497)

P

Palmer System numbering of permanent teeth in each quadrant (p. 574)

palpate feel (p. 290)

paralysis the loss of movement and sensation in a part of the body (p. 201)

parenteral route any route of drug administration other than oral (p. 318)

parliamentary procedure a set of rules to follow in order to conduct a meeting in an efficient manner (p. 16)

participate take part in (p. 379)

passive personality a person who tends to put the needs of others ahead of his or her own needs (p. 369)

passive range of motion exercise performed on the patient by the healthcare employee that moves the joints through their available range (p. 536)

pathogens disease-producing microorganisms (p. 28)

pathology the study of disease (p. 190)

patient care technician (PCT) one who provides assistance to doctors, nurses and other support staff while also interacting directly with the patient (p. 421)

periapical tissue tissue surrounding the apex of the root of a tooth (p. 567)

perineum the area of the body around the genitals and rectum (p. 432)

period amount of time (p. 418)

Glossary

periodontal disease disease of the supporting and surrounding tissues of the teeth (p. 567)

peristalsis contraction and expansion in wavelike motions (p. 172)

permanent dentition permanent teeth that begin to erupt at age six (p. 569)

personal protective equipment (PPE) gloves, gowns, masks, face shields, etc., that are worn when workers are exposed to blood and body fluids (p. 72)

pharmacist a professional who is licensed to prepare and dispense drugs (p. 476)

pharmacognosy the study of drugs that are naturally derived from plants or animals (p. 308)

pharmacokinetics the study of four processes that affect the plasma concentration of drugs (p. 321)

pharmacology the study of the effects of chemical compounds on living things (p. 312)

pharmacotherapeutics the study of the effects of drugs (p. 310)

pharmacy aide one who helps the licensed pharmacist with clerical duties (p. 476)

pharmacy technician one who works in hospitals or retail pharmacies under the direction of a pharmacist (p. 476)

phlebitis an inflammation of the veins (p. 433)

phlebotomy tests and procedures involving an incision, or cut, that is made into a vein or capillary in order to draw blood (p. 613)

physical relating to the body (p. 238)

pinna external ear (p. 156)

pit a small, deep depression on the surface of a tooth (p. 570)

placenta a special organ that acts as an exchange area between mother and fetus (p. 407)

plaque an accumulation of biofilm or bacteria on teeth (p. 581)

pleura double layer of membrane around the lungs (p. 168)

point-of-care test test done on the spot that provides quick, reliable results (p. 624)

policy insurance coverage (p. 45)

policyholder the insured person (p. 694)

popliteal on the thigh (p. 297)

portal of entry means for pathogens to get into the host or the environment (p. 70)

portals of exit escape routes in humans that allow microorganisms to leave (p. 69)

portfolio a collection of materials that exhibits your efforts, progress, and achievements (p. 377)

posterior at the back of the mouth (p. 569)

posterior tibial on the lower leg (p. 297)

postmortem care care provided after a patient dies to help maintain dignity (p. 471)

Preferred Provider Organization (PPO) a group of doctors, hospitals, and other healthcare providers who have contracted with an insurer or administrator to provide healthcare at reduced rates (p. 47)

prefix (P) used at the beginning of a medical term to describe, modify, or limit the term (p. 107)

premenstrual dysphoric disorder (PMDD) similar to premenstrual syndrome, but including more severe mental and emotional symptoms (p. 219)

premenstrual syndrome (PMS) a group of symptoms that appear three to 14 days before the onset of menstruation (p. 219)

premium amount paid to an insurance company for coverage (p. 45)

presbyopia farsightedness that develops with age (p. 253) the inability of the eye lens to focus incoming light (p. 676)

prescription medication drug that can only be dispensed with a doctor's written order (p. 484)

preventive maintenance (PM) inspection of equipment to prevent problems and keep it working properly (p. 772)

primary first-appearing (p. 192)

primary assessment initial evaluation of a client's condition (p. 89)

principal main (p. 718)

principal diagnosis the main reason for the patient's visit (p. 718)

priority importance (p. 494)

privileged communication information that is held private within a protected relationship (p. 342)

process handle information (p. 150)

professional a person trained to work in a specific field (p. 29)

proportion the relation of parts of a whole (p. 244)

proprioception awareness of posture, movement, and change in equilibrium (p. 535)

prosthesis an artificial body part (p. 565)

prosthetic device see prosthesis (p. 766)

protected health information (PHI) health information that must be kept private (p. 346)

protein groups of amino acids that help the body grow, repair itself, and fight disease (p. 268)

proximal surface tooth surface next to an adjacent tooth (p. 570)

puberty physical changes that take place usually between the ages of about 11 to 14 years of age (p. 246)

pulmonary related to the heart and lungs (p. 160)

pulp the innermost tissue of a tooth (p. 571)

pulp canal pulp in the root of a tooth (p. 571)

pulp chamber pulp within the crown of a tooth (p. 571)

pulse a wave of blood flow created by the contraction of the heart (p. 290)

pulse oximeter a device that measures how saturated the red blood cells are with oxygen (p. 495)

Q

qi life force within the body (p. 547)

quality control procedures to ensure that requirements are met (p. 616)

R

radial referring to a pulse felt on the inside of the wrist (p. 290)

radiograph two-dimensional image on X-ray film (p. 661)

radiolucent referring to a contrast substance that X-rays can pass through (p. 662)

radiopaque referring to a contrast substance that X-rays cannot pass through (p. 662)

range a measure between certain limits (p. 289)

range of motion degree to which a muscle or joint is able to move (p. 149)

range-of-motion (ROM) exercises activities that move joints through their full range of motion (p. 516)

react respond (p. 154)

reagent chemical that reacts to other substances (p. 625)

reality orientation helping a patient become aware of his or her surroundings, the date and time, and other information about his or her present situation (p. 469)

receptors proteins found in cells that are stimulated by drugs (p. 310)

reciprocity acceptance by one state licensing authority of a valid license from another state (p. 339)

recommended daily allowance (RDA) amounts of specific nutrients needed by individuals (p. 275)

records management system method of handling patient records (p. 700)

recover return to normal state (p. 205)

rectal in the rectum (p. 288)

region area (p. 136)

register record (p. 668)

registration a listing in an official registry or record as having satisfied the standards for a certain healthcare occupation (p. 339)

reimbursement repayment (p. 696)

relapse recurrence of a disease (p. 207)

relax become less tense or rigid (p. 169)

release let go of (p. 316)

remission the disappearance of a disease (p. 207)

research experiments or studies (p. 416)

reservoirs humans, insects, food, and water that provide food for microorganisms and allow them to multiply (p. 69)

residents clients who are cared for in long-term care facilities (p. 37)

resorb dissolve (p. 569)

resource a service or asset needed for an activity (p. 392)

respiration the act of breathing (p. 135, p. 294)

response reaction to (p. 199)

restore recreate or give back (p. 513)

restrain keep from moving (p. 606)

résumé a brief representation of your credentials (p. 375)

retina the layer of cells at the back of the eye where light is converted into neural signals sent to the brain (p. 676)

rhythm a repeated pattern or beat (p. 291)

RICE rest, ice, compression, and elevation (p. 197)

risk assessment determination of the likelihood that harmful effects will occur from exposure to a harmful substance or circumstance (p. 786)

root the part of a tooth that is embedded in the bone (p. 570)

route of administration the way used to get a drug into the tissues of the body (p. 317)

S

Safe Medical Devices Act (SMDA) law that sets safety guidelines for medical devices (p. 765)

safety freedom from harm or injury (p. 53)

sanitizing destroying bacteria and viruses that may be present after the cleaning process (p. 750)

saturated fat fat that is solid at room temperature (p. 269)

scale device that measures weight in pounds and/or kilograms (p. 261)

scalpel a surgical instrument for cutting (p. 447)

schedule assign a time for (p. 689)

scope of practice acceptable activities based on job description, level of training, and qualifications (p. 339)

secondary assessment evaluation of a client's head, neck, chest, abdomen, pelvis, legs, arms, and back that is performed when there is no immediate need for first aid (p. 90)

sexual harassment an unwanted communication or act of a sexual nature (p. 372)

sexually transmitted disease (STD) disease transmitted through sexual contact and exchange of body fluids (p. 221)

shelter-in-place a room in a facility with few or no windows, in which to take refuge when evacuation is too dangerous (p. 83)

shock a condition that occurs when too little oxygen and nutrients reach the body's cells, tissues, and organs (p. 99)

side effect any effect caused by a drug other than its intended effect (p. 312)

sign something you see, hear, feel, or smell (p. 395)

significant meaningful (p. 459)

similar comparable to (p. 444)

simple mask a device that fits over a patient's nose and mouth and provides a reservoir of oxygen (p. 497)

sleep apnea a halt in breathing during sleep (p. 492)

specific particular or exact (p. 364)

sphygmomanometer instrument used to measure blood pressure (p. 297)

spores microorganisms with a thick protective outer wall (p. 735)

sprain a tear in a ligament (p. 532)

stable in an unchanging state (p. 162)

standard of care the level of performance expected of a healthcare professional in carrying out his or her duties (p. 339)

standard precautions guidelines to minimize the spread of diseases (p. 72)

standards framework of basic knowledge and skills for professionals (p. 5)

statement invoice detailing the service provided and the amount owed for that service (p. 697)

stent a device placed inside a blocked blood vessel to act as a bridge and keep the vessel open (p. 639)

stereotype preconceived idea applied to all things in a group (p. 372)

sterile field an area free of microorganisms that will be used as a work area during a procedure (p. 791)

sterilization the process of killing or removing all microorganisms and their spores (p. 62)

stethoscope an instrument used to hear body sounds (p. 290)

strabismus a condition where one eye focuses properly, but the other eye strays (p. 678)

strain injury to a muscle (p. 532)

strength muscular ability (p. 528)

stroke (a) a condition where an artery supplying blood to the brain becomes blocked, cutting off oxygen and nutrients (b) the bursting of a blood vessel in the brain (p. 93)

structure an arrangement of parts (p. 133)

subcutaneous (subcut) into the soft tissue beneath the skin (p. 450)

subcutaneous layer the layer of skin between the dermis and the body's inner organs (p. 140)

subjective comment statement based on opinion or perception (p. 362)

subluxated out of place (p. 544)

subscriber the insured person (p. 694)

suffix (S) word ending that affects the meaning of a term (p. 106)

superbill a form used to record the patient's illness or condition, the diagnosis, and the procedure received during each office visit (p. 693)

supplement additional nutrients (p. 217)

support services creating a safe and healthful environment for clients and other healthcare professionals (p. 11)

supragingival calculus scale deposits on upper part of teeth (p. 579)

surgical asepsis sterilization of any item that penetrates the skin or comes into contact with a normally sterile part of the body (p. 71)

survive continue to live (p. 746)

sutures stitches that hold a wound or incision together (p. 449)

symptoms problems a patient has that can be seen or measured (p. 212)

synapse a space between neurons (p. 150)

systemic related to the entire body (p. 160)

systolic blood pressure (SBP) pressure exerted on the arteries during the contraction phase of the heartbeat (p. 296)

T

tape measure device to determine length (p. 261)

tasks work to be done (p. 699)

technical relating to information with specific and precise meaning (p. 277)

technique means of accomplishing something (p. 459)

technology practical application of knowledge to accomplish a task (p. 9)

telemedicine transmitting patient images and information to a distant site (p. 772)

teleradiology transmission of an X-ray image to a distant site (p. 772)

temperature a vital sign indicating level of heat in the body (p. 288)

temporal on the side of the forehead near the temple (p. 288)

tendons bands of fibrous tissue connecting muscles to bones (p. 147)

therapeutic class a group of drugs that produce their effects in the same way (p. 310)

therapeutic communication communicating with patients in terms that they can understand (p. 459)

therapeutic diet a special eating plan used to treat or control a condition or disease (p. 752)

therapeutic range the range of concentration of a drug that produces a therapeutic effect without causing harm (p. 321)

therapeutic services providing services to clients over time (p. 9)

the three Cs characteristics (courtesy, compassion, and common sense) that are related to providing competent, courteous healthcare to clients (p. 352)

thrombophlebitis a blood clot in the vein (p. 433)

tickler report a way of tracking when to contact patients or the insurance company about payments (p. 697)

tinnitus ringing in the ear (p. 514)

TJC (The Joint Commission) the organization responsible for accrediting hospitals (p. 772)

tort a civil wrong committed against a person or property, excluding breach of contract (p. 336)

tracing an electrocardiogram printout (p. 634)

transfer (gait) belt a band of fabric or leather that is positioned around a patient's waist during transfers or ambulation (p. 518)

transform change (p. 322)

transmission-based precautions activities that prevent the spread of highly infectious agents (p. 75)

transmit send or convey (p. 644)

transport move or carry along (p. 125)

trauma injury (p. 196)

trigger cause (p. 316)

24-hour dietary recall remembering all foods and beverages consumed in a 24-hour period (p. 755)

tympanic in the ear canal (p. 288)

U

umbilical cord a cordlike structure that links the fetus and the placenta (p. 407)

unconscious unresponsive (p. 88)

undersecretion the release of too little of a hormone (p. 216)

United States Pharmacopeia (USP) national listing of medications (p. 483)

unsaturated fat fat that is liquid at room temperature (p. 269)

urethra tube of smooth muscle with a mucous lining that carries urine out of the body (p. 178)

urinalysis a series of tests performed on urine (p. 607)

urinary tract infection (UTI) infection in the bladder or urethra (p. 215)

U.S. Department of Health and Human Services (DHHS) the national agency that deals with health in the United States (p. 42)

USDA Food Guide an aid to applying the *Dietary Guidelines* that puts foods into groups (p. 277)

use employment of (p. 346)

V

vasoconstriction a narrowing of blood vessels (p. 313)

vastus lateralis a muscle in the mid-thigh (p. 451)

veins vessels that carry blood toward the heart (p. 159)

venipuncture puncturing of a vein with a needle that is designed for blood collection (p. 613)

ventricular fibrillation (VF) an abnormal heart rhythm (p. 93)

verbal communication spoken information (p. 359)

Veterinary Technician National Examination (VTNE) a comprehensive examination to become a veterinary technician (p. 602)

vial a small glass bottle with a rubber stopper (p. 450)

vision sight (p. 682)

visual acuity the ability to see (p. 682)

vital signs indicators of events occurring within the body (p. 288)

vitamins vital nutrients that help regulate body processes (p. 270)

VO2 max test analysis that gauges cardiovascular fitness by assessing an athlete's efficiency of oxygen consumption and cardiac output (p. 534)

voiding excreting urine (p. 178)

volume amount, especially inside a container (p. 324)

voluntary consciously controlled (p. 147)

W

waived test more simple analyses performed by medical laboratory assistants (p. 616)

walker a support device with a frame, handgrips, and four points at the bottom (p. 518)

wellness a state of good health (p. 227)

widespread very common or frequent (p. 213)

word root (WR) the basic meaning of a medical term (p. 106)

workers' compensation insurance that covers accidents, injuries, or diseases that occur in the workplace (p. 47)

World Health Organization (WHO) an international agency that directs and coordinates international health issues (p. 43)

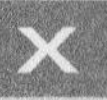

X

X-ray an electromagnetic wave that has a wavelength much shorter than that of visible light (p. 661)

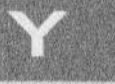

Y

yang part of the life force, *qi*; the "male" principle (p. 550)

yin part of the life force, *qi*; the "female" principle (p. 550)

Z

zoonosis disease that can be passed from an animal to a human (p. 602)

zygote a fertilized ovum (p. 230)

Index

Index

Index

Index

Index

Index

N

Index

P

Index

Index

S

Index

U

V

W

X

Y

Z